Principles and Practice of
PODIATRIC
MEDICINE

Principles and Practice of
PODIATRIC MEDICINE

Edited by

Leonard A. Levy, D.P.M., M.P.H.

Founding Dean and Professor
College of Podiatric Medicine and Surgery
University of Osteopathic Medicine and Health Sciences
Des Moines, Iowa

Vincent J. Hetherington, D.P.M., M.S.

Chairman and Professor
Department of Surgery
Ohio College of Podiatric Medicine
Cleveland, Ohio
Former Professor and Associate Dean for Clinical Affairs
College of Podiatric Medicine and Surgery
University of Osteopathic Medicine and Health Sciences
Des Moines, Iowa

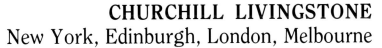

CHURCHILL LIVINGSTONE
New York, Edinburgh, London, Melbourne

Library of Congress Cataloging-in-Publication Data

Principles and practice of podiatric medicine / edited by Leonard A.
   Levy, Vincent J. Hetherington.
         p.   cm.
      Includes bibliographical references.
      ISBN 0-443-08534-X
      1. Podiatry.   I. Levy, Leonard A.   II. Hetherington, V. J.
      [DNLM: 1. Foot — surgery. 2. Foot Diseases.   WE 880 P957]
RD563.P74   1990
617.5'85 — dc20
DNLM/DLC
for Library of Congress   89-22135
                                                              CIP

Distributed in the United Kingdom by Churchill Livingstone, Robert Stevenson House, 1–3 Baxter's Place, Leith Walk, Edinburgh EH1 3AF, and by associated companies, branches, and representatives throughout the world.

Accurate indications, adverse reactions, and dosage schedules for drugs are provided in this book, but it is possible that they may change. The reader is urged to review the package information data of the manufacturers of the medications mentioned.

The Publishers have made every effort to trace the copyright holders for borrowed material. If they have inadvertently overlooked any, they will be pleased to make the necessary arrangements at the first opportunity.

Acquisitions Editor: *Kim Loretucci*
Production Supervisor: *Sharon Tuder*
Production services provided by Bermedica Productions

Printed in the United States of America

First published in 1990

*To
the late Marvin D. Steinberg, D.P.M.,
and
the late Arnold Karpo, D.P.M.*

Contributors

Dennis Anderson, D.O., Comdr. M.C., U.S.N.R.
Surgical Pathologist, Bethesda Naval Hospital, Bethesda, Maryland

Allan M. Boike, D.P.M.
Assistant Professor, Department of Surgery, Ohio College of Podiatric Medicine;
Director, Residency Training Program, Cleveland Foot Clinic, Cleveland, Ohio

Myron C. Boxer, D.P.M.
Director, Department of Podiatry, Gouverneur Hospital, New York, New York

Kenneth G. Canter, D.P.M.
Chief, Podiatry Section, Veterans Administration Medical Center, Minneapolis,
Minnesota

Jeffery Carnett, D.P.M.
Assistant Professor, College of Podiatric Medicine and Surgery, University of Osteopathic Medicine and Health Sciences, Des Moines, Iowa

Jose Castillo, M.D.
Plastic and Reconstructive Surgeon, Private Practice, Philadelphia, Pennsylvania

Edward L. Chairman, D.P.M.
Private Practice, Philadelphia, Pennsylvania

Angel L. Cuesta, D.P.M.
Podiatric Surgery Resident, Metropolitan Hospital, Metropolitan Division, Philadelphia, Pennsylvania

J. Colin Dagnall, L.H.D., F.Ch.S.
Consultant Chiropodist, Cheadle Royal Hospital, Cheadle, Chesire, England; Chiropodist, War Pensioners Service, Blackpool, England

Gregory S. Duncan, D.P.M.
Surgical Staff, Davenport Medical Center; Private Practice, Davenport, Iowa

Eric Goldenberg, D.P.M., M.S.
Private Practice, West Des Moines, Iowa

Gerald A. Gorecki, D.P.M., M.P.H.
Head, Podiatry Section, Orthopaedic Department, Naval Hospital Groton, Groton, Connecticut; Chief, Podiatry Section, Veterans Administration Medical Center, West Haven, Connecticut

Franz Grill, M.D.
Primarius, Pediatric Orthopaedic Department, Speising Hospital; Medical Director, Orthopaedic Hospital Speising, Vienna, Austria

George S. Gumann, Jr., D.P.M.
Staff Podiatrist, Orthopedic Service, Martin Army Hospital, Fort Benning, Georgia

Lawrence Harkless, D.P.M.
Clinical Professor of Podiatric Medicine, Department of Orthopedics, University of Texas Health Science Center at San Antonio, San Antonio, Texas

Arthur E. Helfand, D.P.M.
Professor and Chairman, Department of Community Health and Aging, Pennsylvania College of Podiatric Medicine; Adjunct Professor, Department of Orthopedic Surgery, Thomas Jefferson University Hospital, Jefferson Medical College of Thomas Jefferson University, Philadelphia, Pennsylvania

Vincent J. Hetherington, D.P.M., M.S.
Chairman and Professor, Department of Surgery, Ohio College of Podiatric Medicine, Cleveland, Ohio; Former Professor and Associate Dean for Clinical Affairs, College of Podiatric Medicine and Surgery, University of Osteopathic Medicine and Health Sciences, Des Moines, Iowa.

John J. Holewski, D.P.M.
Clinical Assistant Professor, California College of Podiatric Medicine; Clinical Instructor, Department of Medicine, University of California, San Francisco, School of Medicine; Research Investigator, Rehabilitation Research and Development Service, Veterans Affairs, San Francisco, California

Bonnie Johng, D.P.M.
Assistant Professor, Department of Surgery, Ohio College of Podiatric Medicine, Cleveland, Ohio

Ronald E. Johnson, D.P.M.
Associate Professor and Associate Dean for Clinical Affairs, College of Podiatric Medicine and Surgery, University of Osteopathic Medicine and Health Sciences, Des Moines, Iowa

Gary Peter Jolly, D.P.M.
Senior Consultant, Podiatry Service, Department of Surgery, West Haven Veterans Hospital; Private Practice, West Haven, Connecticut

Warren S. Joseph, D.P.M.

Assistant Professor, Department of Medicine, and Chief, Section of Infectious Diseases, Pennsylvania College of Podiatric Medicine; Consultant in Podiatric Infectious Diseases, St. Joseph's Hospital, Philadelphia, Pennsylvania

Anthony S. Kidawa, D.P.M.

Professor, Department of Medicine, Pennsylvania College of Podiatric Medicine; Chief, Vascular Medicine Section, Foot and Ankle Institute, Pennsylvania College of Podiatric Medicine, Philadelphia, Pennsylvania

Wayne A. Krueger, Ph.D.

Professor, Department of Anatomy, University of Osteopathic Medicine and Health Sciences, Des Moines, Iowa

John E. Laco, D.P.M.

Assistant Professor, College of Podiatric Medicine and Surgery, University of Osteopathic Medicine and Health Sciences, Des Moines, Iowa

Mark E. Landry, D.P.M., M.S.

Clinical Associate Professor, College of Podiatric Medicine and Surgery, University of Osteopathic Medicine and Health Sciences, Des Moines, Iowa; Clinical Instructor, Department of Orthopedics, Truman Medical Center, University of Missouri at Kansas City, School of Medicine; Director, Lakeside Hospital Podiatric Residency Program, Kansas City, Missouri

Eric Lauf, D.P.M.

Private Practice, Alexandria, Virginia

Janis Lehtinen, D.P.M.

Assistant Professor, Department of Podiatric Surgery, Ohio College of Podiatric Medicine, Cleveland, Ohio

Leonard A. Levy, D.P.M., M.P.H.

Founding Dean and Professor, College of Podiatric Medicine and Surgery, University of Osteopathic Medicine and Health Sciences, Des Moines, Iowa

Vincent J. Mandracchia, D.P.M.

Staff, Metropolitan Hospital, Springfield Division, Springfield, Pennsylvania; Private Practice, Philadelphia, Pennsylvania

Daniel J. McCarthy, D.P.M., Ph.D.

Chief, Podiatric Section, Surgical Services Veterans Administration Medical Center, Baltimore, Maryland

Thomas F. McCloskey, D.P.M.

Chief, Podiatric Service, Keller Army Community Hospital, West Point, New York

John P. McDonough, C.R.N.A., Ed.D.

Adjunct Associate Professor, University of Osteopathic Medicine and Health Sciences; Attending Anesthetist, Des Moines General Hospital, Des Moines, Iowa

Stephen J. Miller, D.P.M.

Active Staff, Island Hospital; Private Practice, Anacortes, Washington

Gerit D. Mulder, D.P.M.

Clinical Professor, Departments of Surgery and Orthopedics, and Clinical Instructor, Department of Family Medicine, University of Colorado Health Sciences Center; Assistant Chief, Podiatry Section, Veterans Administration Medical Center; Director, Dermal Ulcer Clinic, Veterans Administration Medical Center; Director, Wound Healing Institute, Denver, Colorado

Joon B. Park, Ph.D.

Professor, Department of Biomedical Engineering, College of Engineering, University of Iowa, Iowa City, Iowa

Phillip Perlman, D.P.M.

Associate Professor, College of Podiatric Medicine and Surgery, University of Osteopathic Medicine and Health Sciences, Des Moines, Iowa

Robert D. Phillips, D.P.M.

Associate Professor and Orthopedic Residency Director, College of Podiatric Medicine and Surgery, University of Osteopathic Medicine and Health Sciences, Des Moines, Iowa

Steven R. Quam, D.O.

Anesthesiologist, Des Moines General Hospital, Des Moines, Iowa

Roche P. Ramos, M.D.

Associate Professor, Department of Pathology, University of Osteopathic Medicine and Health Sciences, Des Moines, Iowa

William Sprague, D.P.M.

Clinical Associate Professor, College of Podiatric Medicine and Surgery, University of Osteopathic Medicine and Health Sciences, Des Moines, Iowa

Gunther Steinböck, M.D.

Consultant and Director of Education, 1. Allgemeine Orthopaedische Abteilung at the Orthopedic Hospital of Vienna, Vienna, Austria

Richard M. Stess, D.P.M.

Assistant Professor, High Risk Foot Center, University of California, San Francisco, School of Medicine; Associate Clinical Professor, Department of Biomechanics, California College of Podiatric Medicine; Chief of Podiatry, Veterans Administration Medical Center, San Francisco, California

Walter W. Strash, D.P.M.

Podiatric Surgery Resident, Metropolitan Hospital, Springfield Division, Springfield, Pennsylvania

Susan J. Tokarski, D.P.M.

Private Practice, Brooklyn, New York

Rodney L. Tomczak, D.P.M.
Associate Professor and Surgical Residency Director, College of Podiatric Medicine and Surgery, University of Osteopathic Medicine and Health Sciences, Des Moines, Iowa

Harold W. Vogler, D.P.M.
Professor, Department of Surgery, Pennsylvania College of Podiatric Medicine; Chairman, Department of Foot and Ankle Surgery and Traumatology, St. Joseph's Hospital; Director of Residency Training in Reconstructive and Traumatological Surgery of the Foot and Ankle, St. Joseph's Hospital, Philadelphia, Pennsylvania

Lee E. Wentworth, Ph.D.
Adjunct Associate Professor, Department of Anatomy, University of California, San Francisco, School of Medicine; Adjunct Associate Professor, Department of Restorative Dentistry and Stomatology, University of California, San Francisco, School of Dentistry; Professor, California College of Podiatric Medicine, San Francisco, California

Alan K. Whitney, D.P.M.
Professor, Department of Podiatric Orthopedics, Pennsylvania College of Podiatric Medicine, Philadelphia, Pennsylvania

Kendrick A. Whitney, D.P.M.
Instructor, Department of Podiatric Orthopedics, Pennsylvania College of Podiatric Medicine, Philadelphia, Pennsylvania

Preface

Principles and Practice of Podiatric Medicine represents a collaborative effort between podiatric physicians and representatives of other medical and surgical disciplines, such as orthopedics, anesthesiology, pathology, and plastic surgery. It attempts to bring together in one volume a comprehensive consideration of current podiatric medical practice. At the same time, it does not presume to take the place of textbooks devoted exclusively to surgery, radiology, dermatology, or other segments within the podiatric profession.

The book's very existence is a tribute to the growth of podiatric medicine over the last two or three decades, and its size demonstrates the broad spectrum of knowledge which now encompasses the profession. In addition, the book's content demonstrates the interdependence of podiatric medicine within the mainstream of health care.

It is a clinically oriented textbook, written primarily by authorities on the foot who practice in a clinical setting. However, it attempts to provide mechanisms and concepts which hopefully contribute to understanding the pathogenesis of diseases and disorders affecting the pedal extremity.

We believe the text will be useful for the practicing podiatric physican as well as other health professionals who feel a need to expand their knowledge about foot disorders or who may be interested in another point of view. It also should be a major resource for podiatric medical students and residents who have sought such a publication. It hopefully will also stimulate the reader to continue his or her self-education throughout professional life.

The editors feel that podiatric medicine, while being a scientific discipline, is also an art, applying anatomy, physiology, biomechanics, microbiology, pathology, biochemistry, and pharmacology to the needs of the patient. With that concept in mind, we are pleased to present *Principles and Practice of Podiatric Medicine*.

Leonard A. Levy, D.P.M., M.P.H.
Vincent J. Hetherington, D.P.M., M.S.

Acknowledgments

We acknowledge with gratitude the many contributors to this text who not only gave up their time to prepare many of the chapters, but who also were the target of our often incessant prodding in order to meet our publisher's deadlines.

Our wives, Eleanore Levy and Josefa Hetherington, and our children, Andrew and Sarilyn Levy and Nancy Hetherington, put up with our inattention during the many countless hours it took to produce this book. One of the editors (VJH) also acknowledges the inspiration of his late brother, Ronald Hetherington, M.D.

In addition, we must acknowledge Candice Arnberg who prepared most of our manuscripts.

Finally, the staff at Churchill Livingstone was so very supportive. A special tribute needs to be given to our editor, Kim Loretucci, who, while being a tough taskmaster, believed in our text and encouraged us to complete it.

Contents

Section III. CLINICAL DISORDERS AND THE SPECIAL PATIENT

Section I

PRINCIPLES

Podiatric Medicine: The Evolution of Practice and Formal Education

1

Leonard A. Levy, D.P.M., M.P.H.

A CHRONOLOGIC HISTORY

Perhaps when compared to the long history of the profession of medicine, podiatric medicine is in a formal sense a relatively new discipline. However, the demand for foot health care obviously has existed since the beginning of humankind, and evidence of provision of such care can be traced to the ancient civilizations of the Egyptians, the Assyro-Babylonians, and the Greeks. Evidence of advice about foot care appears as far back as 2500 B.C. in ancient Egyptian tombs as well as in the famous Ebers Papyrus (circa 1500 B.C.), which promotes the application of olive oil and cow fat to corns. Biblical references to ministrations to the foot include quotes from King Asa, who was alleged to have said, ". . . seek not the Lord, but the physician for foot trouble." (2 chronicles, Ch. 16, verse 12) Mosaic law included principles of hygiene that emphasized foot washing.

Treatment of corns was mentioned in writings by Theophrastus (born circa 372 B.C.). Hikesios of Smyrna (circa 60 B.C.) employed plaster preparations in treating these lesions. The ash of willow bark (salicin) was promoted for corns by Celsus, who lived during the reign of Tiberius Caesar. Wild boar or swine dung was another remedy for this condition, advocated by Pliny the Elder (circa 23–79 A.D.), who also suggested, "Whoever, when he sees a shooting star, soon afterwards pours a little vinegar upon the hinge of a door is sure to get rid of his corns." Other remedies advocated for corns or calluses during the same period included the application of wheat meal, a treatment recommended by Dioscorides, who served under Nero as a Greek army surgeon.

Among the writings of Hippocrates (circa 460–377 B.C.) are references to clubfoot as well as calluses. A surgical approach to the care of corns and calluses is described by Paul of Aegina (circa 615–690 A.D.). He directs, "Wherefore having scarified around the clavus or corn and taking hold of it with the forceps we cut it out by the roots with a sharp-pointed scalpel or lancet for bleeding. So in order that it may not grow again, apply heated cauteries." "Brass filings, old soap and oil" were Anglo-Saxon remedies for the care of hangnails.

By the 14th century in northern Europe the Guild of Barber-Surgeons was established. Its members pulled teeth, did bloodletting, cut corns, applied leeches, and made preparations for the relief of pain. It is postulated that the surgeon, the dentist, and the podiatrist evolved from this group.

In the last quarter of the 17th century, Dagnall referred to a superior class of practitioner who frequented the coffeehouses and baths and who came

3

over from Holland to England when William III ascended to the throne in 1689.

Medical specialization began in France and England in the 18th century with Pierre Fauchard's book *Le Chirurgien dentiste* in 1728. In 1714, Daniel Turner published what may have been the first text in dermatology. Turner included a chapter on diseases of the hands and feet, which included extensive writings on "whitlaws, kibes, warts and corns." He warned of dangers resulting if blood from the cutting of corns and warts fell on sound skin. He attributed corns to a disturbance of the humors of the skin and failed to recognize its traumatic or biomechanical origins.

Rousselot, a French surgeon, began to specialize in what we call podiatric medicine and wrote the first book on the subject, *Mémoire sur les cors des pieds* (Dissertation on Corns of the Feet), in 1755. He was influenced greatly by Daniel Turner's book and indeed added little to Turner. However, Rousselot gave what may be the first description of using caustics in treating skin cancer. On his death in 1770, Turner's notes and practice were passed on to Nicholas Laurent LaForest, who had no medical qualifications and called himself a chirurgien-pedicure. LaForest published a book in 1781 and a second edition in 1782 depicting instruments and foot conditions, including the first depiction of hallux valgus. Nail clippers and several scalpels that he designed are still used today. His text was called *L'Art de soigner des pieds* (The Art of Foot Care). He described the cause of corns as "A thick and sticky humor, hardened in the pores of the skin by a constant pressure which finally forms a hornified mass." LaForest also wrote of the difficulty of curing corns, "because the cause always exists" unless the patient can be persuaded to wear shoes suitable to the condition of the feet.

LaForest treated the poor for free, condemned quacks, and established a school to train soldiers in foot care. He held an appointment to Louis XVI. LaForest's practice disappeared during the French Revolution and he ended his career as a grocer.

Petrus Camper, who held several chairs in medicine, anatomy, and surgery in Holland, published a book in Amsterdam in 1781 entitled *Over den besten schoen* (On the Best Form of Shoe). It dealt with the effect of shoes on the feet and was written to prove to his students that something worthwhile could be written even on the most humble subject.

Camper wrote on what we now refer to as biomechanics. One of the practices he described was the ancient Chinese custom of foot binding, which, performed in infancy, rendered the women of the upper social class relatively inactive but supposedly more sexually attractive.

Corn cutting did not develop as part of the practice of physicians and surgeons. Surgeons considered it beneath their dignity to care for these lesions. Corn cutters sometimes combined this trade with tooth pulling.

An innkeeper, D. Low, produced in 1785 a book entitled *Treatise on the Causes of Corns, Warts, Bunions and Other Painful and Offensive Cutaneous Excrescences.* It was in large part plagiarized from LaForest. Low was the first person to use the term *chiropodist*, believing that it glamorized his work.

Heyman Lion was a German who settled in Edinburgh in the last half of the 18th century. He was first a dentist and corn operator and then what he called a chiropedist. In 1802 Lion published a book called *Treatise Upon Spinae Pedum* (the term he used for the corns). He is regarded as the father of British chiropody.

A book entitled *The Art of Preserving the Feet or Practical Instructions for the Prevention and Cure of Corns, Bunions, Callosities, Chilblains, etc. with Observations on the Dangers Arising From Improper Treatment, Advice to Pedestrians, etc . . . To Which Are Added Directions for the Better Management of the Hands and Nails* was published by a person who simply listed himself as "An Experienced Chiropodist," in London in 1818. This author argued that *podology* and *podologist* were better terms than *chiropody* and *chiropodist*.

Solomon Abraham Durlacher lived between 1757 and 1845. He was a German who came to England from Baden in southern Germany. In 1809 he was listed in the directory of Bath, England, as "Dr. Surgeon Dentist and Corn Operator." He trained his son, Lewis Durlacher, who started practice as a surgeon-chiropodist in London in 1816, eventually becoming chiropodist to George IV, William IV, and Queen Victoria. In 1826, Lewis Durlacher was invited to demonstrate his method of treating ingrowing nails at the Hospital for Surgery. A full account appeared in the prestigious English medical journal *The Lancet* in 1826, which called it the most important improvement in this department of operative surgery. In 1845 Lewis

Durlacher wrote a book called *A Treatise — Corns, Bunions, the Diseases of Nails and the General Management of the Feet*, which contained the first description of plantar digital neuritis, the first illustrations of onychocryptosis (infected ingrowing nail), and the first detailed account of plantar warts. Lewis Durlacher is considered the probable founder of chiropody, which became podiatric medicine. His book in itself established the profession, according to some.

About 1830 "corn doctors" were making rounds in large American cities. They promised to pull out corns by the roots. Actually they would often use concealed fishbone or catgut and then produce it after removing corn tissue. Minor ailments of the foot were often treated by such itinerant operators, who learned their practice through apprenticeships, as was often the case in other medical specialties.

Around 1840, members of a family headed by Nehemiah Kenison of Allentown, New Hampshire, were traveling around New England treating the feet of mill employees in cotton and shoe factories. The family's Boston office displayed a sign with a foot and a legend reading, "Corns Extracted Without Pain, 25 cents." Elected to the New Hampshire state legislature, Nehemiah Kenison was given the honorary title of doctor. The Kenison family established themselves in St. Louis; Philadelphia; Columbia, South Carolina; Duluth, Minnesota; and Washington, D.C. In New York in 1843, John Littlefield opened an office and became the first practitioner in America to use the designation "chiropodist."

Duchenne, a French physician, wrote in 1855 on the relationship of muscle imbalance in the leg to the function of the foot. His classic text, *Physiologie des mouvements*, is still used as a reference.

In 1860, Issachar Zacharie published a book called *Surgical and Practical Observations on the Diseases of the Human Foot with Instructions for Their Treatment to Which is Added, Advice on the Management of the Hand.* Zacharie unsuccessfully tried to form a chiropodial service for the Union Army. Much of his book was plagiarized from Durlacher and another English chiropodist named Eisenberg. Zacharie claimed to be an M.D. and a former pupil of Sir Astley Pasten Cooper, the eminent London surgeon, although Zacharie was only 14 when Cooper died. Beginning in 1862 Zacharie

served as a confidant to Abraham Lincoln as well as the president's chiropodist.

In 1879, the *Journal of the Illinois State Medical Society* published the first podiatric bibliography, entitled "The Chiropodist" and compiled by Edmund Andrew, M.D. In 1895, a small group that included Charles S. Levy, Howard Levy, Lonie Rosenberg, and George Erff founded the Pedic Society of New York and petitioned the New York state legislature for a bill that led to the first law regulating the field. In 1907 the society began to publish the journal *Pedic Items*, which included matters of clinical and professional interest. In 1908 New Jersey legally regulated chiropody practice.

In 1910, George Erff, President of the Pedic Society of New York, and its 166 members proposed the establishment of podiatric educational facilities, with physicians as chief instructors and Board of Regents examinations for candidates. A code of ethics was proposed. Around the same time, the National Association of Chiropodists (NAC) began to evolve. It was established in July 1912 after a proposal in *Pedic Items*, since a similar association had helped obtain better recognition for osteopathy. The NAC was the forerunner of the American Podiatric Medical Association.

Shortly after its formation, the NAC Committee on Standards and Ethics stressed that members of the profession should not perform operations below the skin; should not use titles not lawfully theirs; should not use men carrying sandwich boards or glaring feet on windows or signs for advertising or share offices with manicurists, hairdressers, beauty specialists, or barbers; and should not dispense or use remedies for which they do not know the formulas.

In 1911 the first school was established in New York; called the New York School of Chiropody, it was the forerunner of the New York College of Podiatric Medicine. Shortly thereafter, in the fall of 1912, the Illinois College of Chiropody and Orthopedics was established. It eventually became the Scholl College of Podiatric Medicine.

In 1912, Maurice J. Lewi, M.D., Secretary of the New York Board of Medical Examiners, drafted successful legislation whereby chiropodists would be licensed by the New York State Board. It required graduation from a chiropody school headed by a medical practitioner. That same year Lewi became president of the New York School of Chiropody, which granted the degree Master of Chiropody (M.Cp.). It was a one-year full-time course requiring one year of high school.

In 1914, EC Stanaback of the NAC advocated direct requests to every state for laws regulating the practice of chiropody. He warned that chiropodists should not use the title "Doctor" on professional cards since to do so would antagonize physicians. By 1915, New York, New Jersey, and Pennsylvania had laws regulating practice. Chiropody societies had been formed in 15 states. Iowa chiropodists in 1916 suggested abandoning the term *chiropody* since it sounded so much like *chiropractic.*

On September 19, 1914, the California College of Chiropody was established in San Francisco; it later became the California College of Podiatric Medicine. Two years later the Ohio College of Chiropody, later to become the Ohio College of Podiatric Medicine, was founded. Also in 1916, the California College of Chiropody was permitted to grant the degree of Doctor of Surgical Chiropody (D.S.C.).

When the United States entered World War I in 1917, chiropodists failed to gain commissioned officer status in the military. The U.S. Marine Corps recruited chiropodists at the rank of Sergeant Fourth Class.

In 1918 the Council on Education of the NAC was formed. It was the forerunner of the Council on Podiatric Medical Education, which accredits all U.S. podiatric medical schools and residency programs. Also in 1918 Felix Von Defele coined the term *podiatry.* During the same year the New York School of Chiropody raised its admission requirement to a high school diploma. In 1923 the First Institute of Podiatry, formerly the New York College of Chiropody, and the California College of Chiropody required a high school diploma and two years of full-time day study. In 1925 the Council on Education set a requirement of 2,100 class hours in the medical sciences and 1,000 hours in practical fields.

The NAC in 1921 purchased *Pedic Items* and changed its title to the *Journal of the National Association of Chiropodists.* This was the forerunner of the *Journal of the American Podiatric Medical Association.* At that time 25 states had laws regulating practice. There were 3,784 practitioners and 10 schools teaching chiropody, half of which were

proprietary. Practice privileges extended mainly to the removal of excrescences from the skin of the foot, treatment of abnormal nails, and the care of mechanical problems with padding, shielding, and strapping.

In 1930 Reuben Gross, a New York podiatrist, demonstrated the surgical removal of a corn and the underlying bursa at the NAC convention in Detroit. This was a significant event and perhaps established the beginning of surgical care as an integral part of podiatric practice. During the same period, the use of arch supports and devices molded to the foot as well as physical therapy was introduced into the profession.

The American Association of Colleges of Chiropody–Podiatry was formed in Washington on August 4, 1932. In February of the same year, the magazine *Medicine Economics* recommended that general practitioners in medicine struggling during the Great Depression take podiatry courses and become foot specialists.

In 1934 the Council on Education required a curriculum consisting of three years of full-time coursework plus one year of preprofessional college. This was one of the earliest recognitions by podiatric medicine that it was becoming a so-called "learned profession," a term often reserved for medicine and the law.

In May 1938, Illinois Medical Society members petitioned the House of Delegates of the American Medical Association (AMA) to prohibit AMA members from affiliating with chiropody schools. However, the Judicial Council of the AMA stated, "Chiropody is not a cult as is osteopathy, chiropractic, or Christian science, which have non-scientific bases of treatment, chiropody is an ancillary to medical practice in a limited field considered not important enough for the physician and, therefore, too often neglected, and fills a gap in the medical profession."

In 1940 the Secretary of War opposed the establishment of a Chiropody (Podiatry) Corps as requested by a bill in Congress. The bill died in committee mostly because of physician opposition. However, in January 14, 1941, the U.S. Navy commissioned a limited number of chiropodists. In 1944 there were 58 commissioned practitioners in the Navy.

The American College of Foot Surgeons was organized in 1942. One year later the Michigan State

Supreme Court ruled in favor of podiatrists using narcotics in treatment (*Fowler* v. *State Board of Pharmacy*). The ability of podiatrists to use postoperative analgesics allowed them to perform more surgery.

An organization of orthopedic surgeons recommended in 1949 that podiatrists receive warrant officer rank rather than full commissions in the military. In the same year the American College of Surgeons proposed subdepartments in hospitals for chiropodists. Also in 1949, all podiatric colleges had four-year curricula and required one year of college for admission, but in 1950 podiatrists were still classified as technicians by the Civil Service Commission.

In the Korean War in 1951, the U.S. Army did not recruit podiatrists. The Navy recalled some commissioned podiatrists. The Civil Service Commission reclassified podiatry as a professional occupation. However, it was during the Korean conflict that the opportunity for podiatrists to acquire commissioned officer status in the military was first provided. The Armed Forces Medical Policy Council recommended that the Surgeon-General commission podiatrists as the need arose. In 1953 the Joint Commission on Accreditation of Hospitals (JCAH) informed the NAC that hospitals would not be penalized if they granted podiatrists the same privileges as dentists.

On September 1, 1954, two years of college was made a requirement for admission to all podiatric colleges. New York State in 1957 allowed podiatrists to use the title "foot specialist" on stationery and office signs. The New York State Education Department in 1957 permitted podiatrists to use injections of all sorts for treating skin and allergic conditions; to give sensitivity tests, superficial roentgen therapy, and tetanus antitoxin; to diagnose foot injuries by x-ray, to include the ankle and the lower 3 inches of the leg; and to do all necessary laboratory work. In the same year the first podiatric residency program began in Philadelphia at St. Luke's and Children's Medical Center (now James C. Giuffré Medical Center).

On January 1, 1958, the name of the profession was officially changed to podiatry, and its journal to the *Journal of the American Podiatry Association*. Shortly thereafter, in 1960, the Selden Report was issued recommending changes in podiatric medical education, including improved basic science in-

struction and more full-time professors as well as improved libraries. In 1962 the National Board of Podiatric Medical Examiners administered its first examination. This two-part examination, given at the end of the second year of podiatric medical school in the basic sciences, and at the end of the fourth year in the clinical areas, is part of the requirement for licensure in 43 states and the federal services. The Pennsylvania College of Chiropody was established in 1960, opening in September 1963 and eventually becoming the Pennsylvania College of Podiatric Medicine.

By 1964, podiatric medical schools, which before had issued as many as two or three different degrees upon completion of their programs, now only granted the degree of Doctor of Podiatric Medicine (D.P.M.). The first two residencies approved by the Council on Podiatry Education were granted that designation in 1965. In 1966, podiatrists entered the U.S. Army as first lieutenants and became captains in 6 months, bringing the profession closer to parity with medicine and dentistry. Also in 1966 the terms *chiropody* and *chiropodist* were eliminated from the constitution of the American Podiatry Association.

By 1967, 31 states had Blue Shield plans that covered podiatric services. By 1979, with the addition of North Dakota, all states included Blue Shield coverage for care rendered by podiatrists. Bulletin 44 of the Joint Commission on Accreditation of Hospitals, issued in April 1967, permitted podiatrists to operate in hospital operating rooms without the presence of a gowned, scrubbed M.D. or D.O. surgeon. Podiatric medicine appeared in the standards of the JCAH in 1970 for the first time. Medicare included podiatry in 1968 and defined D.P.M.s as physicians within the scope of podiatric practice.

The Health Professional Educational Assistance Act was amended in 1965 to include podiatric medical schools. This act and subsequent amendments provided funds for construction of new facilities, supported educational innovations, and provided additional money based on the number of students enrolled in the colleges. The Health Professions Loan and Scholarship Program offered scholarship and loan monies to podiatric medical students in financial need.

The Podiatric Health Section of the American Public Health Association was established in 1972.

The American Board of Podiatric Surgery was also established that year, initiating a movement toward board certification in several areas of the profession, which now include surgery, orthopedics, and public health.

In April of 1977 the American College of Surgeons recognized podiatrists as practitioners permitted to perform hospital surgery. In the same year the AMA recognized the right of qualified podiatrists to have practice privileges in hospitals based on their education, training, and experience. JCAH standards in 1976 recognized podiatric house staff (residents).

In 1978 the Medical College Admissions Test (MCAT) was required of applicants to podiatric medical schools. In that same year, all of the podiatric medical colleges required a minimum of three years of college before entry.

In 1985, the American Podiatric Medical Association charged an independent commission with the task of determining how podiatric medicine could best meet the foot health needs of the American people in the year 2000. The Project 2000 Commission made 19 recommendations, some of the most important of which focused on the area of education and training for the profession. Perhaps the most important of these was the recommendation that the existing colleges of podiatric medicine "work diligently toward affiliation or association with academic health science centers."

The commission referred to the 1961 Selden Report and its 26 recommendations. It emphasized that the most important recommendations of the Selden Report not yet fully implemented included those dealing with affiliation of the colleges of podiatric medicine with academic health science centers. The commission noted that nonaffiliation had affected podiatric medical education negatively during the previous 25 years.

THE EVOLUTION OF PODIATRIC MEDICINE AND ITS RELATIONSHIP WITH MEDICINE

Podiatric medicine is not the only profession that provides medical and surgical foot care. Orthopedic surgery also provides care for foot disorders, and other specialties such as family practice and dermatology treat a considerable number of patients with foot problems. Surveys show that, in general, more foot care is provided by podiatric physicians. However, whereas podiatrists perform more surgical procedures for certain common foot disorders such as hallux valgus, hammer toes, and other deformities of the forefoot, orthopedic surgeons are more involved with the care of fractures and dislocations of the pedal extremity. This may be explained to some extent by the fact that a large percentage of patients in most podiatric medical practices are those receiving long-term, conservative care for forefoot disorders. In cases where such care is no longer adequate and surgery becomes an appropriate option, these patients are more likely to have the podiatrist, with whom they have developed a long-term relationship, perform the necessary procedures. The episodic nature of trauma, given existing referral systems in the United States, is more likely to result in patients with such problems being treated by an orthopedist. These factors, combined with a health care system that still permits considerable free choice of physicians, provide patients with several options for foot care. Podiatric physicians, however, restrict themselves to foot care. This is very rarely the case for orthopedists and even less so for other medical specialists. As a result, in the United States podiatrists see the largest number and percentage of patients with problems affecting the foot.

The evolution of the podiatric medical profession, particularly in the last 30 years, has led to licensure for the podiatrist, which permits the provision of any preventive, diagnostic, medical, or surgical procedure for the care of the foot in any of the United States. This has resulted in the creation of a physician whose education and training focus on one anatomic area, in a manner analogous to other medical specialists. Licensure of other physicians (e.g., M.D.s and D.O.s) is unrestricted, but current medical practice, with its continuing concern about such issues as malpractice liability, standards of care in the community, quality of care, and the impossibility of anyone being knowledgeable about all aspects of medicine, has virtually restricted the physician to one aspect of practice (e.g., general surgery, ophthalmology, orthopedics, dermatology, or family practice). Podiatric medical practice, on the other hand, has by license been restricted to the practice of its medical and surgical specialty. The evolution of the profession and this simple difference in licensure, however, continues to contribute to interprofessional disputes, which probably are economic in origin and to some degree the result of strong feelings of tradition. The controversy is often clouded by arguments about who is qualified to do what in the ongoing battle for professional turf.

Over the years, however, improved educational and training programs in podiatric medicine and surgery, ongoing discussions between medical and podiatric medical groups, increased governmental recognition, and other factors have resulted in vastly improved relations between organized general medicine and podiatric medicine. History tells us that this dynamic process will probably continue and that the greatest benefactor will be the patient.

PODIATRIC MEDICAL EDUCATION AND TRAINING

Tables 1-1 to 1-3 chronologically outline the rapid evolution of education and training in podiatric medicine. These advances have been particularly dramatic since World War II.

Podiatric medical schools today are characterized by large, modern facilities, expanded full-time faculties, complex curricula, and students who must look forward to up to a decade or more of education and training. There is only a slight resemblance to what existed before the 1960s. The podiatric medical school of the 1930s and 1940s had the less complex task of preparing individuals for a career that was narrower in scope than current podiatric medical practice. Surgery, for example, was virtually unheard of, as were hospital privileges of any kind. Education and training programs were far shorter than today, and postgraduate residencies were nonexistent.

Those preparing for podiatric medical practice today usually look toward completing a four-year undergraduate degree in a premedical sequence, taking the MCAT examination, obtaining a D.P.M. degree upon completion of another four years of full-time study, and then undertaking a residency

Table 1-1. Modern History of Podiatric Medical Schools in the United States

1911	First podiatric medical school, the New York School of Chiropody, is set up in New York City. It is the forerunner of the New York College of Podiatric Medicine.
1912	Dr. William M. Scholl College of Podiatric Medicine (originally the Illinois College of Chiropody and Orthopedics) is established in Chicago.
1914	California College of Podiatric Medicine opens in San Francisco.
1916	Ohio College of Podiatric Medicine is founded in Cleveland.
1963	Pennsylvania College of Podiatric Medicine succeeds the defunct Temple University School of Chiropody, which had closed three years earlier.
1974	School of Podiatric Medicine in the Health Science Center of the State University of New York at Stony Brook becomes the first podiatric medical program in an academic health science center, but closes two years later because of a fiscal crisis in New York State.
1981	College of Podiatric Medicine and Surgery of the University of Osteopathic Medicine and Health Sciences becomes the first viable podiatric medical program in an academic health science center.
1985	Barry University establishes a School of Podiatric Medicine in Miami Shores, Florida.

of two or even three years' duration. At the end of this training the podiatrist is eligible to complete the requirements for board certification in either podiatric surgery, podiatric orthopedics, or public health, which also entail passing written and oral examinations and accumulating appropriate documented experiences (i.e., certain numbers and types of cases).

Table 1-4 lists the major studies influencing podiatric medical education and their recommendations. It is obvious that the podiatric medical education of the future will be dramatically influenced by rising health care costs, new ways of financing and organizing the delivery of care, and a much greater influx of biotechnology and computerization. A more health-minded public will demand health services as a basic right regardless of socioeconomic status. Growing complexities in all fields of health care, including podiatric medicine, will no doubt make it more difficult for the practitioner to establish an independent practice. One can expect that the solo practitioner of today will begin to be supplanted by multidisciplinary practice arrangements in profit or nonprofit corporations of considerable size. Such arrangements will have a profound effect not only on how students and residents are prepared for practice, but also on what

Table 1-2. History of Educational Requirements for the Podiatric Medical Degree in the United States[a]

College	High School				Preprofessional College			Podiatric Medical College			
	1	2	3	4	1	2	3	1	2	3	4
Barry University[b]							1985				1985
California College of Podiatric Medicine	1916			1923	1938	1953	1978	1915	1923	1938	1946
Dr. William M. Scholl College of Podiatric Medicine	1916	1917	1923	1926	1938	1964	1978	1915	ca. 1925	ca. 1935	1940
New York College of Podiatric Medicine	1912	1917	1919	1921	1932	1940	1968	1912	ca. 1924	ca. 1932	1952
Ohio College of Podiatric Medicine				1916	1938	1964	1978	1917	ca. 1925	ca. 1935	ca. 1945
Pennsylvania College of Podiatric Medicine						1963	1978				1963
University of Osteopathic Medicine and Health Sciences[c]							1981				1981

[a] Year given is the year in which the minimum requirement was implemented.
[b] Established in 1985.
[c] Established in 1981.
Sources: Podiatry Education in the 1960's, Status and Opportunities, Report of the Special Commission on Status of Podiatry Education. p 50. American Podiatry Association, Washington, DC, 1961. Levy LA: The history of a college of podiatric medicine —Index of a growing profession. J Podiatr Med Educ 1(2):22–9, 1970. Bates JE, Holloway LM: A Fast Pace Forward, and Chronicles of American Podiatry, American Podiatric Medical Association (75th Anniversary). p. 55. Pennsylvania College of Podiatric Medicine, Philadelphia, 1987.

Table 1-3. Significant Dates in the College Entrance Testing, National Licensing Examinations, Board Certification, and Residency Training in Podiatric Medicine

1919	Establishment of the Council on Podiatric Medical Education, the nationally recognized accrediting body for evaluating podiatric medical education.
1957	First postgraduate residency program established at St. Luke's and Children's Medical Center, Philadelphia.
1962	National Board of Podiatric Medical Examiners gives its first examination. The examination is currently administered by the Educational Testing Service, Princeton, NJ, and recognized for licensure in 43 states and 3 Canadian provinces, and by the U.S. Army and Navy.
1968	Colleges of Podiatry Admissions Test (CPAT) required of all applicants to podiatric medical schools.
1975	American Board of Podiatric Surgery is established, initiating the process of board certification in the profession.
1978	Medical College Admission Test (MCAT) replaces the CPAT as the examination required of all applicants to podiatric medical schools.
1978	American Board of Podiatric Orthopedics is established.
1987	American Board of Podiatric Public Health becomes the third certifying board for the profession.

type of person will enter the profession. Students looking toward a career as entrepreneurial professionals may begin to be replaced with others who will be equally comfortable as employees of larger health care organizations.

SELECTED READINGS

Dagnall JC: 50th anniversary issue. Br J Chiropody 48(7):137, 1983

Dagnall JC: Economy of the hands and feet. The ClioPedic Items—Bulletin of the Center for the History of Foot Care and Foot Wear, Pennsylvania College of Podiatric Medicine, 2:2, 1987/88

American Podiatric Medical Association, Department of Professional Affairs: History and Current Practice of Podiatric Medicine. American Podiatric Medical Association, Washington, DC, 1984

Table 1-4. Major Studies Influencing Podiatric Medical Education Since 1960

Year	Study	Comments
1960	Selden Report (Special Commission on the Status of Podiatry Education in the 1960s)	Recommends expansion and improvement of facilities at colleges, increased prerequisites for entrance; enlargement of full-time faculty; improved basic science education; affiliation with universities; more research efforts.
1970	Blauch Report (The Podiatry Curriculum: Association of Colleges of Podiatric Medicine)	Detailed examination of the podiatric curriculum, with comprehensive guidelines for education and training of podiatric medical student; designed for the colleges, faculty, and licensing bodies in the profession.
1986	Project 2000 Commission—Comprehensive Foot Care (The Report of the National Commission on Podiatric Medicine—American Podiatric Medical Association)	Recommends that any new and existing podiatric medical schools be affiliated with academic health science centers. Quality of students should improve. Podiatric surgical residencies should be at least 2 in length. Recommends strengthening instruction in aging, ethics, and behavioral sciences. More community leaders should be included on college boards of trustees. A more organized approach to research is advocated. Colleges should reduce dependence on student tuition and determine appropriate number of faculty and improve their salaries.

American Podiatry Association: Podiatry in the '70's—A Report to the Membership—A Decade of Progress 1969–79. American Podiatry Association, Washington, DC, 1979

Bates JE, Holloway LM: A Fast Pace Forward & Chronicles of American Podiatry, American Podiatric Medical Association (75th Anniversary). Pennsylvania College of Podiatric Medicine, Philadelphia, 1987

American Podiatric Medical Association: 75th Annual Meeting and Exhibit Program—Celebrating 75 years. American Podiatric Medical Association, Washington, DC, 1987

Anatomy of the Foot

2

Wayne A. Krueger, Ph.D.
Vincent J. Hetherington, D.P.M., M.S.
Jeffery Carnett, D.P.M.

There are many excellent published descriptions of foot anatomy (see Selected Readings). Rather than replicate a classic description, we have decided to present illustrations of the sectional anatomy of the foot, which effectively depict numerous relationships that are of vital importance to the clinician.

Three feet obtained from previously embalmed cadavers were frozen at −20°C for 2 to 3 weeks before sectioning. Sections 0.9 to 1.3 cm thick were cut with a commercial band saw. Sagittal sections of the left foot were cut from one specimen, oriented as shown in Figure 2-1. Figures 2-2 through 2-4 show the medial surfaces of three sections from this series, arranged from most medial (Fig. 2-2) to most lateral (Fig. 2-4).

Cross sections of the right foot, oriented as shown in Figure 2-5, were cut from a second specimen. Seven of these sections (Figs. 2-6 through 2-12) are illustrated, arranged from most inferior (Fig. 2-6) to most superior (Fig. 2-12). By convention, these transverse sections are viewed from below.

Coronal sections of the right foot, oriented as shown in Figure 2-5, were cut from a third specimen. Figures 2-13 through 2-28 illustrate this series. They are arranged from most anterior (Fig. 2-13) to most posterior (Fig. 2-28), and the anterior surface of each section is shown.

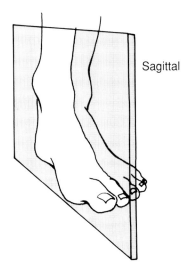

Fig. 2-1. Orientation of sagittal sections cut from a left foot. Figures 2-2 through 2-4 show sagittal sections cut from one specimen, arranged from most medial (Fig. 2-2) to most lateral (Fig. 2-4). The medial surface of each section is shown.

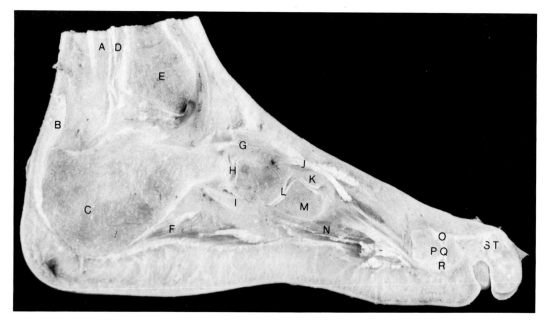

Fig. 2-2. Sagittal section.

Key

A. Peroneus longus
B. Tendo calcaneus (Achilles tendon)
C. Calcaneus
D. Peroneus brevis
E. Fibula
F. Abductor digiti minimi
G. Extensor digitorum brevis

H. Calcaneocuboid joint
I. Peroneus longus tendon
J. Extensor digitorum brevis tendon
K. Base of fourth metatarsal
L. Cuboideometatarsal joint
M. Base of fifth metatarsal
N. Flexor digiti minimi

O. Extensor expansion
P. Head of fourth metatarsal
Q. Metatarsophalangeal joint
R. Glenoid ligament
S. Proximal interphalangeal joint
T. Middle phalanx

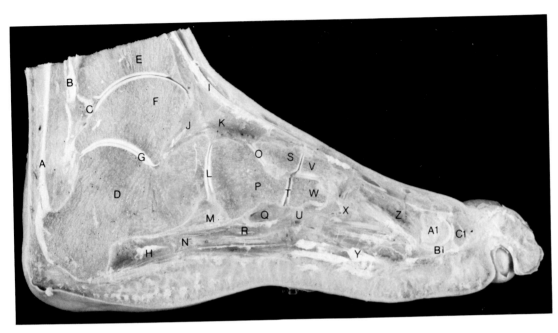

Fig. 2-3. Sagittal section.

Key

A. Tendo calcaneus
B. Flexor hallucis longus
C. Posterior tibiotalar ligament
D. Calcaneus
E. Tibia
F. Talus
G. Talocalcaneal joint
H. Flexor digitorum longus
I. Extensor digitorum longus
J. Cervical ligament (interosseous talocalcaneal ligament)
K. Extensor digitorum brevis
L. Calcaneocuboid joint
M. Plantar calcaneonavicular (spring) ligament
N. Lateral plantar vessels

O. Cuneocuboid joint
P. Cuboid bone
Q. Peroneus longus
R. Flexor hallucis brevis
S. Lateral cuneiform bone
T. Cuboideometatarsal joint
U. Oblique head of adductor hallucis
V. Base of third metatarsal
W. Base of fourth metatarsal
X. Plantar interosseous muscle
Y. Flexor digitorum brevis tendon
Z. Dorsal interosseous muscle
A1. Head of third metatarsal
B1. Glenoid ligament
C1. Proximal phalanx

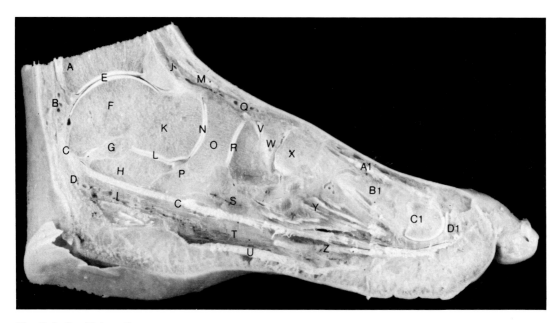

Fig. 2-4. Sagittal section.

Key

A. Tibia
B. Posterior tibial vessels
C. Flexor hallucis longus
D. Lateral plantar vessels
E. Ankle joint
F. Talus
G. Interosseous talocalcaneal ligament
H. Sustentaculum tali
I. Medial plantar vessels
J. Anterior medial malleolar artery
K. Neck of talus
L. Talocalcaneal joint
M. Extensor hallucis longus
N. Talonavicular joint
O. Navicular bone

P. Plantar calcaneonavicular (spring) ligament
Q. Dorsalis pedis artery
R. Medial cuneonavicular joint
S. Flexor hallucis brevis
T. Flexor digitorum brevis
U. Plantar aponeurosis
V. Intercuneiform joint
W. Intermediate cuneiform bone
X. Base of second metatarsal
Y. Oblique head of adductor hallucis
Z. Flexor digitorum longus
A1. Extensor digitorum longus
B1. Dorsal interosseous muscle
C1. Head of second metatarsal
D1. Base of second phalanx

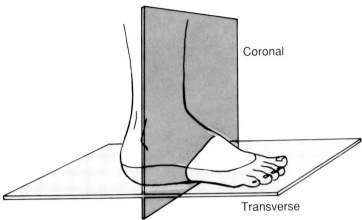

Coronal

Transverse

Fig. 2-5. Orientation of transverse and coronal sections cut from right foot specimens. Figures 2-6 through 2-12 show transverse sections of one specimen, arranged from most inferior (Fig. 2-6) to most superior (Fig. 2-12). The inferior surface of each section is shown. Figures 2-13 through 2-28 show coronal sections of a different specimen. These sections are arranged from most anterior (Fig. 2-13) to most posterior (Fig. 2-28). The anterior surface of each section is shown.

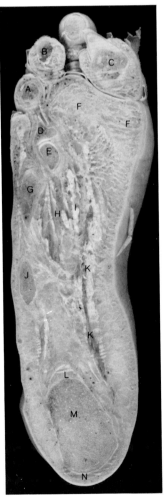

Fig. 2-6. Transverse section.

Key

A. Distal phalanx of fourth digit
B. Distal phalanx of third digit
C. Distal phalanx of first digit
D. Proximal phalanx of fourth digit
E. Fourth metatarsal
F. Fat
G. Fifth metatarsal
H. Flexor digiti quinti
I. Flexor digitorum longus
J. Styloid process of fifth metatarsal
K. Abductor hallucis
L. Flexor digitorum brevis
M. Calcaneus
N. Tendo calcaneus

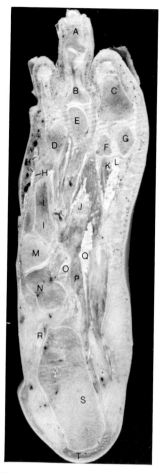

Fig. 2-7. Transverse section.

Key

A. Middle phalanx of second digit
B. Proximal phalanx of second digit
C. Proximal phalanx of hallux
D. Third metatarsal
E. Second metatarsal
F. Lateral sesamoid bone
G. Medial sesamoid bone
H. Extensor digitorum longus tendons
I. Fourth metatarsal
J. Oblique head of adductor hallucis
K. Flexor hallucis brevis
L. Flexor hallucis longus
M. Base of fifth metatarsal
N. Cuboid bone
O. Peroneus longus
P. Quadratus plantae
Q. Flexor digitorum longus
R. Peroneus brevis
S. Calcaneus
T. Tendo calcaneus

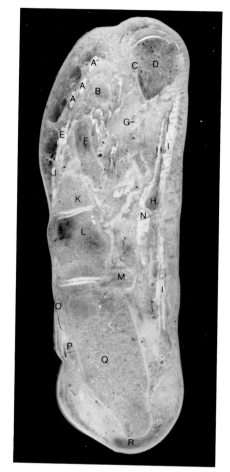

Fig. 2-8. Transverse section.

Key

A. Extensor digitorum longus tendons
B. Second metatarsal
C. Extensor hallucis brevis
D. First metatarsal
E. Extensor hallucis brevis tendon
F. Third metatarsal
G. Plantar metatarsal artery
H. Flexor hallucis brevis
I. Abductor hallucis
J. Peroneus tertius tendon
K. Fourth metatarsal
L. Cuboid bone
M. Short plantar ligament
N. Tibialis posterior tendon
O. Peroneus brevis tendon
P. Peroneus longus tendon
Q. Calcaneus
R. Tendo calcaneus

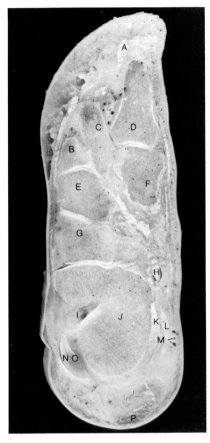

Fig. 2-9. Transverse section.

Key

A. Extensor hallucis brevis tendon
B. Base of third metatarsal
C. Second metatarsal
D. Base of first metatarsal
E. Lateral cuneiform bone
F. Medial cuneiform bone
G. Cuboid bone
H. Tibialis posterior tendon
I. Sinus tarsi
J. Calcaneus
K. Flexor hallucis longus tendon
L. Flexor digitorum longus tendon
M. Posterior tibial vessels
N. Peroneus longus tendon
O. Peroneus brevis
P. Tendo calcaneus

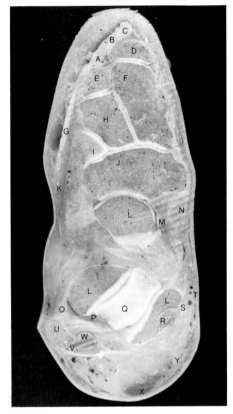

Fig. 2-10. Transverse section.

Key

A. Deep plantar artery
B. Extensor hallucis brevis tendon
C. Extensor hallucis longus tendon
D. First metatarsal
E. Second metatarsal
F. Medial cuneiform bone
G. Extensor digitorum longus tendons
H. Intermediate cuneiform bone
I. Lateral cuneiform bone
J. Navicular bone
K. Peroneus tertius
L. Talus (labeled in three places)
M. Plantar calcaneonavicular (spring) ligament
N. Tibialis posterior tendon
O. Talofibular ligament
P. Subtalar joint
Q. Calcaneus
R. Flexor hallucis longus tendon
S. Tibial nerve
T. Posterior tibial vessels
U. Fibula
V. Peroneus brevis
W. Peroneus longus
X. Tendo calcaneus
Y. Plantaris tendon

19

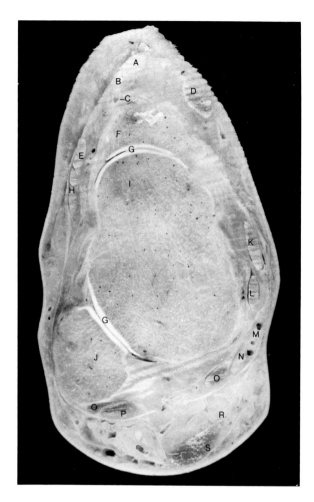

Fig. 2-11. Transverse section.

Key

A. Extensor hallucis longus tendon
B. Extensor hallucis brevis tendon
C. Anterior tibial artery
D. Tibialis anterior tendon
E. Extensor digitorum longus tendon
F. Tibia
G. Ankle joint
H. Peroneus tertius tendon
I. Talus
J. Fibula
K. Tibialis posterior tendon
L. Flexor digitorum longus tendon
M. Posterior tibial vessels
N. Tibial nerve
O. Peroneus brevis tendon
P. Peroneus longus tendon
Q. Flexor hallucis longus tendon
R. Fat
S. Tendo calcaneus

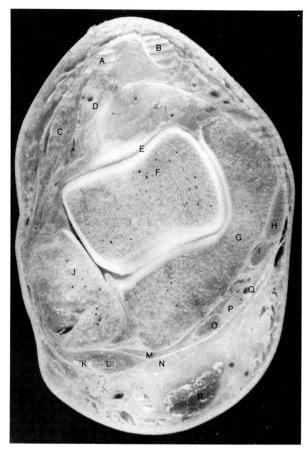

Fig. 2-12. Transverse section.

Key

A. Extensor hallucis longus tendon
B. Tibialis anterior tendon
C. Extensor digitorum longus tendon
D. Anterior tibial artery
E. Ankle joint
F. Talus
G. Tibia
H. Tibialis posterior tendon
I. Flexor digitorum longus tendon
J. Fibula
K. Peroneus brevis tendon
L. Peroneus longus
M. Peroneal artery
N. Fat
O. Flexor hallucis longus tendon
P. Tibial nerve
Q. Posterior tibial vessels
R. Tendo calcaneus

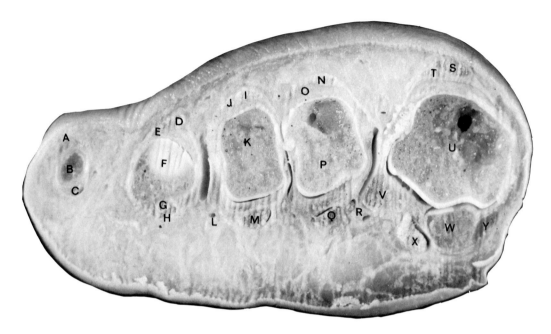

Fig. 2-13. Coronal section.

Key

A. Extensor digitorum longus
B. Fifth metatarsal
C. Flexor digiti minimi brevis
D. Extensor digitorum longus
E. Extensor digitorum brevis
F. Fourth metatarsal
G. Flexor digitorum longus
H. Flexor digitorum brevis
I. Extensor digitorum longus
J. Extensor digitorum brevis
K. Third metatarsal
L. Plantar metatarsal artery
M. Flexor digitorum longus

N. Extensor digitorum longus
O. Extensor digitorum brevis
P. Fourth metatarsal
Q. Flexor digitorum longus
R. Plantar metatarsal artery
S. Extensor hallucis longus
T. Extensor hallucis brevis
U. First metatarsal
V. Lateral sesamoid bone
W. Medial sesamoid bone
X. Flexor hallucis longus
Y. Abductor hallucis

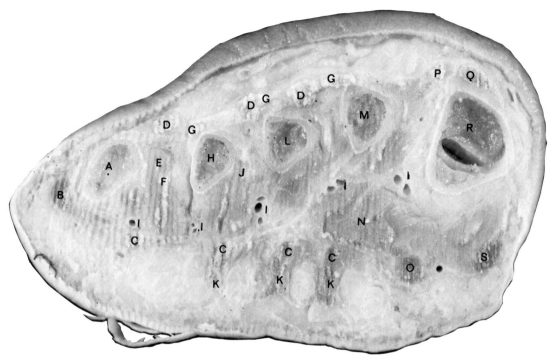

Fig. 2-14. Coronal section.

Key

A. Fifth metatarsal
B. Abductor digiti minimi
C. Flexor digitorum longus
D. Extensor digitorum brevis
E. Dorsal interosseous muscle
F. Plantar interosseous muscle
G. Extensor digitorum longus
H. Fourth metatarsal
I. Plantar metatarsal vessels
J. Plantar interosseous muscle

K. Flexor digitorum brevis
L. Third metatarsal
M. Second metatarsal
N. Oblique head of adductor hallucis
O. Flexor hallucis longus
P. Extensor hallucis brevis
Q. Extensor hallucis longus
R. First metatarsal
S. Abductor hallucis

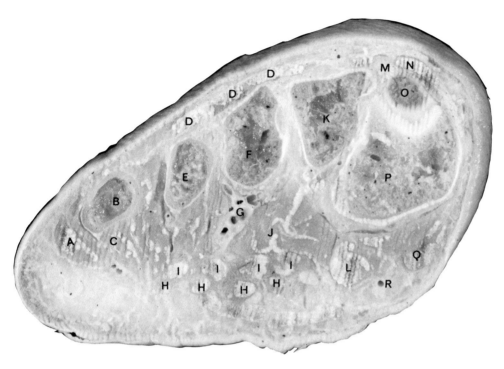

Fig. 2-15. Coronal section.

Key

A. Abductor digiti minimi
B. Fifth metatarsal
C. Flexor digiti minimi
D. Extensor digitorum longus
E. Fourth metatarsal
F. Third metatarsal
G. Lateral plantar vessels
H. Flexor digitorum brevis
I. Flexor digitorum longus

J. Oblique head of adductor hallucis
K. Second metatarsal
L. Flexor hallucis longus
M. Extensor hallucis brevis
N. Extensor hallucis longus
O. Medial cuneiform bone
P. Base of first metatarsal
Q. Abductor hallucis
R. Medial plantar artery

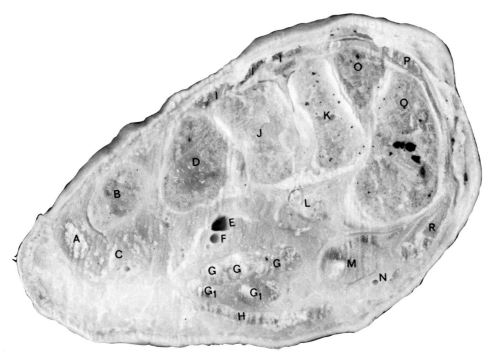

Fig. 2-16. Coronal section.

Key

A.   Abductor digiti minimi
B.   Fifth metatarsal
C.   Flexor digiti minimi
D.   Fourth metatarsal
E.   Lateral plantar vein
F.   Lateral plantar artery
G.   Flexor digitorum longus tendon
G_1.   Flexor digitorum brevis
H.   Plantar fascia
I.   Extensor digitorum longus

J.   Third metatarsal
K.   Second metatarsal
L.   Peroneus longus tendon
M.   Flexor hallucis longus
N.   Medial plantar artery
O.   Intermediate cuneiform bone
P.   Extensor hallucis longus
Q.   Medial cuneiform bone
R.   Abductor hallucis

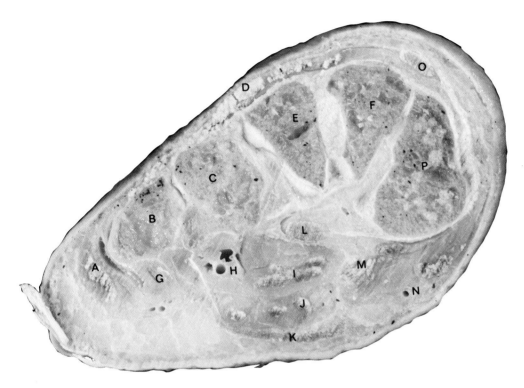

Fig. 2-17. Coronal section.

Key

A. Abductor digiti minimi
B. Fifth metatarsal
C. Fourth metatarsal
D. Extensor digitorum longus
E. Lateral cuneiform bone
F. Intermediate cuneiform bone
G. Flexor digiti minimi
H. Lateral plantar vessels

I. Flexor digitorum longus
J. Flexor digitorum brevis
K. Plantar aponeurosis
L. Peroneus longus tendon
M. Flexor hallucis longus
N. Medial plantar artery
O. Extensor hallucis longus
P. Medial cuneiform bone

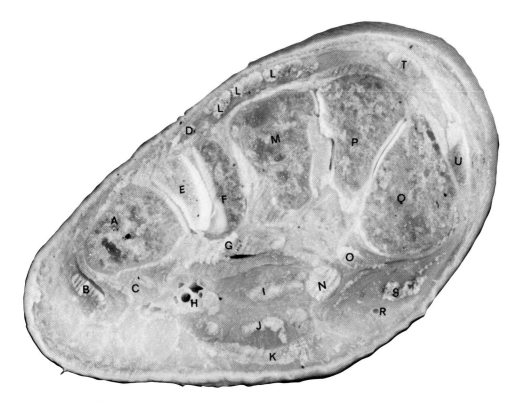

Fig. 2-18. Coronal section.

Key

A. Fifth metatarsal
B. Abductor digiti minimi
C. Flexor digiti minimi
D. Extensor digitorum brevis
E. Base of fourth metatarsal
F. Cuboid bone
G. Peroneus longus tendon
H. Lateral plantar vessels
I. Quadratus plantae
J. Flexor digitorum brevis
K. Plantar aponeurosis

L. Extensor digitorum longus
M. Lateral cuneiform bone
N. Flexor digitorum longus
O. Flexor hallucis longus
P. Intermediate cuneiform bone
Q. Medial cuneiform bone
R. Medial plantar artery
S. Abductor hallucis
T. Extensor hallucis longus
U. Tibialis anterior tendon

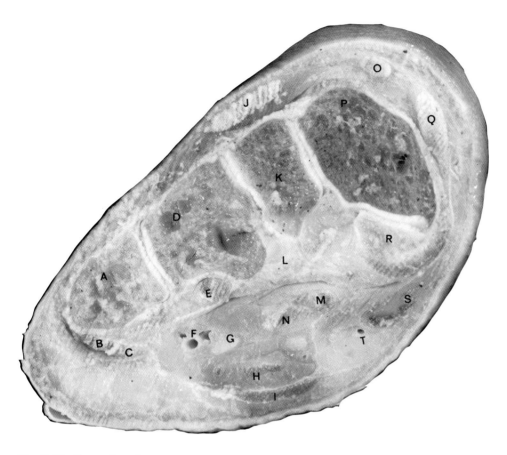

Fig. 2-19. Coronal section.

Key

A. Base of fifth metatarsal
B. Abductor digiti minimi
C. Flexor digiti minimi
D. Cuboid bone
E. Peroneus longus
F. Lateral plantar vessels
G. Quadratus plantae
H. Flexor digitorum brevis
I. Plantar aponeurosis
J. Extensor digitorum longus

K. Lateral cuneiform bone
L. Flexor hallucis brevis
M. Flexor hallucis longus
N. Flexor digitorum longus
O. Extensor hallucis longus
P. Navicular bone
Q. Tibialis anterior
R. Medial cuneiform bone
S. Abductor hallucis
T. Medial plantar artery

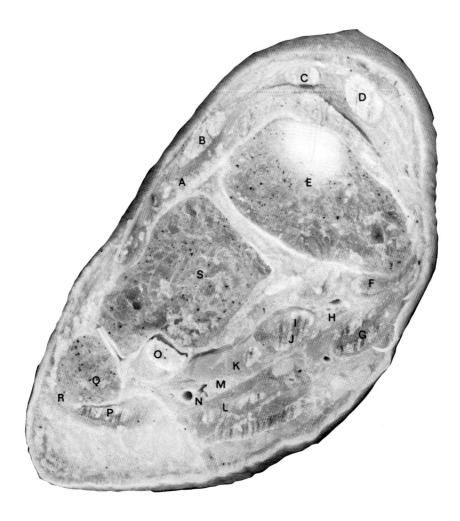

Fig. 2-20. Coronal section.

Key

A. Extensor digitorum brevis
B. Extensor digitorum longus
C. Extensor hallucis longus
D. Tibialis anterior
E. Navicular bone
F. Tibialis posterior
G. Abductor hallucis
H. Medial plantar vein, artery, and nerve
I. Flexor hallucis longus
J. Flexor digitorum longus

K. Quadratus plantae
L. Flexor digitorum brevis
M. Lateral plantar nerve
N. Lateral plantar vein and artery
O. Peroneus longus
P. Abductor digiti minimi
Q. Tuberosity of fifth metatarsal
R. Peroneus brevis
S. Cuboid bone

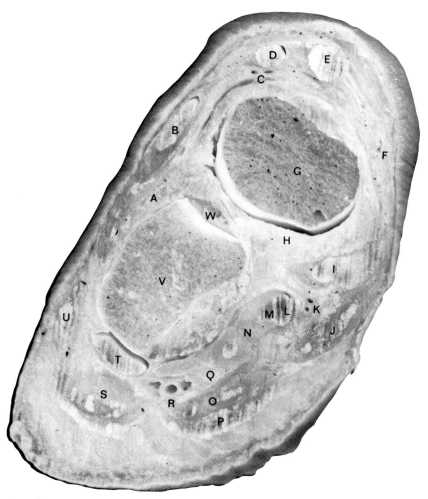

Fig. 2-21. Coronal section.

Key

A. Extensor digitorum brevis
B. Extensor digitorum longus
C. Dorsalis pedis
D. Extensor hallucis longus
E. Tibialis anterior
F. Saphenous vein
G. Talus (head)
H. Plantar calcaneonavicular (spring) ligament
I. Tibialis posterior
J. Abductor hallucis
K. Medial plantar vein, artery, and nerve
L. Flexor digitorum longus

M. Flexor hallucis longus
N. Quadratus plantae
O. Flexor digitorum brevis
P. Plantar aponeurosis
Q. Lateral plantar nerve
R. Lateral plantar vein and artery
S. Abductor digiti minimi
T. Peroneus longus
U. Peroneus brevis
V. Cuboid bone
W. Calcaneus

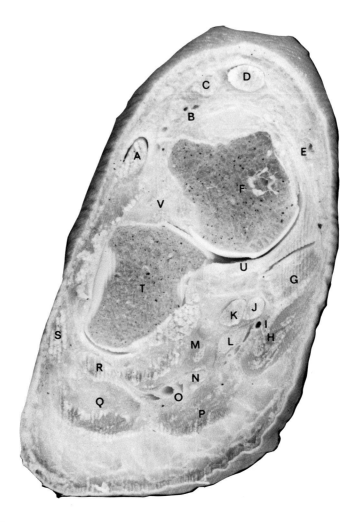

Fig. 2-22. Coronal section.

Key

A. Extensor digitorum longus
B. Dorsalis pedis
C. Extensor hallucis longus
D. Tibialis anterior
E. Great saphenous vein
F. Talus
G. Tibialis posterior
H. Abductor hallucis
I. Medial plantar vein and artery
J. Flexor digitorum longus
K. Flexor hallucis longus

L. Lateral plantar nerve
M. Quadratus plantae
N. Lateral plantar nerve
O. Lateral plantar vein and artery
P. Flexor digitorum brevis
Q. Abductor digiti minimi
R. Peroneus longus
S. Peroneus brevis
T. Calcaneus
U. Plantar calcaneonavicular (spring) ligament
V. Interosseous talocalcaneal ligament

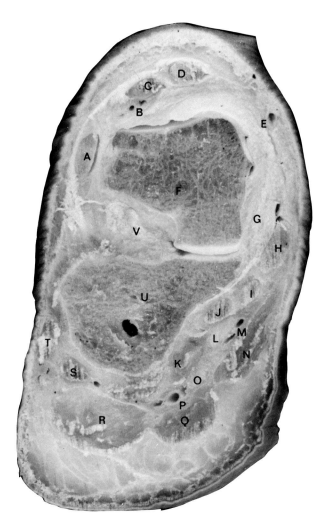

Fig. 2-23. Coronal section.

Key

A. Extensor digitorum longus
B. Dorsalis pedis
C. Extensor hallucis longus
D. Tibialis anterior
E. Great saphenous vein
F. Talus
G. Deltoid ligament
H. Tibialis posterior
I. Flexor digitorum longus
J. Flexor hallucis longus
K. Quadratus plantae

L. Medial plantar nerve
M. Medial plantar vein and artery
N. Abductor hallucis
O. Lateral plantar nerve
P. Lateral plantar vein and artery
Q. Flexor digitorum brevis
R. Abductor digiti minimi
S. Peroneus longus
T. Peroneus brevis
U. Calcaneus
V. Interosseous talocalcaneal ligament

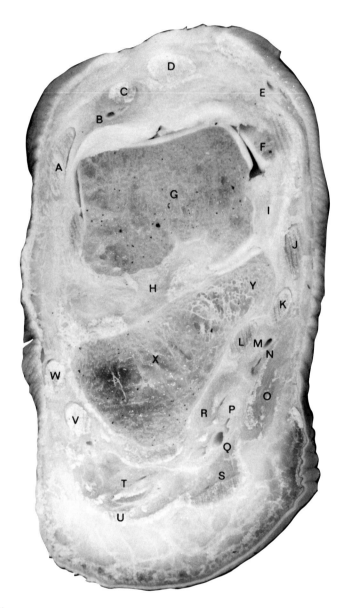

Fig. 2-24. Coronal section.

Key

A. Extensor digitorum longus
B. Dorsalis pedis
C. Extensor hallucis longus
D. Tibialis anterior
E. Great saphenous vein
F. Medial malleolus
G. Talus
H. Interosseous talocalcaneal ligament
I. Deltoid ligament

J. Tibialis anterior
K. Flexor digitorum longus
L. Flexor hallucis longus
M. Medial plantar nerve
N. Medial plantar vein and artery
O. Abductor hallucis
P. Lateral plantar nerve
Q. Lateral plantar vein and artery
R. Quadratus plantae

S. Flexor digitorum brevis
T. Abductor digiti minimi
U. Plantar aponeurosis
V. Peroneus longus
W. Peroneus brevis
X. Calcaneus
Y. Sustentaculum tali

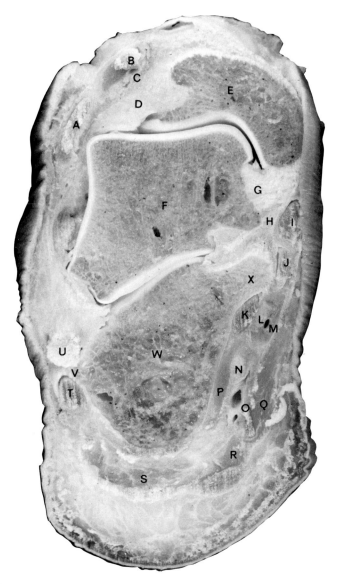

Fig. 2-25. Coronal section.

Key

A. Extensor digitorum longus
B. Extensor hallucis longus
C. Dorsalis pedis
D. Anterior inferior tibiofibular ligament
E. Tibia
F. Talus
G. Anterior tibiotalar ligament (part of the deltoid ligament)
H. Tibiocalcaneal ligament (part of the deltoid ligament)

I. Tibialis posterior
J. Flexor digitorum longus
K. Flexor hallucis longus
L. Medial plantar nerve
M. Medial plantar artery
N. Lateral plantar nerve
O. Lateral plantar vein and artery
P. Quadratus plantae
Q. Abductor hallucis
R. Flexor digitorum brevis

S. Abductor digiti minimi
T. Peroneus longus
U. Peroneus brevis
V. Trochlea peronealis
W. Calcaneus
X. Sustentaculum tali

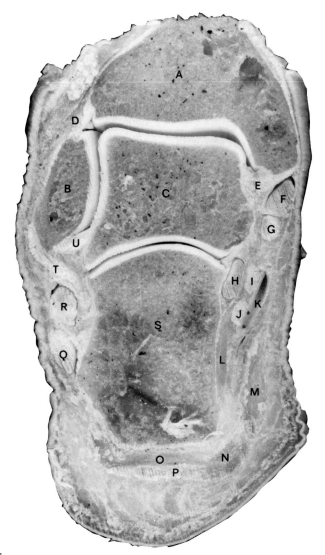

Fig. 2-26. Coronal section.

Key

A. Tibia
B. Fibula (lateral malleolus)
C. Talus
D. Interosseous tibiofibular ligament
E. Posterior tibiotalar ligament (part of the deltoid ligament)
F. Tibialis posterior
G. Flexor digitorum longus
H. Flexor hallucis longus
 I. Medial plantar nerve
J. Lateral plantar nerve
K. Posterior tibial artery with medial calcaneal branches

L. Quadratus plantae
M. Abductor hallucis
N. Flexor digitorum brevis
O. Abductor digiti minimi
P. Plantar aponeurosis
Q. Peroneus longus
R. Peroneus brevis
S. Calcaneus
T. Calcaneofibular ligament
U. Anterior talofibular ligament

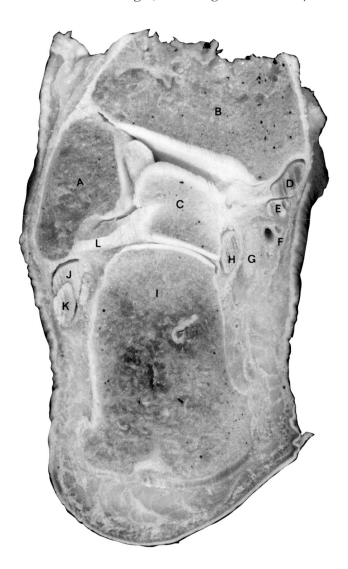

Fig. 2-27. Coronal section.

Key

A. Fibula
B. Tibia
C. Talus
D. Tibialis posterior
E. Flexor digitorum longus
F. Posterior tibial artery

G. Tibial nerve
H. Flexor hallucis longus
I. Calcaneus
J. Peroneus brevis
K. Peroneus longus
L. Posterior talofibular ligament

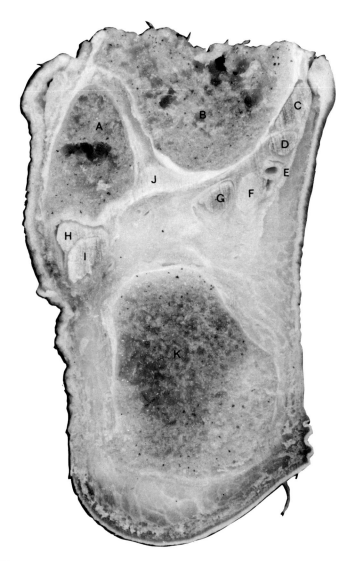

Fig. 2-28. Coronal section.

Key

A. Fibula
B. Tibia
C. Tibialis posterior
D. Flexor digitorum longus
E. Posterior tibial vein and artery

F. Tibial nerve
G. Flexor hallucis longus
H. Peroneus brevis
I. Peroneus longus
J. Posterior inferior tibiofibular ligament

ACKNOWLEDGMENTS

We would like to thank Troy Boffeli, Bob Eckerstorfer, Jeff Pellersels, Marc Trzeciak, and John Volpe for their help in assembling this chapter.

SELECTED READINGS

Bo WJ, Wolfman N, Krueger WA, Meschan I: Basic Atlas of Cross Sectional Anatomy — A Clinical Approach. 2nd Ed. W.B. Saunders, Philadelphia, 1989

Clemente CD (ed): Gray's Anatomy. 30th American Ed. Lea & Febiger, Philadelphia, 1985

Crafts RC: Textbook of Human Anatomy. 3rd Ed. Wiley, New York, 1985

Crouch JE: Functional Human Anatomy. 4th Ed. Lea & Febiger, Philadelphia, 1985

Draves DJ: Anatomy of the Lower Extremity. Williams & Wilkins, Baltimore, 1986

Moore L: Clinically Oriented Anatomy. 2nd Ed. Williams & Wilkins, Baltimore, 1985

Romanes GJ (ed): Cunningham's Textbook of Anatomy. 12th Ed. Oxford University Press, New York, 1981

Sarrafian SK: Anatomy of the Foot and Ankle. JB Lippincott, Philadelphia, 1983

Williams L, Warwick R (eds): Gray's Anatomy. 36th British Ed. Churchill Livingstone, Edinburgh, 1980

Biomechanics of the Lower Limb 3

Robert D. Phillips, D.P.M.

All bodies in the universe, no matter how large or small, move according the laws of nature. The science of physics has been developed to describe the past, present, and future movement and interactions of those bodies. Biomechanics is the science of incorporating the laws of physics to describe the normal and the abnormal function of the body as the mind dictates to it what activities it desires to perform. Whenever any part of the body is subjected to a force that is above the limits it was made to withstand, then an injury must take place. Most of the time these injuries are low grade in nature and are quickly healed by the body's natural processes. Sometimes the injury is great enough that pain is produced. This may be the result of a very large force that produces gross disruption of body tissues, or a small repetitive force that is frequent enough that the injured portion does not have time to heal before the next insult. This will result in an inflammatory response that will produce pain. Sometimes there is no actual injury; however, the energy expended by the body produces less motion than if the energy could be directed in a different direction — that is, the body is not utilizing its energy efficiently.

Podiatric biomechanics analyzes the forces and resultant movements of the joints of the lower extremities. Because the foot is the body's foundation for most activities, it is extremely important to medicine that a segment of health professionals devote themselves to analyzing whether an individual is ambulating in a way that will minimize tissue injury and maximize efficiency of movement. This requires that the foot care specialist have a thorough understanding of anatomy, kinesiology and the physics laws that are applied to produce walking, running, jumping and other forms of human locomotion without producing abnormal forces that will predispose the individual to injury and or deformity.

NEWTON'S LAWS OF MOTION

Podiatry as well as many other physical sciences must give Sir Isaac Newton the credit for establishing many of the basic laws of biomechanics. His laws of motion are still the basic guides to understanding human locomotion. Most of the musculoskeletal pathology of the lower extremity is due to the human body attempting to violate these laws of motion. Therefore it is important for the podiatrist to be well versed in these laws. The better he or she is able to apply these laws, the better he or she will understand the causes of musculoskeletal injuries, and the more accurate he or she will be in applying treatment regimens that will allow the body to heal itself.

Newton's First Law

Newton's first law of motion states that all bodies stay in a constant state of motion — that is, a body at rest stays at rest and a body in motion stays in motion unless it is acted upon by a force. In speaking of linear motion, all bodies have *momentum,* which is conserved, and this momentum remains constant unless a force acts upon that body. The definition of momentum is:

$$momentum = mass \times velocity$$

Since the mass of a body usually does not change, and its momentum does not change, it follows that the velocity must also remain unchanged unless a force acts upon that body.

Velocity is a vector. This means it has both magnitude and direction. Therefore a body continues to move at a constant speed in a straight line unless a force acts upon it. If a force pushes on the body in the same direction it is moving, the body will increase its velocity. If the force is applied exactly opposite the direction the body is moving, then the body will slow down. If the force is applied perpendicular to the direction the body is moving, then it will maintain a constant speed but will change its direction of movement. If the force is applied at an angle that is neither parallel nor perpendicular to the direction of motion, then it can be broken down into two vectors — one vector that is parallel to the direction of motion, which will increase or decrease the speed, and one vector that is perpendicular to the direction of motion, which will change its direction of motion (Fig. 3-1).

All bodies also have angular momentum. This means they are rotating around an axis (usually passing through the center of object) at a certain speed. *Angular velocity* is a measure of the how much of an arc the body rotates through per unit of time. It is expressed as radians or degrees per unit of time. Such terms as "60 degrees per second" or "1 radian per second" are used to express angular

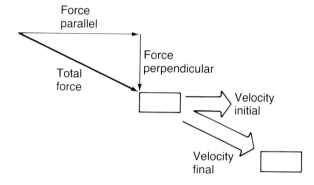

Fig. 3-1. When a force acts on a moving body, it can be broken down into one force parallel to the initial velocity, which increases or decreases the speed of the body, and one force perpendicular to the initial velocity, which changes the direction the body is moving.

velocity. The formula for angular momentum is very similar to that for linear momentum. The term *angular momentum* has been substituted for momentum, the term *angular velocity* has been substituted for velocity, and the term *moment of inertia* has been substituted for the term *mass.* Thus the formula reads:

$$angular\ momentum = moment\ of\ inertia \times$$
$$angular\ velocity$$

Moment of inertia is that property of a body that is a measure of its resistance to change in its angular velocity. If a body has a high moment of inertia then it takes much more force to increase or decrease its angular velocity than if it has a low moment of inertia. The formula for determining moment of inertia is:

$$moment\ of\ inertia = \Sigma[mass \times (radius)^2]$$

The means that the moment of inertia is equal to the summation of each tiny point of mass times the square of the distance of that tiny point of mass from the axis of rotation. The further the mass of a body is spread out from the axis of rotation, the greater will be its moment of inertia, and the closer the mass is concentrated to the axis of rotation the less will be its moment of inertia. A mass that is shaped like a sphere will have a lower moment of inertia than if the same mass were a flat disk, and the flat disk would have a much lower moment of inertia than if the same mass were constructed like

Fig. 3-2. A comparison of the moment of inertia for several types of objects all having the same mass. The solid disk has 50 percent of the moment of inertia of a hoop, and the sphere has 40 percent of the hoop's moment of the inertia. The rod rotating at one end has 33 percent of the moment of inertia if it has the same length as the hoop diameter, and a rod rotating in the center has 8.33 percent of the hoop's moment of inertia, four times less than the rod rotating at its end. (From Stipes JG: The Development of Physical Theories. p. 76. McGraw-Hill Book Company, New York, 1967, with permission.)

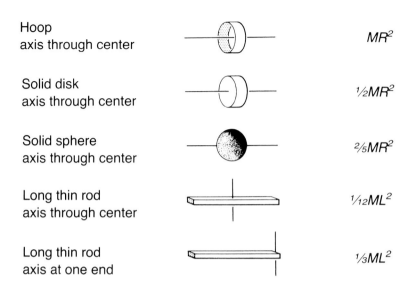

Hoop axis through center	MR^2
Solid disk axis through center	$\frac{1}{2}MR^2$
Solid sphere axis through center	$\frac{2}{5}MR^2$
Long thin rod axis through center	$\frac{1}{12}ML^2$
Long thin rod axis at one end	$\frac{1}{3}ML^2$

a bicycle wheel, with only a few thin spokes connecting most of the mass on the perimeter with the axis of rotation (Fig. 3-2).

As can be seen from Figure 3-2, the moment of inertia is dependent on the axis of rotation. If we consider any long bone in the body, it is easier to start a bone rotating around an axis at its center than around an axis at one end. Likewise it is easier to stop a bone from rotating around an axis as its center than around an axis at one end. This is because the moment of inertia of bone around its center of mass is one-fourth the moment of inertia when it rotates around an axis at one end. This increase in the bone's moment of inertia is an advantage in stabilizing a bone around a joint; however, it is a disadvantage in starting and stopping a bone that is moving around that axis. As will be seen later, stabilization of the joints of the lower extremity is just as important (to produce gait) as moving them.

Most of the long bones are shaped such that the mass is larger at the ends and smaller in the center. By spreading the mass further from its center, the moment of inertia around its center of mass is increased. This means that it takes a greater force to start and stop the bone rotating around its center of mass than if the bone was narrow at its ends and thick in the middle. This can help prevent injury to the bone if an abnormal force is applied to it.

Another simple example of moment of inertia is to consider two feet that have the same mass, but one is short and wide while the other is long and narrow. The short, wide foot will have a lower moment of inertia, whereas the long, narrow foot will have a higher moment of inertia. Therefore it takes less force to produce a change in the angular momentum in the short, wide foot than in the long, narrow foot.

Just as linear momentum remains constant unless a force acts upon it, so angular momentum remains constant unless a force acts upon it. If a body is jointed such that the moment of inertia may be changed, then a change in the body's moment of inertia will be accompanied by a change in the angular velocity. If the moment of inertia increases, the angular velocity decreases, and if the moment of inertia decreases the angular velocity increases. An example of a change in moment of inertia is the person who walks with his or her arms held further away from their body than normal. Holding the arms away from the body will increase the body's moment of inertia around its center of body mass. This means that if the body mass center starts falling to one side, it will fall much slower than if the arms were held close to the body. Therefore the person will be more stable against forces that would tend to tip them to one side or the other.

Another example of a change in moment of inertia is the ice skater who is spinning on the ice. The skater can produce an increase in speed of rotation by decreasing his moment of inertia. He or she does this by pulling his or her arms inward toward the center of rotation. Likewise, he or she may slow the speed of rotation by increasing the moment of inertia. He or she does this by stretching his or her arms outward away from the center of rotation.

Newton's Second Law

Newton's second law states that **force = mass × acceleration**. This is usually written as F = ma. This law means that any time a force is applied to an object, the object accelerates. Since acceleration is the change in velocity divided by the change in time, a force applied to any object will produce a change in the object's velocity — and when the velocity changes, the momentum of the object changes. We may substitute these concepts back into the above equation to say:

$$\text{Force} = \frac{\text{change in momentum}}{\text{change in time}}$$

Because velocity is a vector, this means that it has both magnitude (which is usually called speed) and direction. A positive or negative change in the magnitude of velocity is one type of acceleration. This acceleration is produced by a force that is parallel to the direction of motion. If the force is directed the same way the body is moving, the speed increases; if the force is directed the opposite way, the speed decreases. Another type of acceleration occurs when the direction the object is moving changes without changing the speed. This change in the direction of motion must also be produced by a force; however, the force must be perpendicular to the direction of motion. While this force is being applied, the object moves in an arc until the force is removed, after which it continues moving in a straight line. If a force is constantly applied perpendicular to the direction of motion, then the body will move in a perfect circle, the size of the circle being determined by the magnitude of the force and the speed of the object. If the forces is applied neither parallel nor perpendicular to the direction of motion, then the force vector can be expressed as the sum of two component vectors that are perpendicular to each other. The first component is parallel to the direction of motion and produces an increase or decrease in the speed of the object. The second component is perpendicular to the direction of motion and produces a change in the direction of motion.

The second law of motion must be applied when a person desires to change either the speed or the direction of his or her movement. If the person wants to change speed he or she must generate a force parallel to the direction of motion. If the person wants to change direction of motion, he or she must generate a force perpendicular to the direction of motion. While generating the desired forces, the person accelerates until the force is removed, after which he or she continues moving in a straight line at a constant speed until another force acts upon him or her that changes speed or direction of motion.

Because force is a vector, having both magnitude and direction, all of the forces acting on a body may be added together to find the resultant force on the body. If all of the forces added together equal zero, then no acceleration is produced on the body. One force that is acting upon us at all times is the force of gravity. This force would cause us to accelerate toward the center of the earth if there were no other force present. To keep us from accelerating straight down, an equal force must be acting upon us exactly opposite to the force of gravity. This force is produced by the ground resistance to compression. The concept of weight is a measure of how hard the ground is pushing up to keep us from accelerating downward.

The astute observer will notice that whenever the human body changes speed, it leans forward if it is accelerating and it leans backward if it is decelerating. The reason for this is that, in order to increase the forward velocity of the body, the ground must push the body forward. At the same time it must also push upward to resist gravity. The addition of these two vectors produces a final force vector that points in the direction that the body must lean (Fig. 3-3A). If the body leans further forward than this, then it will fall over forward. If the body leans less than this, then the feet will go out from under the body and the body will fall backward. This same concept holds when the human body is changing directions; however, this time the ground must push the body perpendicular to its direction of motion. The sideways push of the ground plus the upward force of the ground to resist gravity are added together to produce a vector that is angled to the ground (Fig. 3-3B). The body must lean in this direction, which is toward the

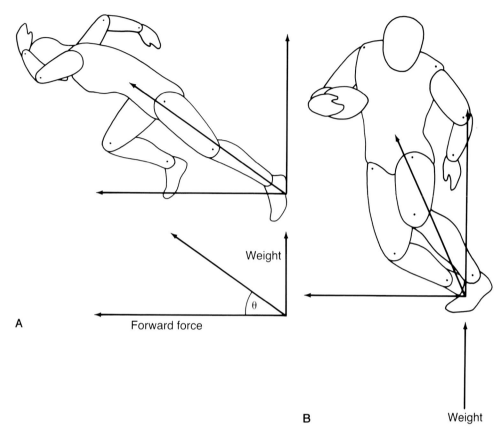

Fig. 3-3. (A) The forward lean of the racer is determined by adding the force of the ground pushing upward, resisting gravity, and the shear force of the ground, increasing the forward velocity of the racer. **(B)** The side lean of the football player changing directions is determined by adding the upward force of the ground, resisting gravity, and the sideward shear force of the ground, changing the player's direction of motion.

center of the circular path it is turning, to prevent falling. If the body leans more than this, then it will fall in the direction of the movement. If the body does not lean enough, then the feet will slide toward the center of the circle and the body will fall away from the center of the circle.

When talking about changing the angular velocity of an object, or in other words creating angular acceleration or deceleration, instead of just applying a force, a *torque* must be applied. The second law of motion is easily modified to account for the production of angular acceleration:

Torque = moment of inertia × angular acceleration

Torque is different from force in that it is equal to the actual force applied times the distance from the

point where the force is applied to the axis of rotation. This is expressed by the formula:

Torque = force × lever arm

Therefore if two forces are equal, but one force is applied twice as far from the axis of rotation as the other, then the first force will produce twice the torque that the second will, and thus the angular acceleration produced by the first force will be twice the acceleration produced by the second force (Fig. 3-4).

To produce motion around an axis, the force must be applied perpendicular to the axis. If the force is parallel to the axis of motion then no torque can be exerted. If the force is oblique to the joint axis (i.e., neither parallel or perpendicular) then it can be subdivided into two components, one com-

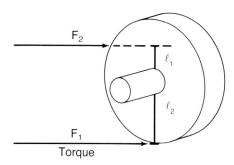

Fig. 3-4. Because torque = force × lever arm, the torque exerted by F_1 is half the torque produced by F_2 even though the two forces are equal. This is because the lever arm of F_1 is one-half the lever arm of F_2. The result of applying both of these forces simultaneously would be a counterclockwise rotation of the wheel.

ponent perpendicular to the axis of rotation and one component parallel to the axis (Fig. 3-5). The component perpendicular to the axis may be calculated by multiplying the total force times the sine of the angle between the force and the axis. The formula for total torque then must be modified to read:

$$\text{Torque} = \text{force} \times \text{lever arm} \times \sin \theta$$

where θ is the angle between the axis and the force.

Instead of referring to a torque being applied to a rotating body, we more commonly say that a *moment* is being applied. Throughout this chapter, this term will be used to describe any torque being

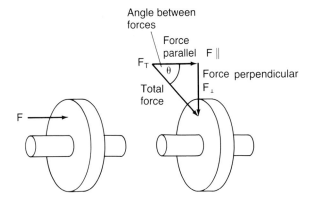

Fig. 3-5. If F is applied parallel to the axis then no torque is produced. If F is making an angle (θ) with the axis then it can be expressed as the summation of $F_\parallel$ and $F_\perp$ to the axis. $F_\perp = F_T \sin \theta$.

applied to a joint. Please do not confuse the term *moment* with the moment of inertia that any body or part of the body has.

Moments and Countermoments

Almost all joint motions occur around a joint axis. Therefore, when talking about motion in the human body, we must talk about angular momentum, angular velocity, angular acceleration, and moments. For a joint to start at rest, move to a new position, and come to rest again, it starts with an angular momentum of zero, then it must be acted upon by a moment to produce angular acceleration until it reaches its maximum angular velocity. When the moment is removed, the joint then moves at a constant angular velocity until an opposite moment acts upon it to produce angular deceleration until its angular momentum is again zero. These moments that produce angular acceleration and deceleration may come from a wide variety of sources. We commonly think of muscles as providing moments, and their importance cannot be underestimated; however, moments may also result from the tension in a ligament, or from the contact of one bony surface with another bony surface, or from the intermolecular and intercellular bonding strength within a body tissue, or from the force of gravity, or from the resistance of the ground or any other object to compression, or from the force of friction from the ground or any other object. In summary, any time a body part changes its angular velocity, a moment can always be shown to produce that change in angular velocity.

At any instant of time there are usually many different moments on a joint that may be added together to find the resultant moment. For example, if muscle A produces a clockwise moment of 5 newton-meters (Nm) on a joint and muscle B produces a counterclockwise moment of 4 Nm, the resultant torque on the joint will be 1 Nm in the clockwise direction. The joint will continue to accelerate in the clockwise direction until the clockwise moments equal the counterclockwise moments. At this point the angular velocity will remain constant until the counterclockwise moments become greater than the clockwise moments, which will cause the joint to decelerate. Sometimes the counterclockwise moment can be

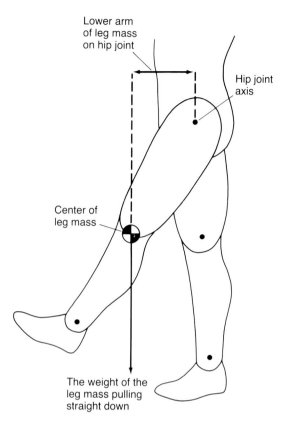

Lower arm of leg mass on hip joint

Hip joint axis

Center of leg mass

The weight of the leg mass pulling straight down

Fig. 3-6. When the leg is off the ground the force of gravity pulls the hip downward with a moment equal to the weight of the leg times the distance between the center of gravity (CG) of the leg and the hip joint axis (HJA).

Gravity will pull the leg toward the ground and help produce motion in the frontal and sagittal planes because these axes are parallel to the ground; however, gravity will not create any transverse plane motion because this axis is perpendicular to the ground.

Another example of the moment placed on a joint by gravity is to consider the moment on the ankle joint of a 70-kg male with a size 10 foot. The center of mass of the foot is approximately 8 cm anterior to the ankle joint and the weight of each foot is approximately 0.5 kg. When the foot is off the floor, the plantar-flexion moment that gravity will place on the ankle joint is calculated by multiplying the force (1 kg = 9.8 newtons) times the lever arm (0.08 meters). In this case the plantar-flexion moment will be equal to 0.39 Nm. To resist this moment, the ankle joint dorsiflexors have to provide a 0.39-Nm dorsiflexion moment on the ankle joint. Since the anterior tibial tendons are approximately 3 cm anterior to the ankle joint axis, this means that they must exert approximately 13 newtons of force to prevent the ankle joint from plantar flexing (Fig. 3-7A).

When weight is on the foot, gravity still places a moment on the ankle joint; however, it is the entire body that is free to move instead of the foot. If the center of body mass is posterior to the ankle joint axis, gravity pulls the body backward, which plantar flexes the ankle joint, and if the body mass center center is anterior to the ankle joint axis then gravity pulls the body forward, which dorsiflexes the ankle joint. In the case of the above person standing on his or her foot, if the center of body mass falls 1 mm posterior to the ankle joint axis, then the plantar-flexion moment on the ankle joint will be 0.68 Nm. Again the ankle joint dorsiflexors must resist this plantar-flexion moment on the ankle joint; therefore they must also place a 0.68-Nm dorsiflexion moment on the joint. This means that they must contract with a force of approximately 23 newtons to prevent the ankle joint from plantar flexing (Fig. 3-7B).

The moment that a muscle places on a joint is equal to the force of contraction times its lever arm times the sine of the angle between the tendon and the axis of motion. Therefore an individual may increase the moment on a joint by actually increasing the strength of the muscle, or by increasing the

exerted by increased force from an antagonist muscle. Sometimes the counterclockwise moment can be exerted by the ligaments of a joint. Sometimes the counterclockwise moment can be exerted by an outside object such as a rock or a wall, which may cause pain.

Gravitational force is constantly applying a moment to each joint. The quantitation of this moment can be computed by multiplying the weight of the body segments on the least supported side of the joint times the distance of the center of mass of those body segments from the axis times the sine of the angle between the joint axis and the force of gravity (Fig. 3-6). Only if the joint axis is perpendicular to the ground will gravity not place a moment on a joint. For example, consider the hip joint, which has three independent axes of motion.

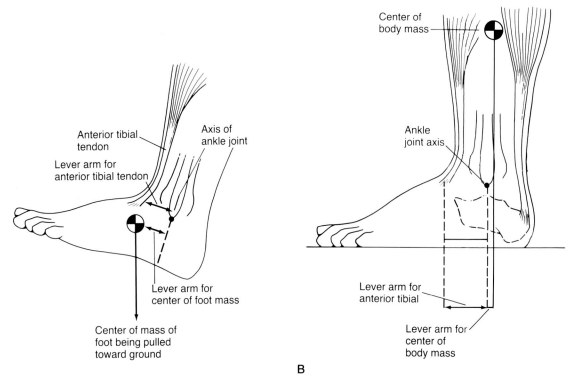

Fig. 3-7. (A) When the 0.5-kg foot is off the ground there is a plantar-flexion moment of 0.39 Nm. The ankle joint dorsiflexors resist this by contracting with a force of 13 N. **(B)** When standing on the ground, each 1 mm that the body's center of gravity falls posterior to the ankle joint axis increases the plantar-flexion moment on the ankle by 0.68 Nm. To counteract the center of mass falling 1 mm posterior to the ankle, the anterior muscle group must contract with a force of 23 N.

lever arm of the tendon or by bringing the muscle tendon closer to being perpendicular to the axis of motion. Likewise a muscle moment may be weakened not only by muscle atrophy but also be decreasing the moment arm of the muscle or by bringing the muscle force vector more parallel with the axis of motion. Therefore when the clinician evaluates why a muscle is not performing its function adequately, he or she must evaluate not only muscle strength but also its direction of pull in relationship to the joint axis and also its lever arm.

Levers

The study of moments and countermoments must also include a discussion of levers. A lever is a rigid beam that has an axis (also called the fulcrum) and two moments: a resistance moment and a moment that is trying to overcome the resistance (the work moment). The moments are calculated again by multiplying each force times its lever arm. If the

moments are equal then no change in the angular momentum will occur. If the resistance moment is greater than the work moment, then the desired movement of the resistance load will **NOT** be accomplished. Only when the work moment is greater than the resistance moment will the desired movement be accomplished. All of the muscles exhibit lever action on the joints to produce desired movement. A short discussion of each type of levers follows.

A *first-class lever* has its fulcrum in the middle of the lever with the resistance and work forces on opposite sides of the fulcrum. Everyone has played with the classic first-class lever, the child's teeter-totter. There are very few first-class levers in the body because most of the muscle tendons insert on the same side of the joint as the resistance load. One first-class lever in the foot is the ankle joint (Fig. 3-8A). When the body weight is centered in front of the ankle joint, it is resisted by the tension in the Achilles tendon, which is posterior to the

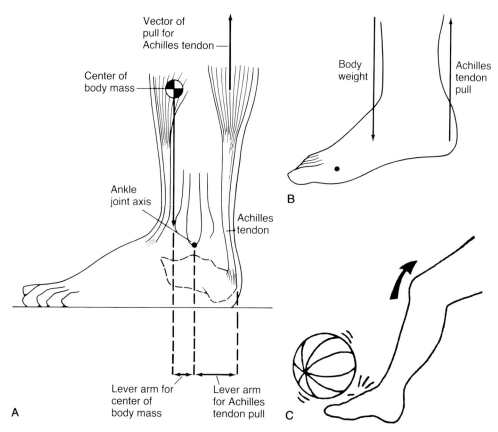

Fig. 3-8. (A) The body weight falling forward around the ankle joint, resisted by the Achilles tendon is an example of a first class lever. **(B)** The Achilles tendon pulling the calcaneus up while body weight is posterior to the first metatarsophalangeal joint is an example of a second-class lever. **(C)** The quadriceps femoris muscles extending the knee to kick a ball is an example of a third-class lever. (Part C from Cochran,[1] with permission.)

ankle joint. A contraction of the triceps surae will pull the calcaneus superiorly and the forefoot inferiorly. Likewise when the body weight is centered behind the ankle joint, it is resisted by the tension in the anterior muscles of the leg, pulling the forefoot superiorly and the calcaneus inferiorly.

A *second-class lever* has its fulcrum at one end of the lever with the resistance in the middle of the lever and the work force on the other end. This is always a very efficient lever because the work force lever arm is always longer than the resistance lever arm. Thus the resistance force can always be overcome with a smaller force. A wheelbarrow and a nutcracker are second-class levers. There are many second-class lever systems in the body. One is exhibited when a person stands on his or her toes (Fig. 3-8B). The metatarsophalangeal joints act as the fulcrum, the body weight is behind the metatarso-

phalangeal joints, and the force lifting the body weight is from the Achilles tendon at the most posterior aspect of the foot.

A *third-class lever* also has its fulcrum at the end; however, the resistance is at the other end while the work force is in the center. In terms of energy expenditure, this is a much less efficient lever than the second-class lever because the resistance lever arm is always longer than the work lever arm; thus the resistance force can only be overcome by a greater work force. The advantage of a third-class lever is that a resistance force can be moved through a large distance by a force moving through a small distance. There are many third-class lever systems in the body. The biceps lifting a weight held by the hand is a third-class lever. The quadriceps femoris kicking a football is also a third-class lever (Fig. 3-8C).

Newton's Third Law

Newton's third law of motion states that for every action there is an equal and opposite reaction. Another way of stating this would be that for every change in the momentum of a body, there is an equal and opposite change in the momentum of the body that acted on the first. Whenever an object acts to change the momentum of a portion of the body, that portion of the body produces an equal but opposite change in the momentum of the object. Taking the extreme example of this, whenever the foot pushes in a posterior direction, the earth pushes the foot in an anterior direction. If the earth pushing the foot anteriorly changes the momentum of the foot so that it moves forward with a certain velocity, the foot has likewise changed the velocity of the earth in the opposite direction; however, because of the extremely large mass of the earth compared to the mass of the body, the change in the velocity of the earth will be so small that it could not be measured.

On a more realistic scale, a ballistic fired from a rifle starts with a momentum of zero and accelerates until it has a new momentum equal to its mass times its velocity. Likewise the rifle has an initial momentum of zero and after the firing it has an equal but opposite momentum of the forward-traveling ballistic. To determine the recoil velocity of the rifle, the momentum of the ballistic is divided by the mass of the rifle. Therefore if you wanted to decrease the recoil of the rifle, you could decrease the forward velocity of the bullet, you could decrease the mass of the bullet, or you could increase the mass of the rifle.

Another example is a baseball player hitting a baseball. When he or she makes contact with the ball, the momentum of the ball changes markedly. The change in the momentum of the ball must be accompanied by an equal and opposite change in the momentum of the player. To counter this opposite change in momentum the player is taught to keep applying force forward, which continues his or her swing after the ball has left the bat. This is known as the followthrough.

It should be noted that every muscle has an origin and an insertion. Whenever the muscle contracts and changes the momentum of the body part distal to the joint, an equal change in the momentum occurs in the body part proximal to the joint. Usually a relative movement is noted only in the body segment that has the smaller mass; however, if that smaller body part has another force acting on it such that it cannot move, then the larger body part must move. An example of this is the contraction of the gastrocnemius muscle. It inserts into the calcaneus and lifts the heel, but it also inserts into the femur and pulls it posteriorly. Therefore when it contracts and increases the plantar-flexing momentum of the forefoot, it also decreases the forward momentum of the femur. If the body weight is close enough to the metatarsophalangeal joints, then a contraction of the gastrocnemius will produce an observed lift of the heel off the floor; however, if the body weight is such that the heel is being forced down onto the ground, then a contraction of the gastrocnemius will produce a posterior acceleration of the leg.

BASICS OF JOINT MOTION

All the joints of the lower extremity move around at least one axis of motion. Some of the joints have more than one axis of motion. Some have axes of

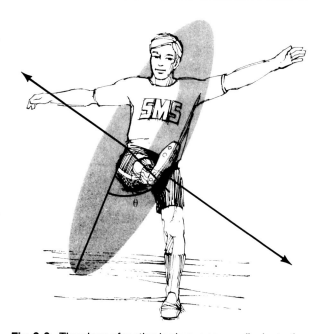

Fig. 3-9. The plane of motion is always perpendicular to the axis of motion. (From Northrip JW, Logan GA, McKinney WC: Introduction to Biomechanic Analysis of Sport. p. 18. William C. Brown Company Publishers, Dubuque, IA, 1974, with permission.)

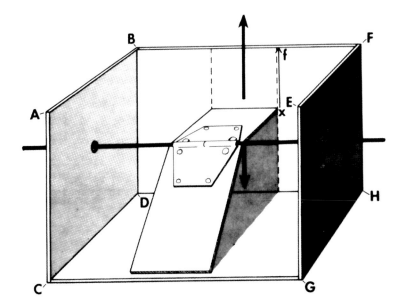

Fig. 3-10. When the observer's eyesight is in the plane of motion, he will see the distal part slide against the proximal part, but no change in the angle between the two parts will be observed. (From Root et al.,[4] with permission.)

motion that have special properties. The important aspect to realize is that when a joint moves around its axis, its angular displacement is measured in a plane that is perpendicular to the axis of motion (Fig. 3-9). If an observer tries to measure motion in a plane that is parallel to the axis of motion, he or she will observe the part that is distal sliding in relationship to the proximal part; however, there will be no change in the angle between the distal and proximal segments (Fig. 3-10). Therefore when we talk about joint motion, we say that motion occurs in a plane that is perpendicular to the axis of motion.

If the axis is perpendicular to the frontal plane, which means it is formed by the intersection of the transverse and sagittal planes, then angular motion occurs only in the frontal plane. When this motion occurs at the hip joint we call it abduction if the leg moves away from the midline of the body, and we call it abduction if the leg moves toward the midline of the body. If frontal plane motion occurs in the foot we say that the foot is inverting if the plantar aspect is turning to face the midline of the body, and we say that the foot is everting if the plantar aspect is turning to face away from the midline of the body.

If the axis is perpendicular to the sagittal plane, which means it is formed by the intersection of the frontal and transverse planes, then angular motion occurs only in the sagittal plane. When this motion occurs at the hip joint, we say that the hip is flexing if the femur is moving anteriorly in relationship to the trunk, and that the hip is extending if the femur is moving posteriorly in relationship to the trunk. When sagittal plane motion occurs at the knee joint we say that the knee is flexing if the tibia is moving posteriorly in relationship to the femur, and we say that the knee is extending if the tibia is moving anteriorly in relationship to the femur. The knee is maximally extended when the tibia and femur form an angle of 180 degrees. An attempt by the knee to extend further is called hyperextension. When sagittal plane motion occurs in any of the foot joints, we say the joint is dorsiflexing if the distal portion of the joint moves in a cephalad direction, and we say the joint is plantarflexing if the distal portion moves toward the plantar side of the foot.

If the axis is perpendicular to the transverse plane, which means it is formed by the intersection of the frontal and sagittal planes, then angular motion occurs only in the transverse plane. When this motion occurs at the hip or knee joint we say the leg segments are externally or internally rotating. When the foot joints are moving in the transverse plane, we say the joint is adducting if the distal portion is moving toward the midline of the body, and we say the joint is abducting if the distal portion is moving away from the midline of the body.

Biplane Motion

Most of the joint axes in the foot are not perpendicular to one of the cardinal planes. This means that they form an angle with at least two of the

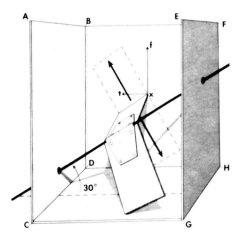

Fig. 3-11. The joint axis is angulated 45 degrees to the bottom and side of the box; however, it is parallel to the back of the box. When 10 degrees of motion occurs around the axis, 7.1 degrees of motion will be observed on both the side of the box and the bottom of the box. (From Root et al.,[4] with permission.)

cardinal planes, and most of the time with all three of the cardinal planes. First, consider a joint axis that is angulated with just two planes. This means that it is still parallel with one plane. When the joint moves around this axis, an angular change will be noted in both of the planes with which the axis forms an angle and no angular change will be noted in the plane that is parallel with the axis. If the axis is angulated 45 degrees with the two planes, then equal angular motions will be noted in both of the planes. The converse statement is also true: if motion is observed in one of the cardinal planes, an equal amount of motion must be observed to occur in the other cardinal plane to which the axis is angulated (Fig. 3-11). The amount of motion observed in each cardinal plane is equal to the amount of motion that occurs in the plane that is perpendicular to the axis of motion times the sine of the angle between the axis and the cardinal plane being observed. Therefore the closer the axis is to being perpendicular to the cardinal plane, the greater will be the observed angular motion in that cardinal plane; conversely, the closer to axis lies to being parallel with the cardinal plane, the less will be the observed angular motion in that cardinal plane.

An example of two-plane motion would be to consider the motion of a hypothetical foot joint whose axis is angulated 30 degrees with the transverse plane and 60 degrees with the frontal plane. If this joint were to move 10 degrees around its axis, an observer of the frontal plane would see an angular change of 10 degrees times the sine of 60 degrees, which would be 8.7 degrees, whereas an observer of the transverse plane would see an angular change of 10 degrees times the sine of 30 degrees, which would be 5.0 degrees. Therefore the two observers would find that there was approximately 1¾ times more frontal plane motion than transverse plane motion. If the frontal plane observer placed a wedge under the foot to limit the frontal plane motion by 5 degrees, the transverse plane observer would see the transverse plane motion limited by almost 3 degrees. Likewise if the transverse plane observer placed a wedge under the foot to increase the transverse plane motion by 5 degrees, the frontal plane observer would see an increase of 8.75 degrees of motion.

Triplane Motion

The above arguments may be applied if the joint axis is angulated to all three body planes. The closer an axis is to being perpendicular to a given cardinal plane, the greater will be the percentage of motion in that plane, and the closer an axis is to being parallel to a given cardinal plane, the less will be the percentage of motion in that plane. Previous research papers have expressed the various angulations of the joints in what is known as spherical coordinates, and therefore spherical coordinates are the commonly used reference system when describing how an axis is deviated in relationship to the cardinal planes. For this system two angles are given, the first (α) is the angle between the sagittal plane and the axis when the axis is projected onto the transverse plane. The second angle (β) is the angle between the transverse plane and the axis of motion (Fig. 3-12). The formulas given for two-plane motion can be rearranged using the nomenclature of spherical coordinates to determine how much motion will be observed in each of the cardinal body planes when the joint moves (μ degrees):

Transverse plane motion $(T_p) = \mu \times \sin \beta$
Frontal plane motion $(F_p) = \mu \times \cos \alpha \times \cos \beta$
Sagittal plane motion $(S_p) = \mu \times \sin \alpha \times \cos \beta$

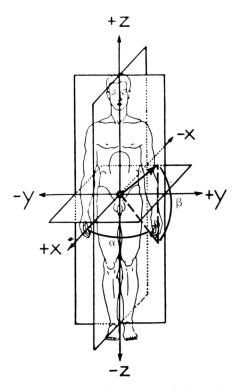

Fig. 3-12. α is the deviation of the axis from the sagittal plane, and β is the deviation of the axis from the transverse plane.

An example of this would be to consider motion around the average subtalar joint axis, which is angulated 16 degrees with the sagittal plane and angulated 42 degrees with the transverse plane. If this joint moves 10 degrees, then, applying the above formulas, the frontal plane observer would see the joint move 7.1 degrees, the transverse plane observer would see the joint move 6.7 degrees, and the sagittal plane observer would see the joint move 2.0 degrees. If the frontal plane observer tried to increase the observed motion by 5 degrees, the transverse plane observer would notice an increased motion of 4.7 degrees and the sagittal plane observer would notice an increased motion of 1.0 degrees. Conversely, if the transverse plane observer tried to decrease the observed motion by 5.0 degrees, the frontal plane observer would notice a decreased motion of 5.3 degrees and the sagittal plane observer would notice a decreased motion of 1.5 degrees. Therefore a change of motion in one plane *must* be accompanied by proportional changes in the motion in the other two planes, and the clinician must be aware that if he or she tries to change abnormal motion in one cardinal plane, he or she will also effect a change in the other two cardinal planes.

Using the above formulas, a clinician could observe the angular change in the three body planes when a joint moves, and determine the degree to which the joint axis is angulated with the sagittal and transverse planes. Using the terms F_p, T_p, and S_p to represent the angular changes on the frontal, transverse, and sagittal planes, it is possible to determine α, β, and μ by the following formulas:

$$\alpha = \tan^{-1}(S_p/F_p)$$
$$\beta = \tan^{-1}(T_p \times \cos \alpha/F_p)$$
$$\mu = T_p/\sin \beta$$

PROPERTIES OF BIOLOGIC MATERIALS

In considering the function of the lower extremity, a short discussion must also be made of the general properties of the various biologic tissues that are subjected to force. The major goal of the podiatric physician is to heal and prevent injury to these tissues. The ability of these tissues to withstand the forces placed upon them is a major consideration when determining proper treatment regimens.

Properties of Bone

Bone provides the major degree of stability to the human body. It allows each body part to assume many different postures and it is the substance to which all of the muscles and ligaments are either directly or indirectly attached. The terms that may be used to describe its properties are nonhomogeneous, anisotropic, viscoelastic, and brittle.

Nonhomogeneity

Bone is not homogeneous on either the micro- or macroscopic level. On the microscopic level it is noted to be composed of lacunae of osteocytes around a Haversian canal. The longitudinal running Haversian canals communicate by the transverse running Volkmann's canals. This microscopic architecture means that the bone will resist different types of forces differently. On the macroscopic level, bones have a dense cortex and loosely arranged cancellous bone or a medullary canal within. Because of the differences in the thickness of the cortices and medullary canals, and the differences between the shapes of the bones, each bone will have its own specific function and will exhibit a different pattern on its ability to resist injury.

Anisotropy

Bone must be able to resist three types of force: *compression, tension,* and *shear* (Fig. 3-13). Bone must also resist bending and torsional forces; however, the processes of bending and torsion are only combinations of the previous three forces. Bone is **anisotropic** because it resists these different forces differently. Its microscopic structure makes bone most resistant to compression forces, moderately resistant to tension forces, and least resistant to shear forces.

The measure of a bone's ability to resist bending is known as its *area moment of inertia.* The process of bending a bone involves one side developing a concave appearance and the opposite side developing a convex appearance. The concave side develops a compression along its length while the convex side develops a tension along its length (Fig. 3-14). The greatest compression and tension develop at the point of maximum deflection. Because

bone is weaker when placed under tension than when placed under compression, the bone will fail first on the tension side, with the crack propagating toward the compression side.

The shapes of the various bones make them resist bending to various degrees. Construction workers have long known that approximately six times more force is needed to bend an I beam than to bend a solid rod of equal cross-sectional area. However the I beam has this high resistance only to forces applied parallel to the long direction of the I, and that the beam has just a little more than one-half the resistance of a solid rod when the forces are applied in the direction of the short segments of the I. On the other hand a perfectly round, hollow rod has a little more than five times the resistance to bending than a solid rod with the same mass, and this resistance is the same no matter what direction the forces are applied (Fig. 3-15). Therefore a perfectly round, hollow tube is the ideal shape for the bones that must resistant bending moments. The more a bone deviates from this perfectly round shape, the lower will be its area moment of inertia and the greater will be its susceptibility to fracture from a bending moment applied at this point. If the tubular continuity is interrupted across any section of the bone, such as that created by a screw hole, this area will lose 50 percent of its area moment of inertia[1] and be much more easily disrupted by a bending moment.

A measure of the bone's ability to resist torsion is known as its *polar moment of inertia.* It is a function of how far from the central axis of the bone the mass is distributed, and is proportional to the fourth power of the radius of the bone (r^4).[1] This means that doubling the diameter of a bone will increase its resistance to torsion by a factor of 16. Therefore the bone shape with the greatest resistance to torque is a hollow bone with a large diameter. When torsion is applied to a bone, with one end of the bone being twisted one direction and the other end of the bone being relatively twisted in the opposite direction, spiral lines of tension, shear, and compression are set up along the surface of the bone. Since bone is more resistant to compression than it is to shear or tension, the bone will fracture in the area of its smallest diameter in a spiral pattern following the tension lines (Fig. 3-16).

Bone exhibits different *stress-strain curves* under

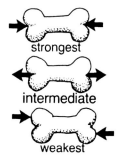

Fig. 3-13. Bone resists compression best *(top)* tension moderately, *(middle)* and shear force least *(bottom)*. (From Cochran,[1] with permission.)

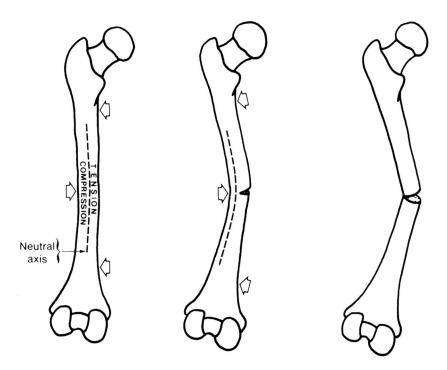

Fig. 3-14. When a bone bends, there is compression on one side and tension on the other. Because bone resists compression better than tension, it will break on the tension side first. (From Gozna ER, Harrington IJ: Biomechanics of Musculoskeletal Injury. p. 4. Williams & Wilkins, Baltimore, 1982, with permission.)

Solid rod		1
Flat beam (on end)		3.5
I beam (on end)		6
I beam (on side)		.6
Hollow cylinder		5.3

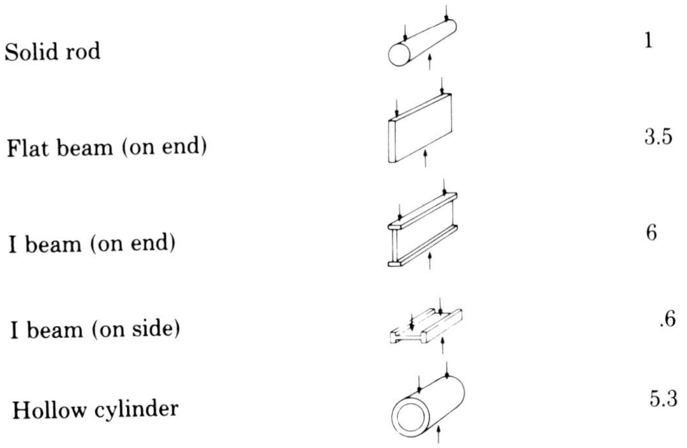

Fig. 3-15. The ability of masses of various shapes to resist bending forces. The I beam has the greatest resistance, but only to forces in one plane. The hollow cylinder is almost as strong in all planes. (From Gozna ER, Harrington IJ: Biomechanics of Musculoskeletal Injury. p. 13. Williams & Wilkins, Baltimore, 1982, with permission.)

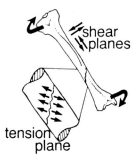

Fig. 3-16. Bone, under a torsional load, fractures in a spiral manner along the plane of tension, starting at the area of smallest diameter. (From Cochran,[1] with permission.)

various types of loads. The actual force exerted on the bone is known as the *stress.* The distorting or bending of the bone without disrupting it is called *strain.* Whenever a force is place on a bone, it will always undergo a certain degree of strain before it starts to fracture. Strain is always expressed as a percentage of the original length of the bone when no stress was placed on it. The stress-strain curve represents the degree of strain that a material will undergo with varying amounts of stress (Fig. 3-17). The area under the stress-strain curve is a measure of the amount of potential energy that the material has absorbed or stored within it.

All stress-strain curves have certain features. At the far left of the curve, it is noted that the curve is a straight line. This is known as the elastic region. In this region there is a linear relationship between the amount of stress applied and the amount that the material deforms. In addition, when the force is removed the material returns to its original shape and size. At the yield point there is a sharp turn and the curve becomes much flatter. This means that it takes very little increase in stress to produce a marked increase in the strain. This is known as the plastic region of the curve and denotes molecular slippage and the breaking of some of the molecular bonds. If the bone (or any material) enters this region microfractures occur, and it will not return to its original shape once the stress has been removed. Finally, the failure point is reached where the curve drops suddenly back to zero and clinical fracture of the material occurs, releasing all of the potential energy it has stored.

Viscoelasticity

One of the important properties of bone is that it is **viscoelastic.** This means that it can absorb various amounts of energy before it fails, depending on the rate at which force is applied. If the force is applied very quickly, the slope of the stress-strain curve is much higher than if the force is applied more slowly (Fig. 3-18). In both instances the bone breaks when it reaches a certain strain; however, it takes much more force to reach this degree of strain when the force is very rapid than when the force is applied much slower. When the strain limit is reached, however, there is much more energy re-

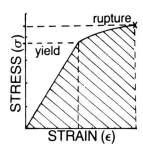

Fig. 3-17. Typical stress-strain curve. The area under the curve is the potential energy the material has stored within it. (From Cochran,[1] with permission.)

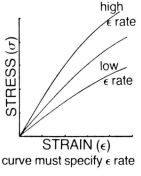

curve must specify ε rate

Fig. 3-18. Bone is viscoelastic. At a high speed of stress application the bone can store more potential energy than at low-speed application, although it will fracture when the failure strain is reached at all speeds. (From Cochran,[1] with permission.)

leased by the bone failing under high-velocity loads than under low-velocity loading, which causes more damage to the bone and soft tissue. Therefore a low-grade force applied over a longer period of time will still produce the same deformation necessary to produce failure as a higher force over a shorter period of time.

Another aspect of viscoelasticity is that bone exhibits a phenomenon called *creep*. If a force is applied to create bone strain without failure, and if that force is kept at a constant level, then the bone will continue to deform without disrupting (Fig. 3-19). Early experiments into viscoelasticity showed that a bone could deform over 150 percent more if a force was applied over a 50-day period than if the same force was applied for only 2 minutes.[2] When the force is released, the bone has an initial elastic response of returning to 50 percent deformation of its original length. Then over the next several weeks the bone again creeps back the last 50 percent, until it is again its original shape.

The above described experiments on the viscoelasticity of bone were performed in vitro; however, bones in vivo also exhibit a phenomenon that is referred to as *Wolff's law*. This law notes that bone can change and adapt its shape according to the forces placed on it. It should be noted that the Haversian canals are oriented in the direction of the compression forces. If a constant force is exerted on a bone that creates a constant strain with-

out the bone reaching failure, then the Haversian canals will redirect themselves to orient again with compression forces. Osteoclastic activity will be noted on one side of the bone while osteoblastic activity will be noted on the other side to create a gradual change in the bone shape. An example of this is when a fracture occurs and the alignment of the two pieces is not perfect, so that the bone is not completely straight after it has healed. After a year or so, if the bone is x-rayed again, the clinician will usually note that much of the malalignment has reduced to give the bone a shape much closer to its original shape.

Bone also adapts itself to resist the amount of stress placed on it. If the stress on a bone is gradually increased the diameter and mineral content of the bone will increase, thus rendering it stronger.[2] Likewise a decrease in stress on the bone will cause a gradual loss in the diameter and strength of the bone. This is why exercise is so important for maintaining bone strength, especially in the elderly.

Brittleness

A bone is termed *brittle* because of the relatively high slope of the stress-strain curve. This high slope means that there is very little strain that the bone can take before it enters the plastic zone and then very little strain within the plastic zone before it reaches the failure point. The degree of brittleness is determined by the ratio of hydroxyapatite to collagen. Patients with a high ratio of protein to mineral will have a high degree of elasticity in the bone, which means the bone can undergo much more strain before it fails. Children usually have the highest ratio of protein to mineral, which means their bones are much more easily deformed without breaking. Patients with a low ratio of protein to mineral will have a high degree of brittleness, which means that the bone can undergo much less strain. Elderly people usually fall in this category, which leads to a higher number of fractures in the elderly, usually with much less stress.

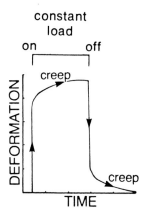

Fig. 3-19. If a bone undergoes a strain from a certain stress and if that stress is maintained, then bone undergoes the phenomenon of creep. (From Cochran,[1] with permission.)

Properties of Tendons and Ligaments

Tendons and ligaments are composed of linearly arranged collagen fibrils that are organized into groups called fibers, and groups of fibers called bundles. The collagen fibers are also interlaced with elastic fibers and have a wavy configuration when they are relaxed. The elastin content of all tendons is about 2 percent, whereas the elastin content of ligaments is variable but generally much higher, as high as 60 percent in the ligamentum flavum.

The function of ligaments is only to withstand tension. They do not effectively resist compression or shear forces. Tension exists in tendons whenever the muscle contracts against a load or whenever the muscle is stretched beyond its resting length. The purpose of ligaments is to stop the joint from moving further than its normal range of motion and to prevent motions that are not in the normal planes of motion. When the joint is between its ends of the range of motion, there should be no tension on the joint ligaments unless there is a moment attempting to move the joint in an abnormal plane. The tension strength of tendon is approximately one-half the tension strength of bone; however, it is considered nonbrittle because its elasticity is approximately 10 times that of bone. Elastin has approximately 200 times the elasticity of bone; therefore the ligaments are more elastic than the tendons because of their higher elastin content.

The normal stress-strain curve for tendons and ligaments is a little different than that for bone (Fig. 3-20). In the stress-strain curve for tendons, the far left of the curve is a fairly flat region, known as the toe portion of the curve, in which there is approximately 1 percent elongation with very little tension applied. This is because when tension is first applied, the wavy configuration of the fibers first must straighten out. The next portion of the curve is the straight elastic region that is due to the collagen portion of the structure. This permits 3 to 4 percent elongation. The third area, between the yield point and the failure point, is the plastic region in which the cross links between the fibrils begin to break. This plastic region allows another 4 percent of elongation; however, the amount of stress needed to deform the tendon from 4 to 8 percent of strain is much less than the stress needed to deform the tendon from 1 to 4 percent. Finally, when a tendon reaches approximately 8 percent of strain, total disruption of the tendon occurs.[3] The ligament stress-strain curve is similarly shaped, although the amount of strain that can occur before disruption may be 15 percent or even more.[1]

Tendons and ligaments also show viscoelastic properties similar to those exhibited by bone.

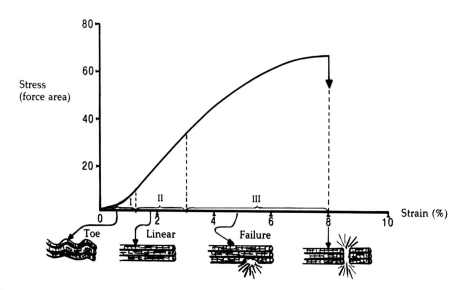

Fig. 3-20. A typical stress-strain curve for tendon. Area I is the toe region, area II is the elastic region, and area III is the plastic region. Failure occurs between 8 and 10 percent strain. (From Curwin and Stannish,[3] with permission.)

When the force is applied rapidly, they act as if they are more brittle; that is, the slope of the stress-strain curve is higher than if the force is applied more slowly. However, the increase in the slope of the curve is not as fast as that in bone during fast loading rates. If a very fast load is applied across a joint the ligament is more likely to fail, whereas if a slower load is applied across a joint an avulsion fracture is more likely to be seen (Fig. 3-21).

Ligaments and tendons show creep and relaxation properties that are more pronounced than bone. If a structure is held for a time at a constant degree of strain, after time it takes less force to hold it at that degree of strain. This property is known as *relaxation*. An example is attempting to provide corrective changes with a cast. After some time in the cast, with the structures under strain, the cast is applying less stress to the structure than when it was first applied. Creep is the corollary of relaxation. If a constant stress is applied to the structure then it will continue to elongate. These properties of relaxation and creep may be used advantageously when attempting to correct pathology using serial casts and stretching exercises; however, they may also be a disadvantage when a constant abnormal stress is being applied to a joint that must be resisted by the ligaments and/or tendons. In this case constant abnormal stress will cause the restraining tissues to elongate, thus causing a continually increasing subluxation and deformity of the joint. Because of this, ligaments and tendons should normally be subjected to abnormal stresses only for brief moments of time.

Properties of Muscle

Muscles are nonhomogeneous on scopic level, being composed of the proteins actin and myosin. Complex biochemical interactions occur between these proteins such that the actin and myosin slide against one another to produce contraction and elongation of the muscle. The maximum muscle contraction is 57 percent of its maximal length. When no energy is being expended between the actin and myosin complexes a muscle maintains whatever length it had just before it stopped its last contraction. If a tension force is placed on that muscle, it continues lengthening until the force ceases or until the muscle starts creating a counterforce, which is registered as tension in the muscle and tendon.

The *length-tension curve* for a muscle is the tension that can be developed in a muscle-tendon unit at various muscle lengths. On the x axis the muscle length is given and on the y axis the tension is expressed. The total length-tension curve can be subdivided into the active curve and the passive curve (Fig. 3-22). The active curve shows the maximum tension that a muscle can develop when it is at various lengths. This is a bell-shaped curve that shows that a muscle is able to develop very little tension as a result of active contractions when it is at its short-

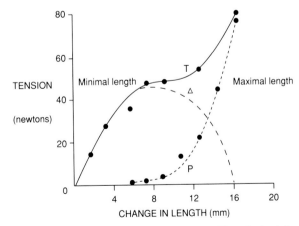

Fig. 3-22. Typical length-tension curve. The *dashed line* represents the active length-tension curve, the *dotted line* represents the passive length-tension curve. The *solid line* is the summation of the passive and active curves. (From Ralston et al: Am J Physiol, 151:612, 1947, with permission.)

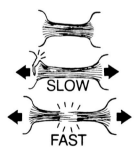

Fig. 3-21. Because the stress-strain slope increases more for bones under fast loads than ligaments under fast loads, a ligament is more likely to rupture under fast loads, whereas an avulsion fracture is more likely under a slowly applied load. (From Cochran,[1] with permission.)

est and longest lengths. Its maximum contractile force can be developed at a point midway between its shortest and longest length, called the *resting length*. The active curve is only the maximum tension possible. It is always possible to develop less than maximum tension at any particular muscle length.

The passive length-tension curve is the tension that naturally exists in the muscle-tendon unit at various muscle lengths when no active muscle contraction is occurring. From its shortest length to its resting length, there is no tension in the muscle when it is not actively contracting; however, from its resting length to its maximally elongated length, there is always a certain degree of tension. This degree of tension increases in an exponential fashion, so that when a muscle is at its maximal length, although it is hardly able to develop any tension as a result of active contraction, there is considerably more tension in the muscle-tendon unit than could be developed in it when it was at its resting length. The passive length-tension curve is fixed for each muscle, and whenever the muscle is at a length that is longer than its resting length, there must be at

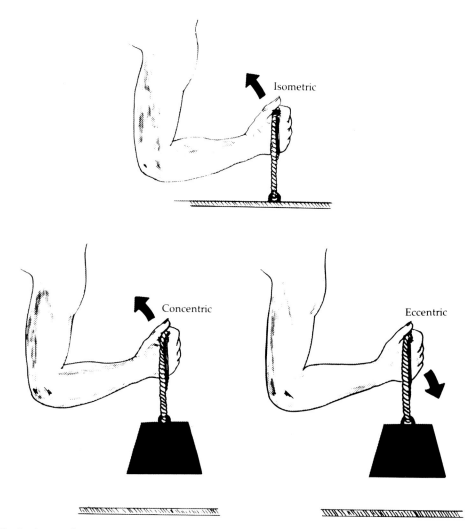

Fig. 3-23. An isometric contraction occurs when the muscle neither shortens nor lengthens. If the muscle shortens it is known as a concentric contraction; if it lengthens it is known as an eccentric contraction. (From Curwin and Stannish,[3] with permission.)

least this much tension in the muscle. Therefore the total tension created by a muscle equals the tension found on the passive length-tension curve, plus whatever active tension the muscle itself can generate at that length. From this curve it is easy to understand why a muscle is able to develop more force when it is contracting during elongation than when it is contracting while shortening.

Muscles may exhibit one of three types of contractions (Fig. 3-23). The first is an *isotonic* or *concentric contraction.* This means that while the muscle is expending energy contracting, it is undergoing shortening and the distance between the origin and insertion of the muscle is decreasing. One of the most common types of concentric contractions is the biceps brachii contracting so that the person may lift an object upward. Likewise, in the leg a concentric contraction of the triceps surae will produce heel lift.

A second type of contraction is the *isometric contraction.* This means that the muscle is expending energy contracting, but it is neither shortening nor lengthening. This means that there is an opposing moment on the joint that is exactly equal and opposite to the moment applied by the muscle. An example of an isometric contraction is the biceps brachii contracting to hold an object at a constant height above the floor. Likewise when a patient is standing still, the gastrocnemius muscle must be in a constant state of contraction to prevent the ankle joint from dorsiflexing as a result of body weight falling anterior to the ankle joint.

The third type of contraction is the *eccentric contraction.* This means that the muscle is expending energy contracting, but is undergoing lengthening. This is a very important type of muscle function because it is responsible for decelerating joint momentum or joint acceleration in the opposite direction. Returning to the biceps brachii again, in order for a person to set an object down slowly, or even at a constant velocity, the biceps must undergo an eccentric contraction. If it did not, the weight would cause angular acceleration of the elbow joint while it was undergoing extension, stopping when tension developed in the anterior ligaments of the elbow, which could produce an injury to the ligaments. A very important eccentric contraction in the lower leg when a person is walking is that of the gastrocnemius and soleus during midstance. At this

time, the center of body mass is anterior to the ankle joint, which places a dorsiflexion moment on the ankle joint. The contraction of the triceps surae keeps the velocity of dorsiflexion constant, and without it, the ankle joint dorsiflexion would be an accelerating motion.

OVERVIEW OF THE GAIT CYCLE

When we discuss ambulation, we usually refer to a patient walking. The time period between the patient contacting the ground with the reference foot and contacting the ground again with the same foot is known as one gait cycle (Fig. 3-24). This gait cycle is divided into two components: the stance phase and the swing phase. The stance phase comprises 65 percent of the entire gait cycle and the swing phase comprises the other 35 percent. This means that during part of the stance phase the opposite foot is swinging through the air — referred to as the single-support phase — and during part of the stance phase the opposite foot is on the ground — known as the double-support phase. Therefore, the gait cycle for each foot is composed of a double-support phase for the first 15 percent of the cycle, a single-support weight-bearing phase for the second 35 percent of the cycle, a double-support phase for the next 15 percent of the cycle, and a swing phase for the final 35 percent of the cycle.

A closer look at the stance phase shows that it is divided into three phases: contact phase, midstance, and propulsive phase. The contact phase comprises the first 17.5 percent of the gait cycle (27 percent of the stance phase), and it starts with heel contact and ends with the forefoot accepting weight. The first 15 percent of the contact phase is a double-support phase and only the final 2.5 percent of the cycle is single support. The midstance phase comprises the next 26 percent of the gait cycle (40 percent of the stance phase), and it starts with the forefoot accepting weight and ends the moment the heel lifts from the ground. It is only a single-support phase. The propulsive phase comprises 21.5 percent of the gait cycle (33 percent of the stance phase), and it begins with heel lift and

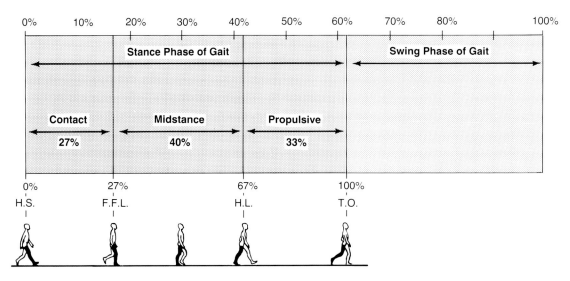

Fig. 3-24. The gait cycle. (From Root et al.,[4] with permission.)

ends with the toe leaving the ground. The first 6.5 percent of the propulsive phase is still a single-support phase, and the last 15 percent of this phase is a double-support phase.[4]

Movements of the Center of Body Mass During Gait

All of the joint movements of the lower extremity during ambulation are angular movements. The combination of all these angular movements produces almost a pure forward linear movement for the center of body mass, with just mild oscillations from a straight line in the direction of motion.

When viewing the center of body mass on the sagittal plane, a gentle up-and-down oscillation is noted twice within each gait cycle (Fig. 3-25). The peaks occur at the middle of midstance of each single-support phase and the valleys occur the middle of each double-support phase. The distance from the bottom to the top of the oscillation is approximately 5 cm for the average-sized adult.[5]

When viewing the center of body mass on the transverse plane, a gentle side-to-side oscillation is noted once within each gait cycle. The maximum lateral displacement occurs at the middle of mid-

stance to the weight-bearing side, followed by a maximum displacement to the opposite side during the middle of its midstance phase.

When viewing the center of body mass on the frontal plane, the combined lateral displacement once to each side and twice up and down during each gait cycle will produce a figure-eight movement of the center of mass during each cycle. The important thing to note about these mild oscillations of the body mass center in all three body planes is that during the whole gait cycle the center of mass should still stay within the pelvis. If body mass center is ever outside the pelvic region while walking in a straight line, then a pathologic situation should be considered to be present.

THE HIP JOINT

The hip joint is a ball-in-socket joint, which means that it has three independent axes of motion that are perpendicular to each other. When this situation occurs, the joint has full freedom of move-

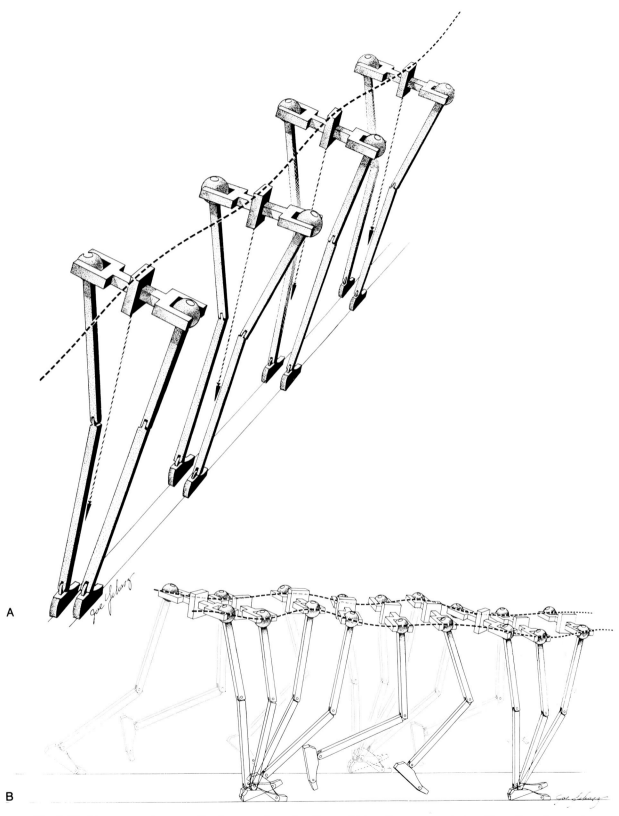

Fig. 3-25. Movement of center of body mass viewed on the sagittal and transverse planes. (From Saunders et al: J Bone Surg [Am], 35:552, 1953, with permission.)

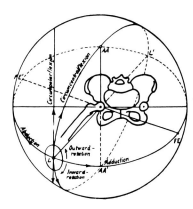

Fig. 3-26. The hip has three axes of motion perpendicular to each other, which allows for full freedom of movement. (From Steindler,[12] with permission.)

ment on the transverse plane, frontal, and sagittal planes. The frontal plane motion is abduction or adduction, the transverse plane motion is internal or external rotation, and the sagittal plane motion is flexion or extension. Therefore the hip joint may exhibit any combination, to any degree, of the three cardinal plane movements (Fig. 3-26).

The range of motion of the hip joint is determined by the edges of the articular surfaces or by the ligaments and/or tendons that cross the joint. The three basic ligaments that cross the joint are the iliofemoral (which is the strongest ligament in the body), the ischiofemoral, and the pubofemoral ligament. These three ligaments are all taut when

the hip is extended and are the major structures limiting hip extension, whereas they are all lax when the hip joint is flexed. When the hip joint is extended, the ileofemoral ligament limits external rotation of the hip, and the ischeofemoral ligament limits internal rotation. Therefore if a patient has a contracture of the ileofemoral ligament, he or she would have limited external rotation when the hip is extended, and if a patient has a contracture of the ischiofemoral ligament, he or she would have a limited internal rotation when the hip is extended.

During normal walking, the major motions of the hip joint occur on the transverse and sagittal planes. On the transverse plane, the entire pelvis starts internally rotating as the foot leaves the ground to start the swing phase. This coincides with the beginning of the midstance phase of gait on the opposite foot and the pelvis starting to externally rotate on the single-support side. During the swing, not only is the pelvis internally rotating, but the femur is internally rotating faster than the pelvis. This internal rotation continues through the entire swing phase and through the contact phase of the next step. As the opposite foot leaves the ground, the midstance phase begins and both the pelvis and the femur start their external rotation, although again the femur externally rotates faster than the pelvis.[6] (Fig. 3-27).

It is important to remember that the rotation of the hip must be accompanied by an equal and opposite rotation of the trunk and arms such that the

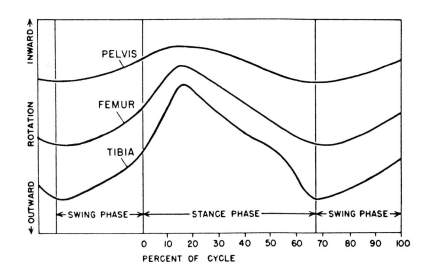

Fig. 3-27. Transverse rotations of bony segments of lower extremity during walking cycle. (From Lehmkuhl and Smith,[6] with permission.)

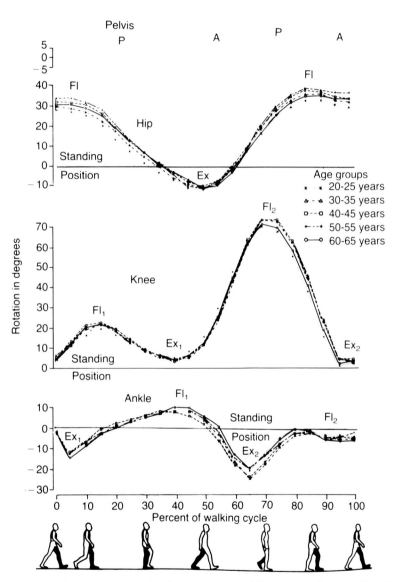

Fig. 3-28. Mean patterns of sagittal rotation for five age groups, 12 men in each group, two trials for each man. (From Lehmkuhl and Smith,[6] with permission.)

angular momentum of the lower half of the body is equal and opposite the angular momentum of the upper half of the body. In this way the person can maintain the body mass proceeding forward in a relatively straight line. If, during single-support phase, the upper body momentum is less than the lower body momentum (e.g., if the angular momentum of the lower extremity rotating to the right is greater than the angular momentum of the trunk and upper extremity rotating to the left), then the line of progression will deviate to the right. If the angular momentum of the upper body rotating to the left is greater than the angular momentum of the lower extremity rotating to the right, then the line of progression will deviate to the left.

On the sagittal plane, the hip is at its maximally extended position at the moment that the heel comes off the ground (Fig. 3-28). It now starts slowly flexing until the toe leaves the ground, then flexes more quickly during the entire swing phase. When the heel strikes the ground again it is at its maximally flexed position. It now begins to extend as the body starts moving over the foot, and this extension motion continues until the heel is ready to leave the ground again.

On the frontal plane, the hip has very little motion during the gait cycle. During the single-support phase there is about a 5 degree drop of the pelvis on the non-weight-bearing side. This means that there is about 5 degrees of hip adduction during midstance. This reduces after the opposite foot has started its contact phase. During swing phase, the hip over the weight-bearing foot has now adducted 5 degrees and the swinging hip must mildly abduct to continue its straight forward motion.

Forces on the Hip During Gait

To understand phasic muscle activity, the biomechanics student must understand the forces acting on the joints. Therefore we will first discuss the forces on the hip joint placed by gravity and the ground. A vertical force from the ground is present any time the foot is in contact with the ground. During swing phase gravitational force is always present, attempting to pull the center of mass of the leg around the hip joint axis of motion into a line that is perpendicular to the ground. During support phase, gravity attempts to pull the body mass center closer to the ground, which means that if the body mass center is posterior to the joint axis then it will be pulled backward, and if the body mass center is anterior to the joint axis then it will be pulled forward.

In addition to the vertical forces from gravity and the resistance of the ground to compression, the ground also provides shear forces in both the anterior or posterior direction, and the medial or lateral direction. These shear forces are really a function of the coefficient of friction between the ground and the foot. If the leg is trying to move forward, and the foot is in contact with the ground, the friction between the ground and the foot prevents the foot from moving forward with the leg; therefore there is a posteriorly directed shear force produced by the ground.

The vertical ground force begins at the moment of heel contact and ends at the moment of toe-off (Fig. 3-29). At heel contact the foot is anterior to the center of the hip joint; therefore the ground pushing up against the foot will attempt to flex the hip (Fig. 3-30). The degree of this flexion moment is determined by the weight of the person and also the length of the step. The greater the step length, the longer the lever arm and the greater the flexion moment on the hip during heel contact. As the body moves forward over the foot, the flexion moment on the hip decreases until the hip joint is directly over the center of the foot. From this point in time, until the toe leaves the ground, the hip joint is anterior to the foot. Therefore the vertical ground force is placing an extension moment on the hip joint. This extension moment again is proportional to the weight of the individual as well as the stride length. The longer the stride length, the greater will be the extension moment on the hip during propulsion.

When viewed on the frontal plane, the foot is usually slightly medial to the center of the hip joint (Fig. 3-25). Therefore the vertical ground force will be constantly placing a slight to mild adduction force on the hip joint. This is not very significant during the double-support phase because the center of body mass is directly between the two feet and the mild adduction forces present on both hips, when added together, produce a direct vertical force to support the body. It is during single-

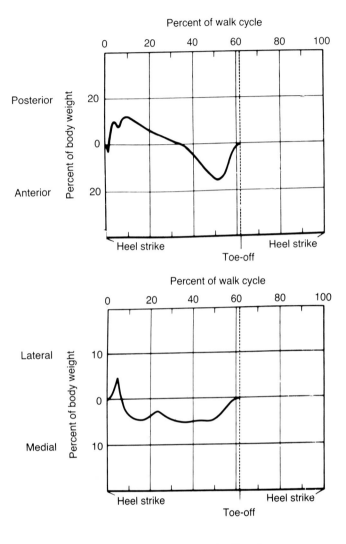

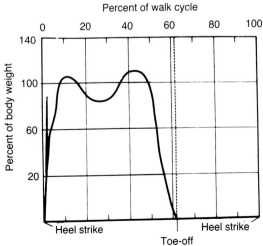

Fig. 3-29. *(Top,)* The shear force the ground places on the foot anteriorly or posteriorly versus time. *(Middle,)* The shear force the ground places on the foot medially or laterally versus time. *(Bottom,)* The vertical force the ground places on the foot versus time. (From Mann,[25] with permission.)

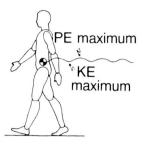

Fig. 3-30. At heel contact, the vertical force on the foot from the ground places a flexion moment on the hip. The center of body mass is still posterior to the hip joint, and gravity pulling it down places an extension moment on the hip. (From Cochran,[1] with permission.)

support phase that the adduction force on the hip becomes quite significant. This is because the center of body mass, although it has moved toward the weight-bearing side, is still quite a distance medial to the hip joint axis. Therefore gravity pulling the center of mass downward places a significant adduction moment on the hip during the single-support phase (Fig. 3-31).

The anterior and posterior shear forces of the ground provide important moments, especially during the contact and propulsive phases of gait. During swing phase the leg has forward velocity,

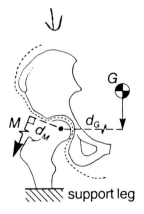

Fig. 3-31. During single-support phase, the ground pushing upward places a slight adduction moment on the hip joint, and the center of mass falling medial to the hip joint also places an adduction moment on the hip joint. (From Cochran,[1] with permission.)

and when the foot contacts the ground this forward velocity must be reduced to zero. The posterior shear of the ground provides the force to reduce the velocity to zero. Since acceleration or deceleration is equal to the change in velocity divided by the time interval over which this change occurs, it is easy to see that the faster the leg is moving forward, the greater must be the deceleration of the leg at heel contact. The amount of force needed to bring the foot to a stop is equal to the mass times the amount of deceleration needed. The average posteriorly directed shear force by the ground is approximately 10 percent of body weight for an average speed of walking[7] (Fig. 3-29). Therefore, the heavier the person the greater will be the posterior shear force during contact, and, more importantly, the faster a person is moving the greater will be the posterior shear force of the ground during contact.

During propulsion the ground must apply an anterior shear force strong enough to accelerate the leg and body forward. This shear force is generated by the leg pushing posteriorly against the ground. For a person walking at an average speed, the anteriorly directed shear is approximately 15 percent of body weight.[7] The faster the person wants to move, the stronger the anterior shear force is during propulsion. The anterior shear force of the ground places a very mild flexion moment on the hip joint during propulsion.

In order for the ground to produce a shear force, there must be friction between the patient's foot, shoe, and the ground. The amount of friction present is dependent on the coefficient of friction between the two surfaces, that is, how they resist sliding against each other when a certain pressure exists between the surfaces. If the coefficient is too low, then, when the leg makes contact with the ground, the posterior shear is decreased and the leg will fail to decelerate fast enough. Because the upward force of the ground flexes the hip, and there is no posteriorly directed force that would decrease the flexion moment on the hip, the person will fall backward with the leg in front of the body. This is the condition when a person steps from a normal surface onto ice. There are several compensations that may be made for this. One is to decrease the length of the stride, which decreases the lever arm for the flexion moment on the hip joint by the vertical ground force. Another is to

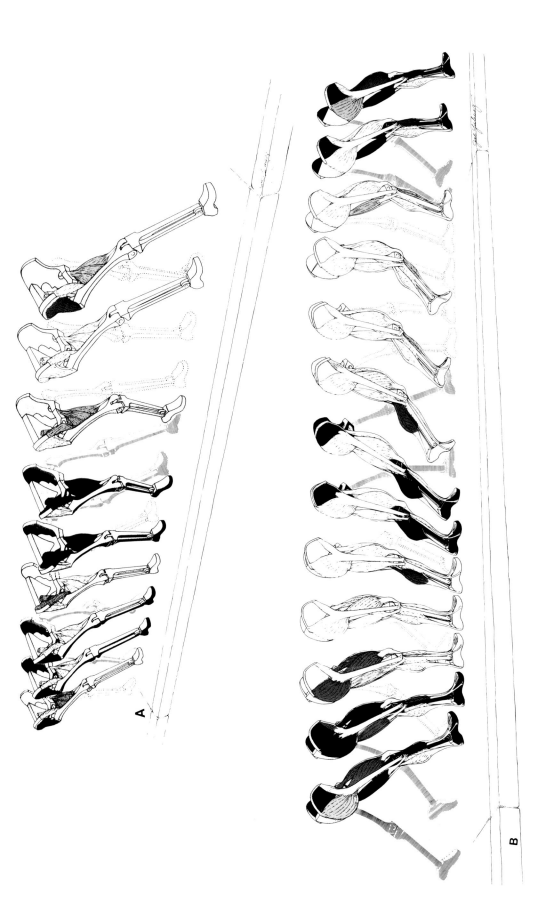

Fig. 3-32. Phasic action of all major muscle groups, shown combined in **A** and **B**. Note that most of the muscles are active at the beginning and end of swing and stance phases. During midstance and midswing, there is minimal muscle activity, although this is the period of maximal angular displacement. It seems that the principal action of the muscles is to accelerate and decelerate the angular motions of the legs. (From Inman et al., 1981, with permission.)

increase the contraction force of the hip extensors during heel contact.

Muscle Activity Around the Hip Joint

The purpose of a muscle is to counteract other forces, and thus either slow down a motion, prevent a motion, or help accelerate a motion. Therefore, in this text, all of the muscle actions are related to the forces acting on the joint and the forces that must be applied to produce the desired motions during the various phases of the gait cycle.

The vertical ground force places a flexion moment on the hip joint while the posterior shear of the ground places a slight extension moment on the hip joint during contact phase. The longer the stride the greater the flexion moment, whereas the faster the leg moves during swing the greater will be the extension moment on the hip. It is important that the extension moments be greater than the flexion moments so that the hip starts its extension movement at heel contact. The extension moments are supplied by the hip extension muscles, the hamstrings and the gluteus maximus (Fig. 3-32). The hamstrings begin contracting about halfway through swing phase, thus slowing the forward speed of the leg. Just slightly before the heel touches down, the gluteus maximus starts its contraction to provide additional extension moment, to withstand the flexion moment produced by vertical ground force. Both muscles relax once the center of the hip joint is directly over the center of the foot.

Once the center of the hip passes over the center of the foot, the vertical ground force is now providing an extension moment on the hip and the hip extension muscles are no longer needed. While it is desirable for the hip extension to continue until heel-off, this extension motion must be kept at a constant velocity; therefore some degree of flexion moment must be provided to keep the hip extension from accelerating too fast. This flexion moment is provided mainly by the iliopsoas muscle, and begins as an eccentric contraction during the second half of the stance phase and then continues as a concentric contraction, actively flexing the hip, during the first half of the swing phase. It is also assisted during the first half of the swing phase by the rectus femoris.

As discussed above, there is a significant adduction moment on the hip joint during the single-support phase of gait. Without a force to counteract this moment, the weight-bearing hip would adduct, and the swing side of the pelvis would drop. The abducting force on the hip during midstance is supplied by the hip abductors, the gluteus medius assisted by the tensor fascia lata; therefore these muscles provide isometric contractions during the single-support phase of gait (Fig. 3-32).

The adductor muscles of the hip are a much more poorly understood group of muscles, and there have been some differences reported as to the nature of their phasic activity. These muscles start their strongest contraction during the propulsive phase of gait, from the time the heel leaves the ground until a little after the toe leaves the ground. This strong contraction occurs mainly in the adductor longus, although the adductor magnus is assisting.[8] This corresponds with the contact phase of the opposite foot. They assist the iliopsoas in flexing the hip joint from its fully extended position; however, as the hip flexes, the flexion moment provided by the adductors decreases. The iliopsoas is a better flexor of the hip when the hip is already flexed. A more important function of the adductors during propulsion is to slow the external rotation of the femur during propulsion and to initiate internal rotation of the femur during the first part of the swing phase.[9]

During the initiation of heel contact the adductors again fire. This time the adductor magnus is the primary contractor, functioning mainly as a hip extender. It should therefore be noted that the adductors contract bilaterally simultaneously during the double-support phase of the gait cycle, with no activity on the support side and little activity on the swing side during single-support phase. Of all of the muscle groups around the hip, loss of the adductors will produce the smallest change in the gait cycle compared to loss of any of the other muscle groups.

THE KNEE JOINT

The knee joint is a complex hinge joint composed of two separate articular surfaces between the tibia and the femur and also a two-sided articular surface

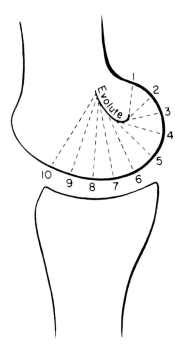

Fig. 3-33. The axis of the knee joint moves posteriorly along the line drawn above as the knee joint moves from extension to flexion. (From Lehmkuhl and Smith,[6] with permission.)

between the femur and the patella. It has its basic axis of motion perpendicular to the sagittal plane, which allows sagittal plane motion of flexion or extension. Full extension is reached when the tibia and femur form an angle of 180 degrees. The joint should have enough motion to allow it to flex at least 120 degrees from full extension. The knee joint, however, is not a pure hinge joint with one degree of motion. Instead it is described as a ginglymus joint with certain reservations. These reservations are:

1. The convex surfaces of the femoral condyles are not perfectly round when viewed on the sagittal plane (Fig. 3-33). The anterior portions of the condyles have a larger radius of curvature than the posterior aspects. This means that the transverse axis of the knee joint moves anteriorly when the knee joint is extended, and it moves posteriorly when the knee joint flexes.
2. The patella is the largest sesamoid in the body, and is part of the joint movement. It is tethered by the patellar retinaculum on the superior, an-

terior, medial, and lateral sides and it is anchored inferiorly by the patellar tendon to the tibial tuberosity. Most of its posterior surface is composed of an articular surface that is divided into two facets by a vertical ridge. The lateral facet is broader and deeper, to articulate with the lateral condyle of the femur, and the medial surface is narrower and shallower, to articulate with the narrower medial condylar articulation on the femur. When the joint is in full extension, the inferior portions of the medial and lateral articular surfaces are making greatest contact with the femur, whereas when the joint is flexed the superior aspects of the articular surfaces are making greatest contact with the femur.[10] When the joint is flexed more than 90 degrees, only the superior medial side of the articular surface makes contact with its femoral articulation.[11]

3. The medial and lateral condyles of the femur are not symmetric. The medial articular surface is longer and narrower and the lateral articular surface is shorter and broader. This means that the two surfaces rotate differently as the knee joint flexes and extends, especially within 30 degrees of full knee extension. As the knee joint is moving from flexion to full extension, when it reaches about 160 degrees (i.e., it is said to be 20 degrees flexed) the lateral condyle starts gliding and rotating inward around a vertical axis, while the medial condyle continues to rotate in the sagittal plane. This motion is very small at first, but as the knee joint progresses from 170 to 180 degrees (i.e., during the last 10 degrees of extension), the inward rotation of the femur becomes quite significant, such that the tibia is observed to externally rotate 0.5 degree for every 1 degree of sagittal plane motion. In other words, the last 10 degrees of extension is accompanied by 5 degrees of external rotation of the tibia on the femur. Likewise, if the knee is in full extension and starts to flex, the tibia wil be observed to internally rotate against the femur during the first 20 degrees of the flexion motion. This rotation of the tibia against the femur as the knee joint moves between 180 and 160 degrees, either extending or flexing, is known as "the screw home mechanism" (Fig. 3-34). If the tibia is not allowed to externally rotate as the knee is trying to extend, then the knee joint

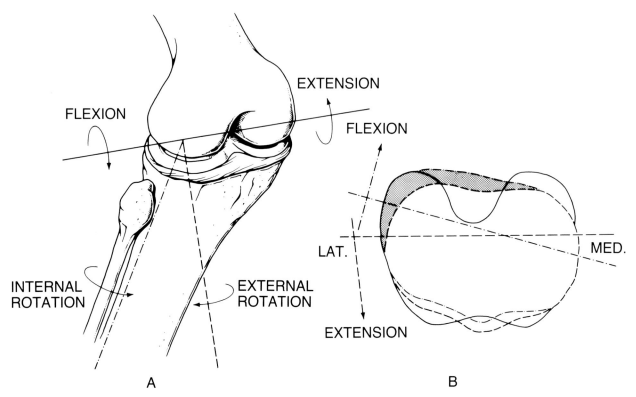

Fig. 3-34. The last 10 degrees of knee extension is accompanied by 5 degrees of external tibial rotaion. Likewise the first 10 degrees of knee flexion is accompanied by 5 degrees of internal tibial rotation. (From Frankel and Nordin,[11] with permission.)

cannot complete its full extension motion. If the tibia is prevented from internally rotating as the knee is starting to flex, then the knee will not be able to start its sagittal plane motion. The screw home mechanism is an important fact to remember in analyzing the pathologic forces that can be placed on the knee joint during gait.

The knee joint is a very unstable joint because it depends only on the tensions in the muscles and ligaments that cross it to maintain its stability. There are no osseous restraints that prevent the knee from being dislocated in one or more directions. The collateral ligaments function to resist abnormal frontal plane motion, and also to resist transverse plane motion when the knee joint is extended. When the knee joint is flexed, there is up to about 40 degrees of transverse plane motion of the tibia against the femur, whereas in full extension there should be no more than about 5 degrees of transverse plane motion. The medial and lateral

collateral ligaments have their origin on the medial and lateral epicondyles of the femur and attach to the medial condyle of the tibia and the head of the fibula, respectively. These are the structures that prevent medial and lateral frontal plane motion of the knee joint. The medial ligament is flatter and is attached to the capsule and the medial meniscus. The lateral ligament is rounder and has no attachments with the capsule or the meniscus. The lateral ligament is tight only when the knee joint is extended more than 150 degrees, and it tightens more when the tibia attempts to externally rotate on the femur. The anterior fibers of the medial collateral ligament are tight when the knee joint is in flexion, while the shorter oblique-posterior fibers are tight when the knee joint is in extension. These oblique-posterior fibers also become tighter when the tibia attempts to internally rotate on the femur with the knee joint extended.

The cruciate ligaments function to mainly resist sagittal plane hypermobility or subluxation of the knee joint. The anterior ligament arises from the anterior intercondylar area on the superior surface of the tibia and courses superiorly-posteriorly-laterally to insert on the medial-posterior aspect of the lateral femoral condyle. When the knee is in full extension, the tibia is articulating with the anterior portions of the femoral condyles, thereby tightening up the anterior cruciate ligament. The ligament then acts as a very strong resistor of any further anterior motion of the tibia on the femur. As the knee joint flexes and the tibia moves posteriorly on the femur, the anterior cruciate relaxes; however, once the knee joint starts flexing more than 90 degrees, the anterior cruciate again begins to tighten up. The posterior cruciate ligament arises from the posterior intercondylar area on the tibia and it courses superiorly-anteriorly-medially to insert on the lateral-anterior aspect of the medial femoral condyle. When the knee joint is fully extended this ligament is relaxed; however, as the knee joint flexes more than 30 degrees, and as the tibia starts moving posteriorly on the femur, it starts tightening up. Its primary function is to prevent the tibia from being dislocated in a posterior direction.

Normal Motion of the Knee

The knee motion during gait is primarily in the sagittal plane, although the transverse plane motion described above must simultaneously occur (Fig. 3-28). At the moment of heel contact, the knee joint is fully extended (180 degrees). As the foot contacts the ground the knee joint starts to flex, and it continues flexing until it is approximately 15 to 20 degrees flexed at the end of the contact phase. At the beginning of the midstance phase of gait the knee joint starts reextending. It continues extending through midstance until it reaches full extension just before heel lift. At the moment of full extension, the heel rises off the floor and the knee joint again starts flexing. During the first part of propulsion, which is the remaining part of the single-support phase, the knee joint flexes approximately 20 degrees. During the double-support phase of propulsion, the knee joint continues to flex, at the same angular velocity, until it is approximately 50 degrees flexed. At this point the toe comes off the ground and swing phase begins. During the swing phase, the knee joint initially continues flexing another 10 to 15 degrees, until the foot has dorsiflexed enough to clear the floor. The knee joint now begins to reextend until it has reached full extension at the moment of heel contact.

In order for the knee joint to undergo its normal flexion and extension motions, it must undergo the normal transverse plane motions according to the screw home mechanism discussed above. Therefore, during the contact phase, when the knee joint is moving from an extended position to a mildly flexed position, the tibia must internally rotate in relationship to the femur. Since the femur is also internally rotating during this phase of gait because of the normal transverse plane motion in the hip, this means that the tibia must internally rotate faster than the femur during the contact phase (Fig. 3-27). If the tibia does not undergo this transverse plane motion in relationship to the femur, then, if the knee is fully extended at the moment of heel contact, it will not be able to flex during the contact phase. In this situation, the only way for the knee to undergo flexion motion during contact is for it to already be somewhat flexed at the moment of heel contact. If the knee is unable to undergo its normal flexion motion during contact phase, there will be a loss of shock absorption by the knee during contact phase, which shock must then be absorbed by the hip and spine.

Just as the tibia must internally rotate in relationship to the femur during contact phase, so during the midstance phase, in order for the knee to fully reextend before heel-off, the tibia must externally rotate in relationship to the femur. Since the normal hip joint motion causes the femur to externally rotate during midstance, the tibia must then externally rotate faster than the femur during midstance. If it does not, then the knee joint will be unable to reach full extension before the heel comes off the floor. Once the heel comes off the floor, the knee joint may then be noted to "snap" into full extension, which will increase the stress on the posterior knee ligaments and knee flexor muscles to prevent the knee from hyperextending.

Forces on the Knee During Gait

The knee joint ligaments and muscles are responsible for resisting all of the forces on the knee joint. Therefore in this section the external forces on the

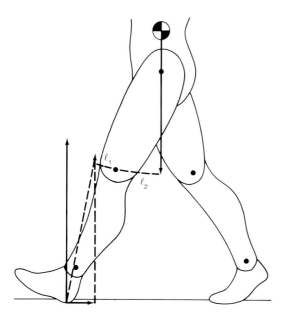

Fig. 3-35. The moments on the knee joint at heel contact. The force of the ground times its lever arm places an extension moment on the knee. The body weight times its distance from the knee joint axis places a flexion moment on the knee.

knee joint are discussed first, and the following section discusses the function of the muscles and ligaments to provide stability and normal movement of this joint.

At heel strike, the upward force of the ground on the heel, which is anterior to the knee joint, places an extension moment on the knee joint. This extension moment is equal to the contact force vector, which is equal to the vertical force of contact plus the posterior shear vector, times its lever arm with the knee joint axis (Fig. 3-35). As can be seen, the lever arm may be increased by a longer leg or a longer stride length, and can be decreased by a shorter leg or a shorter stride length. However, if the leg has a faster forward velocity, then the posterior shear force is greater at contact, and an increase in the posterior force vector will decrease the lever arm of the total ground force vector on the knee. The other strong moment on the knee joint during contact is the strong flexion moment placed on it by gravity pulling the body mass center downward while it is posterior to the knee joint axis. The flexion moment is equal to the weight of

the body mass that is superior to the knee joint times the distance the center of the body mass is behind the knee joint. Because the femur is usually longer than the tibia, increasing the stride length will mean that the lever arm of the center of body mass posterior to the knee joint axis will increase more than the lever arm of the heel anterior to the knee joint axis. Therefore increasing the stride length actually increases the flexion moment on the knee more than it increases the extension moment on the knee during contact phase.

At the end of contact, the knee joint axis is very close to being vertical with the center of force under the foot; therefore there is a very small extension moment on the knee joint. The center of body mass, however, is still a relatively long distance posterior to the knee joint axis; therefore the gravitational pull on the body still places a very strong flexion moment on the knee joint during early midstance. During midstance the body moves

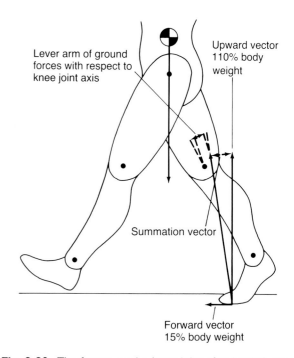

Fig. 3-36. The forces on the knee joint after heel lift. The center of the body mass is still anterior to the knee joint, but its lever arm is decreasing; therefore the extension moment on the knee is decreasing. Meanwhile the ground force pushing up behind the knee joint is placing a flexion moment on the knee.

forward in relationship to the knee joint, and as a result the flexion moment decreases until it is zero when the center of body mass is directly over the center of the knee joint. From this point on, as the body mass continues moving forward, the body weight is anterior to the knee joint axis, which places a strong extension moment on the knee for the rest of the midstance phase.

After heel lift, the knee travels forward faster than the center of body mass; therefore the moment arm of the body anterior to the knee joint decreases, which decreases the extension moment on the knee (Fig. 3-36). As the knee joint axis moves forward of the metatarsal heads and toes, the upward force of the ground behind the knee joint places a flexion moment on the knee, which increases through the propulsive phase of gait.

On the frontal plane, the femur is angulated lateralward from the line of the tibia. This is known as the Q angle, and is approximately 10 degrees. This means that the center of mass of the thigh is mildly lateral to the center of the knee joint, which would produce a very mild tension force on the medial side of the knee, and a very mild compression force on the lateral side of the knee (Fig. 3-37A). Therefore a very mild valgum force is on the knee during the double-support phase of gait. During the single-support phase, the body mass center is falling medial to both the knee and the hip; therefore a varus moment force is placed on the knee when the

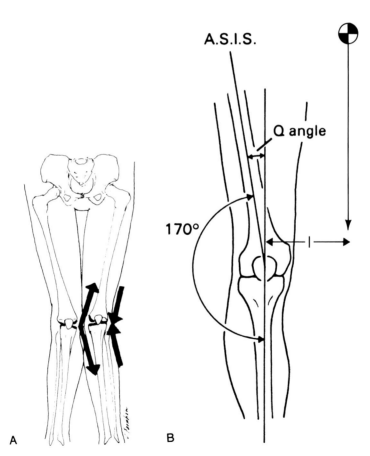

Fig. 3-37. **(A)** During double-support phase, the center of body mass can be divided in two parts, half on each side of the mean sagittal plane. The center of each half of body mass falls lateral to the knee joint, which places a valgus moment on the knee joint. (From Norkin CC, Levangie PK: with permission.) **(B)** During single-support phase, the center of body mass falls medial to the knee joint center, which places a varus moment on the knee. (From Lehmkuhl and Smith,[6] with permission.)

hip joint is adequately stabilized against adduction force during this phase of gait (Fig. 3-37B).

Muscle Activity Around the Knee

The contact phase of gait shows the greatest amount of muscle activity around the knee joint. The knee is fully extended, but needs to flex approximately 15 degrees. To initiate flexion, the tibia must internally rotate against the femur. The popliteus muscle has its origin on the lateral femoral condyle and courses medially-inferiorly, to insert along the popliteal line of the tibia. It is this muscle that contracts during heel contact to initiate internal rotation of the tibia so that the knee joint may flex.

The combination of body weight posterior to the knee joint axis, plus the posterior shearing force of the ground, plus the contraction of the hamstrings during contact phase, creates a flexion moment on the knee that is far greater than the extension moment created by the vertical ground force. Therefore the greatest force of muscle contraction around the knee during contact is that exerted by the quadriceps femoris. These four muscles begin their contraction just before heel contact and end their contraction at midstance when the body weight passes over the center of the knee joint axis. They thereby enable the femur to continue its forward progression during the first half of the stance phase of gait. Contraction by the quadriceps is not necessary during the last half of midstance, because knee extension is accomplished by the center of

body mass falling anterior to the knee joint axis, thus extending the knee. The soleus also plays a role in extending the knee, but this is discussed later.

It should be noted that each of the quadriceps muscles has a slightly different direction of pull. The vastus lateralis is the largest of the quadriceps, and it pulls the patella in a superior-lateral direction. The vastus medialis obliquus is the major muscle for providing a medially directed vector of pull (Fig. 3-38A); however, the lateral pulling vector of the vastus lateralis is usually larger than the medially pulling vector of the vastus medialis. Therefore when the entire quadriceps group contracts, the patella is always pulled in a slightly lateral direction. The more anteriorly projecting lateral condyle of the femur helps to counteract this lateral pull, keeping the patella tracking in the patellar groove. It is important, however, that the vastus medialis obliquus be developed enough so that the patella is not subluxed laterally when the quadriceps contracts.[1]

When viewed on the sagittal plane, when the quadriceps muscles contract, the patella is pulled superiorly. However, the patellar tendon, being anchored to the tibial tuberosity and the patella, and having very little stretch, pulls the patella inferiorly. If the knee joint is completely extended, the superior pull of the quadriceps is 180 degrees to the inferior pull of the patellar tendon, and these equal and opposite pulls result in a vector pull on the patella equal to zero. However, if the knee joint is flexed then the equal pulls of the quadriceps pulling the patella superiorly and the patellar ten-

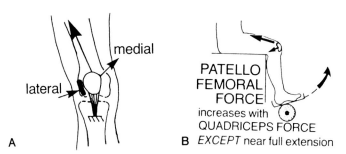

Fig. 3-38. **(A)** Contraction of the quadriceps results in a slight lateral pull of the patella. The vastus medialis obliquus is responsible for neutralizing this laterally directed pull. **(B)** Contraction of the quadriceps results in a compression between the patella and the femur. The amount of compression is proportional to the degree that the knee is flexed. (From Cochran,[1] with permission.)

don pulling the patella inferiorly, when added together, result in a vector that compresses the patella into its femoral articulation (Fig. 3-38B). If the knee joint is flexed 15 degrees, the patellofemoral compression force is 0.13 times the tension force in the quadriceps. If the knee joint is flexed 90 degrees then the patellofemoral compression force is 0.71 times the tension force in the quadriceps. When the knee joint is flexed, the tibia is internally rotated against the femur. Logic would dictate that this would increase the tension in the lateral side of the patellar tendon and decrease the tension in the medial side of the patellar tendon, so that when the quadriceps contracts with the knee joint flexed, the compression between the femur and the patella is greater under the lateral articular surface than under the medial articular surface.

Because there is a mild adduction force on the knee joint during the midstance, there would normally be some stress on the lateral collateral ligaments during this phase of gait. However, this stress on the lateral ligaments is reduced by the tension of the iliotibial band, which inserts on the lateral tibial tubercle just lateral to the tibial tuberosity. The tensor fascia lata, which is providing part of the abduction moment on the hip joint during single-support phase, creates tension along the entire length of the iliotibial band to also stabilize the knee on the lateral side. Because the iliotibial band inserts on the lateral-anterior aspects of the tibia, tension in the band places an external rotation moment on the tibia; thus it can provide some assistance to help the tibia externally rotate faster than the femur during midstance, which would aid in the knee joint reextending during midstance.

At heel-off, the knee joint starts flexing. Because body weight is anterior to the knee joint axis, which tends to keep the knee joint extended, muscle force is needed to start the knee joint flexing. The primary knee joint flexor in early propulsion is the gastrocnemius, which is also lifting the heel from the floor. As was noted above, after heel-off, the knee joint axis starts moving anteriorly faster than the center of body mass; therefore the extension moment created on the knee by the center of mass being anterior to the knee joint axis starts decreasing until it is just about zero at the time the toe leaves the ground. The gastrocnemius starts relaxing about halfway through propulsion,[4] while the short head of the biceps femoris fires, continuing the flexion moment during the latter part of propulsion.[9] There is also a mild contraction of the quadriceps femoris during the latter part of propulsion, which is evidently an eccentric contraction to keep the knee joint flexing at a constant angular velocity.

After the toe leaves the ground, gravity pulls the lower leg downward, which places an extension moment on the knee. This is initially resisted by the continued contraction of both heads of the biceps femoris, which do not relax until the anterior leg muscles have sufficiently dorsiflexed the ankle joint so that the toes can clear the ground. All of the muscles then relax as the knee starts its forward extension moment, and there is no more muscle activity controlling the knee joint until the swing phase is approximate three-quarters through. It is evident that the knee joint continues to reextend while the tibia is posterior to the knee because of the gravitational pull on the leg, which gives the tibia a faster forward velocity than the femur. The continuation of the knee joint reextension, once the leg is past being perpendicular to the ground, is evidently a continuation of its extension momentum. The hamstrings start contracting at about 75 percent of the swing phase, which slows the reextension of the knee, followed by contraction of the quadriceps femoris at about 90 percent of the swing phase, which provide the final amount of force needed for the knee to reach full extension just at heel contact.

THE ANKLE JOINT

The ankle joint is composed of three articular surfaces, the transverse tibiotalar, the medial tibiotalar, and the lateral talofibular articulation. The largest of these is the transverse tibiotalar articulation between the convex superior surface of the talus and the inferior articular surface of the tibia, which is known as the tibial plafond. The medial tibiotalar articulation is composed of a tear-shaped surface on both the talus and the tibia that are continuous and 90 degrees to their respective trans-

OBLIQUITY OF ANKLE AXIS

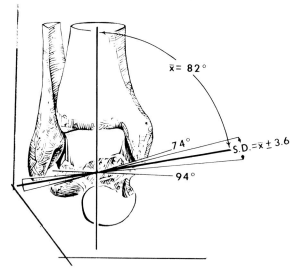

$\bar{x} = 82°$

$74°$

S.D. $= \bar{x} \pm 3.6$

$94°$

Fig. 3-39. The axis of the ankle joint lies just inferior to the distal tips of the medial and lateral malleoli. (From Inman,[5] with permission.)

verse tibiotalar articular surfaces. The talofibular articulation is a triangular-shaped surface between the lateral aspect of the talus, which is continuous with the dorsal articular surface, and the medial surface of the inferior tip of the fibula.

The ankle joint is one of the most stable joints in the lower extremity. It can be viewed as an open-ended, box-shaped joint, which is often referred to as the ankle mortise. The strong syndesmosis between the tibia and the fibula and the bony projections of the malleoli inferiorly around the medial and lateral sides of the talar dome prevent the talus from sliding medially or laterally and also from rotating around a vertical axis within the mortise. The posterior aspect of the tibial plafond projects more inferiorly than the anterior aspect and this blocks the talus from sliding posteriorly within the mortise. The talus is prevented from sliding anteriorly out of the mortise by the strong collateral ligaments.

The three ankle joint surfaces combine to form a ginglymus joint, whose axis passes through two points just inferior to the tips of medial and lateral malleoli (Fig. 3-39). It should be noted that the inferior aspect of the fibular malleolus is a little lower than the inferior aspect of the tibial malleolus. Therefore, when viewed on the frontal plane, the axis is slightly angulated with the transverse plane, an average of about 8 degrees. When viewed on the transverse plane, the axis is angulated with the frontal plane, an average of about 15 degrees.[5] This means that while the major motions of dorsiflexion and plantar flexion occur in the sagittal plane, there is a small component of frontal plane angular movement and an even smaller amount of transverse plane angular movement. Therefore when the ankle joint dorsiflexes it also shows a small degree of talar eversion and abduction, which three motions fit the definition of "pronation," and when it plantar flexes it also shows a small degree of talar inversion and adduction, which fits the definition of "supination."

It should be noted that the medial to lateral distance across the dome of the talus is greater at the anterior aspect than at the posterior aspect. It has been argued by a number of authors that this makes the talus fit tighter within the ankle mortise when it is dorsiflexed and makes it fit looser when the talus is plantar flexed. Inman refuted this idea, noting that the talus was as tight within the mortise when it is plantar flexed as when it is dorsiflexed. His observations and measurements led him to conclude that the dome of the talus can be geometrically described as being a section of a cone, whose axis is identical to the observed axis of motion previously described and whose apex is medial to the talus and forms an apical angle of between 12 and 36 degrees[5] (Fig. 3-40). This means that when the ankle joint dorsiflexes and plantar flexes the lateral side of the talar dome moves further than the medial side, the same as if a cone was rolled on a table. This increases the observed transverse plane motion of the talus toward the midline of the body as it plantar flexes and away from the midline of the body as it dorsiflexes.

The movements of the ankle joint during the gait cycle are referred to as dorsiflexion or plantar flexion, although the reader is already aware that the joint is technically pronating or supinating. Within the context of this discussion about normal joint function, the statement that the ankle joint is "dorsiflexed" means that the ankle is positioned such that the foot and leg form an angle that is less than 90 degrees when viewed from the sagittal plane. Likewise, the statement that the ankle joint is

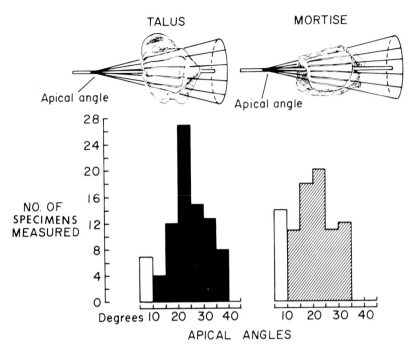

Fig. 3-40. The slope of the talar dome matches the surface shape of a cone with its apex medially. (From Inman,[5] with permission.)

"plantar flexed" means that the ankle is positioned such that the foot and leg form an angle that is greater than 90 degrees when viewed from the sagittal plane. To describe the degree that the ankle is dorsiflexed or plantar flexed, a number that indicates how many degrees the foot is deviated from being perpendicular to the leg is used. For example, the statement that the ankle is dorsiflexed 5 degrees means that the foot and leg form an angle of 85 degrees, and the statement that the ankle is plantar flexed 5 degrees means that the foot and leg form an angle of 95 degrees.

Motions of the Ankle Joint in Gait

As the foot contacts the ground, the ankle joint is dorsiflexed about 5 degrees. The forefoot immediately starts falling toward the ground, plantar flexing the ankle joint until the joint is approximately 10 degrees plantarflexed halfway through the contact phase. During the rest of the contact phase, the ankle joint starts dorsiflexing such that by the time the midstance phase begins, it is in a 5 degree plantar-flexed position. During the entire midstance phase, the ankle joint continues its dorsiflexion motion at a constant angular velocity, until it reaches a 10 degree dorsiflexed position, which marks the end of midstance and begins the propulsive phase of gait as the heel begins rising off the floor. Once the heel starts rising off the floor, the ankle joint again reverses direction and plantar flexes during propulsion, until it is approximately 20 degrees plantar flexed when the toes start leaving the ground. As the leg begins swing phase, the ankle joint starts dorsiflexing until it is again about 5 degrees dorsiflexed at the time the foot clears the ground and passes the opposite support leg. It now stays in this position through the second half of the swing phase until the beginning of the new contact phase.

Forces on the Ankle Joint During Gait

As the foot strikes the ground, the ground contact point against the posterior lateral aspect of the heel is directly beneath the axis of the ankle joint. This means the upward force of the ground applies no moment because its moment arm is zero; how-

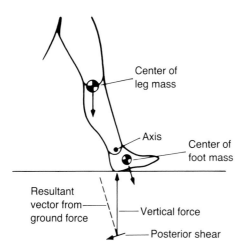

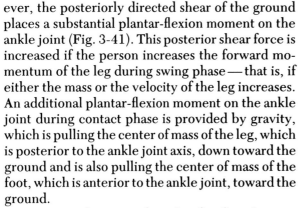

Fig. 3-41. Nonmuscular moments on the ankle joint during contact phase.

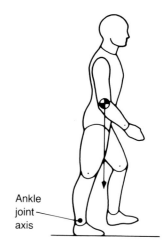

Fig. 3-42. The body mass center falling anterior to the ankle joint in later midstance places a strong dorsiflexion moment on ankle joint.

ever, the posteriorly directed shear of the ground places a substantial plantar-flexion moment on the ankle joint (Fig. 3-41). This posterior shear force is increased if the person increases the forward momentum of the leg during swing phase — that is, if either the mass or the velocity of the leg increases. An additional plantar-flexion moment on the ankle joint during contact phase is provided by gravity, which is pulling the center of mass of the leg, which is posterior to the ankle joint axis, down toward the ground and is also pulling the center of mass of the foot, which is anterior to the ankle joint, toward the ground.

During midstance, after the forefoot has accepted body weight, the body's center of mass falling posterior to the ankle joint continues to place a plantar-flexion force on the ankle joint; however, this decreases as the quadriceps femorae pull the body mass center foreward. Once the center of body mass is anterior to the ankle joint axis, then the body weight falling foward places a strong dorsiflexion moment on the ankle joint. Therefore the last two-thirds of the midstance shows that the only force needed to keep the ankle joint dorsiflexing is the body weight moving anterior to the ankle joint axis (Fig. 3-42).

During the single-support phase of gait, the center of body mass is medial to the ankle joint. Body weight falling medially, pulling the leg me-

dially because of normal function of the abductor hip muscles, would place an inversion moment on the ankle joint. The further medial to the ankle joint the body's center of mass is, the greater will be this inversion moment on the joint. Therefore an inversion moment is greater in people that have genu valgum and in overweight people, and it is less in people that have genu varum or when people are running.

If the center of the weight-bearing surface of the plantar aspect of the calcaneus is directly under the center of the ankle joint, then the ground pushing upward will not place a frontal plane moment on the ankle joint. However, if the center of the weight-bearing surface on the plantar calcaneus is lateral to the center of the ankle joint, then the ground will be placing an eversion moment on the ankle joint. Therefore when the foot is pronated, which causes the calcaneus to move lateral to the leg, the eversion moment on the ankle joint increases.

Muscular Control of the Ankle Joint

The phasic activity of all of the lower leg muscles is shown in Figure 3-43. In discussing the muscle function as related to ankle joint function, the dorsiflexion and plantar-flexion muscles are the most

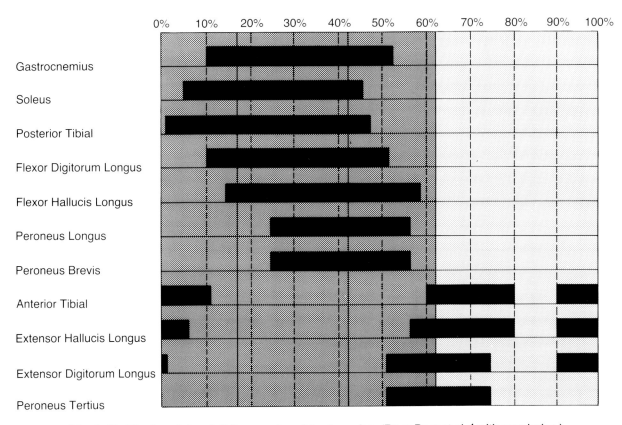

Fig. 3-43. Phasic activity of all the muscles of the lower leg. (From Root et al.,[4] with permission.)

important to discuss. At heel contact there is a large plantar-flexion moment on the ankle joint, and during contact phase it undergoes a high plantar-flexing angular velocity. This plantar-flexing velocity averages 1.5 degrees for every percent of the gait cycle, which is about three times the dorsiflexion velocity that occurs during midstance. Therefore the plantar flexion must be kept at a constant velocity during early contact, and it must be slowed down during late contact for full forefoot loading, to avoid shock absorption injuries to the metatarsals. The anterior muscles of the leg are the only muscles that can provide the dorsiflexion moment for the smooth forefoot contact; therefore they eccentrically contract during the first half of the contact phase to control the rate of forefoot contact with the ground.

The extensor digitorum longus relaxes about 10 percent into contact phase and the extensor hallucis longus relaxes about 35 percent into contact

phase. The anterior tibial finishes contracting about 65 percent through the contact phase, at which time the ankle joint has just stopped its plantar-flexion moment and is barely starting its dorsiflexion motion. At this point in time, when the anterior tibial ceases its contraction, the body center of mass is still a little posterior to the ankle joint axis. This means that there is still a mild plantar-flexion moment on the ankle joint; however, the plantar-flexion velocity has been slowed down to zero, and there is now a slight dorsiflexion velocity. The reason that the ankle joint is able to continue its dorsiflexion velocity before the body mass center moves anterior to the ankle joint axis is because the quadriceps femoris are still actively contracting, pulling the body mass center anteriorly, and the opposite foot is finishing its propulsion, which adds additional forward momentum to the body mass center. Thus the ankle joint can continue its slow dorsiflexion movement of about 0.5 degree per percent of the gait cycle through the last one-third of the contact phase and the first one-third of the midstance phase. The contraction of the soleus begins about one-third through contact phase. While it places a plantar-flexion moment on the ankle joint, it also assist the quadriceps in keeping the knee joint from flexing, while body mass center is posterior to the knee joint axis, and thus it helps to pull the body mass center forward over the foot. The gastrocnemius starts contracting about 60 percent through the contact phase and slows the forward momentum of the femur, thus helping to bring the body mass center over the femur. This process of bringing the body mass center over the foot is the primary method of overcoming the plantar-flexion moment on the ankle joint and starting the ankle joint dorsiflexing during the late contact phase.

Once the body mass center has passed anterior to the ankle joint, there is a strong dorsiflexion moment on the joint, and the longer the moment arm becomes by the body mass moving further anteriorly, the stronger will be that dorsiflexion moment. As was pointed out above, the ankle joint dorsiflexion proceeds through the entire midstance phase at a fairly constant velocity of about 0.5 degree per percent of the gait cycle. Therefore the gastrocnemius and soleus are extremely important eccentric contractors, to ensure that the ankle joint dorsiflexes at a constant velocity through the midstance phase. Without them the ankle joint dorsiflexion would be an arithmetical acceleration, which would produce a geometrical increase in dorsiflexion velocity. Therefore, the more the ankle joint dorsiflexes, the more tension is needed within the Achilles tendon to ensure a constant ankle joint dorsiflexion velocity.

The mechanism of heel lift is mediated by the gastrocnemius and soleus muscles. To produce heel lift, two joints must simultaneously move: the ankle joint must plantarflex and the first metatarsophalangeal joint must dorsiflex, leaving only the digits and metatarsal heads on the ground. Therefore the plantar-flexion moment must exceed the dorsiflexion moment on the ankle joint *and* the dorsiflexion moment must exceed the plantar-flexion moment on the metatarsophalangeal joints (Fig. 3-44). We have already discussed how body weight anterior to the ankle joint produces a dorsiflexion moment while tension in the Achilles ten-

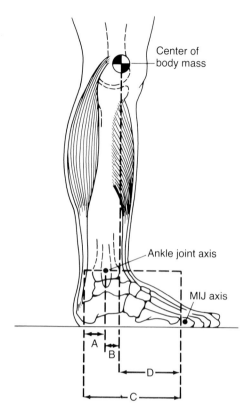

Fig. 3-44. "A" is the lever arm of the Achilles tendon, producing a plantar-flexion moment on the ankle joint. "B" is the lever arm of the center of body mass on the ankle joint. "C" is the lever arm of the Achilles tendon, producing a dorsiflexion moment on the metatarsophalangeal joints. "D" is the lever arm of the center of body mass on the metatarsophalangeal joints.

don produces a plantar-flexion moment. It should also be remembered that as the body weight moves forward of the ankle joint, the dorsiflexion moment increases in linear proportion to the increase in the lever arm; however, the ankle joint dorsiflexion increases the stretch on the Achilles tendon, which increases its tension geometrically (refer to sample length-tension curve, Fig. 3-22). Thus a certain point is reached at which the tension in the Achilles tendon times its distance from the ankle joint becomes greater than the weight of the body times its distance anterior to the ankle joint.

The second criterion that must be met for heel lift is that the dorsiflexion moment on the first metatarsophalangeal joint must be greater than the plantar-flexion moment on the joint. If this criterion is *not* met, and the previously described condition has been met, then one of two things will happen: either the tibia will move posteriorly, which would produce a hyperextended knee, or an abnormal dorsiflexion movement will occur at the midtarsal joint, which will lift the heel and leave the metatarsophalangeal joints extended. When the second situation occurs, the person is said to have an equinus. It should be noted that the dorsiflexion moment on the metatarsophalangeal joints is produced by the ankle joint plantar-flexion muscles, the triceps surae being the most prominent, times their distance from the metatarsophalangeal joint axes. The plantarflexion moment is produced by the body weight falling posterior to the metatarsophalangeal joints times its distance from the joint axes. Once body weight falls anterior to the metatarsophalangeal joints then it is also placing a dorsiflexion moment on the joints.

The soleus muscle quits firing about 15 percent of the way into propulsion. This is because the plantar-flexion moment on the metatarsophalangeal joints is zero, so that only the gastrocnemius firing provides sufficient dorsiflexion moment, and also it permits the tibia to move forward and allow the knee joint to flex during propulsion. The gastrocnemius quits firing about 50 percent into propulsion. At this time the body weight should be far past the metatarsophalangeal joints, thus continuing to provide a dorsiflexion moment through the rest of the propulsive phase.

At the moment that the gastrocnemius quits firing, the extensor digitorum longus begins firing. This is followed by the extensor hallucis longus beginning to fire approximately 75 percent of the way into propulsion, and finally the anterior tibial beginning to fire approximately 90 percent into propulsion. Even though the metatarsophalangeal joints are dorsiflexing during propulsion, the two extensor muscles are functioning in an eccentric manner because the ankle joint continues to plantar flex even after the gastrocnemius muscle has quit firing. The reason for this is that the leg moving forward during propulsion pulls the calcaneus forward, and the only way for the calcaneus to move forward and still leave the digits on the ground is for the ankle joint to plantar flex.

Once the anterior tibial begins firing just before the toes leave the ground, a marked deceleration of ankle joint plantar flexion begins, and just after the hallux leaves the ground the ankle joint dorsiflexion begins. The four anterior muscles now provide a strong concentric contraction to quickly dorsiflex the ankle joint so that the foot may clear the ground through swing. After the foot has cleared the ground, the ankle joint dorsiflexors are quiescent from about 50 percent of the swing phase to about 75 percent of the swing phase. During this time the ankle joint dorsiflexion velocity decreases, but does not completely stop because of the short period of time that the deceleration occurs. During the last 25 percent of the swing phase, the anterior muscles again begin firing and keep the ankle joint dorsiflexing, but at a much slower velocity, preparing it for the next heel contact phase, during which the muscles will again provide eccentric contraction.

THE SUBTALAR JOINT

The subtalar joint is sometimes called the talocalcaneal-navicular joint. It is a complex joint made up of three articular facets between the talus and the calcaneus. The largest of these is the posterior facet, which has a convex surface on the calcaneus that articulates with a concave surface on the inferior talus. Looking at it from superiorly, the facet appears rectangular and is oriented with its long axis running from posterior-medial to anterior-lateral. Looking at it from the sagittal plane, the convexity is noted with the most posterior aspect higher and the most anterior aspect lower, and the most anterior aspect ending at the sinus tarsi. This articular facet has its own separate joint capsule.

The middle facet is between the superior aspect of the sustentaculum tali and the inferior aspect of the neck of the talus. It is mildly concave on the calcaneal surface to match the mild convexity of the inferior neck of the talus. The anterior facet is the smallest facet anterior and lateral to the middle facet, and it articulates with the posterior-inferior-lateral aspect of the talar head. The calcaneal anterior articular facet is continuous with the middle facet in about two-thirds of the population, and is separate in about one-third.[7] Some people include the talonavicular joint in the subtalar joint complex because the middle and anterior facets of the talus are continuous with the talar articular surface for the talonavicular joint, and so is the joint capsule; however, talonavicular joint function is discussed in the section on the midtarsal joint. It should be noted that the talocalcaneal joint may move without any movement between the talus and navicular; however, to do so requires movement of the calcaneocuboid joint. Likewise the talocalcaneal joint may move without any movement between the calcaneus and cuboid, but to do so would require movement between the talus and navicular.

In most of the literature, the subtalar joint has been described as a ginglymus joint with one axis of motion that proceeds from inferior-posterior-lateral to superior-anterior-medial. The average deviation of this axis from the sagittal plane of the foot is about 16 degrees and the average deviation from the transverse plane is about 42 degrees (Fig. 3-45). All researchers do report that there is considerable deviations from these averages in the population. It should also be noted that all of the published data have been from in vitro studies. From discussions above, it will be noted that because of the orientation of the axis to all three body planes, when the joint moves, angular motion will be detected on all three body planes. Using the previously discussed formulas we can calculate that if a person has an average joint axis, if the joint moves 10 degrees in the plane that is perpendicular to its axis of motion, an observer of the frontal plane would observe 7.1 degrees of angular motion, an observer of the transverse plane would observe 6.7 degrees of angular motion, and an observer of the sagittal plane would observe 2.0 degrees of angular motion.

Pronation and supination are the proper terms to describe motions in the subtalar joint. When the joint pronates, the calcaneus everts, abducts, and dorsiflexes in relationship to the talus, and when the joint supinates the calcaneus inverts, adducts, and plantar flexes in relationship to the talus. This is the type of movement that is observed when no weight is being borne by the foot; in other words, these are the observations when the foot is in "open kinetic chain."

When the foot is bearing weight, it is said to be in

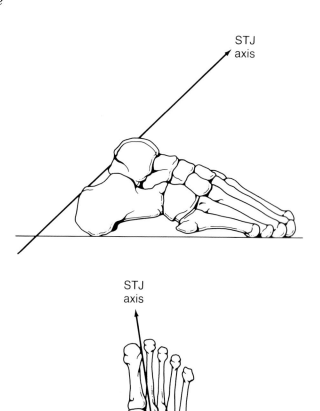

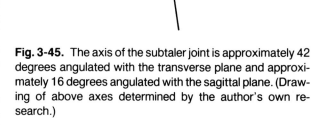

Fig. 3-45. The axis of the subtaler joint is approximately 42 degrees angulated with the transverse plane and approximately 16 degrees angulated with the sagittal plane. (Drawing of above axes determined by the author's own research.)

"closed kinetic chain,"[12] and totally different observations are noted when the subtalar joint pronates or supinates. In closed kinetic chain there is a very strong friction between the foot and the ground, and instead of the distal segment moving on the proximal segment, the proximal segment moves on the distal segment. Therefore when the subtalar joint pronates, instead of the calcaneus dorsiflexing and abducting, the talus plantarflexes and adducts. It should be noted that because of the shape of the ankle joint mortise, the talus can plantar flex independent of the tibia, but when it adducts it carries the tibia and fibula with it; therefore the lower leg is noted to internally rotate. On the frontal plane, when the subtalar joint pronates, the above reasoning would dictate that the talus would invert with the lower leg; however, the leg mass also moves medial to the center of the calcaneus, and this places an eversion moment on the calcaneus. Thus the calcaneus is observed to still evert to the ground and no frontal plane motion is observed between the talus and the ground. Just as closed kinetic chain pronation produces talar plantarflexion and adduction with calcaneal eversion in relationship to the ground, so the same arguments may be used to describe closed kinetic chain supination of the subtalar joint. In this case the talus is observed to dorsiflex and adduct, and the calcaneus is observed to invert in relationship to the ground. Again, the talus moves independent of the tibia in its dorsiflexion movement, but it carries the talus with it on the transverse plane; thus the lower leg is observed to externally rotate when the subtalar joint supinates.

Although the talus might be able to plantarflex or dorsiflex within the ankle joint independent of the tibia and fibula, it cannot move in the transverse or frontal planes independent of the lower leg. Therefore there are very close relationships between movements of the lower leg in the transverse and frontal planes and movements of the subtalar joint in closed kinetic chain. If the lower leg internally rotates, the talus adducts with it and forces the subtalar joint to pronate; thus the calcaneus must evert and the talus must also plantarflex. If the lower leg externally rotates, the talus abducts with it and forces the subtalar joint to supinate; thus the calcaneus must invert and the talus must also dorsiflex. On the other hand, if the calcaneus is forced to evert, it causes the subtalar joint to pronate, and the talus must simultaneously plantarflex and adduct, which will force the lower leg to internally rotate. Likewise, if the calcaneus is forced to invert, it causes the subtalar joint to supinate, and thus the talus must simultaneously dorsiflex and abduct, which will force the lower leg to externally rotate.

In vitro testing has shown a wide variation in the deviations of the axis of the subtalar joint from the sagittal and transverse planes. The deviation from the transverse plane has been reported to vary from about 20 to about 60 degrees.[5] It is important to recognize how this type of variation can affect the coordination between foot and leg motion. If a person has a subtalar joint axis that is only 20 degrees angulated with the transverse plane (assuming there is a normal deviation from the sagittal plane) then calculations predict that when the subtalar joint moves 1 degree in the plane of motion, the frontal plane angular change is 0.90 degree while the transverse plane angular change is 0.34 degree. In other words, every degree of calcaneal eversion produces 0.38 degree of internal rotation of the lower leg and every degree of internal rotation of the lower leg produces 2.65 degrees of calcaneal eversion.

On the other hand, if a person has a subtalar joint axis that is 60 degrees angulated with the transverse plane (assuming again that there is a normal deviation from the sagittal plane) then calculations predict that when the subtalar joint moves 1 degree in the plane of motion, the frontal plane angular change is 0.48 degree while the transverse plane angular change is 0.87 degree. In other words, every degree of calcaneal eversion produces 1.81 degrees of internal rotation of the lower leg and every degree of internal rotation of the lower leg produces 0.55 degrees of calcaneal eversion.

A specific point between the extremely pronated and extremely supinated positions of the subtalar joint is called the *neutral position.* Several descriptions of this neutral position exist. It is commonly described as that position where there is greatest congruity and maximum contact between the talar, calcaneal, and navicular articular surfaces.[13] Others note that it exists at a point at the bottom of an arc, where it takes equal energy to supinate or pronate the joint; that is, if the joint is supinated from the neutral position, then it takes less energy to pronate it than to supinate it, and if the joint is pronated, then it takes less energy to supinate it than to pronate it. It has been noted that this "neutral position" is at a point that is approximately two-thirds from the fully supinated position and one-third from the fully pronated person.[14] Fol-

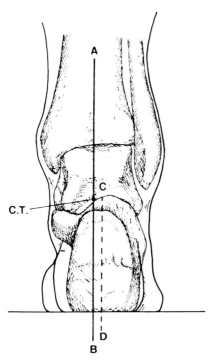

Fig. 3-46. When the subtalar joint is in its neutral position: (a) the sagittal plane of the calcaneus should be parallel with the longitudinal axis of the leg, (b) the center of the calcaneus should lie directly under the center of the leg, and (c) the calcaneus should be perpendicular to the ground. (From Root et al.,[4] with permission.)

lowing these various descriptions, most researchers agree that when the subtalar joint is in its neutral position, the sagittal plane of the calcaneus should be parallel to the longitudinal axis of the leg and perpendicular to the ground, and the center of mass of the calcaneus should be almost directly under the longitudinal axis of the lower leg[4] (Fig. 3-46).

The subtalar joint has very little stability that can be ascribed to the joint geometry. The floor of the sinus tarsi does provides osseous stability by restricting anterior motion of the talus on the calcaneus. This will provide some restriction to pronation. When viewed from the sagittal plane, the posterior facet is between 55 and 75 degrees angulated with the superior surface of the calcaneal body.[7] If the calcaneus is highly angulated with the ground in stance, and if the facet shows a small angle with the superior surface, the facet may be

almost parallel to the ground. This would mean that the force of gravity would create a high degree of compression between the talus and the calcaneus with very little force to cause the joint to slide. If the calcaneus has very little inclination in relationship to the ground, and if there is a large angle between the posterior facet and the superior surface of the calcaneus, then the posterior surface of the subtalar joint may be almost perpendicular to the ground when the patient stands. In this situation, gravity would place a much smaller compression force between the talus and the calcaneus, and instead would pull the talus forward, pronating the joint, until the anterior lip of the posterior articular surface on the talus contacts the floor of the sinus tarsi. The sliding of the talus against the calcaneus medially or laterally or rotation by abduction or adduction is only stopped by the ligamentous structures around the subtalar joint.

Motion of the Subtalar Joint During Gait

Because of the very close ties between motion in the subtalar joint and motion of the leg during closed kinetic chain, the normal motion of the subtalar joint must coordinate with the normal motion of the leg during gait. Failure of this coordination results in many pathologies in both the feet and the legs. At heel contact, the subtalar joint starts between 2 and 4 degrees supinated from its neutral position (Fig. 3-47). As the leg is internally rotating during contact phase, the subtalar joint coordinates by also pronating about 6 to 8 degrees, so that by the end of contact phase the subtalar joint is about 4 degrees pronated from its neutral position. This subtalar joint pronation during contact phase is essential for proper knee joint function. At the initiation of heel contact, the knee is fully extended and must flex approximately 10 to 15 degrees during contact. This requires that the tibia internally rotate faster than the femur. The pronation of the subtalar joint during contact phase, which causes the talus to adduct, helps create a smooth knee joint flexion movement during contact phase by helping the tibia to internally rotate faster than the femur. If the talus is prevented from an adduction motion during contact phase, then the knee joint

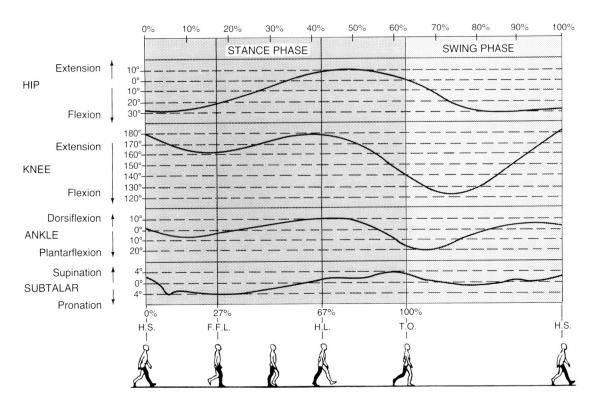

Fig. 3-47. Motion of the subtalar joint in gait. (From Root et al.,[4] with permission.)

must start its flexion motion before heel contact, or it will stay extended through contact phase.

At the end of the contact phase of gait, the leg starts externally rotating. The subtalar joint coordinates by simultaneously starting its supination motion. During the entire midstance phase, the joint is slowly resupinating until it reaches its neutral position just before heel lift. Simultaneously the knee joint is also reextending, which requires that the tibia externally rotate faster than the femur is externally rotating. If the subtalar joint does not supinate during midstance, then the tibia has difficulty externally rotating faster than the tibia, which interferes with the knee joint reaching full extension before heel lift.

During the propulsive phase of gait, the subtalar joint continues its supination motion past neutral position, until it is about 4 degrees supinated at toe-off. During the swing phase of gait, the subtalar joint first pronates so that the joint is a couple of degrees pronated at the time the foot clears the ground, then resupinates so that it is in the supin-

ated position for heel strike again. It should be pointed out that once the heel comes off the ground, the subtalar joint is in open kinetic chain. This means that the calcaneus is free to move against the talus instead of forcing the talus to move against it. Therefore the muscular forces between the foot and leg are able to very quickly externally rotate the tibia faster than the femur and produce knee joint extension. This is often seen when the subtalar joint stays pronated through midstance, and then as soon as heel-off occurs the knee joint suddenly reextends, appearing to "snap" into extension.

Nonmuscular Forces on the Subtalar Joint During Gait

Heel contact occurs by striking the ground on the most posterolateral aspect of the heel. This area of contact is just slightly lateral of being directly under the axis of the subtalar joint. It should be pointed out that anytime the ground pushes up on a part of the foot that is lateral to the axis of the subtalar joint, it produces a pronation moment on the joint, and anytime the ground pushes up on a part of the foot that is medial to the axis of the subtalar joint, it produces a supination moment on the joint.[15] Therefore, the inverted foot, striking the ground slightly lateral to the axis of the subtalar joint, produces a vertical ground force that puts a pronation moment on the joint and starts pronation acceleration. The heel starts everting, bringing more of the medial heel in contact with the surface. When equal amounts of heel surface medial and lateral to the axis of the subtalar joint are in contact with the ground, then the pronation moments due to vertical force are equal to the supination moments. This moment usually occurs when the calcaneus becomes perpendicular to the ground. At this time pronatory acceleration of the subtalar joint reaches zero so that its pronation velocity continues at a constant speed. As the calcaneus everts past perpendicular, more vertical ground force is being exerted medial to the axis than lateral to the axis. Therefore the supination moments begin exceeding the pronation moments. When the supination moment is greater than the pronation moment, the pronation velocity starts decreasing until it reaches zero. At this point in time the joint can start resupinating at the beginning of the midstance phase of gait.

The axis of the subtalar joint is about 15 degrees adducted to the sagittal plane of the foot; however, the sagittal plane of the foot is usually about 10 to 15 degrees abducted to the mean sagittal plane of the body and to the line of progression.[16] Therefore the subtalar joint axis is almost parallel to the line of progression. The ground, placing a posteriorly directed shear to stop forward progression of the foot striking the ground, puts a moment on the subtalar joint that is directly proportional to the sine of the angle between the posteriorly directed force and the axis. If the posterior shear is parallel to the axis, then it can create no moment on the subtalar joint because the sine of 0 degrees is zero. If the axis is slightly adducted to the line of progression, then the posterior shear of the ground places a slight supinatory moment on the subtalar joint. If the axis is abducted to the line of progression, then the posterior shear of the ground will provide an addi-

tional pronation moment on the subtalar joint during contact.

During swing phase, the entire leg and foot is internally rotating. As the heel comes into contact with the ground, a friction is set up between the foot and the ground, with the ground pushing in a lateral direction to the foot to prevent it from internally rotating with the leg. This laterally directed shear during contact phase is normally about 5 percent of body weight,[7] but it places a fairly strong pronation moment on the subtalar joint during contact because it is almost perpendicular to the axis of motion. This pronation moment may be increased by increasing the internal rotational velocity of the leg at heel contact. One example of this would be if the person has a tight semitendinosus muscle that internally rotates the femur and is firing at the moment of heel contact.

It will be noted by an examiner that if the subtalar joint is supinated, the plantar aspect of the calcaneus moves medially, and if the subtalar joint is pronated the plantar aspect of the calcaneus moves laterally. All researchers indicate that the subtalar joint axis is *not* a sliding axis, but is fixed in its relationship with the talus and superior aspect of the calcaneus. Therefore, when the subtalar joint pronates, the plantar aspect of the calcaneus moves laterally and also has an abductory rotation, such that more of the weight-bearing surface of the foot lies lateral to the subtalar joint axis and less lies medial (Fig. 3-48). With more surface area lateral to the axis and with the center of this pressure further from the axis of the subtalar joint, the pronation moment produced by vertical ground force increases, while, with less surface area medial to the axis and with the center of this pressure closer to the axis, the supination moment from vertical ground force decreases. Therefore, with each degree of subtalar joint pronation, the pronation moment on the subtalar joint increases and the supination moment decreases. This means that if there is no supination force applied, the pronation acceleration will increase as the joint pronates, and an increasing pronation acceleration means that pronation velocity increases in an exponential fashion. Therefore for each degree that the subtalar joint pronates, an increasing supination muscle force is needed to provide the moments necessary to reverse the pronation motion during contact phase.

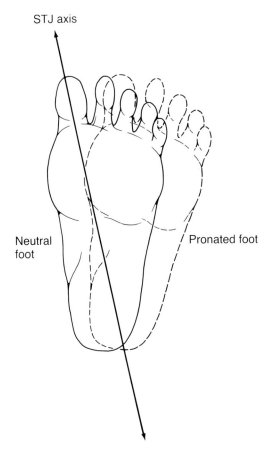

STJ axis

Neutral foot

Pronated foot

Fig. 3-48. The axis of the subtalar joint lies just lateral to the first metatarsal head. When the subtalar joint pronates, the foot abducts and moves laterally. This means that the subtalar joint axis is lying more medial and has a greater angulation with the sagittal plane of the foot when the foot is pronated.

Muscular Forces on the Subtalar Joint During Gait

As the foot contacts the ground, there are a number of pronation moments applied to the subtalar joint that cause the joint to pronate during contact phase, and with each degree of pronation the pronation moment produced by the ground on the subtalar joint increases, which would cause the joint to exponentially increase its pronation velocity. This would be an unacceptable situation because it would mean that the joint would reach the end of its range of pronation movement traveling at a very high velocity. At this point, to keep the joint

from dislocating, the joint ligaments would have to exert a very strong restraining force. While this may be an appropriate occasional function of ligaments, such repetitive stress and strain on the ligaments with each step will produce injury and/or plastic deformity of the ligaments. Therefore, the supination musculature of the subtalar joint must counterbalance this increasing pronation torque on the subtalar joint during contact phase.

The posterior tibial muscle is the strongest of the supination muscles of the subtalar joint. It has the longest lever arm and is more perpendicular to the joint axis than any of the other supination muscles (Fig. 3-49). It is the first of the stance phase muscles to start contracting, beginning almost immediately at heel contact (Fig. 3-43). It provides a strong eccentric contraction to keep the subtalar joint pronating at a fairly constant speed during the first half of contact phase. If the posterior tibial is weakened then it will fail to keep the pronation motion from accelerating, and by the time the other muscles begin firing to help provide the strong supination moments needed to decelerate the pronation, the joint is already pronating at such a high velocity that it will continue pronating until it reaches the end of its range of motion, where the joint ligaments will be abnormally stressed in bringing the pronation velocity back to zero.

If the subtalar joint pronates to the end of its range of motion during contact phase, then it cannot resupinate during the midstance phase of gait. The reason for this is that the plantar aspect of the foot has moved so far lateral to the subtalar joint axis that all of the metatarsal heads lie lateral to the axis, including the first, which means that the ground pushing up against any of the metatarsal heads places a pronation moment on the subtalar joint. Because the function of midstance is to transfer weight onto the forefoot so that the heel can lift from the ground, in the patient who is maximally pronated at the subtalar joint, as weight moves onto the forefoot an ever-increasing pronation moment is placed on the subtalar joint. In this situation, the body cannot generate enough force in the deep posterior leg muscles to start the subtalar joint supinating.

The soleus begins firing about one-third of the way through the contact phase. It is not as strong a subtalar joint supinator as the posterior tibial be-

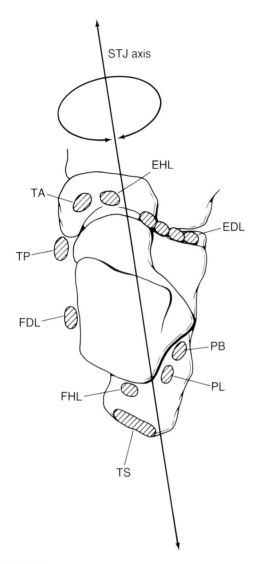

STJ axis

EHL

TA

EDL

TP

FDL

PB

PL

FHL

TS

Fig. 3-49. The tendons of the muscles of the lower leg in relationship to the subtalar joint axis when the joint is in its neutral position. *TA,* tibialis anterior; *EHL,* extensor hallucis longus; *EDL,* extensor digitorum longus; *PB,* peroneus brevis; *PL,* peroneus longus; *TS,* Achilles tendon; *FHL,* flexor hallucis longus; *FDL,* flexor digitorum longus; *TP,* tibialis posterior. (Adapted from Sarrafian.[7])

cause it has a short lever arm, and it is more parallel to the subtalar joint axis. It is joined at about 60 percent of the contact phase by the flexor digitorum longus and the gastrocnemius. The flexor digitorum longus is a weaker supinator of the subtalar joint than the posterior tibial, but stronger

than the soleus. The gastrocnemius is a much weaker supinator than the soleus because it inserts more to the lateral side of the posterior calcaneus than the soleus. Therefore its supination lever arm is much shorter than the soleus, and in some people it has no lever arm on the subtalar joint axis. The final supination muscle to begin firing during contact phase is the flexor hallucis longus, just before midstance phase begins. The major function of these posterior muscles beginning their contraction during contact phase is to provide the deceleration of the subtalar joint pronation and to stop it before it reaches the end of its range of motion. If these muscles do not provide enough force to decelerate the pronation, then the ligaments must provide the tension force to stop the pronation movement. When the ligaments are called upon to provide this amount of supinatory force with every step, it many times leads to ligament deformation and chronic symptoms.

The anterior tibial muscle continues its swing phase contraction into the first two-thirds of contact phase to slow the rate of ankle joint plantarflexion, and it also provides assistance to the posterior tibial during early heel contact in keeping pronation velocity under control. It is important that this muscle not exert too strong a force, because too strong a pull would not allow the ankle joint to plantarflex fast enough during contact phase. It is also noted that as the subtalar joint pronates, the insertion of the anterior tibial moves laterally, closer to the subtalar joint axis. Therefore, during contact, the anterior tibial loses its supinatory lever arm such that, by the end of contact, the insertion of this muscle may lie directly over or even slightly lateral to the subtalar joint axis.

Midstance phase begins as the subtalar joint starts its resupination movement. The resupination velocity during midstance is much slower than the pronation velocity during the contact phase. All of the supination muscles of the posterior leg fire all of the way through the midstance phase to provide supination movement. The soleus and gastrocnemius are the least important supinators during midstance, and any supination function would be only in the early midstance phase of gait before the center of body mass passes anterior to the ankle joint. Once the center of body mass passes anterior to the ankle joint, the triceps surae are responsible for allowing body weight to be borne by the metatarsal heads. It is noted (Fig. 3-45) that even when the subtalar joint is in its neutral position, all of the lesser metatarsal heads are lateral to the axis of the subtalar joint. Therefore, when the ground pushes up against the lesser metatarsal heads, it is putting a pronation moment on the subtalar joint. Thus the triceps surae provides a weak direct supination moment and a strong indirect pronation moment during midstance.

In open kinetic chain, the peroneus longus provides a direct pronation force on the subtalar joint; however, in closed kinetic chain midstance it may assist in resupinating. It begins its contraction about 30 percent of the way through the midstance phase. Because of its insertion to the plantar base of the first metatarsal, it pulls the first metatarsal head down against the ground. In turn, the ground resists this plantar-flexion force and pushes upward, which should be on the medial side of the subtalar joint axis, thus providing additional supination moment and counteracting the indirect pronation moment produced by the triceps surae.

All of the above stance-phase supination muscles continue contracting until after heel lift. The soleus muscle relaxes first, about 15 percent of the way through propulsion. It is followed by relaxation of the posterior tibial at about 25 percent of the propulsive phase, and then the gastrocnemius and flexor digitorum longus at about 50 percent through propulsion. At this point in time, the peroneus brevis is transferring body weight toward the medial side of the forefoot, thus decreasing the ground force upward against the lateral metatarsal heads, which have the longest pronation lever arms on the subtalar joint, and increasing the force against the first metatarsal head, which should have a supinatory lever arm. The flexor hallucis longus and peroneus longus continue firing, providing the moments needed to keep the joint supinating until the peroneus longus quits firing about 70 percent through propulsion, and the flexor hallucis longus relaxes at about 80 percent of propulsion.

The peroneus tertius and extensor digitorum longus begin their contractions about 50 percent through propulsion. These muscles produce a direct pronation moment on the subtalar joint; however, the contractions of the medial column propulsive muscles and the dorsiflexion of the metatarsophalangeal joints keep the joint supinating. The extensor hallucis longus begins contracting about 75 percent through propulsion, which produces a slight direct supination force if the subtalar joint is already supinated, and also an additional indirect supination force because it keeps the first metatarsophalangeal joint dorsiflexed, which helps to produce a plantar-flexion force on the first metatarsal. Finally, the anterior tibial begins contracting just after the flexor hallucis longus finishes its contraction, which provides a strong supination force on the subtalar joint.

The first part of swing phase shows the subtalar joint pronating in order to clear the ground. It is evident that the lateral anterior muscles have the strongest contraction and provide the greatest moment on the subtalar joint during this initial part of swing phase, because they are the only force that could produce subtalar joint pronation at this time. Just before the foot clears the ground, the two lateral anterior muscles relax, and the two medial muscles continue contracting until the toes fully clear the ground. These two muscles, contracting without any antagonistic activity, slow the subtalar joint pronation to zero. Once the foot clears the ground, all of the muscles relax for about the next 25 percent of the swing phase; then, during the last 25 percent of the swing phase, the anterior tibial and the two long extensor muscles, without the peroneus tertius, begin contracting again. It is evident that these three muscles produce a net supination moment on the subtalar joint, because there is a supination movement by the joint to prepare for the next heel contact.

THE MIDTARSAL JOINT

The talonavicular joint is a ball-in-socket joint, with the medial-to-lateral dimension greater than the superior-to-inferior dimension. The calcaneocuboid joint is a saddle-shaped joint, sometimes described as a partial hourglass shape,[17] having a convex surface medial to lateral, with the medial side much more posterior than the lateral, and having a concave surface from dorsal to plantar, with the dorsal aspect projecting more anterior than the plantar aspect. The posteriorly projecting medial side of the calcaneocuboid joint lies under the anterior facet of the subtalar joint. The cuboid and navicular are connected by very strong ligaments such that the navicular and cuboid maintain a constant distance, and one cannot move in space without the other. These two separate articulations, the talonavicular joint and the calcaneocuboid joint, are considered together as the *midtarsal joint,* sometimes known as the transverse tarsal joint[18] or Chopart's joint. The function is very complex and very poorly understood because of the very limited amount of research that has been done.

Movements of the Midtarsal Joint

The first description of the movements of the midtarsal joint was by Manter.[18] His observations were later confirmed by Hicks.[19] The two joints are described as one functional joint with two independent axes of motion, both being oriented from posterior-inferior-lateral or anterior-superior-medial. This means that movement around either axis may be described as pronation or supination.

One of the midtarsal joint axes is known as the longitudinal axis because it is almost parallel with the longitudinal axis of the foot, averaging only 9 degrees of deviation from the sagittal plane and 15 degrees of deviation from the transverse plane[18] (Fig. 3-50). In a person who has an average longitudinal axis, if the joint pronates 10 degrees there would be 9.5 degrees of eversion observed on the frontal plane, 2.6 degrees of abduction observed on the transverse plane, and 1.5 degrees of dorsiflexion observed on the sagittal plane.

The other midtarsal joint axis is known as the oblique axis because of its high angulation with both the transverse and sagittal planes. The average angulation with the transverse plane is about 52 degrees and the average deviation from the sagittal plane is about 56 degrees.[4] This means that in a person who has an average oblique midtarsal joint axis, if the joint pronates 10 degrees, there would be 3.4 degrees of eversion observed on the frontal plane, 7.9 degrees of abduction observed on the transverse plane, and 5.1 degrees of dorsiflexion observed on the sagittal plane. The clinician will observe that frontal plane motion is the smallest component of motion around the oblique axis. He or she will also observe in the clinic that there is a wide variation between patients in the ratio of the amount of sagittal plane motion to the amount of transverse plane motion. Some individuals will show almost pure transverse plane motion and almost no sagittal plane motion, which would mean that the oblique axis is almost perpendicular to the ground, whereas other individuals will show almost pure sagittal plane motion and almost no transverse plane motion, which would mean that the oblique axis is almost parallel to the ankle joint axis. These variant joint axes will produce different stresses and strains on the foot and the leg; however, a discussion of such is not within the scope of this chapter.

The motion in the midtarsal joint may be described as pronation or supination. If the foot is in open kinetic chain, the pronation may be described as the navicular and cuboid dorsiflexing, abducting and everting against the rearfoot, and supination may be described as the forefoot plantar flexing, adducting and inverting against the rearfoot. Closed kinetic chain function, however, is very similar to that seen with the subtalar joint; the friction of the foot against the ground prevents the distal segments from moving against the proximal segments, and therefore the greater tarsus must move against the lesser tarsus. This means that when the midtarsal joint pronates in closed kinetic chain, the talus and calcaneus, moving together, adduct, plantar flex, and invert. Because of the shape of the ankle joint, the plantar flexing of the talus can occur independent of the tibia; however, the frontal and transverse plane motions cannot. Thus the tibia also inverts and internally rotates when the midtarsal joint pronates in closed kinetic chain. The motions of the tibia during closed kinetic chain motion of the midtarsal joint are usually considered only when talking about motion around the oblique axis. As is further explained below, motion around the longitudinal axis of the midtarsal joint is mainly a frontal plane motion to ensure that all of the metatarsal heads make contact with the ground. When supination around the longitudinal axis occurs, the lesser tarsus usually inverts against the greater tarsus.

The term *locking of the midtarsal joint* is often

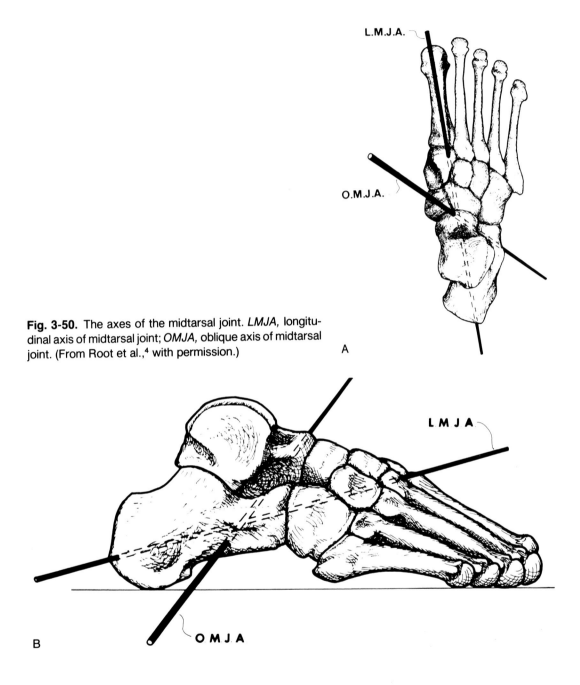

Fig. 3-50. The axes of the midtarsal joint. *LMJA*, longitudinal axis of midtarsal joint; *OMJA*, oblique axis of midtarsal joint. (From Root et al.,[4] with permission.)

used in describing whether the midtarsal joint is functioning correctly or incorrectly. This term arises from the fact that when the heel lifts off the ground, the foot now acts as a second-class lever. The ground is pushing up against the metatarsal heads, which act as the fulcrum. The body weight is attempting to bend the foot, pushing the center of the foot toward the ground while the Achilles tendon is lifting the heel. In other words, the body weight, pushing down between the lifting force and the fulcrum, is attempting to dorsiflex the forefoot against the rearfoot. The less strain that occurs between the lifting force and the fulcrum, the more efficient the foot will be, acting as a lever. Therefore, to have a foot that is rigid during propulsion, the forefoot should already be dorsiflexed (i.e., pronated) to the end of its range of motion, relying on the restraining mechanisms that create that pronatory end of the range of motion. Therefore when the midtarsal joint has reached the pronation end of its range of motion around both axes of motion, then the joint is said to be "locked".[4,20] This locking of the midtarsal is essential for efficient heel lift. Various theories have been advanced about the actual mechanism that stops the midtarsal joint pronation motion, some based on the shape of the calcaneocuboid articular facet,[17] some based on the combination shapes of the talonavicular and calcaneocuboid joints,[21] some based on the keystone architecture of the arch,[22] and some based on the ligamentous structures of the two joints.[23] There has never been any final proof for any of these restraining mechanisms.

The midtarsal joint may move independently of the subtalar joint; however, the subtalar joint may not move independently of the midtarsal joint. If the subtalar joint moves with the calcaneocuboid joint staying motionless, then motion still must occur in the talonavicular joint. If the subtalar joint moves without any motion between the talus and the navicular, then motion must occur between the calcaneus and the cuboid.

Another relationship that exists between the subtalar joint and the midtarsal joint is that the range of motion in the midtarsal joint is dependent on the position of the subtalar joint. When the subtalar joint is supinated and the midtarsal joint reaches the end of its range of motion in the pronatory direction (i.e., when it is in its locked position), the forefoot is less abducted, dorsiflexed, and everted than when it is locked with the subtalar joint in its neutral position. Likewise, the forefoot is more abducted, dorsiflexed, and everted to the rearfoot when the midtarsal joint is locked with the subtalar joint pronated than when the midtarsal joint is locked with the subtalar joint in its neutral position. Phillips and Phillips measured the eversion component of this phenomenon and discovered that the average forefoot was 2 degrees more everted to the rearfoot when the subtalar joint was neutral than when it was fully supinated, and it was 11 degrees more everted to the rearfoot when the subtalar joint was fully pronated than when it was

neutral.[20] It appeared that this increase in the range of motion of the midtarsal joint as the subtalar joint is pronated is an exponential increase.

Motions of the Midtarsal Joint During Gait

As the foot strikes the ground, before the forefoot contacts the ground, the midtarsal joint is pronated around the oblique axis and is supinated around its longituindal axis. While the subtalar joint is pronating during contact, the fifth metatarsal contacts the ground first, followed by the fourth, the third, the second, and finally the first. The ground contacting the fifth metatarsal head places a pronation moment on both the oblique and longitudinal axes, which causes pronation around both axes during contact. The reader will note that it was just stated that the oblique axis was already fully pronated at heel contact and may wonder how it can pronate more during the forefoot loading stage. The reason is that the range of motion of the midtarsal joint increases as the subtalar joint undergoes its pronation movement during contact phase.

Pronation around the oblique axis is seen by the rearfoot moving medially, internally rotating and plantar flexing during contact phase. Because the oblique midtarsal joint axis has a greater angulation with the transverse plane than the subtalar joint axis, the internal rotation of the leg is greater around the oblique midtarsal joint axis than around the subtalar joint axis. The tibia has to internally rotate at least 10 degrees after the heel contacts the ground. The subtalar joint pronation allows approximately 4 degrees of internal rotation; therefore it is up to the pronation around the oblique axis of the midtarsal joint to allow the remaining 6 degrees of internal tibial rotation during contact phase. The fact that tibial rotation may be effected during closed kinetic chain movement by either the subtalar joint or oblique midtarsal joint means that leg symptoms caused by abnormal leg rotations may sometimes be alleviated by controlling motion only around the oblique midtarsal joint axis.

At the end of the contact phase, the subtalar joint is pronated approximately 4 degrees and the oblique axis of the midtarsal joint is fully pronated, which shows the forefoot more abducted and dorsiflexed in relationship to the rearfoot than it would be if the midtarsal joint was fully pronated with the subtalar joint neutral. The metatarsal heads are now all in contact with the ground but the longitudinal axis is not fully pronated, because if it was the forefoot would be everted to the ground.

The midstance phase begins with the subtalar joint starting to resupinate. This resupination of the subtalar joint forces the oblique axis of the midtarsal joint to also start resupinating, although it still stays fully pronated around this axis. This may seem contradictory unless one remembers that when the midtarsal joint is kept fully pronated, the forefoot becomes more inverted, plantarflexed, and adducted to the rearfoot as the subtalar joint is moved from a more pronated position to a less pronated position. Therefore the leg is externally rotating as a result of closed kinetic chain subtalar joint resupination, and also closed kinetic chain midtarsal joint resupination around the oblique axis. This resupination around the oblique axis continues at a fairly constant velocity until the end of the midstance phase.

During the midstance phase, the longitudinal axis of the midtarsal joint is pronating. This is because the supination of the subtalar and oblique midtarsal joints would tend to lift the medial metatarsal heads off the ground. However, by pronating around the longitudinal midtarsal joint axis, the forefoot is able to maintain full contact with the ground.

At the end of the midstance phase of gait, just prior to heel lift, the subtalar joint has reached its neutral position. The midtarsal joint has stayed at the end of its pronation range of motion around its oblique axis (even though it has shown supination movement of the forefoot against the rearfoot), and the longituinal axis has pronated until it has also reached the end of its range of motion. The midtarsal joint therefore has reached its *locked position,* which means that a rigid beam effect can be set up between the forefoot and rearfoot for heel lift.

After heel lift, during propulsion, the longitudinal axis of the midtarsal joint stays fully pronated. The oblique axis of the midtarsal joint does supinate more than it normally would if the subtalar joint supinated and the midtarsal joint stayed locked. This supination of the oblique axis helps the leg to

continue its external rotation.[17] It also plantarflexes the forefoot, which assists in creating normal dorsiflexion of the metatarsophalangeal joints during propulsion.

Swing phase movements of the midtarsal joint are inconsequential except for preparing to make contact with the ground. This means that the longitudinal axis must fully supinate, which it does during the last part of the swing phase. The action of all of the anterior muscles of the leg ensure that the oblique axis stays as pronated as the subtalar joint will permit during swing.

Nonmuscular Forces on the Midtarsal Joint During Gait

During contact phase, before the forefoot makes contact with the ground, the only nonmuscular force acting on the midtarsal joint is gravity pulling the forefoot down to the ground. This means that gravity would place a supination moment on the oblique axis of the midtarsal joint, and a slight supination moment on the longitudinal axis. Because of the low weight of the forefoot, these moments are very insignificant compared to moments produced by muscle activity prior to ground contact.

The first part of the forefoot to make contact with the ground is the fifth metatarsal head, followed by contact of the fourth, then the third, the second, and finally the first. The vertical force from the ground against any metatarsal head will always place a pronation moment on the oblique axis of the midtarsal joint. On the other hand, a vertical force against the fourth or fifth metatarsal heads will produce a pronation moment on the longitudinal axis, a vertical force against the third metatarsal will produce a very slight supination moment,[24] and a vertical force against the second or first metatarsal will produce a strong supination moment. Therefore as the forefoot starts to make contact, first a pronation moment is placed on the longitudinal axis, but as the medial side of the forefoot makes contact, a supination moment is placed on the longitudinal axis until the pronation moments equal the supination moments and the entire forefoot makes contact with the ground. If at any time the force increases under the lateral metatarsals, then the forefoot will attempt to pronate around the longitudinal axis. If the force increases under the medial metatarsal heads, then the forefoot will attempt to supinate around the longitudinal axis.

As the forefoot makes contact with the ground there is still a significant amount of external torque shear exerted by the ground.[25] This laterally directed shear against the forefoot places a strong abduction force against the midtarsal joint, which is a strong pronation moment on the joint. The closer to vertical the oblique midtarsal joint axis lies, the stronger will be the pronation moment placed by this shear force during contact phase. The closer the axis lies to the transverse plane, the smaller will be the pronation moment by the lateral shear from the ground on the midtarsal joint during contact phase.

The change in position of the forefoot to the rearfoot during contact phase also affects the moment on the subtalar joint placed by the ground. During contact phase, the pronation of the subtalar joint allows the forefoot to abduct, dorsiflex, and evert more than it can when the subtalar joint is neutral. When the oblique axis of the midtarsal joint undergoes this motion, the forefoot becomes more abducted to the rearfoot; therefore more of the forefoot is lateral and less is medial to the subtalar joint axis than when the subtalar joint is neutral (Fig. 3-48). Because vertical force from the ground lateral to the subtalar joint axis places a pronation moment on the subtalar joint and vertical force medial to the axis places a supination moment on the joint, this means that with the increased abduction of the forefoot against the rearfoot, the pronation moment on the subtalar joint from the vertical ground force increases, and the supination moment decreases. If the forefoot abducts so far that the subtalar joint axis moves medial to the center of the first metatarsal head, then the entire vertical force from the ground against the forefoot will place a pronation moment on the subtalar joint. This pronation moment is usually so much greater than the supination moments on the subtalar joint that the subtalar joint pronates to the end of its range of motion.

During the midstance phase, the vertical ground force keeps the midtarsal joint at the end of its range of motion around its oblique axis, although the subtalar joint supination is forcing the forefoot into a more supinated position. The vertical ground force supinates the longitudinal axis if the forefoot attempts to evert to the ground and it pronates the longitudinal axis if the forefoot attempts to invert to the ground.

After heel lift, gravity attempts to pull the heel down to the ground, which would plantar flex the forefoot against the rearfoot. This would be considered a supination moment on the oblique axis of the midtarsal joint; however, the tension of the Achilles tendon, placing a vertical ground force against the metatarsal heads, places a strong pronation moment on the oblique axis. The more the heel rises from the ground the closer to the metatarsophalangeal joints the oblique axis moves, which decreases the lever arm of the vertical ground force, thus decreasing the pronation moment from this force.

The longitudinal axis has a fairly strong pronation moment placed upon it during propulsion. This is because the subtalar joint continues to invert, which increases the force under the lateral metatarsal heads; thus the ground force increasing under the fourth and fifth metatarsal heads places a strong pronation moment on the longitudinal axis.

Muscle Function Around the Midtarsal Joint During Gait

Most of the muscle function around the midtarsal joint has been mentioned or alluded to previously. During the swing phase of gait, the anterior muscles of the lower leg are all active. All of these muscles place a pronation moment on the oblique axis of the midtarsal joint. Although no information is available about the actual movement around the longitudinal axis during early swing, it is assumed that it stays pronated around its longitudinal axis because the foot is pronated around the axis during propulsion, and the lateral two anterior muscles provide a pronation moment around the longitudinal axis that is about equal to the supination moment provided by the two medial anterior muscles, which should produce no net movement around the axis during early swing. During the last part of the swing phase, the peroneus tertius does not contract, which means that there is a net supination moment around the longitudinal axis, and thus the forefoot inverts to the rearfoot to prepare for contact with the ground.

During contact phase, the anterior muscles of the leg relax, starting with the most lateral and moving medially. The anterior tibial muscle places a very strong supination force on the longitudinal axis of the midtarsal joint; therefore, even though the ground is placing a strong pronation force against the longitudinal axis of the midtarsal joint, the anterior tibial muscle, contracting eccentrically, makes sure that the joint pronates very slowly around this axis, allowing the metatarsal heads to contact the ground smoothly, from lateral to medial.

The posterior tibial muscle also provides a strong eccentric supination force on the oblique axis of the midtarsal joint during contact phase. Without this muscle, the subtalar joint moves very quickly to the end of its range of motion and the forefoot completely pronates around the midtarsal joint until the navicular makes contact with the ground. During the midstance phase, the posterior tibial provides an important concentric contraction to assist in the resupination around the oblique midtarsal joint axis. The long flexor muscles also assist the posterior tibial in these contact and midstance phase functions.

Both of the peroneal muscles are strong pronators of the oblique axis of the midtarsal joint; however, the peroneus brevis is a pronator around the longitudinal axis while the peroneus longus, plantar flexing the first metatarsal against the ground during closed kinetic chain, provides a supination moment around the longitudinal axis. Therefore the contraction of the peroneus longus must also be accompanied by an antagonistic contraction of the peroneus brevis during late midstance and early propulsion, to keep the midtarsal joint locked while increased pressure is developing under the first metatarsal head. Without this contraction, the ligaments of the midtarsal joint alone would not be able to withstand the bending moments across the joint as the heel comes off the ground. The peroneus brevis therefore plays an important part in lifting the lateral side of the foot during propulsion. If the midtarsal joint is not locked at heel lift, then the peroneus brevis must contract with greater force to lift the lateral column of the foot. This increased contraction will then produce a subtalar joint pronation during propulsion, which will have

the adverse effect of decreasing the rigid lever effect of the foot, but will at least push body weight over to the medial side of the foot. The destabilizing effect this has on the first metatarsal is discussed below.

The plantar intrinsic muscles of the foot — the abductor hallucis, the flexor digitorum brevis, the abductor digiti quinti, and the quadratus plantae — all cross the midtarsal joint plantar to the joint axes. All of these muscles are very close to being parallel with the longitudinal axis; therefore they provide almost no moment on this axis. Because they all provide a force to plantar flex the forefoot against the rearfoot, they are said to provide a supination moment on the oblique axis of the midtarsal joint. The medial muscles have a longer lever arm to the oblique axis than the lateral muscles; therefore it is logical that the medial intrinsics would be able to provide a stronger moment on the oblique axis than the lateral intrinsics. Although no electromyographic studies have confirmed it, it is argued that the quadratus plantae must be the first of these intrinsics to fire, during very early midstance, to stabilize the tendon of the flexor digitorum longus.[4] (Fig. 3-51). This is followed by the abductor digiti quinti and the abductor hallucis during the middle of midstance. Finally, the flexor digitorum brevis starts firing at the start of propulsion. All of the plantar intrinsics continue to concentrically contract through propulsion, assisting in the supination movement around the oblique axis.

If the subtalar joint does not supinate before and after heel lift, then the midtarsal joint cannot plantarflex around the oblique axis during propulsion. This means that the plantar intrinsic muscles are forced into a state where they alone provide the supinatory moments around the oblique axis during late midstance and propulsion, and their contraction would be considered to be isometric or even eccentric. When this occurs the patient often complains of arch pain and fatigue.

The gastrocnemius and soleus muscles are responsible for placing pressure on the metatarsal heads. If there were no tension in the Achilles tendon, the center of body mass would have to stay behind or directly over the axis of the ankle joint to prevent the person from falling forward, and as a result the only weight that would be on the metatarsal heads would be that of the weight of the foot

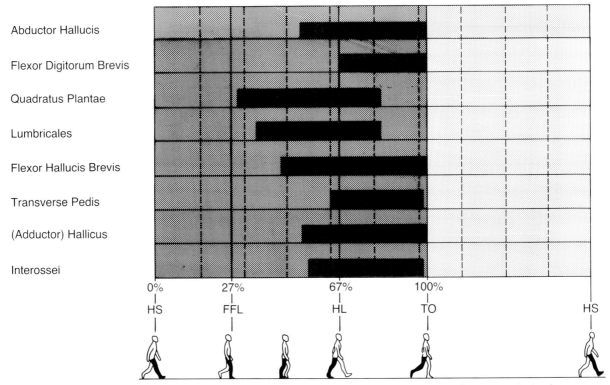

Fig. 3-51. Phasic activity of the intrinsic muscles of the foot. (From Root et al,[4] with permission.)

distal to the midtarsal joint. Therefore tension on the Achilles tendon, with the body weight anterior to the ankle joint axis, places vertical ground force against the metatarsal heads that is a pronation moment on the oblique axis of the midtarsal joint. There is a critical point, although no one has yet determined what that point is, when the dorsiflexion moment on the midtarsal joint, caused by vertical ground force on the metatarsal heads, is greater than the "locking mechanism" (probably ligamentous) can withstand. When this occurs, the midtarsal joint starts pronating further than the locking mechanism should allow, which causes the subtalar joint to also pronate to allow this midtarsal joint pronation. This situation occurs when the Achilles tendon is short, such that the critical point for abnormal midtarsal joint pronation is reached before the body mass center is far enough forward to facilitate metatarsophalangeal joint dorsiflexion. Other factors that can mimic this include: too much tension in the hamstring muscles, an osseous block preventing ankle joint dorsiflexion, generalized ligamentous laxity, and an oblique midtarsal joint

axis that is too far deviated from the sagittal plane, such that it is close to being parallel with the ankle joint axis.

THE FIRST RAY

The first cuneiform and first metatarsal are commonly called the *first ray*,[19] and are discussed as one unit when discussing function. Motion in the first ray comprises motion in the first cuneonavicular joint, the first-second intercuneiform joint, the second metatarsal–first cuneiform joint, the first metatarsocuneiform joint, and the first-second intermetatarsal joint. The exact way each of these joints contributes to the total motion of the first ray has not been described yet.

Each of the first ray joints is fairly flat, and it would appear that by themselves each joint would be a sliding movement, yet the motion of the first ray has been described to occur around an axis of motion that is directed from posterior-medial and slightly superior to anterior-lateral and slightly inferior.[19] The angulation of this axis with the sagittal plane has been estimated to be 45 degrees which means that it is also about 45 degrees angulated with the frontal plane. The angulation with the transverse plane has been estimated to be slightly downward as the axis proceeds from proximal to distal (Fig. 3-52). If this is true, then it means that for every degree of sagittal plane motion, 1 degree of frontal plane motion will be observed. It also means that there is almost no angular motion observed on the transverse plane when the first ray moves.

No words have been coined to describe the motion of a joint with an axis that is oriented the way the first ray axis is oriented. The first ray will be observed to either dorsiflex, invert, and move slightly toward the second metatarsal (i.e., abduct away from midline of the body), or to plantar flex, evert, and slightly move away from the second metatarsal (i.e., adduct toward the midline of the body). Therefore, for the purpose of this chapter,

the first ray either "dorsi-inverts" or it "plantar-everts."

The more that the axis of the first ray in angulated with the transverse plane, the more transverse plane motion will be observed when the first ray moves. If the first ray axis proceeds from proximal-medial-inferior to distal-lateral-superior, then when the first ray dorsi-inverts, it will move away from the second metatarsal instead of toward it. It should be noted that when the tarsal bones evert to the ground, the axis of the first ray changes from being slightly tilted down as it proceeds from proximal to distal to being tilted upward. This means that if there is abnormal dorsiflexion of the first metatarsal during stance, it will move away from the second metatarsal instead of moving a little bit toward it.

Observation of clinical motion of the first ray when the second metatarsal and the other tarsal bones are immobilized shows that there is an average of 10 to 12 mm of sagittal plane displacement of the head of the first metatarsal when the first ray moves through its entire range of motion.[26] This displacement has never been translated into angu-

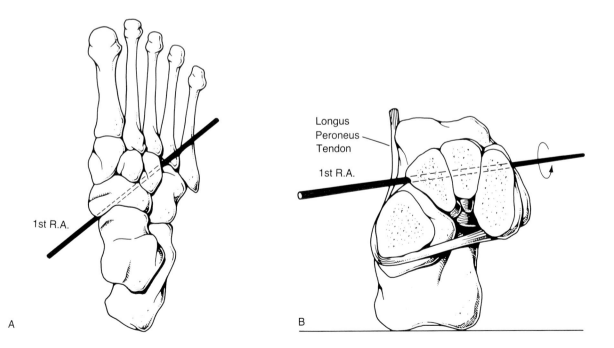

Fig. 3-52. The axis of motion of the first ray. (From Root et al,[4] with permission.)

lar motion around its axis, although angular motion has been described to be over 20 degrees by some authors.[19] It is generally thought that the neutral position of the first ray is halfway between its maximally dorsiflexed and maximally plantar-flexed positions.[14] This definition has been derived from the concept that when the subtalar joint reaches its neutral position with the midtarsal joint locked just before heel lift, the first metatarsal should be on the same plane as the second metatarsal, and should be neither maximally dorsiflexed nor maximally plantar flexed. This would allow the hallux to sit in its neutral position, neither dorsiflexed nor plantar flexed. Motion of the hallux against the first metatarsal as a function of first ray position is discussed later.

Motions of the First Ray During Gait

During gait, the first metatarsal head is the final aspect of the forefoot to contact the ground. At the time it makes ground contact, the lesser tarsus is mildly everted to the ground because of the pronation of the subtalar joint and oblique axis of the midtarsal joint during contact phase. Therefore the first metatarsal is at first a little dorsiflexed and abducted away from the second metatarsal. During the midstance phase of gait, the subtalar joint and oblique midtarsal joint are resupinating, causing the lesser metatarsal heads to invert a little to the ground, and the first metatarsal begins its plantar-flexing–everting motion, although the degree to which it plantarflexes during midstance is very small. It is not until propulsion that the first metatarsal starts plantar flexing significantly. This it must do in order to facilitate normal dorsiflexion motion of the hallux for propulsion. Although the dorsiflexion motion of the first metatarsophalangeal joint can be reproduced in open kinetic chain by concomitant plantar-eversion of the first ray, in the closed kinetic chain the hallux and sesamoids remain fixed in their relationship with the ground while the first metatarsal rolls in a posterior direction[27] (Fig. 3-53). By the time the first metatarsophalangeal joint is fully dorsiflexed just before heel lift, the first ray is in its maximally plantar-flexed position. After heel lift it is suddenly dorsiflexed by the anterior tibial muscle, where it stays through swing phase.

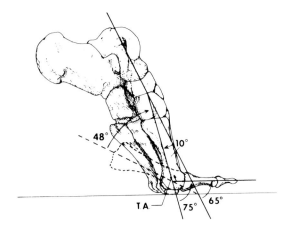

Fig. 3-53. During closed kinetic chain dorsiflexion of the first metatarsophalangeal joint, the hallux and sesamoids stay fixed while the first metatarsal rolls upward and posteriorly, creating about a 10 degree plantar-flexion angle with the talus and navicular. (From Root et al,[4] with permission.)

Nonmuscular Forces on the First Ray During Gait

The first metatarsal head acts as one of the three points of balance for the entire foot. In addition it has a greater diameter than any of the other metatarsal bones, and therefore is able to bear twice the weight of any of the other metatarsals.[28]

Vertical force from the ground against the first metatarsal should be a significant part of helping the subtalar joint resupinate during midstance phase of gait. This is because this is the only metatarsal head that lies medial to the subtalar joint axis,[15] and therefore the only supination moment that can be placed on the subtalar joint by the ground when weight is transferred onto the forefoot is the vertical force under the first metatarsal head. If the first metatarsal head is dorsiflexed, then the lateral metatarsal heads are forced to accept weight, and since the lateral metatarsal heads are usually lateral to the subtalar joint axis, an increased vertical ground force against them, with a decreased vertical ground force under the first, places a pronation moment on the subtalar joint. The pathologic condition known as "metatarsus primus elevatus" is where the neutral position of the first metatarsal lies above the level of the second metatarsal. This leads to pathologic pronation

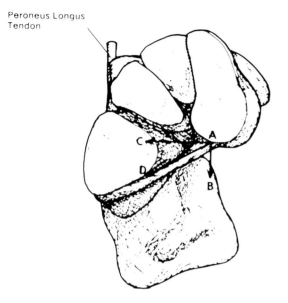

Peroneus Longus
Tendon

Fig. 3-54. The pull of the peroneus longus is the only effective stabilizing force on the first ray. *Vector B,* plantar pull of peroneus longus; *Vector C,* lateral pull of peroneus longus; *Vector D,* plantar and lateral pull of peroneus longus.

of the subtalar joint during midstance and propulsion because of the lack of vertical force that can be generated under the first metatarsal head.

If the first metatarsal is plantarflexed in relationship to the second, then the opposite situation occurs. The ground force is increased against the first metatarsal head, which places an inversion moment on the foot until the eversion moment produced by pressure against the lateral metatarsal heads equals the inversion moment. In this situation, however, the first joint that will have an inversion moment placed upon it will be the longitudinal axis of the midtarsal joint. This is because the longitudinal axis of the midtarsal joint is closer to being perpendicular to the vertical ground force, and because the increased vertical ground force under the first metatarsal head has a longer moment arm on the longitudinal midtarsal joint axis than on the subtalar joint axis. However, once the inversion moment on the longitudinal midtarsal joint axis becomes less than the inversion moment on the subtalar joint axis, or the longitudinal axis reaches the supination end of its range of motion, then the subtalar joint will supinate.

Just as the first metatarsal places effective moments on the foot joints proximal to it, so motions of

the proximal foot joints caused by other forces on those joints can create positional changes on the first metatarsal. Whenever the calcaneus is inverted to the ground, the normal forefoot will also be inverted to the ground. Gravity, then, pulls the first metatarsal into a plantarflexed position. If the calcaneus is fixed by another deformity to stay inverted to the ground, then the first metatarsal will probably become fixated in a plantarflexed position. Conversely, when the calcaneus is everted, if the midtarsal joint is to stay locked, then the forefoot will also be everted to the ground. This increases the vertical ground force against the medial column and may be compensated by either the midtarsal joint supinating around its longitudinal axis and/or by the first ray dorsiflexing. If the first ray dorsiflexes, then it also inverts, leaving the sesamoids and hallux valgus rotated at the first metatarsophalangeal joint. This dorsi-inversion compensation by the first metatarsal is the primary etiology of many cases of hallux abductovalgus.

Muscular Forces on the First Ray

In order for the ground to apply pressure upward against the first metatarsal head, the first ray must push down with an equal and opposite force. There are two ways for the first ray to develop this force. One is for the restraining ligaments of the first ray to be put on tension, preventing the first ray from moving dorsally when the ground pushes upward. This is a very poor mechanism except for the briefest of moments of time because chronic tension on the first ray plantar ligaments will result in discomfort for the patient and also subluxation of the joint over time as a result of ligament creep and relaxation. The most efficient way of producing first ray plantarflexion force is muscular contraction of the peroneus longus.

The peroneus longus enters the foot at the lateral side of the peroneal groove of the cuboid, and then courses in a superior-medial-distal direction to insert at the plantar proximal aspect of the base of the first metatarsal and the contingent aspect of the first cuneiform. When the peroneus longus contracts it produces a vector of force in the direction that the tendon is coursing, and this vector can be expressed as the summation of three orthogonal vectors: the posteriorly directly force vector plus

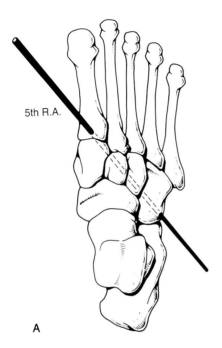
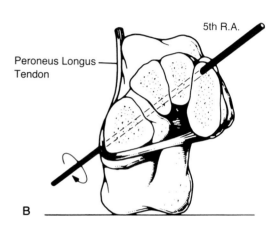

Fig. 3-55. The fifth ray axis has been described as being 35 degrees deviated from the sagittal plane and 20 degrees deviated from the transverse plane. (From Root et al,[4] with permission.)

the plantarly directed force vector plus the laterally directed force vector (Fig. 3-54). The magnitude of the vector that is directed plantarly is equal to the tension within the tendon times the sine of the angle the tendon makes with the ground as it courses from lateral to medial. As one can easily see, if the medial arch is very close to the ground, then there is a very small angle between the ground and the tendon when viewed on the frontal plane; thus only a very small plantarly directed force can be exerted by the first metatarsal, even when the peroneus longus contracts very forcefully. For example, if there is a 10 degree drop between the medial and lateral side of the foot, the plantar pull of the peroneus longus will be 17.6 percent the total tension in the tendon. If there is a 20 degree drop, then the plantar pull of the peroneus longus will be 36.4 percent of the tension in the tendon, which is twice the plantar force that could be achieved in the first case. If the drop is 30 degrees then the plantar pull of the peroneus longus will be 57.7 percent of the tension in the tendon, which is three times the plantar force. As one can see, the

greater the difference in height between the plantar base of the first metatarsal and the lateral side of the cuboid, the greater will be the plantarflexion force of the first metatarsal when the peroneus longus contracts, and as a result the greater will be the supination force exerted on the subtalar joint by the ground pushing upward against the first metatarsal head.

THE FIFTH RAY

Although virtually nothing is known about the motions of the central three metatarsals, it is known that the fifth metatarsal has independent motion at the fifth metatarsal–cuboid joint. This motion occurs around an axis that is directed from inferior-lateral-proximal to superior-medial-distal. In the experiments of Hicks, the axis of motion is described as proceeding from the superomedial border of the foot at the first metatarsal–cuneiform joint to a point that is 1.5 cm above and behind the styloid process of the fifth metatarsal.[19] Root et al. set this axis as being 20 degrees deviated upward from the transverse plane and 35 degrees deviated medially from the sagittal plane[4] (Fig. 3-55). Because of the direction of the axis, the joint motions are pronation (i.e., the fifth metatarsal dorsiflexes, abducts, and everts) or supination (i.e., the fifth metatarsal plantar flexes, adducts, and inverts). If the deviation numbers are correct, then it means that if the joint were to move 10 degrees, 7.7 degrees of sagittal plane motion would be observed, 5.4 degrees of frontal plane motion would be observed, and 3.4 degrees of transverse plane motion would be observed.

The clinical evaluation of the range of motion of the fifth ray has been to stabilize the third and fourth metatarsals in their dorsiflexed position, and to find how many millimeters above and how many millimeters below the level of the fourth the fifth metatarsal is free to move.[4] The total range of motion may be as small as 2 to 3 mm or as great as 10 to 12 mm. It is generally considered that this range of motion should be equally divided so that the fifth metatarsal may move equal distances above and below the level of the fourth metatarsal. This half-way point between the ends of the range of motion is considered to be the neutral position and should be at the level of the plane that the third and fourth metatarsal heads lie in.

Function of the Fifth Ray in Gait

The movements of the fifth metatarsal in gait have not been studied in any detail and can only be conjectured from the very limited understanding that exists of the forces on the fifth metatarsal and the movements of the rest of the foot. As the forefoot contacts the ground, the longitudinal axis of the midtarsal joint is supinated. This means that a plane should exist between metatarsal heads one and five that is inverted to the ground. Because the peroneus tertius does not contract during the last half of swing phase, gravity should plantarflex the

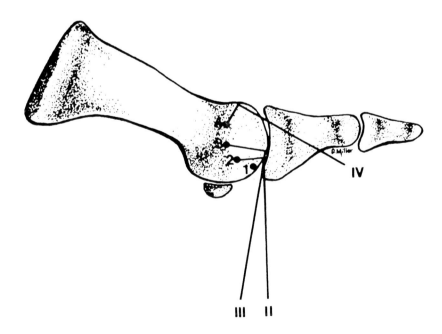

Fig. 3-56. The horizontal axis of the first ray is at the joint surface (point 1) when the proximal phalanx is neutral. As the joint dorsiflexes, the instantaneous center of rotation moves in an arc described by points 2, 3, and 4. (From V. Hetherington, with permission.)

metatarsal prior to the contact until it is at its maximally supinated position. The fifth metatarsal therefore contacts the ground before the fourth metatarsal head. It is logical to assume that the vertical ground force would pronate the fifth metatarsal until the fourth metatarsal contacts the ground. It should stay in this pronated position, a little above its neutral position, until the second metatarsal contacts the ground. At this point in time, gravity should pull the fifth ray back to its neutral position. If the central metatarsal heads evert to the ground, gravity will dictate that the fifth metatarsal be pulled into a somewhat supinated position in relationship to the other metatarsal heads. If the central metatarsal heads invert to the ground, vertical ground force will try to pronate the fifth metatarsal in relationship to the other metatarsal heads.

As the midstance phase progresses, more weight is being transferred to all of the metatarsal heads. In addition, the midtarsal joint is supinating around its oblique axis and pronating arounds its longitudinal axis to develop stability. The vertical force under the fifth metatarsal head should therefore increase significantly during the latter half of the midstance phase; however, it does not increase quite as much as the force under the fourth metatarsal head.[28] There are several reasons for this. The first is that the fifth metatarsal is usually much shorter than the fourth metatarsal; therefore in order for the fifth to bear the same weight as the fourth, the fifth metatarsal must have its base lower than the fourth (which it usually does) and/or it must have a greater inclination angle to the transverse plane. The second reason is that there is very poor muscle stabilization of the fifth metatarsal against the ground. Without some type of plantar pull, or resistance to upward pressure, the metatarsal head cannot register any force between it and the ground. This resistance against upward ground pressure appears to be dependent on the plantar ligaments of the fifth metatarsal–cuboid joint, with some possible assistance from the abductor digiti minimi, the flexor digiti minimi brevis and opponens digiti quinti, and the fourth dorsal interosseous, pulling the fourth and fifth metatarsals toward each other when they contract. All of these small muscles contract during the latter part of midstance and into the first part of propulsion.

During propulsion the fifth ray is the first metatarsal to lose its weight-bearing function, which occurs approximately one-third of the way through the propulsive phase.[4,25] This occurs just about the time the peroneus tertius, which is a major dorsiflexor of the fifth metatarsal, begins to fire. It is assumed that the fifth metatarsal then dorsiflexes during the rest of the propulsive phase and stays dorsiflexed through the first 35 percent of the swing phase when the peroneus tertius relaxes. During the rest of the swing phase it probably plantarflexes again, preparing itself for the next contact phase.

THE FIRST METATARSOPHALANGEAL JOINT

The first metatarsophalangeal joint is a modified ball-in-socket joint that functions as a ginglymus joint with certain reservations. The head of the first metatarsal has a high convexity when viewed from the sagittal plane and a very mild convexity when viewed from the transverse plane. The articular surface proceeds far more proximal on the plantar aspect than on the dorsal aspect. This articular surface is for articulating with the sesamoids. When viewed on the frontal plane, the head of the first metatarsal and the base of the proximal phalanx have a medial-to-lateral dimension that is greater than the superior-to-inferior dimension. Motion at the first metatarsophalangeal joint can occur around any one of the three axes of motion.

The primary motion at the first metatarsophalangeal joint is the sagittal plane motion, denoted as dorsiflexion or plantar flexion. Just as the knee joint is a ginglymus joint with certain reservations, so the sagittal plane motion of the first metatarsophalangeal joint may be described as a ginglymus joint with certain reservations. These are:

1. The axis of the first metatarsophalangeal joint is a sliding axis. New research by Heatherington et al.[27] demonstrates that when the joint is at neutral, the instantaneous axis of rotation is at the joint surface of the center of the first metatarsal head. As the first proximal phalanx moves dorsally, the joint axis moves in a proximal-dorsal direction, describing a concave arc that faces

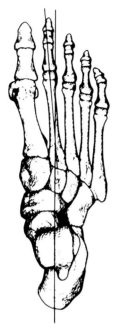

Fig. 3-57. With the first metatarsal dorsi-inverted, the lever arm between the tibial sesamoid and the vertical axis is less than the lever arm between the fibular sesamoid and the vertical axis. (From Hetherington VJ: Motion of the first metatarsal phalangeal joint. J Foot Surg, 28, 1989, with permission.)

a dorsal-distal direction (Fig. 3-56). This arc coincides with the shape of the heaviest cancellous bone in the first metatarsal head when viewed on a sagittal plane x-ray.

2. More than 20 degrees of dorsiflexion of the first proximal phalanx requires that the first metatarsal plantarflex. In this way, the axis can slide in a dorsal-proximal direction. This plantar flexion of the first metatarsal may occur at the joints of the first ray, or at the oblique axis of the midtarsal joint. The exact amount of first metatarsal plantarflexion needed as a function of first proximal phalanx dorsiflexion has not been described; however, as was previously noted, significant plantarflexion occurs around both the oblique midtarsal joint axis and the first ray axis during propulsion. Failure of the first metatarsal to plantarflex will result in the proximal phalanx attempting to continue to dorsiflex around an axis that is too far distal and plantar flexed. This will result in the dorsal edge of the proxi-

mal phalanx compressing and digging into the articular surface of the first metatarsal head, producing damage to the articular cartilage. If this process goes unchecked, then bony proliferation will occur in this region, which will result in a structural limitation of joint dorsiflexion.

3. The joint has two sesamoids that slide in the grooves under the first metatarsal head. The sesamoids are attached to the plantar base of the proximal phalanx by the plantar sesamoidal ligaments. When the proximal phalanx dorsiflexes, the sesamoids are pulled anteriorly. When the muscles that are attached to the sesamoids contract, they pull the sesamoids proximally, which plantarflexes the proximal phalanx.

The second axis that the first metatarsophalangeal joint moves around is a vertical axis that passes directly through the center of the first metatarsal head, exactly between the two sesamoid, thus allowing for a small amount of abduction or adduction. The abduction or adduction needed for normal gait is very small; however, more may be needed for other types of nonlinear weight-bearing activities. The amount of abduction or adduction is limited by the tension in the collateral ligaments, and also by the compression of the sesamoids against the crista under the plantar first metatarsal head, which separates them.

Frontal plane motion around a longitudinal axis through the shaft of the first metatarsal is also possible, and a small amount is needed during gait. This is because when the first metatarsophalangeal joint dorsiflexes, the first metatarsal plantar-everts. The proximal phalanx, if it is to maintain its constant relationship to the ground, must dorsiflex and invert to the metatarsal head. Likewise, plantarflexion of the metatarsophalangeal joint must be accompanied by dorsi-inversion of the first ray, which means that the proximal phalanx really plantarflexes and everts in relationship to the first metatarsal head.

The neutral position of the first metatarsophalangeal joint occurs when the hallux is parallel to the ground with the subtalar joint neutral, the midtarsal joint locked, and the first ray in its neutral position. When the average foot is bearing weight in this position, the first metatarsal is approximately 20 degrees plantar flexed in its attitude with the ground.[29] This means that the hallux is about 20 degrees dorsiflexed to the longitudinal axis of the first metatarsal when it is in its neutral position. From here on, when the text states that the first metatarsophalangeal joint is dorsiflexed, it is in reference to its neutral position, not in absolute relationship to the longitudinal axis of the first metatarsal. Thus "the hallux is 10 degrees plantarflexed" means that the hallux is 10 degrees plantarflexed from its neutral position, even though the hallux is still about 10 degrees dorsiflexed in relationship to the longitudinal axis of the first metatarsal.

Function of the First Metatarsophalangeal Joint in Gait

The function of the first metatarsophalangeal joint during the gait cycle is described in terms of its sagittal plane motion, although the reader should be cognizant that sagittal plane motion requires motion of the sesamoids, motion of the first ray, and also some degree of frontal and a slight degree of transverse plane motion. During the swing phase of gait, the extensor hallucis longus provides a fairly strong dorsiflexion force on the first metatarsophalangeal joint. Because the first metatarsal is also being dorsiflexed by the anterior tibial muscle during swing and contact phase, the force of the extensor hallucis longus keeps the hallux only about 20 degrees dorsiflexed through the swing and the first part of contact.

The extensor hallucis longus relaxes about one-third of the way through contact phase, thus allowing the hallux to plantarflex until it purchases the ground. The hallux now stays in contact with the ground until toe-off, although significant motion at the joint occurs because of the motions more proximally. The anterior tibial keeps the first ray dorsiflexed during the middle one-third of contact, and the rearfoot pronation during the last third of contact phase keeps the first ray dorsi-inverted in relationship to its neutral position until the end of contact, which means that the first metatarsophalangeal joint is a little plantar-everted in relationship to the first metatarsal during the last two-thirds of the contact phase.

During the midstance the first metatarsal undergoes a mild degree of plantar-eversion to its neutral position, which means that the proximal phalanx is undergoing a mild degree of dorsiflexion-inversion, until it is in its neutral position just before heel lift. As the hallux is reaching its neutral position, it begins to bear significant weight.[4] The only way for it to register more force under it than the actual weight of the toe is for the flexor muscles to pull the toe down against the floor. In this way the floor can push upward with an equal and opposite force, thus registering weight under the great toe.

It should be noted that significant body weight does not begin under the hallux until the heel rises from the floor. As long as the center of body mass is proximal to the metatarsophalangeal joints, body mass is providing a plantar-flexion moment on the metatarsophalangeal joints. The dorsiflexion moment on the joints is provided by the tension in the Achilles tendon, thus creating a second-class lever at heel lift. Once the center of body mass passes distal to the metatarsophalangeal joint, then the body weight starts creating a dorsiflexion moment on the metatarsophalangeal joints. The flexor muscles create the plantar-flexion moments to keep the toe dorsiflexing at a constant velocity, until the hallux is about 45 degrees dorsiflexed to the transverse plane of the foot (which means that it is about 75 degrees dorsiflexed to the longitudinal axis of the first metatarsal), at which time the hallux comes off the ground.

Muscle Function Around the First Metatarsophalangeal Joint

The flexor hallucis longus is the first hallux muscle to start contracting, beginning just before the start of the midstance phase of gait. Its main function in the early part of midstance is to assist the posterior tibial and flexor digitorum longus in creating resupination of the subtalar and midtarsal joints. The flexor hallucis brevis and extensor hallucis brevis begin contracting simultaneously, about halfway through the midstance phase. These appear to give equal and opposite dorsiflexion and plantar-flexion force to the metatarsophalangeal joint, stabilizing it in a proximal direction and producing a proximally directed shear against the ground, and in return the ground begins its forward directed shear.

The abductor hallucis and adductor hallucis muscles begin their contractions simultaneously, about two-thirds of the way through the midstance phase of gait. The abductor hallucis inserts into the tibial sesamoid and its pull provides a plantarflexion moment and also an adductory (meaning toward the midline of the body) moment around the vertical axis. The adductor hallucis inserts into the fibular sesamoid and its pull provides a plantarflexion moment and also an abductory (meaning away from the midline of the body) moment around the vertical axis. If the adductory moment equals the abductory moment, then these two muscles combine to produce a straight plantarflexion moment on the joint. However, if there is a difference in the moments these muscles produce, either the two muscles are not of equal strength or their moment arms in relationship to the vertical axis are not equal. In this case, then, a transverse plane motion is created during propulsion. The most common imbalance occurs when the first ray is abnormally dorsi-inverted as it enters propulsion, such as occurs when the calcaneus is everted to the floor. In this case the hallux is everted in relationship to the first metatarsal, and the tibial sesamoid is a little closer to the vertical axis than is the fibular sesamoid (Fig. 3-57). Therefore the moment arm of the abductor is smaller than the moment arm of the adductor muscles, and as a result there is a transverse plane motion of the hallux toward the lesser digits when these two muscles contract. Over time, there is a contracture of the ligaments on the lateral side of the joint and the hallux becomes fixed in this laterally deviated position. This is the most common pathway for the development of hallux abductovalgus.

REFERENCES

1. Cochran GVB: A Primer of Orthopaedic Biomechanics. Churchill Livingstone. New York, 1982
2. Currey JD: The mechanical properties of bone. Clin Orthop Related Res, 73:210–231, 1970
3. Curwin S, Stanish WB: Tendonitis: Its Etiology and Treatment. The Collamore Press, DC Heath and Co, Lexington, MA, 1984
4. Root ML, Orien WP, Weed JH: Normal and Abnormal Function of the Foot. Clinical Biomechanics Corporation, Los Angeles, 1977
5. Inman VT: The Joints of the Ankle. Williams & Wilkins Co, Baltimore, 1976
6. Lehmkuhl LD, Smith LK: Brunnstrom's Clinical Kinesiology. 4th Ed. FA Davis Co, Philadelphia, 1983
7. Sarrafian SK: Anatomy of the Foot and Ankle. JB Lippincott Co, Philadelphia, 1983
8. Green DR, Carol A: Planal dominance. J Am Podiatry Assoc 74:98–103, 1984
9. Close JR: Functional Anatomy of the Extremities, Some Electronic and Kinematic Methods of Study. Charles C Thomas Publishing, Springfield IL, 1973
10. Warwick R, Williams PL: Gray's Anatomy. 35th British Ed. WB Saunders Co, Philadelphia, 1973
11. Frankel VH, Nordin M: Basic Biomechanics of the Skeletal System. Lea & Febiger, Philadelphia, 1980
12. Steindler A: Kinesiology of the Human Body, Under Normal and Pathological Conditions. Charles C Thomas Publisher, Springfield, IL, 1964
13. Bailey DS, Perillo JT, Forman M: Subtalar joint neutral, a study using tomography. J Am Podiatry Assoc, 74:59–64, 1984
14. Root ML, Orien WP, Weed JH, Hughes RJ: Biomechanical Examination of the Foot. Clinical Biomechanics Corp, Los Angeles, 1971
15. Kirby KA: Methods for determination of positional variations in the subtalar joint axis. J Am Podiatr Med Assoc, 77:228–234, pages 228–234.
16. Sgarlato TE: The angle of gait. J Am Podiatry Assoc, 55:645–650, 1965
17. Bojsen-Moeller F: Calcaneocuboid joint and stability of the longitudinal arch of the foot at high and low gear push off. J Anat, 129:165–176, 1979
18. Manter JT: Movements of the subtalar and transverse tarsal joints. Anat Rec, 80:397–410, 1941
19. Hicks JH: The mechanics of the foot. I. The joints. J Anat, 87:345–357, 1953
20. Phillips RD, Phillips RL: Quantitative analysis of the locking position of the midtarsal joint. J Am Podiatry Assoc, 73:518–522, 1983
21. Elftman H: The transverse tarsal joint and its control. Clin Orthop, 41–45, 1960
22. Hicks JH: The mechancis of the foot. II. The plantar aponeurosis and the arch. J Anat, 88:25–31, 1954
23. McPoil T, Cameron JA, Adrian MJ: Anatomical characteristics of the talus in relation to the forefoot

deformities. J Am Podiatr Med Assoc, 77:77–81, 1983

24. Root ML, Weed JH, Orien WP: Neutral Position Casting Techniques. Clinical Biomechanics Corp, Los Angeles, 1971

25. Mann RA: Surgery of the Foot. 5th Ed. CV Mosby Co, St. Louis, 1986

26. Kelso SF, Richie DH, Cohen IR et al: Direction and range of motion of the first ray. J Am Podiatry Assoc, 72:600–605, 1982

27. Hetherington V, Carnett J, Patterson BA: Motion of the first metatarsophalangeal joint. Unpublished research paper, 1988

28. Stott JRR, Hutton WC, Stokes IA: Forces under the foot. J Bone Joint Surg [Br], 55:335–343, 1973

29. Hlavac HF: Differences in x-ray findings with varied positioning of the foot. J Am Podiatry Assoc, 57:465–471, 1967

SELECTED READINGS

Atkins KR: Physics. John Wiley & Sons, Inc, New York, 1967

Basmajian JV: Muscles Alive, Their Functions Revealed by Electromyography. 2nd Ed. Williams & Wilkins, Baltimore, 1967

Burns MJ: Biomechanics. Chpt. 2. In McGlamry ED (ed): Fundamentals of Foot Surgery. Williams & Wilkins, Baltimore, 1987

Cailliet R: Knee Pain and Disability. FA Davis Co, Philadelphia, 1973

Close JR, Inman VT, Poor PM, Todd FN: The function of the subtalar joint. Orthopaed Clin Related Res. 50:159–179, 1967

Gozna ER, Harrington IJ: Biomechanics of Musculoskeletal Injury. Baltimore, Williams & Wilkins, 1982

Green DL, Morris JM: Role of adductor longus and adductor magnus in postural movements and in ambulation. Am J Phys Med, 49:223–240, 1970

Inman VT, Ralson HJ, Todd F: Human Walking. Williams & Wilkins, Baltimore, 1981

Kapandji IA: The Physiology of the Joints. Vol. 2. 5th Ed. Churchill Livingston, New York, 1987

McGuigan TM: The biomechanics of the knee. Arch Podiatr Med Foot Surg, supp., 1:35–42, 1978

Norkin CC, Leavangie PK: Joint Structure and Function, A Comprehensive Analysis. FA Davis Co, Philadelphia, 1983

Reilly DT, Burstein AH: The mechanical properties of cortical bone. J Bone Joint Surg [Am], 56:1001–1022, 1974

Seibel MO: Foot Function, A Programmed Text. Williams & Wilkins, Baltimore, 1988

Simon SR, American Academy of Orthopaedic Surgeons: Orthopaedic Science, A Resource and Self-Study Guide for the Practitioner. The American Academy of Orthopaedic Surgeons, Park Ridge, IL, 1986

Sutherland DH: Gait Disorders in Childhood and Adolescence. Williams & Wilkins, Baltimore, 1984

Thomas GB, Jr.: Calculus and Analytic Geometry. Addison-Wesley Publishing Co, Reading, MA, 1968

Section II

PATIENT EVALUATION

The Podiatric History and Examination

4

Myron C. Boxer, D.P.M.
Susan J. Tokarski, D.P.M.

THE HISTORY

The history and physical examination are the sine qua non for establishing a proper diagnosis. The diagnostic process begins with the taking of the history, which consists of several sections, each designed to elicit certain information about the patient and his or her problem.

First the patient's vital statistics are obtained. Included are the patient's name, address, date of birth, telephone number, marital status, and referral source of the patient.

Next the examiner elicits the chief complaint, which is the primary problem for which the patient is seeking help. There may be more than one chief complaint. At times it may be advantageous to record the chief complaint in the patient's own words, which may convey the information better than any paraphrase. The examiner should then immediately obtain the history of the chief complaint, including its onset, duration, course, and any previous therapy and its results, as well as any factors influencing the chief complaint.

The medical and surgical histories are obtained next. The medical history consists of all past and present medical problems as well as their sequelae.

Information should be obtained about childhood diseases as well as problems during adulthood, and about any allergies, hospitalizations, and medications that the patient is currently taking. The surgical history should reveal any previous surgical procedures and their complications and sequelae if any. Any reactions to anesthetics should be noted here as well.

Questions about social history should elicit information concerning personal habits, social status, occupation, and recreational habits. Included in personal habits should be questions relating to smoking, alcohol consumption, and the use of drugs. If the patient smokes, the examiner should ascertain how many packs per day and for how many years. If the patient drinks alcoholic beverages, the kind and quantity consumed should be known. Other questions include: Does the patient have any problems referable to sleeping? Does the patient use medication to fall asleep? Does the patient sleep during the day? Does the patient eat a well-balanced diet? Are there any food allergies? Does the patient exercise on a regular basis? How much leisure time does the patient have? Does the patient use any drugs? Is there a problem of addiction? Is the patient married? Are there any marital problems? An occupational history should be taken since certain occupations may create health hazards. The social history should include a record of all past and present occupations and working conditions and whether there was exposure to dangerous or harmful chemicals or other substances.

A concise description of the patient's family medical history should be obtained, since there are family patterns to certain illnesses such as allergies, hemophilia, hypertension, emotional problems, heart disease, gout, and the arthritides. Determining the cause of death of a family member may help in the diagnosis of hereditary diseases.[1]

Finally, the examiner should perform a review of systems. This portion of the history serves as a catchall. Each organ system is reviewed to make sure that no information was omitted during the history up to this point.

First, the patient should be asked about his or her overall general health. Has there been any loss or gain of weight? Have there been any recent recurrent infections, fevers, night sweats, or fatigue that might signal a systemic illness? The review then proceeds to the specific organ systems.

Skin. Has the patient noticed any changes in skin color, temperature, or texture? Has there been any change in hair distribution on the extremities? Have any rashes developed? Has there been any bruising of the skin or pruritus? Have the nails become discolored, brittle, deformed, or softened? Have there been any gross changes in moles or nevi?

Head. Has the patient sustained any recent injuries to the head? Has there been a problem with headaches? Have there been any subcutaneous lumps or areas of alopecia?

Eyes. Is the patient myopic or hyperopic? Does the patient have a history of glaucoma, diplopia, discharges, cataracts, or blurring of vision? Is the patient color blind? Does the patient use corrective lenses?

Ears. Has there been any loss of hearing? If so, is it unilateral or bilateral? Does the patient have ringing of the ears? Does the patient experience vertigo? Has there been any discharge from the ears? Does the patient experience earaches? Has the patient had any infections? Is there a history of prior ear surgery?

Nose. Does the patient have any sinus problems? Is there a history of nasal discharge, frequent colds, loss of smell, or problems with breathing? Is there a history of previous nasal surgery?

Mouth and Throat. Are there any lesions in the oral cavity? Do the gums bleed? Has there been a loss of teeth? Has the patient noticed a loss of taste? Has there been any hoarseness? Is there a history of tonsillitis? Have there been any problems with dysphagia?

Neck. Has there been any swelling, stiffness, or pain? Is there limitation of motion in the patient's neck?

Cardiovascular. Is there a history of cardiac disease? Has the patient experienced any palpitations or arrhythmias? Is there a history of chest pain, shortness of breath on exertion, or paroxysmal nocturnal dyspnea? Is there a history of hypertension or hypotension? Has the patient had rheumatic fever? Has the patient noticed any cyanosis or coldness of the extremities? Has there been any pedal or ankle edema? When was the last electrocardiogram performed, and what was the result?

Respiratory. Does the patient experience any difficulty breathing? Is there any wheezing or cough? Does the patient bring up blood when coughing (hemoptysis) or excessive amounts of sputum? Has there been a history of bronchitis, tuberculosis, asthma, emphysema, pneumonia, or excessive upper respiratory infections? Has the patient had a recent chest x-ray examination or tuberculin skin testing?

Gastrointestinal. Has the patient experienced any recent change in weight? Is the appetite good? Is there any problem with digestion? Are bowel movements normal? Has there been any rectal bleeding? Does the patient have a history of hemorrhoids?

Genitourinary. If the patient is male, has he had any problems with impotency or with his prostate? If female, are there any menstrual problems such as irregular bleeding, excessive bleeding, or persistent discharge? The number of pregnancies as well as deliveries, including any complications, abortions, or miscarriages, should be ascertained. Does the patient practice contraception? If so, what type? Is there a history of urinary tract infections, renal calculi, or bladder problems?

Nervous System.   Is there a history of recurrent headaches, seizures, fainting spells, or convulsions? Does the patient experience episodes of dizziness? Is there a problem with tremors or balance? Has the patient ever experienced any paresthesias involving the extremities? Is there a history of cerebrovascular accident?

Psychiatric.   Has the patient ever suffered from any psychiatric problems such as anxiety, mood disorders, or depression? Does the patient use any psychotherapeutic medications?

Musculoskeletal System.   Does the patient experience any arthralgias or arthritis? Is there any history of fractures, sprains, or strains? Does the patient have any gait problems (e.g., is the gait antalgic, ataxic, or spastic)? Is muscle weakness present? Is there a history of previous musculoskeletal injuries or surgical procedures?

Hematopoietic.   Is there a history of any blood dyscrasias or bleeding disorders? Does the patient fatigue or bruise easily? Has the patient been on any type of anticoagulant therapy?

Endocrine.   Is there a history of polyuria, polydipsia, or polyphagia? Is there a history of thyroid disease? Has the patient had hyperglycemia or glycosuria?[2]

THE VASCULAR EXAMINATION

It is imperative that an accurate history be taken before one begins the vascular examination. In many instances, the history alone will give valuable clues to the severity of a vascular problem.

A common symptom associated with peripheral vascular disease is pain. Valuable information about the vascular status of a patient may be obtained from the degree and nature of the pain with which the patient presents. Pain that occurs at rest and is nonrelenting usually indicates severe arterial embarrassment. This type of pain is referred to as pretrophic or rest pain and most often is due to

severe ischemia. Elevation of the extremities will invariably make this type of pain worse, since the aid of gravity in moving blood to the lower extremities is lost. Patients with rest pain will report that their pain comes on and intensifies when they are in bed. The discomfort of rest pain is quite severe and usually precedes the onset of ulceration and gangrene.

Pain associated with sudden arterial occlusion, on the other hand, characteristically has a very acute onset and is accompanied by changes in skin temperature and color. This acutely painful condition is often the result of a thromboembolic phenomenon.

The pain of intermittent claudication is due to ischemia of a muscle brought on by exercise. The exercise does not have to be strenuous and may be as mild as simple walking. Rest usually relieves the pain, and it is more readily tolerated than pretrophic pain. It is an indication of advanced arterial disease. Typically, the posterior crural muscles cramp upon walking a specific distance. The pain of claudication may also occur in the muscles of the thigh, the buttocks, and the intrinsic muscles of the foot.

The vascular examination of the patient should include a check of the following pulses for their symmetry and quality (Fig. 4-1):

1. The dorsalis pedis artery on the dorsum of the foot
2. The posterior tibial artery behind the internal malleolus
3. The popliteal artery in the popliteal fossa
4. The superficial femoral artery in the groin
5. The abdominal aorta just to the left of the umbilicus.

If pedal pulses are not palpable, one should go further up the vascular tree to the popliteal area, the groin, or even the abdomen to try to isolate the level of an occlusion.

The color changes of the skin are basically influenced by two factors: the amount of blood, and the color of the blood. Normally, the skin should be warm and fairly pink in color. It is warm because the flow is rather fast, and it is pink in color because the blood supply is abundant with fully oxygenated blood. Skin that is warm and deep red in color gen-

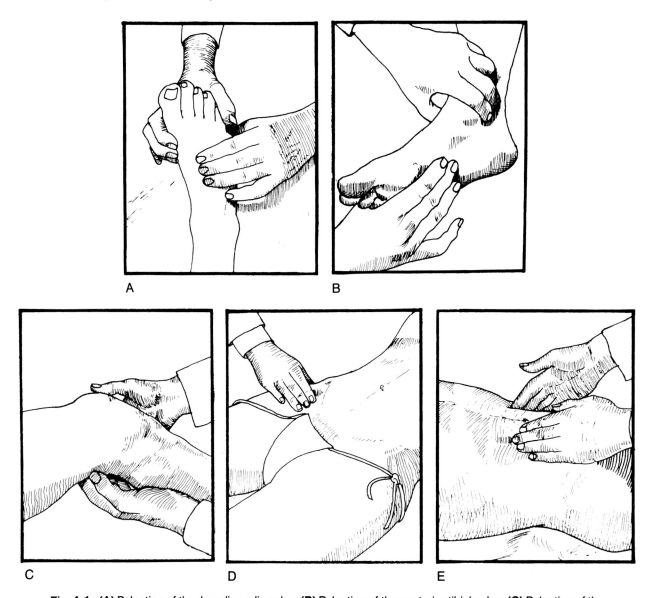

Fig. 4-1. (A) Palpation of the dorsalis pedis pulse. **(B)** Palpation of the posterior tibial pulse. **(C)** Palpation of the popliteal pulse. **(D)** Palpation of the femoral pulse. **(E)** Palpation of the abdominal aorta. (From McRae,[9] with permission.)

erally indicates rapid flow and a state of inflammation. Skin that is warm and deeply cyanotic tends to indicate blood flow that is somewhat imperfect and in which the skin has been warmed by some external source. Cold, pale, cyanotic skin indicates very slow or absent blood flow. Cold, deeply colored red skin indicates blood flow in which perfusion is not good and there may be damage to the small vessels.

The elevation dependency color change test is useful in identifying occlusive arterial disease. This is so because color changes of the skin that occur with a change in posture occur only in occlusive arterial disease. Normally, on elevation of an extremity, normal pink color should be maintained. Pallor of the skin on elevation indicates arterial embarrassment. Normal color should also be noted when the extremity is in the dependent position. A deep rubor on dependency may indicate venous incompetence and/or poor arterial flow.

Trophic changes of the skin such as loss of hair and atrophy of the skin and subcutaneous structures will occur when the arterial supply is compromised. These should be looked for when doing the vascular examination.

Skin temperature is also an excellent indicator of vascular status. Normally, the skin temperature should be in the range of 82° to 90°F. Cold skin may indicate either functional vasospasm or organic occlusive vascular disease. The temperature normally should decrease as one goes distally down the limb. In cases of inflammation within the foot, this temperature gradient may be diminished or even reversed. In severe arterial disease where the foot is arterially embarrassed, the temperature drop-off will be rather rapid and the temperature gradient is increased.

Capillary return is a measure of small vessel competency. The test is performed by simply pressing and releasing the tip of one of the digits and measuring how long it takes for the blood to refill the capillary bed. Capillary return should normally be within 1 second. The longer the capillary bed takes to fill after being compressed, the greater the arterial embarrassment to the part.

One of the most valuable tests in the vascular examination is the venous filling time, which measures the amount of time it takes for the blood to flow from the arterial side, through the capillary bed, and over to the venous side. If the arteries are occluded, or if the small vessels of the capillary network are diseased or occluded, the venous filling time will be increased.

The venous filling time is tested by first lowering the limb and picking out a vein that is fairly prominent on the dorsum of the foot. The limb is then elevated for 1 minute and milked to drain the selected vein. Then the limb is lowered into a dependent position, and the time that it takes for the first visible sign of the vein beginning to fill is measured. Normally the vein should begin to fill within 10 seconds. This test measures both small vessel and large vessel competency. The test is invalid in the presence of varices because of blood reflux.

One of the diagnostic instruments of value in the vascular examination is the oscillometer. The oscil-

lometer measures the amplitude of the pulse wave underneath a cuff that is applied around the leg. The oscillometer can be used to measure the vascularity of one limb against another and to compare one limb to itself at a later date. An oscillometer can also be used to isolate the level of an occlusion, since pulses will be recorded above the level of an occlusion but will not be found below the occlusion. It should be remembered that the oscillometer is a qualitative instrument and cannot be used to take quantitative measurements.

The oscillometer consists of a sensitive aneroid capsule and an arbitrary scale. The aneroid capsule records small volume changes in the limb. These changes are shown on the scale of the oscillometer. They are proportional to the amount of blood flowing into the peripheral arteries during cardiac systole. Decreased lumen sizes are reflected as smaller oscillometric readings. If there is complete occlusion of the arteries by a clot or plaque, an oscillometric reading of zero will be noted. The patient should be examined in a relaxed, supine position. The cuff of the oscillometer is snugly wrapped around each of four levels of the lower leg: the thigh, above the knee, below the knee, and above the ankle. The cuff is inflated to just above the patient's systolic blood pressure and is then lowered by increments of 10 mm Hg. At each increment of 10 mm Hg, the range of motion of the needle should be noted. The most important reading is found at the greatest excursion of the needle. Normally the excursion of the needle will be within a range of 5 to 15 units or higher at the level of the calf and 3 to 8 units above the ankle. The excursion of the needle should be approximately the same for similar sites on both lower extremities. Lower readings at specific sites over time indicate progression of an occlusive process.

Oscillometry has its limitations. It can be used to determine whether occlusion exists, and it may grossly localize the level of an occlusion. It measures the overall progression of the occlusive disease. It does not indicate whether collateral circulation is developing, and it cannot predict the future status of the limb. Misleading results can be caused by a brawny edema of the leg or by a vasospastic problem. If a vasospastic problem is suspected, the vasospasm should be relieved by clinical means and the readings taken again. If phlebothrombosis of the calf is suspected, oscillometry should not be done at that level.[3]

Another valuable instrument is the Doppler ultrasound machine. The ultrasound beam vibrates at a specific frequency and is reflected back with a change in frequency that is proportional to the velocity of the flow. The modified beam is displayed as a wave form or transmitted as a sound. The patient is examined in the supine position. The head of the bed should be raised 20 to 30 degrees to produce pooling of blood in the lower limbs. The patient should be relaxed. The Doppler probe should be held at a 45-degree angle to the artery and tilted toward the direction of blood flow. Ultrasound coupling gel is applied to the patient's skin. The pulse sound is located by using the Doppler probe. Arterial signals have a relatively high frequency, are pulsatile, and vary with the cardiac cycle. Venous signals are relatively low frequency sounds, vary with the respiratory cycle, and are not pulsatile. When the Doppler probe is placed directly over an area of stenosis, the signal will have an abnormally high pitched frequency. If the Doppler probe is placed proximal to an area of stenosis, and if there is good collateral circulation between the probe and the point of stenosis, the signal will sound normal. If there is no collateral circulation, the signal will be harsh. Absence of a signal indicates either complete occlusion or a very slow flow of blood through the area.

With the Doppler device, segmental arterial systolic pressures can be obtained from several arteries, including the common femoral artery, the superficial femoral artery, the popliteal artery, the posterior tibial artery, and the dorsalis pedis artery. A tourniquet should be placed in the upper thigh region, above the knee, below the knee, and above the ankle. A Doppler probe should be placed somewhere distal to the tourniquet, and a systolic pressure reading is taken by lowering the cuff pressure until the first sound of blood flow is heard (systolic pressure). Pressure drops of 30 mm Hg or more between segments in one leg indicate abnormalities. Normally, systolic pressures should drop by approximately 10 mm Hg at each level as one goes distally down the leg.

There are four elements to the normal wave form of a peripheral artery: It has multiphasic pulsatility, sharp upstroke and downstroke during systole, and a variable reverse flow during diastole followed by oscillations. The large proximal arteries, like the common femoral artery, show these characteristics better than the smaller, more distal arteries such as the dorsalis pedis artery. Monophasic, one-sound pulsatility or an absence of pulsatility indicates severe stenosis or complete occlusion of the vessel proximal to the probe. The flow to the area is derived from collateral circulation. Milder degrees of proximal stenosis causing decreased arterial compliance are indicated by an absence of the dicrotic notch; a smaller, lower systole upstroke; a slower systole downstroke; and fewer diastole oscillations. A flat recording indicates multilevel occlusion leading to a total loss of blood flow during systole.

Another important measure of vascularity is the ankle/brachial index. This is the ratio of the ankle systolic pressure to the brachial systolic pressure. Normally the ankle pressure should be equal to or greater than the brachial pressure. Hence an ankle/brachial index of 1.0 or greater excludes the possibility of arterial occlusive disease. Ankle/brachial indices between 0.6 and 0.8 are associated with claudication, indices between 0.4 and 0.6 are associated with rest pain, and indices of less than 0.4 are associated with ulcers and gangrene.

Ankle systolic pressures generally reflect the overall degree of occlusion in the more proximal arteries. An important source of error is calcification of the arterial wall, which causes very high pressure measurements. In some cases of proximal stenosis, resting measurements may therefore be normal.

Ankle systolic pressures have been used to predict healing. Minor toe amputations have been found to heal with ankle pressures of 40 to 70 mm Hg. Patients with infected paronychiae with pressures of 70 to 90 mm Hg have been found to have an excellent chance to heal.[3-5]

DOPPLER ANALYSIS OF VENOUS FLOW

The normal venous signal obtained with the Doppler probe has five important characteristics: it is spontaneous, it is phasic with respiration, it augments with limb compression, it is competent with proximal limb compression or Valsalva maneuvers, and it exhibits nonpulsatility. Abnormal venous signals include an absence of flow, absence of phasicity with respiration, and attenuated or absent augmentation and incompetency and pulsatility. The Doppler instrument can be used to examine the superficial, communicating, and deep veins of the lower extremity. The patient should be rested in the supine position with the head of the bed elevated. The posterior tibial vein is examined first. Ultrasound gel is applied to the area, and the Doppler probe is held at a 45-degree angle to the skin. The artery is located first using the Doppler instrument. The vein is found next to the artery. The venous sound is a high-pitched sound that resembles the noise of strong wind. The calf muscles should be compressed to establish the competency of the posterior tibial vein valves. Upon release of the calf compression, augmentation of venous flow sounds should occur if the calf veins are patent. The attenuation instead of augmentation is the most reliable sign of calf vein thrombosis. The posterior tibial vein on the other leg should also be evaluated and compared, and the greater saphenous vein should also be evaluated. Increased flow velocity in the saphenous vein may indicate calf vein thrombosis, with collateral circulation through the superficial vein. The common femoral vein, the superficial femoral vein, and the popliteal vein should also be evaluated. The communicating veins of the limb may be evaluated by applying a rubber tourniquet to the leg. This prevents reflux through incompetent superficial veins. The calf should then be compressed, and the sites of venous reflux should be evaluated above the level of the tourniquet.[3]

Plethysmography records changes in the dimension of the limb associated with each heartbeat or in response to temporary occlusion of venous return (venous occlusion plethysmography). The volume changes may be sensed in many different ways, by strain gauge, photoelectric, air, or pulse volume recordings among others. The resulting wave forms will all be similar in appearance. Analysis of the pulse contour is a useful indicator of peripheral arterial circulation.

Strain gauge plethysmography uses mercury-filled Silastic tubing placed around a limb or digit to measure volume changes in the area with each cardiac cycle.

The pulse volume recorder is a qualitative plethysmograph that uses cuffs placed on a body part.

It emits infrared light from a diode to the underlying skin, and the back-scattered light is received by a photodetector. Wave forms are then obtained and may be used to assess digital blood pressure and the extent of ischemia.

A normal pulse contour shows a steeply rising upslope (anacrotic limb), with a sharp peak and a downslope (catacrotic limb) that curves toward the base line and has a dicrotic notch. A mildly obstructed artery will show loss of the dicrotic notch and a slight bowing of the downslope away from the base line. As the obstructive process continues and becomes moderate, there develops a delay in the upslope and a rounded peak. A severe obstruction shows wave forms of low amplitude. The amplitude of the pulse volume tracing has a clear relationship to the degree of arteriosclerotic disease as well as to local blood pressure, arterial competence, and the number of arteries in the segment being tested. The pulse volume recorder may also be used to obtain segmental pressures. Both segmental pressures and wave form analysis can be used to arrive at a diagnosis.

Photoplethysmography records toe cutaneous blood content in the capillary networks. The photoplethysmograph consists of a transducer with an infrared light-emitting diode and a phototransistor receiver. The pulse wave that is obtained may be used to evaluate qualitatively the vascularity of the part being examined.[3,5,6]

Plethysmography may be used to evaluate venous disease. In venous outflow plethysmography, the lower extremity is elevated above the level of the atrium, and a plethysmograph transducer is placed around the calf. The pneumatic cuff on the thigh is inflated above the peripheral venous pressure (30 to 50 mm Hg) for 1 to 2 minutes until the increase in calf volume stabilizes. The cuff is then deflated, and the rate of decrease in calf volume is measured with the plethysmograph. This rate of emptying is proportional to the patency of the deep veins. This technique is not sensitive to venous thrombosis of the calf and can not distinguish superficial venous disease from deep venous disease.[3]

Trendelenburg's test is a test of valvular competency. While the leg is elevated a tourniquet is applied to the midthigh. The examiner waits 20 seconds. Then the patient is asked to stand, and the examiner notes the time it takes for the superficial veins below the tourniquet level to fill up. Immediate filling indicates an incompetent valve at the saphenofemoral junction. Absence of immediate filling indicates a competent valve at the saphenofemoral junction. Perthes' test is a test of the competency of the valves of the saphenous and communicating veins and is also used to determine if there is thrombosis of the deep veins. The test is performed with the leg in a dependent position. A tourniquet is applied to the thigh to compress the long saphenous vein. The patient then ambulates. If the superficial leg varices become less prominent, the communicating veins below the tourniquet level are competent. If the superficial veins remain filled or become more prominent, there is incompetence of both the superficial veins and the communicating veins. If the leg vein becomes more prominent, the skin becomes dusky, and the patient complains of discomfort in the leg, there is impairment of the deep venous system with incompetence of the communicating veins.[1]

The Allen test is used to detect occlusive lesions of the dorsalis pedis or the posterior tibial artery distal to the ankle. The foot is elevated, and the examiner compresses the dorsalis pedis artery with the thumb. The foot is then placed in a dependent position with the dorsalis pedis artery still compressed. A return of color to the foot indicates a patent posterior tibial artery. The test is then repeated with the examiner compressing the posterior tibial artery. This tests the patency of the dorsalis pedis artery.[3,7]

THE ORTHOPEDIC EXAMINATION

General Examination

The orthopedic examination begins as soon as the patient enters the room. This is a good time to quickly check for the presence of an antalgic gait or the use of ambulatory aids. The examiner observes the patient carefully, watching the ease or lack thereof with which the patient removes his or her shoes and stockings and gets into the examining chair. How much assistance does the patient require?

It is necessary to assess both function and structure. Through the history and examination, the examiner must evaluate the patient's ability to carry out his or her daily routine as well as make a diagnosis of the presenting complaint. This is best done by developing a standardized, disciplined examination, the extent of which is dictated by the chief complaint and the condition of the patient.[8] The examination is conducted by the traditional steps of inspection, palpation, range of motion testing, and gait analysis. The sequence may be varied so as to perform an efficient examination without needless repositioning and movement of the patient.

Inspection

The examiner notes the general appearance of the foot and any obvious deformity. The presence of bunions, calcaneal or cuneiform exostosis, and deformities that may indicate old fractures is noted.[9] The relative lengths and positions of the digits are observed. Do the digits under- or overlap, or are they contracted? One should always check the hands, as they are often involved if the patient has arthritis. Note the presence of redness or swelling. Swelling is usually due to underlying inflammation. It can be produced by thickened synovium, increased joint fluid, or local edema. The "window sign," with wide separation of the toes, is produced when there is thickening of the metatarsophalangeal joint synovium. Joint swelling or deformity can also be due to bursae, inflamed tendons, or osteophytes.[10]

The surfaces of the foot, as well as the skin between the toes, must be inspected for hyperkeratoses, which indicate bony deformity, abnormal weightbearing, or ill-fitting shoes.[8] The patient's shoes should always be inspected, noting the heel height, the wear pattern from heel to toe, the overall shape of the shoe (narrow pointed toes, inadequate toe box, or breakdown of the medial or lateral counter), and the presence of orthotic or other supportive devices.[11]

Palpation

By palpation the examiner detects the presence of swelling and tenderness. A knowledge of topographic anatomy is necessary to know what structures are being palpated.[10] A common mistake is not to use sufficient force in palpating. A good rule is to use enough force so that the examiner's thumbnail blanches. Of course, common sense dictates that an inflamed, swollen joint is not examined with this much pressure.[10] Always palpate the less symptomatic side first, and always compare it with the opposite foot.

In a symptomatic patient the following structures can be palpated in the foot: the anterior surface of the ankle, which is facilitated by plantar flexion of the joint; the distal ends of the medial and lateral malleoli, noting especially the attachments of the medial and lateral collateral ligaments; the area of the sinus tarsi, which is deeply palpated; the insertion of the Achilles tendon on the calcaneus, checking for tenderness or nodules along the length of the tendon; and the dorsum of the midtarsal joint. The metatarsals can be compressed as a group and palpated individually. Note any tenderness and the presence of a bursa over the dorsal or medial aspect of a bunion. Palpate each metatarsophalangeal joint and the interphalangeal joint of each digit.

When palpating the metatarsophalangeal joints it is important to be able to distinguish between joint pain and pain in the surrounding structures. True joint pain hurts on both sides of the joint. Palpate the dorsal and plantar surfaces but do so on both the medial and lateral aspects of the joint. If the pain is present on only one side, the pathology may be in the interspace structures. This is helpful, for example, in distinguishing between joint pain and pain from a neuroma in the web space.

Check also for tenderness of the first metatarsal sesamoids. Note the absence or anterior displacement of the plantar fat pad, a common source of metatarsal pain. Palpate the entire length of the plantar fascia, noting tenderness and areas of fibrous nodules. Again, always check the hands as they are commonly involved.[9]

Range of Motion

With passive manipulation the major articulations of the foot are checked for limitation, contractures, deviation from normal, crepitation, and painful movement.[11] The quality of motion as well as the actual range of motion of all joints should be noted. It is important to note any asymmetry of motion between the right and left sides. Good quality of motion means that a joint can be moved smoothly through a full range with an abrupt termination at either end.[12] There should not be any pain, crepitus, or limitation. Crepitus, a dry grating or crackling that may be either heard or felt, is caused by roughened articular cartilage or, in cases of advanced arthritis, by bone rubbing against bone. Limitation of motion can be due to bony ankylosis, patient guarding, muscle spasm, fibrosis, adhesions, capsular contractions, subluxation or dislocation, ruptured or inflamed tendons, or an intra-articular loose body.[10] An abnormal increase in range of motion may suggest ligamentous rupture on general ligamentous laxity.

The following joints are taken through a range of motion: the ankle joint, the subtalar joint, the midtarsal joint, and the first metatarsophalangeal joint. In addition, the first ray position, the calcaneal position, the malleolar position, tibial varum, leg length, hip position, and arch morphology are noted.

The ankle joint is put through a full range of dorsiflexion and plantar flexion. Measurement of the range of dorsiflexion is made with the patient supine and the knee fully extended. The foot is put in the neutral position, and the examiner dorsiflexes the ankle joint. The measurement is made from the lateral aspect using the angle made by the long axis of the leg with the lateral border of the foot, from the heel to the fifth metatarsal base (Fig. 4-2). The patient should have at least a few degrees of dorsiflexion available beyond the vertical and,

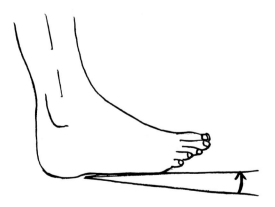

Fig. 4-2. Measurement of the range of dorsiflexion.

ideally, a minimum of 10 degrees of dorsiflexion. If not, remeasure with the knee flexed to remove the influence of the gastrocnemius. If dorsiflexion is still inadequate, one assumes there is soleus shortening or a bony block at the ankle.[13] This must then be assessed radiographically.

Plantar flexion of the ankle is checked for quality of motion. The normal range is 55 degrees.

Although average values for ranges of motion are usually given, an average individual is difficult to find. Therefore, the examiner must evaluate any biomechanical variations discovered in light of whether or not the patient is functioning adequately.[11]

To evaluate the subtalar joint the patient lies face down with the feet hanging over the edge of the table. The leg to be examined is positioned so that the heel is parallel to the floor. The lower third of the leg is bisected, making sure not to use the Achilles tendon as a reference. The posterior surface of the calcaneus is also bisected, using the bony margins as a guide. The heel is firmly grasped and the subtalar joint inverted and everted, as the examiner notes the angle made between the two bisections (Fig. 4-3). The average range of motion is 30 degrees, with twice as much inversion as eversion. The foot is then placed in the neutral position and the relationship of the calcaneus to the leg, or neutral rearfoot position, is measured. The average value is 3 to 4 degrees of varus.

While the patient is still prone, the midtarsal joint is assessed, both the oblique and the longitudinal axis. The oblique axis is examined by placing the foot in the neutral position and grasping the foot just distal to the midtarsal articulation. The joint is then moved through a range of motion basically in the direction of dorsiflexion and plantar flexion; the examiner notes whether the range is adequate or limited. All limited range of motion should be noted as to whether it is marked, moderate, or mild.[12] The longitudinal axis is examined by noting the relationship of the forefoot to the rearfoot. This is done by placing the foot in the neutral position and, with the thumb on the fourth and fifth metatarsal heads, dorsiflexing just to the point of resistance.[13] A measuring device is placed on the previously marked bisection of the calcaneus and carried down so it is imposed on the plane of the forefoot (second through fourth metatarsals; Fig. 4-4). The device will either be parallel to the forefoot or make an angle. In a normal individual the forefoot should be parallel or within about 2 degrees of varus in relationship to the rearfoot.

The first ray consists of the first metatarsal and the medial cuneiform bone. The range and direction of motion of this segment are measured by placing the foot in the neutral position and grasping

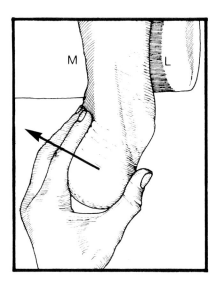

Fig. 4-3. Measurement of subtalar joint range of motion. (From McRae,[9] with permission.)

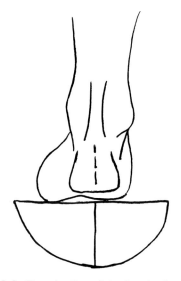

Fig. 4-4. Examination of the longitudinal axis.

the lesser metatarsal heads between the thumb and forefinger of the hand to stabilize them. With the same fingers of the opposite hand the examiner holds the first metatarsal head so that it can be moved through a range of motion above and below the plane of the lesser metatarsals (Fig. 4-5). The neutral position, plantar flexion, and dorsiflexion of the first ray may be visually estimated by viewing the position of the examiner's thumb, either above or below, in relationship to the opposite thumb, which is on the lesser metatarsals. The range of motion should be the same both above and below the second metatarsal level.[12]

The average range of motion of the first metatarsophalangeal joint is 65 degrees of extension and 40 degrees of flexion.[9] This is measured with the patient seated and the foot not bearing weight (Fig. 4-6). As with all joints, limited and painful motion should be noted. Here it is important to distinguish between true joint pain and pain from the pressure of the examiner's fingers over a tender bunion or bursa.

Measurement of tibial torsion or internal tibiofibular rotation is made with reference to malleolar position.[14] The normal value for an adult is 13 to 18 degrees from the external malleolar position. For most purposes this measurement may be visually estimated by noting the position of the malleoli in relation to one another.

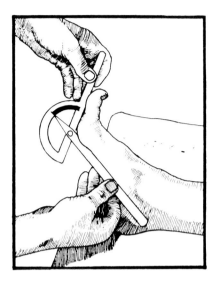

Fig. 4-6. Measurement of range of motion of the first metatarsophalangeal joint. (From McRae,[9] with permission.)

Equality of limb length is quickly assessed by having the patient sit with hips flat against the back of the examining chair and the knees fully extended. In the normal patient the internal malleoli should be at the same level. If there is shortening, the patient is positioned to lie squarely supine on the table, and a measurement of total leg shortening is made. The tip of the tape measure is placed on the anterior superior iliac spine and pressed down until it hooks under the inferior edge of the spine. From here a measurement is made to the middle or inferior edge of the internal malleolus (Fig. 4-7). Always compare both sides and repeat the measurements until consistent. This measurement gives no indication as to the site of the shortening,[9] which is further investigated by measurements at different levels of the hip, thigh, and leg.

Internal and external rotation at the hip is about equal in both directions in the normal adult. The average range is 45 degrees in either direction. This examination is performed with the patient in both the supine and sitting positions, with the knee fully extended. The center of the patella is marked as a reference point and related to time on a clock while the leg is rotated internally and externally to the end of its motion. A detectable difference between the flexed and extended hip positions indicates a restrictive soft tissue influence at the hip. A

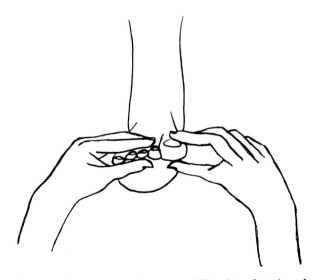

Fig. 4-5. Measurement of range and direction of motion of the first metatarsal and the medial cuneiform.

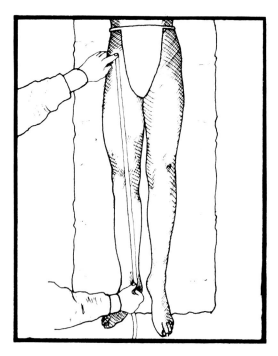

Fig. 4-7. Assessment of equality of limb length. (From McRae,[9] with permission.)

more accurate assessment can be made by having the patient lie prone with the knees flexed. The examiner moves the feet and legs laterally while the patient keeps the knees together to check internal hip rotation. The examiner then crosses the patient's feet and legs to assess external hip rotation (Fig. 4-8A & B). This is repeated with the patient supine and both hips and knees flexed (Fig. 4-8C & D). These maneuvers allow a sensitive comparison of the two sides.[9]

The height of the arch is noted as high, medium, or low while the foot is not bearing weight. The patient then stands for the remainder of the examination, and the effect of weightbearing on arch morphology is noted. The flexibility of the foot is assessed by asking the patient to rise on his or her toes. The arch should rise and the rearfoot supinate because of the windlass effect of the plantar fascia.[14] Failure of the heel to invert upon this maneuver indicates a rigid or weak foot.

The amount of tibial varum is checked by having the patient stand with his or her back to the examiner and briefly march in place to demonstrate the patient's usual angle and base of gait. The foot is put in the neutral position, and the angle made by the previously marked bisection of the lower leg with the vertical is measured (Fig. 4-9). The normal range is 2 degrees.

To determine calcaneal position, the examiner views the patient from behind and notes whether the heels are inverted or everted. This can be quantified by measuring the angle made by the bisection of the heel with the vertical.

Gait Analysis

Gait analysis may properly be performed either before or after the static examination. Less experienced examiners may find it helpful to first conduct the static examination and use the findings to help assess problems that may be expressed more subtly in gait. The patient should be observed, both barefoot and in shoes, over a fair distance and viewed from the front, back, and side. It is important to note any asymmetry between the two sides. Arm swing should be symmetric. The examiner should note whether there is a tilt of the head or a drop to either side of the shoulders or pelvis. Obvious abnormalities such as a limp or unequal step length are noted.[11] If the patient is wearing trousers, these must be pulled up securely over the knees to observe the position of the patellae and the degree of genu varum or valgum. Heel strike and heel rise are examined in regard to position of the heel when it contacts the ground, and the presence of early heel rise is noted. Early heel rise is most often due to tightness of the gastrocnemius and soleus muscles.[11] The degree of intoe and outtoe is observed along with the position of the patellae to help detect the level of abnormality. Note the degree of pronation and where it occurs in the gait cycle. Finally, observe whether the patient has a propulsive or a flatfooted, apropulsive gait.

THE NEUROLOGIC EXAMINATION

"Disease of the peripheral nervous system stands as one of the most difficult subjects in neurol-

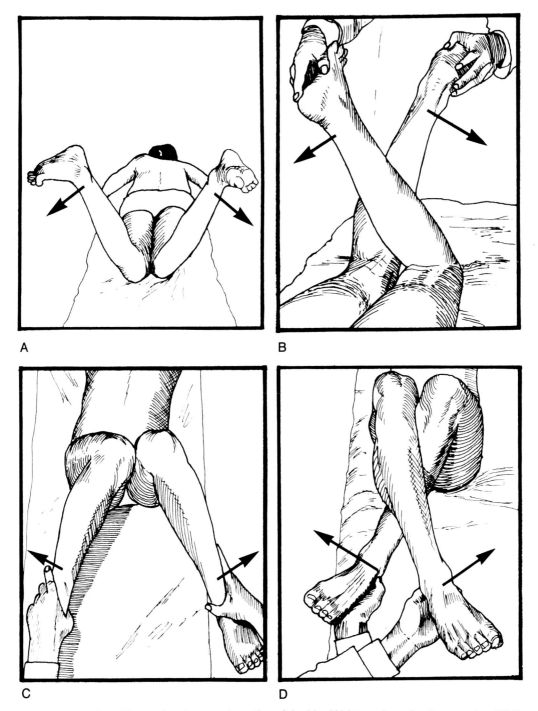

A

B

C

D

Fig. 4-8. Examination of internal and external rotation of the hip. **(A)** Internal rotation in extension. **(B)** External rotation in extension. **(C)** Internal rotation at 90 degrees flexion. **(D)** External rotation at 90 degrees flexion. (From McRae,[9] with permission.)

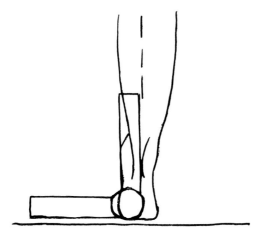

Fig. 4-9. Measurement of the amount of tibial varum.

ogy."[15] Therefore, it is not surprising that the lengthy and seemingly complex neurologic examination is often the most intimidating for the novice to perform and interpret. Inability or reluctance to perform an adequate examination may result in failure to detect neurologic disease. Developing an orderly and methodical examination ensures thoroughness and keeps both the patient's and the examiner's effort to a minimum. The information gathered through a comprehensive history and examination may be sufficient for diagnosis. More sophisticated testing such as electromyography, nerve conduction velocity, and nerve or muscle biopsy should only be performed with a specific purpose in mind, as they are expensive and time consuming for the patient. The results of these procedures do not give a specific clinical diagnosis but only aid in diagnosis. Therefore, these procedures should be used only to gain information otherwise unobtainable that will help to clarify the clinical problem.[16]

An understanding of the basic organization of the nervous system into upper and lower motor neurons will provide important leads to the neurologic diagnosis. The examiner must be familiar with the functions carried in the ascending and descending tracts and the final common pathway of the peripheral nervous system in order to correctly interpret the findings of the examination and determine the nature and location of any disease. Whatever is being tested, the examiner should try to form a mental picture both of the pathway that a particular sensation follows from the site of stimulation and of the relationship of that pathway to neighboring nervous structures.

The extent of the examination is directed by the chief complaint, but includes muscle, reflex, and sensory testing. Additional and perhaps repeated testing is warranted in the following situations:

1. Trophic changes of the nails or skin (hyper- or hypohidrosis, discoloration, increased or decreased hair growth) or trophic or malperforans ulcers.
2. Specific presenting neurologic complaint (pain, numbness, paresthesias, or weakness) or a family history of neurologic complaint or neurologic disease.
3. Metabolic disease or deficiency, such as diabetes mellitus, hypothyroidism, or alcoholism, that affects the peripheral nervous system; muscle atrophy or Charcot-type joint changes.

Muscle Testing

Examination of muscle requires thorough knowledge of anatomic origins and insertions and muscle actions. The lower limbs are examined for muscle actions, muscle size, tone, involuntary movements, and strength. As with all parts of the physical examination, one inspects, palpates, and compares with the opposite limb.

Muscle Size

Muscle size varies considerably with age, sex, body type, nutritional state, occupation, and athletic activity.[17] Muscle wasting or atrophy accompanies disuse and is also characteristic of a number of lower motor neuron disorders, including amyotrophic lateral sclerosis, peroneal muscular atrophy, Aran-Duchenne atrophy, and Wohfart-Kugelberg-Welander disease.[18,19] Muscle hypertrophy, an increase in muscle size or bulk, is found with prolonged repetitive exercise and in some forms of myopathy.[20] If indicated, measurements may be made to compare the limbs. However, small differences in size may only reflect asymmetric development, which is not uncommon in the calf muscles.[17]

Muscle Tone

Tone is the slight resistance offered by a resting limb to passive movement.[14] The examiner should test muscle tone by passive range of motion of the joints and note the resistance offered to movement. Spasticity, or hypertonia, points to a lesion somewhere along the course of the corticospinal pathway.[20] Flaccidity, or hypotonia, occurs where there is injury or disease of the anterior horn cells or their axons.[21]

Involuntary Movements

The examiner should note the presence or absence of involuntary movements such as tics, tremors, athetosis, or choreic movements.[22] Fasciculations are seen as twitches in a resting muscle as the result of an involuntary contracture of muscle fibers of a motor unit. These intrinsic muscle movements may be seen through the skin and occur in certain disorders of the lower motor neuron such as amyotrophic lateral sclerosis and progressive spinal muscle atrophy. However, benign fasciculations may occur in normal persons, particularly in the calves and hands.[23]

Muscle Strength

Muscle power is graded as shown in Table 4-1.

The ability to assess muscle strength properly is gained through repeated testing of weak and strong patients to learn the limits of normality. The generally preferred method of testing is to have the patient resist pressure exerted by the examiner. This method is easy for the patient to understand and therefore ensures better cooperation. Pressure should be applied slowly and smoothly and gradually increased to a maximum.[17]

The strength of dorsiflexion and plantar flexion at the ankle is tested by asking the patient to pull up

Table 4-1. Grading of Muscle Strength

Grade	Response
5	Normal power; movement against gravity and full resistance
4	Movement against gravity and partial resistance
3	Movement against gravity
2	Movement with gravity eliminated
1	Slight contraction; no movement
0	No contraction

and push down, respectively, against the examiner's resistance. These movements may also be tested by asking the patient to walk on the heels and on the toes. Similarly, the patient is asked to invert and evert the foot against resistance to test the muscles controlling these movements. Unless there is demonstrated weakness, this testing of muscle groups is adequate to assess muscle power about the foot and ankle. In certain instances, testing of individual muscles may be necessary to isolate an area of weakness. When testing isolated muscles it is important to be able to recognize compensation by other muscles that perform the same movements. Therefore, it is necessary to palpate as well as observe the muscle and its tendon.[17]

Reflex Testing

The important deep tendon reflexes to be tested in the lower extremity are the patellar and Achilles tendon reflexes. A deep tendon or myotatic reflex is elicited by sharply striking an already partially stretched tendon. A reflex arc is completed when the suddenly stretched muscle sends a signal to the spinal cord via a sensory nerve fiber. There is synapses with an anterior motor neuron, and a signal is transmitted via the motor fiber back to the original muscle.[24] The examiner should also check for the presence of pathologic reflexes and ankle clonus.

To test the deep tendon reflexes, the examiner should tell the patient to relax and not to aid in the examination. The patient must also be properly positioned so that the muscle is under a mild stretch. The tendon is struck briskly with the small end of a reflex hammer. If reflexes are absent or diminished, reinforcement is used by having the patient lock the fingers and pull one hand against the other while the examiner attempts to elicit a reflex. This is known as Jendrassik's maneuver. It may be helpful to distract the patient.

Reflexes are usually graded as shown in Table 4-2. One should remember, however, that hyperactivity in the presence of a normal plantar response is considered a normal finding.

Patellar Reflex

To elicit the patellar reflex (L2–L4 and the femoral nerve), the patient may either be seated with

Table 4-2. Grading of Reflexes

Grade	Response
4+	Hyperactive (often characteristic of disease; associated with clonus)
3+	Brisk (may be normal but suggestive of disease)
2+	Average (normal)
1+	Diminished (low normal)
0	Absent; no response

the legs hanging loosely or supine with the examiner's arm supporting the flexed knee and the heel resting lightly on the table.[12] The patellar tendon is located by palpation and struck briskly just below the patella.

Achilles Reflex

The Achilles reflex (S1–S2, tibial nerve) is elicited with the patient seated by slightly dorsiflexing the ankle and striking the Achilles tendon with a reflex hammer. It may be elicited with the patient supine by flexing the limb at the hip and the knee and rotating it externally so that it rests across the opposite shin. Again, the examiner dorsiflexes the ankle and strikes the Achilles tendon. Alternatively, the patient may kneel on a chair with the feet and ankles hanging over the edge.

The clinical significance of absent or hyperactive reflexes must be interpreted in light of the findings of the complete neurologic examination. Abnormal responses are most significant when found only on one side. Absent or diminished reflexes may result from an interruption in the reflex arc at the level of the anterior horns, the anterior roots, the peripheral nerves, or the posterior roots. Exaggerated reflexes occur with lesions of the corticospinal tracts. Rarely, normal individuals are found who are areflexic or who demonstrate hyperactivity, including sustained clonus.[17]

Plantar Response

Along with hyperactive reflexes, pathologic reflexes are also seen with disease of the corticospinal tracts. The Babinski sign, or extensor plantar response, consists of extension of the great toe and fanning (flexion and abduction) of the lesser toes. When this sign is present it almost always signifies disease of the central nervous system. However, this response may also be elicited in normal infants up to 6 months of age, in the intoxicated or sleeping adult, or after a generalized seizure.[21]

The patient should be positioned with the knee slightly flexed and the thigh externally rotated. The plantar response is elicited by lightly stroking the lateral aspect of the plantar surface of the foot from the heel to the metatarsal head area and then medially across the ball.

Too much pressure will cause a voluntary withdrawal, which may be confused with a Babinski response. When the results are equivocal or the sole is very sensitive, there are several other methods of obtaining the plantar reflex (Table 4-3). Each has the same significance as the Babinski response but is less reliable.

Ankle Clonus

Ankle clonus may also be elicited in patients with hyperactive reflexes. The examiner supports the knee with one hand in a partially flexed position and with the other hand sharply dorsiflexes the patient's foot. Clonus appears as rhythmic oscillations between dorsiflexion and plantar flexion. Sustained clonus indicates upper motor neuron disease, but a quickly exhaustible clonus may be normal.[19]

Table 4-3. Methods of Eliciting Pathologic Reflexes in the Lower Extremity

Reflex	Stimulus	Response
Babinski	Stroking of the lateral edge of the plantar surface of the foot	Extension of the hallux and fanning of the lesser toes
Chaddock	Stroking of the lateral aspect of the foot below the fibular malleolus	Babinski-like
Oppenheim	Firm, almost painful downward stroking of the tibia starting at the knee	Babinski-like
Gonda	Flexion followed by sudden release of the third or fourth toe	Dorsiflexion of the hallux
Schäffer	Squeezing of the Achilles tendon	Babinski-like
Gordon	Firm compression of the calf muscle	Babinski-like

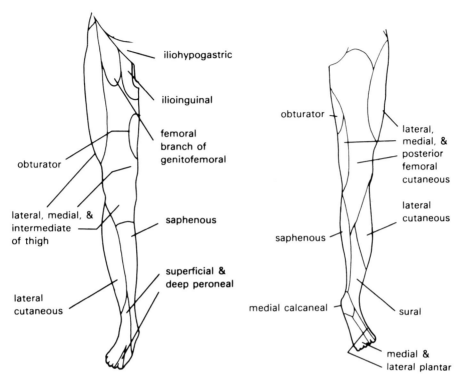

Fig. 4-10. Innervation by the sensory nerves. (Modified from Romero-Sierra C: Neuroanatomy: A Conceptual Approach. Churchill Livingstone, New York, 1986, with permission.)

Sensory Testing

Sensory testing is one of the most difficult and time-consuming parts of the neurologic examination. The patient's response to a stimulus is often difficult for the examiner to evaluate objectively. In addition, the testing presumes cooperativeness, alertness, and a certain level of intelligence on the part of the patient.[25]

It is important to conduct a thorough but efficient examination to avoid testing to the point of fatigue, when the patient's responses may become unreliable. It is better to retest at the next visit than engage in prolonged testing. A clear explanation and demonstration of the test should also be given so the patient knows what is expected of him or her. The patient should be instructed to close the eyes during the testing and to respond with a simple "yes" or "sharp" or "dull" every time he or she perceives the stimulus. One always compares sensation in symmetric areas on both lower extremities.

A basic screening examination of sensation,

when no deficit is suspected, includes sensation of light touch, pain, vibration, and position. Sensation is classified as either superficial (light touch, pain, and temperature) or deep (deep pressure and pain, position sense, passive motion, and vibration).[25]

The ability to interpret altered or decreased sensation requires a basic knowledge of the distribution of innervation by sensory nerves and dermatomal patterns (Figs. 4-10 and 4-11). Although cutaneous innervation may vary slightly from person to person, the basic pattern is relatively constant. Patterns of dermatomes are also variable, and it is not necessary to memorize their exact details as there is considerable overlap.

When testing reveals regions of abnormal superficial sensation, the borders of such regions should be mapped out on the skin and then recorded in a chart.[17] Abnormalities of sensation are described as analgesia (complete absence of sensitivity to pain), hypalgesia (diminished sensitivity to pain), hyperalgesia (increased sensitivity to pain), anesthesia (complete loss of sensation, especially pain), hypesthesia (decreased sensitivity to stimuli), hyper-

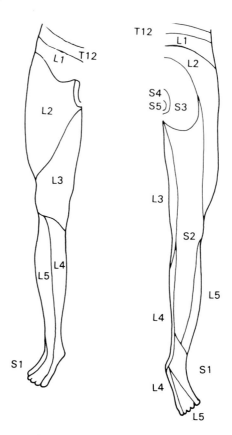

Fig. 4-11. Dermatomal patterns. (Modified from Romero-Sierra C: Neuroanatomy: A Conceptual Approach. Churchill Livingstone, New York, 1986, with permission.)

esthesia (increased sensitivity to stimuli), and paresthesia (abnormal or perverted sensation, such as burning, prickling, or formication).[26]

Light Touch

The patient's ability to perceive light stroking of the skin is tested. The fibers that carry this superficial sensation ascend in both the opposite ventral spinothalamic tract and the dorsal fasciculi of the same side. Light touch is tested by a wisp of cotton, with which the examiner covers all dermatomes in a random, unpredictable order to prevent anticipation of the stimulus.[17] The thick skin of the soles will require a heavier stimulus and the hairy areas a lighter one.[25] The patient is instructed to respond "yes" when the stimulus is perceived.

Superficial Pain

Both superficial and deep pain, along with temperature, ascend in the lateral spinothalamic tract. As with light touch, this test should be conducted in seemingly random fashion using the head and the pointed end of a sterile pin or needle. After a brief demonstration, the patient should be instructed to answer quickly either "sharp" or "dull" upon feeling the touch of the pin. The pinpricks should be delivered no more rapidly than one per second, or the effects may be summated and excessive pain may result.[25] The patient should be informed that he or she may change the answer if necessary. This instruction will help to uncover delayed pain appreciation, which can be found in the legs of those with peripheral neuritis or tabes dorsalis.[17]

Vibration

Vibratory sense is a composite sensation of touch and rapidly alternating deep pressure.[25] This form of temporally modulated tactile sensation ascends in both the posterior and the lateral funiculi.[21] It is important to demonstrate the sensation of vibration by placing the tuning fork on the bony prominence of the wrist or the forehead if necessary. The patient is instructed to respond "yes" upon feeling a "buzzing" and then inform the examiner when it stops. This is done to make sure the patient is responding to the vibration and not just to pressure. Testing is initiated distally at the interphalangeal or the metatarsophalangeal joint of the hallux. If there is no impairment, more proximal parts are omitted.[8] It is advisable to begin with a silent control, as persons with peripheral neuritis and combined system disease may have a constant tingling in the feet and legs.[25] The length of time that the patient feels the vibration is noted. If the patient no longer feels the vibration while the fork is still in motion, the fork is quickly moved to the opposite limb for comparison. Symmetry of any deficit is important. There is diminution of vibratory sense with increasing age, and over the age of 50 there may be some deficit. After age 65 some deficit at the ankles is common. This decrease due to aging should be relatively symmetrical.

Position Sense

Position sense and appreciation of passive movement are carried in the dorsal fasciculi, and tested in the lower extremities by passive vertical movements of the toes, which the patient must determine as either up or down. So that the patient cannot use pressure on the skin as a clue to the direction of the movements, the examiner should grasp the toe firmly by the sides. The examiner demonstrates with large movements and then tests for the smallest detectable change.[18]

Position sense can be tested further by asking the patient to stand with the feet together, first with the eyes open and then with the eyes closed. Although even the normal patient may sway slightly with the eyes closed, a conspicuous difference in balance with the eyes open and closed constitutes a positive Romberg's sign.[25]

Gait may be evaluated by having the patient open the eyes and walk naturally, then in tandem heel-to-toe fashion. The examiner notes the smoothness of movement and whether there is ataxia or tremor.

ACKNOWLEDGMENT

The assistance of Dr. Marcia Bienenstock in the preparation of this chapter is gratefully acknowledged.

REFERENCES

1. Prior JA, Silberstein JS: Physical Diagnosis. CV Mosby, St Louis, 1963
2. Health Assessment Handbook. Springhouse Corp, Springhouse, PA, 1985
3. Abramson D: Circulatory Problems in Podiatry. Karger Basel, Switzerland, 1985
4. Bernstein EF, Fronek A: Current status of noninvasive tests in the diagnosis of peripheral arterial disease. Surg Clin North Am 62:468, 1982
5. Lennihan R Jr, Mackereth M: Ankle pressures in arterial occlusive disease involving the legs. Surg Clin North Am 53:657, 1973
6. Bernstein E (ed): Noninvasive Diagnostic Techniques in Vascular Disease. CV Mosby, St Louis, 1978
7. Wilson RC: Clinical diagnostic tests in podiatric medicine. Can Podiatrist (October):6, 1979
8. Bates B: A Guide to Physical Examination. 2nd Ed. JB Lippincott, Philadelphia, 1979
9. McRae R: Clinical Orthopaedic Examination. 2nd Ed. Churchill Livingstone, Edinburgh, 1983
10. McCarty DJ: Differential diagnosis of arthritis; analysis of signs and symptoms. p 36. In McCarty DJ (ed): Arthritis and Allied Conditions. 9th Ed. Lea & Febiger, Philadelphia, 1979
11. Mann RA: Principles of examination of the foot and ankle. p 31. In Mann RA (ed): Surgery of the Foot. 5th Ed. CV Mosby, St Louis, 1983
12. Root ML, Orien WP, Weed JH, et al: Biomechanical

Examination of the Foot. 1st Ed. Vol. 1. Clinical Biomechanics Corp, Los Angeles, 1971

13. Wernick J, Langer S: A Practical Manual for a Basic Approach to Biomechanics. Vol. 1. Langer Acrylic Laboratory, New York, 1972

14. Tax HR: Podopediatrics. 2nd Ed. Williams & Wilkins, Baltimore, 1985

15. Adams RD, Asbury AK: Diseases of the peripheral nervous system. p 2156. In Petersdorf RG, Adams RD, Braunwald E, et al (eds): Harrison's Principles of Internal Medicine. 10th Ed. McGraw-Hill Book Co, New York, 1983

16. Adams RD, Chiappa KH, Martin JB, et al: Diagnostic methods in neurology. p 2010. In Petersdorf RG, Adams RD, Braunwald E, et al (eds): Harrison's Principles of Internal Medicine. 10th Ed. McGraw-Hill Book Co, New York, 1983

17. Mayo Clinic and Mayo Foundation, Department of Neurology and Department of Physiology and Biophysics: Clinical Examinations in Neurology. 3rd Ed. WB Saunders, Philadelphia, 1971

18. Richardson EP, Adams RD: Degenerative diseases of the nervous system. p 2118. In Petersdorf RD, Adams RD, Braunwald E, et al (eds): Harrison's Principles of Internal Medicine. 10th Ed. McGraw-Hill, New York, 1983

19. Chusid JG: Correlative Neuroanatomy and Functional Neurology. 6th Ed. FA Davis, Philadelphia, 1971

20. Alpers BJ, Mancall EL: Clinical Neurology. 6th Ed. FA Davis, Philadelphia, 1971

21. Carpenter MB: Core Text of Neuroanatomy. 2nd Ed. Williams & Wilkins, Baltimore, 1978

22. Walton JN: Brain's Diseases of the Nervous System. 8th Ed. Oxford University Press, New York, 1977

23. Young RR, Bradley WG, Adams RD: Approach to clinical myology. p 2169. In Petersdorf RG, Adams RD, Braunwald E, et al (eds): Harrison's Principles of Internal Medicine. 10th Ed. WB Saunders, Philadelphia, 1971

24. Guyton AC: Textbook of Medical Physiology. 6th Ed. WB Saunders, Philadelphia, 1981

25. Victor M, Adams RD: Disorders of sensation. p 113. In Petersdorf RG, Adams RD, Braunwald E, et al (eds): Harrison's Principles of Internal Medicine. 10th Ed. WB Saunders, Philadelphia, 1971

26. Dorland's Medical Dictionary, Shorter Edition. W.B. Saunders, Philadelphia, 1980

Radiographic and Other Diagnostic Methods

5

Gerald A. Gorecki, D.P.M., M.P.H.

The computer has made it possible to see much that was heretofore invisible. Computer-generated pictures allow multidimensional views of organs, often revealing warning signs of occult disease and obviating exploratory surgery. This new vision is made possible by the processing of a staggering amount of digital data.

Many of these new computerized techniques are costly, and their usefulness in certain organ systems is not clear. However, many will eventually prove advantageous, and will have indications for use in the lower extremities. This chapter presents a cursory view of the scientific background of medicine's new "eyes," to allow podiatric physicians to visualize the indications for the lower extremities. Some of the traditional diagnostic instruments are also presented. It must be pointed out that these "new" technologies will most likely become standard clinical tests by the time this text is printed.

COMPUTED TOMOGRAPHY

Since Roentgen's discovery of x-rays in 1895, radiologic images have been displayed in a two-dimensional (planar) format on either emulsion film or a cathode ray tube (CRT).[1] The continuous-tone two-dimensional radiograph provides useful information, but the superimposition of images in different planes often produces a problem of interpretation when one attempts to envision a three-dimensional representation of an anatomic structure.[2]

In computed tomography (CT) a computer is used to reconstruct a complete cross-sectional body plane or reformatted planar image (Figs. 5-1 and 5-2) from multiple x-ray absorption measurements taken about the body's periphery.[2] Thus, the digital computer made possible a quantum leap in the evolution of radiologic imaging.[3] Information is now available for the computer reconstruction of anatomic structures in three dimensions.[1,4,5,6] One of the most exciting applications of three-dimensional CT imaging is in the field of reconstructive surgery, as milling machines use CT data to reconstruct plastic models of various anatomic areas. With these models, rehearsal surgery may be performed to determine the precise size of replacement parts such as implants and bone grafts. The most likely use for these models will be in the rearfoot, the ankle, the hip, the spine, and the skull.[4,5,6]

Most important for podiatry has been the application of the knowledge gained from CT to the ankle joint. CT has been predicted to have value in three areas[4]: (1) three-dimensional images should

129

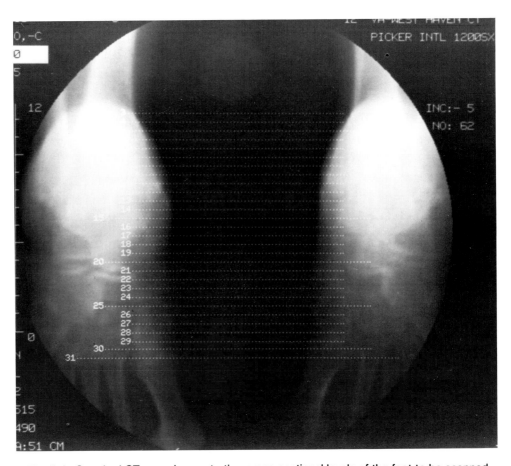

Fig. 5-1. Standard CT scan demonstrating cross-sectional levels of the foot to be scanned.

improve the physician's ability to diagnose conditions affecting the ankle joint, such as intra-articular or osteochondral fractures; (2) complex osteotomies or other surgical procedures may be planned preoperatively by preparation of solid models of the bones and performing rehearsal surgery on the models; and (3) custom bone implants such as plates or joint replacement prostheses may be manufactured through a computer-aided design/manufacturing (CAD/CAM) system using the exact three-dimensional anatomy to determine design and size requirements.

Woolson has pointed out that the limitations of this technology relate largely to metallic scatter artifact; until CT algorithms that eliminate metallic artifact are developed, scanning of bones adjacent to large metallic implants will not yield good three-dimensional images.[4]

MAGNETIC RESONANCE IMAGING

Magnetic resonance imaging (MRI) has created considerable excitement in the medical field because of its ability to diagnose and characterize many different disease processes. Many studies have been published on the diagnostic use of MRI in such organ systems as skeletal muscle, the brain, the liver, and the cardiovascular system, as well as

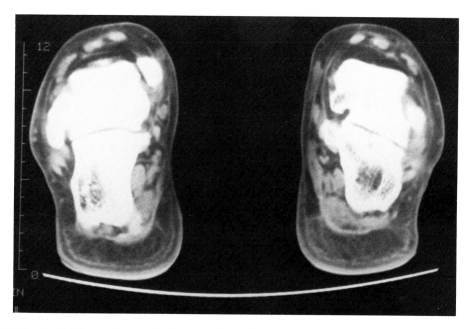

Fig. 5-2. Standard CT scan demonstrating nonunion of an attempted subtalar joint fusion in the left foot.

in oncological diagnosis.[7] MRI is now at an evolutionary stage, and it may be that not all of the high expectations it has aroused will be met, especially regarding the possible applications to podiatry. Nevertheless, it is worthwhile to describe its basic principles, applications, and current limitations so as to allow each podiatric physician to determine its potential usefulness to the lower extremities.

Nuclear magnetic resonance (NMR) was first demonstrated independently by Purcell et al. and by Bloch and colleagues.[7-9] The first spatially oriented, nonbiologic magnetic resonance image was produced by Lauterbur in 1973.[10] Essentially, NMR is the absorption and reemission of radiofrequency electromagnetic energy by certain nuclei when placed in a magnetic field. Since nuclei have a unit of electrical charge, they have a magnetic field or moment. This naturally occurring magnetic field allows the use of an external magnetic field to manipulate the nuclei, producing NMR. The stable iostopes of hydrogen, phosphorus, and carbon are capable of displaying resonance. The physics involved in MRI, such as the production of macroscopic magnetic moments or magnetization, polarization of magnetic nuclei, signal, pulse sequences,

and image acquisition, as well as instrumentation (types of magnets), site planning, installation, and other considerations have been thoroughly described by Johnston and colleagues.[11]

Because MRI is similar to CT scanning in identifying structural disorders, and because it is more costly and difficult to use than CT, the usefulness of MRI must be judged against that of CT before MRI can become an accepted investigative tool. At present, MRI has demonstrated diagnostic superiority over CT in a limited number of important, mostly neurologic disorders, and is complementary to CT in the diagnosis of certain other disorders.[11] For most of the remaining organ systems its usefulness is not clear, but the absence of ionizing radiation and the ability of MRI to produce images in any tomographic plane may eventually prove advantageous. Sierra and colleagues have reported on a case of avascular necrosis of the talus after trauma.[12]

The potential hazards of MRI relate to the effects of the static magnetic field, radiofrequency heating effects, and the effects of currents induced either by rapidly switched magnetic field gradients or by movement through the magnetic field.[7] This certainly presents a danger to patients with cardiac pacemakers or implanted ferrous objects (screws, plates, etc.); however, there is as yet no verified evidence of any detrimental effects of a static magnetic field.

SINGLE PHOTON EMISSION COMPUTED TOMOGRAPHY

Single photon emission computed tomography (SPECT) is being used with increasing frequency in nuclear medicine. It is performed with the use of rotating gamma cameras. Initial problems were encountered in the interfacing of computers and software from one company with gamma cameras from other companies; today, however, every manufacturer of SPECT equipment provides both the computer and the software for the imaging studies. SPECT has been used to image practically every radiopharmaceutical available. Its potential best use is expected to be with technetium-99m-labeled radiopharmaceuticals that reflect blood flow or metabolic function in such organs as the brain, heart, liver, lung, and bone.[12]

The potential use of SPECT in podiatric medicine will be in bony structures, since SPECT produces excellent images where there is substantial superimposition of bones.[13] To date, bone studies using SPECT have mainly involved patients with suspected disease of the hips, lumbar spine, temporomandibular joints, or facial bones.[13] Bone SPECT was found to be the most sensitive noninvasive test for evaluating the extent of arthritis in 27 patients with chronic knee pain examined by conventional radiography, bone scanning, and subsequent arthroscopy.[13]

Collier and colleagues evaluated conventional radiography, arthrography, SPECT, and planar bone imaging in 36 patients with temporomandibular joint dysfunction who were undergoing preoperative evaluation.[14] SPECT imaging had a 94 percent sensitivity, comparable to that of arthrography (96 percent) and much better than planar bone imaging (76 percent) or lateral radiography (4 percent). Bone SPECT imaging appears to be a

very sensitive method for evaluating patients with internal derangement of the temporomandibular joint, and thus could prove to be a very useful diagnostic tool for midtarsal and rearfoot pathology.

BONE SCANNING

The science of nuclear medicine began in the early 1900s but did not progress rapidly until the mid-1930s, when Hevesy successfully used radiophosphorus for the study of metabolism in healthy patients.[15] The development of bone scanning began in the 1940s and early 1950s with the use of calcium-45 and strontium-89 for studying bone metabolism. This was followed in the 1960s by the use of calcium-47, strontium-85, strontium-87 m, and fluorine-18.[15] Since the advent of 99m-technetium-labeled phosphorus-containing compounds (Fig. 5-3), gallium-67 citrate (Fig. 5-4), indium-111, and thallium-201 in the 1970s, diagnoses have become increasingly accurate.

Scintigraphy has many indications, including the staging of malignant bone disease, differentiating of monostotic from polyostotic disease, and differentiating of pain that is not clearly nonskeletal in origin (especially ill-defined or diffuse pain). It is also useful in the study of metabolic bone disorders, viability of bone, skeletal trauma (including stress fractures), osteomyelitis, the arthritides, vascular bony hyperemia secondary to inflammation, thrombophlebitis, sympathectomy, osteomyelitis, and congenital developmental disorders, as well as infection of the lung and kidney and several other nonmalignant and inflammatory lesions (thyroiditis, Duchenne muscular dystrophy, and renal amyloidosis). It can also be used to predict ischemic ulcer healing, especially of the foot.[15-17]

Bone scintigraphy for infection is most widespread in podiatric medicine and certainly is not a new concept. However, the debate continues as to whether idium-111-labeled white blood cells (WBC), gallium-67, or technetium-99m-MDP scintigraphy (Figs. 5-5 to 5-7) is more accurate in the diagnosis of bone infections.[18,19] Certainly the literature is replete studies of with sequential tech-

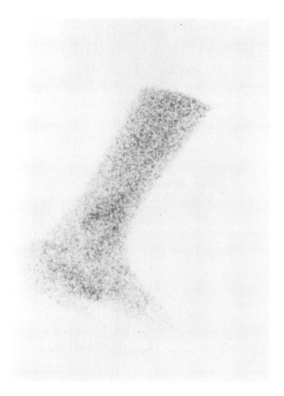

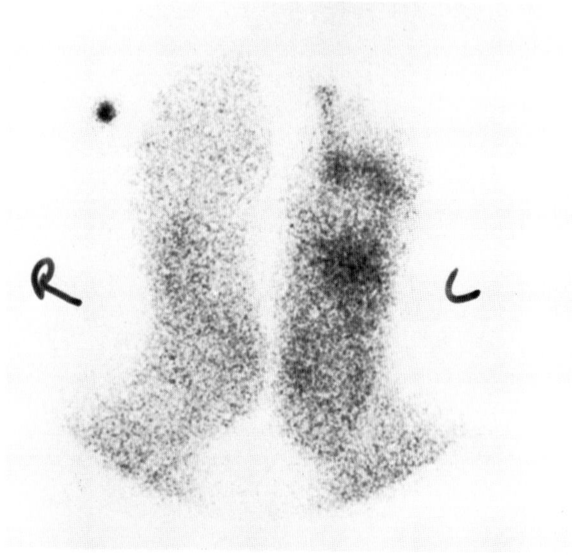

Fig. 5-4. Twenty-four-hour plantar gallium-67 scan compatible with osteomyelitis of the left hallux and first metatarsal head. (Courtesy of L Soldano, M.D., Veterans Administration Medical Center, West Haven, CT.)

Fig. 5-3. Technetium-99m-MDP scan demonstrating nonperfusion of the distal left foot, clinically compatible with dry gangrene. (Courtesy of L Soldano, M.D., Veterans Administration Medical Center, West Haven, CT.)

netium-gallium imaging; however, indium-111 WBC scintigraphy may prove to be superior and may replace sequential technetium-gallium imaging.[19] Further clinical and laboratory investigation into the specificity and accuracy of each technique is warranted.

tic technique is performed the podiatric physician may be alerted to the possibility that their patient's children could have congenital or other deformities or anomalies, as clubfoot often may be a component of neuromuscular disorders, skeletal dysplasias, or karyotypic abnormalities. This may prove to be a possible indication for amniocentesis if clubfoot is identified.[24] One then may be prepared to treat or assist in treating significant congenital deformities.

ULTRASONOGRAPHY

Ultrasonography (ultrasound) is a diagnostic procedure most often associated with the field of obstetrics, and it is within this context that 35 cases of antenatal sonographic diagnoses of club foot have been described.[20-24] Although not all pregnant women who are podiatric patients are candidates for diagnostic ultrasound, when this diagnos-

THE LIXISCOPE

The lixiscope is essentially a portable x-ray fluoroscope (the name is in part an acronym for *l*ow *i*ntensity *x*-ray *i*maging). It was originally conceived by Yin and Seltzer for use in x-ray astronomy where single-photon imaging is required[25,26] (Fig. 5-8). Its high sensitivity and high gain permit a reduction in the amount of radiation compared to certain standard diagnostic fluoroscopic proce-

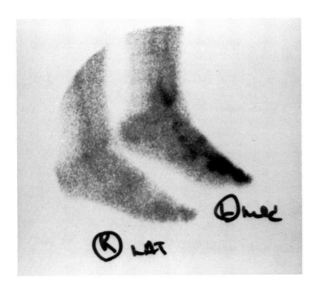

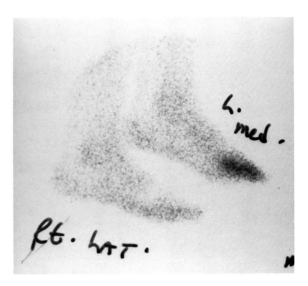

Fig. 5-5. Technetium-99m-MDP scan compatible with osteomyelitis of the left hallux and first metatarsal head. (Courtesy of L Soldano, M.D., Veterans Administration Medical Center, West Haven, CT.)

Fig. 5-6. Forty-eight-hour gallium-67 scan of the patient in Figure 5-5, demonstrating less intense activity in the first metatarsal ray of the left foot. (Courtesy of L Soldano, M.D., Veterans Administration Medical Center, West Haven, CT.)

dures. The lixiscope produces a visible light image, which can be recorded on fast instant processing films or other devices such as a video recorder.

The radioactive point source is iodine-125, which emits about 28 keV x-rays.[26,27] The photons generated by the radioactive isotope are collimated to strike a scintillator screen; an x-ray image is formed by the differential attenuation of the body's tissues. The x-ray image is then converted to visible light. The scintillator screen is located outside the vacuum envelope of a high-gain microchannel plate (MCP) visible light image intensifier and is made of fiberoptics to prevent image degradation and to enhance the ruggedness of construction.[27] The visible light image is converted to an electron image by a photocathode. Several additional technical steps occur whereby ultimately the fiberoptic output plate displays an intensified image on the output surface of the MCP. The image intensifier is powered by two C-size alkaline batteries.

The lixiscope is a low-dose, compact, rugged, and fully portable x-ray intensifier system for use in laboratory and clinical settings (Figs. 5-9 and 5-10) and in the field. The unit is autoclavable and is therefore useful in the operating room for evaluating procedures involving osteotomies, metallic fix-

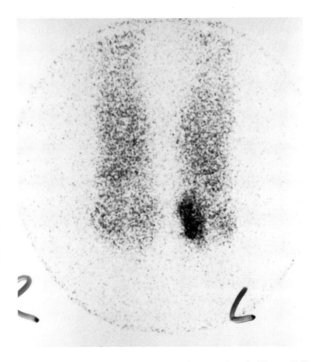

Fig. 5-7. Indium-111 WBC scan of the patient in Figure 5-5, compatible with osteomyelitis of the left hallux. (Courtesy of L Soldano, M.D., Veterans Administration Medical Center, West Haven, CT.)

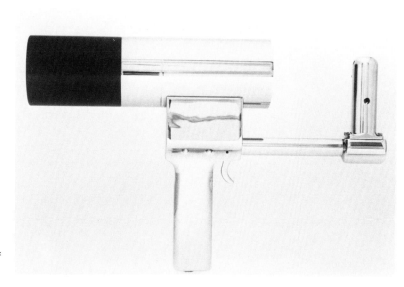

Fig. 5-8. Lixi Imaging Scope. (Courtesy of Lixi, Inc., Downers Grove, IL.)

ation, internal fixation, implants, foreign body removal, or minimal incision surgery.[26] In sports medicine, the examination can be performed on the playing field or in the field house to ascertain the presence of fractures or dislocations.[27] The lixiscope facilitates the internal fixation of fractures in the emergency room, especially when percutaneous fixation devices are used or open reduction, further reduction, or additional internal fixation devices are needed.[27]

PERIPHERAL VASCULAR ANALYSES

Noninvasive tests in peripheral arterial occlusive and venous diseases offer the podiatrist a valuable supplement to subjective clinical assessment, which can be difficult and sometimes unreliable.[28] A clinical technique for noninvasive arterial visualization was first introduced in 1971 by Mozersky and colleagues and was termed "ultrasonic arteriography." This technique produced noninvasive images of carotid, iliac, femoral, and popliteal vessels.[29] In principle, the Doppler technique tests the blood's velocity and direction at a given location but cannot be used to determine flow volume, which is a function of the cross-sectional area of the

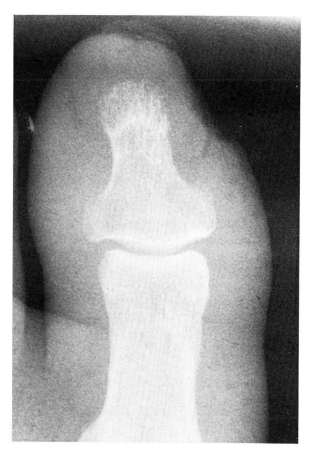

Fig. 5-9. Standard dorsoplantar radiograph of the left hallux with medial ulcerative erosion of the soft tissue. (From Gorecki et al.,[26] with permission.)

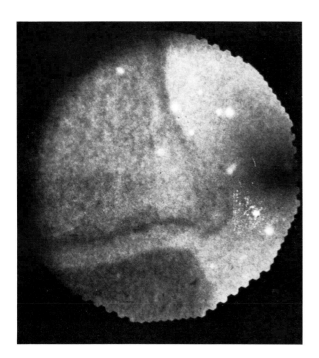

Fig. 5-10. Polaroid photograph of the left hallux through the lixiscope demonstrating medial erosion of the base of the proximal phalanx consistent with osteomyelitis. (From Gorecki et al.,[26] with permission.)

mine segmental systolic blood pressures, allowing for the localization of arterial stenosis. In 1970, Yao introduced the ankle/brachial index, which is the ratio of the brachial systolic pressure to the ankle systolic pressure. This index may be useful in determining healing abilities in the foot and ankle.[30]

Another noninvasive test of interest to the podiatric practitioner is a simple physiologic index of tissue perfusion, the transcutaneous oxygen tension ($TCPO_2$). $TCPO_2$ may be used together with Doppler systolic pressure measurements to improve diagnostic accuracy (Figs. 5-11 and 5-12).

$TCPO_2$ is measured by means of electrodes which detect oxygen molecules diffused through the skin. $TCPO_2$ measurements in the lower extremities may be made on the anteriomedial aspect of the calf, the dorsum of the foot, the anterior aspect of the thigh, and in proximity to any lesions.

vessel. The velocity and direction in simplest terms are determined by the use of a probe with two crystals, one of which transmits a spectrum of ultrasonic impulses (frequencies) while the other receives the impulses. The time lag from transmission to reception is directly related to the velocity of blood flow within the lumen. Many variables may interfere with the signal frequency, such as the incident angle of the ultrasonic beam, changes in cross-sectional diameter of the vessels, variations in blood viscosity, edema, excessive fibrosis, and calcific deposits. The addition of an oscilloscope allows one to visually interpret the waveform created by the pulse of moving blood. Such interpretation is less prone to error than the interpretation of characteristic sounds, which is limited by examiner experience and auditory acuity. The normal arterial waveform is triphasic, whereas the normal venous waveform is monophasic. Venous signals are also characteristically lower in pitch and are not related to heart rate.

The Doppler technique may be used to deter-

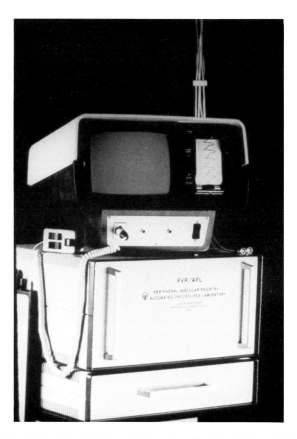

Fig. 5-11. The Peripheral Vascular Registry/Automated Procedures Laboratory (PVR/APL). (Courtesy of Life Sciences, Inc., Greenwich, CT.)

These measurements are compared to measurements from the chest to arrive at an index.[28]

Although a clear advantage of $TCPO_2$ has been reported in some cases, other hemodynamic tests such as Doppler, ultrasound, photoplethysmography, and angiography should also be implemented and may aid in the anatomic location of disease.[28] For instance, hemodynamic tests may detect mild disease in cases where $TCPO_2$ is still normal. $TCPO_2$ measurements may also be limited and influenced by edema, hyperkeratosis, cellulitis, and obesity, all of which can reduce thermal conductivity, capillary flow, and therefore the transmission of oxygen.[28]

Angiography is the radiographic visualization of the arterial tree by the injection of a contrast medium. It remains an essential preliminary step in the planning of revascularization procedures (Fig. 5-13). Wagner described the angiogram as a "road map" for delineating areas of occlusion, the degree of collaterization, the degree of damage to the traumatized artery, and areas of aneurysmal dilation.[31] Wagner further pointed out that angiography is not without some hazards and complications,

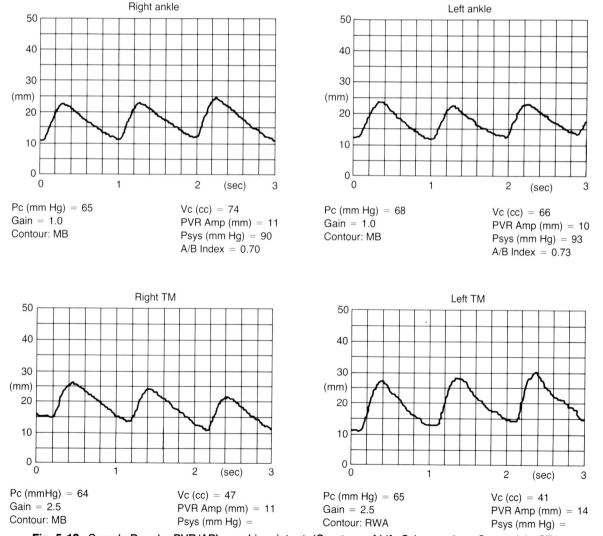

Fig. 5-12. Sample Doppler PVR/APL graphic printout. (Courtesy of Life Sciences, Inc., Greenwich, CT.)

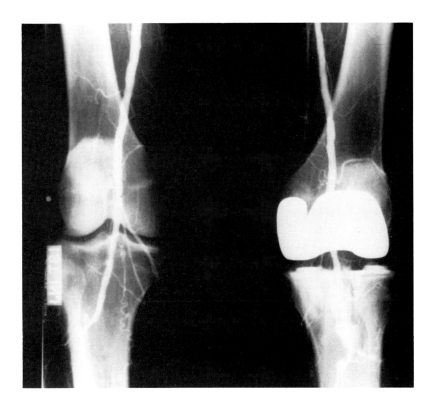

Fig. 5-13. Arteriogram demonstrating occlusion of major vessels into the leg with poor collateral flow and runoff.

such as allergic response to the medium, local extravasation of the medium, injury to the arterial wall, thrombosis, infection at the injection site, bleeding, vasospasm, and renal failure.[31] The podiatric practitioner must therefore have a thorough understanding of both noninvasive and invasive diagnostic methodologies in dealing with the peripheral circulation on a daily basis and recognizing vascular pathology.

XERORADIOGRAPHY

Xerography, first developed by Carlson in 1937, is based on the principle of photoconductivity, whereby combining a photoconductor (selenium), electrostatic charges, and light exposure produces a permanent image.[32] Xeroradiography is the recording of x-ray images obtained with a standard roentgenographic camera by the xerographic process rather than by the photochemical one used in conventional roentgenography.

Xeroradiography uses standard x-ray equipment and special xerographic equipment developed by the Xerox Corporation. The xeroradiographic plate consists of an aluminum sheet with a thin layer of the photoconductor, vitreous selenium, which is held in a protective cassette to shield it from exposure to ambient light. This plate is then inserted below a high-voltage wire, establishing a voltage potential, which results in a positive electrostatically charged surface. The plate is then exposed to conventional x-rays, resulting in a discharge on the photoconductor. The discharge is proportional to the tissue densities in the anatomic part traversed by the x-rays, producing a pattern of the part being examined. The plate is then specially processed to produce a powder image on the plate surface, which is then transferred to a plastic-coated paper and fixed by heat to provide a permanent record. The plates may be reused after treatment by a special conditioner-processor developed by Xerox (125 Xeroradiographic System). The white-appearing areas on a conventional radiograph appear deep blue on the xeroradiographic image, whereas other densities of the film appear between white and light blue.

There are many applications of xeroradiography, such as identification of the borders of masses (edge enhancement) and fractures (Fig. 5-14), especially hairline cortical fractures; visualization of trabecular patterns (Fig. 5-15), soft tissue damage, joint effusions, hematomas, and the biceps, gastrocnemius, and achilles tendons (Fig. 5-16); detection of most nonmetallic foreign bodies; and visualization of joint replacement prostheses.[32]

Tenography

Tenography (tenosynoviography) is a diagnostic modality whereby a radiopaque contrast medium (dye) is injected into a tendon sheath and provides a permanent radiographic record for assessing the extent of soft tissue pathology.[34] The introduction of the contrast material into the tendon sheath should be performed in less than 7 days, as an organized hematoma may seal a pathologic region and result in inaccurate assessments. This test is not without risks; however, adverse reactions are reported in fewer than 5 percent of cases.[35] Reinherz

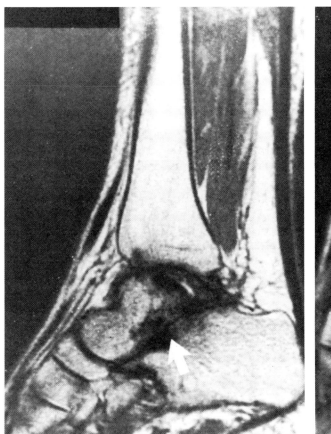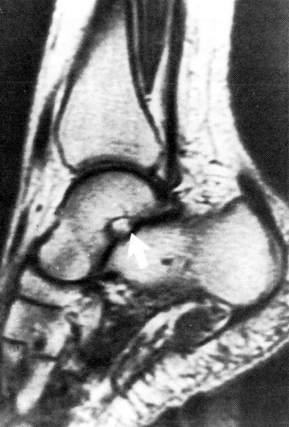

Fig. 5-14. Xeroradiograph of an osteocartilaginous body within the subtalar joint secondary to trauma. (Courtesy of C Jones, D.P.M., Chicago, IL).

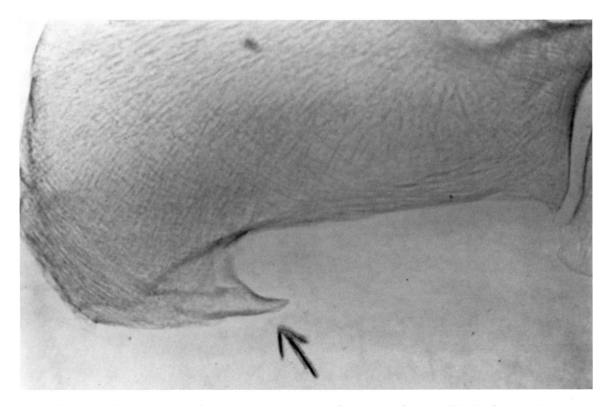

Fig. 5-15. Xeroradiograph of a plantar calcaneal spur. (Courtesy of C Jones, D.P.M., Chicago, IL.)

and colleagues have pointed out a variety of indications for tenography; these include abnormalities within tendon complexes (e.g., lipoma), peroneal tenosynoviography for calcaneofibular ligament pathology, evaluation of status after trauma (adhesions, tendons trapped beneath fractures, hypertrophic bone healing, etc.), inflammatory tendon conditions (rheumatoid arthritis, gout, etc.), and mechanical stress factors.[34] Tenosynoviography is thus a valuable adjunct in assessing and identifying soft tissue pathology about the ankle.

In the standard procedure, the appropriate tendon is identified, a 20 to 25 gauge needle is used to inject 4 to 25 ml of contrast medium mixed with local anesthetics to alleviate postprocedural pain. The needle is advanced into the tendon sheath until resistance from the tendon is felt. Sometimes saline is injected first until flow proceeds smoothly, and then the dye is injected. Reinherz and colleagues have advocated the following technique, which adds little risk while improving the accuracy of sheath penetration: A linear 1.0-cm incision is made over the tendon, followed by a stab incision in the dorsum of the sheath. A 19 gauge lumbar/caudal-epidural catheter with stylet is inserted as far distally as possible, and the dye is infiltrated.[34]

ARTHROGRAPHY

Arthrography was first introduced by Wolff in 1940.[36] As applied in the ankle, it consists of the injection of a radiopaque dye via a 22 to 25 gauge needle after scrubbing the ankle with iodophor solution. After the joint is entered, serosanguinous fluid is removed, and 1 to 5 ml of a local anesthetic is injected to reduce postprocedural pain. This is followed by injection of a commercially available radiopaque dye.[36,37] Anteriorposterior, lateral, and oblique x-ray films are taken immediately, with additional anteroposterior views taken with the ankle

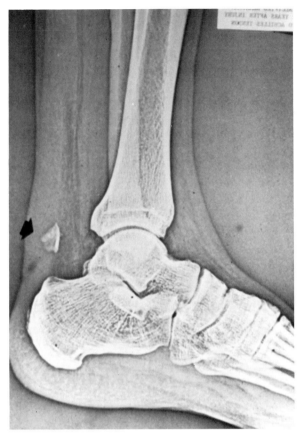

Fig. 5-16. Xeroradiograph of a calcified mass in the Achilles tendon. (Courtesy of C Jones, D.P.M., Chicago, IL.)

in forced inversion and supination. A normal ankle arthrogram reveals no extravasation of dye except for occasional filling of the tendon sheaths of the flexor hallucis longus and/or the flexor digitorum longus (20 percent) and the peroneal tendons (14 percent).[36] All other extravasations are considered pathologic.

In a rupture of the distal tibiofibular ligaments, contrast medium may penetrate proximally into the tibiofibular joint, but this finding is considered normal as long as the dye does not cross the proximal margin of the ankle mortise and extravasate between the tibia and the fibula above this level.[36] Complete rupture of the deltoid ligament occurs rarely, with the anterior portion mostly affected, and will demonstrate massive extravasation of contrast medium about the medial malleolus.[36] Rup-

tures of the anterior talofibular ligament demonstrate extravasation of dye around the tip of the distal tibia and up along the fibula and usually present with a dye-free zone between the tibiofibular syndesmosis and the extra-articular accumulation.[36] No dye-free zone occurs with ruptures of the tibiofibular ligaments, allowing for a differentiation between the two conditions when massive extravasation of contrast medium is present.

Calcaneofibular ligament ruptures are invariably associated with anterior talofibular ruptures and demonstrate similar extension of contrast medium about the fibular tip. Posterior talofibular ligament rupture is rare and is associated with rupture of the other two lateral ankle ligaments.[36]

ANKLE ARTHROSCOPY

The value of arthroscopy in the diagnosis and treatment of knee disorders is well established, but ankle arthroscopy was considered impractical until the development of the small-bore arthroscope (1.7 mm diameter with a cannula diameter of 2.2 mm) in 1970 by Watanabe.[38-41] The more recent literature expounds on the usefulness of ankle arthroscopy. Five portals of entry are recognized. Ankle arthroscopy differs from knee arthroscopy principally in that it requires higher pressure to distend the joint capsule and vigorous joint manipulation and distraction to obtain adequate visualization.[40]

The major intra-articular structures that may be visualized are the distal tibia, the tibial and fibular malleolus, the talar dome, the tibiofibular synovial recess and fringe, the anterior and posterior talofibular ligaments, the anterior tibiotalar ligament, the anterior ankle capsule, and the synovial lining.[39] Areas that have been found difficult to visualize include the trochlear talar surface and the distal tibiofibular articulation, as well as potentially the anterior and posterior talofibular ligaments.[38]

Indications for ankle arthroscopy include osteochondritis dissecans of the talus, post-traumatic or degenerative ankle arthritis, persistent undiagnosed synovitis, osteochondral bodies (loose bodies), rheumatoid arthritis, tophaceous gouty arthritis, preoperative evaluation of the unstable ankle, adhesive capsulitis, osteochondral fractures, persistent undiagnosed pain, and intra-articular adhesions.[38,41] The major contraindications are local or systemic infections and acute inflammation of the joint (rheumatoid, gouty, or pseudogout attacks). The presence of joint prostheses and ankylosis are relative contraindications.[40,41] Possible and reported complications of ankle arthroscopy are extravasation of fluid into the soft tissue, instrument breakage, damage to the extra-articular neurovascular structures, infection, and iatrogenic joint damage.[38,40,41]

Arthroscopic instrumentation consists of the optical system (telescope, fiberoptic cables, etc.), a light source, and an irrigation system.[40,41] The procedure is performed under strict aseptic technique in an operating room (inpatient or outpatient) and may or may not require the use of a tourniquet. Details of specific techniques are presented in many journal articles as well as in textbooks. Undoubtedly, a major factor in the successful use of ankle arthroscopy is the surgeon's experience and knowledge of the ankle's anatomy.[40,41]

Electrodiagnosis

The electrodiagnosis of neuromuscular disorders is primarily made by electromyography (EMG) and electroneurography (ENG; also called nerve conduction velocity [NCV] studies). These studies provide information about the motor and sensory portions of the peripheral nervous systems.

EMG of skeletal muscle can be compared with electrocardiography, which uses surface electrodes to detect the electrical activity of the cardiac muscle. In EMG, a needle electrode is inserted directly into the muscle to provide the degree of sensitivity needed to record the often low amplitude action potentials. The electrical activity of the muscle fibers may be amplified electronically and displayed on a cathode ray oscilloscope, projected through a loudspeaker, stored on magnetic tape, or recorded on light-sensitive paper.[42] Standard text-

books describe the specific techniques for different muscles. Essentially, the muscle is examined in four different stages of activity: during the insertion of the electrode, at complete rest, during a minimal contraction of the muscle, and during maximal contraction.[42]

NCV studies provide information primarily about the myelination of the fastest conducting myelinated fibers. They measure the latency of motor nerve conduction, which is the time from stimulation of a nerve to the evoked muscle response to the onset of the first negative deflection of the response. The NCV is obtained by stimulating several points along a nerve, measuring the distance between these stimulation points (proximal and distal latency), and dividing by the differences in latencies. In addition to the latency, the shape, amplitude, and duration of the evoked response should be noted, as any or all of these parameters may be necessary to make an accurate diagnosis.[42]

The primary clinical applications fall into two broad classifications: those diseases primarily affecting the Schwann cell and the myelin sheath (with the axon remaining relatively intact), and those affecting the axon.[42] Most neuropathies tend to be predominantly of one type or the other, although some show characteristics of both. Some examples are isoniazid and nitrofurantoin toxicity and porphyria.[42] Demyelinating neuropathies (diabetes, Guillain-Barré syndrome, lead poisoning, diphtheria, etc.) are another category of clinical neuropathies. A third category consists of those diseases that predominantly affect the interstitial connective tissue of nerve. These include leprosy, amyloidosis, Charcot-Marie-Tooth disease, Déjérine-Sottas disease, and Friedreich's ataxia.[42] The last category of neuropathies, those that are traumatic in origin, includes neuropraxia, axonotmesis, and neurotmesis. Each has different prognoses and different diagnostic criteria. The anterior horn cell disease of most importance to podiatrists is poliomyelitis, although amyotrophic lateral sclerosis is the most common, occasionally presenting with complaints involving the foot (foot-drop and ankle instability).

The most important entrapment syndromes known to podiatrists are the tarsal tunnel syndrome and the traumatic neuroma (Morton's neuroma). When a specific etiology can be identified, tarsal tunnel syndrome is most commonly the result of fracture, dislocation, or chronic ligamentous strain; however, rheumatoid arthritis, diabetes mellitus, gout, and myedema have also been implicated as causative factors.[43]

In 1979, a technique called near-nerve sensory nerve conduction was introduced, which used surface electrodes as the recording electrodes and ring electrodes to stimulate the first and fifth toes.[44] This technique improved the diagnostic sensitivity of the terminal latency from 54 percent to 90.5 percent of cases, and thus provided a superior method of diagnosing this nerve compression syndrome.[44,45] This technique also allowed for the recording of sensory compound nerve action potentials orthodromically in the interdigital nerves of the foot and for confirming the diagnosis of interdigital neuropathy (Morton's neuroma) electrophysiologically.[46]

Electrodynography

Electrodynography (EDG) is a method of recording, organizing, quantifying, and displaying, via graphic waveforms, electronically acquired data concerning sequential vertical forces exerted at discrete segmental points on the soles of the feet. It was solely conceived by Langer and developed by podiatric physicians.[47-49] Polchaninoff is considered the father of the Electrodynogram System (Langer Biomechanics Group, Deer Park, NY).[47] The development of EDG allowed the opportunity to determine the degree of structural aberration or deformity in the feet and legs by using commonly defined, neutral position reference points when making static measurements or segmental motions and positions.[47] While the EDG was technologically a concept, the force plate was the state-of-the-art apparatus for measuring forces; however, it still possessed the following disadvantages[47]: foot forces were represented as averages as opposed to discrete segmental forces, force values were measured between the shoe and the plate, and force plates were permanently mounted.

Thus, the following considerations for a technical foot force data acquisition system were considered essential[47]:

1. Force sensors required the capability of registering certain segments and discrete location signals.
2. Signals had to be individually calibrated and quantified with regard to force amplitude, time of occurrence, duration and cessation of force, and time of occurrence of peak force.
3. Force sensors had to be comfortable, hygienic, and nonrestricting, and have no influence on gait.
4. Force/time data had to be accurate, reliable, and reproducible within acceptable parameters.

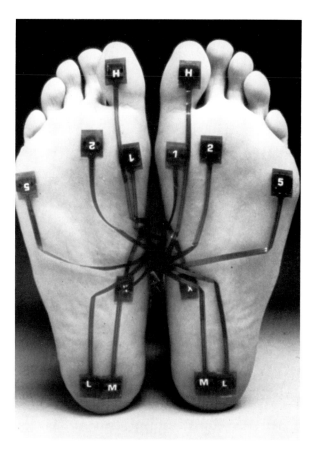

Fig. 5-17. EDG 1184 sensors in place. (Courtesy of the Langer Biomechanics Group, Inc., Deer Park, NY.)

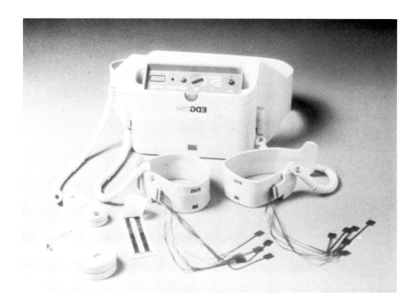

Fig. 5-18. EDG 1184 assembly. (Courtesy of the Langer Biomechanics Group, Inc., Deer Park, NY.)

5. Patients had to be able to wear any kind of shoes during data acquisition.
6. Force/time data had to be obtainable on any surface and at any time of the day.
7. Force/time data had to be capable of being placed in commonly understood clinical contexts.

EDG data may be used to diagnose aberrant biomechanical functions of the legs and feet[47] (Fig. 5-17). Thus, clinical EDG represents a major tool in the diagnostic and therapeutic armamentarium of practitioners engaged in the analysis of foot and gait function, including the surgeon, the rehabilitation specialist, the physical therapist, researchers, academicians, and specialists in diabetic and vascular disease (Figs. 5-18 and 5-19).

The principles of EDG and techniques of EDG clinical examination and data analysis are discussed in detail elsewhere.

A clear implication of this review of diagnostic techniques is that computers have significantly enhanced the techniques of medical diagnosis and will continue to do so, enabling medical personnel to make better and more comprehensive judgments. Many of these new diagnostic devices are

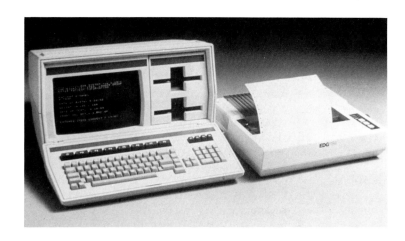

Fig. 5-19. EDG 1184 data processor and printer. (Courtesy of the Langer Biomechanics Group, Inc., Deer Park, NY.)

costly, however, and their use in the extremities has yet to be clearly defined. It is up to the profession itself to determine the future of these new diagnostic instruments in the practice of podiatry.

REFERENCES

1. Woolson ST, Dev P, Fellingham L, Vassiliadis A: Three dimensional imaging of bone from computerized tomography. Clin Orthop 202:239, 1986
2. Melincoff R: Computerized tomography: the "CT" scanner. J Am Podiatry Assoc 70:161, 1980
3. Hounsfield GN: Computerized transverse axial scanning. Br J Radiol 46:1016, 1973
4. Woolson ST, Dev P, Fellingham L, Vassiliadis A: Three-dimensional imaging of the ankle joint from computerized tomography. Foot Ankle 6:2, 1985
5. Viraponge C, Shapiro M, Gmitro A, Sarwar M: Three-dimensional computed tomographic reformation of the spine, skull, and brain from axial images. Neurosurgery 18:53, 1986
6. Viraponge C, Gmitro A, Sarwar M: The spine in 3D-computed tomographic reformation from 2D axial sections. Spine 11:513, 1986
7. Chan L: The current status of magnetic resonance spectroscopy–basic and clinical aspects. West J Med 143:773, 1985
8. Bloch F, Hansen W, Packard M: Nuclear induction. Phys Rev 69:127, 1946
9. Purcell E, Torrey H, Pound R: Resonance absorption by nuclear magnetic moments in a solid. Phys Rev 70:460, 1946
10. Lauterbur P: Image formation by induced local interactions: examples employing nuclear magnetic resonance. Nature 242:190, 1973
11. Johnston D, Liu P, Wismer G, et al: Magnetic resonance imaging: present and future applications. Can Med Assoc J 132:765, 1985
12. Sierra A, Potchen E, Moore J, Smith H: High-field magnetic resonance imaging of aseptic necrosis of the talus. J Bone Joint Surg 68A:927, 1986
13. Coleman R, Blinder R, Jaszczak R: Single photon emission computed tomography (SPECT), part II, clinical applications. Invest Radiol 21:1, 1986
14. Collier B, Carrera G, Messer E, et al: Internal derangement of the temporomandibular joint. Detection by single-photon emission computed tomography. Radiology 149:557, 1983
15. Clark W, Fann T, McCrea J, Venson J: Uses of bone scanning in podiatric medicine. J Am Podiatry Assoc 68:621, 1978
16. Hoffer P: Gallium infection. J Nucl Med 21:484, 1980
17. Ohta T: Noninvasive technique using thallium-201 for predicting ischemic ulcer healing of the foot. Br J Surg 72:892, 1985
18. Al-Sheikh W, Sfakianakis G, Mnaymneh W, et al: Subacute and chronic bone infections: diagnosis using In-111, Ga-67 and Tc-99mMDP bone scintigraphy and radiology. Radiology 155:501, 1985
19. Merkel K, Brown M, Dervanjee M, Fitzgerald R: Comparison of indium-labeled-leukocyte imaging with sequential technetium-gallium scanning in the diagnosis of low-grade musculoskeletal sepsis. J Bone Joint Surg 67A:465, 1985
20. Miskin M, Rothberg R, Rudd N, et al: Arthrogryposis multiplex congenita: prenatal assessment with diagnostic ultrasound and fetoscopy. J Pediatr 95:463, 1979
21. Chervenak F, Tortora M, Hobbins J: Antenatal sonographic diagnosis of clubfoot. J Ultrasound Med 4:49, 1985
22. Hashimoto B, Filly R, Callen P: Sonographic diagnosis of clubfoot in utero. J Ultrasound Med 5:81, 1986
23. Benacerraf B, Frigoletto F: Prenatal ultrasound diagnosis of clubfoot. Radiology 155:211, 1985
24. Benacerraf B: Antenatal sonographic diagnosis of congenital clubfoot: a possible indication for amniocentesis. J Clin Ultrasound 14:703, 1986
25. Yin L, Seltzer S: The lixiscope. A pocket size x-ray imaging system (NASA Technical Memorandum 78064). National Aeronautics and Space Administration, Greenbelt, MD
26. Gorecki G, Weisman S, Kidowa A: Lixiscope. A podiatric evaluation. J Am Podiatry Assoc 72:304, 1982
27. Van Pelt B, Plevak J: The lixiscope: a portable x-ray fluoroscope. Nuclear Instruments and Methods in Physics Research A242:531, 1986
28. Cina C, Katsamouris A, Megerman J, et al: Utility of transcutaneous oxygen tension measurements in peripheral arterial occlusive disease. J Vasc Surg 1:362, 1984
29. Mozersky D, Baker D, Strandness D: Ultrasonic arteriography. Arch Surg 103:663, 1971
30. Yao S: Haemodynamic studies in peripheral arterial disease. Br J Surg 57:761, 1970
31. Wagner F: The dysvascular foot: a system for diagnosis and treatment. Foot Ankle 2:76, 1981
32. Winiecki D, Biggs E: Xeroradiography and its appli-

cation in podiatry. J Am Podiatry Assoc 67:393, 1977

33. Campbell C, Roach J, Jabbur M: Xeroroentgenography: Evaluation of uses in diseases of the bones and joints of the extremities. J Am Bone Surg 41A:271, 1959

34. Reinherz R, Zawada S, Sheldon D: Tenography around the ankle and introduction of a new technique. J Foot Surg 25:357, 1986

35. Shehadi W, Toniolo G: Adverse reactions to contrast media. Diag Radiol 137:288, 1980

36. Stepanuk M: Arthrography of the ankle joint in the diagnosis of acute ankle sprains. J Am Osteopath Assoc 76:528, 1977

37. Zang K: Traumatic Ankle Conditions. Futura, Mt. Kisco, NY, 1976

38. Drez D, Guhl J, Gollehon D: Ankle arthroscopy: Technique and indications. Foot Ankle 2:138, 1981

39. Lundeen R: Arthroscopic anatomy of the anterior aspect of the ankle. J Am Podiatry Assoc 75:367, 1985

40. Aldrich M, Arenson D: Ankle joint evaluation—an overview of arthroscopic technique. J Foot Surg 24:349, 1985

41. Lubell J, Fallot L: Ankle joint arthroscopy. J Foot Surg 25:128, 1986

42. Reischer M, Delagi E: Electrodiagnosis. p 68. In Jahss M (ed): Disorders of the Foot. WB Saunders, Philadelphia, 1982

43. Kuritz H, Sokoloff T: Tarsal tunnel syndrome. J Am Podiatry Assoc 65:825, 1975

44. Oh S, Sarala P, Kuba T, Elmore R: Tarsal tunnel syndrome: electrophysiological study. Ann Neurol 5:327, 1979

45. Oh S, Kim H, Ahmad B: The near-nerve sensory conduction in tarsal tunnel syndrome. J Neurol Neurosurg Psychiatry 48:999, 1985

46. Oh S, Kim H, Ahmad B: Electrophysiological diagnosis of interdigital neuropathy of the foot. Muscle Nerve 7:218, 1984

47. Langer S: Welcome to the future—electrodynography. Langer Biomechanics Newsletter 10:1, 1982

48. Langer S, Polchaninoff M, Hoerner E: Principles and Fundamentals of Clinical Electrodynography. Langer Biomechanics Group, Deer Park, NY, 1982

49. Polchaninoff M: Gait analyses using portable, microprocessor-based segmental foot force measurement system. In Proceedings of the Seventh Annual Symposium on Computer Applications in Medical Care. IEEE Computer Society Press, Silver Spring, MD, 1983

Sensory Evaluation

John J. Holewski, D.P.M.
Lee E. Wentworth, Ph.D.

The majority of neurologic disorders associated with the lower extremity involve poor or abnormal sensation, gait disorders, and certain neuropathies. Although this chapter concentrates on the anatomy, physiology, and evaluation of the somatosensory system, it is important to remember that sensory and motor functions are interdependent at all levels of the nervous system, from the peripheral nerves to the cerebral cortex, and that impairment of sensation can affect all aspects of motion — volitional, reflex, postural, tonic, and phasic.

The somatosensory systems are organized to receive, process, and relay stimulus information. They consist of serial chains of neurons extending from the periphery to the spinal cord, the brain stem, the thalamus, and the cerebral cortex. Knowledge of the structure, function, and distribution of sensory receptors in the skin and deeper structures; the organization and distribution of peripheral nerves and spinal roots; and the pathways by which sensory impulses are conveyed centrally through the spinal cord and brain stem to the thalamus and cerebral cortex is necessary to evaluate and understand sensory dysfunction. Symptoms and signs of sensory dysfunction reflect deficits due to failure at some level along the sensory channel from the receptor to the decoding regions in the brain. The neuron has a stereotypical reaction to injury; therefore, localization of the lesion generally will help establish the differential diagnosis.

SPINAL AND PERIPHERAL NERVES

Distribution

Dorsal and ventral roots attach to the spinal cord by a series of filaments. The roots penetrate the dura to reach the intervertebral foramen, where the dorsal root enlarges to enclose the dorsal root ganglion, containing the cells of origin for the dorsal root afferent fibers. The dorsal and ventral roots unite distal to the ganglion to form a mixed spinal nerve, or common nerve trunk, containing both afferent (sensory) and efferent (motor) fibers. Each spinal nerve divides into four branches, meningeal ramus, a ramus communicans, and a dorsal and a ventral primary ramus. The ventral rami innervate the limbs and the ventrolateral part of the body wall.

147

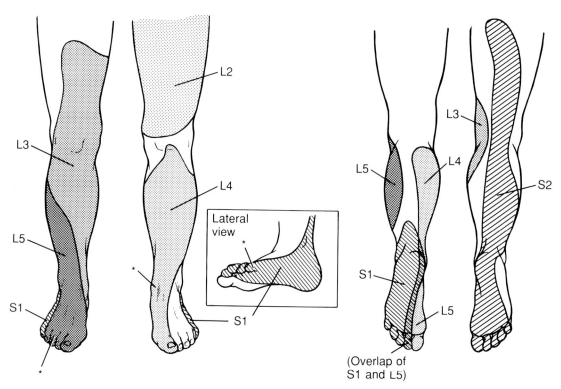

Fig. 6-1. Degree of overlap in the segmental and dermatomal innervation of the lower extremity. Asterisked sites represent autonomous zones, which can be used for sensibility measurements for the fourth and fifth lumbar and first sacral nerve roots. (From Foerster.[3])

In the cervical and lumbosacral regions, the ventral rami intermingle and form plexuses from which the major peripheral nerves emerge. Thus, the peripheral nerves generally contain fibers derived from more than one ventral ramus. Because of this mixing, the segmental or dermatomal maps indicating peripheral areas of the limbs innervated by individual dorsal roots do not correspond to the cutaneous maps indicating areas innervated by peripheral nerves (Figs. 6-1 and 6-2). (*Segmental* refers to the spinal cord segment with which the spinal roots connect, whereas *dermatomal* refers to the area of skin innervated by the sensory fibers of a single dorsal root.) There is some overlap, so that a region of skin will usually be innervated by parts of three adjacent roots. Complex dermatomal maps have been drawn, based on physiologic experimentation and the study of neurologic disorders and surgical sections of spinal roots and nerves. However, the maps are not identical; differences result from individual variation, overlap, and dif-

ferences in method. Variation can result from intersegmental rootlet anastomoses adjacent to the cervical and lumbosacral spinal cord,[1] and from individual differences in plexus formation and peripheral nerve distribution.[2]

The dermatome maps in Figure 6-1 show the degree of overlap in adjacent dermatomes. These maps are based on Foerster's studies[3,4] of a large number of human patients by a combination of methods, and have been found to be clinically useful.[2,5] The three asterisked sites added to Figure 6-1 are selected as autonomous zones for the dermatomes supplied by the fourth and fifth lumbar and first sacral nerve roots.[6] They are consistently depicted as being innervated by these nerve roots on dermatomal diagrams developed by the most widely accepted authorities.[3,7] The cutaneous maps in Figure 6-2 depict a general innervation pattern based on dissections of nerves in the lower extremity and do not show the degree of overlap or variations that exist. (For further discussion on

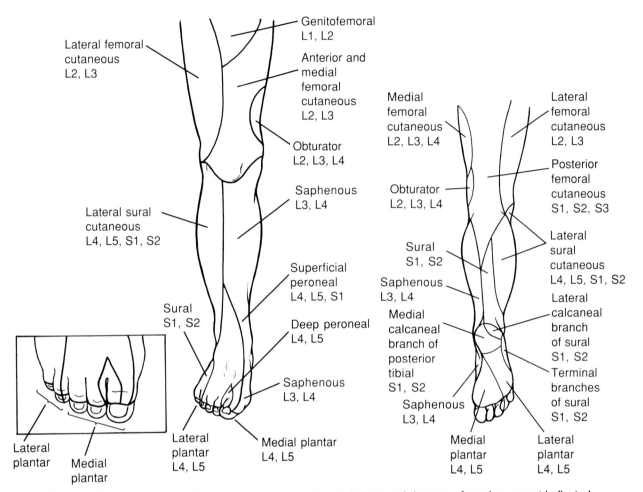

Fig. 6-2. Cutaneous innervation of the lower extremity. Variations and degrees of overlap are not indicated.

variations in innervation patterns in the lower extremity, see refs. 8–12.)

It is important to realize that the maps depict presumably normal distribution. Spinal cord sensitivity may be altered by root sections in such a way as to affect the size of the dermatome being tested by peripheral stimulation.[2] Cutaneous nerve maps are similar to dermatome maps only in the trunk, and there is less overlap in the peripheral nerve distribution than in the spinal nerves. Peripheral nerves vary in their course and distribution, and adjacent nerves may interact with each other.[13,14] This may account for unexpected residual sensation or movement after section of a nerve. If a peripheral nerve is cut, the muscles supplied by the nerve are greatly weakened or completely paralyzed, autonomic dysfunction occurs, and sensa-

tion is lost in the central part of the area of distribution of the peripheral nerve and diminished at the edges because of overlap of adjacent peripheral nerves. Also, several peripheral nerves pass through osteofibrous canals, where they may be subjected to compression. Smorto and Basmajian[15] have summarized the chief sites of compression and discuss related literature.

Nerve Fiber Classifications

There are two major classifications of nerve fibers, based on fiber diameter, conduction velocity, threshold to electrical stimulation, nature of the electrical record, and type of nerve being studied. One classification, initially proposed by Erlanger and Gasser,[16] is based on the conduction speeds in frogs' nerves. It includes motor and sensory fibers and categorizes nerve fibers into three groups. The large, heavily myelinated, and fastest conducting A group is subdivided into α, β, and γ subgroups. In mammals an Aδ subclass of fibers is added containing fibers which are not finely myelinated preganglionic autonomic fibers, but are similar to the B fibers in conduction velocity. The C fibers are unmyelinated and have the slowest conduction velocities. In mammals, approximately 75 percent of axons in cutaneous and dorsal spinal nerves are unmyelinated, as are 50 percent in muscle nerves and 30 percent in ventral spinal nerves.[17]

Lloyd[18] proposed a classification based on a study of dorsal root afferents; thus it is used only with sensory fibers. The myelinated fibers are divided into three groups: I for large, heavily myelinated fibers; II for moderately myelinated fibers; and III for thinly myelinated fibers. The nonmyelinated fibers form group IV (Tables 6-1 and 6-2).

The conduction velocity of a fiber has important clinical significance. Whereas an Aβ fiber conducting at 50 m/sec conveys information to the central nervous system (CNS) in 0.02 second, a noxious input carried by a C fiber conducting at 0.5 m/sec can take 2 seconds or more to carry information to the CNS, and this time delay can result in tissue damage before the CNS can process the information.

CENTRAL PATHWAYS FOR AFFERENT IMPULSES

The Dorsal Column-Medial Lemniscal System

There are two major pathways for the conscious perception of somatosensory stimuli: the anterolateral system and the dorsal column-medial lemniscal system. The central processes of primary or first-order neurons of the larger myelinated afferents (Aα and Aβ groups) conduct via the ipsilateral dorsal columns somatotopically, with sacral fibers running medial to more rostral levels. These fibers synapse somatotopically in one of the dorsal column nuclei of the caudal medulla, with fibers for the lower body synapsing in the nucleus gracilis, and fibers for the upper body synapsing in the nucleus cuneatus. Second-order neurons of the dorsal column nuclei project their axons across the midline to ascend in the contralateral medial lemniscus to the ventral posterior lateral nucleus (VPL) of the thalamus. VPL neurons project their axons through the posterior limb of the internal capsule to terminate somatotopically in the somatosensory cortex (postcentral gyrus). The distinguishing feature of this dorsal column-medial lemniscal system is that information concerning location, quality, shape,

Table 6-1. Classification of Peripheral Nerve Fibers

Sensory and Motor Fibers	Sensory Fibers	Fiber Diameter (μm)	Conduction Velocity (m/sec)	Functional Classification	
Myelinated					
Aα	Ia	12–20	70–120	Motor:	Extrafusal motor (α motoneurons)
				Sensory:	Primary afferents of muscle spindle (Ia)
	Ib			Sensory:	Golgi tendon organs
Aβ	II	6–12	30–70	Motor:	Fusimotor collaterals of α motoneurons
				Sensory:	Flower spray of muscle spindle; mechanoreceptors
Aγ		2–8	10–50	Motor:	Intrafusal motor (γ motoneurons)
Aδ	III	2–6	4–30	Sensory:	First pain (fast, pricking pain); cold
B		<3	3–30	Motor:	Preganglionic autonomic
Unmyelinated					
C	IV	0.2–1.5	0.3–2	Motor:	Postganglionic autonomic
				Sensory:	Second pain (slow, burning pain), temperature

Table 6-2. Characteristics of Myelinated and Unmyelinated Fibers

Fiber	Local Anesthetic Sensitivity	Electrical Excitability	Reaction to Pressure Block
Thickly myelinated	Low	High	Early
Unmyelinated	High	Low	Late

and temporal sequence of stimuli is transmitted with great fidelity at each synaptic site along the pathway.[19]

The Anterolateral System

The anterolateral system is composed of separate ascending pathways that together play a major role in pain and temperature sense and only a minor role in touch and proprioception. This system is different from the dorsal column-medial lemniscal system in that it is phylogenetically older and less precise; it has a large component of uncrossed ascending fibers, and crossing occurs in the spinal cord instead of the brain stem; the cells of origin for the anterolateral system are located in the dorsal horn and are postsynaptic to primary afferents, whereas the fibers in the dorsal columns are mostly collaterals of primary afferents. The anterolateral fibers terminate throughout the brain stem as well as in the thalamus. The anterolateral system contains three major pathways, classified on the basis of their site of termination, and two of these are concerned with the transmission of pain sensations. The fibers of the spinothalamic tract mediate fast pain sensations relayed from the periphery by Aδ fibers. The spinothalamic fibers terminate in the ventral posterolateral nucleus of the thalamus, as do those of the medial lemniscus. The spinoreticular tract mediates slow pain sensations via C fibers from the periphery and terminates on neurons in the reticular formation of the brain stem, which relay information rostrally to nuclear groups in the thalamus and to the periaqueductal gray matter of the midbrain. Neurons in the thalamus then project to the cortex.

These two somatosensory systems are examples of parallel sensory pathways, each serving somewhat different but overlapping functions. This par-

allel organization is important clinically, because if only one pathway is damaged, residual sensory capabilities can still be processed by the remaining pathway. In addition to these pathways for conscious perception, information about the stimulus is passed directly, or indirectly via interneurons, to motor neurons for reflex response, or unconsciously to other supraspinal centers such as the cerebellum.

SENSORY RECEPTORS

The peripheral sensory receptors are concerned with transducing various forms of energy into neuronal activity. This activity, if it is of sufficient intensity, results in the discharge of nerve impulses whose pattern and frequency constitute the neural code, which is interpreted by the CNS as a sensory experience. Natural stimuli are complex and generate neural activity that is fractionated into separate sensory channels by the filtering properties of the receptors. "Sensation is an abstraction, not a replication of the real world," as afferent fibers accentuate some stimulus features and neglect others.[20] Each type of sensory receptor is responsive to different characteristics of a stimulus (such as cold, wet, coarse sand), from steady indentation to high-frequency vibration for mechanoreceptors, from cold to warm for thermal receptors, static or dynamic limb position for proprioceptors, and potentially harmful input for nociceptors. The appreciation of these qualities of sensibility depends on such factors as the diameter of the first-order neuron, the properties of the sensory receptor, the size and population of the receptive field, and the threshold for the sensory unit.[21] Usually, the modality of sensation mediated by a particular axon is specific for each axon, and the type of stimulus to which it is particularly sensitive is the adequate stimulus (light touch, warmth, deep pressure). Different sensations occur through combinations of axons transmitting impulses. Qualities such as wetness and roughness are thought to involve activation of the entire set of receptors mediating touch-pressure, and receptors mediating pain sensation may also be responsible for the perception of itch and tickle. Appreciation of qualities of sensibility also depend on the integrated neural mechanisms of the CNS.

Sensory Input

From the multiple sensory impulses generated in many different kinds of sensory receptors and nerve endings, the CNS derives precise information concerning the quality, intensity, and locus of stimuli and their spatial and temporal patterns.

Threshold

The thresholds for sensory units vary according to several factors, such as site tested, age, sex, circulation in the area, temperature in the area, attention and cooperation of the individual, etc.[22] The adequate stimulus, or the stimulus with the lowest threshold for activating the receptor, provokes graded generator potentials across the membrane of the sensory terminal, and a propagated action potential if the generator, or receptor, potential reaches the threshold of the trigger zone of the afferent fiber.[21] Generator potentials from different afferent endings differ in duration and rate of adaptation. A continuous stimulus may result in a generator potential that is tonic, or slowly adapting (toothache or joint position sense), or one that is phasic or rapidly adapting (some touch receptors).

The absolute sensory threshold is the lowest stimulus intensity detected. Threshold is statistically determined from several series of stimuli of different intensities, and is defined as the stimulus intensity detected in 50 percent of trials. In addition to measuring a subject's threshold for a particular stimulus, it is possible to measure the threshold of a particular class of afferent fibers to the same stimulus. Although psychophysical observations are usually obtained from human subjects and afferent fiber recordings from experimental animals, Vallbo and his colleagues,[23-25] using percutaneously inserted intraneural electrodes, found that the absolute sensory threshold from a mechanical stimulus sometimes coincided with the threshold of a single afferent fiber in the fingertips, but the psychophysical detection threshold was considerably higher in the center of the palm. Although the absolute sensory threshold may sometimes coincide with the threshold of the afferent fiber, generally the psychophysical threshold, or that perceived by the subject, is higher than that recorded for the afferent fiber.

Studies have shown that sensory thresholds are not fixed and can be modified by the context of expectation in which the stimulus is detected. A subject is more likely to report the presence of a stimulus when it is absent (false alarm) if it is important not to miss the occurrence of a stimulus (e.g., a soldier in a foxhole ducking in response to gunfire). On the other hand, thresholds increase when the response is less important (e.g., the threshold for pain often increases when one is competing in a sporting event). These changes in sensory threshold result from changes in the thresholds of neurons within the CNS (facilitation or inhibition from other sources within the CNS), and not from changes in receptor threshold in the periphery. Interpretation of threshold can also be influenced by other factors. Thus, temperature change will produce a mechanoreceptive illusion, such that weights feel heavier when cold than when warm, for example. Sensibility can also be affected by storage in the sensory cortex. An example of this is the reaction of patients with neurovascular cutaneous island pedicle transfers. The patient can be trained to interpret a sensory experience as occurring in the recipient site of pedicle transfer, but in an emergency such as a burn to the recipient area, the training is lost and the patient reacts by moving the donor area.[26]

Spatial Density

Spatial discrimination is explained by receptor innervation density and receptor field size. The awareness of spatial aspects of sensory experience includes the ability to localize the site of stimulation and the ability to distinguish two closely spaced stimuli. The capacity to resolve two stimuli is quantified by measuring the distance between two stimuli — the two-point threshold. This ability is related to the receptor innervation density of an area, is greater distally, and decreases as more proximal parts of the body are tested.[19] As the two-point threshold increases, there is a corresponding decrease in the accuracy with which a subject is able to localize the site of stimulation. The smaller the size of the receptive field, the greater the number of sensory units in a given body area and the greater the somatotopic representation of that body part in the cerebral cortex.[22]

The population of sensory receptor units also varies considerably. Cold sensors are more numerous than warm ones by a ratio of 4 : 1 to 10 : 1, with both types more common on the hands and face than elsewhere. The superficial tissues of the hand are more densely innervated than are more proximal cutaneous regions of the upper extremity, and may have as many as 2,500 nerve endings in a single square millimeter of tissue.[19] The peripheral branches of ectodermal sensory units overlap with the branches of adjacent sensory units, so that the activity of sensory units gradually changes with a moving stimulus. However, the degree of overlap varies with the type of receptor and body area.

Intensity

Intensity is coded in terms of frequency of action potentials. Increased numbers of action potentials can occur from increased frequencies in a single fiber or from increased numbers of activated endings. Suprathreshold stimuli lead to receptor (or generator) potentials with faster rates of rise and greater amplitude, which then evoke chains of action potentials at progressively higher frequencies. Thus, the discharge frequency of an afferent fiber increases with increasing stimulus intensity, and this is known as the frequency code for stimulus intensity. Stronger stimuli also activate a greater number of receptors, so that stimulus intensity is also encoded in the size of the responding population, or the population code. Thus, the stimulus intensity is encoded in two ways, by the frequency of action potentials and by the population of activated afferent fibers.[21]

Detection of the magnitude of stimuli is important for the ability to discriminate between stimuli and to estimate the stimulus intensity. The capacity to distinguish stimuli that differ only in magnitude depends on the size of the stimuli. As the intensity of the reference stimulus increases, the difference in magnitude necessary to perceive a second stimulus as different also increases. Thus, one can distinguish a 1-kg weight from a 2-kg weight, but not usually a 50-kg weight from a 51-kg weight, although the difference is still 1 kg.[21]

Location

Location coding is considered segmentally, and dorsal root fibers entering each spinal segment transmit information to the CNS from a specific skin region (dermatome), from a specific muscle (myotome), and from a specific bone or joint region (sclerotome). These regions are similar in the neck and trunk regions, but do not correspond to each other in the head and limbs.

Modality

Sensory modality is related to the method of stimulation (pinprick, vibration) and the receptors in the region being stimulated. To activate a receptor, a stimulus must be of suitable quality and intensity (greater than threshold). Most sensory receptors are modality specific; that is, each receptor responds preferentially to a given type, or modality, of stimulus, such as light touch or warmth. Other stimuli might activate the receptor, but one kind of stimulus, the adequate stimulus, has the lowest threshold for activating the receptor. Single receptors and the afferent fibers to which they connect elicit the same sensation whether a receptor is activated by a natural (or adequate) stimulus or whether its afferent fiber is activated by an artificial (e.g., electrical) stimulus. This is known as labeled-line coding, and almost all the coding in sensory systems is done by labeled line. There is also labeled-line coding of the quality of sensations so that a given type of receptor will always produce the same modality of sensation regardless of the kind of stimulus. Thus, stimulation of a photoreceptor, even by mechanical pressure, will produce the sensation of light. In the same way, under appropriate conditions, stimulation of a cold receptor by intense heat will result in a sensation of cold.[21]

Classification of Sensory Receptors

Sensory receptors have been classified in several ways, for example, by function (somatic and visceral receptors, proprioceptors, chemoreceptors, photoreceptors, and audioreceptors), or by the source of the stimulus (exteroceptors, proprioceptors, and interoceptors). An anatomic classification based on the structure of the terminal portion of the peripheral process divides receptors into free nerve endings, expanded tip endings, and encapsulated endings. Free nerve endings are the most frequently occurring type in this classification. They form the majority of sensory receptors in the skin, are present in almost all epithelia, and are also present in connective tissue, muscle, and serous membranes. They are the terminal branches of peripheral processes that lose all their coverings and end without specialization in the innervated area. They are derived from small unmyelinated or finely myelinated axons, and a single fiber often branches profusely over a wide area. Expanded tip endings are found in the Merkel touch corpuscles and the cold receptors of the skin, where the terminal portion of the afferent ending expands as it contacts an epithelial cell. Receptors with encapsulated endings have a connective tissue sheath surrounding the nerve terminal and include the pacinian corpuscle, Ruffini endings, Meissner's corpuscle, muscle spindles, and Golgi tendon organs.

Several modalities of somatic sensation can be consciously perceived separately from the rest, and in most cases there is a separate receptor or group of receptors associated with each modality. Thus, somatic receptors can also be classified, on the basis of their selective response to stimuli, into nociceptors, thermoreceptors, mechanoreceptors, and proprioceptors. Table 6-3 lists the primary receptor types in human glabrous (nonhairy) skin, the classifications to which they belong, and their major characteristics.

Nociceptors

Nociceptors are receptors that are preferentially sensitive to noxious or to potentially damaging stimuli. Morphologically, nociceptors are free nerve endings and are connected to axons of two fiber classes: Aδ and C. In cutaneous nerves, 10 percent or more of the myelinated fibers and 50 percent or more of the unmyelinated fibers are nociceptive, depending on the species and the part of the body studied.[27] Although nociceptors respond preferentially to noxious stimuli, some may also mediate some aspects of crude touch. Some Aδ receptive afferents respond with only a few impulses to gentle stroking, but increase their frequency and have a more prolonged response to noxious stimuli.[28] When the dorsal columns, mediating information from touch-pressure mechanoreceptors, are damaged, individuals still have some sensibility to crude touch. This crude touch sensation presumably results from activation of pain and thermal receptors and is transmitted to higher centers by way of the anterolateral system.

The thinly myelinated nociceptive afferents have a wide range of conduction velocities, and the receptive fields vary in size, with smaller zones located more distally on the limbs.[27] Subclasses of Aδ nociceptors have been described and include high-threshold mechanoreceptors (HTMs), which respond only to intense mechanical stimuli, and mechanoheat receptors (AMHs), which respond to

Table 6-3. Classification and Major Characteristics of the Primary Receptor Types in Glabrous Skin

Classification	Subclass	Afferent Fiber	Adequate Stimulus
Nociceptor	HTM	Aδ	Intense mechanical
	AMH	Aδ	Intense mechanical or noxious heat
	Polymodal	C	Intense mechanical, noxious heat, or irritant chemical
Thermoreceptor	Cold	Aδ and C	Decreases in temperature of 0.5°C (between 10° and 35°C)
	Warm	C	Increases in temperature (between 30° and 46°C)
Mechanoreceptor	FA I (Meissner's corpuscle)	Aβ	Sinusoidal skin displacement (tapping) at frequencies from 8 to 64 Hz
	FA II (Pacinian corpuscle)	Aβ	Sinusoidal skin displacement (vibration) at frequencies > 64 Hz
	SA I (Merkel cell neurite complex)	Aβ	Pressure
	SA II; (Ruffini nerve ending)	Aβ	Stretch

intense mechanical stimuli or noxious heat (greater than 45°C).[29] It is not yet known whether Aδ cold receptors play a role in pain discrimination.[30]

The most common unmyelinated cutaneous nociceptor is the C-polymodal nociceptor, which is excited by intense mechanical stimuli, noxious heat, and irritant chemicals. It represents more than 90 percent of C fibers in human cutaneous nerves, although the morphology is not yet determined.[24] The threshold for activating C polymodal nociceptors with von Frey's hairs has been reported to range from 0.7 to 13 grams. They also respond to intense stimuli such as a needleprick, and a few respond to cooling of the skin below 20°C, heating above 40°C, and chemical stimuli such as itch powder, nettle leaves, and bradykinin.[31,32] A few C fiber "warm" receptors have been identified,[33] but the low-threshold C mechanoreceptors responding to noxious cooling in the rabbit[34] have not yet been described in humans. As with the Aδ nociceptors, the discharge rate of C nociceptors increases with increased stimulus intensity.[24] Receptive fields for C nociceptors vary in size and are often complex, with pointlike receptive regions surrounded by relatively insensitive areas. The spots of different C units may overlap, so that even a pointed stimulus can activate several C nociceptors.[35]

In compression block experiments where A fiber transmission is blocked, depriving the subject of awareness of the exact location, depth, and type of stimulus, chemical and mechanical noxious stimuli are perceived as a delayed, uncomfortable stinging or burning. Stimuli activating C nociceptors usually also evoke impulses in A fibers, which then induce sensation resulting from integrative actions in the CNS. Some C nociceptors are excited by stimuli perceived as heat or itch, and it has been suggested that these nociceptors contribute to a painful component of such sensation, which probably results from activation of more than one type of receptor.[31,32] The pain induced by electrical stimulation of C fibers can be reduced considerably by stimulation of A fibers with vibration, and sometimes also by pressure on or cooling of the skin within the projected pain area.[36] There is spatial and temporal summation of input from primary afferents at CNS levels, and the CNS plays a modulating role in inhibiting or summating information from peripheral receptors.[29]

Cutaneous inflammation results in primary hypalgesia at the site of injury, and this has been explained by sensitization of nociceptors, probably due to local release of chemical mediators in the inflamed area (such as metabolites of arachidonic acid and bradykinin). The pain of acute arthritis may be accounted for by similar inflammation-induced changes in response properties of fine articular afferents, and possibly also by release of substance P from primary afferents. Secondary hypalgesia in regions surrounding an injury is not yet understood and probably results from changes in both the periphery and the CNS.[29] The pathophysiology of chronic pain is still unclear.

There are two types of pain. Fast, localized pain (also called first pain) is a sharp, stinging pain corresponding to a pinch or pinprick. It is mediated by Aδ fibers. Slow pain (also called second pain) is a burning, aching pain that is felt after fast pain and may last for seconds or hours. It is mediated by more slowly conducting C fibers.

Thermoreceptors

Usually, thermoreceptor units preferentially sensitive to cold are innervated by Aδ fibers, and those for warmth by C fibers. The receptive fields of warm units appear to be single spots, whereas those of cold units can have multiple spots separated by relatively unresponsive areas.[37] The threshold and intensity of warm and cold sensations depend on the absolute temperature of the skin, the rate of change, and the stimulus area. The average indifferent temperature is about 29°C,[38] and both warm and cold units have a resting discharge at normal temperatures. Cooling thermoreceptors are sensitive to decreases in skin temperatures, and their discharge frequency increases when the temperature decreases by as little as 0.5°C.[37,39–42] They respond with a higher frequency to sudden lowering than to more gradual lowering of skin temperature, and they adapt during a maintained stimulus and show a transient inhibition to warming.[38] The sensitivity of the receptor to cold is about the same as what human subjects report when the temperature probe is placed on the skin. These receptors respond best between 30° and 10°C. Paradoxical cold is seen when a heat stimulus of 45°C is applied to a cold receptor. This stimulus would ordinarily be painful when applied to diffusely innervated areas of skin, but when applied to a single cold spot it is experienced as cold, not hot. This is an example of labeled-line coding, and the quality of the sensation is determined by which "line" is stimulated, not necessarily by what kind of stimulus is being used to turn on the activity.[21]

Only a few human cutaneous thermoreceptors mediating warmth have been studied. Fibers are spontaneously active from 32°C and show an increase in frequency as the skin is moderately warmed at a rate from 0.5°C/sec to 1.5°C/sec, whereas cooling causes a transient inhibition of discharge.[43] Although sensation of warmth is mediated by unmyelinated C fibers, the initial pain associated with intense heat is mediated by heat nociceptors (Aδ). Human sensation of warmth parallels that of the warm receptors at temperatures between 30° and 45°C. For warm receptors, an increase in temperature produces an increase in the firing rate of the fiber up to temperatures at or above 45°C, when the firing rate rapidly declines to zero. At 45°C tissue damage may start to occur, so that very hot stimuli (greater than 45°C) are considered noxious, and this sensation is mediated by separate nociceptors and is considered to be a part of the sensation of pain. Thus, only for warm stimuli (less than 45°C) is there a strong correlation between discharge properties of warm fibers and estimations of warmth. Above 45°C the discharge of heat nociceptors correlates well with perceived heat pain, but not with perceived warmth.[21]

The underlying function of thermoreception is still unresolved. At 33°C both cold and warm receptors are statically active, but no conscious temperature sensation is felt. Conscious sensation begins when a relatively high number of thermal impulses per unit of time reaches the CNS, suggesting that the threshold of thermal sensation is dependent to some extent on the signal-to-noise ratio and integrative aspects of the CNS.[44]

Mechanoreceptors

Mechanoreceptors are generally connected to afferent fibers in the Aβ range and convey information about tactile sensation, or the direction, speed, and shape of mechanical deformation of the skin.

They are classified according to the size and shape of their receptive fields (large or small, sharp or obscure borders) and by their adaptation response (rapidly or slowly adapting).[25] Fast-adapting (FA) mechanoreceptors respond to a moving stimulus and only at the onset and perhaps termination of a long-lasting stimulus, whereas slowly adapting (SA) mechanoreceptors respond continuously for long periods to an enduring stimulus. The most sensitive areas of the skin to touch (fingertips and tongue) have the smallest receptive fields and the largest number of receptive fields per unit area of the skin, and thus the greatest cortical representation.[21] Although different mechanoreceptors mediate the subjective quality of simple tactile sensations (e.g., tapping, pressure), natural stimuli are usually complex and activate different combinations of mechanoreceptor classes at the same time.

Four types of low-threshold mechanoreceptor units with large afferent fibers have been identified in the glabrous skin of the human hand: FA I, FA II, SA I, and SA II. On the basis of morphologic and functional data in other species, the four types of units are believed to be the Meissner's corpuscle, the pacinian corpuscle, the Merkel cell neurite complex, and the Ruffini nerve endings, respectively.[24,25,45–51] The Meissner's corpuscles are usually found in the dermal papillae on the frictional surfaces of digits. Meissner's corpuscles are abundant in young individuals and decrease with age. Pacinian corpuscles are widespread and are found subcutaneously over the entire body, especially in the hand and the foot, and in numerous other connective tissue sites. The Ruffini ending is sometimes seen in the subcutaneous tissue of the pulp of the finger but is more commonly seen in joint capsules. The Merkel cell neurite complex is found in the deeper portion of the germinative layer along the dermal papillae. They too are numerous at birth and decrease in number with age.[27,52,53]

Spatial acuity is maximal at the fingertips and reasonably parallels the density of FA I and SA I units. The electrical threshold of the FA I and FA II units have been found to match the psychophysical thresholds when minute touch stimuli were applied to the fingertips while impulses from single nerve fibers were being recorded. However, the psychophysical thresholds of the SA units were much higher. A single impulse in a single FA I unit could often reach consciousness with both mechanical and electrical microstimulation. A series of impulses was usually required for FA II units to be consciously perceived.[48]

The FA I units respond best to intermittent tapping or sinusoidal skin displacement at frequencies from 8 to 64 Hz, whereas FA II units respond best to frequencies above 64 Hz. The SA I units give graded responses to steady indentations, and on intraneural stimulation give rise to the sensation of pressure. On intraneural stimulation to individual SA II units, no particular sensation has been reported. The SA II units have a tendency to spontaneous activity and are responsive to lateral skin stretching, often with directional sensitivity, and thus can provide detailed information on the magnitude of direction and rate of change of tensions within the skin as well as between the skin and deeper structures.[50,54]

FA I and SA I units have extensively overlapping, multiple, small receptive fields with sharp boundaries (as measured with von Frey's hairs at 4 to 5 times threshold) with relatively uniform sensitivity. Their density increases distally, with an abrupt increase from the main part of the finger to the fingertip. The spatial distribution and receptive field properties of FA I and SA I units make them well suited for tactile spatial analysis, and these factors are believed to account for the increase in two-point discrimination capacity from the palm to the fingertip. The extensive overlapping also may prevent drastic alterations in discrimination capacity with moderate loss of peripheral units in aging or pathologic processes.[50,55]

The FA II and SA II units have large receptive fields with obscure boundaries and a single zone of maximal sensitivity, and are almost evenly distributed over the glabrous skin of the hand. The sensitivity of these units declines very slowly with distance, so the units are also sensitive to remote stimuli. It has been suggested that FA II and SA II units may also play a role in proprioceptive functions. The SA II units in the nail regions of the hand have been found to discharge with increased frequency in response to increased joint movement, and it is thought that the influence of joint angle on the unit response may be mediated by simultaneous alterations in skin tension.[50,54]

Hairy skin has not been studied in detail in humans. Specialized and encapsulated receptors are not common in hairy skin, and the primary innervation is from free nerve endings and endings associated with hair follicles. Single-unit recordings from myelinated afferents in human hairy skin have been made primarily from the superficial branch of the radial nerve supplying the dorsum of the hand, and findings in this area may not be typical for hairy skin because large areas are covered with transitional skin. The data are from a small sample and are not as specific as for glabrous skin, as the samples were considered in two general groups, slowly adapting and rapidly adapting, which included hair follicle receptors. Tests with von Frey's hairs indicated thresholds from less than 0.1 to 4.5 grams.[24] The peritrichous endings of the hair follicles are activated by hair movement and vary considerably in complexity. The smallest hair follicles have at least two stem nerve fibers, which form an inner longitudinally palisading plexus and an outer circular plexus.[52]

Proprioceptors

Proprioception includes the sense of balance, movement, and position of the limbs. Balance is mediated primarily by the specialized receptors of the vestibular apparatus. Perception of the stationary position of the limb (position sense) and the speed and direction of limb movement is possibly mediated by mechanoreceptors in joint capsules, mechanoreceptors of the skin, and mechanoreceptors in muscle. Joint afferents do not appear to play a dominant role in sensing the position of the limb at rest, but rather are sensitive at extremes of joint angles and respond to pressure changes in the joint capsule. It is unclear whether joint receptors play a role in sensation of limb movement, because patients with total hip replacements (and thus no innervation to the joints) can still detect the direction of passive limb movement, although the threshold is elevated. Cutaneous receptors are also not necessary for accurate assessment of limb position or movement, and anesthetizing the skin around the knee joint has no effect on estimates of joint angle.[21] Matthews, Burgess, and their colleagues found that vibration of the biceps muscle increased muscle spindle activity and gave the illusion that the arm was more extended. They thus concluded that joint angle appears to be estimated from information about muscle length provided by muscle spindle receptors.[56,57]

Skeletal muscle contains the highly organized encapsulated muscle spindles, the encapsulated Golgi tendon organs, and free nerve endings. The muscle spindles are found in all human skeletal muscle, but their number varies from muscle to muscle depending upon the degree of CNS control. Muscles capable of delicate movements and under a high degree of CNS control have the most spindles. Each ovoid spindle consists of a connective tissue capsule; one or two long, thick nuclear bag intrafusal fibers; and several smaller and thinner nuclear chain intrafusal fibers, which traverse the spindle. The spindle is in parallel with the extrafusal fibers, and the primary and secondary endings are activated by muscle stretch, which then lengthens the intrafusal bundle. The primary endings respond most to the dynamic phase of the stretch (dynamic sensitivity), whereas the secondary endings are more sensitive to maintained stretch (static sensitivity). Thinly myelinated γ, or fusimotor efferent nerve fibers that end on the striated portions of the intrafusal fibers near both poles of the capsule, also innervate the spindles. The fusimotor activity causes the intrafusal fibers to contract and stretch the nonstriated part of the fiber carrying the sensory endings. This causes increased sensitivity of the sensory ending so that they discharge more readily and at increased rates when their muscle is stretched.[21,58]

Golgi tendon organs are thinly encapsulated receptors found primarily at musculotendinous junctions. They are in series with 15 to 20 extrafusal skeletal muscle fibers that enter the fibroelastic capsule, and terminate in musculotendinous junctions that give rise to collagen fiber bundles. Both contraction and stretching of the muscle cause the collagen bundles to straighten and compress the sensory fibers; thus, the Golgi tendon organs can register small changes in muscle tension. As they are stimulated during muscle contraction, when the tendon is under tension, they can register active contraction of muscle, which the afferents in the muscle spindle are unable to do.[21,58]

SENSORY EXAMINATION OF THE LOWER EXTREMITY

Sensation is the conscious appreciation and interpretation of stimuli. The integrity of certain aspects of the afferent system can be ascertained through the elicitation of various reflexes or by electrophysiologic recording of propagated action potentials. However, sensation is a subjective function and requires a conscious and cooperative subject for its expression.[59]

The importance of an adequate sensory examination is not fully appreciated by many. Often this portion of the foot examination is very crude or is deferred totally. Crude evaluations can usually detect only gross deficits and do not provide an indicator of the performance of a patient's sensory system that can be compared with other patients or with the same patient over time. Quantitative methods to evaluate sensory thresholds are now available, making it possible to obtain valuable information on how a patient's sensory system is functioning. These quantitative tests are being used to detect and characterize neuropathy, but their value in setting minimal criteria for the diagnosis of neuropathy and for staging severity remains inadequately studied.

Sensory Threshold Determination

Classically, the sensory threshold is measured by determining the stimulus intensity required for a sensation to be just detectable. That is, the examiner presents a stimulus that evokes a sensory experience in the patient. The patient then compares its magnitude with an internal standard and decides whether or not he or she has detected the stimulus. This signal detection theory assumes the constant presence in sensory channels of neural activity uncorrelated with any external stimulus. This random activity or "noise" adds to the neural activity evoked by a stimulus. The patient's task therefore is to decide, within the limits of probability, whether neural activity at any moment is sufficiently above the noise base line to justify the belief that an external stimulus made a contribution to that neural activity.[60] To make such a decision, the patient adopts a criterion. Whenever neural activity exceeds this criterion level the patient reports a stimulus as "present," and when the activity is below criterion the patient reports a stimulus as "absent." This criterion level has been shown to vary with any one of several different nonsensory, motivational variables and leads to the problem of subjectivity in sensory evaluation.[61]

Methods of Threshold Determination

There are several methods of eliciting sensory thresholds from patients, each offering advantages over the others. Table 6-4 lists the techniques of threshold determination and compares their features. These distinctions are important to understand when employing techniques for testing different sensory modalities.

Threshold Method. In the threshold method, the patient is instructed to report honestly whether or not he or she feels a stimulus as the physician gradually increases the stimulus. This method does not include null trials for determination of the false alarm rate. Many times the patient reports feeling stimuli that actually occurred only in their imagination. This of course gives a false low threshold. On the other hand, patients will often pass their true threshold level (false high threshold) if they are uncertain whether what they felt was actually the stimulus.

Yes/No Procedure. In the yes/no procedure the patient is told to inform the examiner whether a stimulus was applied ("yes") or not applied ("no") after the examiner gives a command to respond. The stimulus is applied randomly on only half the trials. The advantage of this technique is the inclu-sion of null trials, which provide information to the examiner as to whether the patient actually felt a stimulus and is not responding to background alone (false alarm). As with the threshold technique, the patient still must decide whether the stimulus is perceived or adopt a criterion level, which unfortu-nately makes these two techniques very subjective.

Two-Alternative Forced-Choice Method. The two-alternative forced-choice method eliminates individual criterion levels in patients, thus elimi-nating subjectivity. The patient is informed that two intervals will be announced about 2 seconds apart and that very shortly after one of the an-nounced intervals the patient will be given the stimulus. The stimulus is randomly applied at ei-ther the first or the second interval. To eliminate the influence of voice inflection, a clicker device is used to announce the intervals: one click for inter-val 1 and two clicks for interval 2. The patient is to report which of the two intervals they thought the stimulation followed. Patients are thus forced to choose an interval and make their best guess, even if they are not sure. Conducting many trials will allow sufficient data to determine statistically whether the number of correct responses was only due to guessing, or whether the stimulus was actu-ally perceived. Usually this technique is computer assisted in order to quickly tabulate a sufficient number of trials and analyze probabilities. Thresh-old level is the level at which the stimulus can be felt 50 percent of the time. This corresponds to a correct response rate of 75 percent in forced-choice testing, because at threshold, a correct re-sponse will occur by sensation 50 percent of the time and by chance in half of the remaining trials in which no sensation occurs.

Often, the up-and-down transformation rule (UDTR) of Wetherill and co-workers is used in

Table 6-4. Summary of Testing Methods for Sensory Threshold Determination

Procedure	Incorporation of False Alarm	Elimination of Nonsensory Factors	Simplicity of Method
Threshold	No	No	Simple
Yes/no	Yes	Limited	Simple
Two-alternative forced choice	Yes	Establishment of internal criterion prohibited	Lengthy trials necessary
Interval comparison[a]	Yes	Some	Simple

[a] Not recommended for finely graded stimuli.

determining detection thresholds.[62] This rule or algorithm provides a method for adjusting stimulus intensity to estimate sensory thresholds based on mathematical theory. Stimulus intensity is decreased if the patient's responses are accurate; likewise, if the responses are inaccurate the stimulus intensity is increased (Fig. 6-3). Threshold levels can be approximated by completing testing after the occurrence of six changes of direction and calculating the mean of the six levels at which the changes occurred.[63] Variations of this algorithm include terminating after eight changes in direction and calculating the mean of the last six reversals,[64] and terminating after five errors and averaging values for the five errors combined with the five lowest correct score.[65,66]

Interval Comparison Method. The interval comparison method is a modification of the two-alternative forced-choice technique. When patients are tested using graded stimuli that vary by large increments (e.g., logarithmic differences as exist between Semmes-Weinstein aesthesiometry filaments), a drop in stimulus intensity occurs to a stimulus level that the patient can not discern. In this modification, patients are strongly encouraged to select an interval, but are not forced to do so if they have no idea in which interval the stimulus occurred.[67] In a forced-choice method, even in this

situation where the stimulus has reached a point below the patient's threshold, the patient would be forced to guess. Many trials are therefore required to rule out guessing. This modification simplifies testing by allowing testing to terminate when patients have reached a stimulus level below their threshold.

Unfortunately, one can argue that including a third, no-choice option, may allow patients to set an internal criterion. This technique is therefore not as pure as the two-alternative forced-choice method, but is more practical when a computer is not available for handling data from many trials, and for stimulus intervals that are not finely graded. This method differs from the yes/no procedure in that during a given test period patients are always offered an interval with a stimulus and an interval without a stimulus. Patients can always compare and choose one interval, instead of sometimes getting a stimulus and reporting when they think they may have felt it as in the yes/no procedure.

Control of Variables in Testing

Every effort should be made to control those variables that contribute to the subjective nature of sensory testing. These variables include environ-

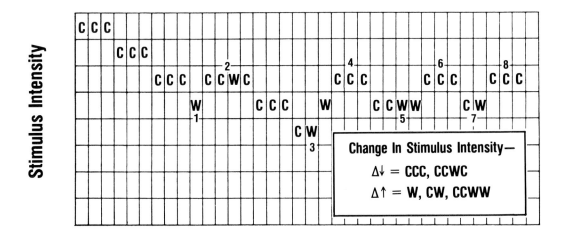

Fig. 6-3. Use of the up-and-down transformation rule for determining detection thresholds. Note the direction of change in stimulus intensity for each sequence of wrong (W) and correct (C) responses. (Adapted from Bertelsman et al.[64])

mental effects, patient-related variables, instrument variation, method-related variables, and examiner-related variables. Callahan has described these variables, which are summarized in Table 6-5.[68] The examiner's knowledge of these variables and attempts to control them will help make testing more accurate and reliable. All examinations, when possible, should be conducted in a quiet room providing a comfortable and distraction-free environment. The examiner should try to keep the subject's attention focused during the test as well as to convey clear information regarding what is expected of the subject during the test. Instruments should be calibrated and checked regularly. When possible, the two-alternative forced choice method of testing should be used. When patients are followed sequentially, it is best to have the same examiner collect the data.

Sensory Testing

The range of apparatus available and the techniques employed vary with the sensory modality being evaluated. This discussion begins with what is currently available for testing each sensory modality and then describes more sophisticated systems available only in research centers. Only the following modalities are presently quantifiable for a lower extremity evaluation: vibratory, light touch and pressure, temperature, proprioception, and two-point discrimination. Pain is too complex a

Table 6-5. Variables Contributing to the Subjective Nature of Sensibility Testing

Environment-related variables
  Background noise distracts patient and tester
  Noises that accompany stimulus may provide clues
Patient-related variables
  Patient attitude
  Level of concentration and anxiety
  Calloused skin
Instrument-related variables
  Instrument variation
Method-related variables
  Consistency of instructions given
  Application of stimulus
  Time interval between applications and duration of stimulus
Examiner-related variables
  Experience of examiner
  Examiner's attention to detail and concern for adherence to methods
  Examiner's level of concentration and fatigue

perception to allow standardization, and stereognosis is not practical for the lower extremity. Methods involving direct nerve stimulation, including conduction studies of sensory nerves and transcutaneous nerve stimulation, are briefly described. Quantitative sensory testing is a new area of research under constant development. Information learned in this field of neurology will lead to improved sensory testing in the future, replacing the crude testing methods presently in use.

Temperature

A portable thermal sensitivity tester (NTE-2, Sensortek, Inc., Clifton, NJ) is available which has two identical nickel-coated copper plates that can be set and maintained over a wide range of temperatures (Fig. 6-4). Thermal electrical cooling or heating is achieved, allowing temperatures to be set within $0.1\,°C$ over a $50.0\,°C$ range and changed at a rate exceeding $1.0\,°C/sec$. The use of two plates allows thresholds to be determined using the two-alternative forced-choice algorithm. Arezzo et al.[65] reported the mean thermal threshold for the great toe in 100 subjects free of any history of neurologic disease or diabetes as $1.01\,°C$, with a standard deviation of $0.61\,°C$. With age there are apparent increases in both threshold and variance, but these are not statistically significant. Data using the Computer Assisted Sensory Examination system (described later) shows a stronger trend toward decreasing thermal sensitivity with age.[63] Another thermal sensitivity tester, the Marstock stimulator (Somedic, Stockholm, Sweden), has only one plate.[69] Patients are asked to press a switch as soon as the plate is felt to be either warm or cool. Once the switch is pressed, the direction of the current and therefore the direction of the temperature change is reversed. This is repeated for 2 minutes and a temperature range is measured.[69] Unfortunately, with this technique the variable of patient reaction time needs to be considered, unlike in the two-alternative forced-choice method. Both testing techniques have been very valuable in early detection of sensory deficit in diabetic subjects.[66,69,70]

When instrumentation is not available to provide surfaces at different temperature for testing, metal or glass tubes can be heated or cooled with water to

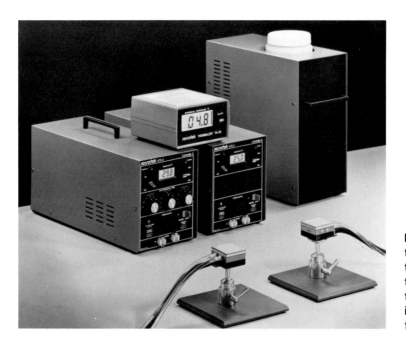

Fig. 6-4. The NTE-2 thermal sensitivity tester provides a means of measuring a patient's ability to discern small ranges of temperature differences in the feet. The temperature difference between two plates is sensed, and patients report which plate feels cooler.

provide surfaces with distinct temperature differences. Exact temperatures are hard to maintain, making it difficult to achieve smaller temperature ranges. With this crude method, only gross temperature ranges or the ability to perceive hot and cold can be tested. For example, with extremes of running tap water at 45° and 110°F (10° and 43°C) only a 65°F (33°C) difference is tested, although patients should be able to perceive much smaller differences in temperature. It is more accurate to test a patient's ability to perceive a zone difference of less than 5°C in the cold and hot regions of the temperature scale.

Patients' ability to feel noxious levels of temperature is due to the triggering of pain fibers. These noxious levels of thermal sensitivity are not routinely tested due to the danger of tissue damage to the patient. Measurements of heat and cold pain can be performed using the Marstock stimulator. The patient presses the temperature direction change switch as soon as a painful sensation is perceived. According to Ziegler and associates,[71] the maximal levels for heat pain (to avoid burning) and cold pain thresholds are 50°C and 0°C, respectively. At these levels the change in temperature is automatically reversed. Normal values (mean ± SEM) of 44.1° ± 0.3°C for heat pain and 14.7° ±

0.7°C for cold pain were obtained from 70 healthy volunteers ages 17 to 64 years on the right lateral aspect of the dorsum of the foot.[71]

Vibratory Sense

Perception of vibratory stimuli has been grossly evaluated by applying a vibrating tuning fork to bony prominences on the body and asking the patient if he or she can identify vibration. Patients report when the sensation ceases as the investigator slows or stops the stimulus. The bony prominences most conveniently tested in the lower extremity are the dorsal aspects of the terminal phalanges of the great toes, the plantar aspects of the first and fifth metatarsal heads, the plantar aspect of the heel, the styloid process of the fifth metatarsal, the metatarsal tuberosity of the navicular, the malleoli, and the tibial tuberosities.

Bickerstaff[72] recommends when testing with a tuning fork that the vibration of the fork be tested first by the examiner to be sure it is vibrating enough; a bony point must be used; unless the test is clearly explained, many patients think it is the sound that they are meant to detect (do not use the word "humming"). Unfortunately, the vibration of tuning forks varies with the force used to strike the

A

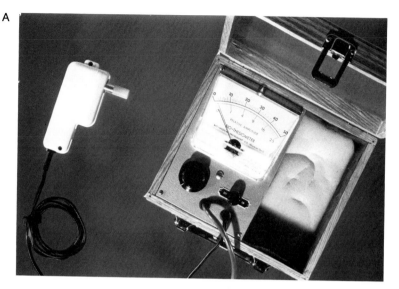

B

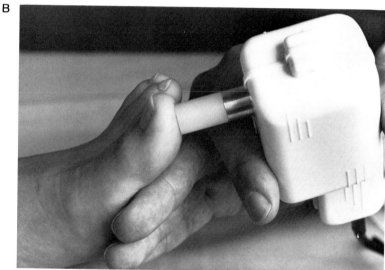

Fig. 6-5. (A) The biothesiometer is a portable device allowing quantitative measurement of vibratory detection thresholds in the feet. **(B)** Care is taken to properly support the testing probe on the testing surface, providing a consistent pressure on the skin.

fork and declines with time, not allowing any effective quantitation of threshold.

A biothesiometer (Biomedical Instruments, Cleveland, OH) is available which provides a method of quantifying vibratory detection thresholds (Fig. 6-5A). Varying the current with a rheostat allows the examiner to control the amplitude of vibrations in the testing probe. The amount of vibration can be expressed as absolute units based on a 50-volt meter or as microns of motion at the vibratory tip (which can be calculated from absolute units). Pressure from the vibratory tip can alter the threshold level; increased pressure decreases

thresholds.[73] One hand-held biothesiometer, the Vibrameter (Somedic, Stockholm, Sweden) has a pressure indicator allowing control of this factor. Proper technique for holding the stimulation surface to the testing site can also help control this variable (Fig. 6-5B). One instrument, the Vibratron II (Sensortek, Clifton, NJ), provides two independent testing surfaces, allowing incorporation of the two-alternative forced-choice testing technique (Fig. 6-6).

The threshold of vibratory sensation has a strong positive correlation with age, and males have slightly increased thresholds over females when

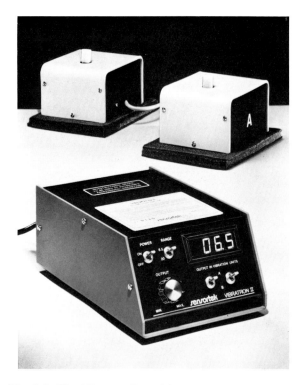

Fig. 6-6. The Vibratron II provides two separate vibrating rods, which allow the two-alternative forced-choice procedure to be used for determination of vibratory detection thresholds.

measurements are obtained at the pulp of the great toe.[74,75] Sosenko et al. have shown a correlation with body stature, which may account for the difference between sexes.[76] The pulp of the great toe has been the location used for measurement in most studies in the lower extremity. Calculated means of vibratory perception thresholds of the pulp of the great toe for age groups 15, 35, and 55 years old were 8.8, 12.9, and 19.9 volts for males and 8.3, 10.8, and 14.6 volts for females,[74] respectively.

Touch and Pressure

Originally, horse hairs of varying thickness were used by von Frey to exert forces of varying strength according to the thickness and length of the hairs used.[77] This apparatus was modified in the 1960s by Semmes, Weinstein, et al., who used nylon monofilaments (Fig. 6-7).[78] These filaments (Fig. 6-8) exert a consistent force at the surface of the skin when the filament buckles. A maximal vertical force is achieved upon buckling of the filament, and any additional force is exerted horizontally. By using filaments of different diameter or length it is possible to determine patients' cutaneous pressure sensation thresholds. The Semmes-Weinstein aesthesiometer set (Fig. 6-7) consists of a precisely calibrated series of nylon monofilaments of equal length (35 mm) and varying diameters set into indi-

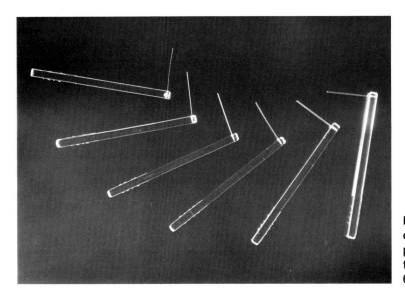

Fig. 6-7. Semmes-Weinstein aesthesiometer set with individual nylon monofilament probes are calibrated to represent (from left to right) 3.61, 4.31, 5.07, 6.10, 6.45, and 6.65 log (0.1 mg) force.

A

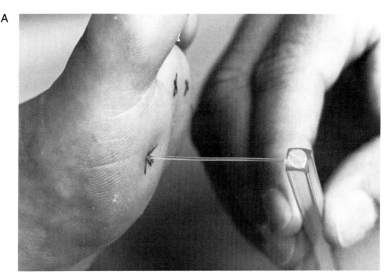

B

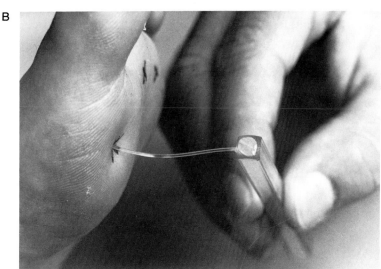

Fig. 6-8. (A) Application of an aesthesiometer probe to a site on the foot. **(B)** Bowing of the filament limits the amount of pressure exerted by the probe.

vidual Lucite handles (Research Designs, Inc., Houston, TX). The common logarithm of the force exerted by these filaments is an approximate linear function of diameter, providing an interval scale for the computation threshold, and has been expressed by Semmes et al. in units of log (0.1 mg) force. This value represents the common logarithm of 10 times the force in milligrams required to bow the monofilament.[79] The Semmes-Weinstein pressure aesthesiometer has been used in following the rehabilitation of nerve injuries of the hand[80] and in mapping sensitivity diminutions and losses in patients with Hansen's disease.[81] This method has

also demonstrated sensory deficits in the lower extremities of diabetic patients.[67,81] The following guidelines for testing cutaneous pressure sensation of the foot were developed by the Rehabilitation Research and Development Department at the Veterans Administration Medical Center in San Francisco.[67] The recommended range of filaments for testing the foot includes filaments calibrated to represent 3.61, 4.31, 5.07, 6.10, 6.45, and 6.65 log (0.1 mg) force.

Generally, testing is done in a descending direction, starting with a strong stimulus that is perceived by the patient (usually the 6.10 probe) and continuing until the patient is unable to detect the stimulus. If the patient cannot detect the 6.10 probe, testing is restarted with the 6.65 probe. Testing of multiple sites is better than monitoring of one single site. The plantar forefoot sites are generally the most accurate in discriminating between normals and patients with foot ulcers. The six sites of the plantar forefoot include the five metatarsal heads (sites 1 to 5) and the plantar hallux pulp (site 6); areas of callus are avoided. In patients with diffuse or nucleated callus, the region just distal to the metatarsal heads and proximal to the plantar sulcus is usually devoid of callus and is within the same dermatome distribution. These sites beneath the metatarsal heads are also more prone to ulceration because of local pressure factors and the mechanics of neurotrophic ulcer formation.

The interval comparison method is performed as follows. With the aid of a random number data sheet, the filament is applied randomly to each site during only one of two consecutively announced time intervals A and B. Care is taken to be consistent, with no change in voice inflections to provide any additional clues when the stimulus is applied. A clicking device can be used to announce the intervals. This method provides one interval of background with no stimulus and another interval of stimulus. The patient is then asked whether any sensation was felt after test interval A or test interval B. Subjects are encouraged to select the test interval in which they felt the stimulus, but are allowed to report that they cannot determine at which interval the stimulus was applied. These instructions are explained to the patient and demonstrated on the patient's forearm to be sure the patient understands the testing procedure. One of the following three results is recorded: the subject has selected the correct test interval for the stimulus, the subject has selected the wrong test interval, or the subject was unable to select a test interval (could not feel the probe). A sensitivity threshold level (STL) is determined by selecting the smallest filament that elicits at least two correct interval responses in a triplicate repetition set.

Monitoring STLs can be useful to determine whether patients are insensate and may be at risk to develop problems. Progressive sensory loss in patients with diabetic peripheral neuropathy can lead to the development of neurotrophic ulceration. Identifying a danger zone of sensation loss may provide a risk discriminator level to determine whether the patient is likely to develop problems. When patients reach this risk discriminator level, proper intervention should be taken to prevent complications from occurring as a result of their sensory loss. One study comparing STLs in diabetic patients with and without ulceration to normals suggests that three of the six plantar forefoot sites should have an STL greater than 5.07 log (0.1 mg) force to best discriminate between normal subjects and patients with foot ulcers.[67] That is, patients who cannot accurately identify the correct interval in which a 5.07 filament was applied in at least three sites in one foot are considered at risk. This risk discriminator level must be tested prospectively to determine its ability to accurately predict the risk of development of neurotrophic ulcers.

Two-Point Discrimination

The objective of the two-point discrimination test is to determine whether the patient can discriminate between being touched with one or with two points and the minimum distance at which two points touching the skin are recognized as such. A small pair of calipers or a compass with blunt ends is required to conduct the test. Measuring scales incorporated into these instruments make them convenient to use. A paper clip is not recommended since often a sharp barb is present at one end, which the examiner must be careful to apply away from the skin to avoid stimulation of pain receptors.[68] The points of the caliper are set at 45 mm and progressively brought together as accurate responses are obtained. The pressure from the testing instrument should not produce ischemia at the area tested; it should stop just at the point of blanching. When the two points are applied they should contact the skin simultaneously, and the line between the points should parallel the longitudinal axis of the extremity. An interval of 3 to 5 seconds should be allowed between applications. The testing distance is decreased until the patient is unable to correctly identify the number of points applied. At least 7 out of 10 responses must be accurate in order for a measurement to be recorded. Normal thresholds for two-point discrimination distance have been reported as 15 to 30 mm for the sole of the foot,[82] 30 to 40 mm for the dorsum of the foot,[83] and 40 to 50 mm below the knee.[84] This test is more useful on the hand, where surgeons have documented more detailed discrimination norms (normal is less than 6 mm, fair is 6 to 10 mm, and poor is 11 to 15 mm).[85] In the hand, two-point discrimination is the classic test of functional sensibility, because it is generally acknowledged to relate to the ability to use the hand for fine tasks.[86,87] This test is not commonly performed on the foot because the foot is generally not involved in fine discriminatory tasks.

Proprioception

The assessment of position or joint sense is made by moving the great toe in a vertical plane and asking the patient, whose eyes are closed, to describe the direction of movement each time the digit is moved. After perception of an initial movement of substantial amplitude is tested, it must be determined whether the patient can appreciate finer movements. An interphalangeal joint requires 5 to 10 degrees of passive movement for recognition, unlike the shoulder joint, where less than 1 degree of passive movement can normally be recognized and a given position can be reproduced within 2 degrees.[22] Care must be taken to grasp the digit on the sides so as to not provide any additional clues about the direction of movement. Quick movements are more stimulating than slow movements; an average middle speed is preferred. Each move should be identified by the patient with the single word "up" or "down" in relation to the previous stationary position and not in relation to the neutral or midposition.

Ankle joint position sense can be measured by having the patient match the angular displacement of a passively positioned reference foot. Berenberg and associates measured the precise angular position of the ankle by means of calibrated potentiometers connected to a microcomputer.[88] In their ankle measurements of 22 men and women between 21 and 50 years old, with no neurologic disease, subjects made accurate matches over a wide range of positions, with an average error of about 3 degrees.[88]

Direct Nerve Stimulation

Direct nerve stimulation provides an objective quantitative assessment of nerve function. Nerve conduction testing is the classic technique used for the quantitative evaluation of neuropathy. The diagnostic interpretation of the electrically evoked nerve compound (action) potential includes an analysis of sensory and motor conduction velocities, response amplitudes, and latencies. The standard nerve conduction velocity measurement is obtained from the peak of this evoked compound action potential, and is therefore primarily an index of the integrity of the largest, most rapidly conducting myelinated fibers.[89] Electrodiagnosis of the sensory nerves is usually conducted on the medial plantar and sural nerves with varied techniques.[90–93] These examinations can be very uncomfortable to patients. Nerve conduction testing is one of the recommended tests for documentation of peripheral neuropathies.[94,95] Nerve conduction testing is not recommended as a screening tool.

A transcutaneous neurostimulator (Fig. 6-9) is available which allows easy evaluation of direct nerve stimulation of sensory nerves (Neurometer, Neurotron, Inc., Baltimore, MD). The stimuli produced are not as noxious to the patient as those used in nerve conduction studies, providing better patient cooperation and feasibility for use as a screening tool. The instrument provides three different frequencies (5, 250, and 2,000 Hz) of stimulation by continuous sine wave current. The apparatus includes switches that allow ease of conducting the two-alternative forced-choice technique. Sensors are applied directly to the skin with a conductive gel. Studies have shown a correlation of transcutaneous nerve stimulation with other clinical findings[96] and with electrodiagnosis.[97] More studies are needed to correlate the different frequencies with different fiber types that are being stimulated. Usually the trigeminal (face), median (index finger), and peroneal nerves (dorsum of the great toe) are evaluated. Current per-

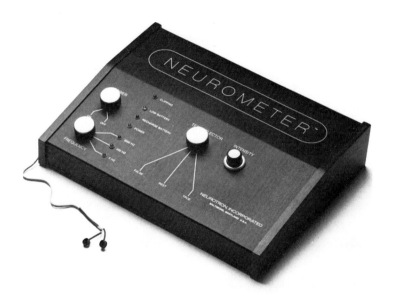

Fig. 6-9. The Neurometer provides non-aversive transcutaneous electrical stimulation, automatically compensating for variations in resistance. Current perception thresholds are determined for three distinct populations of nerve fibers by testing with three sinusoidal frequencies. The test selector switch allows easy incorporation of the two-alternative forced-choice testing procedure.

ception threshold measures of the dorsum of the great toe (mean ± SD) based on a study of 60 neurologically healthy subjects were 77 ± 35 mA at 5 Hz, 110 ± 33 mA at 250 Hz, and 332 ± 66 mA at 2,000 Hz.[98,99]

Computer Assisted Sensory Examination

The Computer Assisted Sensory Examination (CASE) is a superior system for the evaluation of cutaneous sensations of touch and pressure, vibration, and thermal sensitivity.[100] This battery of tests is computer assisted and is not subject to the problems of hand-held instrumentation. The design of the system allows the two-alternative forced-choice testing method to be used, so that a sufficient number of repetitive trials can be tabulated. This system and its advantages have been described in detail by Dyck and co-workers.[100,101] Another computer-assisted sensory examination has been described by Potvin and Tourtellotte.[102] Unfortunately these computer-assisted systems are at present available only in research centers.

Clinical Considerations

Sensory evaluation cannot be considered in isolation from motor status or other physical findings in arriving at a proper diagnosis. Hyperesthesia (excessive sensibility to sensory stimuli), hypesthesia (diminished sensibility), and paresthesia (abnormal spontaneous sensation) can all indicate nerve pathology. The extent or location of sensory loss can help identify the etiology. A localized sensory abnormality following the distribution of cutaneous nerves may reflect nerve compression (nerve entrapment), traumatic injury (nerve laceration or microtraumatic neuropathy), or other focal nerve lesions (neuritis or neuroma). Sensory abnormality following a dermatome distribution or spinal nerve root involvement (L4, L5, or S1) may be indicative of radiculopathy. Patchy hypesthesia usually not following either of these patterns can be found in Hansen's disease. A generalized stocking distribution may represent metabolic (diabetes or uremia), toxic (alcohol, drug, or chemical), ischemic, hereditary, or acquired peripheral neuropathies.

The sensory system in the lower extremity functions to provide sensory feedback and enable locomotion and protective capabilities. Protective sensibility is defined as the conscious appreciation of pain, cold, warmth, and pressure before tissue damage results from the stimulus.[22] Evaluation of these systems is important to determine lack of protective sensation and the risk of developing tissue damage from abnormal pressure or temperatures, so that proper preventative measures can be taken.

REFERENCES

1. Pallie W: The intersegmental anastomoses of posterior spinal rootlets and their significance. J Neurosurg 16:188, 1959
2. Gardner, E. Bunge RP: Gross anatomy of the peripheral nervous system. In Dyck PJ, Thomas PK, Lambert EH, Bunge R (eds): Peripheral Neuropathy. Vol. 1. p 11. WB Saunders, Philadelphia, 1984
3. Foerster O: The dermatomes in man. Brain 56:1, 1933
4. Foerster O: Symptomatologie der Erkankungen des Ruckenmarks und seiner Wurzeln. In Bumke I, Foerster O (eds): Handbuch der Neurologie. Vol. 5. Springer, Berlin, 1936
5. Fender FA: Foerster's scheme of the dermatomes. Arch Neurol Psychiatry 41:688, 1939
6. Weise MD, Garfin SR, Gelberman RH, et al: Lower-extremity sensibility testing in patients with herniated lumbar intervertebral discs. J Bone Joint Surg 67A:1219, 1985
7. Keegan JJ: Neurosurgical interpretation of dermatome hypalgesia with herniation of the lumbar intervertebral disc. J Bone Joint Surg 26:238, 1944
8. Bardeen CR: Development and variation of the nerves and the musculature of the inferior extremity and of the neighboring regions of the trunk in man. Am J Anat 6:259, 1907
9. Goss CM: Anatomy of the Human Body, by Henry Gray. Lea & Febiger, Philadelphia, 1973
10. Prutkin L: Normal and anomalous innervation patterns in the lower extremity. p 100. In Omer GE, Spinner M (eds): Management of Peripheral Nerve Problems. WB Saunders, Philadelphia, 1980
11. Sarrafian SK: Anatomy of the Foot and Ankle. JB Lippincott, Philadelphia, 1983
12. Stevens CL: Lumbosacral plexus lesions. p 1425.

In Dyck PJ, Thomas PK, Lambert EH, Bunge R (eds): Peripheral Neuropathy. Vol. 1. WB Saunders, Philadelphia, 1984
13. Gardner E, Gray DJ, O'Rahilly R: Anatomy. 4th Ed. WB Saunders, Philadelphia, 1975
14. Hollinshead H: Anatomy for Surgeons. 2nd Ed. Hoeber Medical Division, Harper and Row, New York, 1971
15. Smorto MP, Basmajian JV: Clinical Electroneurography. Williams & Wilkins, Baltimore, 1977
16. Erlanger J, Gasser HS: Electrical Signs of Nervous Activity. University of Pittsburgh Press, Philadelphia, 1937
17. Williams PL, Warwich R (eds): Gray's Anatomy. 36th Ed. WB Saunders, Philadelphia, 1980
18. Lloyd DPC: Conduction and synaptic transmission of the reflex response to stretching in spines of cats. J Neurophysiol 6:317, 1943
19. Mountcastle VB: Medical Physiology. 13th Ed. CV Mosby, St Louis, 1974
20. Mountcastle VB: The view from within: pathways to the study of perception. Johns Hopkins Med J 1236:109, 1975
21. Kandel ER, Schwartz JH (eds): Principles of Neural Science. 2nd Ed. Elsevier Biomedical, New York, 1985
22. Omer GE: Sensibility testing. p 3. In Omer GE, Spinner M (eds): Management of Peripheral Nerve Problems. WB Saunders, Philadelphia, 1980
23. Vallbo AB, Johansson RS: Skin mechanoreceptors in the human; neural and psychophysical thresholds. p 185. In Zotterman Y (ed): Sensory Functions of the Skin in Primates. Pergamon Press, Oxford, 1976
24. Vallbo AB, Hagbarth KE, Torebjork HE, Wallin BG: Somatosensory, proprioceptive, and sympathetic activity in human peripheral nerves. Physiol Rev 59:919, 1979
25. Torebjork HE, Vallbo AB, Ochoa JL: Intraneural microstimulation in man: its relation to specificity of tactile sensations. Brain 110:1509, 1987
26. Omer GE Jr, Day DJ, Ratliff H, Lambert P: The neurovascular cutaneous island pedicles for deficient median nerve sensibility: new technique and results of serial functional tests. J Bone Joint Surg 52A:1181, 1970
27. Light AR, Perl ER: Peripheral sensory systems. p 210. In Dyck PJ, Thomas PK, Lambert EH, Bunge R (eds): Peripheral Neuropathy. Vol. 1. WB Saunders, Philadelphia, 1984
28. Burgess PR: The physiology of pain. Am J Clin Med 2:121, 1974
29. Raja SN, Meyer RA, Campbell JN: Peripheral

mechanisms of somatic pain. Anesthesiology 68:571, 1988

30. Price DD, Dubner R: Neurons that subserve the sensory discriminative aspects of pain. Pain 3:307, 1977

31. Torebjork HE: Afferent C units responding to mechanical, thermal and chemical stimuli in human non-glabrous skin. Acta Physiol Scand 92:374, 1974

32. Torebjork HE, Hallin RG: Skin receptors supplied by unmyelinated (C) fibres in man. p 475. In Zotterman Y (ed): Sensory Function of the Skin in Primates. Pergamon Press, Oxford, 1976

33. Konietzny F, Hensel H: The dynamic response of warm units in human skin nerves. Pfluegers Arch 370:111, 1977

34. Shea VK: Normal and Regenerated Cutaneous Sensory Receptors With Unmyelinated (C) Fibers in Rabbit's Ear. Unpublished doctoral dissertation, University of North Carolina, 1982

35. Hallen RG, Torebjork HE: Methods to differentiate electrically induced afferent and sympathetic C unit responses in human cutaneous nerves. Acta Physiol Scand 92:318, 1974

36. Bini G, Cruccu G, Hagbarth KE, et al: Analgesic effect of vibration and cooling on pain induced by intraneural electrical stimulation. Pain 18:239, 1984

37. Sumino R, Dubner R: Response characteristics of specific thermoreceptive afferents innervating monkey facial skin and their relationship to human thermal sensitivity. Brain Res Rev 3 (Brain Res 228):105, 1981

38. Jarvilehto T, Hamakinen H: Touch and thermal sensations: psychophysical observations and unit activity in human skin nerves. p 279. In Kenshalo DP (ed): Sensory Functions of the Skin of Humans. Plenum Press, New York, 1979

39. Hensel H, Iggo A, Witt I: A quantitative study of sensitive cutaneous thermoreceptors with C afferent fibers. J Physiol (Lond) 153:113, 1960

40. Hensel H, Andres KH, von During M: Structure and function of cold receptors. Pfluegers Arch 352:1, 1974

41. Iggo A: Cutaneous thermoreceptors in primates and sub-primates. J Physiol (Lond) 200:403, 1969

42. Hensel H, Boman KK: Afferent impulses in cutaneous sensory nerves in human subjects. J Neurophysiol 23:564, 1960

43. Konietsny F, Hensel H: The dynamic response of warm units in human skin nerves. Pfluegers Arch 370:111, 1977

44. Hensel H: Cutaneous thermoreceptors. p 79–110.

In Iggo A (ed): Handbook on Sensory Physiology. Vol. 2, Somatosensory System. Springer, Heidelberg, 1973

45. Knibestol M, Vallbo AB: Single unit analysis of mechanoreceptor activity from the human glabrous skin. Acta Physiol Scand 80:178, 1970

46. Knibestol M: Stimulus-response functions of slowly adapting mechanoreceptors in the human glabrous skin area. J Physiol (Lond) 245:63, 1975

47. Johansson RS, Vallbo AB: Tactile sensory coding in the glabrous skin of the human hand. Trends Neurosci 6:27, 1983

48. Vallbo AB, Johansson RS: Properties of cutaneous mechanoreceptors in the human hand related to touch sensation. Human Neurobiol 3:3, 1984

49. Iggo A, Muir AR: The structure and function of a slowly adapting touch corpuscle in hairy skin. J Physiol (Lond) 200:763, 1969

50. Johansson RS: Tactile sensibility in the human hand: receptive field characteristics of mechanoreceptive units in the glabrous skin area. J Physiol (Lond) 281:101, 1978

51. Hagbarth KE, Torebjork HE, Wallin BG: Microelectrode recordings from human skin and muscle nerves. p 1016. In Dyck PJ, Thomas PK, Lambert EH, Bunge R (eds): Peripheral Neuropathy. Vol. 1. WB Saunders, Philadelphia, 1984

52. Carpenter MB, Sutin J: Human Neuroanatomy. 8th Ed. Williams & Wilkins, Baltimore, 1983

53. Quilliam TA: The surface texture of human skin. J Audiov Media Med 1(1):25–7, 1978

54. Johansson RS, Vallbo AB: Tactile sensibility in the human hand: relative and absolute densities of four types of mechanoreceptive units in glabrous skin. J Physiol (Lond) 286:283, 1979

55. Vallbo AB, Johansson RS: Tactile sensory innervation of the glabrous skin of the human hand. p 29. In Gordon G (ed): Active Touch: The Mechanism of Recognition of Objects by Manipulation. Pergamon Press, Oxford, 1978

56. Matthews PBC: Muscle spindles: their messages and their fusimotor supply. p 189. In Brooks VV (ed): Handbook of Physiology. Section I: The Nervous System. Vol. II, Motor Control. American Physiological Society, Bethesda, MD, 1981

57. Burgess PR, Wei JY, Clark FJ, Simon J: Signaling of kinesthetic information by peripheral sensory receptors. Annu Rev Neurosci 5:171, 1982

58. Weiss L (ed): Histology: Cell and Tissue Biology. 5th Ed. Elsevier Biomedical, New York, 1983

59. Lindblom U, Ochoa J: Somatosensory function and dysfunction. p 283. In Asbury AK, McKhann GM, McDonald WI (eds): Diseases of the Nervous

System. Clinical Neurobiology, Vol 1. Armore Medical Books, Philadelphia, 1986

60. Green DM, Swets JA: Signal Detection Theory and Psychophysics. John Wiley & Sons, New York, 1966

61. Sekuler R, Nash BA, Armstrong R: Sensitive, objective procedure for evaluating response to light touch. Neurology 23:1282, 1973

62. Wetherill GB, Chen H, Vasudeva RB: Sequential estimation of quantal response curves: a new method of estimation. Biometrika 53:439, 1966

63. Dyck PJ, Karnes J, O'Brien PC, Zimmerman IR: Detection thresholds of cutaneous sensation in humans. p 1103. In Dyck PJ, Thomas PK, Lambert EH, Bunge R (eds): Peripheral Neuropathy. Vol. 1. WB Saunders, Philadelphia, 1984

64. Bertelsman FW, Heimans JJ, Weber EJM, et al: Thermal discrimination thresholds in normal subjects and in patients with diabetic neuropathy. J Neurol Neurosurg Psychiatry 48:686, 1985

65. Arezzo JC, Schaumburg HH, Laudadio C: Thermal sensitivity tester: device for quantitative assessment of thermal sense in diabetic neuropathy. Diabetes 35:590, 1986

66. Sosenko JM, Kato M, Soto RA, et al: Specific assessments of warm and cool sensitivities in adult diabetic patients. Diabetes Care 11:481, 1988

67. Holewski JJ, Stess RM, Graf PM, Grunfeld C: Aesthesiometry: quantification of cutaneous pressure sensation in diabetic peripheral neuropathy. J Rehabil Res Devel 25:1, 1988

68. Callahan AD: Sensibility testing: clinical methods. In Hunter JM, Schneider LH, Mackin EJ, et al (eds): Rehabilitation of the Hand. CV Mosby, St Louis, 1984

69. Guy RJ, Clark CA, Malcolm PN, Watkins PJ: Evaluation of thermal and vibration sensation in diabetic neuropathy. Diabetologia 28:131, 1985

70. Levy DM, Abraham RR, Abraham RM: Small and large-fiber involvement in early diabetic neuropathy: A study with the medial plantar response and sensory thresholds. Diabetes Care 10:441, 1987

71. Ziegler D, Mayer P, Wiefels K, Gries FA: Assessment of small and large fiber function in long-term type 1 (insulin-dependent) diabetic patients with and without painful neuropathy. Pain 34:1, 1988

72. Bickerstaff ER: Neurological Examination in Clinical Practice, 4th Ed. p 157. Blackwell Scientific Publications, Oxford, 1980

73. Lowenthal LM, Hockaday DR: Vibration sensory thresholds depend on pressure of applied stimulus. Diabetes Care 10:100, 1987

74. Steiness IB: Vibratory perception in normal subjects. Acta Med Scand 158:315, 1957

75. Bloom S, Till S, Sonksen P, Smith S: Use of a biothesiometer to measure individual vibration thresholds and their variation in 519 non-diabetic subjects. Br Med J 288:1793, 1984

76. Sosenko JM, Gadia MT, Fournier AM, et al: Body stature as a risk factor for diabetic sensory neuropathy. Am J Med 80:1031, 1986

77. von Frey M: Untersuchungen Über Die Sinnes Functionen der Menschlichen Haut. In: Abhandlungen der mathematisch-physischen Classe der königlich sachsischen Gesellschaft der Wissenchaften. 23:208, 1897

78. Semmes J, Weinstein S, Ghent L, Teuber HL: Somatosensory Changes after Penetrating Brain Wounds in Man. p 4. Harvard University Press, Cambridge, MA, 1960

79. Levin S, Pearsall G, Ruderman RJ: von Frey's method of measuring pressure sensibility in the hand: an engineering analysis of the Weinstein-Semmes pressure aesthesiometer. J Hand Surg 3:211, 1978

80. Bell JA: Light touch/deep pressure testing using Semmes-Weinstein monofilaments. p 399. In Hunter JM, Schneider LH, Mackin EJ, et al (eds): Rehabilitation of the Hand. CV Mosby, St Louis, 1984

81. Birke JA, Sims DS: Plantar sensory threshold in the ulcerative foot. Lepr Rev 57:261, 1986

82. Ruch TC, Patton HD (eds): Physiology and Biophysics. WB Saunders, Philadelphia, 1965

83. Mayo Clinic, Department of Neurology and Physiology and Department of Biophysics: Clinical Examinations in Neurology. 5th Ed. p 180. WB Saunders, Philadelphia, 1981

84. Omer GE Jr: The assessment of peripheral nerve injuries. In Cramer LM, Chase RA: Symposium of the Hand. Vol. 3. CV Mosby, St Louis, 1971

85. American Society for Surgery of the Hand: The hand, Examination and Diagnosis. American Society for Surgery of the Hand, Aurora, CO, 1978

86. Moberg E: Objective methods for determining the functional value of sensibility in the hand. J Bone Joint Surg 40B:454, 1958

87. Onne L: Recovery of sensibility and pseudomotor activity in the hand after nerve suture. Acta Chir Scand 300:1, 1962

88. Berenberg RA, Shefner JM, Sabol JJ Jr: Quantitative assessment of position sense at the ankle: a functional approach. Neurology 37:89, 1987

89. Lambert EH, Dyck PJ: Compound action potential of sural nerve in vitro in peripheral neuropathy. In

Dyck PH, Thomas PK, Lambert EH (eds): Peripheral Neuropathy. WB Saunders, Philadelphia, 1975

90. Burke D, Skuse NE, Lethlean AK: Sensory conduction of the sural nerve in polyneuropathy. J Neurol Neurosurg Psychiatry 37:647, 1974

91. Murai Y, Kuroiiwa Y: Sural nerve conduction velocity in peripheral neuropathies and subacute myelo-optico-neuropathies (SMON). J Neurol Sci 20:339, 1973

92. Guiloff RJ, Sherratt RM: Sensory conduction in medial plantar nerve. J Neurol Neurosurg Psychiatry 40:1168, 1977

93. Eves ML, Seigler DE, Ayyar DR, Skyler JS: Medial plantar sensory response. Am J Med 76:842, 1984

94. Consensus Statement—Report and Recommendations of the San Antonio Conference on Diabetic Neuropathy. Diabetes Care 11:592, 1988

95. Dyck PJ: Detection, characterization, and staging of polyneuropathy: assessed in diabetics. Muscle Nerve 11:21, 1988

96. Bleecker ML: Quantifying sensory loss in peripheral neuropathies. Neurobehav Toxicol Teratol 7:305, 1985

97. Weseley S, Katims J, Leibowitz B: Neuropathy of uremia: assessment by nerve conduction times vs current perception thresholds. Paper presented at the Tenth International Congress of Nephrology, 1986

98. Katims JJ, Naviasky EH, Rendell MS, et al: Constant current sine wave transcutaneous nerve stimulation for the evaluation of peripheral neuropathy. Arch Phys Med Rehab 68:210, 1987

99. Operating Manual for Neurometer Diagnostic Neurostimulator. Neurotron, Inc., Baltimore

100. Dyck PJ, Zimmerman IR, O'Brien PC, et al: Introduction of automated systems to evaluate touch-pressure, vibration and thermal cutaneous sensation in man. Ann Neurol 4:502, 1978

101. Dyck PJ, Thomas PK, Ashbury AK, et al: Diabetic Neuropathy. WB Saunders, Philadelphia, 1987

102. Potvin AR, Tourtellotte WW: Quantitative Examination of Neurologic Functions. Vol. 2. CRC Press, Boca Raton, FL, 1985

Pruritus in Podiatric Practice

7

Leonard A. Levy, D.P.M., M.P.H.

In addition to pain, swelling, and deformity, itching in the lower extremity is one of the symptoms that brings people to the podiatric physician for care. Apart from some qualitative terms about its severity, it is often far more difficult for patients to describe the nature of their pruritic symptoms. However, because pruritus is such a common dermatologic phenomenon affecting the foot, it is essential that the podiatrist understand its pathophysiology and accept the often difficult challenge of developing a management plan to treat the condition causing the itching sensation, if it is known.

PATHOPHYSIOLOGY

A number of theories have been put forward as to whether there are specific end organs for the various sensations that skin may experience, including itching. As yet, however, a morphologically distinct end organ has not been positively identified.[1] Denman questioned whether pruritus, which is so closely related to pain, is not in fact a subthreshold level of pain.[2] This theory is partly supported by Kinkle and Chapman,[2] who pointed out that patients with congenital absence of pain sensation

also do not perceive itch. They also noted that persons whose spinothalamic tract has been sectioned lose sensation of pain and itch, but still perceive touch.[3]

It is also interesting to note that, during induction of lumbar anesthesia, a pinprick causes itching even after pain is no longer perceived and that, at deeper stages of analgesia, itching disappears while touching and temperature sensation persists. This evidence has led some to conclude that itching is a submodality of pain.[4] However, since in clinical situations pain and pruritus are easy to distinguish, and itch also evokes a scratch reflex, Denman concluded that itch is better considered a primary sensory modality rather than subthreshold pain.[1]

Stimuli that may result in itching are both physical and chemical in nature. Physical stimuli that have been used, for example, include thin wire, electrical stimuli, and heat. Chemical stimuli that may precipitate pruritus include histamine, kinins, and perhaps bile salts.[5] Dry skin is often associated with itching, as are prostaglandins, but these are not considered stimuli of themselves. Rather they are thought to lower the threshold for evoking pruritus.[6] Itch receptors have been described by Cauna as being free, unmyelinated, penicillate nerve endings associated with the epidermis.[7] Itch apparently is conveyed on unmyelinated C fibers, which if electrically stimulated result only in itching but not pain.[8] The afferent C fibers enter the dorsal horn of the spinal cord, synapse, cross the midline, and ascend in the spinothalamic tracts closely associated with pain fibers. The stimulus is transmitted via the spinothalamic tract to the thalamus and the sensory cortex.

Although histamine is not the only peripheral mediator for pruritus, it is considered to be the classic mediator. The method and amount of administration of this substance and the age of the patient govern the response to it. For example, intravenous injection does not cause itch, but superficial cutaneous injection does. Small doses given intradermally yield pruritus, whereas large doses result in burning pain. In persons over age 50 there appears to be a decreased response to intradermal histamine injection in spite of the appearance of a flare or wheal formation.[9]

Davies and Greaves suggested that histamine may cause itching by activating other mediators such as substance P or prostaglandins.[10]

CLINICAL EXPRESSION

Examples of skin diseases frequently associated with pruritus, which may be localized in the foot and ankle and therefore seen in podiatric practice, are listed in Table 7-1.

Since pruritus may be associated with many different causes and skin diseases, it is essential to acquire a careful history and perform a meticulous examination of the skin of the lower extremities, other easily exposed areas, and, when necessary, other parts of the body. Consultation with a dermatologist or internist is often invaluable.

When local or systemic organic causes of itching are not in evidence, psychogenic factors may well be the primary cause of pruritus. In addition, a number of preexisting organic diseases, such as urticaria, psoriasis, and atopic eczema, may be exacerbated by an emotional disorder. Some feel that localized neurodermatitis has its origin in emotional stress and is characterized by severe, persisting, and paroxysmal pruritus. It is often correlated with episodes of tension and stress, of which the

Table 7-1. Skin Diseases in Which Pruritus May Be a Symptom

Xerosis or dry skin
Fungal infections
Scabies
Atopic dermatitis and nummular eczema
Insect bites
Creeping eruption
Pediculosis
Contact dermatitis
Psoriasis
Diabetes
Hodgkin's disease
Lichen planus
Urticaria
Folliculitis
Lichen simplex chronica
Sunburn
Fiberglass dermatitis
Fixed drug eruption
Dyshidrosis
Lichen amyloidosis
Herpes simplex

patient may be aware. Labeling itching as a psychosomatic disorder, however, should be done with care, since an undiagnosed somatic disorder may exist concurrently.[11]

Pruritus not uncommonly occurs when no local or systemic cause is demonstrated, especially in the elderly and particularly in the lower extremities. In diabetics, itching is the most common skin symptom, especially on the legs. It is also found in many other systemic diseases such as polycythemia vera, lymphoma, myeloma, hypo- and hyperthyroidism, obstructive biliary disease, and chronic renal failure. These diseases are found more frequently in the elderly. Pruritus occurs in 10 to 25 percent of cases of Hodgkin's disease and usually begins on the legs. It may precede internal symptoms by a year or more.

Aging of the skin and its associated pruritus may be initiated and accelerated by environmental factors. Although such itching can occur at any time, fall and winter are the seasons when it is most common, probably because of lower humidity and overheated homes. The elderly are particularly susceptible because aged skin has less moisture. In diabetes, decreased perspiration due to impairment of the cutaneous nerves may be a factor leading to dryness or asteatosis and, as a result, pruritus.[12]

MANAGEMENT

In addition to treating the responsible systemic disease or local cause, one should hydrate dry skin by bathing it for about 15 to 30 minutes in lukewarm water and then immediately applying a lubricating cream or ointment. Using a humidifier to increase the amount of water in the air and avoiding hot water and soap as much as possible are also helpful.

In general, however, pruritus is difficult to manage. In addition to trying to remove the cause, one hopes to eliminate scratching since this may lead to erythema, fissures, excoriation, ulcers, wheals, lichenification, and pigmentation. Lichenification is the most common effect of chronic, paroxysmal pruritus and is characterized by leathery thickening of the skin due to prolonged rubbing and scratching.[13]

Topical therapy may include the application of ice bags or hot water bottles. However, in patients with peripheral vascular disease or diabetes, this ancient but sometimes effective treatment should be avoided, or used only with extreme caution if it appears to be the only effective therapy. Topical phenol, usually in concentrations of 0.5 to 2.0 percent, has been very effective but can be systemically toxic because of absorption. It has also been reported to sometimes induce gangrene. Agents such as lidocaine, benzocaine, and procaine in 5 percent preparations have been reported to be effective, but some have warned against contact sensitization after prolonged use.[13] Other topical preparations sometimes used include liquor carbonis detergens, 2 to 8 percent lotions, tincture of benzoin, chloral resorcinol, olive oil, alcohol, and acetic acid.

Probably the most popularly used topical agents are the corticosteroids, particularly when the itching is due to inflammation. These are available in sprays, lotions, creams, and ointments. Intralesional injections are often very effective. These are available in suspension form, including such preparations as triamcinolone suspension, and are especially helpful when localized inflammation or lichenification is present. Use of lower potency corticosteroids such as hydrocortisone 1 percent or fluorinated quarter-strength corticosteroids topically, under plastic-wrap occlusion, is effective and rarely produces adrenal suppression or side effects.[14]

Skin should be protected from external irritants, and sudden temperature change should be avoided. When emotional tension and stress are a significant factor associated with pruritus, stimulants that may aggravate such tension, such as caffeine and theobromine, which are found in coffee, tea, chocolate, and cola drinks, and should be avoided. In some cases, alcohol should be avoided.

Oral treatment of itching with agents such as the antihistamines sometimes needs to be used. Some of those that have been employed include promethazine (Phenergan), trimeprazine (Temaril), diphenhydramine (Benadryl), and methdilazine (Tacaryl). Cyproheptadine (Periactin) and antiserotonin drugs have been used, and in urticarial eruptions, hydroxyzine (Atarax or Vistaril) is helpful.[13]

REFERENCES

1. Tuckett RP, Denman ST, Chapman CR, et al: Pruritus, cutaneous pain and eccrine gland and sweating disorders. J Am Acad Dermatol 11:1000, 1984
2. Denman S: A review of pruritus. J Am Acad Dermatol 14:376, 1986
3. Kunkle EC, Chapman WP: Insensitivity to pain in man: a research. Nerv Ment Dis Process 23:100, 1943
4. Rothman S: Pathophysiology of itch sensation. p 189. In Montagna W (ed): Advances in Biology of Skin. Vol. 1. Pergamon Press, Oxford, 1960
5. Shelly WB, Arthur RP: The neurohistology and neurophysiology of the itch sensation in man. Arch Dermatol 76:296, 1957
6. Hagermark O, Strandberg K, Hamberg M: Potentiation of itch and flare responses in human skin by prostaglandins E2 and H2 and a prostaglandin endoperoxide analog. J Invest Dermatol 69:527, 1977
7. Cauna N: Morphological basis of sensation in hairy skin. Prog Brain Res 43:35, 1976
8. Torebjork HE, Ochoa JL: Pain and itch from C fiber stimulation. Soc Neurosc Abstr 7:228, 1981

9. Keele CA, Armstrong D: Substances Producing Pain and Itch. p 288. Edward Arnold, London, 1964

10. Davies MG, Greaves MW: The current status of histamine receptors in human skin: therapeutic implications. Br J Dermatol 104:601, 1981

11. Linder EF, Kamenetz HL, Dorfman W: The lower extremities and systemic disease. p 32. In Clinical Review of Disorders of the Lower Limbs, Scicom, Stamford, CT, 1972

12. Samitz MH: Cutaneous Disorders of the Lower Extremities. 2nd Ed. pp 102, 142. JB Lippincott Co, Philadelphia, 1981

13. Domonkos AN, Arnold HL Jr, Odom RB: Andrew's Diseases of the Skin Clinical Dermatology. 7th Ed. p 56. WB Saunders Co, Philadelphia, 1982

14. Roenigk HH: Office Dermatology. p 53. Williams & Wilkins, Baltimore, 1981

The Weak and Paralytic Foot

8

Mark E. Landry, D.P.M., M.S.

The muscles of the human foot may be weak (paretic) or paralytic from a partial or complete disruption of their motor supply. These disorders may indicate dysfunction anywhere from the cerebral cortex to the neuromuscular junction. The insult may be vascular, traumatic, neoplastic, metabolic, or inflammatory. As with any illness, the history, the presenting symptoms, associated disease, and the review of systems are critical to the formulation of a diagnosis. However, the development of the neurologic diagnosis is simplified by determining the possible level of the lesion or disease process. Primary muscular disease (dystrophy) must also be ruled out.

By far the most dramatic disorder is the acute neurologic deficit. Its effect on the individual is obvious and profound. Numerous lesions at any level of the central or the peripheral nervous system may initially present with the symptom of foot-drop from a weakened pretibial muscle group. A subtle weakness and inability to lift one's foot when stepping up onto a curb or stairstep may be the first clue to a neurogenic weak foot. The patient may have associated paresthesias in the contralateral limb, a minor eye disturbance, or an annoying urinary incontinence, all of which the patient felt too insignificant to pursue further, but may be elicited in the podiatric history and physical examination.

A patient with a weak foot secondary to poor skeletal alignment may present with even more subtle subjective and objective symptoms.[1] The patient may have had a relatively withdrawn and inactive life-style as a child. By no means is a subtle weak foot confined to the flail foot and flatfoot. Loss of the intrinsic musculature in the foot has been recognized as an etiology of pes cavus for over a century.[2]

This chapter reviews the more common causes of the weak and paralytic foot, with emphasis on diagnosis of the general anatomic level(s) of the neurologic lesion or disease. Neurologic testing of myotomes, dermatomes, and reflexes are incorporated in the routine biomechanical and gait analysis. Case illustrations are given to better illustrate the clinical significance of the neurologic examination when examining the limb, ankle, and foot (Figs. 8-1 to 8-3).

ANATOMIC LEVEL

The evolution of the motor system represents a process of encephalization whereby an increasing number of functions within the central nervous

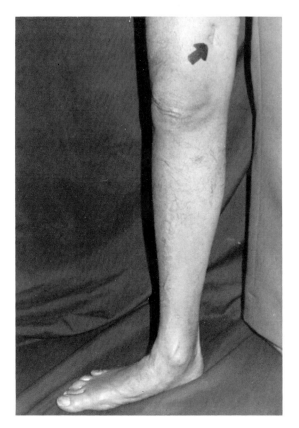

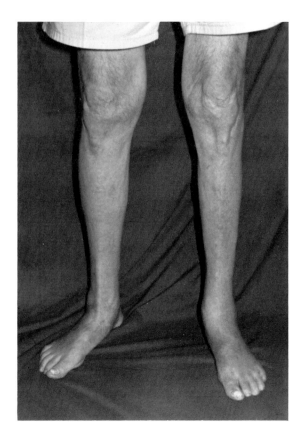

Fig. 8-1. Traumatic mononeuropathy of the sciatic nerve left this World War II veteran with a hyperpronated footdrop. The arrow points to the scar of the original shrapnel injury. The patient presently uses a polypropylene ankle-foot orthosis.

Fig. 8-2. This 70-year-old man had a 2-year history of left low back, hip, and leg paresthesia. Note the atrophied left calf and pronated foot. Clinical testing of the reflexes, dermatomes, and myotomes localized the anatomic level of the spinal lesion to L4-L5.

system became dependent on the cerebral cortex for operation. A hierarchy of motor activity is present in the human nervous system. Volitional activity starts with ideation at the level of the cerebral cortex. Initiation of movement patterns is influenced and generated by the basal ganglia. Most of the activity of the limbs, feet, and toes originates in the anterior portion of the paracentral lobule adjacent to the falx cerebri. This movement pattern is modified by the cerebellum. Meanwhile there is modulation of the activity by the somatosensory cortex and final refining of the outgoing motor impulse at the level of the spinal cord.[2]

The Corticospinal System

The corticospinal or pyramidal tract originates in the precentral gyrus of the frontal lobe of the cere-

bral cortex (primary motor cortex). The corticospinal tract (CST) fibers from the precentral gyrus converge and descend through the posterior limb of the internal capsule, the midportion of the crus cerebri of the midbrain, the pons, and the pyramids of the medulla. The pyramids are located in the anterior portion of the medulla and appear as two longitudinal paramedian ridges. At the caudal end of the medulla, at the level of the foramen magnum, most of the fibers (approximately 85 percent) cross (decussate) to the opposite side of the spinal cord. All of the corticospinal fibers affecting the lower extremity cross to the contralateral side at this level. Hence, lesions to one side of the CST, cerebrum, or brain stem would affect the musculature of the contralateral limb. The crossed CST fibers descend in the lateral funiculus as the lateral corticospinal tract (LCST). At the appropriate level for

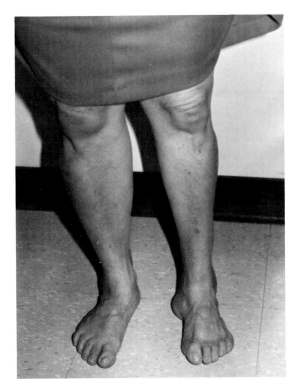

Fig. 8-3. This 45-year-old woman gave a history of right cortical injury in infancy. The contralateral limb was delayed and atrophied in growth. Note the cavus foot. Babinski's sign was present on the left.

motor innervation the fibers leave the tract and synapse on intermediate neurons and some ventral horn cells.[3]

The motor system is more than the CST, however.[4] The rubrospinal, reticulospinal, and vestibulospinal tracts comprise additional descending influences. The basal ganglia and the cerebellum also strongly influence the system. The sensory system (i.e., proprioception) also affects normal movement. A descriptive rather than functional division of the pyramidal from the extrapyramidal system is commonly used. The pyramidal system includes the CST and the corticobulbar pathway (to the motor nuclei of the brain stem). All other motor pathways such as the rubrospinal and reticulospinal tracts are part of the extrapyramidal system. Parkinson's disease is a familiar example of a disease process that is located largely in the extrapyramidal system.

The pyramidal tract (CST) is associated with skilled volitional movements of the distal limbs.

Therefore, isolated lesions of the CST often produce paresis and clumsiness of the distal limb (the upper more than the lower; see Fig. 8-3). The extrapyramidal system is involved in crude, stereotyped associative movements of the proximal limb and axial musculature, such as swinging the arms while walking. The vestibular system primarily influences the axial musculature, whereas the reticular formation influences all of the muscle groups by its effect on the γ motor neurons and the basic spinal circuits.

The Cerebellum

Cerebellar disorders are more obvious if the lesion is unilateral and other signs of upper or lower motor neuron disease are absent. The cerebellum can be divided into three functional zones[5]: the midline or vermian region primarily connects with the vestibular system and the spinal cord, the paravermian region involves both the spinal cord and cerebral cortex, and the lateral zone receives extensive input from the motor regions of the cerebral cortex.

Lesions of the lateral aspects of the cerebellar hemispheres cause ataxia, hypotonia, intention tremor, and cerebellar dysarthria (speech impairment) on the ipsilateral side. Lesions of the paravermian or intermediate zone cause gait ataxia but not upper limb ataxia. A 10-year-old boy with a slow-growing tumor in the intermediate zone may present with a 2-month history of a stumbling and incoordinated gait. The only other sign might be frequent headaches.[5]

The Spinal Level

Quite often, lesions within the spinal cord affect both motor and sensory tracts (e.g., Brown-Séquard's syndrome). It is, however, certainly possible to have a small lesion of the LCST below the level of the pyramidal decussation that affects only motor activity on the ipsilateral side. Bilateral lesions of the LCST in the high cervical region result in upper motor neuron weakness or paralysis of all limbs (quadriplegia), whereas bilateral lesions in the lower thoracic levels affect only the lower extremities (paraplegia). The cervical and T12–L1 spinal cord segments are more susceptible to injury in car accidents and sports because of their motion and vulnerability to ischemic necrosis. In multiple sclerosis, demyelination of the axonal fibers of the CST in the spinal cord takes place. Other tracts and the brain stem are affected as well. The disease may present as patchy areas of hypesthesia coupled with spastic weakness distal to the level of demyelination.

The Anterior Motor Neurons

The motor neurons for the lower extremities are located in the anterior gray horns of the spinal cord from T12 to S4. Diseases affecting these levels of the nervous system include amyotrophic lateral sclerosis (ALS), poliomyelitis, and certain genetic disorders such as myelomeningocele and the hereditary motor neuron diseases (see Chapter 23). In ALS, signs of both lower and upper motor neuron disease may be present.

In poliomyelitis, the segmental level for L4 is frequently affected. Since the anterior tibial muscle is largely supplied by this segment, poliomyelitis of L4 results in foot-drop with a steppage gait. Lesions of the motor neurons in the anterior horn of the spinal cord are termed lower motor neuron diseases. Flaccid paralysis, atonia, areflexia, and fasciculations are classically associated with lower motor neuron disease. In contrast, lesions of the upper motor neurons including the CST often present with spastic paralysis, hypertonia, hyperreflexia, and latent disuse atrophy (see Table 8-1).

Many lower motor neurons participate in basic spinal reflex arcs. The fundamental reflex arc includes the sensory afferent fiber entering the spinal column via the dorsal root, an internuncial neuron, and the motor efferent fiber exiting via the ventral root. Motor neurons in the anterior ventral horn receive information from both upper motor neurons as well as the numerous reflex arcs in that segment and others.[6]

The Nerve Roots

The nerve roots supplying the lower extremities arise from T12 to S4. Herniated discs, osteoarthritis, and spondylolisthesis are frequently associated with nerve root damage (radiculopathy). Distal weakness, paresthesias, and a loss of reflexes may result. Knowledge of the distribution and significance of the myotomes, dermatomes, and reflexes can help to locate the precise segmental level (see Fig. 8-2). Approximately 85 percent of lumbar disc protrusions occur at the L4-L5 and L5-S1 levels, 10 percent at the L3-L4 level, and only 5 percent at higher levels.[3]

The Peripheral Nerves

Peripheral neuropathy may have motor weakness or sensory loss or both as predominant features. It may also either involve one nerve and its distal parts as a mononeuropathy (Fig. 8-1) or affect many of the peripheral nerves as a polyneuropathy. In diabetic polyneuropathy, sensory loss predominates, whereas in Guillain-Barré syndrome and Charcot-Marie-Tooth disease motor

Table 8-1. Tests and Signs Associated With Anatomic Lesions of the Nervous System

Test or Sign	Corticospinal	Cerebellum	Ventral Motor Neuron	Nerve Root	Nerve(s)	Neuromuscular Junction	Muscle
Gait	+	++	+	+	+	+	+
Power	↓	−	↓	↓	↓	↓	↓
Tone	↑	−	↓	↓	↓	−	−
Reflexes	↑	−	↓	↓	↓	−	−
Babinski	+	−	−	−	−	−	−
Dysthesias	Possible	−	+	++	++	−	−
Atrophy	−[a]	−	++	+	+	−	−
Fasciculations	−	−	+	+	+	−	−
Lasègue	−	−	−	+	−	−	−
Fatigue	+	−	+	−	−	++	+
Heel-knee-shin	−+	+	−	−	−	−	−

[a] Later disuse atrophy is seen.

loss is more common. The damage may be axonal or demyelinating. With partial injury or insidious disease the sensory symptoms often prevail. With more rapidly occurring or complete nerve damage severe muscle weakness or paralysis is seen.[7]

Trauma is the most common cause of mononeuropathy.[7] The patient in Figure 8-1 incurred a shrapnel wound to his posterior thigh in World War II. This damaged both the peroneal and tibial components of the sciatic nerve. The resulting anesthetic foot-drop with severe hyperpronation required the use of a polypropylene ankle-foot orthosis.

The Neuromuscular Junction

Muscle weakness may also occur at the level of the neuromuscular junction. Myasthenia gravis is one of the more common examples, although it more often occurs in the muscles of the upper extremities and face (e.g., the eyelids). Disorders at the neuromuscular level result in motor deficits only. No sensory impairment accompanies the weakness. Tick paralysis and botulism are other examples of disease at this level.

Primary Muscle Disease

Genetic muscle disease presents at birth, with generalized weakness and hypotonia, or soon after. It is usually nonprogressive or slowly progressive compared to the more rapidly progressive spinal (anterior motor neuron) muscular atrophy seen in Werdnig-Hoffmann disease. More commonly, hypotonia with lack of normal maturation signs is seen in cerebral palsy. Among the acquired muscle diseases is idiopathic polymyositis. The pelvic muscles are usually first involved. The patient has difficulty climbing stairs and getting out of a chair, or might complain of an inability to raise the arms above the shoulders.

Etiologies of a weak or paralytic foot include trauma, vascular lesions or accidents, neoplasms, and metabolic, degenerative, endocrine, and infectious diseases. Again, the clinical manifestation is determined by the anatomic location. Once the

Table 8-2. Differential Diagnosis of Muscle Weakness According to Neuroanatomic Localization

Location	Vascular	Trauma	Neoplastic	Degenerative-Metabolic-Toxic	Inflammatory
Motor cortex	Thrombosis Embolus	Laceration Subdural or extradural hematoma	Meningoma Metastasis Glioma	—	—
Internal capsule	Thrombosis Embolus Hemorrhage	—	Glioma Metastasis	—	Abscess Infarction
Brain stem	Thrombosis Hemorrhage	"Contusion"	Astrocytoma	+	MS
Spinal cord	"Ant. spinal artery syndrome"	Spinal fracture Spondylosis	Astrocytoma Ependymoma Metastasis (extramedullary)	ALS SCD PA	MS (Incl. transverse myelitis)
Cranial and spinal motoneurons	Thrombosis Hemorrhage	Glioma Neurilemmoma Meningeal carcinoma and leukemia	Infiltration	ALS	Meningitis
Peripheral nerves	Mononeuropathy Polyarteritis	Laceration Compression	Compression Infiltration Remote effect	Lead	Leprosy Guillain-Barré syndrome
Neuromuscular junction	—	—	Eaton-Lambert syndrome	Botulism	Myasthenia gravis
Muscle	—	—	Remote effect	Muscular dystrophies	Polymyositis/ dermatomyositis

SCD, spinocerebellar degeneration; PA, pernicious anemia; ALS, amyotrophic lateral sclerosis; MS, multiple sclerosis.
(From Swanson,[7] with permission.)

location of the lesion is established, a differential diagnosis can be determined (Table 8-2).

THE CLINICAL HISTORY

The age, nature of onset, and any preexisting disease facilitate the clinical diagnosis and underlying etiology of the weak or paralytic foot.[2,4-8] The history of trauma will often be obvious. However, in some instances additional probing by the examiner may be necessary. Minor head trauma in the elderly can cause subdural hematoma, precipitating a gradual and mild hemiparesis occurring over a period of weeks,[5] often accompanied by headaches.

The age of a patient colors the clinician's palette of possible diagnoses. The elderly harbor degenerative processes affecting the nervous system. In the child, consideration must be given to the prenatal and birthing history. Metabolic and endocrine disorders can cause neuropathy, diabetes being one of the more common diseases seen. Nutrition and the general state of health must be considered. Vitamin B_{12} deficiency leads to posterior column disease, where there is loss of proprioception affecting the patient's gait. The family history must be reviewed. Was a relative confined to a wheelchair in later years because of severe pes cavus or weak calves? Are there any associated symptoms?

A comprehensive history starts with the necessary statistics, including date and place of birth, sex, weight, height, and source of referral. The presenting or chief complaint is then recorded. Was the onset abrupt or insidious? Obtain the exact date whenever possible and have the episode described fully: What was its location? What was its course? its character? its frequency? its duration? What has happened since the onset of the chief complaint? Are the symptoms the same, worse, or improved? Are there any factors that aggravate or alleviate the symptoms? Bending over may increase cerebral pressure, causing a transient headache, a symptom associated with a space-occupying lesion or inflammatory process. Low back or leg pain associated with coughing or Valsalva's maneuver may be present with a herniated disc syndrome. Have there been remissions and exacerbations? any prior diagnostic tests or treatments? What is currently being done by the patient? by another physician?

Cerebral vascular accidents in the elderly are usually sudden, affecting one limb or side of the face. The arterial occlusion affects the hands and face more often than the lower extremity. The podiatrist more often sees the geriatric patient after a severe stroke. The onset of a stroke may follow administration of a general anesthetic in an elderly patient. Of course, depending on the location of the vascular occlusion or hemorrhage, the symptoms can involve any of the following: dysphagia, impaired vision, weakness or paralysis, intense headaches, loss of consciousness, convulsions, or difficulty in swallowing and breathing.

A transient ischemic attack, on the other hand, might be revealed in the patient's history or in casual conversation. The elderly patient may well ignore these early warning signs. A temporary motor weakness anywhere generally lasts less than 12 minutes, but may be present for up to 24 hours. The transient attacks often precede more serious vascular accidents. Therefore a patient relating an 8-minute episode of foot-drop, aphagia, or loss of vision should be encouraged to receive immediate medical care.

Patients with hypertension can develop spontaneous hemorrhage affecting the motor fibers of the internal capsule. Sudden hemiplegia results. Headaches are more common in vascular hemorrhage than in arterial occlusion. Atherosclerosis of vessels (e.g., the middle cerebral artery) supplying the motor system commonly results in thrombosis or embolism. Small infarcts can specifically damage only the motor pathways. When the brain stem is affected, damage to the cranial nerves can be manifested (e.g., by constricted pupils).

Sudden paralysis of both legs could also be due to advanced atherosclerotic disease involving the anterior spinal artery. A loss of sensation occurs as well. However, the posterior column is spared as its arterial supply is different. Therefore, proprioception, vibration, and touch remain intact.

Weakness in one or both legs is seen in meningioma, a relatively common brain tumor, especially where it involves the central falx cerebri. Meningioma has a predilection for this area, where the motor activity for the foot and leg originates.[5] Monoparesis can also result from metastatic carcinoma, most commonly from bronchial carcinoma. Progressive hemiplegia is seen with infiltrating tumors, especially astrocytoma or oligodendroglioma, affecting the internal capsule.

When symptoms of progressive hemiplegia, headache, and fever are present, a brain abscess must be considered. Meningitis will occasionally cause chronic arachnoiditis, resulting in spinal compression and progressive spastic weakness of the legs. Arachnoiditis may also follow back surgery. The scarring can affect patients variably, but leg pain and dysfunction can be associated with activity. In older patients, narrowing of the lumbar spine (spinal stenosis) will prevent walking because of associated leg pain. Tarsal pulses will be normal. Cauda equina compression also variably affects the legs and feet.

The patient may report gait disturbances. Does a quick turn cause the patient to stumble and reel? Does the patient have difficulty climbing stairs? An early symptom of Parkinson's disease, a less agile gait, might first be noted by the patient.[4]

History taking for a child with a possible neurologic weak foot includes a prenatal and birth history.[8-10] Was gestation uneventful? What was the general health of the mother? Were fetal movements present by the fifth month? An absence of these movements might suggest Werdnig-Hoffmann disease.[8] Was the child carried to term? Was there an attempt at self-induced abortion? How many pregnancies had the mother had, and were there any previous abortions? What was the birth presentation? Was delivery prolonged and the child hypoxic? What type of anesthesia was given? Was the child unresponsive at birth? Were sucking and feeding normal? Was there any evidence of head trauma? Was the child given oxygen? Was any asymmetry present?

The developmental history of the child must also be explored. When did the child first hold the head up? smile? roll? sit up? grasp? stand? speak? Were there any delays in the child's walking or running? Can the child rise from the ground quickly? When did the child begin to climb stairs? Are there any existing problems with the siblings or other relatives?

CLINICAL EXAMINATION

Salient tests for neurologic disorders should be included in the routine podiatric biomechanical and gait analysis. These include tests for coordination, power, reflexes, and sensations. The following is an outlined approach to the podiatric gait analysis and examination using standardized forms (Figs. 8-4 and 8-5). By no means is the outline all-inclusive, and the forms can be modified to each clinician's practice. The forms are not intended for use with the infant, as the examination of the neonate and infant requires special tests of neurologic maturation. Myelination of the spinal cord largely occurs in the first 6 months of infancy. Neurologic responses related to the myelination process include the grasping and stepping reflexes at birth as well as the timely appearance of the righting and tilting responses. More on these special tests for infants are presented later in this chapter. Nevertheless, the forms in Figures 8-4 and 8-5 should serve as a model for the evaluation of a child or an adult, especially when there is suspected weakness.

The patient is examined in stance and in gait and then while sitting, supine, and prone. The child or adult should be fitted with a pair of boxer shorts kept on the premises or brought with the patient. The boxer shorts can be easily brought down to the level of the posterior superior iliac spines (PSIS) for inspection in sitting, stance, and gait. Men need not wear a shirt; women can wear a bathing suit top. Infants may be examined under less modest circumstances as indicated.

Stance and Gait Analysis

In the adult and older child the examination is initiated with a general observation of the patient while standing (in stance). Is the patient steady on his or her feet? Can the patient balance on one foot (Trendelenburg's sign)? Can the patient perform repeated toe raises on one foot? Does this compare equally with the other foot? Can partial knee-bends be done on each leg without difficulty? The last 20 degrees of extension requires the most mus-

```
                          R                              L
                              GAIT ANALYSIS
_____ Head Position _____
_____ Shoulders _____
_____ Handedness _____
_____ Spine _____
_____
_____ PSIS _____
_____ Hip _____
_____ Thigh _____
_____ Knee _____
_____ Knee Extensions (L2-4) _____
_____ Tibiae _____
_____ Toe Walk (S1) _____
_____ Hindfoot _____
                              Heel Walk
_____ (w/FF Sup. L4) _____
_____ (w/digits ext. L5) _____
_____ Angle of Gait _____ Base: _____
_____


Coordination: _____
Tone: _____
Power: _____
Atrophy: _____
Other: _____
_____
_____
```

Fig. 8-4. Podiatric gait analysis.

cular exertion. Does the arch reconstitute itself on toe raise?

Evaluation of selected myotomes of larger muscle groups of the lower extremities should be done first in the stance and gait analysis. The repeated toe raises will more accurately reveal any relative calf weakness. Similarly, the partial knee-bends are most helpful for detection of quadriceps weakness.

The spine should be inspected and palpated for any curvature of point tenderness. If any is found, at what segmental level is it? Is there single or double curvature? Are the legs bowed or knocked? Which foot is more flaccid and flat? Does one leg appear smaller than the other? Do the calves appear atrophic compared to the thighs? With the patient bending forward, does one side of the thorax appear higher than the other? Is there asymmetrical paravertebral muscular development or spasm?

Gait analysis is then done to perceive any gross variation from the usual tandem (heel-to-toe) walk. A number of neurologic gaits are characteristic. Some of the common ones are reviewed first. The determinants of "normal" gait should be familiar to the reader.[8]

The scissorlike gait of spastic paraplegia is seen in patients with spastic cerebral palsy. Depending on the severity, the knees are flexed and adducted, appearing to knock and roll around each other as the legs slide forward. Often the foot is markedly pronated, but it may be supinated with a toe-to-toe cycle depending on the muscles affected with the spasticity. The patient may also circumduct the leg to prevent the knees from knocking.

Steppage gait is seen where paralysis of the anterior tibial muscle is present. The dangling foot is swung through the swing phase; the hip flexor and leaning body assist in lifting the entire limb. The

SITTING:

R   L

REFLEXES

	Quad DTR (L4)	
	PTib DTR (L5)	
	Achilles DTR (S1)	
	Babinski's	

DERMATOMES

	Thigh (L123, S2)	
	Ankle (L45, S1)	
	Sole (S1)	

MYOTOMES

	Iliopsoas (T12, L123)	
	Quad (L234)	
	Ant Tib (L4)	
	Long Extensors (L5)	
	Peronei (S1)	
	Intrinsics (S23)	

SUPINE:
(Myotomes, Cont.)

| | Glut Med (L5) | |
| | Addtrs (L234) | |

(Length and Girth)

	True Leg Length	
	Apparent Leg Length	
	Calf	
	Patella	
	4 cm Thigh	
	20 cm Thigh	

(Torsion & Joint Alignment)

	Femur	
	Tibia	
	STJ	
	MTJ	
	Digits	

(Flexibility)

	Lig Laxity	
	Gastrocnemius	
	Soleus	
	Hamstrings	
	Psoas	

(Other)

	Fasciculations	
	Heel-Knee-Shin	
	Sit-up (T5-12, L1)	

PRONE:
(Myotomes, Cont.)

	Quadriceps (L234)	
	Med Hamstrings (L5)	
	Biceps Femoris (S1)	
	Gluteus Maximus (S1)	

OTHER: _____

SUMMARY: _____

Fig. 8-5. Podiatric examination.

foot then slaps the ground, initially supinated, yielding only too soon to the body weight and pronating. Steppage gait can be seen in both lower and upper motor neuron disorders, but predominates in peripheral nervous system dysfunction. As already noted, it can be a component of trauma to the motor area of the cerebral cortex specific for the lower limb. The anterior tibial muscle is largely supplied by L4 and to a lesser degree by L5; hence, common root lesions at L4-L5 may present with steppage gait. In middle-aged persons with a history of poliomyelitis steppage gait may be seen.

Stomping with a wide base of gait is seen in patients with posterior column disease.[4] The loss of proprioception requires the patient to constantly look down at the feet to check their placement. This spinal ataxia is more profound with the patient's eyes closed. Stomping is seen in multiple sclerosis among many other diseases and lesions affecting the posterior column and proprioception.

Cerebellar disease, on the other hand, can produce ataxia with the patient's eyes open or closed. In early or subtle forms of cerebellar ataxia, the patient may appear to walk relatively normally; however, when the patient is suddenly asked to turn right or left, incoordination and stumbling may become apparent. An awkward and clumsy child may have a milder dyspraxia without disease. Cerebellar dysfunction also results in a mildly broad-based gait. Multiple sclerosis and Friedreich's ataxia among other diseases can present with both spinal spasticity and cerebellar ataxia; this has been called "jiggling."[2]

The term *apraxic gait* refers to the loss of gait often seen in patients with senile dementia, although no firm etiology has been found. The feet may appear glued to the ground, and the patient may have difficulty initiating gait. The senile patient is seen to take smaller and shorter steps, to the point where he or she may completely lose the ability to walk.

Loss of agility in walking may be one of the first signs of extrapyramidal disease (e.g., Parkinson's disease).[4] In more advanced stages of Parkinson's disease, the patient initiates the gait slowly with small steps *(marche à petits pas)*, but then takes increasingly quicker steps. This is known as "snowballing" or festination.

Waddling with compensatory lordosis is seen in congenital myopathy and acquired myositis. Proximal muscle groups are more often involved; hence the associated difficulty in rising from a chair or from the floor (Gowers' sign). The patient may place the hands on the thighs to help extend the knee and assist a weakened quadriceps, especially when walking up an incline. A paralyzed gastrocnemius-soleus group will produce a calcaneus gait. An insufficient heel-lift posteriorly displaces the tibia at the ankle joint to enhance the leverage of the foot.

Not all neurologic disorders leading to a weak or paralytic leg will be evident from the patient's history or gait analysis. Moreover, the patient may relate vague symptoms he or she may feel are attributable to poor circulation, a short leg, or running style, when in fact an early neuromuscular disorder is present — all the more reason to include the neurologic observations in the gait analysis and the biomechanical examination. Each of the parameters in the gait analysis and podiatric examination will be discussed with reference to Figures 8-4 and 8-5.

The position of the head is observed in gait. Does it list to one side? The shoulder is usually lower on the dominant side. The handedness is noted. Any other irregularities of the spine are noted. The PSIS and the hip swing more to the higher side if any leg length discrepancy exists. Trendelenburg gait is ruled out; a significant drop of the hip opposite the paralyzed gluteus medius is seen. Weakness of the psoas (hip flexor) and ipsilateral pretibial musculature can be detected in gait. Hip flexion is therefore noted. The thigh is observed for internal and external rotation: Does the knee remain internally rotated? Is there any apparent atrophy or weakness in the vastus medialis? in the proximal thigh? If any weakness is suspected, the patient is asked to do several partial knee-bends. Are the lower legs thin compared to the thighs, as is seen in hereditary peroneal muscular atrophy (Charcot-Marie-Tooth disease)? The patient is asked to walk on tiptoes to check the S1 myotome, and then asked to walk with the feet supinated. This isolates the activity of the anterior tibial muscle (L4) and its usually visible tendon. The patient then heel-walks with the toes extended (L5). The angle and base of the patient's usual gait are then recorded.

When suspected, posterior column disease can

be differentiated from cerebellar disease by having the patient close the eyes (Romberg's test). Although not a conclusive test by itself, vision can mask and compensate the loss of proprioception seen in diseases affecting the posterior column.

Power, tone, coordination, and any atrophy can be assessed from the initial gait analysis. Any other symptoms or signs involving the upper extremity, the neck, and the face should be noted and correlated with the findings of the lower extremity, and followed up with appropriate consultation. Other standard neurology texts (e.g., ref. 4) provide a comprehensive review of testing for the cranial nerves and other helpful tests of the upper extremities.

The Seated Examination

The Reflexes

The patient is asked to sit on the edge of the examining table. The blood pressure can be taken if this has not been done already. Deep tendon or muscle stretch reflexes (DTRs) of the lower extremities and Babinski's responses are first checked (Fig. 8-5). The quadriceps and triceps surae (Achilles tendon) are routinely checked. The posterior tibial muscle, although difficult to elicit, is also checked.

The reader should be familiar with other superficial, deep, and pathologic reflexes, but they are not necessarily included in the routine podiatric examination. More common superficial reflexes include the corneal, sucking, and pharyngeal gag reflexes.

Specific to the lower extremities are the cremasteric (L1–L2), anal (S3–S5), and abdominal (T6–L1) superficial reflexes. Although tests of these reflexes are not routinely performed on the podiatric patient, knowledge of them can be helpful in assessing acute spinal trauma, radiculopathy, and early motor loss in multiple sclerosis.[3]

Superficial reflexes are segmental reflexes normally present. These include the normally elicited flexor response of the Babinski test. Pathologic responses include the extensor response or Babinski's sign and clonus.

The Babinski test is extremely useful in detecting suprasegmental or upper motor neuron disease. When any noxious or painful stimulus is applied to the foot, both foot and limb typically retract from the stimulus. Thus, especially in the supine patient, the knee and hip may flex in addition to the response in the foot. Babinski's sign is also seen in the infant up to 18 months of age. With the ensuing maturation of the myelination in the spinal cord, the upper motor neurons effectively suppress the more primitive extensor Babinski reflex. Unless disease is present, the response is "flexor" in the adult; Babinski's sign is absent. Babinski's sign includes hyperextension of the hallux with fanning (abduction and slight flexion) of the lesser toes.

A Babinski's sign is elicited by stroking the sole of the foot with a relatively sharp object. The motion should be slow, deliberate, and painful—to the point of eliciting a response. This may occur after drawing the metal end of the neurologic hammer only 1 inch forward from the lateral sole of the foot. Ordinarily the stroke starts from the lateral sole of the heel and is brought slowly forward, eventually crossing over to the first metatarsophalangeal joint. The best response occurs the first time it is tested.

Other noxious stimuli can similarly produce a flexor or extensor response, but with less reliability. Chaddock's test uses a sharp stroke drawn from the inferolateral malleolus along the lateral edge of the foot to the distal fifth metatarsal. Oppenheim's test uses firm and painful pressure from the knuckles of the examiner's hands astride the tibial crest. The knuckles bear down into the paratibial muscles and slowly descend along the tibia from its tubercle to the ankle. Gordon's stimulus is a firm grasp to the belly of the gastrocnemius. Stransky's test is a forceful abduction of the fifth digit, which is held for a couple of seconds and then released. Gonda's reflex occurs when the third and fourth digits are distracted and plantarflexed, held, and then released. Of these additional reflexes, Chaddock's and Oppenheim's are the most reliable.[2]

Reflexes are also altered in upper and lower motor neuron diseases. In the lower limb, L4, L5, and S1 are commonly tested. The quadriceps is supplied by the femoral nerve originating from the second, third, and fourth lumbar segments. However, L4 is predominantly tested.[11] The pointed end of the neurologic hammer is used. The patellar tendon is palpated. Often it is positioned slightly lateral to the midline when the patient is sitting. If the patient is bedridden and supine, the knee can be flexed about 30 degrees while the thigh is held off the bed. If the DTRs cannot be obtained, the reflex is facilitated or "reinforced" by Jendrassik's maneuver: the patient is asked to grasp one hand with the other and pull while the tendon is percussed. The DTRs should be graded and, more importantly, compared to those of the contralateral limb.

Grading commonly is from zero to four. If there is no reflex present even with reinforcement, the grade is zero. A trace reflex is one that is present with facilitation. The physiologic range is from 1+ to 3+. Of course, this grading is somewhat subjective, but differences between right and left DTRs are significant. A grade of 4+ is used for hyperreflexia associated with pathology (i.e., clonus).[7]

Clonus, associated with suprasegmental lesions, is a response to sudden, gentle and sustained stretching of selected muscle groups. The gastrocnemius and soleus muscles are commonly tested. The response consists of repetitive beats persisting as long as the calf is stretched. Rapidly pushing the patella distally on an extended leg will also produce an available clonus in the quadriceps. With the patient sitting, the forefoot can be lifted by the examiner, with the fingers under the ball of the foot. The fingers then are tapped with the neurologic hammer, and an Achilles reflex may be seen with a sustained clonus. An easier method to check further for clonus is used later when the patient is prone: the knee is flexed about 45 degrees and the foot is then quickly dorsiflexed at the ankle.

The Achilles DTR tests S1 predominantly. Although the tibial nerve innervates both the gastrocnemius and the posterior tibial muscles, the nerve roots vary. The Achilles DTR has components from L5 to S2, with S1 the major segmental supply.

The Achilles tendon is stretched by gently holding and lifting the foot. The tendon is then tapped with the blunt end of the neurologic hammer. If the response is zero, the reflex can be checked later in the examination when the patient is prone. In the prone position the knee is flexed 90 degrees, the forefoot is again dorsiflexed, and the Achilles tendon tapped.

Several variations of the Achilles DTR test exist for use in the bedridden patient. With the patient supine, the lower leg can be crossed over its counterpart, the foot dorsiflexed, and the reflex elicited. Another alternate means of suddenly stretching the Achilles is to tap the blunt end of the hammer against the fingers of the examiner as described above when checking for clonus.

Functional testing of the reflex for the L5 segment can be done as follows (Fig. 8-6): The posterior tibial tendon is stretched by pronating the relaxed and dependent foot. The tendon becomes visible or palpable between the navicular bone and the medial malleolus. Again, the pointed end of the neurologic hammer is used to elicit a response. Testing for the L5 response requires considerable practice and appears to be easier in pes cavus feet. A smaller percentage of fibers from the S1 segment also feed the posterior tibial muscle via the tibial nerve.

The Dermatomes

The dermatomes of the lower extremity are readily checked with a common sewing pinwheel.[3] Two pinwheels can be used at the same time in the following manner: The pinwheels are drawn down the anterior thigh, crossing the dermatomes for L1, L2, and L3. A longitudinal strip at the posterior thigh is innervated from the S2 segment, and this should also be tested. Crossing the pinwheels from the extreme medial to the lateral ankle will include the dermatomes for L4, L5, and S1. Innervation of the sole of the foot is quite variable but includes sensory information to S1 to S4.[3]

Tests for posterior column disease include vibratory, proprioception, and stereognosis. These should be checked in diabetics among others suspected of having posterior column disease.

The Myotomes

The size and strength of most of the muscle groups of the lower extremity mandate observation first in stance and then in gait, after which the manual examination can be meaningful. The hip flexor (psoas) is easily checked. The seated patient is asked to lift the thigh against an examiner's hand that is applying a downward force at the knee. The point of application of the force of the examiner's hand is at a considerable distance from the axis of

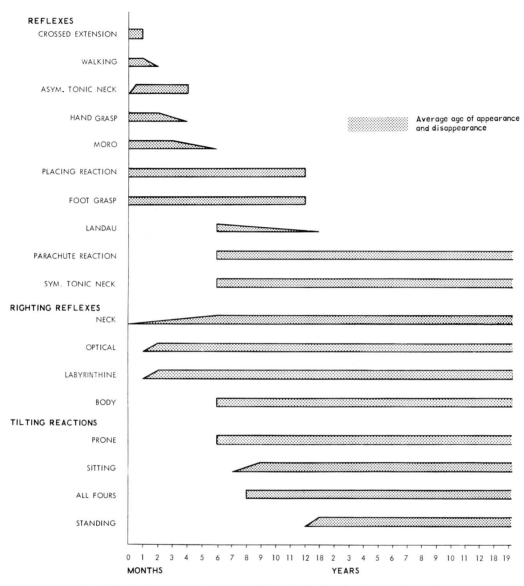

Fig. 8-6. Reflex maturation chart. (From Tachdjian,[8] with permission.)

rotation of the hip. Moreover, the weight of the lower leg adds to the force applied by the examiner's hand at the knee. This combined use of a long lever arm and the weight of a body part in the application of force against the muscle being tested helps to validate the manual examination of musculature in the lower extremity. In selected patients, further isokinetic testing can be done using me-

chanical measurements when necessary to compare very subtle differences between specific muscle groups of each limb.

When manual force blocks hip flexor activity on one or both sides relatively easily, significant disease may be present. The iliopsoas muscle group receives multiple innervation from the T12, L1, L2, and L3 segments. The disease process must involve most of these nerve roots in order to produce a clinically observed weakness of the hip flexor.[3] Compare this to a local disease process of L4. The anterior tibial muscle normally fires during the swing phase of gait, lifting the forefoot adequately to clear the ground. Since the anterior tibial is mostly supplied by L4, a local disease of L4 produces a profound and overt foot-drop.

The quadriceps can also be checked in the sitting position (Fig. 8-5). However, this should be done to substantiate any weakness observed in the static and gait examination. To test the quadriceps, the patient extends the knee while the examiner's hand applies opposing force at the lower end of the tibia. Then the patient is asked to invert and evert the foot against the examiner's application of force at the forefoot. The short flexors and extensors are also tested and compared with each other and their long counterparts. In pes cavus, abduction of the fifth digit may be absent.

The peroneus longus muscle is more difficult to block manually. The patient is asked to pronate the forefoot against the examiner's application of force. The examiner pushes up against the head of the first metatarsal. The peroneus brevis, however, is easily outleveraged by the examiner; therefore manual examination is more valid here. The peroneus longus muscle and tendon can be visually observed and palpated in the static examination when the patient stands on the ball of the foot.

Activity of the posterior tibial muscle can be isolated in the following manner: The seated patient crosses the leg to be tested "man style." The patient is then asked to invert the heel, being careful not to lift his forefoot and thus recruit the anterior tibial muscle. Chronic pronators will have difficulty using the posterior tibial muscle alone. The tendon is ordinarily visible.

The Supine Examination

The patient is next placed in a supine position. The hip abductors (L5 for the gluteus medius) and adductors (L2–L4) are also checked isotonically. The examiner's hands apply force at the ankles, and the patient is then asked to abduct and adduct the extended legs. This test is more valid and useful in children because of the size relative to the examiner.

The supine examination includes more biomechanical measurements, including those for limb length, joint motion, limb torsion, and alignment (Fig. 8-5). Limb length is first measured as standardly taught (see Chapter 4). The girth of both limbs is measured at four locations and compared. Many neurologic conditions of the lower extremity eventually diminish the size of the limb.

To measure the calf, the knee is flexed to 45 degrees. The tape measurement is taken at the apparent maximum girth. The knee or patellar level is next measured. The girth is then taken 4 cm above the superior pole of the patella to specifically evaluate the relative mass of the vastus medialis. Finally, with the knee still flexed at 45 degrees, the girth at 20 cm above the patella is recorded.

Torsion and range-of-motion measurements can be expressed as a fraction; for example, if the subtalar joint has 10 degrees of eversion and 20 degrees of inversion, this is recorded as 10/20. The neutral positions can be calculated after the clinical examination. In a pronated weak foot, the midtarsal joint untwists and becomes inverted; this inversion is often measured in degrees. Pes cavus feet are more often seen with a valgus torque to the midtarsal joint, again measured and expressed in degrees with standard podiatric instrumentation.

Flexibility

A number of tests can be used to evaluate ligamentous laxity, which is not to be equated with muscle flexibility. However, a quick thumb-to-wrist test may be sufficient. Loose-jointed individuals can bring their thumbs all the way to their wrists, whereas tight-jointed individuals may have 3 inches of space between thumb and wrist. The average measurement, however, is 2 inches.

Flexibility of more common muscle groups is tested, including the major antigravity muscles (Fig. 8-5). A tight psoas can be associated with low back disorders. When the knee is brought to the chest, the contralateral thigh should remain on the table. If, however, the contralateral thigh lifts off the table (again this movement is measured in degrees), a tight psoas is likely. When stretching the calf, clonus can be reevaluated.

The examiner should observe any fasciculations

in the limbs of the supine patient. Also while the patient is supine a brief coordination test specific for the lower extremities is done. The heel-knee-shin test requires the patient to place one foot on the opposite tibial tuberosity and then brush the foot down the shin to the ankle. The patient affected with a cerebellar disorder specific to the lower extremities will falter on doing this.

Finally, at the end of the supine examination the patient is asked to do a slow sit-up. If there is radiculopathy at any of the higher spinal segments (T5–T12, L1), the abdomen will be asymmetrically flexed (Beevor's sign).

The Prone Examination

The final part of a neurologic examination for weak foot includes evaluation of additional myotomes in the prone position. The knees of the patient are flexed 90 degrees, and the examiner applies resistance to check both the quadriceps and the hamstrings. The biceps femoris is largely supplied by the S1 nerve root. This can be compared with any calf weakness, which also involves S1. The gluteus maximus, also supplied by S1, is checked by having the prone patient lift the thigh against the examiner's resistance.

With the patient in the prone position, some measurements can be repeated as necessary. The Achilles reflex is best tested with the patient prone, and biomechanical measurements also are often taken in the prone position.

The Pediatric Examination

A suspected weak foot seen in infancy requires special testing for neurologic maturation. Cerebral palsy often involves delayed motor development and can be suspected when maturation levels are not reached at the expected time (Fig. 8-6). Some of the more important reflexes will be described here. For more detailed information on specific tests, Tachdjian's[8] text is recommended. Jordan[11] has reviewed normal locomotion in the infant, and Sharp[12] has provided a review of normal motor development in the infant.

In the neonate, subcortical activity prevails. Early motor behavior is "stereotyped, without definite purpose, poorly controlled, and reflexively patterned."[12] During the first 2 years of life the cells of the cortex and respective motor pathways become myelinated and mature. Hence the emergence of cortical dominance is exhibited by planned movement and suppression of the haphazard movements of the infant.

Maturation occurs in a cephalocaudal direction. Consequently, the Babinski extensor response and the foot placement and foot grasping responses persist to about 18 months of age, whereas the hand grasping reflex is lost by 5 months.

Other common reflexes at birth include the crossed extension, walking, asymmetric tonic neck, and Moro reflexes. These reflexes should be absent by 9 months of age. Other maturation reflexes occur anytime from birth (the neck righting reflex) to after 12 months of age (the tilting reaction when standing). Most of the maturation reflexes that occur after birth are present from 6 months on (see Fig. 8-6).

The Moro reflex is normally present in the infant up to 6 months of age. The test is performed by supporting the child's head while the child is in a supine position, and then suddenly releasing the support. The startled infant extends the limbs, then flexes and adducts them.

During the first month, the crossed extension or Phillipson's reflex should be present. It is elicited by application of a painful stimulus to one leg, producing abduction and flexion of the contralateral limb followed by adduction and extension. It almost appears as if the neonate is attempting to push away the stimulus.[12] Firm pressure anywhere on the limb should produce the reflex. Absence of this reflex suggests a partial or incomplete spinal lesion. The Babinski test ordinarily produces withdrawal of the limb, with flexion occurring at the knee and the hip. Light stimulation of the sole of the foot will produce the foot grasping reflex, similar to the hand grasping reflex.

The placing reaction and the walking or stepping reflex can be checked at the same time. The infant is supported at the waist; the anterior ankle is brushed against the corner of the examining table. The child reacts by lifting the foot and leg, attempting to place the foot on a firm surface. The stepping reflex is next tested by holding the child over the examining table and lightly touching the soles to the table as the child is moved forward. The child will take steps. The stepping or walking reflex is present only for about a month or two, whereas the placing reaction persists through the first year. Absence of these reflexes suggests brain damage.

Postural reflexes include the asymmetric and symmetric neck reflexes. The asymmetric neck reflex should appear in the first month of life. When the head of the supine infant is turned to one side, arm extension is produced on the side toward which the head was turned while flexion occurs in the contralateral arm. This response disappears by 6 months, but the symmetric neck reflex appears about this time.

The symmetric neck reflex is tested as follows: The infant is held prone in the examiner's lap, and the head and neck are flexed. Symmetric arm flexion occurs. Persistence or even exaggeration of the asymmetric neck reflex is seen in infants with cerebral palsy. Absence of the symmetric neck reflex also suggests delayed motor development.

The Landau test also tests delayed reflex maturation. Instead of supporting the child in the lap as in the symmetric neck reflex test, the examiner supports the child by the abdomen, so that the child is suspended horizontally. The head, neck, back, and hips should hyperextend ("Superman's flight"). This reaction should be present at 6 months, diminishing by 18 months.

The body will right itself when turned or tilted. The earliest of the righting reflexes occurs shortly after birth. The neck righting reflex causes the body of the infant to turn after the head has been turned and held. The body of the supine infant will be seen to turn as a whole. Beyond 6 months, the body turns segmentally in a cephalocaudal direction (the body righting reflex).

In a 3-month-old, the examiner should see the labyrinthine and the optical righting reflex. When the infant is held and tilted to one side, the head and neck will normally seek an upright position. Blindfolding differentiates the labyrinthine from the optical reflex.

After 6 months, tilting reactions should be observed. If the child is tilted to one side when prone, sitting, or on all fours, limb abduction and extension will occur to counter the tilt. Of course, this reaction continues through life. Another test of equilibrium maturation, the standing tilt reflex, is useful in ruling out cerebral palsy and other disorders of motor control. The child is supported while standing and tilted to the point of losing balance. The 12- to 18-month-old will hop to react to the apparent fall. The affected patient will simply lean his or her weight into the examiner's arms.

REFERENCES

1. Ganley JV: Calcaneovalgus deformity in infants. J Am Podiatry Assoc 65:5, 1975
2. Mayo Clinic, Department of Neurology and Department of Physics and Biophysics, Mayo Clinic; Clinical Examinations in Neurology. 5th Ed. WB Saunders, Philadelphia, 1981
3. Hoppenfeld S: Orthopaedic Neurology: A Diagnostic Guide to Neurologic Levels. JB Lippincott, Philadelphia, 1977
4. Ross RT: The Nervous System. 2nd Ed. Medical Examination Publishing, New York, 1985
5. Montgomery EB, Wall M, Henderson VW: Principles of Neurologic Diagnosis. Little, Brown, Boston, 1986
6. Liveson JA, Spielholz NI: Peripheral Neurology: Case Studies in Electrodiagnosis. FA Davis, Philadelphia, 1979
7. Swanson PD: Signs and Symptoms in Neurology. JB Lippincott, Philadelphia, 1984
8. Tachdjian M: Pediatric Orthopedics. WB Saunders, Philadelphia, 1972
9. McCrea JD: Pediatric Orthopedics of the Lower Extremity. Futura, Mount Kisco, NY, 1985
10. Tax HR: The systemic significance of the posturally poor foot position in the infant and child. Clin Podiatry 2(4), 1985
11. Jordan RP: The neuromotor development of bipedal location in the normal infant. J Am Podiatry Assoc 71:2, 1981
12. Sharp JT: Assessment of normal motor development in the child. J Am Podiatry Assoc 71:2, 1981
13. Ganley JV: Podopediatrics. Clin Podiatry 1(3):725, 1984

Edema

9

Lawrence Harkless, D.P.M.
Thomas F. McCloskey, D.P.M.

Edema of the feet and lower leg is a very common initial complaint brought to the podiatric physician. The diagnosis is usually very easy to make with proper utilization of the fundamentals of clinical medicine, the history and physical examination, but occasionally it can be occult and elusive. The cause is usually within the vascular system; however, systemic causes must also be considered.

PATHOPHYSIOLOGY

Guyton defines edema as excessive interstitial fluid within the tissues.[1] An understanding of the production and reabsorption of interstitial fluid is paramount to understanding edema. Intracapillary blood pressure and osmotic pressure of pericapillary material cause flow from the plasma, whereas interstitial fluid pressure and plasma osmotic pressure favor reabsorption. When transmural pressure is greater than osmotic pressure at the arterial end of a capillary, fluid extravasation results. As the blood continues along the capillary loop there is an increase in plasma osmotic pressure and a decrease in interstitial osmotic pressure due to fluid or electrolyte transfer from plasma to the interstitial space. As the intracapillary pressure drops, the balance reverses, causing fluid reabsorption of the same amount. Alteration of this balance causes fluid retention in the tissues until the molecular concentration is altered so that a balance can be achieved between osmotic effect and the rise in interstitial pressure.[2]

Traditionally, lymphatic flow was thought to be the result of fluid not reabsorbed at the venous end of the capillary. The lymphatic system then carried this fluid centrally. This concept may be too simple, however. Lymphatics may be essential for the transfer of proteins and "foreign cells"[2] from the interstitial space. The needed volume of lymphatic flow would then be that volume necessary to keep this material in solution.[2]

Edema can result from various mechanisms (Fig. 9-1). These include:

1. Increased capillary pressure. Pitting results from the collection of normal interstitial fluid. This is seen in heart failure and venous obstruction.
2. Increased osmotic pressure of the pericapillary material. This occurs when the capillary wall is

193

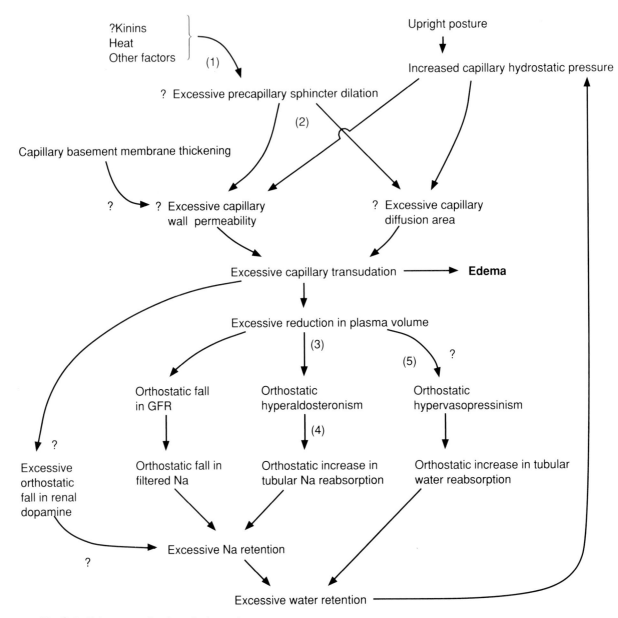

Fig. 9-1. Primary mechanisms in the pathogenesis of edema. Since all mechanisms result in leakage of fluid from the vascular into the extravascular space, the extent of edema would be limited by the fall in blood pressure with developing hypovolemia were it not for secondary mechanisms (not depicted), which result in renal retention of sodium and water: for example, secondary aldosteronism, possible vasopressin release, and intrinsic renal changes (e.g., a fall in the glomerular filtration rate). (From Streeten,[3] with permission.)

damaged, resulting in the leakage of protein, as in infection, trauma, and urticaria. If the lymphatic system is damaged, resulting in the collection of protein, edema develops. As the protein content of fluid increases, coagulation occurs and the edema becomes nonpitting.

3. Reduction of plasma osmotic pressure. Pitting results as the fluid resembles interstitial fluid.

This condition is seen in hypoproteinemic states.[2]

BILATERAL EDEMA

Edema of both extremities usually indicates a systemic process and not the simultaneous occurrence of a unilateral problem or process (Table 9-1). When edema of systemic origin is suspected, a characteristic clinical pattern is usually present. The onset is insidious with no history of a precipitating event. Edema begins simultaneously in both legs and advances to the same degree in each leg. Although pain is not generally a complaint in edema of systemic origin, it may be indicative of the underlying disease process. Clinical examination usually reveals a soft, pitting edema in the feet, ankles, and lower leg, often extending to the knees (Fig. 9-2).

Idiopathic Cyclic Edema

Idiopathic cyclic edema is very poorly understood. The diagnosis is one of exclusion of all other known causes of lower extremity edema. Clinical features include swelling of the face, hands, feet, legs, and the abdomen in women. The episodes have no relationship to the menstrual cycle. There is a typical weight gain of 1 to 2 kg/day, but gains of up to 6 kg have been noted. The swelling subsides at night. Anxiety, depression, headache, and irritability are also associated with this problem. The

Table 9-1. Causes of Bilateral Leg Edema

Congestive heart failure
Nephrotic syndrome
Acute glomerulonephritis
Hepatic cirrhosis
Hypoproteinemia
Idiopathic cyclic edema
Dependent position
Lipedema
Drugs
Primary lymphedema
Exposure to severe temperatures

(From Ruschhaupt and Graor,[4] with permission.)

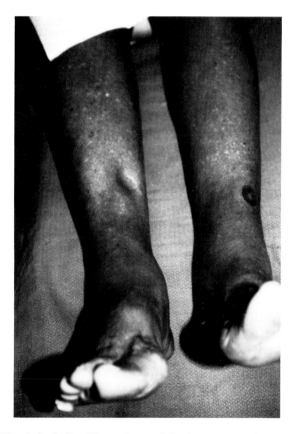

Fig. 9-2. Soft, pitting edema of the lower extremity secondary to edema of systemic origin.

syndrome appears to be self-limited, lasting from 6 months to 20 years. Several mechanisms have been discussed, but the exact cause remains unknown (Fig. 9-3). Young suggests that "most likely, we are seeing a variety of disease with possible unrelated mechanisms that result in edema." A multiplicity of therapies have been suggested, with some success. These include progesterone, weight reduction, spironolactone, salt-losing diuretics, sympatholytics, symphathomimetics, bed rest, restriction of salt intake, Unna boots, and elastic stockings[5] (Fig. 9-4).

Renal Abnormalities

Nephrotic syndrome and acute glomerulonephritis are renal abnormalities that may initiate edema. Laboratory findings of proteinuria, hypoalbuminemia, and hypercholesterolemia are diag-

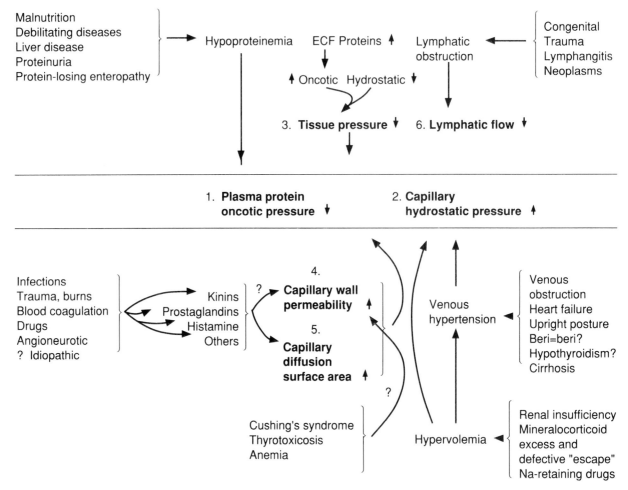

Fig. 9-3. Pathogenesis of the idiopathic edemas. The postulated or established sites of therapeutic or experimental corrective measures are indicated by numbers: *1*, sympathomimetic amines; *2*, external compression of the lower limbs; *3*, subtotal adrenalectomy, sympathomimetic amines; *4*, spironolactone and conventional diuretics; *5*, ethanol. (From Streeten,[3] with permission.)

nostic of nephrotic syndrome. However, a history of nocturia and polyuria may be a clue to the origin of edema despite a paucity of signs or symptoms of uremia.

Edema in a patient with a history of group A β-hemolytic streptococcal infection should raise suspicions of acute glomerulonephritis. When these diseases are suspected, renal biopsy is often used to confirm the diagnosis.[4]

Congestive Heart Failure

The clinical history of patients with congestive heart failure (CHF) may include dyspnea on exer-

tion, orthopnea, paroxysmal nocturnal dyspnea, hyperextension, angina, or previous myocardial infarction (Fig. 9-5). Examination usually reveals rales, rhonchi, jugular venous distention, tachycardia, tachypnea, hepatomegaly, cardiomegaly, and ventricular gallop. Chest radiography will often reveal pulmonary congestion and cardiomegaly.[4]

Liver Disease

The patient with edema due to liver disease can usually be easily recognized clinically. Alcoholism is a common cause of hepatic cirrhosis. A history of jaundice, abdominal swelling, or numbness or

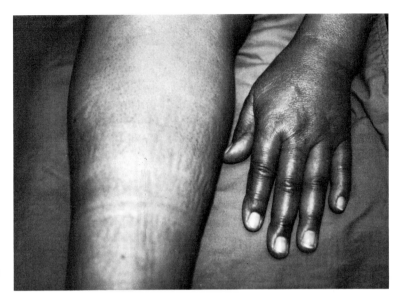

Fig. 9-4. Idiopathic edema of the hands and legs.

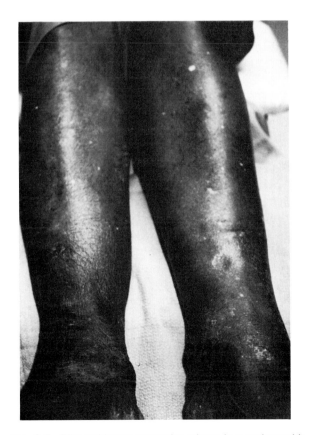

Fig. 9-5. Bilateral lower extremity edema in a patient with congestive heart failure.

burning of the feet along with edema raises the probability of hepatic cirrhosis. We have seen several patients present with a chief complaint of numbness and swelling in the feet. The presence of plantar and palmar erythema, hepatosplenomegaly, ascites, spider angiomas, and jaundice should increase the clinician's suspicion of hepatic dysfunction as the cause of the systemic problem.[6,7]

Lipedema

Lipedema is often mistaken for lymphedema. It is seen primarily in women. The clinical presentation is characterized by the deposition of excess fat in the tissues from the waist down to the ankles; it is familial, bilateral, symmetric, and painless. Usually the feet are spared; however, we have seen numerous patients complaining of swelling in their ankles which proved after careful examination to be fat deposition. This deposition is almost exclusively localized at the level of the lateral malleolus (Fig. 9-6).

Edema is usually not associated with lipedema; however, when pitting occurs it is associated with other problems such as water retention.[5]

There is no satisfactory treatment available. Patients should be cautioned to avoid gaining weight since excessive fat deposits in the buttocks and legs are difficult to reduce by losing weight.[5]

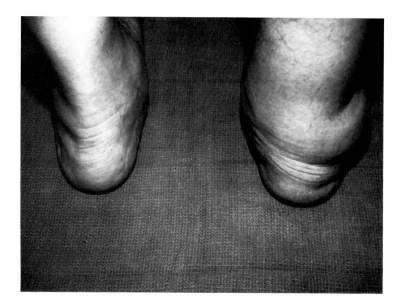

Fig. 9-6. Fatty deposition under the lateral malleoli in a patient with lipedema.

Dependency

Normal individuals who stand or sit for prolonged periods of time will have edema. This can be explained by lack of muscle activity; however, maintenance of a dependent position can also increase capillary blood pressure, causing fluid accumulation. It is very important not to overlook dependency.

Patients who are at increased risk include those who have suffered strokes and those with rheumatoid arthritis or degenerative joint disease. Treatment should include elastic stockings, Jobst stockings, TED hose, Ace bandages, and periodic elevation of the feet.

Hypoproteinemia

Hypoproteinemia is caused by hepatic dysfunction, malnutrition, and chronic malabsorption due to persistent diarrhea.[4]

Drugs

Various medications can cause edema, which is usually soft, pitting, and bilateral, and often similar to the swelling seen in hypoproteinemia and idiopathic cyclic edema.

Antihypertensive drugs that induce edema include nifedipine, methyldopa (Aldomet), guanethidine (Ismelin), hydralazine (Apresoline), diuretics, diazoxide (Hyperstat), and rauwolfia preparations. The nonsteroidal anti-inflammatory medications such as ibuprofen (Motrin), indomethacine, phenylbutazone (Butazolidine), and oxyphenbutazone (Tanderil) have been cited as causing edema as a result of their sodium retention qualities. Certain hormone medications may cause or exacerbate fluid retention. The medications often cited include progesterone, corticosteroids, estrogens, testosterone, and adrenocorticotropins. One should rule out drugs and their abuse as the etiology (Fig. 9-7).[4,5,8,9]

UNILATERAL LEG EDEMA

The presentation of unilateral leg edema necessitates a thorough history and physical examination. A comprehensive understanding of the differential diagnosis of unilateral leg edema as well as its characteristic signs and symptoms are important. Young sums up this concept best: ''swelling, like fever, is not a disease in itself but a sign of an under-

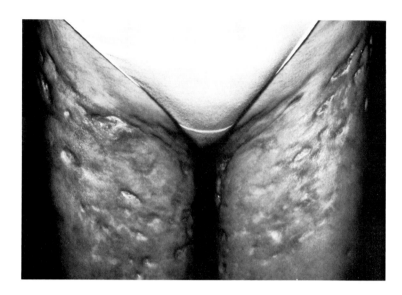

Fig. 9-7. Fibrotic, brawny edema of the lower extremities secondary to pentazocine (Talwin) abuse.

lying disorder."[5] Acute onset with signs of inflammation and predisposing factors suggests thrombophlebitis, whereas a sudden snap in the posterior calf may indicate a gastrocnemius rupture.[4,10] Gradual onset with noted pigmentary changes and varicosities suggests venous disease.

Chronic Venous Insufficiency

Multiple etiologies of unilateral leg edema have been identified (Table 9-2). The most common cause is chronic venous insufficiency, which often results from either symptomatic or asymptomatic deep vein thrombosis. Valves are destroyed and

Table 9-2. Causes of Unilateral Leg Swelling

Chronic venous insufficiency
Deep vein thrombophlebitis
Primary or secondary lymphedema
Infection
Trauma
Dependent position
Vascular anomalies
Tumors
Factitious edema
Gastrocnemius edema
Popliteal cyst
Compartment syndrome
Popliteal aneurysm
Retroperitoneal fibrosis
Angioneurotic edema
Pretibial myxedema
Exposure to severe temperatures

(From Ruschhaupt and Graor,[4] with permission.)

vessel walls weakened, creating increased venous pressures upon dependency and resulting in swelling. Early on, the edema is soft and pitting, but it becomes progressively fibrotic and indurated. In many instances, varicosities, pigmentary changes, stasis dermatitis, and ulcerations develop. These symptoms make up the postphlebitic syndrome. Congenital abnormalities of the venous system may also cause these changes (Table 9-3, Fig. 9-8).[4,5]

Phlebitis, thrombophlebitis, and *phlebothrombosis* are terms that describe the extent of venous disease. Phlebitis represents the inflammation that occurs prior to thrombus production. There is localized pain and tenderness. Thrombophlebitis describes the inflammation, tenderness, and cordlike texture of a vein. Phlebothrombosis describes the presence of a clot within a vein and is not associated with inflammation. A thorough understanding of lower extremity venous anatomy is important as it helps to explain why thrombi develop.

The venous system of the lower extremity is divided into the superficial and deep systems, as seen in Figure 9-9.[12]

The superficial system consists of the following:

1. The great saphenous vein drains the medial aspect of the foot. It joins the femoral vein just below the inguinal ligament. There are many communications with the deep system. This vein has between 10 and 20 valves.

Table 9-3. Predisposing Factors for Development of Thrombosis

Advanced age
Obesity
Pregnancy
Previous thromboembolic problems
Recent diarrhea
Recent inactivity (e.g., due to illness, injury, surgery, child-
  birth, or prolonged travel)
Cancer
Collagen vascular disease
Chronic ulcerative colitis
Chronic pulmonary disease accompanied by elevated hemato-
  crit
Congestive heart failure
Homocystinuria
Myocardial infarction
Stroke
Paralysis
Polycythemia vera
Leukemia
Thrombocythemia
Antithrombin III deficiency
Protein C deficiency
Medications (e.g., diuretics, corticosteroids, estrogens, oral
  contraceptives)

(From Young,[11] with permission.)

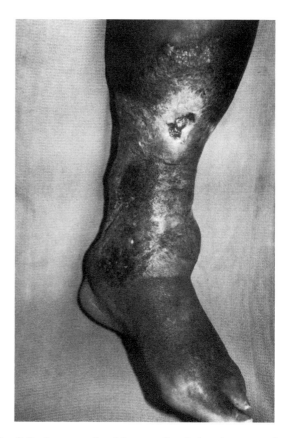

Fig. 9-8. An example of the results of chronic venous insufficiency. Note the fibrotic nature of the skin.

2. The medial marginal vein branches off the great saphenous vein and communicates with the deep posterior tibial vein.
3. The posterior arch veins also connect with the deep posterior tibial vein.
4. The small saphenous vein drains the lateral aspect of the foot and calf. It usually drains into the popliteal vein.

The deep venous system consists of the anterior and posterior tibial veins and the peroneal veins. They follow the arterial system and have multiple anastomoses.

There are also three sets of muscular veins or sinusoids that drain the soleus and gastrocnemius muscles. They are valveless and are often the site of thrombi, as the blood becomes stagnant. Virchow in 1956 presented a triad of factors that he felt described the etiology of thrombi: changes in the vessel wall, alterations of blood coagulability, and changes in blood flow. The two most important factors appear to be blood stasis and activation of the coagulation system. In many patients thrombi seem to develop on normal endothelium.[13] The exact reason why the coagulation system becomes active is unknown, although there are many theories.[12,14,15]

In superficial thrombophlebitis, the superficial veins are involved. Localized edema, tenderness, and a palpable, indurated cord are present. Absent is an elevated systemic temperature. The most common cause is varicose veins. In a young male, superficial phlebitis may suggest thromboangiitis obliterans, whereas in an elderly or middle-aged person without varicosities an occult malignancy must be ruled out. Inflammatory lesions such as erythema nodosum, induration, nodular vasculitis, insect bites, and nonsuppurative panniculitis need to be considered. Most of these lesions are globular rather than linear, and they often ulcerate, whereas superficial thrombophlebitis does not. At times a biopsy may be needed for confirmation.[11] Treatment consists of rest, elevation, moist heat, elastic stockings, and anti-inflammatory drugs.

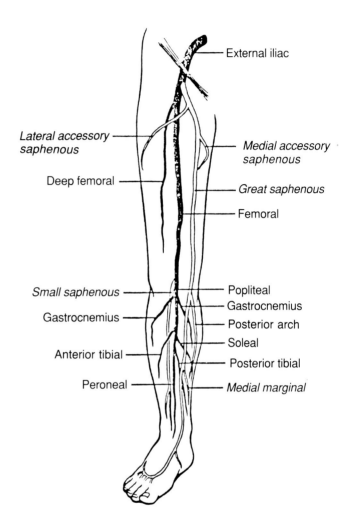

External iliac

Lateral accessory saphenous

Medial accessory saphenous

Deep femoral

Great saphenous

Femoral

Small saphenous

Popliteal

Gastrocnemius

Gastrocnemius

Posterior arch

Anterior tibial

Soleal

Posterior tibial

Peroneal

Medial marginal

Fig. 9-9. The deep and superficial venous systems of the leg. Only single channels of the major veins are shown, although some are normally duplicated and all are complicated by interconnections and variable patterns of communication and drainage. The deep venous system is illustrated by solid lines and the superficial venous system by open lines and italicized labels. (From George,[12] with permission.)

Deep vein thrombophlebitis is more serious, involving severe pain and edema; however, in over 50 percent of patients the physical signs are absent or minimal. A deep cyanotic discoloration may be present along with distended superficial veins. Pitting edema develops rapidly. These patients must be placed on heparin quickly to prevent pulmonary emboli. Doppler, plethysmography, and radioiodinated fibrinogen testing may be used, but venograms are the gold standard to confirm venous disease.[5]

A less common form of venous disease is phlegmasia cerulea dolens, also known as venous gangrene. It is characterized by extensive thrombosis of the iliofemoral vein and its tributaries, producing severe circulatory changes within the limb. Signs of disease include severe pain, cyanotic hue

with petechial lesions, extensive edema of the entire limb, diminished or absent pulses, and gangrene of the foot. Shock may result from the trapping of blood. Phlegmasia cerulea dolens is most commonly seen in patients with advanced metastatic lesions.[5] Connett reported three cases of left common iliac vein obstruction resulting in unilateral edema. The patients ranged in age from 15 to 19 years. Obstruction was due to a congenital band of tissue. A moderate amount of edema was noted. Diagnosis was confirmed with phlebography.[16]

Lymphedema

Primary and secondary lymphedema must always be considered in the differential diagnosis.

The etiologies are numerous, with resulting lymph stasis being either congenital or acquired. Lymphatic vessels become incompetent, and with obstruction intralymphatic pressures rise, causing dilation and valvular insufficiency. Lymphangiograms are often not necessary for diagnosis.

Primary (idiopathic) congenital lymphedema is present at birth, with unilateral swelling. There are two forms of congenital lymphedema: nonfamilial and familial (Milroy's disease).

Lymphedema praecox, or primary acquired lymphedema, appears in women more often than men by a 10:1 ratio between adolescence and 40 years of age. The upper extremities are rarely involved. The etiology is unclear; however, there is evidence of decreased superficial lymphatics in these patients. Swelling occurs spontaneously about the foot and ankle. The edema, which is often nonpitting, worsens after sitting or standing during warm weather and during menses. The edema progresses throughout the lower extremity and in 50 percent of cases becomes bilateral. Twenty-five percent of patients have episodes of cellulitis or lymphangiitis. Bed rest and elevation only offer temporary relief.[2,4] Elastic stockings and diuretics may be used as short-term therapy. Surgery is sometimes necessary to restore tissue tension and lymphatic drainage. Edema with onset after the age of 40 is termed lymphedema tarda.

Secondary obstructive noninflammatory lymphedema may be caused by metastatic lesions of the lymph nodes. It may occur following irradiation. Hawkins et al. reported on 10 patients who developed unilateral leg edema secondary to lymphoma. The edema was most often the initial symptom and often signaled relapse or progression of the disease.[10,17] Young states that prostatic carcinoma is the most common etiology in men after age 40; in women, carcinoma of the genital tract is the most likely cause.

Secondary inflammatory lymphedema is caused by recurrent cellulitis and lymphangiitis. Fever and chills precede the edema. Inflammation of the lymphatic system (lymphangiitis) from thrombosis and fibrosis causes lymph stasis by occlusion. Recurrent attacks are likely. Fungal infection of the digits predisposes patients to attacks of bacterial infection, causing lymphangiitis and cellulitis. Chronic edema may result. The mass effect of infectious processes may cause edema as seen in gas production, abscesses, osteomyelitis, and parasitic infection (filariasis). Maceration between the digits due to chronic tinea infection is a common portal of infection.[4]

Filariasis

Filariasis, also known as elephantiasis, is caused by two types of nematodes, *Wuchereria bancrofti* and *Brugia malayi*. Some 200 million people are estimated to be affected with the parasites, which are widespread throughout the tropical and subtropical areas of South America, Asia, and the Pacific. *Brugia malayi* is seen primarily in Southeast Asia. Infection develops from the bite of the carrier mosquito. Larvae are injected into the skin, migrate to the lymphatic system, and mature within 1 year.

Many infections are asymptomatic, with elephantiasis developing only after prolonged residence in an endemic area. Inflammatory and obstructive symptoms develop as granulomatous reactions from degenerating areas. There is evidence of caseous necrosis. Microfilariae in the blood or body fluids are diagnostic. Serologic tests are not specific, and lymph node biopsy is successful in 25 percent of cases. Biopsies may further worsen the obstruction.[18]

Treatment consists of diethylcarbamazine, which reduces the number of microfilariae. Reactions to the dying parasites may be controlled with antihistamine and lower doses of diethylcarbamazine. The elephantiasis is not reversed. Elastic stockings may help to control edema[19] (Fig. 9-10).

Trauma

Trauma is a common etiology of edema. A history of trauma with clinical presentation of ecchymosis, unilateral edema, and palpable tenderness help to make the diagnosis (Fig. 9-11). The sudden onset of pain following a loud, snapping pop often suggests rupture of the medial head of the gastrocnemius muscle. A ruptured Baker's cyst must be considered in patients with rheumatoid arthritis or knee instability. A venogram may be necessary to rule out deep venous thrombosis, as a ruptured Baker's

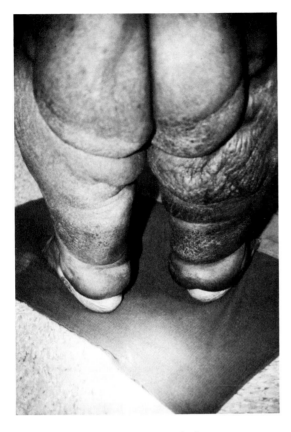

Fig. 9-10. Elephantiasis.

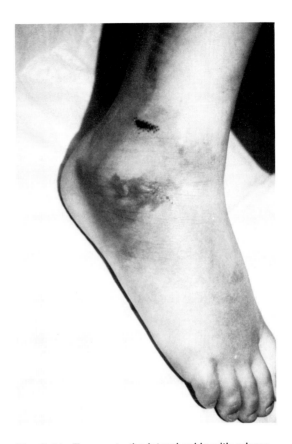

Fig. 9-11. Trauma to the lateral ankle with edema.

cyst may mimic its symptoms. Compartment syndromes from trauma, thrombi, or emboli are possible. Severe edema and pain develop, and a fasciotomy may be necessary to prevent gangrene.[5] Inflammatory arthropathies such as gout and Charcot's disease may present with localized pain, swelling, and warmth (Fig. 9-12).

Vascular Anomalies

Primary arterial disease in the form of an aneurysm may cause unilateral edema. Bates reported an aneurysm of the superficial femoral artery causing pain, swelling, and stasis dermatitis due to compression of the venous system.[20] Others have reported similar symptoms secondary to a popliteal aneurysm.

Arteriovenous fistulas must be considered in the presence of unilateral edema. A history of pene-

trating injury and the presence of a bruit or thrill may suggest a traumatic arteriovenous fistula. A congenital fistula presents with varicosities, hemangiomas, and increased length and circumference of the limb. Arteriography and venous oxygen saturation may be needed for diagnosis.[5]

Neoplasms

Tumors of the lower extremity may cause localized edema. They may be benign or malignant in nature. Lipomas, hemangiomas, sarcomas, and bone tumors are examples of edema-producing lesions.

Pretibial Myxedema

Pretibial myxedema is localized to the pretibial area and dorsum of the foot. It occurs in patients

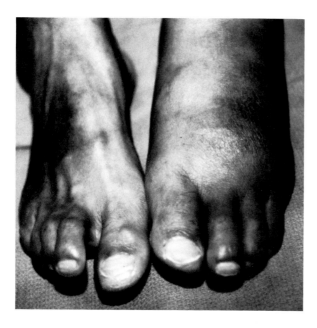

Fig. 9-12. Unilateral edema of the left foot. This patient subsequently went on to Charcot deformity.

with hyperthyroidism and Grave's disease (Fig. 9-13).

Arteriosclerosis

Lower extremity edema is noted in patients with arteriosclerosis secondary to capillary atony. Severe edema often occurs after arterial bypass surgery in the leg because of its capillary atony and disruption of the lymphatic drainage. The disruption of lymphatic drainage would explain the edema in an extremity in which a greater saphenous vein harvest has been performed (Fig. 9-14).

Dependent Positioning

Dependent positioning of the legs increases swelling, as does hot weather. Eugene Landis has described how warm temperature increases edema: "Heat produces peripheral vasodilation, raises capillary blood pressure conspicuously and

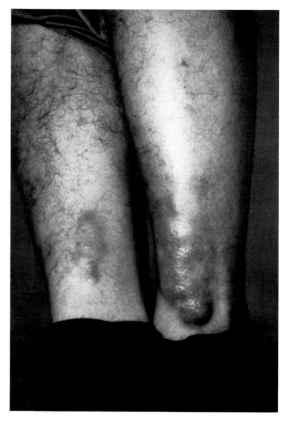

Fig. 9-13. Patient with Graves' disease who presented with pretibial myxedema.

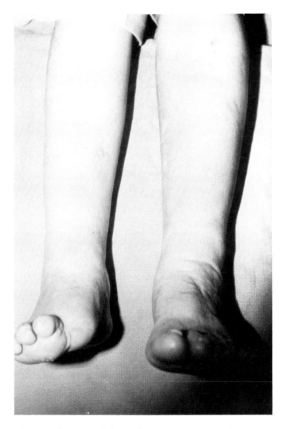

Fig. 9-14. Edema of the left lower extremity is evident in this patient after coronary arterial bypass grafting.

through relaxation of capillaries, increases the area of endothelium available for filtration."[21,22]

Factitious Edema

Ruschhaupt and Graor called factitious edema a "perplexing cause of unilateral swelling." The history of chronic edema that follows no pattern should raise some questions. Astute examination may find the impression of some sort of compressive disease and help to diagnose the problem.[4]

The importance of a thorough history and physical examination is apparent from this discussion. In many instances, laboratory examination should be used to confirm the diagnosis suggested by the onset, duration, and nature of the discomfort.

REFERENCES

1. Guyton AC: Textbook of Medical Physiology. 6th Ed. p 375. WB Saunders Co, Philadelphia, 1981
2. Galloway JMD: The swollen leg. Practitioner 218:676, 1977
3. Streeten DH: Idiopathic edema: pathogenesis, clinical features and treatment. Metabolism 27(3):353, 1978
4. Ruschhaupt WF, Graor RA: Evaluation of the patient with leg edema. Postgrad Med 78(2):132, 1985
5. Young JR: The swollen leg. Am Fam Physician 15(1):163, 1977
6. Helfand AE, Anania WC, Chinkes SL, et al: Screening for the pedal manifestations related to chemical abuse. J Am Podiatr Med Assoc 78(1):15, 1988
7. Albert SF: Electric foot surgery and the alcoholic. J Am Podiatry Assoc 71(1):8, 1981
8. Schooley RT, Wagley PF, Lietman PS: Edema associated with ibuprofen therapy. JAMA 237(16):1716, 1977
9. MacGregor GA, Tasker PRW, DeWardener HE: Diuretic-induced oedema. *Lancet* 1:489, 1975
10. Hawkins KA, Amorosi EL, Silber R: Unilateral leg edema: a symptom of lymphoma. JAMA 244(23):2640, 1980
11. Young JR: Evaluation of the patient with spontaneous thrombophlebitis. Postgrad Med 78(2):149, 1985
12. George JN: Thrombophlebitis. Medicine Grand Rounds, University of Texas Health Science Center at San Antonio, April 11, 1984
13. Sevitt S: The structure and growth of valve-pocket thrombi in femoral veins. J Clin Pathol 27:517, 1974
14. Broze GJ Jr: Binding of human factor VII and VIIa to monocytes. J Clin Invest 70:526, 1982
15. Bach R, Oberdick J, Nemerson Y: Immunoaffinity purification of bovine factor VII. Blood 63:393, 1984
16. Connett MC: An anatomical basis for unilateral leg edema in adolescent girls. West J Med 12(4):324, 1974
17. Kurz L: Unilateral leg edema (letter to the editor). JAMA 246(15):1660, 1981
18. Grove DI, Warren KS, Mahmoud AAF: Algorithms in the diagnosis and management of exotic disease. VI. The Filariases. J Infect Dis

19. Moschella SL, Hurley HJ: Dermatology. 2nd Ed. p 1745. WB Saunders Co, Philadelphia, 1985
20. Bates JD: Unilateral swelling of a lower extremity secondary to primary arterial disease. JAOA 76(9):688, 1977
21. Kissin M: Edema in hot weather (letter to the editor). JAMA 231(11):1135, 1975
22. Landis E: The mechanism of edema formation. Mod Concept Cardiovasc Dis 4(11), 1935

Section II

PATIENT EVALUATION

B. Laboratory Diagnosis

Laboratory Studies and Procedures 10

Roche P. Ramos, M.D.
John E. Laco, D.P.M.

The huge variety and volume of available laboratory tests confronts the podiatrist with a major dilemma. What tests should be ordered on what patients? When, how, how often, at what cost, grouped or individually, and in what sequence? What is the interpretation of the results and what steps then should be taken?

Should the podiatrist order one of each laboratory test on each patient once a lifetime, once a year, once an hour, or never? Many forces influence these decisions. Among them are availability of laboratory service, what the podiatrist knows about the medical need for the test, and economic considerations, such as cost and who makes the profit or takes the loss. Laboratory tests should not be ordered without a plan for using the information gained. What will be done if the test result is normal? High? Low?

Every podiatrist should focus on problem solving by seeking and identifying specific patient problems and pursuing each to its logical conclusion, based on defined goals. It is important to define and obtain an initial comprehensive data base and proceed from there. Many patients are approached best by combining clinical observations and laboratory tests plus observations of clinical course, therapeutic response, and the like. The goal should be to perform every appropriate laboratory test well and economically and to perform none that are not properly indicated.

MULTIPHASIC SCREENING TESTS

Screening tests are designed to "rule in" or "rule out" the presence of a given disease entity in a patient (e.g., a high uric acid level is indicative of gout, but also of many other conditions, such as lymphoma, leukemia, and myeloproliferative diseases). Properties of an ideal screening test are rapid results, high sensitivity, and economy. The limitation of a screening test in general is that it oftentimes cannot be used *alone* to make a definitive diagnosis.

Definitive or diagnostic tests are tests or procedures, the results of which are diagnostic for a given disease entity in a patient. Ideally, this should be a single test or procedure. Frequently there is no single absolutely diagnostic or definitive test for a given disease or disease entity. Usually a group of tests and clinical evaluation of the patient are necessary to make the proper diagnosis.

Multiphasic screening tests are a *group* of tests or procedures designed to "rule in" or "rule out" the presence of a disease. The purpose of the test is to establish the state of health or disease in a patient; to establish the "baseline" values for given parameters in a patient; to assess the effect of treatment or lack of treatment on the progress of disease in the patient; and to indicate which definitive tests should be performed. Proper evaluation and understanding of the multiphasic screening test is very important. Improper use of data provided in multiphasic screening, or by any other means, is a potential source for medicolegal problems. Common sense and clinical judgment must prevail in the interpretation and follow-up of the results of multiphasic screening tests.

HEMATOLOGIC TESTING

The qualitative and quantitative abnormalities found in the peripheral blood are the result of an imbalance between cell production, cell release, and cell survival. In healthy individuals there is a constant balance between the rates of formation and destruction of erythrocytes (red cells), leukocytes, (white cells), and platelets. Disturbance of this critical balance, in terms of either changes in rates of formation, disordered formation, or increased utilization and destruction, is essentially responsible for the final pathologic condition.

Anemia

Anemia is the most common hematologic disorder and is characterized by a multiplicity of conditions that can be complicated and confusing. Anemia is defined as a concentration of hemoglobin in the peripheral blood that is below normal for the age and sex of the patient.

Causes of anemia fall into three major pathophysiologic categories: impaired red cell production, blood loss, or accelerated red cell destruction (hemolysis) in excess of the ability of the marrow to replace these losses. The presence of anemia may be a sign of an underlying disorder whose cause should be identified, since correction may be important to the individual.

The clinical approach to an anemic patient begins with a good history and physical examination. Clues from the history and the physical examination will often save time, pain, and expense in obtaining the diagnosis (Table 10–1). The following are examples of topics that should be investigated:

Diet: Alcoholics are prone to develop folic acid deficiency. Vegetarian diets can result in iron deficiency.

Drug ingestion and exposure to chemicals: Megaloblastic, hemolytic, and aplastic anemias may result from a variety of toxic agents.

Occupation: People working in storage battery factories may develop anemia from lead poisoning.

Bleeding history: Iron-deficiency anemia can result from menorrhagia, multiple pregnancies, and carcinoma of the colon.

Ethnic and racial history: Sickle cell anemia in black patients, thalassemia in patients of Mediterranean and Southeast Asian descent, and pyruvate kinase deficiency in the Amish of central Pennsylvania.

Neurologic symptoms: Patients with Vitamin B_{12} deficiency commonly develop neurologic symptoms, such as distal parasthesias. Jaundice suggests hemolysis or hepatitis. History of other disease producing anemia, such as renal disease, liver disease, or chronic inflammatory diseases.

Anemia may be classified by red cell morphology as macrocytic, normocytic, or microcytic (Table 10–2). Macrocytes (mean corpuscular volume greater than 100 μm^3) are found in accelerated erythropoiesis, chronic liver diseases, folate or vitamin B_{12} deficiency anemia, and some malignancies. Microcytes (mean corpuscular volume less than 80 μm^3) often indicate iron-deficiency anemia, anemia of chronic disease, thalassemia, sideroblastic anemia, lead poisoning, and vitamin B_6 de-

Table 10-1. Elementary Steps in the Diagnosis of Anemia

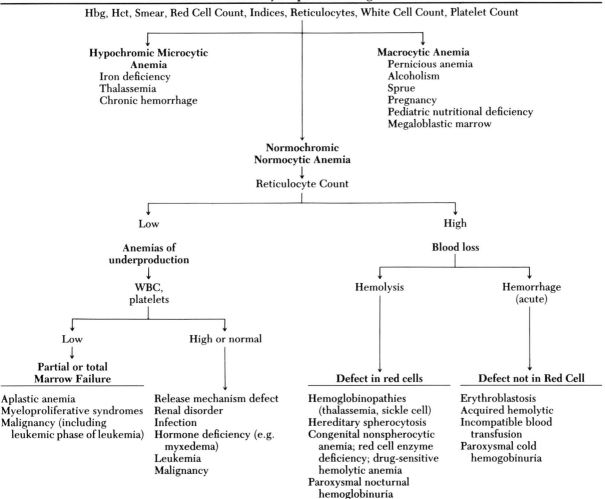

ficiency. Normocytes (mean corpuscular volume of 80 to 90 μm³) in anemia are found in chronic disorders such as chronic infection and rheumatoid arthritis.

Hematologic Patterns of Anemias

Iron-Deficiency Anemia. Anemia is characterized by low mean corpuscular volume (MCV), low mean corpuscular hemoglobin (MCH), serum iron less than 35 mg/dl, total iron-binding capacity (TIBC) more than 350 mg/dl, serum ferritin below 10 ng/ml, and absence of hemosiderin in the marrow. Serum ferritin is an accurate indicator of body iron stored in most patients, except in the presence of liver disease, chronic inflammation, acute leukemia, Hodgkin's lymphoma, and other types of neoplasm.

Thalassemia. Thalassemia has a hematologic pattern similar to that described for iron-deficiency anemia. The incidence of β-thalassemia is high in areas where there are many people of Mediterranean origin, especially Italian, whereas α-thalassemia is more common in Cantonese people (of Chinese origin). The hemoglobin value is usually between 10 and 13 g/dl, but the red blood cell (RBC) count is often higher than normal. The diagnosis of thalassemia minor may be established de-

Table 10-2. Erythrocyte Indices in Anemia

Adult Reference Range	MCV	MCHC
Normocytic, normochromic	$80-100\ \mu m^3$	30–38%
Microcytic, hypochromic	$<80\ \mu m^3$	20–30%
Macrocytic, normochromic	$>100\ \mu^3$	30–38%

MCV increased in:
  Folic acid deficiency (alcoholism, dietary, malabsorption,
    pregnancy)
  Vitamin B_{12} deficiency (pernicious anemia, malabsorption)
  Marked reticulocytosis (acute bleeding, hemolytic anemia)
  Cirrhosis
  Less common causes: malignancy, phenytoin or cytotoxic
    drugs, myxedema, aplastic anemia

MCV decreased in:
  Chronic iron deficiency
  Thalassemia
  Anemia of chronic disease (uremia, rheumatoid collagen
    diseases, severe chronic infection)
  Less common causes: polycythemia, lead poisoning,
    congenital spherocytosis, and some abnormal
    hemoglobins (Hbg E, Hbg Lepore)

finitively by finding an elevated concentration of hemoglobin A_2 or F as determined by hemoglobin electrophoresis.

Megalobastic Anemia. This type of anemia is easily recognized by large oval macrocytes, hypersegmented polymorphonuclear cells, megaloblastic dyspoiesis in the bone marrow findings, and low serum levels of vitamin B_{12} or folic acid.

Hemolytic Anemia. In most long-term hemolytic anemias, the reticulocyte count is elevated (greater than 5 percent) and the indirect serum bilirubin is slightly elevated (greater than 1 mg/dl). The serum lactic dehydrogenese level may be elevated and the heptoglobin absent. Hemosiderinuria can be found in the urine 2 to 3 days after onset of hemolytic anemia. After these general signs of hemolysis are established, specific tests to establish the type of hemolysis should be carried out: osmotic fragility to establish hereditary spherocytosis, Coombs' test to establish autoimmune hemolytic anemia, hemoglobin electrophoresis to diagnose hemoglobinopathy, and enzyme studies to diagnose hereditary nonspherocytic hemolytic anemia. The hemoglobinopathies occur mostly in the black population, but target cells are common to all populations. Sickle cell anemia is the most common hemoglobinopathy in the black population, but other variants, S/C and C/C disease, must be considered.

Absolute Marrow Failure. The normal marrow tissue has been replaced by fat (aplastic anemia), fibrosis (myelofibrosis), or malignancy (lymphosarcoma, multiple myeloma, or leukemia). The platelet count and absolute reticulocyte count are usually low. A bone marrow aspirate and biopsy specimen are essential for specific diagnosis.

Pure RBC Anemia. The diagnosis is suspected in patients with profound anemia with very low reticulocyte counts (less than 1 percent), but normal white blood cell (WBC) and platelet counts and normal RBC morphology. Bone marrow aspiration and biopsy are essential for diagnosis.

Hypersplenism. Hypersplenism is characterized by a large spleen, pancytopenia, and cellular marrow without morphologic abnormalities of the RBCs, WBCs, or platelets. This syndrome is usually secondary to some other disease, for example, cirrhosis of the liver, Gaucher's disease, congestive splenomegaly.

Laboratory Evaluation

The initial laboratory evaluation of anemia should include a RBC count, hemoglobin, hematocrit, red blood cell indices, reticulocyte count, leukocyte count, and platelet count. It is also important to examine the peripheral blood film under the microscope. Examination of the blood smear should include a search for the following cells or bodies that may lead to the diagnosis:

1. Spherocytes indicate hereditary spherocytosis or autoimmune hemolytic anemia.
2. Schistocytes (contracted cells, helmet cells, triangular cells) suggest mechanical damage to blood vessels by fibrin or cancer.
3. Oval cells suggest congenital elliptocytosis, megaloblastic anemia, and occasionally refractory normoblastic anemia or myelofibrosis.
4. Prominent basophilic stippling (young cells whose RNA is precipitated by Wright's stain; these cells are differentiated from reticulocytes whose RNA is precipitated only by supravital stain) suggests lead poisoning or thalassemia minor.
5. Target cells are seen in patients after splenectomy, with jaundice or liver disease, and in many hemoglobinopathies.

Table 10-3. Normal Values for Hematocrit

Men	40–54%
Women	37–47%
Newborn	44–62%

Table 10-5. Normal Values for Reticulocyte Count

Men	0.5–1.5% of total
Women	0.5–2.5% of total
Newborns	2–5 % of total

6. Howell-Jolly bodies (nuclear remnants) are present after splenectomy and frequently in megaloblastic anemia.
7. Sickled RBCs found in sickle cell anemia.

Hematocrit

Hematocrit is the volume of red blood cells (packed cell volume) found in 100 ml of blood (Table 10–3). For example, a value of 46 percent means that there are 46 ml of red blood cells in 100 ml of blood. Hematocrit is a combined measure of the size, capacity, and number of cells present in the blood and, along with the hemoglobin value, establishes the presence and severity of anemia.

Hemoglobin

Hemoglobin is the oxygen-carrying pigment and main component of the red blood cells. It combines with and transports oxygen to body tissues and helps to carry carbon dioxide to the lungs. It establishes the presence of anemia and evaluates the effectiveness of therapy. Normal values are given in Table 10–4.

Reticulocyte Count

Reticulocytes are immature RBCs that circulate in the blood for 1 to 2 days while maturing. Their numbers are reported as a percentage of mature RBC, and reflect bone marrow activity (Table 10–5). The reticulocyte count increases following blood loss or during effective therapy for certain kinds of anemia. It helps to differentiate between hypoproliferative and hyperproliferative anemias. It also assesses blood loss, bone marrow response to anemia, and therapy for anemia.

Erythrocyte Sedimentation Rate

The erythrocyte sedimentation rate (ESR) is the speed at which RBCs settle in well-mixed venous blood (Table 10–6). This rate is increased when the negative charge on the RBC membrane decreases so that there is an increased rouleaux formation. Such would be the case in conditions where there are elevated fibrinogen and globulin levels.

The ESR monitors inflammatory or malignant disease. It can aid in the detection and diagnosis of occult disease (tuberculosis, tissue necrosis, or connective tissue disease). A decreased ESR is found in prolonged standing of the specimen and in many abnormal forms of RBCs, such as in sickle cell anemia, wherein there are large number of irreversibly sickled RBCs. A marked elevation of the ESR is found in monoclonal gammopathies and hyperfibrinogenemias, rheumatoid arthritis, chronic inflammation, and neoplasia.

White Blood Cell (Leukocyte) Count

The white blood cells (WBCs) are the body's first defense against infection. Various types of WBCs serve different functions. When bacteria invade

Table 10-4. Normal Values for Hemoglobin

Men	14–18 g/dl
Women	12–16 g/dl
Newborns	18–27 g/dl

Table 10-6. Normal Values for Erythrocyte Sedimentation Rate[a]

Men	
under 50 years	<15 mm/hour
50+ years	<20 mm/hour
Women	
under 50 years	<20 mm/hour
50+ years	<30 mm/hour
Newborns	0–2 mm/hour
Neonatal to puberty	3–13 mm/hour

[a] Using the Westergren method.

the body, *neutrophils* migrate to the area of inflammation to phagocytize the invading organisms, and the bone marrow is stimulated to produce and release large numbers of mature neutrophils as well as immature forms (bands), which appear in the peripheral circulation.

Eosinophils phagocytize antigen-antibody complexes and foreign particles and appear to defend against helminthic parasites. Therefore, in patients with allergic diseases the circulating eosinophil level is often elevated.

Monocytes are leukocytes that are formed in the bone marrow and migrate into inflammatory exudates to actively phagocytize bacteria, viruses, antigen-antibody complexes, inorganic substances, and erythrocytes. Monocytes may transform into macrophages and multinucleated giant cells. Monocytosis is seen in chronic inflammatory disorders.

Lymphocytes comprise 20 to 35 percent of circulating leukocytes. Their primary responsibility is antibody production, immunologic memory, and cell-mediated immunity. *Basophils* comprise about 0.5 percent of circulating leukocytes. They are considered to be phagocytic and are associated with blood stasis and coagulation, allergic reactions, and anaphylactoid states.

The absolute determination of the number of leukocytes (total white blood cells) gives only partial information. Unless an accurate differential white cell count is done, listing values for each of the five types of leukocyte, significant information or the existence of a pathologic state can be missed. For example, a WBC count may be normal even in the presence of severe sepsis. In such a case, a differential WBC count would reveal a sharp increase in the number of neutrophils with increased immature cells (a shift to the left).

The WBC count is a count of the number of leukocytes per unit volume in a sample of venous blood. Normal values for adults are 5,000 to 10,000/μl, and for newborns 9,000 to 30,000/μl. Mild to moderate leukocytosis (11,000 to 20,000/μl) usually indicates infectious disease, mainly of bacterial etiology. Usually the leukocytosis increases with the severity of the infection, except in elderly or debilitated patients, in whom severe sepsis can coexist with only a modest leukocytosis.

Leukemoid reaction is a marked nonleukemic leukocytosis with immature cells present. Differential diagnosis will depend upon the clinical history, physical examination findings, and other laboratory test such as leukocyte alkaline phosphatase. In the infectious process leukocyte alkaline phosphatase is elevated, whereas in chronic myelocytic leukemia it is usually very low.

The presence of more than 30 percent *blast cells* in the peripheral blood and bone marrow is diagnostic of acute leukemia with or without elevated WBC count.

TESTS FOR HEMOSTASIS

The hemostatic mechanism has two primary functions: confining circulating blood to the vascular bed, and arresting bleeding at the site of an injured vessel. The hemostatic process depends on delicate and complex interactions among at least five components: blood vessels, plasma coagulation proteins, physiologic protease inhibitors, platelets, and the fibrinolytic system.

The hemostatic responses are divided into two steps: primary and secondary hemostasis. The primary response involves interaction between blood vessels and circulating platelets, producing a primary platelet plug. Secondary hemostasis involves interactions of coagulation proteins, which result ultimately in the generation of cross-linked fibrin, which stabilizes the platelet plug.

Clinical Approach

Abnormalities of primary and secondary hemostasis typically present different patterns of bleeding. Abnormalities of primary hemostasis are characterized by bleeding of mucous membranes and many small, superficial ecchymosis. These patients might also give a history of abnormal intraoperative bleeding and oozing from small cuts or wounds. Clinical disorders associated with abnormalities of primary hemostasis include quantitative as well as qualitative abnormalities of platelets, vascular abnormalities, and von Willebrand's disease.

Patients with abnormalities in secondary hemostasis (coagulation factor deficiencies) typically have abnormal bleeding that involves large blood vessels, causing lumpy subcutaneous ecchymosis together with intramuscular hematomata and hemarthrosis. In obtaining a history of bleeding, it is important to question a patient carefully regarding the frequency of bleeding and to ascertain whether episodes of bleeding are associated with trauma. Many patients attribute episodes of bleeding to other illnesses. It is also important to ask about dental extractions, tonsillectomy, appendectomy, circumcision, and other surgical procedures. A history of prolonged postoperative bleeding or transfusions associated with any of these procedures is suggestive of a bleeding problem. It is also important to document the first episode of abnormal bleeding. This history may be particularly helpful in differentiating a hereditary bleeding problem from an acquired abnormality.

A family history of bleeding problems is helpful in establishing a diagnosis of a hereditary abnormality of hemostasis. The pattern of inheritance may have great diagnostic relevance.

Drug history is very important because the number of potential drug-induced bleeding disorders has been increasing. The most common is associated with aspirin. Aspirin affects platelet function and may produce a clinical picture of an abnormality of primary hemostasis. Other drugs often associated with an abnormal laboratory result are chlorpromazine hydrochloride and procainamide. Patients who have taken these drugs for long periods may have a prolonged activated partial thromboplastin time as a result of drug-induced "lupus anticoagulant." Penicillin may affect platelet function or may be associated with specific factor inhibitors. History of anticoagulant therapy should be noted.

Laboratory Procedures

The best screening tests for identifying potential hemostatic problems are thorough personal and family histories. The most important screening procedures used in the laboratory are (1) examination of a peripheral smear, (2) platelet count, (3) determination of bleeding time, (4) prothrombin time, (5) activated partial thromboplastin time and (6) thrombin time.

Examination of a peripheral smear and platelet count may yield much information about a patient. The number of platelets should be established and correlated with the platelet count. Morphologic studies of red blood cells may be helpful in solving a clinical problem. The presence of schistocytes suggests a microangiopathic hemolytic anemia, as seen in patients with acute disseminated intravascular coagulation. The size and morphologic appearance of platelets may also be evaluated. Large platelets have been identified as being younger and more active metabolically as well as physiologically. A lack of granularity of platelets is associated most often with production of dysplastic platelets in patients with underlying myeloproliferative disorders.

Bleeding time is the single best procedure for evaluating primary hemostasis. Patients with an abnormal bleeding time but a normal platelet count arbitrarily are designated as having qualitative abnormalities of platelet function. Such patients include those with von Willebrand's disease, those who have recently ingested various antiplatelet drugs (e.g., aspirin) and those with uremia. To further evaluate such patients, additional platelet function studies are indicated; they include platelet aggregation tests, quantification of the various components of the factor VIII complex, and platelet retention procedures.

Patients with quantitative abnormalities of platelets are evaluated in a different manner. In many laboratories, if a platelet count is less than 50,000 cells/μl, bleeding time is not determined. The next procedure in such patients would be a bone marrow examination. Patients with thrombocytopenia may be divided into those in whom bone marrow production of platelets is decreased and those in whom peripheral destruction of platelets is increased.

Prothrombin Time

Measurement of the prothrombin time (PT) evaluates the extrinsic system. The prothrombin time is an excellent test for monitoring oral anticoagulant therapy because factor VII is the first coagulation factor to be appreciably affected by oral anticoagulants. The prothrombin time may also be prolonged by congenital and acquired deficiencies of factors VII, X, V, and II and fibrinogen. The presence of circulating anticoagulant may also prolong the prothrombin time.

Activated Partial Thromboplastin Time

Patients with a normal prothrombin time but an abnormal activated partial thromboplastin time (APTT) typically have deficiencies of factors that are unique to the intrinsic system (i.e., factors XII, XI, VIII, and IX; Fletcher factor; and Fitzgerald factor). Patients with the lupus type of anticoagulant often present with a normal PT but a prolonged APTT.

The APTT is also widely used for monitoring heparin therapy. Patients who are receiving full-dose heparin therapy ideally have an APTT that is 2½ times longer than the upper limit of the normal range. The patient's baseline APTT may be used as a reference point for determining the prolongation of the APTT.

Thrombin Time

The thrombin time is abnormal when the plasma level of fibrinogen is decreased or when there are circulating anticoagulants, fibrin degradation products, or paraproteins. Patients with hereditary or acquired abnormalities of the fibrinogen molecule (dysfibrinogenemia) have an abnormal thrombin time.

TESTS FOR URINARY TRACT DISEASES

The current diagnostic procedures used in the workup of a patient with urinary tract disease are history, physical examination, and examination of the urine (Table 10–7); imaging techniques (intravenous urogram); and determination of serum creatinine level or creatinine clearance to estimate renal function.

Proper interpretation of the urinary sediment, as well as of the urine culture, requires attention to detail in collecting the urine specimens. All pa-

tients should be well hydrated before the urine is collected for segmentation of the voided stream into its diagnostic part. Examination of the urine may be considered from two general standpoints: (1) diagnosis and management of renal or urinary tract disease, and (2) the detection of metabolic or systemic diseases not directly related to the kidney.

There are certain important considerations to be borne in mind relative to the collection of urine specimens for examination. The urine sample must be collected in a clean, dry container and should be examined when freshly voided (within 1 hour of voiding). Red blood cells, leukocytes, and casts decompose in urine that has been allowed to stand for several hours at room temperature. Casts and neutrophils disappear rapidly in hypotonic and alkaline urines. Bilirubin and urobilinogen will decrease, especially with exposure to light. Glucose is utilized by cells and bacteria. Bacterial contamination regularly occurs, usually resulting in alkalinization of the urine owing to the conversion of urea to ammonia by *Proteus* species. Turbidity develops as bacteria multiply and alkaline precipitates occur. The color will change (usually darken) and the odor will become offensive.

For most routine examinations, a concentrated specimen is referable to a dilute one. The first morning specimen of urine, voided on rising, is the most concentrated specimen. This specimen is the best one to examine for nitrite and protein. Valuable information about the concentrating ability of the kidney may also be gained from the specific gravity of this specimen. However, a randomly collected specimen is often more convenient for the patient and will be suitable for most screening purposes. Random specimens for routine urinalysis should be examined fresh, within 1 hour after voiding, or refrigerated and examined as soon as possible. If delays are anticipated specimens should be refrigerated before delivery. Quantitative creatinine and protein determinations are done on 24-hour urine collections refrigerated between voidings and with no preservative.

In collection of urine for bacteriologic examination, a clean-voided midstream specimen is desirable, but catheterization or suprapubic aspiration of the bladder is sometimes necessary. Bacteriologic culture should be done immediately. When this is not possible, the urine should be refrigerated

Table 10-7. Urinalysis Abnormalities Found in Various Urinary System Diseases

Diseases	Macroscopic Urinalysis	Microscopic Urinalysis
Acute glomerulonephritis	Gross hematuria "Smoky" turbidity Proteinuria	RBCs and RBC casts Epithelial casts Hyaline and granular casts Waxy casts Neutrophils
Chronic glomerulonephritis	Hematuria Proteinuria	RBCs WBCs Occasional blood casts Granular and waxy casts Epithelial casts Tipid droplets
Acute pyelonephritis	Turbid Occasional "odor" Occasional proteinuria	Numerous neutrophils (many in clumps) Few lymphocytes and histiocytes Leukocyte casts Epithelial casts Renal epithelial cells Bacteria RBCs Granular and waxy casts
Chronic pyelonephritis	Occasional proteinuria	Leukocytes Broad waxy casts Granular and epithelial casts Occasional leukocyte casts Bacteria RBCs
Nephrotic syndrome	Proteinuria Fat droplets	Fatty and waxy casts Cellular and granular casts Oval fat bodies and or vacuolated renal epithelial cells
Acute tubular necrosis	Hematuria Occasional proteinuria	Necrotic or degenerated renal epithelial cells Neutrophils and erythrocytes Granular and epithelial casts Waxy casts Broad casts Epithelial tissue fragments
Cystitis	Hematuria	Numerous leukocytes Erythrocytes Transitional epithelial cells Histiocytes Bacteria Absence of casts
Urinary tract neoplasia	Hematuria	Malignant cells Neutrophils Erythrocytes Transitional epithelial cells

Viral infection	Hematuria
	Occasional proteinuria
		Enlarged mononuclear cells
		    or multinucleated cells with prominent
		    intranuclear or cytoplasmic inclusions
		Neutrophils
		Lymphocytes and plasma cells
		Erythrocytes

at 4°C until cultured for a period of not more than 12 hours as a rule, although specimens have been cultured without detriment after 4 days of adequate refrigeration. Clean-voided urine specimens are used for bacterial, mycobacterial, fungal, and viral cultures; 24-hour specimens are used for the detection of schistosoma and onchocerca. Bacteria may or may not be significant, depending on the method of urine collection and how soon after collection of the specimen the examination takes place. Well-mixed uncentrifuged urine may be examined with Gram's stain. If bacteria are identified in the lens, it suggests that more than 100,000 organisms/ml, are present. Yeast cells *(Candida albicans)* are found in urinary tract infections (e.g., in diabetes mellitus), but yeast are also common contaminants from skin and air.

For cytologic examination, a 2-hour collection of urine after initial voiding in the morning will allow the collection of fresh cells from the urinary tract. Urine for evaluation of tumor cells is usually collected into an equal volume of 50 percent alcohol, or urine may be mixed in equal volumes with Saccomano's fixative or Mucolexx. Unfixed urine should be refrigerated immediately upon voiding and should reach the laboratory within 1 hour to prevent cell loss.

SYNOVIAL FLUID TESTING

Synovial fluid (SF) is produced by dialysis of plasma across the synovial membrane and by secretion of a hyaluronate-protein complex by the synovial membrane. The functions of the SF are to provide lubrication and nourishment for articular cartilage. In most cases, SF examination is not highly specific for any particular type of arthritis (Table 10–8). Only in septic or crystal-induced arthritis is SF examination highly sensitive and specific for a single disease entity.

Ideally, the patient should be fasting for 6 to 12 hours before SF aspiration to allow equilibration of glucose between plasma and SF. The appearance of normal SF is crystal clear and pale yellow (Table 10–9). Cloudiness, turbidity, milkiness, purulence, and greenish tinging occur in inflammatory conditions. Grossly bloody SF may occur with fractures, traumatic arthritis, neurogenic arthropathy, hemophiliac arthritis, pigmented villonodular synovitis, or ruptured aneurysm. Black specks can occur (the "ground pepper" sign) in fluid from ochronotic joints.

Viscosity is estimated by allowing SF to form a string by placing a drop on the thumb, touching this with a finger, and separating the finger to form a string. Normal SF forms a string 4 to 6 cm in length. If the string breaks before reaching a length of 3 cm, viscosity is lower than normal. Decreased viscosity may occur in a wide variety of inflammatory conditions, whereas increased viscosity can be seen in effusions from hypothyroid patients.

The total leukocyte count in normal SF is less than 200/ml. A very high leukocyte count (over 100,000/ml) strongly suggests bacterial infection. Occasionally, active gout or rheumatoid arthritis may present with SF leukocytes counts over 100,000/ml. The "routine" differential count usually is reported only as the percentage of neutrophils. The accepted upper limit is 25 percent neutrophils, over 90 percent is suggestive evidence of bacterial arthritis, even if the total cell count and other measurements are within normal limits.

Gram's stain is positive in about 50 percent of patients with joint sepsis. Depending upon the type of infection, cultures may be positive in about 30 to 80 percent of patients with septic arthritis. It is important to remember that septic arthritis can coexist with other types of arthritis, such as lupus,

Table 10-8. Classification of Arthritides[a]

Group I (Noninflammatory)	Group II (Inflammatory)	Group III (Infectious)	Group IV (Crystal-induced)	Group V (Hemorrhagic)
Osteoarthrosis	Rheumatoid arthritis	Bacterial	Gout	Traumatic arthritis
Traumatic arthritis	Lupus erythematosus	Mycobacterial	CPPD[b] crystal deposition	Hemophilic arthropathy
Osteochondritis dessicans	Reiter's syndrome	Fungal	disease	Anticoagulation
Osteochondromatosis	Rheumatic fever		Apatite-associated	Pigmented villonodular
Neuropathic	Ankylosing spondylitis		arthropathy	synovitis
osteoarthropathy	Regional enteritis			Neuropathic osteoarthropathy
Pigmented villonodular	Ulcerative colitis,			Synovial hemangioma
synovitis	psoriasis			

[a] Adapted from Rippey JH: Synovial fluid analysis. Lab Med 10:140, 1979.
[b] *CPPD*, calcium pyrophosphate dihydrate.

Table 10-9. Synovial Fluid Findings by Disease Category[a]

Finding	Normal	Category[b]				
		Group I	Group II	Group III	Group IV	Group V
Appearance	Yellow, clear, or slightly cloudy	Yellow or clear	Yellow, cloudy, turbid, or bloody	Yellow, green, or milky	Yellor or turbid	Red-brown or xanthochromic
WBCs/μl[c]	0–200 (0–0.2 × 10⁹/l)	0–5,000 (0–5 × 10⁹/l)	2,000–200,000 (2–200 × 10⁹/l)	50,000–200,000 (50–200 × 10⁹/l)	500–200,000 (0.5–200 × 10⁹/l)	50–10,000 (0.05–10 × 10⁹/l)
Polymorphonuclear leukocytes (%)	<25	<30	>50	>90	<90	<50
Crystals present	No	No	No	No	Yes	No
RBCs present	No	No	No	Yes	No	Yes
Blood glucose to synovial fluid glucose to ratio (mg/dl)[c]	0–10 (0–0.56 mmol/l)	0–10 (0–0.56 mmol/l)	0–40 (0–2.22 mmol/l)	20–100 (1.11–555 mmol/l)	0–80 (0–4.44 mmol/l)	0–20 (0–1.11 mmol/l)
Culture	Negative	Negative	Negative	Often positive	Negative	Negative

[a] Data from Rippey JH: Synovial fluid analysis. Lab Med 10:140, 1979.
[b] Groups as described in Table 10–8.
[c] Values in parentheses are SI units.

erythematosus, gout, and pseudogout. If sepsis is suspected, but Gram's stain and culture are inconclusive, synovial biopsy may be needed to establish a diagnosis.

Five types of crystal-induced arthritis have been reported: (1) arthritis associated with apatite crystals, (2) gout caused by monosodium urate (MSU), (3) pseudogout caused by calcium pyrophosphate dihydrate (CPPD), (4) chronic arthritis caused by talcum crystals introduced during joint surgery, and (5) acute synovitis caused by intra-articular injection of crystalline corticosteroid preparations. Such crystals may persist in SF for a month or longer following intra-articular injection.

TESTS OF STANDARD LABORATORY PARAMETERS

In this section common causes of abnormal values are listed, with clinical correlation, for several standard laboratory testing parameters. Further information can be obtained from the references listed in the Selected Readings.

Sodium

Causes of Hyponatremia

Sodium loss, renal:
  Diuretic treatment
  Salt-wasting nephropathies
  Adrenal insufficiency
  Bicarbonaturia
  Ketonuria
Sodium loss, extrarenal:
  Vomiting
  Diarrhea
  "Third interspace loss"
  Burns
Excess total body water (edema):
  Nephrotic syndrome
  Cirrhosis
  Cardiac failure
  Acute and chronic renal failure
  Water intoxication (consumed or administered)

Hyponatremia without apparent increase in extra cellular fluid (ECF):
  Hypothyroidism
  Glucocorticoid deficiency (Addison's disease)
  Chronic disease
  Persistent or inappropriate secretion of vasopressin (ADH)

Clinical Comments. Of clinical importance is the large number of patients on diuretic therapy. Technically, sodium is commonly evaluated as a routine chemistry panel for preoperative surgical screenings. Of particular importance is possible water intoxication from administration of excessive amounts of water, causing hyponatremia. This may possibly come into play during administration of intravenous therapy in the hospital.

Causes of hypernatremia

Hypertonic fluid loss, renal:
  Osmotic diuresis (marked glycosuria, mannitol diuresis, urea diuresis due to high-protein tube feeding, high sodium load contributory, chronic renal failure)
Hypertonic fluid loss, extrarenal:
  Profuse sweating
  Diarrhea in children without adequate fluid replacement
Loss of water, renal:
  Central diabetes insipidus
  Nephrogenic diabetes insipidus (etiology may be hypercalcemia and hyperkalemia)
Loss of water, extrarenal:
  Insensible losses from lungs and skin (i.e., fever)
Other causes of hypernatremia:
  Cushing's syndrome
  Hyperaldosteronism
  Excess sodium intake (sodium bicarbonate intake)

Potassium

Causes of Hypokalemia

Intracellular movement from ECF to intracellular fluid (ICF):

Alkalemia
Insulin therapy
Hypokalemic periodic paralysis (familial disease)
Intracellular movement from ECF to ICF from depletion of total body potassium:
Gastrointestinal fluid loss (vomiting, diarrhea, nasogastric suction)
Renal losses:
Diuretics (most common)
Metabolic alkalosis
Renal tubular acidosis
Mineralocorticoid excess
Other causes:
Postoperative fluids without potassium
Antibiotics (carbenicillin, gentamicin, amphotericin B)

Clinical Comments. Signs and symptoms associated with hypokalemia include muscle weakness and hyporeflexia as well as cardiac arrhythmias and increased sensitivity to digitalis. Hypokalemia can also produce changes on an electrocardiogram. From a clinical viewpoint, hypokalemia may be produced from diuretics, and therefore patients relating a history of muscle weakness may need to have their serum potassium checked. Also, patients on diuretic therapy should routinely have their potassium level checked preoperatively because hypokalemia does produce cardiac arrhythmias.

Causes of Hyperkalemia

Movement of potassium from ICF to ECF:
Acidemia
Cellular damage (e.g., fever, hemolysis, rhabdomyolysis, crush injury, extensive infection)
Increase in total body potassium and hyperkalemia:
Acute and chronic renal failure
Mineralocorticoid deficiency (Addison's disease)

Clinical Comments. Extensive infection or extensive trauma, as in a crush injury, may result in hyperkalemia, which may result in alterations in cardiac excitability. An electrocardiogram should be obtained in these particular clinical scenarios with appropriate treatments.

Calcium

Causes of Hypercalcemia

Metastases of malignant neoplasm to bone
Vitamin D–like compounds produced by neoplasms
Malignant tumors secreting parathyroid hormone
Hyperparathyroidism
Thiazide administration
Multiple myeloma
Sarcoidosis
Vitamin D intoxication
Milk-alkali syndrome
Leukemia
Hyperthyroidism
Adrenal insufficiency
Immobilization (Paget's disease)
Diuretic phase of acute tubular necrosis
Acromegaly

Clinical Comments. Of particular importance to podiatry are the symptoms associated with hypercalcemia, which include neuromuscular weakness, arthralgias, severe pruritus, and restless leg syndrome. Arthralgia may be due to gout, pseudogout, calcific tendonitis, and chondrocalcinosis.

Causes of Hypocalcemia

Hypoparathyroidism
Vitamin D deficiency
Vitamin D dependency
Renal tubular disease
Renal failure
Hypomagnesemia
Acute pancreatitis
Hypoproteinemia
Increased calcium utilization
Alkalosis (hyperventilation, vomiting, fistulae)

Clinical Comments. Clinical relevance is that the earliest symptoms of hypocalcemia are paresthesias of the lips, fingers, and toes. The most common characteristic syndrome caused by hypocalcemia is tetany. Hypocalcemia is a fairly infrequent finding in the laboratory.

Uric Acid

Most Common Etiologies of Hyperuricemia

Renal failure
Ketoacidosis
Lactate excess
Use of diuretics
Gout
Early azotemic renal disease
Leukemia
Lymphoma
Macroglobulinemia
Polycythemia
Multiple myeloma
Neuroblastoma
Psoriasis
Frequent in sickle cell anemia
Hemolytic anemia
Diet (high protein)
Medications (thiazides, furosemide)

Clinical Comments. Hyperuricemia is an expected finding in acute gouty arthritis, but is common and may exist with other acute arthropathies. Particular attention has been directed toward the thiazides and furosemide as causes of elevated uric acid. Some drugs, such as salicylate, probenicid, sulfinpyrazone, and phenylbutazone, inhibit uric acid excretion in low doses but have a uricosuric effect in high doses. Ethanol can increase the plasma urate concentration.

Enzymes

Serum Glutamic-Oxaloacetic Transaminase (SGOT)

Elevated in:
Acute myocardial infarction
Hepatic disease
Muscle diseases, trauma, injury
Acute pancreatitis
Biliary disease with opiates
Cholecystectomy
Mesenteric infarction
Pulmonary infarction
Brain infarction
Medications (oxacillin, erythromycin, opiates)

Fifty percent of patients with metastatic carcinoma
Eighty percent of patients with infectious mononucleosis

Serum Glutamic-Pyruvic Transaminase (SGPT)

High elevations in:
Viral hepatitis
Hepatic necrosis
Elevated in:
Acute myocardial infarction
Chronic hepatitis
Cirrhosis
Liver metastases
Congestive heart failure

Clinical Comments. Values of SGPT and SGOT are helpful for early recognition of viral hepatitis as well as toxic hepatitis for patients on hepatotoxic drugs (griseofulvin is a drug used commonly in podiatry). Therefore liver function tests such as SGOT and SGPT should be performed on a periodic basis. SGOT and SGPT tests may be necessary to monitor liver function when patients are on nonsteroidal anti-inflammatories for extended periods of time.

Lactate Dehydrogenase (LDH)

Elevated in:
Megaloblastic anemia
Extensive carcinomatosis
Myocardial infarction (10 to 14 days)
Pulmonary infarction
Granulocyte or acute leukemia
Hemolytic anemia
Infectious mononucleosis
Progressive muscular dystrophy
Hepatitis
Obstructive jaundice
Cirrhosis
Chronic renal disease

Clinical Comments. Lactate dehydrogenase consists of five isoenzymes, LD_1 through LD_5. Various diseases reveal abnormal patterns of isoenzyme composition and these patterns can be useful in determining pathology. The LDH level is useful in determining myocardial and pulmonary infarction.

Alkaline Phosphatase (ALP)

Increased with:
   Osteitis deformans
   Rickets
   Osteomalacia
   Hyperparathyroidism
   Healing fractures
   Osteoblastic bone tumors, primary and secondary
   Growing children and pregnant women in third trimester (physiologically elevated)
   Hepatobiliary disease
   Hyperthyroidism
   Hyperphosphatemia
   Intravenous albumin
   Myocardial infarction
   Pulmonary infarction
Decreased with:
   Hypervitaminosis D
   Milk-alkali syndrome
   Scurvy
   Hypophosphatemia
   Hypothyroidism

Clinical Comments. Elevated levels of alkaline phosphatase indicate bone disease with increased osteoblastic activity. This is especially useful in determining the presence of primary and secondary osteoblastic bone tumors.

Creatine Phosphokinase (CPK)

Elevated with:
   Myocardial infarction
   Progressive muscular dystrophy
   Striated muscle necrosis, acute atrophy
   Alcoholic myopathy
   Delirium tremens
   Hypothyroidism
   Pulmonary infarction
   Pulmonary edema
   Exercise
   Intramuscular injections
   Acute psychotic reactions
   Postoperative state (increased with electrocautery)

Clinical Comments. Useful in the detection of myocardial and muscle disease. Isoenzymes of CPK (MM, BB, and MB) may indicate more specific pathology. Creatine phosphokinase is increased with muscle necrosis and progressive muscular dystrophy, and it should be taken into consideration that exercise, as well as intramuscular injections, will increase the CPK level.

SELECTED READINGS

Berkow R: The Merck Manual. 15th Ed. Merck & Co, Inc, Rahway, NJ, 1987

Henry JB: Clinical Diagnosis and Management by Laboratory Methods. 17th Ed. WB Saunders Company, Philadelphia, 1984

McEntyre RL: Practical Guide to the Care of the Surgical Patient. 2nd Ed. CV Mosby Company, St. Louis, 1984

Rodnan GP, Schumacher HR: Primer on the Rheumatic Diseases. 8th Ed. Arthritis Foundation, Atlanta, 1983

Wyngaarden JB, Smith LH, Jr.: Cecil Textbook of Medicine. WB Saunders Company, Philadelphia, 1985

Skin Biopsy and the Foot 11

Leonard A. Levy, D.P.M., M.P.H.

VALUE OF THE SKIN BIOPSY

Although the foot is so often the site of dermatologic pathology and is easily available for histologic examination, skin biopsies in podiatric medical practice are remarkably infrequent. Certainly, a biopsy is not always necessary to diagnose many common podiatric skin disorders. However, in many circumstances its value cannot be overemphasized.

Freeman[1] reminds us of some of the data that may be obtained from a biopsy specimen:

The extent of the lesion (i.e., its level of invasion)
The stage of a disease process
The specific etiology
The likelihood that a particular lesion has been removed
The likelihood that a particular lesion can be removed
The acquisition of prognostic factors
The response to treatment
The differentiation of malignant from benign lesions and primary from metastatic lesions
The differentiation of a tumor from a cyst or granuloma
The determination of the presence or absence of a vascular invasion in a malignant or other lesion
The establishment or confirmation of a diagnosis

In addition, the biopsy can be curative for certain small lesions and even foreign bodies that may be otherwise difficult to remove (e.g., splinters of glass or steel wool). It can also be an invaluable research tool for the discovery of new disease entities and the clarification of others. Not to be overlooked in a cancer-conscious society is the potential to reassure the patient as well as the doctor of a lesion's benignity. One must also appreciate the medicolegal value that the biopsy can have, including that of sharing responsibility with the pathologist who performs the histologic examination. Certainly the failure to perform a biopsy when indicated can place the podiatric physician at much greater risk of being involved in malpractice litigation.

PUNCH BIOPSY

For most skin lesions a punch biopsy is convenient to perform and suitable for obtaining an adequate specimen for histologic examination. Indeed, it is the procedure used most frequently by the dermatologist.[2] Although for small lesions a punch biopsy may be considered excisional (i.e., it removes the entire lesion), in the case of larger lesions it is a type of incisional biopsy (i.e., removal of a portion of lesion). Shave biopsies are carried out

225

by making a horizontal slice through the skin just below what one expects the depth of the lesion to be. It is designed for conditions in which an elevated lesion is encompassed within the superficial part of the skin. One may misjudge the depth of the pathology, however, and remove less than a full-thickness piece of the lesion, which may be too superficial for adequate identification.

The punch biopsy can be performed as quickly and as easily as a shave biopsy. It is used for lesions that are expected to extend as deep as the lower dermis. The punch is a circular cutting instrument that frees up a plug of tissue from the external epidermis to the subcutaneous layer. In podiatric

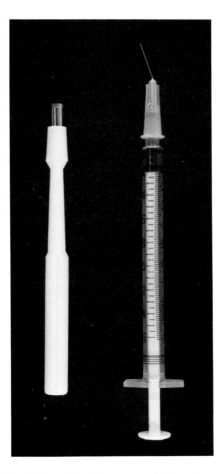

Fig. 11-1. Left to right: Biopsy punch (4 mm) used to remove skin specimen, and 1 cc syringe with 27 gauge ½-inch needle. Note that needle is bent slightly for use as a skin hook. This avoids damaging the specimen.

medicine 4-mm punches are most frequently used; these are inexpensive and available in disposable, individually packaged, sterile packets.

The skin is prepared by washing with soap and water and then wiping the area to be biopsied with alcohol. The circular punch is placed perpendicular to and directly on the skin, and slight downward pressure is applied while the punch is rotated gently so that it cuts a plug of tissue down to the subcutaneous layer. On the plantar surface of the foot this may require penetration almost to the full thickness of the tubular cutting portion of the instrument. On the dorsum of the foot a relatively thin cut is made until free bleeding is seen around the rim of the punch and the tissue appears to be loose in the center of the punch. The skin can then be gently lifted with a 27 gauge ½-inch needle that has been bent to form a hook. This avoids using a forceps or thicker skin hook, which could damage or distort the specimen. The subcutaneous fat under the specimen being removed, which is still attached, is cut with a small scissors (e.g., iris scissors), and the specimen is placed immediately in a bottle containing 10 percent formalin. Usually the amount of formalin should be 20 times the volume of the specimen to make sure the specimen is completely covered with the solution. If the bottled specimen is to be exposed to cold during shipment, a few drops of ethanol should be added to the formalin solution to prevent freezing (Figs. 11-1 and 11-2).

Hemostasis can usually be obtained at the biopsy site with direct pressure using sterile gauze. Rarely are other measures such as electrodessication or styptics necessary. When a 4-mm punch is used it is usually not necessary to use a suture to repair the defect. Caution should be taken when a biopsy needs to be performed on a weight-bearing area. However, if no other lesions are available and there is a suspicion that the lesion may be malignant, the need to perform the biopsy may outweigh the risk of creating a painful scar. Such a scar, which only rarely occurs, may be the necessary price to pay to prevent the loss of a limb or a life.

Obviously, the punch biopsy or any other biopsy requires anesthesia. The needle and anesthetic solution should not be injected into the lesion, but around and/or under it. This can be done in most

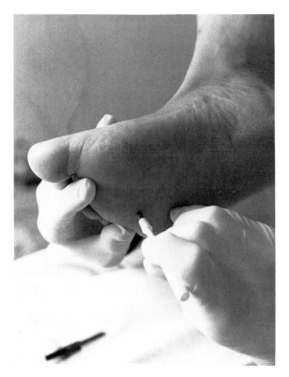

Fig. 11-2. Use of the 4 mm disposable biopsy punch in the removal of a small plantar lesion.

instances with a 1-ml syringe and a ⅜- or ½-inch 26 or 27 gauge needle. The total amount injected rarely exceeds 1 ml. The addition of 1 : 100,000 to 1 : 200,000 epinephrine is preferred to help avoid excessive bleeding.

Rarely do complications arise from a biopsy wound. A dry, sterile dressing over the wound usually is all that is necessary. Sometimes this can be a simple sterile adhesive bandage. The patient should be seen about 3 days postoperatively to make sure no infection has occurred. Patients should be told to keep the wound dry until the area is no longer wet. Most wounds granulate quite well in about 2 weeks, and the eventual result is a flat, painless light scar. Most skin lesions do not have to have adjacent normal skin included in the biopsy. When a biopsy is being done of a blister, however, it is best to take the edge of an early lesion and include a portion of adjacent skin.[3] Scalpel rather than punch biopsy is advised by some for lesions on the toes and overlying joints.[2]

NAIL BIOPSY

Few practitioners see more nail pathology than the podiatric physician, yet the frequency with which biopsies of the nails are performed is surprisingly small.

Norton warned that tumors under and about the nail should be suspected whenever persistent infection, discomfort, or a visible mass is present and has recommended that biopsy be done early and even repeatedly if necessary. Pigmented bands occurring in Caucasians, if not related to drug therapy or Cushing's syndrome, also must be biopsied to rule out malignancy, according to Norton.[4] Although longitudinal pigmented bands under the nails are generally of no significance in blacks, Pack and Oropeza reported that in a series of 72 patients with subungual melanoma, 5 were blacks.[5]

A biopsy punch is a valuable instrument for performing biopsies of the nail bed and plate. After anesthetizing the toe at the base with 1 percent lidocaine hydrochloride and preparing the digit by soap and water scrub followed by an alcohol wash, the nail plate may be penetrated with a 4-mm punch.

It is suggested that, after the nail plate has been fully penetrated, another 4-mm punch be used to complete the penetration through the nail bed. This should result in a circular plug of nail plate attached to the underlying nail bed down to but not into the underlying bone. Unlike a skin biopsy, the base of the specimen usually does not have to be cut with scissors when obtaining a nail biopsy. Postoperative discomfort is generally minor and scar formation is rare.

In the event that the matrix needs to be biopsied, the posterior nail fold can be incised near the lateral and medial nail grooves and retracted proximally to expose the matrix. Then the matrix specimen is obtained using a biopsy punch. The nail fold is then replaced and a few 4-0 or 5-0 sutures are used for closure. A nail matrix biopsy may result in some permanent defects of the nail, and the patient should be informed in advance of this possibility.

THE PATHOLOGIST AND THE PODIATRIC PHYSICIAN

The podiatric physician should provide the pathologist with any information that will be helpful in evaluating the specimen. This should include the age, sex, and race of the patient and the site of the biopsy as well as a description and history of the lesion. If multiple lesions are present, lesions selected for biopsy should appear to be typical of the condition and should not have been infected, treated, excoriated, or otherwise tampered with. It is preferable to remove a lesion or a specimen from a lesion that is well developed and mature, except in the case of blisters, which should be early lesions (preferably less than 24 hours old) with their roof intact. Occasionally it is necessary to take several biopsy specimens in evolving eruptions or in situations when there appear to be several types of lesions.

Specimens should be sent to pathologists who are qualified and experienced in examining biopsy specimens from the skin of the foot. During the past several years laboratories have been established by podiatric physicians who have developed the specialty of podiatric pathology. Because of the function of the foot, certain skin lesions there differ in appearance from the same lesions elsewhere, especially in weight-bearing areas, and the pathologist who lacks a good understanding of these lesions may not be able to provide an adequate and useful report. In addition, certain lesions that may be unique to the foot may not be as well understood by pathologists who have little experience with foot pathology (e.g., certain mechanically induced hyperkeratotic conditions).

BIOPSY AND MALIGNANT MELANOMA

Controversy continues about the appropriateness of performing a punch or other incisional biopsy on a lesion suspected of being a melanoma.

A study of 472 patients at New York University Medical Center and Massachusetts General Hospital showed that there was no significant alteration in the survival rate at the end of 5 and 9 years in patients who had either an incisional or an excisional biopsy. That is, patients whose biopsies consisted of cutting into a melanoma (e.g., a punch biopsy) and those who had the entire lesion excised did not have any difference in survival rates in this large series.[6] Apparently the risk of tumor embolization appears to be more theoretical than real.[7-9]

Since studies show that the diagnosis of melanoma is not easy clinically, with a reported accuracy level of only 64.4 percent of cases, biopsy is a critical examination that must not be avoided.[10] Lederman and Sober have emphasized that incisional biopsy can be of great value in diagnosing these conditions. They indicated that it avoids the need to do extensive initial surgical procedures for large lesions. However, they did recommend that total excisional biopsy be done when possible, since this makes the entire tumor available for histopathologic evaluation.

Lederman and Sober also stated that the prognosis of melanoma appears to depend not on what type of biopsy is done, but rather on the thickness of the lesion. Lesions 1.70 mm or thicker have a poorer prognosis than those less than 1.70 mm thick.[6]

REFERENCES

1. Freeman RG: Handling pathological specimens for gross and microscopic examination in dermatological surgery. J Dermatol Surg Oncol 8:673, 1982
2. Samitz MH: Cutaneous Disorders of the Lower Extremities. 2nd Ed. p 24. Philadelphia, JB Lippincott, 1981
3. Lookingbill DP, Marks JG Jr,: Principles of Dermatology. p 44. Philadelphia, WB Saunders Co, 1986
4. Norton LA: Nail disorders. J Am Acad Dermatol 2:460, 1980
5. Pack GT, Oropeza R: Subungual melanoma. Surg Gynecol Obstet 124:571, 1967
6. Lederman JS, Sober AJ: Does biopsy type influence survival in clinical state I cutaneous melanoma? J Am Acad Dermatol 13:986, 1985

7. Lee YN: Diagnosis, treatment and prognosis of early melanoma: the importance of depth of microinvasion. Ann Surg 191:87, 1985

8. Harris MN, Gumport SL: Total excision biopsy for primary malignant melanoma. JAMA 226:354, 1973

9. Elder DE, Dupont-Guerry IV, Heiberger RM, et al: Optimal resection margin for cutaneous malignant melanoma. J Plast Reconstr Surg 71:66, 1983

10. Kopf AW, Mintzis M, Bart RS: Diagnostic accuracy in malignant melanoma. Arch Dermatol 111:1291, 1975

Podiatric Radiology

12

Ronald E. Johnson, D.P.M.

The use of radiologic techniques and studies is an invaluable tool to the podiatric medical physician. The ability to visualize the osseous structures of the foot and their relationships is essential to the competent diagnosis and treatment of the podiatric patient.

The podiatric physician must be proficient in positioning of the patient as well as producing radiographic images of the foot that will relate accurate information for interpretation. He or she must also have knowledge of foot development and normal podiatric radiologic characteristics if abnormal pathomechanics or pathology of the foot is to be appreciated. Finally, the podiatric physician must possess a high degree of understanding of various abnormal osseous, biomechanical, and structural radiographic presentations to be able to formulate a diagnosis and institute an expedient treatment plan.

The author's intent is to present general introductory information in the area of podiatric radiology, realizing that an in-depth podiatric radiologic work is out of the scope of this book. An attempt is made to provide significant useful information in a clear, succinct manner through the use of radiographs, illustrations, and brief descriptions. The reader is referred to the many fine podiatric and general radiology textbooks available for additional reference and study.

RADIOGRAPHIC POSITIONING

The goal in the production of radiographs is to produce a clear and accurate representation of structures and relationships of structures of the anatomic part being radiographically examined. If this goal is to be accomplished, adequate information will need to be produced radiographically to assist the podiatric physician in diagnosis and ultimately treatment planning.

For the physician to be able to accurately assess a radiograph he or she must select and produce appropriate projections of the anatomic part that is to be examined. These projections must be easily duplicated by each assistant or practitioner and remain standardized throughout the medical profession.

The proper selection of projections will help to minimize patient exposure to radiation and provide information as well as documentation to the podiatric physician. Each projection will provide limited information, and therefore the podiatric physician must be cognizant of each projection with respect to the information each will specifically provide.

The majority of radiographic examinations of the foot will be performed with the foot in a weight-bearing position in the angle and base of gait. The *angle of gait* refers to the angle formed between the feet and the line of progression during ambulation. This can easily be observed by having the patient ambulate a short distance prior to taking the x-ray. The usual angle of gait is between 10 and 15 degrees. The *base of gait* refers to the distance observed between the right and left medial malleoli during ambulation and is approximately 2 inches in the normal patient.

Radiographic positioning is usually described in terms of radiographic views or radiographic projections. These terms generally relate to either the trajectory of the x-ray beam or the relationship of the anatomic part being examined to the x-ray film. It is essential that the podiatric physician and assistant be familiar with both of these terminologies in order that accurate communication will exist. While the terminology of views and projections are both used, it is generally held that projections best define the radiograph.

The term *projection* refers to the anatomic area of the foot or ankle into which the x-ray beam enters (the initial portion of the term) and the anatomic area from which the x-ray beam exists (the second portion of the term) in the description of the projection. For example, a dorsoplantar projection of the foot is one in which the x-ray beam enters the dorsal aspect of the foot and exits the plantar aspect of the foot.

The term *view* refers primarily to the x-ray image and describes the portion of the foot closest to the film. For example, when a dorsoplantar projection as just described is taken, the image produced is a plantardorsal view because the plantar aspect of the foot is closest to the film.

Atlas A: Podiatric Projections and Views

Foot: Dorsoplantar (DP or AP) Projection, Plantar-Dorso View

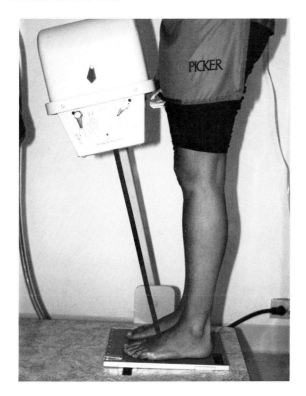

Fig. 12-1. Position for DP projection of left foot.

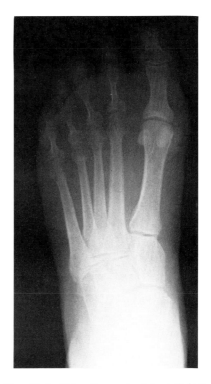

Fig. 12-2. DP radiograph of the left foot.

STRUCTURES DEMONSTRATED: Phalanges, sesamoid bones, metatarsals, and tarsal bones.

PATIENT POSITIONING: One-half of film is blocked off with lead longitudinally. Patient stands with foot upon the exposable one-half of the film in the angle and base of gait.

REFERENCE PART: Base of the second metatarsal to the center of the film.

CENTRAL RAY: Tube angled 15 degrees cephalad (15 degrees from vertical).

**Foot: Lateral Oblique Projection, Medial
Oblique View**

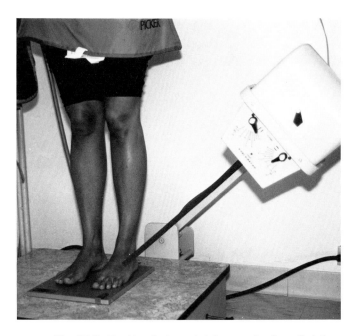

Fig. 12-3. Position for lateral oblique projection of left foot.

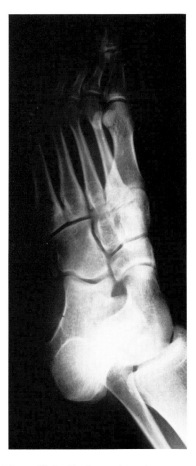

Fig. 12-4. Radiograph of lateral oblique projection of left foot.

STRUCTURES DEMONSTRATED:

Phalanges, metatarsals, tarsals, and sesamoid bones.

PATIENT POSITIONING:

Film cassette flat and lateral aspect of foot is parallel and along edge of cassette nearest tube.

REFERENCE PART:

Third (lateral) cuneiform to center of film.

CENTRAL RAY:

Tube angled 40 degrees with central ray at fourth metatarsal–cuboid articulation.

Foot: Lateral Projection, Medial View

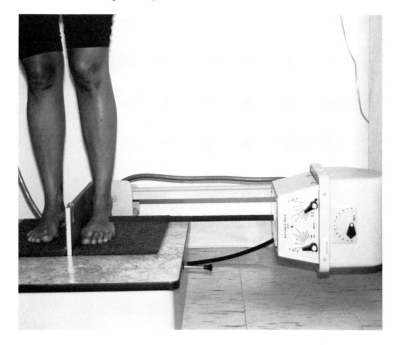

Fig. 12-5. Position for lateral projection of left foot.

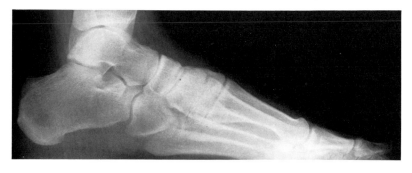

Fig. 12-6. Radiograph of lateral projection of left foot.

STRUCTURES DEMONSTRATED:	First metatarsal, first cuneiform, navicular, talus, and calcaneus.
PATIENT POSITIONING:	Film cassette vertical, one-half of exposable portion in orthoposer slot. Medial aspect of foot next to film and opposite foot in angle and base of gait.
REFERENCE PART:	First (medial) cuneiform to center of the film.
CENTRAL RAY:	Tube angled 90 degrees from vertical (perpendicular to film) and aimed at the fourth metatarsal base.

Foot: Axial Sesamoid Projection, Plantar
Axial View

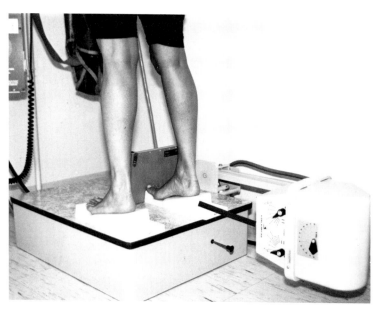

Fig. 12-7. Position for axial sesamoid projection of right foot.

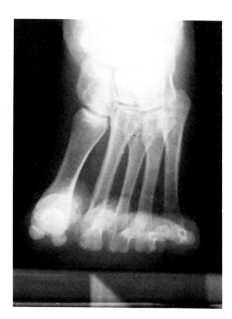

Fig. 12-8. Radiograph of axial sesamoid projection of right foot.

STRUCTURES DEMONSTRATED:

Plantar aspect of first metatarsal head, sesamoid bones, plantar aspect of lesser metatarsals.

PATIENT POSITIONING:

Patient standing in positioning blocks in angle and base of gait. Film placed perpendicular to the floor with end of axial positioning device against film. X-ray only one foot at a time.

REFERENCE PART:

Third metatarsal head to center of film.

CENTRAL RAY:

Perpendicular to film, centered on positioning block at posterior and inferior aspect of calcaneus.

Foot: Coalition Projection, Harris and Beath View

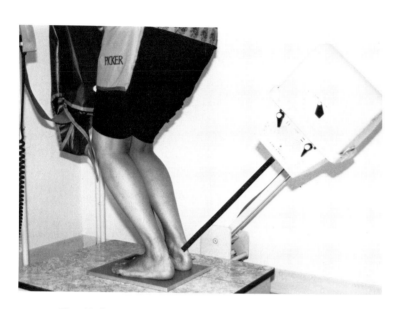

Fig. 12-9. Position for coalition projection of right foot.

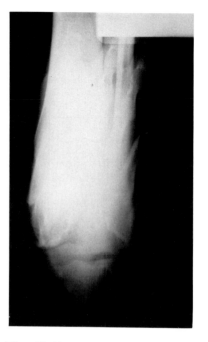

Fig. 12-10. Radiograph of coalition projection of right foot.

STRUCTURES DEMONSTRATED:	Inferior aspect of talus, middle and posterior facets of talocalcaneal articulation, and axial of calcaneus.
PATIENT POSITIONING:	Patient standing on film on orthoposer in angle and base of gait with foot on long axis of film. Knees and ankles flexed.
REFERENCE PART:	Navicular to center of film.
CENTRAL RAY:	Tube angled 35 to 45 degrees entering from posterior at level of talocalcaneal joint, passing through the subtalar joint to the film.

**Foot: Axial Calcaneal Projection, Axial
Calcaneal View**

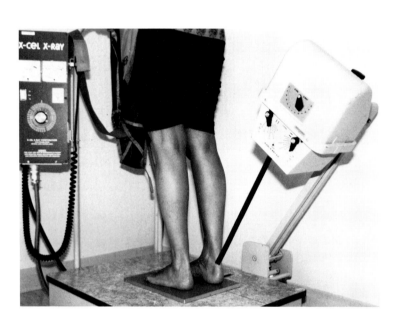

Fig. 12-11. Position for calcaneal axial projection of right foot.

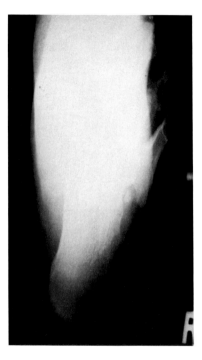

Fig. 12-12. Radiograph of calcaneal axial projection of right foot.

STRUCTURES DEMONSTRATED:	Calcaneus.
PATIENT POSITIONING:	Patient stands on film on orthoposer in angle and base of gait with foot on the long axis of the film with back to the x-ray tube and leans slightly forward.
REFERENCE PART:	Posterior aspect of ankle joint to center of film.
CENTRAL RAY:	Tube angled 25 degrees from vertical and aimed at the posterior aspect of the heel at the approximate level of the talocalcaneal joint.

**Ankle: Anterior-Posterior (AP) Projection,
Posterior-Anterior View**

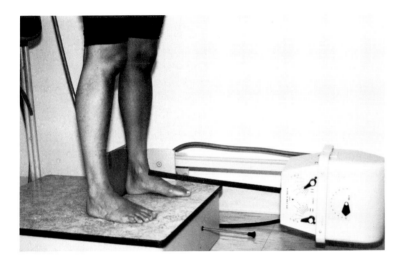

Fig. 12-13. Position for AP projection of left ankle.

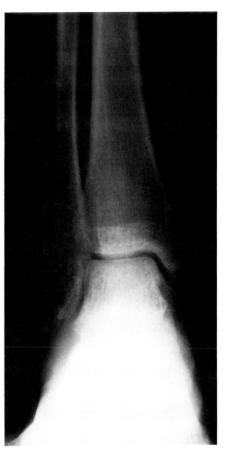

Fig. 12-14. Radiograph of AP projection of left ankle.

STRUCTURES DEMONSTRATED:	Trochlear surface of talus, ankle mortise, medial and lateral malleoli, distal tibia and fibula.
PATIENT POSITIONING:	Film in orthoposer slot. Patient standing in front of film with posterior aspect of calcaneus against the film and foot straight ahead.
REFERENCE PART:	Posterior aspect of ankle in center of film.
CENTRAL RAY:	Perpendicular to the film and entering anterior aspect of the ankle joint midway between the medial and lateral malleoli at center of film.

Ankle: Lateral Oblique Projection, Medial Oblique (MO) View

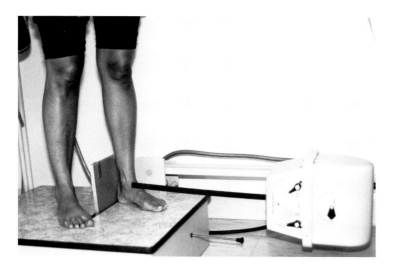

Fig. 12-15. Position of lateral oblique projection of left ankle.

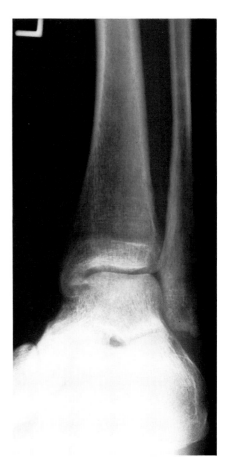

Fig. 12-16. Radiograph of lateral oblique projection of left ankle.

STRUCTURES DEMONSTRATED:	Distal tibia and fibula, ankle mortise and trochlear surface of talus, and tibiofibular syndesmosis.
PATIENT POSITIONING:	Film in orthoposer slot. Patient standing in front of film with posterior medial aspect of calcaneus against film and 45 degrees of internal rotation of the entire leg.
REFERENCE PART:	Posterior aspect of medial malleolus in center of film.
CENTRAL RAY:	Perpendicular to the film and entering the ankle joint medial and anterior to the lateral malleolus.

Ankle: Lateral Projection, Medial View

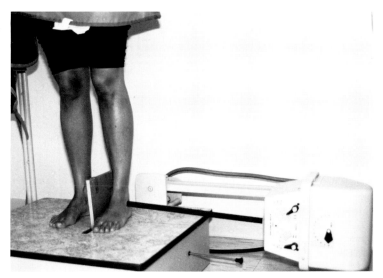

Fig. 12-17. Position of lateral projection of left ankle.

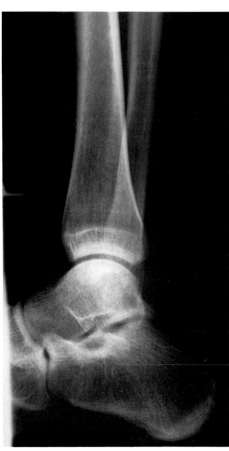

Fig. 12-18. Radiograph of lateral projection of left ankle.

STRUCTURES DEMONSTRATED:	Distal tibia and fibula, talus, and calcaneus.
PATIENT POSITIONING:	Film in orthoposer slot. Patient standing with medial malleolus against center of film.
REFERENCE PART:	Medial malleolus to center of film.
CENTRAL RAY:	Perpendicular to film and entering the lateral malleolus.

PODIATRIC RADIOGRAPHIC CHARTING

Charting of the foot radiograph is the recording of diagnostic information from the radiograph that will enhance the standard written description of findings and conclusions in the radiographic report. This additional documentation involves the determination of lines, reference points, and angles that may be measured, assigned values, and compared. These relationships can therefore be expressed as numeric values and ratios that can be utilized in the assessment of positional relationships and assist in the establishment of diagnostic classification of the foot type as well as evaluate foot pathology.

The various podiatric charting techniques available are numerous. Again, it is not the author's intention to provide the reader the complete list of podiatric radiographic charting techniques, but rather to provide the reader with many of the more commonly used podiatric radiographic charting angles and relationships. The following podiatric charting relationships are provided as well as illustrations of the angles and relationships with normal values when appropriate.

Atlas B: Podiatric Charting Relationships

Transverse Plane Measurements (DP projection)

Hallux Interphalangeal Angle

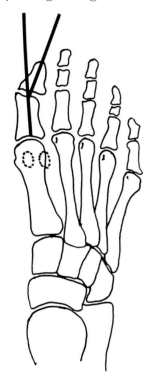

Fig. 12-19. Hallux interphalangeal angle.

1. Relationship between a longitudinal bisection of the distal phalanx of the hallux and a longitudinal bisection of the proximal phalanx of the hallux.
2. Normal = 8 to 10 degrees.

Hallux Abductus Angle

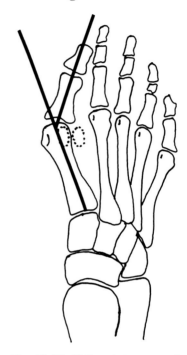

Fig. 12-20. Hallux abductus angle.

1. Relationship between a longitudinal bisection of the proximal phalanx of the hallux and a longitudinal bisection of the first metatarsal.
2. Angle always abducted unless varus deformity of the hallux is present.
3. Normal = 15 to 16 degrees.

Intermetatarsal Angle

Metatarsus Adductus Angle

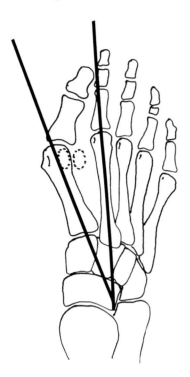

Fig. 12-21. Intermetatarsal angle.

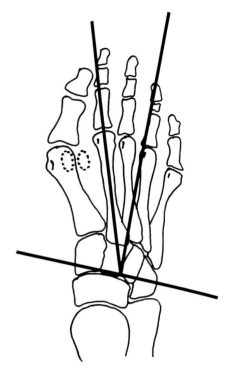

Fig. 12-22. Metatarsus adductus angle.

1. Angle formed by a bisection of the first metatarsal and a bisection of the second metatarsal.
2. Evaluate in conjunction with the metatarsus adductus angle.
3. Normal = 8 to 10 degrees.

1. Angle formed by the metatarsal axis (second metatarsal) and the lesser tarsal axis.
2. Angle is almost always adductory.
3. Normal = 16 to 18 degrees.

Proximal Articular Set Angle (PASA)

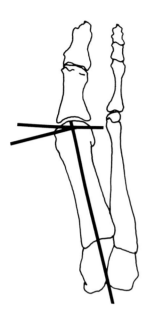

Fig. 12-23. Proximal articular set angle (PASA).

1. Relationship between a longitudinal bisection of the first metatarsal to the effective articulating cartilage of the first metatarsal.
2. Normal = 5 to 7 degrees.

Distal Articular Set Angle (DASA)

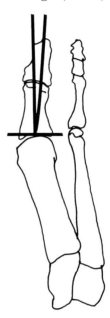

Fig. 12-24. Distal articular set angle (DASA).

1. Relationship between a longitudinal bisection of the proximal phalanx of the hallux to the effective articulating cartilage of the base of the proximal phalanx of the hallux.
2. Normal = 5 to 7 degrees.

Metatarsal Protrusion Distance   *Tibial Sesamoid Position*

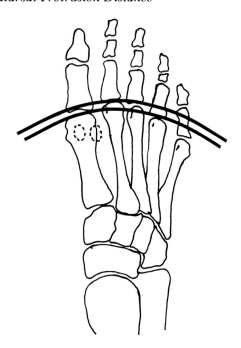

Fig. 12-25. Metatarsal protrusion distance.

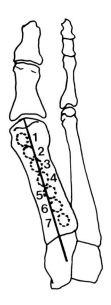

Fig. 12-26. Tibial sesamoid position.

1. Comparison of an arc formed by a compass at the point of the longitudinal bisection of the first metatarsal and an arc at the point of the longitudinal bisection of the second metatarsal.
2. Can be used to compare any two metatarsal lengths.
3. When comparing first to second metatarsal, distance will be positive if first is longer and negative if first is shorter.

1. Relationship of tibial sesamoid bone to the longitudinal bisection of the first metatarsal.
2. Measures displacement of the sesamoid bones in the transverse plane.
3. Represents an indirect measurement of the intermetatarsal angle.

Talocalcaneal Angle

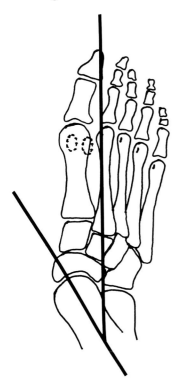

Fig. 12-27. Talocalcaneal angle.

1. Relationship of the longitudinal axis of the talar neck to the longitudinal axis of the rearfoot.
2. Not a bisection of the talus, but a defining of the axis of the talar neck.
3. Normal = 15 degrees.

Cuboid Abduction Angle

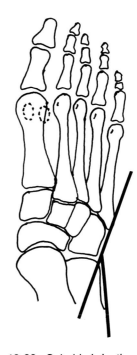

Fig. 12-28. Cuboid abduction angle.

1. Relationship of the lateral border of the calcaneus to the lateral border of the cuboid.
2. Normal = 0 to 5 degrees.

Sagittal Plane Measurements (Lateral Projection)

Calcaneal Inclination Angle

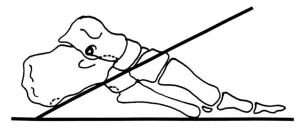

Fig. 12-29. Calcaneal inclination angle.

1. Relationship of the calcaneus to the weight-bearing plane.
2. Index of relative arch height.
3. Normal = 15 to 30 degrees.

Talar Declination Angle

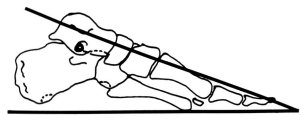

Fig. 12-30. Talar declination angle.

1. Angle formed by the line of the collum tali axis and the plane of support.

Lateral Talocalcaneal Angle

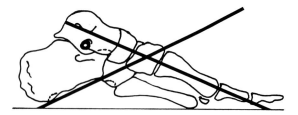

Fig. 12-31. Lateral talocalcaneal angle.

1. Angle formed by the intersection of the bisection of the talar neck axis (collum tali) and the calcaneal axis of inclination.

First Metatarsal Declination Angle

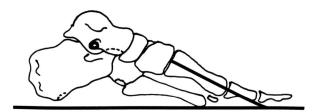

Fig. 12-32. First metatarsal declination angle.

1. Angle formed by a line of the first metatarsal axis and the surface of support.

Bohler's Tuber Joint Angle

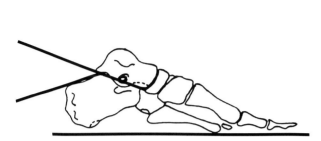

Fig. 12-33. Bohler's tuber joint angle.

1. Relationship between the upper contour of the tuberosity of the os calcis and the line uniting the highest point of the anterior process with the highest point of the posterior articular surface.
2. Overlies the posterior articular facet and is a measurement of the sagittal plane relationship between the talus and calcaneus.
3. Assesses the degree of intra-articular depression of calcaneal facets in calcaneal fractures.
4. Normal = 25 to 40 degrees.

Fowler-Philip Angle

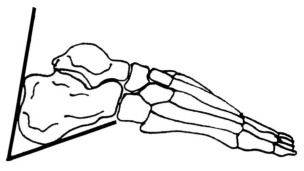

Fig. 12-34. Fowler-Philip angle.

1. Relationship of the posterior aspect of the calcaneus to the plantar aspect of the calcaneus.
2. Helpful in the evaluation of Haglund's deformity of the calcaneus.
3. Normal = 44 to 62 degrees.

RADIOLOGIC DEVELOPMENT OF THE FOOT

When evaluating the pediatric foot radiographically one must have an understanding of the normal development and radiologic appearance of the foot. The development and radiologic appearance of the normal pediatric foot is discussed here, with many of the specific pathologic deformities discussed in more detail in other areas of this book.

A discussion of radiologic foot development must include some generalities and information regarding prenatal and postnatal foot growth and development. It is not this author's intention to present a complete description of foot development and appearance of the foot, but rather to present information leading to a general understanding with respect to neonatal foot development and growth. It is hoped that with a basic understanding of the development of the foot a better appreciation and understanding of radiographs of the pediatric foot will follow.

While it appears that the bulk of foot growth occurs in the period from birth to adulthood, the foot increases in length an average of less than 2 percent of stature from age 1 to 18 years. Relative foot growth is most active prenatally and slows greatly from the period before birth to early adulthood.

Foot length generally doubles in 1 month during the fifth fetal month. In contrast, it takes 4 years for the foot to double its length at birth and 8 years to double the foot length at age 6 months. It generally takes 18 years before the male foot is twice as long as it is when the boy is 1½ years old.[1]

It is also interesting to note that the foot ceases growth before almost any other part of the skeleton. At the age of 10 years females will have reached approximately 90 percent of their foot growth and males will have reached approximately 80 percent of their final foot growth. Generally closure of the epiphyseal centers and cessation of foot growth takes place at approximately 14 years of age in females and 16 years of age in males.

Caution must be used when discussing pediatric age in relation to pediatric development. There are variations in individual child development and rates of development for many reasons. The ages of development are used as guidelines and should be used in evaluation of radiographs in such a manner. There are conditions in which age and radiographic development may not coincide, and these presentations will require a more in-depth workup with comparison of skeletal development in other regions of the body.

The radiologic development of the foot cannot be understood without some knowledge of the prenatal development, chondrification, and ossification of the foot. It is important to bear in mind as development of the foot is discussed that the skeletal structural components of the foot are determined prior to the seventh postovulatory week of intrauterine life.[2]

Stages of Skeletal Development

Mesenchymal Stage

During approximately the fifth postovulatory week the axial mesenchyme condenses, differentiates, and forms the anlage of the foot. Phalangeal models are formed and for a short period of time a thick web remains between the digital rays.

The metatarsals differentiate in the late mesenchymal stage. These metatarsal rays are spread apart, but will gradually approximate with development of the foot.

The differentiation of the tarsus follows that of the metatarsals. The distal ends of the tibia and fibula are also formed during this mesenchymal stage.

Cartilagenous Stage

In approximately the sixth to seventh postovulatory week cartilage cells begin to form in the mesenchymal prochondral anlage. Chondrification advances the skeletal elements with morphogenesis moving toward the adult form occurring. This produces more clearly indentifiable skeletal elements of the foot.

Chondrification of the skeletal elements of the foot occur in 14 stages. The sequence of these stages is:

1. Central three metatarsals
2. Fifth metatarsal and cuboid

3. Calcaneus, talus, lateral cuneiform
4. Middle cuneiform
5. First metatarsal, medial cuneiform
6. Navicular (last tarsal element) Phalanges—proximal to distal sequence:
7. Proximal phalanx (second, third, fourth)
8. Proximal phalanx (fifth)
9. Proximal phalanx (hallux)
10. Middle phalanx (second, third, fourth)
11. Middle phalanx (fifth)
12. Distal phalanx (hallux)
13. Distal phalanx (second, third, fourth)
14. Distal phalanx (fifth)

By the end of this embryologic period proper morphology and relationship of cartilaginous skeletal components are determined and closely resemble those of the adult foot. This is an important consideration when evaluating and studying the pathogenesis of congenital foot deformities. This reiterates the fact that the skeletal structural components are determined by the end of this period, or approximately the seventh postovulatory week of intrauterine life.

Osseous Stage

Ossification is an important stage from a radiologic point of view in that as the skeletal elements of the foot undergo ossification these elements can be identified and evaluated radiographically.

This histologic process of ossification is periosteal and endochondral in the metatarsals as well as the proximal and middle phalanges of the foot.[3] This type of ossification is characterized by the formation of a bone collar around the central area of the cartilagenous diaphysis. This is followed by invasion of a periosteal bud into the cartilagenous shaft, initiating the endochondral ossification. This endochondral ossification then extends in a proximal and distal direction until the skeletal element is ossified.

The distal phalanx of the foot differs in that it ossifies by intramembranous and endochondral ossification. This ossification process is characterized by the formation of a distal "cap" of intramembranous bone formation at the distal end of the cartilagenous distal phalanx. This cap is then converted into a bony "thimble fitting over the cartilagenous phalanx and enclosing it almost up to its base."[4] This process of intramembranous and endochondral ossification begins at the distal tip of the distal phalanx and extends proximally until the phalanx is completely ossified.

It is important to note that the forefoot elements of the foot ossify before the rearfoot elements. The distal phalanx of the great toe is generally the first foot element to ossify and can begin ossification as early as the seventh postovulatory week. Ossification of the forefoot generally occurs between the third and fifth prenatal lunar month. The sequence of ossification of the forefoot is generally as follows[2]:

Distal phalanx of great toe
Second, third, and fourth metatarsals
First and fifth metatarsals
Distal phalanges of lesser toes
Proximal phalanges of hallux and second toe
Third, fourth, and fifth proximal phalanges
Middle phalanges of lesser toes

The rearfoot ossification begins at approximately the third to fourth prenatal lunar month with ossification of the calcaneus. The second rearfoot element to ossify is the talus, with ossification at approximately the eighth prenatal lunar month. Because the talus ossifies late in prenatal development it is not always present radiographically at birth.

The last tarsal element that can exhibit ossification before birth is the cuboid. The cuboid ossification center is present at birth approximately 50 percent of the time and is generally present in 90 percent of foot radiographs by the age of 6 months.

The navicular and the three cuneiform bones ossify in the postnatal period. The ossification centers of all foot elements are usually identifiable on radiographs by 3 to 3½ years of age.

When evaluating radiographs of patients from birth through early childhood one must bear in mind that the basic shapes of the bones of the foot are completely patterned in cartilagenous tissues. Conventional radiographs of a child's foot will only demonstrate areas of bone mineralization or ossification. One should not make the error of thinking that the foot is a homogeneous mass that only becomes differentiated upon ossification.

When visualizing a radiograph of a child's foot one must realize that the complete bone elements are present even though not visible on the radiographs. The only information that may be used when evaluating the radiograph is the actual areas of specific bones that are ossified and thus evident on the radiograph.

Consideration for the type of ossification center present in each osseous element of the foot must be evaluated when interpreting osseous and joint relationships in the pediatric foot.

Bones such as the cuboid and talus will generally present *centric* ossification centers in which the ossification center is located at approximately the geometric center of the bone. These bone elements with a centric ossification center will present a different radiographic development pattern of ossification than will elements such as the calcaneus, which has an *eccentric* ossification center. The eccentric ossification center will have its loci removed from the geometric center of the ossifying bone and thus one region of the bone will appear radiographically to develop before another region. For example, the lack of mineralization in the anterior process area of the calcaneus due to the calcaneal eccentric ossification center placement makes this area ossify later and thus appear visible later in development radiographically.

The talus at this period of development should be in close alignment with the calcaneus. The distal portion of the talus is usually mineralized first while the posterior inferior portion of the talus is usually not visualized radiographically at this stage. Dorsoplantar projection will usually reveal that the head of the talus is advanced beyond the anterior process of the calcaneus because of the early development of the distal portion of the talus and the eccentric location and ossification of the calcaneus. A lateral projection should also reveal this apparent advance of the talus beyond the midtarsal joint line.

Radiologic Stages of Skeletal Foot Growth

The development of the foot from a radiologic perspective exhibits definite characteristics at distinct periods of foot maturation. It is during these periods of chronologic development that one can observe certain common radiographic characteristics of normal foot development.

Birth to 2 Years

It is during this stage of foot development that the vital components of the rearfoot and the midtarsal joint become radiologically evident (Fig. 12-35). The calcaneus, talus, and cuboid, being the foot bones receiving the greatest stress, are solidly configured and easily identified on radiographs.

The body of the calcaneus is the calcaneal region primarily visualized because of early mineralization of that area. Ossification centers of the talus and calcaneus are usually present, as well as differences in areas of ossification of these bones. One must be careful not to interpret the related position of the calcaneus and the talus as coinciding with the placement of the midtarsal joint of the foot.

The cuboid is present radiographically in approximately 50 percent of infants at birth and approximately 90 percent of infants by 6 months of age. The cuboid bone's centric ossification center and pattern of mineralization will place its radiographic appearance in a position generally far removed from the anterior portion of the calcaneus at this stage.

The lateral cuneiform will make its appearance in the form of a small ossification center by approximately 6 to 7 months of age.

The navicular bone in some patients will begin to appear during this stage, with the ossification center at times becoming radiographically visible by 23 to 24 months of age.

2 Years to 5 Years

The ossification center and development of the navicular marks the early period of this stage as well as continued ossification and growth of the talus, calcaneus, cuboid, and lateral cuneiform bones (Fig. 12-36).

The medial and middle cuneiform bones generally appear at approximately 3 years of age and the secondary epiphyses of the phalanges and metatarsals become radiographically apparent about this same time. This period is usually characterized as a period of rapid foot growth, and the physician must be cautious in interpretation of foot radiographs during this period. While osseous elements reveal a significantly increased radiographic development in appearance, the lack of substantially developed bones may lead to misinterpretation with respect to true alignment and relationships.

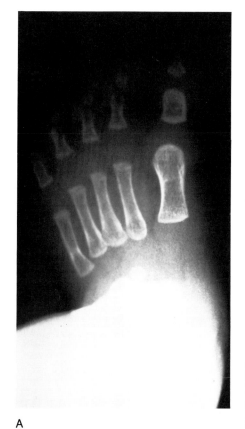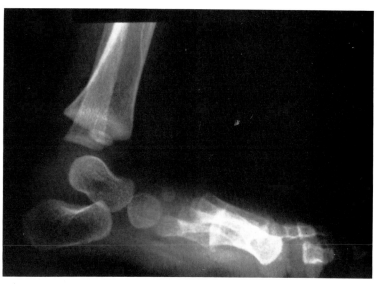

A   B

Fig. 12-35. **(A)** DP projection of left foot, child 18-months-old. **(B)** Lateral projection of left foot, child 18-months-old.

Innumerable variations in ossific centers occur, and multiple ossification nuclei may provide confusion in interpretation. There may be variable growth rates present between tubular long bones and round bones. Gross irregularities in the outline of mineralized zones of the plantar tuberosity of the calcaneus may also give the appearance of a malformed bone when in fact this is normal for development of this bone in some cases.

5 Years to 12 Years

This period continues to be a period of rapid maturation of the foot. The foot growth during this stage is at a spasmodic rate, although it progresses in relatively steady increments. Radiographic features at this point are of significant value for use in interpretation of foot pathoanatomy.

As a result of incomplete mineralization and ossification the distal end of the metatarsal shaft and the articulating phalanx remain widely separated. In spite of this radiographic appearance the foot is completely capable of sustaining stresses applied to the metatarsophalangeal joint areas.

The final secondary center of ossification appears in the foot during this stage with the appearance of the calcaneal epiphysis, or more correctly calcaneal apophysis (Fig. 12-37). This calcaneal growth center will usually appear at approximately 8 years of age in females and approximately 10 to 11 years of age in males.

12 Years to 22 Years

During this stage all osseous elements of the foot are present and continue to mature, culminating in the complete formation of the bones and joints of the foot (Fig. 12-38).

Final fusion of all epiphyseal areas as well as the calcaneal apophysis occurs during this stage. Fu-

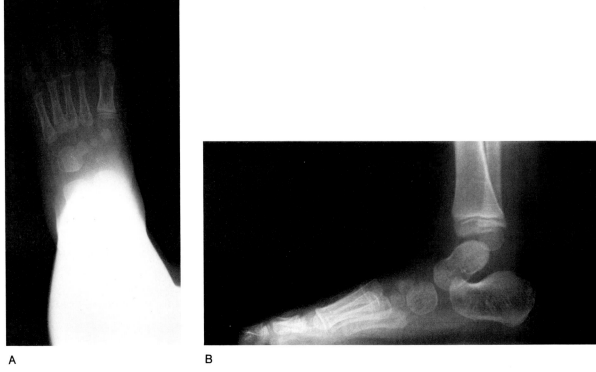

A   B

Fig. 12-36. (A) DP projection of left foot, child 36-months-old. **(B)** Lateral projection of left foot, child 36-months-old.

sion of these epiphyseal areas brings to a close the development of the foot. It is this completely developed foot that we radiographically evaluate as the adult foot.

RADIOGRAPHIC EVALUATION OF THE NORMAL FOOT

The majority of foot function occurs during gait and in stance. In gait normal foot position is best evaluated at midstance, whereas in stance this normal foot position is best evaluated with the feet in the natural angle and base of stance or gait. Therefore weight-bearing radiographs of the feet taken in the natural angle and base of gait will provide the most useful and accurate radiographic evaluation.

The radiographic evaluation should reveal generally normal shapes and relationships of the osseous elements of the foot. These bone shapes and relationships are consistently noted and are therefore deemed to be radiographically noted as normal.

The talus on lateral projection should reveal a rounded dorsal aspect of the talar body or talar dome without evidence of flattening. The posterior process of the talus should not be excessively long or appear separated from the body of the talus. The head of the talus should be rounded and of substantial size (Fig. 12-39).

The calcaneus will usually reveal rounded posterior and plantar tuberosities. The sustentaculum tali should be of large enough size to be easily identifiable and should be oriented parallel with the transverse plane of the subtalar joint. The anterior process of the calcaneus is usually identifiable and of moderate size.

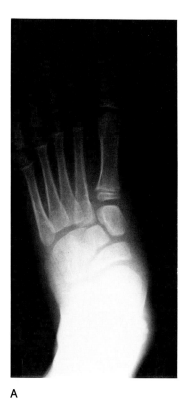

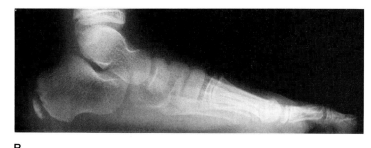

A　　　　　　　　　　　　　　B

Fig. 12-37. (A) DP projection of left foot, child 7-years-old. **(B)** Lateral projection of left foot, child 7-years-old.

The navicular bone in the normal foot should present radiographically as somewhat rectangular in shape. The dorsoplantar projection should reveal approximately equal medial and lateral width of the navicular and should not extend excessively on the medial aspect of the foot (Fig. 12-40). The cuboid should present with good alignment and articulation with the calcaneal articulating surface. The plantar tuberosity of the cuboid appears smooth and somewhat rounded.

The anterior margin of the medial cuneiform should articulate closely with the base of the first metatarsal. The articular margin of the base of the first metatarsal should be perpendicular to its long axis to provide proper articulation of the first metatarsal with the medial cuneiform bone.

Dorsoplantar Projection

The dorsoplantar projection of the foot will reveal bone and joint relationships existing primarily in the transverse plane.

In the normal foot the radiograph will show the head of the talus to be closely bound to the calcaneus and superimposed on the anterior portion of the calcaneus. Normally approximately 75 percent of the talar head will articulate with the adjacent navicular bone (Fig. 12-41). The talus will present with a slight medial deviation of approximately 15 degrees from the long axis of the foot. The lateral border of the calcaneus at its anterior border will usually lie parallel to the long axis of the foot.

The midtarsal joint of the foot, which is comprised of the talonavicular joint and calcaneocuboid joint, functionally joins the rearfoot with the forefoot and can be readily evaluated on the dorsoplantar foot projection. This midtarsal joint relationship can be accessed by evaluating the continuity of a line drawn outlining the articulation of the talonavicular and calcaneocuboid joints, commonly referred to as the cyma line. The midtarsal joint of the normal foot will show continuity or an unbroken cyma line (Fig. 12-42).[5]

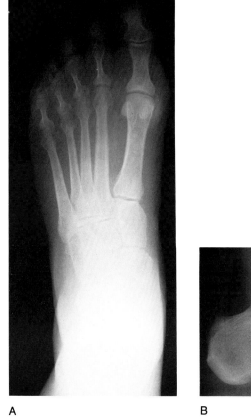

A

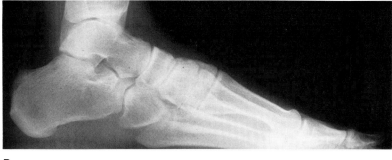

B

Fig. 12-38. (A) DP projection of adult foot. **(B)** Lateral projection of adult foot.

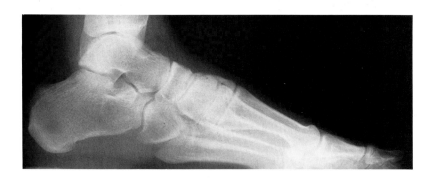

Fig. 12-39. Lateral projection, normal foot.

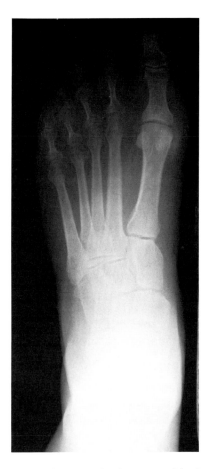

Fig. 12-40. DP projection, normal foot.

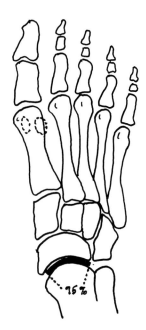

Fig. 12-41. Navicular coverage of talar head.

Lateral View

The lateral projection of the foot will assist in the evaluation of bone and joint relationships existing primarily in the sagittal plane.

In the normal foot the lateral weight-bearing foot projection will reveal a continuous or unbroken cyma line at the midtarsal joint articulation (Fig. 12-43). The sinus tarsi should be distinctly visible and a prominent feature on this view. A line drawn from the posterior talocalcaneal joint through the superior surface of the sinus tarsi should place the body of the talus parallel to the supporting surface.

The plantar tuberosities of the calcaneus should be visible and the calcaneal inclination angle should provide an index as to the height of the foot

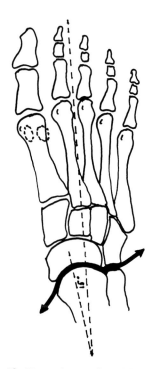

Fig. 12-42. Normal cyma line, DP projection

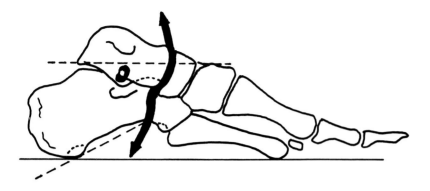

Fig. 12-43. Normal cyma line, lateral projection.

architecture. The calcaneal inclination angle should be comparatively equal in both feet.

The sustentaculum tali should be easily identified as an area of increased density inferior to the sinus tarsi. This sinus tarsi density should not be excessively broad or wide in appearance.

The articulating facet of the cuboid bone should be in even alignment with its corresponding calcaneal articulating facet and the area of the peroneal groove in the inferior region of the cuboid is usually observed as an area of increased density.

The long axis of the first metatarsal bone should generally be in orientation with the axis of the medial cuneiform, navicular, and head of the talus. All articulating surfaces of the talar head, navicular, medial cuneiform, and first metatarsal base should appear evenly aligned without dorsal or plantar gaps or without narrowing.

Accessory Bones of the Foot

Supernumerary or accessory bones are common and numerous in the foot. While accessory bones in many areas of the foot are considered normal findings, care must be taken to differentiate these accessory bones from chip- or avulsion-type fractures. Figure 12-44 shows the names and location of many of the commonly encountered supernumerary and accessory bones of the foot.

Pes Cavus

The pes cavus foot type is characterized by its distinctive high arch morphology. The unusual stress at various points of the foot, faulty weight-bearing loading factors, and limitation of mobility provide the basis of symptoms associated with this foot type.

The cavus foot type is best evaluated radiographically with weight-bearing dorsoplantar and lateral projections in the angle and base of gait. This foot radiographically presents with classic cavus architecture, with more severe forms represented by an exaggeration of this basic pes cavus architecture (Fig. 12-45).

Evaluation of the lateral weight-bearing projection of the cavus foot will characteristically reveal an increased calcaneal inclination angle exceeding 30 degrees. There is also an increased inclination of the first and fifth metatarsals. An accentuation of the subtalar joint region as well as the sinus tarsi is also usually noted, and it is not uncommon to find a calcaneocuboid fault with contracted digits present.

The cyma line in the cavus foot type will appear on the dorsoplantar projection, as well as the lateral weight-bearing projection, as normal with a posterior break in specific instances. An accentuation of the subtalar joint region as well as the sinus tarsi is also usually noted on the lateral weight-bearing projection.

Pes Planus

The pes planus, or pronated foot, will present radiographically with many distinguishing radiographic features. This foot type may be congenital or acquired. It is important not only to recognize this foot type, but to also identify the segment of the foot involved, along with foot faults that may be

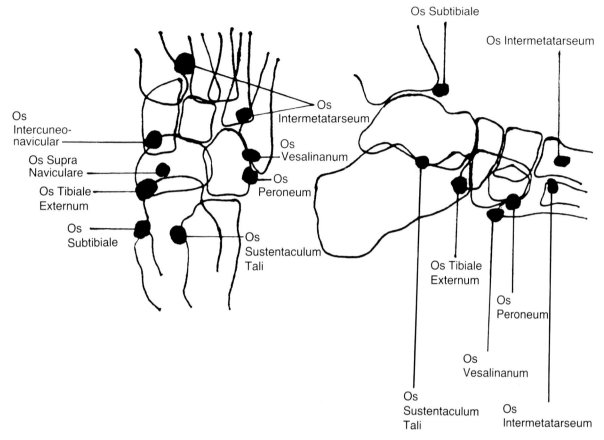

Fig. 12-44. Common accessory bones of the foot. Os vesalianum, Os tibiale externum, Os sustentaculum tali, Os supra naviculare, Os intermetatarseum, Intercuneonavicular bone, Os subtibiale, Os peroneum.

present. A foot fault syndrome is the pathoanatomy of bone abnormality, malposition, or both, occurring in aggregate at a specific part of the foot.[5]

The radiographic evaluation of the pes planus foot type is primarily concerned with the pathoanatomy with respect to subluxations, which in turn create hypermobility and produce the radiographic signs as well as clinical symptoms associated with this foot type. In addition to these subluxations the podiatric physician must be aware of subtle changes in bone position in reaction to the reactive forces of weightbearing and ambulation, as well as abnormalities of bone shape that may restrict or change the normal joint range of motion and allow normal function of the foot.

When the pathologic changes are primarily noted in the rearfoot region, the pathologic radiographic entity referred to as *hindfoot-subtalar-*

midtarsal fault syndrome by Gamble and Yale[5] is radiographically demonstrated. This fault syndrome exhibits specific characteristics that may exist independently or in combination with other fault syndromes of the foot. It should be noted that any single finding alone does not accurately indicate a fault syndrome, but a combination of characteristics will produce the picture or pattern of a given fault syndrome.

The hindfoot-subtalar-midtarsal fault syndrome will usually present with many, if not all of the following characteristics. There will usually be noted an anterior break in the cyma line that defines the normal relationships of the calcaneus, talus, navicular, and cuboid. This cyma line is normally continuous, but becomes anteriorly broken as the foot pronates and the talus plantar flexes and adducts, producing the distal and plantigrade dis-

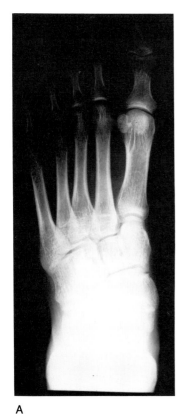

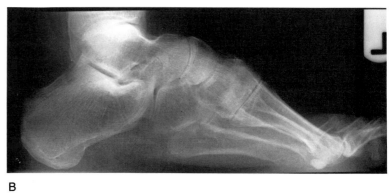

A   B

Fig. 12-45. (A) DP projection of cavus foot. **(B)** Lateral projection of cavus foot.

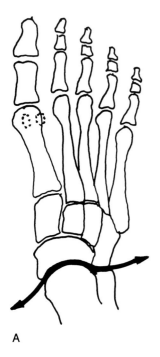

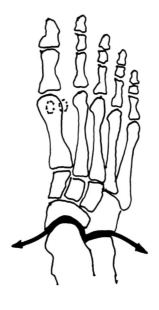

Fig. 12-46. (A) Normal cyma line, DP projection. **(B)** Anterior cyma line break, DP projection.

A   B

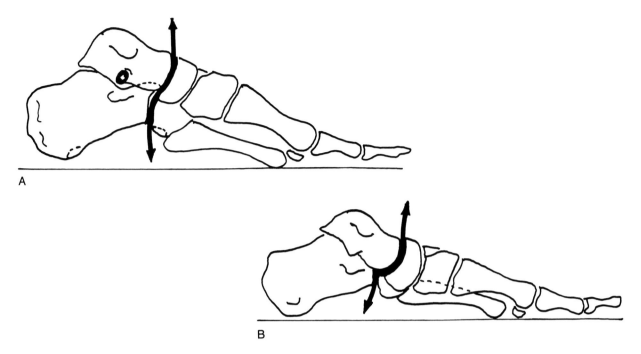

Fig. 12-47. (A) Normal cyma line, lateral projection. **(B)** Anterior cyma line break, lateral projection.

placement noted on the radiograph. This finding appears to be consistent with the pronated foot and appears on the lateral as well as the dorsoplantar weight-bearing projection (Fig. 12-46).

In addition to the anterior cyma line break the lateral weight-bearing projection (Fig. 12-47) will also usually exhibit a low pitch of the calcaneus or a decrease in the calcaneal inclination angle with associated lower height of the foot framework. The area of the sinus tarsi is usually diminished or obliterated and occasionally a pseudo – sinus tarsi may be present as a result of positional changes of the talus in relationship to the calcaneus with pronation of the foot. Eversion of the calcaneus consistent with pronation may be noted by the finding that the lateral tuberosity of the calcaneus is slightly raised from the supporting surface and more visible radiographically. The region of the sustentaculum tali will usually appear lowered and appear as a broader area of density instead of the thin dense line of the normal foot. This appearance radiographically of the sustentaculum tali is a result of the pronated position of the foot and eversion of the calcaneus. Because of this same pronatory rota-

tion the tubercle of the cuboid usually will fail to exhibit the peroneal groove on the radiograph.

The dorsoplantar projection of the weight-bearing pronated foot will, in addition to the anteriorly displaced cyma line, reveal a slight to moderate gap at the midfoot region resulting from the talus appearing loosely bound to the anterior process of the calcaneus. The medial rotation of the talus (increased talocalcaneal angle) usually exceeds 15 degrees, and less than 75 percent of the talar head will appear to articulate with the navicular (Fig. 12-41).

Acquired faults to the medial forefoot segment may appear in conjunction with hindfoot-subtalar-midtarsal faults. The *naviculocuneiform fault* is one of the most common of these medial forefoot segment faults and is best evaluated on lateral weight-bearing projections.

The primary feature on the lateral weight-bearing projection of the naviculocuneiform fault is depression of the navicular cuneiform joint (Fig. 12-48). This is exhibited as a result of the anterior border of the navicular and the posterior border of the medial cuneiform pivoting plantarward. The

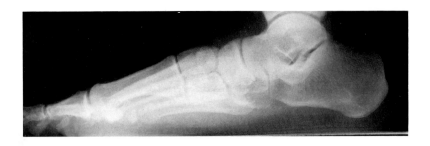

Fig. 12-48. Naviculocuneiform fault.

anterior border of the medial cuneiform thus pivots dorsally, producing a prominence at the base of the first metatarsal–cuneiform joint. In extreme cases of naviculocuneiform fault, the middle cuneiform bone may be visualized as an inverted triangle rising above the articulation of the navicular cuneiform joint.

COMMON ARTHRITIC DISEASES OF THE FOOT

Arthritic disease of the foot accounts for much discomfort and disability. It is therefore imperative that the podiatric physician have a good understanding of the radiologic presentation of arthritic disease and arthritic disease processes. The podiatric physician must also possess the ability to distinguish between the various common arthritic disease entities radiographically.

Degenerative Joint Disease

One of the more common arthritic entities is that of osteoarthritis or degenerative joint disease (DJD). This joint disease presents with clinical features principally affecting the weight-bearing joints of the hip, knees, ankles, and spine as well as the foot. Osteoarthritis or DJD is common in the later decades of life.

The pathology or pathogenesis of DJD is usually a result of one of several factors. These factors may include aging, recent or remote trauma, and slowing of metabolic and reparative process of the cartilage, or the condition may result from laxity or instability of supporting tissues of joints, resulting in eventual fibrillation of cartilaginous joint surfaces.[6] The mechanism of this process begins with minute fissures in the cartilage that penetrate into the subchondral bone. The synovial fluid then gains access to the deeper cells within the cartilage. A reparative process is initiated to some extent at this time, but this fails to keep pace with the progressive depletion of the matrix of the cartilage. Levels of protolytic enzymes and cartilage water content then become increased resulting in a tendency to erosion and flaking of the cartilaginous surface.[7] At times small fragments of cartilage will tend to break away and create what is termed "joint mice." As a result of these cartilaginous changes, blood vessels extend from the subchondral bone to the articular cartilage. Small foci of pseudocystic areas appear with the subchondral bone, and these areas fill with fibrous tissue. As the process proceeds, the cartilage becomes more deeply eroded, and in some areas the subchondral bone becomes completely divided. The loss of cartilage results in a narrowness of the joint space that is observed radiographically.

Small bony outgrowths, or osteophytes, develop from the margins of the articular cartilage extending along the adjoining ligaments and capsular attachments, producing the characteristic bony spurring that is noted in DJD. Degenerative joint disease has a characteristic radiographic appearance (Fig. 12-49). In the early stages of the disease process there are radiographic changes that appear to present as slight squaring or sharpening of the subarticular bony margins of the joint. The sharpening proceeds to marginal osteophyte formation or bony spur formation. As the condition becomes more moderately advanced definite narrowing of the joint is noted that may increase symmetrically or remain asymmetric. The subchondral bone may

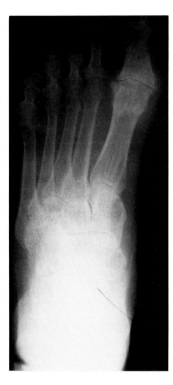

Fig. 12-49. Degenerative joint disease. First metatarsalphalangeal joint left foot.

become considerably eburnated, condensed, and sclerotic. In the very advanced stage a bone spur may become quite large and irregular and the bone spurs at the joint margins may actually meet one another and surround the entire joint. Occasionally joint mice or loose bodies may form within the joint itself.

Neurotrophic Arthropathy (Charcot's Joint)

Charcot's joint is an extreme degree of progression of degenerative osteoarthritis. This entity is usually associated with sensory loss or loss of proprioception in which the normal protective reactions of the joint are not invoked. The resultant altered function in the supporting tissue and structures produces joint instability. This joint instability leads in time to joint trauma that is cumulative, eventually resulting in subchondral fractures, de-

generative changes, and complete joint disorganization.

This arthropathy is radiologically present primarily in two forms. *Atrophic arthropathy,* which is evident with resorption of the bone ends and without osteophytes, sclerosis, or fragmentation present, is the form encountered most often in the upper extremities.

The second form, *hypertrophic arthropathy,* is seen more often in the lower extremities. This form is usually initiated by joint effusion and progression is usually slow, but occasionally may be rapid. There is classically joint narrowing with a marked bony sclerosis present. No osteoporosis is evident, even in the advanced stages. Fractures and fragmentation of the articular surfaces becomes present, with subluxation and dislocation proceeding finally to malalignment of the joint articular surfaces, and eventually total disorganization of the joint (Fig. 12-50).[8]

This type of arthropathy may be associated with neurologic disorders of the vertebral column or spinal column, and may be seen in patients who have sustained injury to posterior nerve roots or peripheral nerves as well as diabetic patients.

Gouty Arthritis

Gouty arthritis is an arthritic entity that is common in nature. The gouty arthritic picture radiographically is usually not evident on initial gouty attacks, but is evident over a period of time in which repeated or persistent gout manifestations have been present.

The general classification of gout includes primary gout, which is usually defined as an underlying disease that represents an inborn error in metabolism. Secondary gout is hyperuricemia, which is usually the result of many other types of disorder, such as renal disease, endocrine abnormalities, hemotologic disease, starvation, obesity, or psoriasis. There is one other gout presentation, which is that of idiopathic gout, which primarily occurs in men and has been reported in a ratio of 20 : 1.[9]

The hyperuricemic entity appears to have a predilection for joints of the lower extremity, particularly the first metatarsophalangeal joints of the foot and joints of the ankles and knees.[10] The inter-

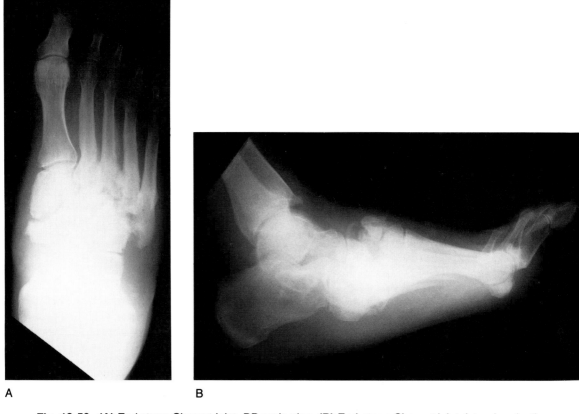

Fig. 12-50. (A) End stage Charcot joint, DP projection. **(B)** End stage Charcot joint, lateral projection.

phalangeal and metatacarpal joints of the hands as well as the joints of the wrists and elbows are also commonly involved areas.

Clinical presentation of gout is that of pain and tenderness with swelling of the joint area. The pain appears to recur, especially at night, and there may be intervals in which the patient is asymptomatic. The patient may over periods of time present with diagnostic gouty tophi that represent deposits of monosodium urate in the tissues. Chronic tophaceous gout will present with urate deposition in either articular cartilage, subchondral bone, synovial membrane, joint capsule, or periarticular tissues. The urates may ultimately penetrate an entire thickness of cartilage and collect in subchondral bone, producing the radiographic evidence of a pseudocyst type of defect. Tophaceous deposits may also occur away from the joints in areas such as the ear, skin of the fingertip, palms, or sole of the foot. Radiographic findings in patients with chronic or uncontrolled gouty arthritis will present as the classical Martel's sign in which there are punched-out margins of the joint region that represent the deposit of monosodium urate crystals in the previously described pseudocystic type of appearance.

Rheumatoid Arthritis

Rheumatoid arthritis is a common chronic disease characterized by nonsuppurative inflammation of the diarthrodial joints, frequently associated with a variety of extra-articular manifestations.[8] The metatarsophalangeal and metacarpophalangeal joints are among the most common sites of involvement. The initial lesion is usually a proliferative synovitis.[11]

The hands and feet as well as wrists and ankle

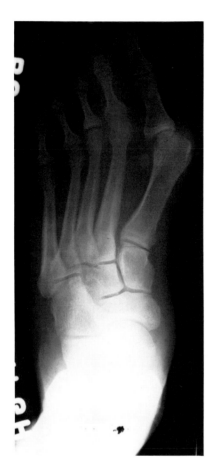

Fig. 12-51. Early rheumatoid arthritis of foot, DP projection.

areas are almost always involved, with these areas frequently being the first joints to become involved. The presentation is usually symmetric, with fusiform swelling of the digits at the proximal interphalangeal joints a characteristic early symptom.[12]

This early symptomatology is a result of an inflammatory synovitis the etiology of which is not clearly understood. This reaction produces hyperemia of the synovia with edema and increase in synovial fluid. This results in enlargement and multiplication of the synovial villi with hyperplasia of all capsular elements. Granulation and fibrosis replace the subchondral bone, producing early osteoporosis of the region.[13] This occurrence leads to two of the earliest radiographic changes seen in rheumatoid arthritis: an increase in the joint space

secondary to the edema present, and juxta-articular deossification.

As the disease progresses pannus formation develops. This pannus formation is the result of granulation tissue protrusions from the synovial fringe and ultimately results in absorption of the cartilage tissue and cartilage degeneration. This stage is associate with more marked osteoporosis and many times pseudocystic bone absorption. Eventually the underlying bone tissue becomes exposed and will reveal erosion on radiographs (Fig. 12-51).

Eventually all cartilage tissue is destroyed and replaced by pannus. Progression of the disease leads to subluxation of the metatarsophalangeal joints with associated fibular deviation, boutonniere deformities, and "swan-neck" appearance on radiographs (Fig. 12-52).

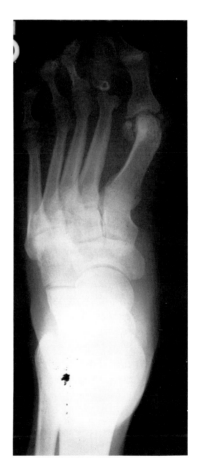

Fig. 12-52. Rheumatoid arthritis of foot in advanced stage, DP projection.

The end stage of this disease process is that of fibrous ankylosis of the joint. This fibrous ankylosis becomes trabeculated and eventually forms a bony ankylosis. This stage is often associated with contractures and positional deformities of the joint.

INFECTION OF BONE

Osteomyelitis

The term *osteomyelitis* appears as early as 1844 in a reference by Nealton to infection of the bone and marrow.[14] The term is generally used in conjunction with bacterial infection of bone, but the condition also may result from viral, mycotic, or parasitic etiology. *Staphylococcus aureus* is the most commonly involved organism.

The clinical presentation of osteomyelitis has been described as acute, subacute, chronic, and residual. Because of the considerable overlap and radiographic, laboratory, and histologic similarities that occur with these presentations, it has been suggested that the terms *initial osteomyelitis* and *recurrent osteomyelitis* might be more appropriate.[15]

Osteomyelitis resulting from direct extension or from hematogenous seeding are the two basic types. Direct extension is the most common type of osteomyelitis and is usually the result of skin ulceration or wounds in which the bacterial infection finally invade the bone.

Hematogenous osteomyelitis is a more indirect method of bone infection in which the bacteria travels in the bloodstream and lodges in the bone, producing infection. This hematogenous bacterial spread may result from a primary source of infection such as an upper respiratory tract infection, urinary tract infection, or other primary lesion or source of infection. It is always necessary to obtain a detailed history in cases of suspected hematogenous osteomyelitis.

It is important to consider that bone responds slowly to inflammation and infection. It is for this reason that many of the classic radiographic signs of osteomyelitis may not be noted for 2 to 4 weeks following infection of the bone tissue. It may also be possible that the osteomyelitis is clinically well controlled, while radiographs give the appearance of unchecked deterioration.[16]

The classic radiographic signs of osteomyelitis include radiolucency, sclerosis, sequestration, involucrum, cloaca, and subperiosteal calcification (Fig. 12-53). *Radiolucency* is nearly always present and usually is seen as regular or irregular areas of decreased density. *Sclerosis*, when present, may be evidence either of advanced bone repair or possibly the opposite finding of dead or nonviable bone.

The classic radiographic findings of sequestrum, involucrum, and cloaca are associated with the accumulation of pus and debris from infection within the bone. The *sequestrum* is actually an area or piece of dead bone that results as the purulent exudate accumulates and eliminates the blood supply to that area or portion of bone. This area may become separated from the surrounding bone and can be seen on x-ray as a sclerotic region or area of increased density.

The *cloaca* is an area of radiographic decreased

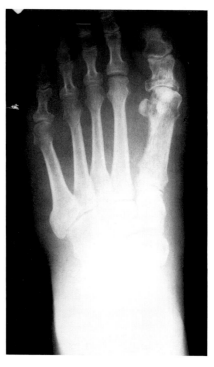

Fig. 12-53. Osteomyelitis involving the first metatarsal of the foot, DP projection.

density usually located at or near the periosteal region of the bone. The cloaca actually represents openings for the discharge of pus and debris from the bone.

The *involucrum* represents an area of new bone production and is a result of pus accumulation beneath the periosteum producing elevation of the periosteum. This lifting of the periosteum stimulates the production of periosteal new bone in much the same manner as periosteal new bone formation is stimulated by fracture or injury to the periosteum. This appears radiographically in osteomyelitis as a region of increased density adjacent to the area of active osteomyelitis.

The common radiographic finding of *subperiosteal calcification* with osteomyelitis is a result of the osseus infection elevating the periosteum of the bone with calcification of the space between the periosteum and the bone.

Acute Hematogenous Osteomyelitis

Acute hematogenous osteomyelitis is more commonly seen in infants and children, but may occasionally be seen in the elderly patient. This type of osteomyelitis is "seeded" into the bone via the bloodstream and most often involves the rich cancellous bone of the medullary region. Because of the anatomic vascular supply of the metaphysis and epiphyseal complex in children this infection commonly is located in the metatarsal region of the long bone. Again, as a result of anatomy and vascular flow the physis will many times act as a barrier to the extension of the infection into the joint. However, this infection may break through the physis or move along the periosteum and extend into the joint space if the infection is allowed to progress unchecked and produce the septic joint.

The earliest radiographic sign in children is usually deep soft tissue edema adjacent to involved areas of bone with early signs of bone destruction in the metaphyseal region of the bone. Periosteal new bone formation forms the involucrum about the involved region, and regional osteoporosis occurs in response to the inflammation in the area as the infection progresses.

Chronic Osteomyelitis

Osteomyelitis in the adult shows a greater tendency to be chronic. This patient is not usually systemically ill, as with hematogenous osteomyelitis. The site of infection usually presents with a local low-grade infection and associated persistent drainage from one or more sinus tracts. There are usually recurrent episodes of localized pain, erythema, and swelling of the involved area.

Chronic osteomyelitis radiographically presents as an area of thickened, irregular sclerotic bone containing several radiolucent areas with elevated periosteum. This presentation of osteomyelitis is usually never completely cured, but the low-grade infection persists and undergoes periods of remission followed by exacerbation of the infection. This may with time produce layers of eburnation of cortical areas radiographically and ultimately produce gross structures changes. This type of osteomyelitis is usually clinically controlled to some degree, but is usually never completely resolved.

ATLAS C: RADIOGRAPHS OF COMMON PODIATRIC PROBLEMS

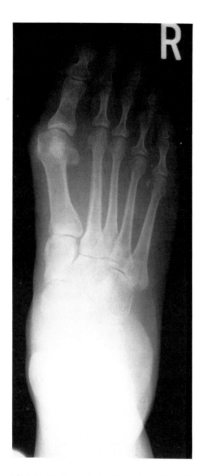

Fig. 12-54. Hallux abducto valgus (moderate).

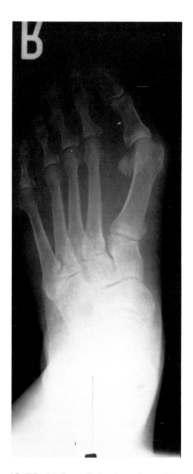

Fig. 12-55. Hallux abducto valgus (severe).

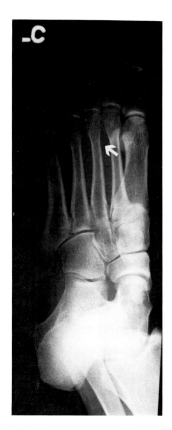

Fig. 12-56. Metatarsal stress fracture (early).

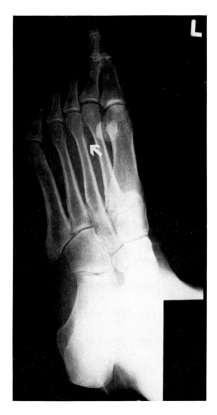

Fig. 12-57. Metatarsal stress fracture (3 to 4 weeks).

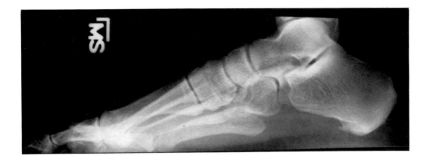

Fig. 12-58. Inferior calcaneal spur left foot.

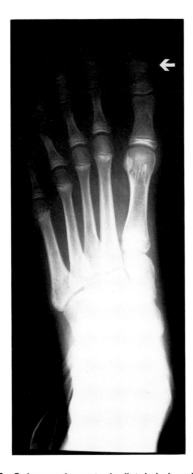

Fig. 12-59. Subungual exostosis distal phalanx left hallux.

REFERENCES

1. Anderson M, Blais M, Green WT: Growth of the normal foot during childhood and adolescence. Am J Phys Anthropol, 14:287–308, 1956
2. O'Rahilly R, Gardner E, Gray DJ: The skeletal development of the foot. Clin Orthop 16:7, 1960
3. Sarrafian SK: Anatomy of the foot and ankle. JB Lippincott, Philadelphia, 1983
4. Dixey FA: On the ossification of the terminal phalanges of the digits. Proc R Soc Lond, 31:63, 1881
5. Gamble FO, Yale I: Clinical Foot Roentgenology. Robert E. Krieger Publishing Co, New York, 1975
6. Meschan I: Roentgen Signs in Diagnostic Imaging. Vol. II. WB Saunders Co, Philadelphia, 1985
7. Mankin HJ, Thrasher AZ: The effect of age on glycosaminoglycan synthesis in rabbit articular and costal cartilage. J Rheumatol, 4:343, 1977
8. Greenfield GB: Radiology of Bone Diseases. 2nd Ed. JB Lippincott, Philadelphia, 1975
9. Resnick D: The radiographic manifestations of gouty arthritis. CRC Rev Diagn Imag, 9:265, 1977
10. Grahame R, Scott JT: Clinical survey of 354 patients with gout. Ann Rheum Dis, 29:461, 1970
11. McMaster M: The natural history of the rheumatoid metacarpophalangeal joint. J Bone Joint Surg [Br], 54B:687, 1972
12. Meschan I: Analysis of Roentgen Signs in General Radiology. WB Saunders, Philadelphia, 1973
13. Weisman SD: Radiology of the Foot. Williams & Wilkins, Baltimore, 1983
14. McGlamry ED (ed): Comprehensive Textbook of Foot Surgery. Vol II. Williams & Wilkins, Baltimore, 1987
15. Waldvogel FA, Vasey H: Osteomyelitis: the past decade. N Engl J Med, 303:360–370, 1980
16. Kehr LE, Zulli LP, McCarthy DJ: Radiographic factors in osteomyelitis. J Am Podiatry Assoc, 67:716, 1977

Section III

CLINICAL DISORDERS AND THE SPECIAL PATIENT

Infections

13

Warren S. Joseph, D.P.M.

Bacterial infections of the foot and leg can manifest themselves in a tremendous variety of forms and require a wide spectrum of diagnostic and therapeutic modalities. A simple, easily treated infected ingrown toenail, or paronychia, may be caused by the same organisms as a full-blown diabetic foot infection requiring major amputation. Likewise, this diabetic foot infection may be caused by the progression of that simple paronychia.

To adequately understand and treat this broad spectrum of diseases, a logical, systematic approach to their diagnosis and treatment must be followed. An understanding of the etiology, pathogenesis, bacterial and host factors, clinical features, and treatment, both antimicrobial and surgical, is necessary.

This chapter utilizes a logical clinical approach to assist in the evaluation and care of the infected podiatric patient. Diagnosis of infection in general, probably the single most important task facing the clinician, is covered in detail. This is followed by a discussion of each of the distinct clinical infectious diseases, with emphasis placed on their individual diagnostic and therapeutic challenges. Finally, selection principles of antimicrobial agents are discussed.

DIAGNOSIS

Diagnosis of any infection can be broken down into four steps: clinical, laboratory, bacteriologic, and radiographic. Individually, each may not yield sufficient information to allow an accurate diagnosis, but when considered together a more complete picture of the disease emerges.

Clinical

A complete history of the patient's current illness and past medical history is the most important first step in making a clinical diagnosis. Although considered a banality by many in this age of high-tech laboratory medicine, an accurate history may make the diagnosis of the infection and even give the clinician a clue as to therapy without seeing the area in question.

The first question asked should be about the precipitating factor. Was it a puncture wound? A corn between the toes that the patient tried to trim with a scissors?

The duration of the signs and symptoms should be questioned next. This can give an idea as to the severity of the infection by indicating the rapidity of the spread. Knowing this progression could also help with the microbiologic diagnosis. For example, *Staphylococcus epidermidis* tends to sequester in postoperative wounds for extended periods of time before progressing slowly. Clostridial gas gangrene progresses much more rapidly than many other forms of necrotizing infections.[1]

Has the patient noted any lumps or pain behind the knee or in the groin? This will give a clue as to systemic involvement of the infection with resultant lymphadenitis. Has lymphangitis, described to the patient as streaks moving up the leg, been noted? Many patients know this as "blood poisoning." Question the patient as to the presence of night sweats or chills, both indications of a systemic spread of the infection. Finally, ask about prior therapy. Has the patient taken any antibiotics, prescribed or unprescribed, for the problem? Drug addicts must be questioned carefully on this point because there is a large street market of oral antibiotics. Prior antibiotic usage can throw off all culture results and lead to false clinical symptoms.

The patient history must also include a history of past illness. Diseases such as diabetes mellitus have distinctive infectious complications, as is discussed in a later section. Of course, other diseases such as peripheral vascular disease will also affect the way in which the patient presents with an infection and is managed. A history of renal or hepatic disease will most likely change the selection of antibiotics. Just as important as what medical problems the patient has, however, is knowledge of the diseases of which he or she has no history. As a case in point, a patient who presents with an unusually severe infection should be questioned as to recent weight loss, polyuria, polydypsia, and the like. More than once, diabetes mellitus has been diagnosed by the presentation of a foot infection.

With the threat of acquired immunodeficiency syndrome (AIDS), the patient's social history becomes of supreme importance. Any history of intravenous drug abuse or homosexual behavior must be culled from the patient. AIDS patients will manifest with a variety of pedal infections ranging from onychomycosis to cellulitis, often with unusual etiologies. Furthermore, any current AIDS therapy, such as Azidothymidine (AZT), must be explored because this will affect the antibiotic therapy of the foot infection.

Physical examination is the second step in making a clinical diagnosis of infection. Does the patient look "sick"? Patients presenting with severe infections have what is called a "septic appearance." In general there is a disheveled, lethargic look to these people. Women will have neither brushed their hair nor put on any makeup. Men will be unshaven. When lying in bed, the sheets may be pulled up over their heads. They respond slowly to questions if at all.

On examination, the classic clinical sign of infection is the presence of cellulitis. Traditionally described as being associated only with some of the gram-positive organisms such as streptococcus,[2] cellulitis can be defined as any inflammatory reaction of the cellular structures, skin, or other connective tissues.[3] This inflammation can be caused by, but is not limited to, bacterial agents. Furthermore, mostly all of the clinically important bacteria can cause this symptom. Cellulitis presents with five cardinal signs: redness (rubor), swelling (tumor), heat (calor), pain (dolor), and loss of function (functio laesa) (Fig. 13-1). These five signs of inflammation are caused by the body's response to the presence of a foreign organism. There is massive capillary dilatation to allow an increased blood flow to the part, thus causing the rubor and calor. This dilatation causes channels to open in the capillary, allowing the migration of the phagocytes and fluid into the perivascular space and causing the tumor. This migration, or chemotaxis, is moderated by factors excreted by the organism that are known as chemotactic factors. Dolor is the result of the massive expansion of the tissues leading to pressure and thus firing of the cutaneous nerve endings. Loss of function is a result of the increased pain and swelling, making joint motion difficult.

The presence of this cellulitis is neither diagnostic of infection, since there are nonbacterial causes of inflammation, nor exclusionary of its absence. Patients who have significant peripheral vascular disease may be unable to mount a significant inflammatory response to infection. These patients will respond to the challenge by necrosis and frank gangrene.[4] Furthermore, some organisms may not cause a classic cellulitic reaction.

What is the extent of the cellulitis if present? Are there palpable lymph nodes in either the popliteal fossa or the groin? The absence of popliteal nodes

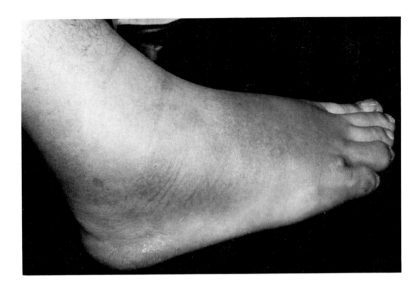

Fig. 13-1. Cellulitis of the foot secondary to an abscess in the fourth interdigital space. Note the loss of normal topography as a result of massive edema.

does not preclude the presence of inguinal nodes. Is there evidence of lymphangitis? All of these will give an idea of the extent of spread of the infectious process.

Many organisms have a distinctive color and or odor to their drainage, knowledge of which may provide an important clue as to the infectious etiology. *Staphylococcus aureus* will present as a creamy yellow pus with little odor (aureus — gold). *Staphylococcus epidermidis* drainage is characteristically white (originally known as *S. albus;* albus — white). Streptococcus often presents with little or no drainage. When present it is more watery in appearance.

To become familiar with the odors of different organisms, a cooperative microbiology lab is invaluable. Cultures of each organism that produce a characteristic odor should be "sniffed" until the organism is easily identified by smell alone (Table 13-1).

Oral temperature should be taken routinely on all patients either suspected of having an infection or with a documented infection. Fever is the body's response to pyrogens, both intrinsic and extrinsic. Many bacteria, especially the gram-negative rods, produce a potent pyrogen, a lipopolysaccharide located on the outer cell wall membrane.[5] This is not sufficient to explain the fever that accompanies all infections, however, since gram-positive organisms do not produce this extrinsic pyrogen. It has

been found, that in the presence of infection, the patient's leukocytes are capable of producing their own intrinsic pyrogen.[6]

There are three types of fever, classified by the pattern of temperature.[5] *Continuous fever* means just that, the temperature is elevated throughout a 24-hour period with small variations only of 1 °C or less. This is usually seen in infections that continuously seed the blood system.

Intermittent fever is defined as elevated for 24 hours but with temperature swings of greater than 1 °C. This is usually characterized by repeated cycles of sweats and chills. This is present in infections that cause intermittent bacteremia, such as abscess formation, and therefore is the most common in podiatric infections.

The final type of fever is *remittent fever.* In this situation the temperature remains normal for anywhere from a few hours to a few days.

Table 13-1. Drainage Characteristics

Organism	Color	Odor
S. aureus	Golden	None
S. epidermidis	White	None
P. aeruginosa	Green	Sweet: "fruity" or "grape"-like
Streptococcus	Little	None
Proteus spp.	White	"Mousey," ammonia
Bacteroides and other anaerobes	Brown-red, watery	Foul, "fetid"

(From Scurran,[82] with permission.)

Fever is useful clinically as a baseline to follow the progress or deterioration of a patient's condition. Further, there is no evidence that fever is harmful; in fact, it may be beneficial. For these reasons, the use of antipyretics should be avoided unless the fever gets dangerously high, above 105°F.[5,7,8]

Occasionally, a patient will present with a resolving infection, or no clinical signs or symptoms of infection, yet will be running a fever. This is referred to as fever of undetermined origin (FUO). In order to determine the cause of the FUO, the patient must first be taken off any antibiotics for at least 48 hours. This will allow a full reculturing of the entire patient, including wound, urine, and sputum. Removing the patient from the antibiotic will not only allow more reliable cultures, but eliminates the possibility of drug fever. To determine the cause of an FUO, even patients with severe infections may need to be removed from antibiotic treatment. Along the same line, if possible patients should be taken off any other medication. Drugs such as phenytoin and phenobarbital are notorious causes of drug fever. A full FUO workup also includes examination of non-drug-related causes.

Laboratory

The single most important blood study used in the evaluation of infections is the complete blood count (CBC) with differential. In acute infectious processes the body responds by markedly increasing the production of polymorphonuclear leukocytes (PMNs). This will lead to an absolute leukocytosis. When the bone marrow production of these cells becomes overwhelmed by the demand, immature cells called band forms are released prematurely into circulation. Therefore, in the presence of an acute bacterial infection, the two parameters to examine most closely are the total white blood cell (WBC) count and the band count. In more chronic infections, there may be a reversal of the ratio between PMNs and lymphocytes; however, the total count should still be elevated. Unfortunately, in the foot, the localized nature of the infection may preclude any abnormalities in the CBC.

Another laboratory value that is used in the management of infection is the erythrocyte sedimentation rate (ESR). The ESR is very nonspecific, being elevated with fever and other inflammatory disorders, including arthritis. Therefore, it is rarely helpful in diagnosis of infection. When taken as a baseline and found to be elevated, however, it may be beneficial in following the progress of therapy. This is especially true in the case of osteomyelitis.

Because of the lack of specificity of the ESR, C-reactive protein (CRP), a protein that is capable of binding to bacterial cell walls and fixing complement, is used in some cases to diagnose infection. Although slightly more sensitive and specific for infection, this is still of questionable diagnostic value. C-reactive protein may also be used to follow the progress of therapy.

Although not directly useful in the actual diagnosis of infection, blood chemistries such as Sequential Multiple Analyzer (SMA)-6, -12, and -24 are necessary to evaluate and treat the patient. These series, which include electrolytes, liver function tests, and renal status tests such as blood urea nitrogen (BUN) and serum creatinine, are helpful in determining antibiotic usage, dosage, and toxicity. Serum glucose levels, also available with the above tests, can be useful for the evaluation of diabetes mellitus or glucose intolerance. Because of the increased stress placed on the body by infection, patients with even mild glucose intolerance will become hyperglycemic in the face of infection.

Bacteriologic

Diagnosis of the causative organism of an infection, or "knowing your bugs," is dependent on three factors: Gram's stain, culture and sensitivity, and an empiric knowledge of what should be causing the infection. *Gram stain* is one of the most important, yet underutilized, techniques available to the clinician. This simple test is easy, inexpensive, and quick to perform, and yields a wealth of information. Along with the most basic information such as gram positive or gram negative, rod or cocci, the Gram stain can help actually identify the organism. Each bacteria has a distinct morphology. *Staphylococcus aureus* appears as gram-positive cocci in grapelike clusters. *Streptococcus* will appear as gram-positive cocci in chains. Even the gram-negative organisms will have individual characteristics. *Pseudomonas aeruginosa* is a long, thin, slightly curved rod. *Klebsiella* is a short, stout rod in diploid-like pairs.

Gram stain is also useful in differentiating an infection from a wound contamination. The presence of PMNs in a smear should lead the clinician to treat the source as being actually infected. Bacteria without the presence of these cells tends to point toward wound contamination.

Diagnosis of anaerobic infection can be aided by the use of a Gram stain. If the smear reveals a plethora of organisms, all with differing morphologies, and the culture report reveals only one or two aerobic organisms, the presence of anaerobes must be suspected. Anaerobic organisms are notoriously difficult to culture unless optimum technique prevails. Therefore, there is a good probability in the above situation that the laboratory could not isolate the more fastidious anaerobic organisms.

Culture and Sensitivity

The microbiology lab can be a clinician's closest ally, or his worst enemy. It seems that report slips are never on the chart when expected, or "no growth at 24 hours" appears with a specimen from a very "messy" wound. Like it or not, most of these results are due to inadequacies on the clinician's part.

Obtaining a good culture specimen is the single most important step in the microbiologic diagnosis. To ensure that the lab has adequate material with which to work, the following rules should be followed. First, scrupulous attention must be paid to the use of aseptic technique. The presence of a contaminant from the skin or the environment can cause confusion in interpretation and lead to improper antibiotic selection. For example, *S. epidermidis* for many years was considered a skin contaminant only. Now it is known to cause infections in special cases such as implant surgery.[9] This organism is frequently methicillin resistant, making correct antibiotic selection imperative. Second, a specimen must be taken from a representative area of infection. Sinus tract cultures are notoriously inaccurate in determining the causative organism in osteomyelitis. There is less than 50 percent con-

cordance between what is found in the sinus and the true infecting organism in the bone.[10] The proper culture would be a bone specimen harvested through a separate incision site. Third, adequate amounts of drainage should be collected. One drop of purulence is not enough for a Gram stain, anaerobic, and aerobic cultures. Fourth, all initial cultures should be taken either before the start of antimicrobial therapy, or with the patient off therapy for at least 48 hours. The presence of any antibiotic can be enough to inhibit the growth of the organism, rendering cultures unreliable. Finally, the specimen must be transferred to the lab in an appropriate medium and in an expedient fashion. This last rule is of particular importance in the special case of anaerobic and surgical specimens.

Anaerobic organisms can be isolated from many podiatric infections. Diabetic foot infections and necrotizing fasciitis immediately conjure visions of anaerobic organisms. Yet, as mentioned above, they are difficult for most laboratories to culture. There are a few steps that a clinician may take to assist the microbiologist. Whenever possible the anaerobic specimen should be the first taken. This is especially important when an abscess is opened for the first time because any exposure to oxygen may be enough to prohibit the growth of an obligate anaerobe. Aspiration of purulence into a syringe or tube will assure adequate quantity, and the syringe or tube can be used for transport to the lab, assuming that this is done quickly. The use of rubber stoppers to seal the tip of the needle is unnecessary and may precipitate inadvertent puncture wounds. Commercially available anaerobic transport media are probably the most commonly used vehicle. These contain a prereduced medium and often include an indicator to assure their usable condition.

Surgical specimens present a special problem when sent for culture and sensitivity testing. Often, the material to be cultured is placed in formalin with the pathologic specimens. Needless to say, this renders it useless. Any material retrieved at the time of surgery that is to be sent for microbiologic evaluation should be either sent as rapidly as possible in a dry, sterile container or (less advisable) in sterile nonbacteriostatic saline.

The microbiologic evaluation of cellulitis was traditionally performed by the aspiration of the leading edge of cellulitis. If no fluid was aspirated, nonbacteriostatic saline was first injected and then withdrawn for culture. Unfortunately this procedure yields poor results. In recent studies only 10 to 14.5 percent of the aspirations were successful in recovering an organism.[11,12]

Blood Cultures

There are three types of bacteremia: transient, intermittent, and continuous. Transient bacteremia occurs in all people on a daily basis. The act of brushing one's teeth, or of eating a hard food, can cause release of the oral microbial flora into the system. A more intensive bacteremia will occur with dental, gastrointestinal, or urinary tract manipulation. This is of little clinical significance except possibly in patients with damaged heart valves. Continuous bacteremia is considered diagnostic of endocarditis unless proven otherwise. Intermittent bacteremia is of the greatest importance to podiatrists because this occurs with the presence of an abscess or other local wound infection. All of these bacteremias are diagnosed by the use of blood cultures. Protocol for ordering blood cultures in the patient who is feared to be bacteremic, or in the face of a FUO, is as follows. Aseptic technique must be observed, with antimicrobial skin preparation performed. Two to three sets of cultures should be drawn in a 24-hour period. Each set must be drawn from a rotating site at least 20 minutes apart. If five to six cultures have been taken over the span of 2 days and no changes are observed in the patient, no further cultures are indicated even in the face of persistent fever. Remember that any number of tubes drawn at the same site and time equals only one culture. Since most bacteremias are of relatively low magnitude, sufficient volume (20 to 30 ml) must be taken at a time. Interpretation of blood culture results can be challenging. If the cultures required a long period of time to become positive, or only a single bottle yields a positive subculture, accurate diagnosis is complicated. The particular bacteria isolated may give a clue as to the validity of the culture. A single bottle isolate of *S. epidermidis* most likely can be read as a contaminated culture from the skin. However, the same organism isolated more frequently

may have to be addressed. *Staphylococcus aureus,* on the other hand, may have to be contended with even if only one bottle is positive.

Empiric Knowledge

The third step in the microbiologic evaluation of an infection is taking what amounts to an educated guess as to what is causing the infection. There are many types of pedal infections that have a statistically high correlation with a particular organism. Postoperative infections tend to be caused by species of staphylococcus most commonly, streptococcus less so, and rarely gram-negative bacteria. A puncture wound infection that develops late infectious complications such as osteomyelitis is most frequently caused by *P. aeruginosa.*[13] Each infection is covered in its own section.

Knowing where the patient acquired the infection will also help in identifying the possible pathogens. So-called community-acquired pathogens tend to be less resistant and therefore easier to treat than their more resistant counterparts, the "nosocomial pathogens." The community-acquired group includes *S. aureus* (not methicillin resistant), varieties of streptococcus, *Proteus mirabilis,* and *Escherichia coli.* The hospital-acquired nosocomial group includes *Enterobacter, Serratia, Acinetobacter, Citrobacter,* and other multiresistant organisms. Having some idea as to which group is responsible will aid in directing the treatment plan.

Radiographic Diagnosis

The radiographic diagnosis of infection is covered in the section on osteomyelitis.

SUPERFICIAL SKIN AND SOFT TISSUE INFECTIONS

Various bacteria are capable of causing specific primary infectious manifestations on the skin. The distinct clinical picture of each is helpful in determining the offending organism and the appropriate treatment. In this section, those with podiatric implications are discussed.

Cellulitis

Cellulitis is defined as an acute spreading infection of the skin and, possibly, deeper connective tissue.[14] It is usually seen following a traumatic episode where the skin defenses have been violated or near the site of concurrent skin infection, such as an ulcer. The trauma may be major, such as a puncture wound, surgery, or laceration, or as seemingly insignificant as an insect bite. Clinically the area becomes markedly red, hot, and swollen. Boundaries are not clearly demarcated. Normal superficial topography is lost because of the tenseness of the skin. These signs can appear from hours to several days following the initial trauma. The patient may present with fever, malaise, chills, or other constitutional signs. Regional lymphadenopathy and lymphangitis may occur as a result of proximal spread. In older patients, cellulitis may precipitate thrombophlebitis, for which it may be confused.

Laboratory tests will reveal a leukocytosis with probable shift to the left. Blood cultures may be positive because of the bacteremia that often results. Material for culture and sensitivity is difficult to collect unless there is a draining sinus from the initial trauma site or skin breakdown occurs as a result of secondary skin necrosis. Gram-negative organisms may colonize these sites, making them unreliable for culture purposes. Aspiration of the advancing edge of the cellulitis with nonbacteriostatic saline has been advocated for microbiologic evaluation. Recently, however, this has been found to result in a low yield of organisms (about 10 percent). Punch biopsy of infected tissues is only slightly more successful.[11]

Group A streptococcus and *S. aureus* are the causative organisms most frequently implicated in cellulitis. Other organisms may cause the syndrome on less frequent occasions. The streptococcal variety will spread more rapidly with a higher incidence of bacteremia. Therefore, if cellulitis is noted occurring shortly (6 to 12 hours) following the precipitating event, this organism should be assumed.

Treatment consists of intravenous antibiotics and incision and drainage where indicated. A penicillinase-resistant penicillin such as nafcillin or oxacillin would be effective against both staphylococcus and streptococcus. Alternatives to these would include a first-generation cephalosporin, such as cefazolin, which is given less frequently and in smaller doses than the penicillins, making it cost effective. If the patient has an anaphylactic history to penicillin, clindamycin is an effective alternate. Erythromycin IV is also an alternative but must be administered carefully because of its propensity to cause venous irritation. If the etiologic agent is known to be streptococcus, then aqueous penicillin G is the antibiotic of choice.

A high frequency of podiatric patients are seen with a history of peripheral vascular disease. Many of these patients have undergone vascular reconstruction. A unique form of cellulitis known as *postsaphenous phlebectomy donor leg cellulitis* has been described in these patients.[15] Anywhere from 1 to 103 months (mean 15 months) following saphenous vein phlebectomy, an acute cellulitis may occur along the donor surgical site. The patient will present with fever, malaise, a leukocytosis, and other signs and symptoms of cellulitis. This may be confused with thrombophlebitis due to calf pain and a positive Homans' sign. Diagnostic testing should include noninvasive venous testing and a venogram to rule out thrombophlebitis.

Group A streptococcus is the most frequently implicated organism in these infections. The etiology is thought to be associated with interdigital tinea pedis allowing organisms to enter the tissues. In one case poison ivy of the foot was the precipitating factor. Once in the tissues the large amount of edema fluid presents a perfect growth medium for the bacteria.

Treatment is the same as for any cellulitis. In addition, local measures, such as topical antifungals, should be instituted to treat the tinea pedis. Without therapy for the tinea, there have been cases of recurrence of the cellulitis.

Paronychia

Paronychia, or inflammation around the nail borders and grooves, is usually a pyogenic infection of bacterial origin. This is possibly the single most frequent infection treated by podiatrists. A nail spicule will lodge itself in the nail groove and act as a foreign body, allowing the development of infection. Clinically, there is marked edema, erythema, and pain immediately around the affected nail border. There may be proximal spread of the cellulitis, although there is rarely any systemic involvement. Depending on the chronicity of the problem, exuberant granulation tissue may be noted in the grooves. Drainage is often present and its character is dependent on the infecting organism.

Traditionally, *Candida* was considered the most common causative organism. In reality, however, staphylococcus species are more frequently seen. Other bacterial causes include streptococcus and gram-negative organisms, including *P. aeruginosa*.

Treatment success is dependent on removal of the offending nail spicule to allow adequate drainage. Further drainage should be promoted by the use of soaks or wet-to-dry dressings. Exuberant granulation tissue should be handled with either excision or the application of 75 percent silver nitrate. The use of oral systemic antibiotics is not indicated except in cases with extensive proximal spread of the cellulitis or systemic signs of infection, or in a compromised host.

Erythrasma

Often misdiagnosed as tinea pedis, erythrasma is a bacterial infection frequently found in the interdigital spaces of the feet. This disease is characterized by maceration of the interspaces that is slowly spreading and pruritic. On Wood's light examination, a "coral red" fluorescence is noted that is practically diagnostic. Gram stain reveals grampositive bacilli. There may be cellulitis of the distal portion of the foot.

The causative organism is *Corynebacterium minutissimum*. Treatment consists of oral erythromycin (1 g/day) for 1 week. Wet-to-dry dressings may help promote drying of the interdigital spaces.

Other bacterial infections may mimic tinea pedis by causing interdigital maceration with subsequent tissue breakdown and cellulitis. Proper diagnosis of this *"gram-negative athlete's foot"* is essential since if treated as a fungal infection it may actually progress. *Pseudomonas aeruginosa* is the most frequently found organism.[16] On Wood's light examination a green fluorescence is noted. If confined to the skin, treatment is strictly topical with the application of wet-to-dry acetic acid dressings. If cellulitis has occurred, proper antipseudomonal antibiotic therapy should be instituted.

Folliculitis

Infection within the hair follicle is termed *folliculitis*. Although not common on the foot, when it does occur, it is found on the dorsum and on the toes. Clinically, small erythematous papules are found. A central pustule may be seen. Causative organisms include *S. aureus, Candida*, and, in the case of "hot tub dermatitis," *P. aeruginosa*.[17] Treatment consists strictly of local care, including compresses and topical antibiotics. The disease may either be self-limiting or progress to a deeper *furuncle* formation with surrounding cellulitis.

Staphylococcus Scalded Skin Syndrome

Caused by *S. aureus* capable of producing an exfoliative exotoxin (phage group II), staphylococcus scalded skin syndrome is a severe, but rare, infection. Usually seen in children, it can affect adults. Occurrence may follow an antecedent *S. aureus* skin infection such as occurs postoperatively. Clinically, fever and skin tenderness may be present. Large, flaccid bullae appear and rupture, exposing the underlying layers of red, scalded-appearing skin. Treatment consists of intravenous antibiotics directed at the organism along with fluid maintenance therapy. Prognosis is good, with lesions clearing in 2 weeks.[14]

Other Skin and Soft Tissue Infections

Other less common skin and soft tissue infections that occur on the foot include *impetigo, ecthyma*, and *erysipelas*. Impetigo, usually caused by Group A streptococcus, is a superficial infection of the

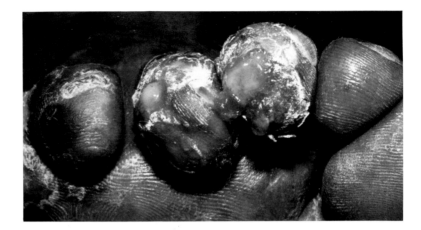

Fig. 13-2. Impetigo of the toes previously misdiagnosed, and treated unsuccessfully, as tinea pedis. Classic honey-colored crusts and Gram stain showing gram-positive cocci are useful in making the diagnosis.

skin. It is characterized by vesicles that become "honey-gold"-colored crusts (Fig. 13-2). This is more frequent in children and is very contagious, spreading easily to other family members. Primarily occurring on the face and other exposed areas, the bacteria can be inoculated onto the foot by scratching. Treatment consists of penicillin, parenteral or oral; erythromycin for allergic patients; and local care. Mupirocin, a new topical antibiotic, has also been found effective.[18]

Ecthyma most frequently occurs on the lower extremities. Initially, the lesions are similar to impetigo but will be much deeper, penetrating the epidermis. These lesions are punched out and crusted-appearing, with greenish yellow crusts. Streptococcus is the most frequent cause, although pseudomonas bacteremia will cause a form of the disease known as *ecthyma gangrenosum*. Treatment of the streptococcal disease is similar to that for impetigo.

A form of cellulitis that includes lymphatic blockage is called erysipelas.[2] Almost always caused by Group A streptococcus, erysipelas presents as a sharply demarcated, advancing edge of cellulitis, with raised borders. Leukocytosis, fever, and pain are common presenting features. Although mostly found on the face, any area with lymphatic blockage, including the lower extremities, may be involved. Treatment, as with any streptococcal disease, is best accomplished with penicillin. Depending on the severity of the case a parenteral antibiotic may be indicated.

PUNCTURE WOUND INFECTIONS

The months of May through October find an increasing number of puncture wounds presenting to offices and emergency rooms. During this time many people, especially children, are outside without shoe gear, increasing the probability of these wounds. In one study, 887 out of 108,648 pediatric visits to emergency rooms were due to punctures of the foot.[19] Most frequently nails are the cause, occurring in 98 percent of reported cases. The remaining 2 percent are the result of stepping on any number of other objects, including glass, rocks, wire, splinters, and sewing needles.

Infectious Complications

Only 10 percent of these puncture wounds become infected.[20,21] Most heal uneventfully with few complications and often little intervention. When complications arise, cellulitis is the most common, occurring 50 percent of the time. *Staphylococcus aureus* and other gram-positive organisms, including *Streptococcus* and coagulase-negative *Staphylococcus*, are the most frequently isolated pathogens in these cases. Other less commonly reported organisms include *E. coli*, *Klebsiella* species, and other gram-negative species.

Other infectious complications of puncture

wound infections, such as deep abscess and septic arthritis, occur less frequently. Osteomyelitis, occurring at a frequency of 0.6 to 1.8 percent, is the least common. In cases that progress to osteomyelitis, *P. aeruginosa* is by far the most likely pathogen, occurring in 90 percent of all cases.[19] Pyarthrosis is a result of an osteomyelitic process that invades the joint space from adjacent bone, or by direct inoculation of the organism into the joint by the penetrating object.

Inadequate primary care is the usual cause of these infectious complications. Most puncture wounds are treated by superficial cleansing of the wound, tetanus prophylaxis, soaks, and broad-spectrum oral antibiotics. The superficial nature of the exploration is inadequate to detect the presence of retained foreign material in the wound. This includes devitalized pieces of skin, soil, corrosion from the penetrating object, and shoe or sock particles. These foreign bodies, occurring in 3 percent of these wounds, may cause infection even in the face of antibiotic therapy. In the series reported by Miller and Semian, of postpuncture wound infections not responding to intravenous antibiotics, 60 percent of the patients who required incision and drainage were found to have retained foreign bodies present.[22]

Prevention of Late Infection

Proper primary care, although not a guarantee, can significantly reduce the incidence of infectious complications in puncture wounds.[23] Taking a complete history is the initial step, by determining the potential for contamination. Where did the injury occur? Barnyard soil flora differs markedly from city street flora, which differs from that found if a patient steps on an object in brackish water. What was the penetrating object and its condition, and how deeply did it penetrate? What footwear, if any, was being worn at the time? Did the patient perform "bathroom surgery" on the wound? If the injury occurred a number of days previously, has there been any exacerbation in symptomatology?

Radiographs should be taken to assess the possibility of retained foreign bodies. Xeroradiograms may demonstrate soft tissues more clearly. Radionuclide scanning may assist in the early diagnosis of osteomyelitis.

Wound care must be aggressive and complete. Surgical débridement under local or regional anesthesia may be necessary to probe the wound deeply. Irrigation is performed with sterile saline and povidone iodine solution or another suitable antiseptic such as chlorhexidine. The wound should be packed open to allow adequate drainage.

Tetanus prophylaxis has virtually eliminated *Clostridium tetani* toxemia as a complication and is standard practice. The patient's inoculation status and wound evaluation determines this therapy.

The final step in the primary care of these wounds is home care instructions. The patient is instructed to rest the foot, keep it elevated, and apply a minimum of weight-bearing. Soaks may promote drainage but should be performed only in sterile water, or water with added antiseptic. The patient should be followed on a regular basis to observe for any changes in wound status.

The use of oral antibiotics is controversial. They should probably not be used in cases of uncomplicated puncture wounds seen within the first 24 hours. Fitzgerald and Cowan[19] found that in 465 patients to whom antibiotics were not given, only two required incision and drainage, and one of those had retained a foreign body. Furthermore, antibiotics may actually serve to select out infections with more resistant organisms, or mask any existing infection. Antibiotics should not supplant adequate initial care. They are ineffective in the face of retained foreign materials. Antibiotics are beneficial in the case of complicated or neglected wounds, and wounds in which there is late cellulitis or other established infections.

Pseudomonas Osteomyelitis

Johanson in his series of 11 children first demonstrated the prevalence of *P. aeruginosa* as a frequent cause of osteomyelitis following puncture wounds.[13] Since then, others have reported similar series in both adults and children.[24] The traditional predilection of this infection for children can be explained in two ways. First, puncture wounds as a whole are more common in children than adults. More importantly, however, *Pseudomonas* has a predilection for cartilaginous structures because of their relative avascularity. These structures, such as epiphyseal plates, are more common in children.[13] This is evidenced not only in pedal infections. *Pseudomonas* has long been associated with infections of the cartilage of the outer ear in diabetics (malignant otitis externa). Siebert et al.[25] discovered that although the disease is remarkably similar in children and adults, the prognosis for complete recovery, even with a delay in diagnosis, is much better in adults. If diagnosis and treatment were delayed more than 3 weeks in children, chronic infection requiring bone resection occurred. The same delay in adults yielded better results.

A number of theories have been advanced to explain the frequency of *pseudomonas* as a cause of osteomyelitis following puncture wounds. The presence of *P. aeruginosa* as a normal flora of the foot has been studied by a few authors. Fritz examined the feet of 85 children and cultured interspaces, arches, and sneakers. He found that out of 370 specimens, only one grew *P. aeruginosa.*[26] A similar study found no *Pseudomonas* out of cultures from 100 individuals.[22] A related theory is that *P. aeruginosa* can be cultured from tap water and soil.[27] Therefore it may be inoculated by the penetrating object, or by the tap water soaks performed by the patient. The third theory involves the use of oral antibiotics. Minnefor et al. speculated that the commonly prescribed oral antibiotics such as cephalexin, ampicillin, erythromycin, and tetracycline have no effect against *P. aeruginosa.* Therefore, these drugs may allow a superinfection with the gram-negative organisms.[28]

The clinical and laboratory presentation of a patient with late *Pseudomonas* infection after a puncture wound appears to be remarkably consistent in

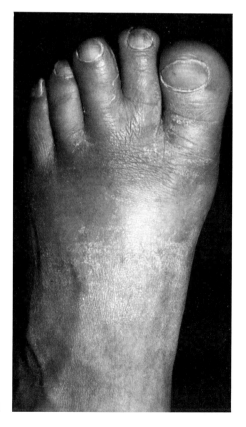
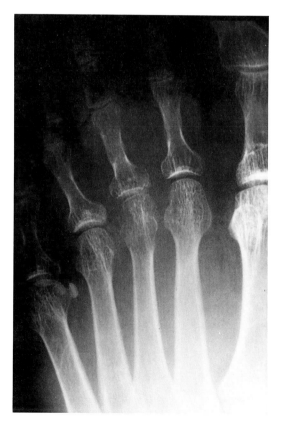

A   B

Fig. 13-3. (A) Patient presenting with cellulitis of the foot following puncture wound of the plantar aspect. Multiple remissions and exacerbations of symptoms while on oral antibiotics suggest a diagnosis of osteomyelitis. **(B)** Destruction of bone, third metatarsal head, confirming the diagnosis of osteomyelitis in the patient in Figure 13-3A.

all reported series.[24] The patient is first seen in the emergency room, where the primary wound care previously described is administered. As a result of the intervention there is an immediate decrease in the signs and symptoms of infection, including pain, erythema, and edema. Anywhere from 3 days to 8 weeks (average 1 to 3 weeks) after the initial injury, there is an exacerbation of these symptoms, although the patient feels well (Fig. 13-3A & B). Laboratory results are often equivocal. A CBC may show little or no leukocytosis and shift to the left. The ESR may only be slightly elevated if at all. Radiograms fail to show any changes initially, but in all cases will eventually become consistent with osteomyelitis.

Diagnosis and Treatment

Early diagnosis and the above-described aggressive local treatment are essential in preventing the late complication of *Pseudomonas* osteomyelitis. Fitzgerald and Cowan found that only 65 of 774 (8.4 percent) patients seen within the first 24 hours following injury presented with cellulitis up to 4 days later. This number increased to 57 percent with a greater delay.[19]

Green and Bruno documented a pattern of infection response and eventual sequelae based on the delay in diagnosis of osteomyelitis.[29] Three categories were differentiated:

Type 1: An early diagnosis with surgical drainage and débridement, followed by adequate antibiotic coverage, resulted in complete healing without any permanent bone and joint damage.

Type 2: If diagnosis and treatment are delayed 9 to 14 days, the infection will be eradicated with débridement and adequate antibiotic coverage, but there may be residual bone and joint damage.

Type 3: If diagnosis and treatment are delayed greater than 3 weeks, the infection becomes chronic, necessitating bone resection for final cure.

Treatment of *Pseudomonas* osteomyelitis, like any osteomyelitis, is both medical and surgical in nature. Adequate surgical bone débridement is necessary (Fig. 13-4). Administration of antibiotics alone may only suppress the infection. As a result, specific anti-*Pseudomonas* parenteral antibiotics must be used in conjunction with débridement.

Traditionally, antibiotic therapy consisted of a combination of an aminoglycoside with an antipseudomonal penicillin (Table 13-2). As always with aminoglycoside therapy, serum creatinine and antibiotic levels must be monitored closely. Because of the toxicities encountered with the use of aminoglycosides, especially for the prolonged period of time needed to treat osteomyelitis, a number of newer, safer agents are being utilized. Ceftazidime, a third-generation cephalosporin, has been employed successfully in this disease. As with any single-agent β-lactam, more widespread experience is necessary to determine formation of re-

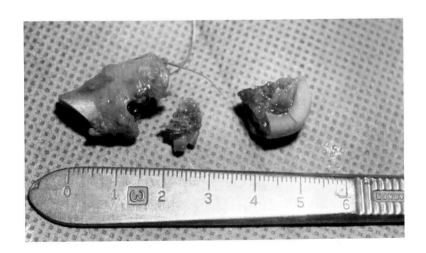

Fig. 13-4. Bone débrided for culture of third metatarsal following puncture wound osteomyelitis.

Table 13-2. Antibiotic Therapy of *Pseudomonas aeruginosa* Infections[a]

Aminoglycosides[b]
  Tobramycin
  Amikacin
  Gentamicin
Antipseudomonal Penicillins
  Piperacillin
  Azlocillin
  Mezlocillin
  Ticarcillin[c]
Cephalosporins
  Ceftazidime
  Cefoperazone
Monobactams
  Aztreonam
Carbapenems
  Imipenem/cilastatin
Quinolones
  Ciprofloxacin (oral)

[a] Drugs in each class are listed by relative efficacy. List is of approved, marketed antibiotics available at the time of compilation.

[b] Aminoglycosides should be combined with a penicillin for synergy. Penicillins should not be used as single agents because of development of resistance. All other drugs on this list have been used effectively as single agents.

[c] Ticarcillin/clavulanic acid cannot be used as a single agent. It is no more effective against *Pseudomonas* than straight ticarcillin.

(From Scurran,[82] with permission.)

sistance. Imipenem and aztreonam are other new agents that may be efficacious in this disease and lack the potential dangers of the aminoglycosides. Another drug that appears especially exciting in the treatment of *Pseudomonas* osteomyelitis is ciprofloxacin, a carboxyquinolone agent that has the unique advantage of being effective when given orally.

As with any discussion of osteomyelitis, the length of therapy is a matter of debate. Siebert et al. treated eight patients for 4 weeks and one patient for 3 weeks after incision and débridement with no sequelae noted.[25] One patient who was treated for 2 weeks subsequently developed chronic osteomyelitis and required a subsequent 4-week treatment course. Jacobs et al. differ in that they suggest that only 10 to 14 days of antibiotics are required following proper débridement.

Marine Puncture Wounds

When a puncture or laceration is sustained while in water, a unique set of organisms may be impli-

cated. Which organism in particular depends on the clinical situation.

Aeromonas hydrophilia, a gram-negative bacillus, may be isolated from a wound cellulitis following swimming or wading in rivers, lakes, or other freshwater sources. The organism is usually sensitive to gentamicin, chloramphenicol, and tetracycline to a lesser degree. Gentamicin in combination with a penicillinase-resistant penicillin is the therapy of choice following freshwater cellulitis.[14]

If the injury is sustained in salt or brackish water, one of the *Vibrio* species should be considered. These infections may be severe and rapidly progressing. Necrotizing fasciitis has been reported.[31] Antibiotic sensitivities are similar to the above. Surgical débridement should be utilized when indicated.

The final marine pathogen is *Mycobacterium marinum*. Found in swimming pools, aquaria, and other freshwater sources, this organism causes a range of disease from suppuration to granuloma formation. Infection usually occurs on the extremities and begins as a small nodule that may progress to an ulceration and then a granuloma. Antibiotic therapy includes rifampin and ethambutol in combination. Tetracycline has also been effective.[32]

DIABETIC FOOT INFECTIONS

It is estimated that over 10 percent of the population of the United States is diabetic. Foot infection is the most common septic cause of hospitalization in these patients. The National Center for Health Statistics, in the 1983 Short Stay Hospital Survey, lists almost 3 million patient admissions for diabetes mellitus. Of these, almost 125,000 were admitted for a concomitant lower extremity infection.

Infections are debatably more common in diabetics than nondiabetics. There is little doubt, however, that once established they are more severe and recalcitrant to treatment. Furthermore, the risk of developing gangrene in these patients is 53 times higher than normal in male diabetics over

40, and 71 times greater in females of the same age group.[33]

Although the past 50 years have seen a number of advances in the treatment of diabetes, the morbidity and social and economic burden of this disease remain tremendous. Amputation is still a frequent result. Because of prolonged hospitalizations, the diagnosis-related payment to the institution is usually exceeded. The patients are frequently relegated to collecting either long-term or permanent disability and rarely return to work. This section examines the pathology leading to these infections, including the triad of immunopathy, neuropathy, and angiopathy. The microbiology and antimicrobial therapy are also discussed.

Immunopathy

The contribution of immunopathy to the development of the diabetic foot infection is somewhat controversial. Most investigators agree, however, that an increase in serum glucose will adversely affect the immune function in these patients.[34]

Humoral immunity appears to remain intact. Normal or increased levels of circulating immunoglobulins have been noted, possibly because of the increased frequency of infection.[35] There is no defect in immune responses or complement fixation. Although earlier data suggested a decreased antibody response to staphylococcus toxin[36] and typhoid vaccine,[37] extrinsic factors such as poor nutritional status may explain this.

The immunologic deficit in these patients appears at the phagocyte level and may be related to the presence of hyperglycemia and the lack of insulin. Mowat and Baum,[38] and more recently Molenaar et al.,[39] have demonstrated a defect in in vitro chemotaxis of PMNs from diabetic patients. This defect was corrected when the cells were incubated with insulin. Phagocytosis and intracellular microbicidal function of the leukocyte are also markedly diminished in the face of hyperglycemia. With proper diabetic control these defects are either partially or totally reversible.

A defect in phytohemagglutinin-induced lymphocyte transformation in poorly controlled diabetics was reported by MacCuish et al.[40] This was not observed in normal controls, pointing to a decrease in cell-mediated immune response in diabetics.

Angiopathy

Vascular disease in the diabetic tends to be more widespread, occur at an earlier age and at a greater frequency, and progress to more advanced stages than in the nondiabetic. Under the age of 40, a patient with diabetes mellitus will have a 25 percent chance of exhibiting severe arteriosclerosis, a number much higher than the 2 to 5 percent incidence seen in nondiabetics. Diabetics greater than 40 years of age exhibit marked vascular changes 50 to 150 times more frequently than nondiabetics.[41] Dinerstein et al.[42] elucidated four major differences between diabetic and nondiabetic angiopathy. The diabetic patient will exhibit a more diffuse and multisegmental lesion. There is an increase in bilateral involvement, the so-called second limb syndrome in which reconstruction or amputation of the contralateral limb occurs two-thirds of the time. Infrapopliteal vessels are more frequently involved than the more proximal vessels. Finally, in part because of this distal involvement, there is a higher incidence of gangrene.

Two major categories of vascular disease contribute to the pathogenesis of diabetic foot infections: microangiopathy and macroangiopathy. Because these topics are covered elsewhere, only their contribution to the development of infection is discussed here.

Microvascular disease is probably the most important in terms of infection, although its very presence has been debated.[43] A number of studies have described narrowing or complete occlusion of capillaries as a late complication of diabetes.[34]

The pathology of these changes is complex. Capillary basement membrane thickening, platelet aggregation, increased blood viscosity, and premature cell aging have all been indicted. More recently, capillary injury due to hyperperfusion and vasodilatation causing an increase in macromolecule deposition has been reported.[44] These changes in the capillaries may further impair the already compromised chemotaxis of the leukocytes, preventing inflammatory response to trauma. In fact, thrombosis and necrosis is the usual diabetic response to tissue stress as opposed to inflammation. There is evidence in some studies that tight glucose control may cause cessation or even reversal of the microvascular changes.[45]

Neuropathy

Neuropathy is the single most important factor in the development of the infected diabetic foot. It has been estimated that as many as 50 percent of all diabetic patients receiving insulin manifest symptomatic neuropathy.[46] Three manifestations of neuropathy have been described: sensory, motor, and autonomic. All three contribute to predisposing the diabetic foot to infection.

The etiology of this neuropathy is not fully understood. Angiopathy of the vasa nervorum causing an ischemia of the nerve was the classic explanation. Although more recently discounted in favor of metabolic explanations, this theory may be regaining support. The metabolic explanations include accumulation of intraneural sorbitol, glycosylation of nerve protein, and reduction of axonal transport. Green et al.,[47] have postulated that a decrease in nerve myoinositol, which occurs with hyperglycemia, will decrease activity of the sodium-potassium–ATPase pump activity. This diminished pump activity decreases the action potential that forms across the axon. All of these metabolic explanations are based on the presence of hyperglycemia. With strict glucose control many of the symptoms can be reversed or retarded.

The signs and symptoms of these neuropathies are covered elsewhere. How they relate to infection is vital to understand (Fig. 13-5).

Motor neuropathy will cause atrophy of the intrinsic musculature of the foot. An imbalance of the long versus the short flexors and extensors results, with subsequent dorsal dislocation of the toes. This places a retrograde downward force on the metatarsal heads. Distal dislocation of the plantar fat pad occurs. The plantar aspect of the foot, and the dorsal aspect of the toes, are exposed to excessive repetitive forces with ambulation, and hyperkeratosis results. Because of increases in collagen cross linking, and a possible accelerated collagenase activity found in diabetic skin, ulceration results. Sensory neuropathy prevents the patient from be-

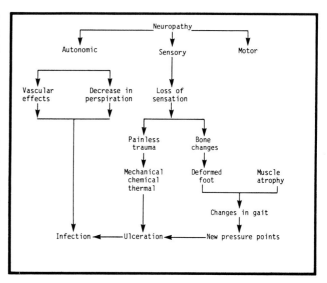

Fig. 13-5. Mechanism by which diabetic neuropathy leads to infection. (From Joseph and LeFrock,[34] with permission.)

coming aware of the situation until often an infectious process has begun. The first indication to the patient of trouble comes with foul odor or visible drainage on the sock.

Autonomic dysfunction impairs sweating and alters vascular responsiveness. This contributes to the formation of hyperkeratotic plaques leading to the above scenario of ulcer formation. Dyshidrosis leads to fissuring of the skin, allowing normal floras to become potentially invasive. Sympathetic failure is associated with vasodilation, arteriovenous shunting, and edema, all of which impair vascular response to infection.

Advanced neuropathic changes can eventually lead to diabetic arthropathy or Charcot's joint. A combination of autonomic, sensory, and motor deficits leads to this complication. The most common sites for Charcot's joint changes include the midtarsal and the tarsal-metatarsal articulations. Clinically, there is a collapse of the normal architecture of the plantar arch, resulting in possible ulceration. Edema, heat, and erythema may also be present, making differentiation from a septic process both difficult and vital to proper therapy.

When neuropathic changes are combined with impaired host immune responses and alteration of local blood supply, the predisposition for infection in these feet becomes obvious. Once established, these factors further combine with the unique microbiology of these infections to make treatment a challenge.

Infection

Because of the "unholy triad" of neuropathy, angiopathy, and immunopathy, infections that diabetics acquire may be more severe and refractory to treatment than similar infections in nondiabetic patients. Further, the severity may be masked by the inability to mount a proper response. Along with common infections, diabetic patients often present with an entirely distinctive spectrum of infections not seen in patients without the disease.

Soft Tissue Infections

Skin and skin structure infections are possibly the most common of all diabetic infections. Greenwood, in 1927, found that 25 percent of diabetic patients gave a history of significant cutaneous infection, and 10 percent of the patients had a current infection.[48]

Dermatophytes

Fungal infections of the feet are reported in 60 to 80 percent of diabetic patients whether symptomatic or not.[49] The most severe form of this disease is acute vesicular tinea pedis (Fig. 13-6). Vesicle formation causes direct erosions into the epidermis and may allow secondary bacterial infection to evolve. A more common form of dermatophytic infection is caused by *Trichophyton rubrum.* Dry, scaling lesions with central clearing are noted in a moccasin distribution over the plantar aspect of the feet. A macerated intertrigo may also be seen. If allowed to progress, skin fissuring may occur, again allowing secondary bacterial invasion. Prevention of this breakdown becomes especially important in the interspaces because of the proximity of multiple tendon sheaths. If secondary infection occurs in this area, proximal spread through the sheaths is possible.

Aggressive local therapy of the dermatophyte infections is usually sufficient. Topical antifungal agents in the proper base are effective. In the case of vesicular disease, wet-to-dry astringent dressings will assist in drying of the tissues. Oral antihistamines are useful in the control of pruritus. Refractory or particularly severe infections may require the short-term use of oral antifungal agents. If secondary bacterial infection ensues, proper antibiotic therapy should be instituted.

Onychomycosis is another commonly occurring infection in the diabetic foot. If the thickening of the nail plate is allowed to continue unchecked, excessive pressure will develop on the nail bed, causing subungual ulceration. Again, secondary bacterial invasion may occur.

Paronychia

Trauma, onychomycosis, or improper nail-cutting technique may lead to an infected ingrown toenail, or paronychia. The common causative or-

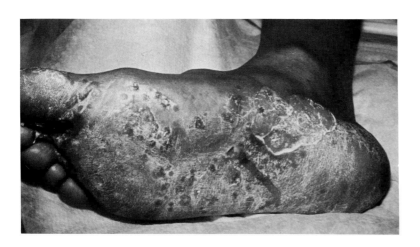

Fig. 13-6. Acute vesicular tinea pedis common in patients with diabetes mellitus.

ganism is usually bacterial and includes staphylococcus species and *Proteus.* Textbooks often refer to *Candida* as being a frequent isolate. Identification of the causative organism is important since empiric antibiotic therapy may aggravate a fungal condition.[50] Paronychia in the nondiabetic patient is manifest by localized inflammation of the nail grooves. Diabetic patients, unable to respond in this fashion, may present with frank necrosis of the toe (Fig. 13-7).

Differential diagnosis of toenail pain is complicated in patients with angiopathy. A patient may present with a chief complaint of "ingrown nails." On careful history it is ascertained that the pain only occurs at night or with elevation of the limb. Pain is relieved with shoe gear and ambulation. The physician who removes this nail may be faced with a gangrenous toe secondary to ischemic rest pain.

Treatment of paronychia in the face of diabetes must be predicated on vascular supply. Primary excision of the offending nail border is the only definitive cure. This should be followed by local care, including wet-to-dry dressings to promote drainage. Topical creams and ointments should be avoided because they may cause maceration of tissue. Because this is usually a localized infection, systemic antibiotic therapy is rarely necessary, but may be indicated in the face of recurrent or recalcitrant infection.

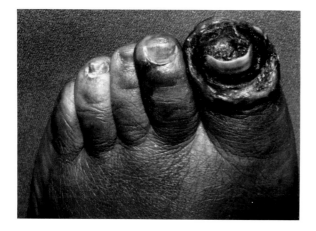

Fig. 13-7. Necrosis with frank gangrene following paronychia in a patient with diabetes.

Plantar Space Abscess

The foot is divided by plantar fascia and muscular septae into six distinct plantar spaces. Four to five are located centrally, one medially, and one laterally. Any soft tissue infection of the foot, whether from a mal perforans, a puncture wound, or an interspace infection, may spread proximally into one or more of these spaces, forming an abscess. Spread will occur along the path of least resistance, including tendon sheaths or small- and medium-sized vessels, causing necrosis. Abscess formation will cause an increase in local pH, and a decreased oxygenation potential (eH), allowing the growth of obligate anaerobes. Furthermore, within the abscess there is a marked decrease in phagocytosis, and diminished penetration of certain antibiotics such as the aminoglycosides. The only effective therapy is aggressive incision and drainage.

Necrotizing Infections

"Gas gangrene" is actually an entire class of infections that represent the most severe form of soft tissue infection. If not treated promptly and aggressively, there is highly associated systemic toxicity and morbidity. Diabetics are highly prone to this disease. LeFrock and colleagues found that of 60 patients with lower extremity infections, 10 (16.7 percent) demonstrated gas in infected tissues.[51]

Clinical signs and symptoms include soft tissue crepitus, a watery, often foul-smelling discharge, and necrosis of the skin. The depth of the necrosis will relate to which disease entity is present. Necrotizing fasciitis is a rapidly progressing, rare infection that is differentiated by its involvement of subcutaneous tissue without affecting underlying muscle. In contrast, synergistic necrotizing cellulitis will also involve the muscle. Pain, although possibly severe, is not a dependable diagnostic criterion because of the anesthesia that may be present secondary to necrosis of superficial nerves. Radiographic findings include the presence of soft tissue emphysema, seen as a radiolucency in the tissue planes.

Although *Clostridium perfringens* causes a rapidly progressing, often fatal variant, it tends to be rare. Any of a variety of organisms are capable of being etiologic. The coliforms, both aerobic and anaerobic, are frequent causes. Gram-positive cocci, including *Peptococcus, Peptostreptococcus,* and *Streptococcus pyogenes,* have also been isolated. Nonbacterial causes of soft tissue gas include trauma with resultant trapped air, and the use of hydrogen peroxide irrigation.

Osseous Infection

Osteomyelitis has a predilection for diabetic patients. Waldvogel et al. found that of 247 cases of osteomyelitis studied, one-third were in diabetics.[52] The disease, however, is not significantly different from that in nondiabetics. It usually occurs later in life, with most cases seen between the ages of 50 and 70. The small bones of the foot are the most frequently involved secondary to the contiguous focus of a mal perforans, or vascular insufficiency–caused gangrene. In most cases, this osteomyelitis is polymicrobial; two or more bacterial or fungal species, including *S. aureus* (the most common), are found.

The most vexing problem with osteomyelitis in the diabetic is the diagnosis. As discussed previously, differentiation from either diabetic osteolysis or Charcot's joint, especially with overlying ulceration, is difficult. Despite advances in radionuclide technique, as discussed in the section on diagnosis of osteomyelitis, bone biopsy remains the definitive diagnostic test.

Microbiology

Culture Techniques

The location from which a culture of the diabetic foot infection is taken is important in isolating the primary pathogens. Deep specimens, harvested from a prepared aseptic site, are the most valuable. Because this is not often practical, superficial specimens may have to suffice. The correlation between superficial and deep culture results has been studied by Sharp and colleagues.[53] Fifty-eight cultures were examined from 52 patients. In only 10 of 58 specimens were identical organisms or combinations isolated. In 34 of 58 cases, organisms from deep tissues could not be cultured from superficial tissues. Sapico et al. examined the three most commonly used culture techniques, ulcer swabs, needle aspiration, and curettage of the ulcer base. Of the three, curettage had the highest concordance and ulcer swab the lowest.[54]

Bacteriology

Through the mid-1970s, the predominant organisms reported to be isolated from the infected diabetic foot included *S. aureus,* group B streptococcus, the facultative gram-negative organisms, the enterobacteriaceae, and *C. perfringens* in the case of gas gangrene.[55,56] This is a polymicrobial infection. More recently, with the advent of sophisticated culturing techniques, Sapico,[54,57] LeFrock,[51] and others have shown that the obligate anaerobic organisms are of great significance in these infections. In Sapico et al.'s series of 32 patients, cultures of deep tissue yielded pure aerobic cultures in six cases, pure anaerobic only once, and mixed cultures in 25 cases. A mean of 4.1 species (2.84 aerobes and 1.97 anaerobes) was isolated from each patient.[57]

The aerobic organisms isolated differ for each center. *Proteus mirablis, S. aureus,* and *E. coli* are consistently reported. Group D streptococcus (enterococcus), and *P. aeruginosa,* reported as very common by some, are found rarely in others. This last point is of significance in determining antibiotic therapy because of the resistance of these organisms to multiple agents.

A range of 4.1 to 5.8 anaerobic species was isolated from each patient. Although the number of species was lower, the anaerobic organisms were found to be in greater quantity than the aerobes. These data are in accord with numerous other studies.[51,53,54,56]

The predominance of anaerobes can be explained in part by the aforementioned formation of abscesses. Other factors contributing to an anaerobic environment include the presence of diabetic immunopathy, leading to an overgrowth of facultative organisms. These organisms utilize the already diminished oxygen, further decreasing the eH and thus enhancing the anaerobic milieu. The frequent presence of necrotic tissue also is fertile breeding ground for these organisms.

The presence of anaerobic bacteria may be detected prior to the results of the culture and sensitivity report. A characteristic foul odor is noted, thus the name "fetid foot." Gas or crepitus, although not diagnostic of anaerobic infections, may be suggestive. A polymicrobial Gram stain with monomicrobial culture results suggests that a number of anaerobic organisms were present but not isolated.

One fairly consistent finding is the presence of *Bacteroides fragilis* and other *Bacteroides* species as the most frequently isolated organisms in the diabetic foot. The importance of this is twofold. *Bacteroides fragilis* is a multiresistant organism. Most anaerobes are susceptible to penicillin, but *B. fragilis* is not. This is due, at least in part, to the ability of *B. fragilis* to form a glycocalyx, protecting its colonies. Furthermore, *B. fragilis* acts synergistically with other organisms, particularly the gram positives, causing more severe infections than either organism would alone.[58] For these reasons the antimicrobial therapy of these infections must be predicated on the drug's ability to treat *B. fragilis* infections.

Treatment

Once a severe infection has become established, aggressive surgical incision, drainage, and débridement becomes the therapy of choice. Localized processes may be best handled by amputation of the affected part (i.e., a toe). If the infection has spread to the plantar spaces, a radical débridement becomes necessary (Fig. 13-8). Meticulous care must be taken to preserve any vital structures while removing all necrotic tissue. All six plantar spaces may require exploration to provide adequate drainage. Once the débridement has been accomplished, the wound should be packed open to promote dependent drainage.

Local wound care should likewise be aggressive and frequent. Twice-a-day dressing changes with bedside débridement on an as-needed basis are useful to keep the wound clean. The use of topical antiseptics such as povidone iodine, sodium hypochlorite (Dakin's solution), or acetic acid, is a matter of personal choice because no good comparative data are available. Subsequent surgical débridement and eventual revision will frequently be necessary. Attention must also be addressed to the functional requirements of the patient. A transmetatarsal amputation may give a better functional result than removal of random toes and metatarsal heads.

In the face of severe infection, antibiotic therapy becomes an important adjunct to the surgical therapy discussed above (Table 13-3). The agent empirically selected must have good activity against the anaerobes, especially *B. fragilis*. It also must be sufficiently broad spectrum to cover the other multiple pathogens frequently isolated. Nephrotoxicity is an important consideration. Because diabetes

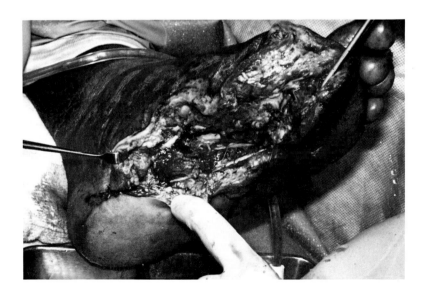

Fig. 13-8. Radical débridement of a plantar space abscess in a diabetic patient. All central plantar spaces have been exposed and drained.

Table 13-3. Initial Empiric Therapy for Diabetic Foot Infections[a]

Infected ulcer (oral)
  Amoxicillin/clavulanic acid
  Clindamycin
  First-generation oral cephalosporin
  Ciprofloxacin + clindamycin (for more severe infection)
Moderately severe infection (parenteral)
  Cefoxitin
  Ticarcillin/clavulanic acid
  Ampicillin/sulbactam[b]
  Cefotaxime
  Ceftizoxime
Severe limb- or life-threatening infection
  Imipenem/cilastatin
  Clindamycin + cefotaxime or ceftizoxime
  Clindamycin + ampicillin + aminoglycoside[c]

[a] Based on clinical presentation and assumption of usual pathogens.
[b] Useful when streptococcus group D *(Enterococcus)* are anticipated.
[c] This traditional "triple-agent therapy" should be used with caution because of the nephrotoxic potential of the aminoglycosides. For this reason, the regimens not containing aminoglycosides are employed whenever possible.

mellitus is a multisystemic disease, most of these patients will present with underlying renal insufficiency.

For the purpose of antibiotic selection, the diabetic foot can be divided into two categories, mild to moderate, and severe life or limb threatening. For the former class, monotherapy with a broad-spectrum agent is usually sufficient. Any one of a number of cephalosporins with antianaerobic activity are useful. Cefoxitin has the most clinical experience and data reported in this type of infection.[59] Cefotaxime, ceftizoxime, cefoperazone, cefotetan, and the combination of ticarcillin/clavulanic acid are other drugs that have been used successfully as single agents.

More severe infections provide a challenge in antibiotic usage because combination therapy is often indicated. Traditionally a triple-agent combination including an aminoglycoside, a penicillin, and an anaerobic agent has been utilized. Although effective, the potential for nephrotoxicity induced by the aminoglycoside while using this combination warrants caution. Double-agent therapy consisting of a third-generation cephalosporin, such as cefotaxime or ceftizoxime, in combination with an antianaerobic agent, such as clindamycin, has been used successfully by this author. Although a costly

combination, there is significantly less chance of toxicity.

The one single agent that may prove effective in these severe life- and limb-threatening infections is imipenem/cilastatin.[60] This antibiotic, the broadest spectrum agent to date, demonstrates excellent activity against all of the pathogens found in the diabetic foot. Its activity against *B. fragilis* is comparable to the specific anaerobic agents such as metronidazole and clindamycin. Although relatively safe, the drug may be epileptogenic in patients with prior history of seizures or with marked renal impairment. In these cases the dosage must be reduced.

BACTERIAL OSTEOMYELITIS

In dealing with bacterial infections of the bones of the lower extremity, definition of terms becomes a priority for understanding and treatment of the disease. *Osteomyelitis*, commonly used to describe all infections of bone, should in the strictest sense of the term be defined as infection of the bone marrow and adjacent structures. This would preclude many common types of bone infections treated by the podiatric physician. "Osteomyelitis" should be differentiated from the more general term *osteitis*, which refers to any inflammatory process of bone, including infection. Semantics aside, although first described in the 1700s,[61] this disease continues to be possibly the most misunderstood, and most difficult to diagnose and treat, infectious disease of the lower extremity.

Because of the increased volume and sophistication of bone surgery being performed on the foot coupled with the use of implantable materials, changes in the pathogens causing the disease and the understanding of the processes involved are occurring. Silastic and metal implants can cause a localized decrease in host defenses. Phagocytic chemotaxis and phagocytosis are decreased in their presence. Fibronectins cause bacterial adherence to the implant, and the glycocalyx shields the organisms from host and chemotherapeutic attack. Chemoprophylaxis is selecting out an entirely different collection of pathogens from those originally described. In this section the classification, diagnosis, and treatment of osteomyelitis (the term that will be used, for the sake of convention) are discussed.

Classification

Traditionally, osteomyelitis has been classified into three categories: hematogenous, direct extension, and secondary to vascular insufficiency.[52] These can then be temporarily divided into acute, subacute, and chronic. Although a number of new classification systems have been proposed and are touched upon here, this breakdown is the most commonly employed.

Hematogenous osteomyelitis is a disease of the very young or the very old. Following an episode of bacteremia, the organisms settle in the metaphyseal region of the long bones of the lower extremity in the young, and in the vertebral bodies of the elderly. In the long bones, the metaphyseal region has a complex vascular plexus that causes sludging of the blood and deposition of the bacteria. Furthermore, the lack of phagocytic lining cells of the afferent loops and the relative inactivity of the lining in the efferent loop of the long bones in children has been implicated in the pathogenesis. This is usually a monomicrobial infection, with *S. aureus* being the most common pathogen. Vertebral hematogenous osteomyelitis is most frequently caused by gram-negative organisms. The bacteremia in these cases is often preceded by a manipulation of the genitourinary or gastrointestinal tracts. A third type of hematogenous disease is seen in intravenous drug abusers. *Pseudomonas aeruginosa* or methicillin-resistant staphylococcus is isolated in these patients, having been directly inoculated into the bloodstream.[62]

Direct extension osteomyelitis occurs most frequently in the middle years. It is the result of infection of the surrounding soft tissues after surgery or trauma. Implantation of organisms into the bone following puncture wounds, implant surgery, or contiguous septic arthritis are all examples of this frequent entity. Common in podiatric practice, direct extension osteomyelitis is a vexing diagnostic and therapeutic disease. Unlike the more easily predicted causative organisms found in hematogenous osteomyelitis, any number of gram-positive or gram-negative bacteria have been implicated. Traditionally, postoperative osteomyelitis following bone surgery or implant arthroplasty presented with *S. aureus* as the primary pathogen. More recently, the coagulase-negative staphylococci, previously considered benign contaminants, have become of major concern. The reason for this shift in bacteriology is not fully understood. Numerous factors, including the increased usage of antimicrobial prophylaxis, have been indicted. These organisms are capable of producing a polyglycolic slime layer that acts to shield the colonies from host defenses.[63] Furthermore, there is a methicillin resistance rate of up to 80 percent in these isolates. This characteristic renders commonly used antibiotics, such as cephalosporins and penicillins, useless. Vancomycin, a very expensive and potentially toxic agent, is the sole drug effective against these bacteria.

The final type of osteomyelitis described by this classification is that "secondary to vascular insufficiency." Occurring after the age of 50, frequently in diabetics, and affecting the small bones of the foot, this disease is common to podiatric practice. The infection tends to be polymicrobial, with both aerobic and anaerobic organisms being isolated. Because of local tissue hypoxia secondary to decreased profusion, circulating antibiotics may reach inadequate levels to treat the disease. Surgical intervention may likewise be unsuccessful.

The differentiation into acute, subacute, and chronic disease by clinical and radiographic criteria further complicates the classification situation and thus the understanding of the processes. There are acute exacerbations of so-called chronic disease and, likewise, there is acute disease of long standing. Osteomyelitis may present acutely years after implant surgery yet radiographically appear chronic. The temporal classification in a case such as this becomes difficult. One possible alternative that has been suggested is the use of the terms *initial* and *recurrent*.

There are a number of more recent systems devised to replace or augment the above. Cierny et al. used the anatomic location of the disease coupled with the physiologic state of the host to define the disease.[64] Once this is determined, a complicated

STAGE III

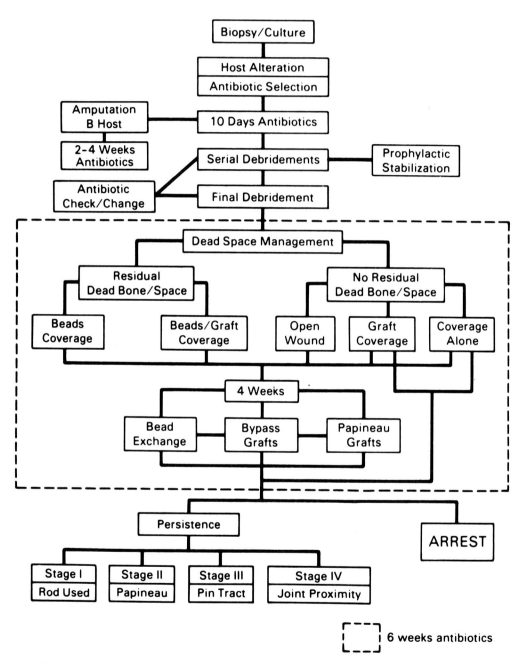

Fig. 13-9. Systemized treatment flowchart for osteomyelitis. (From Cierny et al.,[64] with permission.)

Table 13-4. Classification of Osteomyelitis as Described by Buckholz

Type I Wound Induced	
Type I-A	Open fractures with complete incontinuity graded according to the extent of soft-tissue injury as grade 1, 2, or 3
Type I-B	Penetrating wounds of injury as in puncture wounds, missile wounds, cutaneous ulcers, or reinfection of wound
Type I-C	Postsurgical infections exclusive of implant surgery Type I-B and I-C involve nonfractured bone
Type II Mechanogenic Infection	
Type II-A	Implants of surgery as joint prostheses and stable fixation devices
Type II-B	Contact instability as bone-to-bone appositional movement or implant-to-bone instability
Type III Physeal Osteomyelitis	
Epiphyseal plate infection in children	
Type IV Ischemic Limb Disease	
Arterial deficiency	
Type V Combinations	
Types I through IV as acute bone infections	
Type VI Osteitis with Septic Arthritis	
Co-existing bone and joint infection	
Type VII Chronic Osteitis/Osteomyelitis	
Recurrent infection and infected pseudoarthroses	

(From Buckholz,[65] with permission.)

flowchart is employed to choose the most appropriate therapy (Fig. 13-9). This system does not differentiate acute from chronic, and provides a systematic approach to the treatment, both surgical and medical.

Most recently, Buckholz described a system utilizing the mechanogenesis of the infection coupled with an understanding of the local "vascular defenses" of bone to classify the disease process and determine a therapeutic course.[65] In contradistinction to the Cierny et al. system, a clear differentiation is made as to acute versus chronic disease (Table 13-4). The drawback to both of these newer classifications is that a large number of cases must be applied to assure that the system will be applicable.

Diagnosis

Despite the onslaught of new, sophisticated roentgenographic techniques and laboratory tests, the diagnosis of osteomyelitis continues to be one of the most challenging in podiatric medicine. As with any infectious disease, however, the principles discussed earlier remain valid.

The importance of a complete history cannot be overly stressed. In some cases the history may be practically diagnostic. If a patient relates a 3-week history of a puncture wound to the foot with recent exacerbation of symptomatology, *P. aeruginosa* osteomyelitis can almost be assumed.

Physical examination may or may not be indicative of infection. The cardinal signs of cellulitis may be present or absent. Fever and malaise are also inconsistent findings. In the case of hematogenous osteomyelitis, pinpoint tenderness may be the only physical sign of underlying disease. If bone is exposed through a frankly infected site, the diagnosis of clinical osteomyelitis can be made.

Radiographic changes may be inconclusive. Bone must lose 30 to 50 percent of its mineral content before the loss becomes evident on plain films. Therefore, there is a lag of 2 weeks or greater before changes in the bone may be seen on an x-ray. By this time, the process will have become rather invasive. When evident, common radiographic signs of acute osteomyelitis include soft tissue swelling, cortical erosions, periosteal elevation, and frank bone destruction. In chronic disease new bone formation (involucrum) can be seen along with islands of dead, radiodense sclerotic bone (sequestrum) (Fig. 13-10).

Because of the prolonged lag noted above, a number of nuclear scintigraphic techniques have been advanced to provide a more rapid diagnosis. Changes may be seen on bone scintigraphy within 24 hours of inoculation. Technetium and gallium have been used either individually or sequentially with mixed results. Both of these tests are highly sensitive but relatively nonspecific. Especially in the face of possible diabetic osteoarthropathy, the differentiation by scintigraphy is complicated. Park et al. found in their relatively small series less than an 80 percent specificity with slightly higher positive predictability.[66] Indium-111–labeled leukocyte scanning is a newer technique that showed initial promise as being both sensitive and specific for infection. Although impressive early results raised great expectations, some of the initial enthusiasm has quelled. One recent abstract examines the use of a combination of all three techniques with excellent results.[67]

Standard and computed tomography (CT) may be helpful, especially in cases of chronic disease, to localize sequestrum. Its use otherwise is limited.

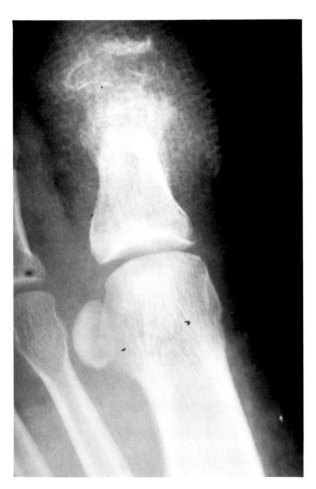

Fig. 13-10. Radiograph of osteomyelitis of the hallux. There is frank bone destruction, periosteal elevation, and sequestrum formation.

The laboratory may be helpful in the diagnosis of osteomyelitis. Although the usual indices of infection — CBC with differential, ESR, or CRP — may be elevated, localized infection of the foot often presents without rises in these parameters. Even if nonspecific for infection in some cases, these tests do provide a baseline set of values to monitor the progress of therapy.

Blood cultures should be obtained on all patients with suspected acute hematogenous osteomyelitis. They can be positive 50 percent of the time. Although hematogenous osteomyelitis is caused by staphylococcus 60 to 90 percent of the time, children with negative blood cultures should undergo

aspiration of bone or surgical biopsy. These two procedures reportedly have a 60 and 90 percent yield, respectively.[68]

Definitive diagnosis should be based on direct surgical culture of bone or aspirated material. Sinus tract cultures are unreliable, with less than a 50 percent concordance with the true infecting organism. The one exception to this rule appears to be *S. aureus*, which may be present in up to 70 percent of the deep bone specimens if cultured from a sinus.[10] Bone specimens must be harvested from a clean surgical site to minimize contamination from extraneous organisms. If possible, the patient should be taken off of all antibiotics, both parenteral and oral, for at least 48 hours prior to the procedure. Any residual bone or tissue levels of antibiotic may render culture results less than reliable. Some success has been reported with the percutaneous needle biopsy technique. Radiographic visualization of the biopsy location will assure proper placement of the needle into infected bone. Bone sent to the microbiology laboratory must be cultured not only for the usual aerobic and anaerobic bacteria, but also for fungi and mycobacteria.

Pathologic evaluation of bone for osteomyelitis cannot be relied upon for diagnosis. Many inflammatory changes in bone, both acute and chronic, may mimic osteomyelitis.

Treatment

Sequestration of organisms in islands of necrotic bone is the major cause of failure in the treatment of this disease. These organisms may remain quiescent in the bone for upwards of 50 years before causing exacerbation of the process. For this reason surgical débridement of bone is the cornerstone in the therapy of osteomyelitis. Antibiotics, while an important adjunct, are rarely successful as sole therapy. The one exception to this is acute hematogenous osteomyelitis. Long-duration therapy of 4 to 6 weeks with adequate dosage of parenteral antibiotics has been successfully employed. Recent literature suggests that the use of 2 weeks or less of parenteral therapy followed by 4 weeks of oral therapy meets with equally good results.[68] Careful patient selection is necessary to assure compliance. If insufficient duration or dosage is used a more chronic, recalcitrant disease may develop.

For other forms of osteomyelitis the importance of antibiotics is rarely debated yet difficult to assess. Because of the varied nature of the disease, controlled clinical studies are difficult to design and evaluate. Animal studies account for the majority of the data addressing important questions such as duration of therapy. Achievable bone levels of antibiotics are often touted by pharmaceutical sales representatives, yet are technically difficult to perform and of questionable value.

When using antibiotics in the treatment of osteomyelitis, general principles of antimicrobial therapy must be observed. The drug should be selected on the basis of proper culture results. Empiric usage may subject the patient to unnecessarily broad-spectrum, expensive, potentially toxic agents. The agent selected should be bactericidal because of the diminished host defenses present in the area. Minimal inhibitory concentrations (MICs) of the drug for the infecting organism should be low enough to be exceeded in the bone by six to eight times. Current thought dictates that a duration of 4 to 6 weeks of parenteral therapy following the definitive débridement is required for the best therapeutic results. With the advent of home health care parenteral therapy the patients need no longer be hospitalized for the entire period. The insertion of a Hickman catheter, a central line, or a heparin lock allows the patient to administer the drug himself at home. Once again proper patient selection is imperative. The development of long-acting antibiotics such as ceftriaxone allows once-daily dosing through either intravenous access or the intramuscular route.

Meticulous débridement of infected, necrotic bone is the hallmark of treatment of osteomyelitis. In the foot, débridement is simplified by the number of bones and joints forming a natural barrier to the spread of the infection. If a distal phalanx is infected, complete removal of the bone effects a cure. With the increasing sophistication of podiatric surgery, however, large bone involvement, including first metatarsal, tibia, and fibula, is becoming an increasing problem. In these bones, "cure" may not be possible. Even with careful débridement and prolonged courses of antibiotic therapy, there is no guarantee that all of the organism is eradicated.

To assure eradication of the organisms, a number of different modalities have been employed to in-crease local concentration of antibiotics. Ingress-egress catheterization has been advocated by some authors. This treatment is controversial, with the advocates pointing to the large local concentration of drug with no associated systemic toxicity. Detractors claim an increase in resistant organism "superinfection" and local tissue toxicities.

More extensively studied is the implantation of antibiotic-impregnated beads into the site of infection. The antibiotic, usually gentamicin, leaches out of the polymethylmethacrylate bead into the surrounding tissue. Supporters of this modality report high local drug levels with no associated toxicity. Furthermore, the dead space that remains following débridement is occupied, thereby decreasing the chances of hematoma formation. Detractors once again point to the possibility of superinfection with resistant organisms. The possibility of elevated serum aminoglycoside levels with subsequent toxicity is also cited. For this reason other antibiotics, including cephalosporins, have also been studied with reportedly good results. Although not "officially" approved by the Food and Drug Administration (FDA), there are enough encouraging data in this area to render the use of beads worthy of consideration.

Another apparently useful modality in the surgical treatment of osteomyelitis is the use of vascularized myocutaneous free flaps to fill debrided spaces. The procedure involves the microvascular removal of a distant muscle and its vascular pedicle, such as latissimus dorsi, with its subsequent placement and revascularization into the dead space. Oxygen tension, and therefore leukocyte function, has been shown to be increased in the presence of these vascularized flaps. This allows the bone to fight the infection more readily, thereby decreasing the amount of time needed to treat the infection and close the soft tissue defect.

It must be pointed out that the above techniques are relatively new. Osteomyelitis is a difficult disease to study in that there are a myriad of variables that cannot, by the nature of the disease, be controlled. Therefore, all of the above studies must be evaluated with a critical eye.

One aspect of the treatment of osteomyelitis that appears to be uniformly accepted is the importance of osseous stability. External or internal rigid fixation will prevent devascularization of the bone and further tissue damage. For this reason, even in the face of local infection stable fixation should be kept in place.

BACTERIAL ARTHRITIS

Septic arthritis is an acute process. Immediate recognition and treatment is essential to reducing the morbidity of the disease. Any delay will adversely affect the prognosis, allowing severe, crippling joint destruction. Despite the development of potent antibiotics, septic arthritis continues to be the most destructive form of arthritis. With proper, timely, therapy, however, a cure will often result.

Microbiology

Ang-Fonte et al. have reported that the incidence of septic arthritis has remained relatively stable in recent years: about 1.3 cases per 1,000 hospital admissions.[69] The spectrum of organisms that are responsible for these cases, however, has changed somewhat. *Neisseria gonorrhoeae* continues to be the most prevalent cause of the disease and probably the most benign and responsive to treatment. This organism is followed closely by *S. aureus* and the streptococci. Where the changes are occurring is in the increasing prevalence of the gram-negative rod infections, especially in drug abusers and hospitalized patients.

Age of the patient is an important factor in determining the probable causative organism. At 2 years or younger, *Haemophilus influenzae* is the most frequently isolated. Over the age of 2 through adolescence, staphylococcus becomes the most prevalent. *Neisseria gonorrhoeae* becomes the major pathogen in sexually active adults. Later in life, staphylococci and the gram-negative rods again take precedence.

Pathophysiology

Like osteomyelitis, the pathophysiology of septic arthritis can be divided into disease of hematogenous origin and that secondary to direct extension. Unlike osteomyelitis, however, hematogenous spread is the most common cause. Because of its rich vascular supply, the synovial joint lining is very susceptible to seeding by blood-borne organisms from concurrent infections. The site of these distant infections varies. In patients with gram-negative septic arthritis, the most common site is the urinary tract. With gram-positive infections, the most common location is a skin or upper respiratory infection. The distant focus is therefore often predictable once the organism is cultured from the joint. The seeding process is facilitated by the presence of a preexisting joint abnormality or in patients with immunodeficiencies. Patients with rheumatoid arthritis have an increased incidence of septic arthritis. The reason for this, although not totally clear, may be part the fact that the bacteria are able to more readily penetrate previously damaged joints. The use of concurrent systemic corticosteroids may also be a factor.

Probably more common from a podiatric standpoint is septic arthritis secondary to a contiguous focus. An osteomyelitic focus at the distal end of a bone may either traverse the cartilaginous plate to enter the joint directly, or break through at a site of attachment of the joint capsule, allowing direct access. Postoperative infections following joint-invasive procedures, including implants, will cause a septic arthritis. Arthroscopy performed on the ankle may cause seeding of the joint with subsequent infection. Finally, any of a number of traumatic events, including puncture wounds and animal bites, have been implicated.

Organisms implicated in these contiguous focus cases differ from those discussed in the hematogenous scenario. *Staphylococcus epidermidis*, previously thought benign, is becoming a frequent pathogen following implant surgery. The treatment of this organism is complicated by a high rate of methicillin resistance, approaching 80 percent. As discussed in an earlier section, *P. aeruginosa* frequently is the causative organism following puncture wound septic arthritis. Animal or human bite infections present with an unusual and distinctive set of organisms. Mixed infections containing *Pasteurella multocida*, a gram-negative rod, are seen in animal bites. Human bites often contain staphylococcus, streptococcus, anaerobic oral flora, and *Eikenella corrodens*. The antibiotic treatment of these infections is complicated by the usual resistance of *Eikenella* and *Pasteurella* to frequently used cephalosporins.

Clinical Presentation

The septic joint uniformly presents with marked increase in local temperature, painful, limited range of motion, and erythema. The patient may present with constitutional signs and symptoms of infection. Goldenberg and Cohen noticed a rectal temperature of at least 100 °F in 90 percent of the patients in their series. However, they noted the fever to be low grade and transient. In the same series, leukocytosis was noted in only 60 percent of the patients.[70] Shaking chills are uncommon except in disseminated gonococcal infections. Any young, sexually active, otherwise healthy patient who presents with acute joint pain should be considered as having gonococcal arthritis until proven otherwise.

Differential diagnosis is difficult. Gout and other crystal-forming arthropathies, acute rheumatoid arthritis, Lyme disease, lupus, seronegative spondyloarthropathies, and trauma must all be considered. Gout is possibly the most common disease to be differentiated from septic arthritis. Aspiration of the joint for microscopic evaluation of crystals, trial courses of colchicine therapy, and disease history are usually adequate to make the diagnosis.

Radiographic findings of septic arthritis can be nonspecific. Soft tissue edema with joint swelling is seen early in the process. If there is progression to osteomyelitis, or joint spread from a contiguous focus, the typical radiographic appearance of that disease will be noted. Following implant arthroplasty, a septic process may present as lucency around the implant, representing loosening.

Definitive diagnosis is made by the isolation of organisms from aspirated synovial fluid, or their demonstration on Gram stain. Unfortunately, Gram stain is fairly unreliable in these cases, with positive results less than 65 percent of the time. This number increases with gram-positive organisms and decreases with the gram negatives. Gonococcus can only be seen 25 percent of the time. Blood cultures should be performed in all cases. This is especially true when hematogenous spread is suspected.

Synovial fluid analysis reveals evidence of severe inflammatory response. White cell count has been reported as high as 900,000 in the fluid.[71] Polymorphonuclear leukocytes are the predominant cell type. Mucin clot formation is poor.

Treatment

The hallmark of successful treatment of septic arthritis is prompt diagnosis. With delay, there is a marked increase in the prevalence of joint destruction and osteomyelitis, necessitating bone resection.

Treatment is predicated on removal of the purulent joint effusions and parenteral antibiotic therapy directed at the causative organism. These effusions can cause rapid destruction to the joint cartilage as a result of increased joint pressure and the presence of leukocyte-released enzymes.

Technique for removing the infected joint fluid is controversial. Two accepted methods include closed joint aspiration and open joint drainage.[71,72] Although both have proven effective in eradicating the infectious process, aspiration may cause less residual joint morbidity. The key to successful aspiration therapy is the use of the technique whenever the joint requires it. This may translate into daily or even twice-daily aspirations at first. With control of the infection, joint effusions should decrease and the frequency diminish. Open drainage is now reserved for joints recalcitrant to aspiration therapy, or as first-line therapy in the infected hip.

Parenteral antibiotic therapy is based on the Gram stain and culture results. Empiric therapy can be based on the clinical presentation, including the age of the patient, sexual history, and the presence of any probable distant foci such as an abscess. The use of intra-articular antibiotics should be avoided because most antibiotics achieve synovial fluid levels equal to or greater than their serum levels with intravenous administration. Furthermore, intra-articular injections may cause a reactive chemical synovitis that is damaging to the joints.[73]

With early diagnosis and proper treatment the results can be satisfactory. Ninety percent of patients with gonococcal arthritis recover completely. This number decreases to 70 percent with *S. aureus*, and further with gram-negative infections.

ANTIBIOTIC SELECTION PRINCIPLES

Antibiotics are seemingly released every week. With each new announcement a hoard of sales representatives appear magically in an unsuspecting, unprepared physician's waiting room. Each is there to espouse the wonders of the new "miracle drug." The competition is never far behind. If they have not yet prepared a new potion, they are sure to tell the doctor, in no uncertain terms, what deficiencies can be found in the new agent.

Welcome to the multimillion dollar world of antibiotic marketing. In 1986, hospital purchases of parenteral antibiotics amounted to over 1.5 billion dollars. Cephalosporins alone accounted for over 800 million of these dollars. With this plethora of both old and new agents, the average physician easily becomes confused as to what is the appropriate drug for each type of infection. Surprisingly, despite all of the advances in antimicrobial chemotherapy, no one drug has emerged as the one to use in all situations. In fact, the selection principles applied to antibiotics today are largely unchanged from when the first agents were released. In this section these principles are reviewed. They include the definition of "drug of choice" (DOC), identity of the organism, susceptibility, and host and drug factors.

Drug of Choice

The drug of choice can simply be defined as that drug with the narrowest spectrum, the least toxicity, and the lowest cost that can be employed in the treatment of a specific infection (Table 13-5). By way of example, penicillin G is still considered the DOC for almost all group A streptococcal infections despite over 40 years in that position. The drug is one of the least expensive on the market, is

Table 13-5. Effective Antibiotics Against Common Lower Extremity Pathogens[a]

Organism	First Choice	Other Usable Agent
Staphylococcus aureus		
Penicillin suscept.	Pen	FGC
Penicillin resist.	PRP, FGC	Vanco, Clinda
Methicillin resist.	Vanco	Cip, TMP/SMX
Streptococcus		
Non–group D	Pen	FGC, Clinda
Enterococcus	Amp, Mezlo	Pen, Vanco
Neisseria gonorrhoeae	TGC	Pen, Tetra, Cip
Proteus mirabilis	FGC	Amp
Proteus vulgaris		
(indole positive)	SGC, TGC	Cip, ESP, Azt
Escherichia coli	FGC	Amp, SGC, Azt
Enterobacter, Citrobacter, Serratia	Cip, TGC[b]	TMP/SMX, ESP, AMG, Azt
Haemophilus influenzae	SGC	Cip, ESP, Azt
Klebsiella species	SGC, TGC	Cip, Azt
Pseudomonas		
(non-*aeruginosa*)	TMP/SMX	APC
Bacteroides fragilis	Met, Imp, Clinda	SGC,[c] TGC[d]
Pseudomonas aeruginosa	(See Table 13-6)	

[a] Abbreviations: *Pen*, penicillin; *FGC*, first-generation cephalosporin; *PRP*, penicillinase-resistant penicillin; *Vanco*, vancomycin; *Clinda*, clindamycin; *Cip*, ciprofloxacin; *TMP/SMX*, trimethoprim/sulfamethoxazole; *Amp*, ampicillin; *Mezlo*, mezlocillin; *TGC*, third-generation cephalosporin; *Tetra*, tetracycline; *SGC*, second-generation cephalosporin; *ESP*, expanded spectrum penicillin; *Azt*, aztreonam; *AMG*, aminoglycoside; *APC*, antipseudomonal cephalosporin; *Met*, metronidazole; *Imp*, imipenem/cilastatin.
[b] May be initially active, but organisms can develop resistance via inducible β-lactamase.
[c] Cefoxitin and cefotetan are the only ones in this group that are active.
[d] Ceftizoxime and cefotaxime may show some anti-*Bacteroides* activity.

very narrow-spectrum for streptococcus, and except in allergic patients is extremely safe.

Identity of the Organism

Identity of the organism can be achieved through a number of clinical and laboratory means outlined in an earlier section. These include Gram stain, culture and sensitivity, and an empiric knowledge of which organisms predominate in a given infection. One method of identification, not used frequently in lower extremity infections, is the enzyme-linked immunosorbent assay (ELISA). The ELISA detects the presence antibodies and antigens in a clinical specimen. It is used most commonly for viral diseases and other difficult-to-isolate or fastidious organisms. Other immunologic tests, such as complement fixation and latex agglutination, are also available for the detection and diagnosis of these organisms. A few of the diseases diagnosed in this fashion include brucellosis, tularemia, and legionellosis. The only organism common in the lower extremity that may be diagnosed by way of immunologic markers is streptococcus, through the use of an antistreptolysin O titer (ASO). The ASO titer may be useful in a case of cellulitis where no organism can be isolated.

Susceptibility of the Organism

Susceptibility of the organism is determined by a number of different methods depending on the laboratory and the clinical situation. This determination becomes necessary since a species of organisms can vary widely in sensitivity to a given antibiotic. For example, *Staphylococcus aureus* may be penicillin sensitive, penicillin resistant, nafcillin sensitive, or even nafcillin resistant.

Trends in susceptibility patterns also develop in a particular community or hospital. Many hospital microbiology laboratories will print an "antibiogram." This useful document lists all of the bacteria isolated over a period of time and documents their percentage of susceptibility to all antibiotics tested (Table 13-6). This knowledge is helpful in determining the use of empiric therapy prior to receiving the final results from the laboratory. The incidence of methicillin-resistant staphylococcus is on the rise. Some centers have infection rates with upwards of 60 percent or more methicillin-resistant *S. aureus*. If the staff are familiar with this statistic in a given hospital, through the use of an antibiogram, empiric therapy of all staphylococcal infections can be determined.

The laboratory susceptibility test found most commonly in hospitals and independent laboratories is the disk diffusion (Kirby-Bauer) method. In this test an antibiotic saturated paper disk is "dropped" onto a plate containing Mueller-Hinton agar streaked with a pure culture of bacteria. After 18 to 24 hours of incubation a "zone of inhibition," or clear area with no bacterial growth, is noted around the disks of some antibiotics. This zone's diameter is then measured and the result compared to a set of standards, prepared by the National Committee for Clinical Laboratory Standards (NCCLS), to determine whether the bacteria is "sensitive," "intermediate," or "resistant." The advantages of this test are its relative low cost and ease. The main limitation of this procedure is that the results are strictly qualitative and not at all quantitative. However, for most commonly encountered lower extremity infections, it yields sufficient information to direct therapy.

More precise information is generated by testing serial dilutions of an antibiotic against an inoculum of the clinical isolate. After incubation of 18 to 24 hours the tube with the least concentration of antibiotic that shows no visible growth of bacteria is identified. This results in the determination of the MIC. The MIC is defined as the minimal concentration of an antibiotic needed to inhibit growth of the organism. The MIC result is expressed in micrograms per milliliter. The resultant MIC is then checked against a series of NCCLS standards called "breakpoints" to determine if the organism is susceptible or not. These breakpoints take into account factors such as peak achievable serum levels and other pharmacokinetic parameters. For example, for cefazolin, a commonly used first-generation cephalosporin, the organism is resistant if not inhibited by a concentration of greater than 16 μg/ml, and sensitive if inhibited by less than or equal to 8 μg/ml.

Following MIC determination, all dilutions of antibiotic that contain no growth of bacteria can then be plated onto antibiotic-free media. After 24

Table 13-6. Antibiogram Showing Bacterial Isolates in Hospital and the Percentage of Each Organism Susceptible to Different Antibiotics

Gram Negative	No. of Isolates	Amikacin	Ampicillin	Cefotaxime	Ceftazadime	Cefoxitin	Cephalothin	Gentamicin	Mezlocillin	Bactrim	Tobramycin
Acine. calcoaceticus var.	76	89	0	22	53	0	0	72	74	80	82
Citrobacter diversus	14	100	0	100	100	100	93	93	100	100	100
Citrobacter freundii	41	100	24	40	79	17	13	99	71	91	99
Enterobacter aerogenes	92	95	1	25	28	3	1	63	32	46	66
Enterobacter cloacae	137	99	4	73	85	9	3	85	70	85	91
Escherichia coli	638	98	67	98	99	98	67	90	73	88	93
Klebsiella pneumoniae	296	99	0	94	95	88	74	86	73	72	87
Morganella morganii	55	100	0	10	10	63	0	98	100	63	100
Proteus mirabilis	357	100	95	100	100	100	100	100	100	92	100
Proteus vulgaris	24	100	0	100	100	100	0	100	100	75	100
Providencia	95	100	33	99	99	84	13	83	65	50	86
Pseudomonas aeruginosa	556	96	21	95	99		82	70			86

Gram Positive	No. of Isolates	Ampicillin	Cefamandole	Erythromycin	Clindamycin	Penicillin	Oxacillin	Trimeth./sulfa	Vancomycin
Enterococcus	456	98							100
Staph. aureus	894		46	42	41	2	46	43	100

hours any growth is then noted. If there is bacterial growth the antibiotic did not kill the organism but only inhibited it while present. The first dilution where there is no formation of colonies is then referred to as the *minimal bactericidal concentration* (MBC). The MBC is defined as the smallest concentration of antibiotic required to kill 99.9 percent of the organisms. The MBC : MIC ratio can be used to interpret whether an antibiotic is bactericidal or bacteriostatic. If the MBC is within two dilutions of the MIC, the antibiotic is considered cidal. Despite this, the clinical significance of this result is questionable.

A less commonly used determination of antibiotic susceptibility, similar in technique to the MIC, is the *serum bactericidal titer* (SBT), also known as the Schlicter test. Following administration of an antibiotic, the patient's serum is drawn and serial dilutions are then made of that serum. An inoculum of the infecting organism is then made into each dilution and incubated. Similarly to the MIC, the greatest dilution without bacterial growth is then determined. Generally, a titer of 1 : 8 correlates well with successful clinical outcome.[74] The SBT historically has not been well standardized. For this reason it is only considered potentially useful for monitoring therapy in osteomyelitis and subacute bacterial endocarditis.

Host Factors

Host factors are individual quirks in a patient that affect the antimicrobial activity, absorption, excretion, and toxicity of an antibiotic. These include age, history of prior adverse reactions, genetic and metabolic factors, renal and hepatic function, pregnancy, immune status, and site of infection.

Age will have numerous effects on the activity of the drug.[75] With increasing age there is a greater likelihood of some of the other host factors being present, such as diminished renal or hepatic function. There is a higher incidence of hypersensitivity reactions in the elderly. Absorption from the gastrointestinal tract may be affected by changes in gastric acidity. Absorption following intramuscular injection may be altered as a result of atrophy of muscle and fat. In young patients drugs such as tetracycline may permanently stain developing teeth and bones.

History of prior adverse reaction must be ascertained in each patient. This should be more in depth than just questioning if the patient is "allergic." Many patients are under the mistaken notion that they have a drug allergy when, in fact, it may be an unrelated reaction. The type and severity of any reaction should be known.

Genetic abnormalities such as glucose-6-phosphate dehydrogenase deficiency may lead to hemolysis when these patients are given sulfonamides. *Metabolic* diseases such as diabetes mellitus will have many effects, ranging from drug interactions between oral hypoglycemic agents and some antibiotics to the effects of the disease on the kidneys, causing alterations in antibiotic excretion.

Renal insufficiency will affect the way many antibiotics are metabolized and excreted, potentially causing toxic levels to build up in the patient. Although the aminoglycosides are the best known examples of this, many other antibiotics from almost all commonly used drug classes can be involved. In the face of renal dysfunction the dosage regimen of many drugs may have to be altered (Table 13-7). These dosage modifications can take the form of decreasing the amount of each dose or increasing the time interval between the doses.

Table 13-7. Antibiotics Requiring Dosage Adjustments in Varying Degrees of Renal Insufficiency

Antimicrobial agents requiring no dosage change regardless of renal function
    Erythromycin, clindamycin, chloramphenicol, doxycycline, cefoperazone, oxacillin, cloxacillin, dicloxacillin, nafcillin, nalidixic acid, rifampin, amphotericin B,[a] sulfadimidine

Antimicrobial agents requiring dosage change only with severe renal failure
    Penicillin G, amoxicillin, ampicillin, methicillin, cephalothin, cephalexin, cefamandole, cefoxitin, cefotaxime, ceftizoxime, piperacillin, lincomycin, isoniazid, ethambutol, trimethoprim-sulfamethoxazole

Antimicrobial agents requiring dosage change with impaired renal function
    Carbenicillin, ticarcillin, cefazolin, moxalactam, streptomycin, kanamycin, gentamicin tobramycin, sisomicin, amikacin, nefilmicin, polymyin B, colistin, vancomycin, flucytosine

Antimicrobial agents contraindicated in renal failure
    Tetracyclines (except doxycycline and possibly minocycline), nitrofurantoin, cephaloridine, long-acting sulfonamides, methenamine, para-aminosalicyclic acid

[a] Even though amphotericin B is excreted primarily by nonrenal means, this drug must be used with caution in patients with impaired renal function because of its nephrotoxicity.
(From Moellering,[77] with permission.)

The amount of alteration can be found in the package insert for the drug, or calculated by using a "dosing nomogram." This nomogram usually takes into account the patient's renal status, age, weight, and sex.

Hepatic dysfunction, although affecting a fewer number of drugs, can have the same problems as with renal insufficiency. The antibiotics most commonly involved are clindamycin, erythromycin, and chloramphenicol. Tetracyclines should also be avoided in these patients.

Although the use of any drug during *pregnancy* or nursing should be avoided, in some cases antibiotics may need to be used. The teratogenic potential of many drugs is unknown. However, most cephalosporins, penicillin, and erythromycin are relatively safe.[76] Only ticarcillin and metronidazole have been shown to be teratogenic in animal studies.[77] Other considerations include the ability of the drug to cross the placenta, causing toxic effects on the fetus; whether a drug is found in breast milk; or direct toxicity to the mother. An example of the latter is tetracycline. Besides its effect on the fetal bones and teeth, tetracycline has been shown to cause a fatty necrosis of the liver and renal destruction in pregnant women that may be fatal.

The patient's *immune status* will determine how the patient handles infecting bacteria. An immunocompromised patient will not be able to adequately kill and then clear the organisms. Furthermore, nonpathogenic contaminating floras may be able to gain a foothold in the patient and become pathogenic. These patients may require multiantibiotic regimens of bactericidal agents to assist their immune systems.

Finally, the *site of infection* will play a determining role in the selection of antibiotic therapy. An adequate level of antibiotic must be able to penetrate into the area and then work effectively. In the presence of an abscess, there is a decreased pH and possibly an anaerobic environment with decreased oxygenation potential. Aminoglycosides are ineffective in this situation. Implanted foreign bodies can cause a local immune compromise. Furthermore, some bacteria are capable of producing adherence factors in the presence of foreign bodies. A slime layer may shield a colony, making it impenetrable to most antibiotics, with the possible exception of clindamycin.

Drug Factors

Each class of antibiotic agents has unique properties with which the clinician should be familiar before using any member of that class. It is beyond the scope of this chapter to cover each of these in detail. Regardless of variation in different types of agents, however, there are basic properties common to all antimicrobials that should be known before any drug is used. These properties include in vitro activity, in vivo activity, potential for development of resistance, toxicity, pharmacokinetics, and cost. This guideline will also be helpful when considering any of the plethora of new antibiotics released onto the market.

In vitro activity refers to the ability of an antibiotic to work against a given pathogen in the laboratory setting. This is usually determined by running MICs and, less frequently, MBCs against large numbers of the entire range of organism for which the drug is targeted. In the literature this is then reported in terms of MIC_{50}, MIC_{90}, and "range" of MICs for each organism. The MIC_{50} can be described as that MIC at which one-half of a number of organisms of the same species are inhibited. This is actually a median number. For example, of 100 *S. aureus* strains are tested, the concentration needed to inhibit 50 of the strains is recorded. Likewise, the MIC_{90} is that concentration needed to inhibit 90 percent of the strains. The "range" is listed as the lowest MIC that was needed for the most susceptible organism of the group to the MIC for the most resistant. Of all of these numbers, the MIC_{90} is probably the most useful. Although usually a higher number than the 50 by two or more dilutions, most clinicians would rather take a 90 percent gamble on a drug's efficacy than a 50 percent one when dealing with a patient. The MIC_{50} is of limited value but seems to be the favorite of the pharmaceutical representative, who can point to significantly lower numbers in an effort to promote his drug.

In vivo activity is the ability of a drug to work against not only a specific organism, but also a specific disease state in the clinical setting. During developmental stages of a new agent the FDA requires large numbers of clinical trials to assess the safety and efficacy of the drug. These studies tend to be well controlled, blinded, randomized, and comparative, with significant numbers of patients enrolled. The data are then reviewed for statistically significant trends. Practitioners reviewing the data for applicability to their patients should keep in mind the comparability to their situation from both a microbiologic and a clinical standpoint. Although the organisms found in an intra-abdominal abscess may be similar to those found in the diabetic foot infection, the data showing efficacy in one may not be applicable to the other. Specific local factors, such as anatomic variation and circulatory deficiencies, may be present in one infection and not the other.

The development of *resistance* of an organism to an antibiotic is generally mediated in one of two ways. The bacteria can go through a chromosomally mediated genetic alteration that changes factors such as cell penetration ability and antibiotic binding. An example of this type of resistance has recently become of great clinical importance. Some staphylococcus species will alter one of the penicillin-binding proteins (PBP 2a) on their cell walls. This confers resistance to all penicillinase-resistant penicillins and cephalosporins. These organisms have become known as methicillin-resistant staphylococcus. The other method is through the production of enzymes that inactivate the antibiotic. The most common example of this is the production of β-lactamase, which will cleave the β-lactam bond of the penicillins and the cephalosporins, rendering them inactive.

The inappropriate use of antibiotics has been responsible for much of the resistance problems now encountered. If too low a dose of drug is given for too short a period of time, the bacteria may be exposed to "subinhibitory levels." Continued passes through these levels may cause an organism to become resistant to that agent. Some organisms have the ability to produce "inducible β-lactams." When exposed to β-lactam antibiotics, Gram-negative organisms such as *Enterobacter, Citrobacter,* and *serratia,* which may be initially reported as susceptible, can begin to produce β-lactams to inactivate the drug.

Toxicity, or adverse reactions, is a potential problem with all antibiotic agents. Each class has its own unique spectrum of untoward reactions (Table 13-8). There are, however, risk factors that may increase the incidence of reactions. These include

Table 13-8. Adverse Reactions of Antibiotics

Drug Class	Reactions
Penicillins	Allergy Neutropenia Seizures Platelet dysfunction Interstitial nephritis[a] Diarrhea
Cephalosporins	Allergy Bleeding[b] Alcohol intolerence[b] Diarrhea[c]
Thienamycins	Seizures[d]
Aminoglycosides	Nephrotoxicity Ototoxicity Neuromuscular blockade
Clindamycin	Diarrhea Allergy Hepatotoxicity
Vancomycin	Ototoxicity Nephrotoxicity[e] "Red man syndrome"[f]
Erythromycin	Allergy Thrombophlebitis (IV) Nausea Diarrhea Cholestatic hepatitis
Tetracyclines	Allergy Staining—teeth and bones Photosensitivity Thrombophlebitis Nausea Diarrhea Superinfection Renal Hepatic—fatty necrosis
Metronidazole	Alcohol intolerence Seizures
Rifampin	Red staining of soft contact lenses and urine
Sulfonamides	Allergy Gastrointestinal Hematologic Crystalluria

[a] Usually related to methicillin.
[b] Any drug that contains the methylthiotetrazole moiety.
[c] Most common with cefoperazone.
[d] Seen mostly in patients with prior history of seizures or with impaired renal function.
[e] Less common with newer preparations. Synergistic nephrotoxicity seen with concurrent aminoglycoside usage.
[f] Related to histamine release with too-rapid dosing.

severity of infection, previous recent exposure to an antibiotic, preexisting renal or liver disease, and increased age.

The *pharmacokinetics* of a particular antibiotic

will help to determine its frequency of dosing and efficacy in particular situations. Pharmacokinetic parameters include the half-life ($t_{1/2}$), tissue penetration, protein binding, peak and trough serum levels, volume of distribution, route of elimination, and rate of elimination, to name but a few. These all vary for each individual drug and are what is responsible for making each antibiotic unique. The clinical significance has been well documented for some of these parameters (half-life, elimination) but for others is speculative (protein binding).

Cost of antibiotics has become more important in this age of prospective payments to hospitals. The cost of giving an antibiotic can be divided into three areas: drug cost, dosing cost, and monitoring. Drug cost is the price paid for the antibiotic dose alone. This can vary from as little as $0.40 for 80 mg of gentamicin to over $30 for 1 g of some newer β-lactams. Even within a given class, such as the cephalosporins, costs can range from $2/g to as much as $25/g. The acquisition price of an antibiotic can be misleading. A drug with a prolonged $t_{1/2}$ that can be given one or twice a day, although costing more on a gram-per-gram basis, may prove less expensive to administer. Each time a drug is dosed in a hospital there is expense to prepare and give the agent to the patient. This includes pharmacy time, nursing time, bottles, and solutions. Estimates range from $5 to $10 additional cost for these services. Therefore, a drug dosed twice a day may be upwards of $20 cheaper than one dosed four times a day. The final cost is that for monitoring therapy. The best example of this is the need to measure serum levels and renal function in a patient receiving aminoglycosides. Although the antibiotic acquisition cost may be low, these drugs can prove very costly to use.

SPECIAL TOPICS IN THE USE OF ANTIBIOTICS

Antibiotic Combinations

With the new broad-spectrum antibiotics on the market, most infections in the lower extremity can be treated with the use of a single agent. There are, however, some situations in which a clinician may wish to combine two or more drugs for a variety of reasons.

There are three possible sequelae when antibiotics are combined: Synergistic activity, antagonistic activity, or indifferent (additive) activity may result. *Synergy* can be defined as the combination of drugs A and B yielding *better* activity than would be expected by their combined sum of activity. *Antagonism* is the combination of drugs A and B yielding *less* activity than would be expected from their sum. *Additive activity* is defined as the situation in which the activity of the combination yields the same as that of the sum. Unfortunately, the in vitro result of combining antibiotics can be technically difficult to demonstrate. Therefore, the activity of some combinations is not well known.

Indications

The possible use of combination therapy is indicated when one or more of the following goals is in mind: preventing resistance, using "shotgun" therapy for severe infections, if a polymicrobial infection is suspected, and if synergy can be demonstrated.

Prevention of Resistance.   The best example of this is the use of the antistaphylococcal drug rifampin. Rifampin when used alone against staphylococcus is extremely effective for a short period of time. Very rapidly the organism becomes resistant unless the rifampin has been given with another agent.

"Shotgun" Therapy.   Prior to knowing the results of the culture and sensitivity test a broad range of organisms may be covered. This is done in the hope of covering the possible pathogen from the start. The need for this type of therapy is obviated by the use of diagnostic principles covered early in this chapter. With most lower extremity infections, the probable pathogen can be determined empirically through a Gram stain, the history, the physical, and an "educated guess."

Polymicrobial Infection.   If two or more organisms are causing an infection it may be potentially difficult to cover them all with one agent. This indication is becoming less important with the advent of newer broader spectrum drugs.

Synergy.   If synergy can be determined for a combination against a particular organism, combination therapy may be indicated. The best example of this is the synergy seen by the combination of a penicillin with an aminoglycoside against *Enterococcus*. This has been demonstrated in the treatment of endocarditis, but its relevancy to lower extremity infections remains unclear.

Contraindications

Contraindications to combination therapy include antagonism, cost, and adverse reactions.

Antagonism. There are two possible antagonistic reactions that can occur when antibiotics are combined: *direct antagonism* and *microbial antagonism*. The direct type occurs before the drugs come into contact with an organism. If penicillin and an aminoglycoside are mixed together in the same container, the aminoglycoside may be inactivated. For this reason, when these two are combined they are kept in separate containers and dosed at different times. Microbial antagonism occurs when one antibiotic causes the organism to become resistant to the other. A theoretical example of this is the use of two β-lactams in combination. Because of the possibility of one drug causing inducible β-lactamases to be produced by the cell, the second β-lactam may be destroyed.

Cost. The use of two or more agents will significantly increase the cost of therapy not only because of drug cost, but also because of dosing and monitoring costs (discussed above). This increased cost of combination therapy serves to make a relatively expensive single-agent regimen cost effective.

Adverse Reactions. As stated above, all antibiotics are capable of producing adverse effects. The combination of two or more of these agents may expose the patient to a greater likelihood of this occurring. Furthermore, it may be difficult to determine which agent is causing the reaction.

Antibiotic-Associated Diarrhea

Antibiotic-associated diarrhea is mediated by two major mechanisms. Many antibiotics achieve levels in the gastrointestinal (GI) tract either through excretion directly into the gut or by metabolism in the liver. This active drug found in the GI system can cause alterations in normal gut flora, changing the way in which food is digested. These flora alterations can cause diarrhea.

The second mechanism is by the production of an enterotoxin by *Clostridium difficile*, a gram-positive obligate anaerobe sometimes found as a normal flora in the gut. Because of the production of plaques or "pseudomembranes" on the mucosa of the bowel, this variant is commonly referred to as pseudomembranous colitis. Clinically, the patient can have severe diarrhea with abdominal cramping and fever. The diagnosis of true pseudomembranous colitis must be made by proctoscopic or endoscopic examination of the bowel to demonstrate the formation of the plaques. False-negative results are possible because these plaques may form at a more proximal level beyond the reach of the scope. Stool samples can be examined for WBCs and blood, and sent for a *C. difficile* titer. Unfortunately, titers can be elevated in any patient receiving broad-spectrum antibiotics.

Treatment of antibiotic-associated diarrhea is determined by the severity of the infection and the diarrhea. If possible antibiotic therapy should be discontinued. In many cases this alone is sufficient to alleviate the diarrhea without further treatment. It is interesting to note that up to one-third of patients may not develop diarrhea until after the antibiotic has been stopped. If antibiotics must be continued specific therapy for the diarrhea should be started. In the face of positive *C. difficile* titers this specific therapy involves the use of oral vancomycin (125 mg every 6 hours) or metronidazole (500 mg every 8 hours). Vancomycin is considered the treatment of choice in severe cases because of its reliability. The intravenous form has been shown to be ineffective. The major drawback to vancomycin is its high cost. For this reason, oral metronidazole has become the drug of choice in some institutions. Therapy should be continued for 5 to 7 days.

The use of antidiarrheal agents is contraindicated. By slowing bowel motility significant levels of the toxin can build, causing a toxic megacolon.

Antibiotic Prophylaxis

Prophylaxis means pretreatment! If pretreatment is impossible, we should wait to see what happens to patients and only come to their aid when they show overt signs of infection, which we can treat specifically.[78]

The above statement by Allgower et al., from Basel, Switzerland, is included to define the overused and frequently abused term *prophylaxis*. Prophylaxis must be differentiated from *therapeutic*, by far the most common use for antibiotics. Indeed prophylaxis does mean pretreatment. If infection is already present this constitutes therapy. The first rule of prophylaxis is that the antibiotic must be at optimum levels at the time of insult or injury. The antibiotic selected should be directed against common organisms found in the infections. The organisms and their susceptibility patterns can vary in different locations. Duration of therapy remains an open question, with 24 hours appearing to be equally efficacious to longer durations.

Two arenas where prophylaxis is often considered in the lower extremity are surgery and trauma. Because the indications differ, each is covered separately. The final area in which prophylaxis is often misused is in the patient with cardiac compromise.

Surgical

The postoperative infection rate for clean, elective bone surgery is often quoted as being only 1 to 2 percent.[79] Because this is not a very common occurrence, there is a paucity of data on large enough study populations to make any definitive statement as to the necessity for prophylactic antibiotic usage in lower extremity surgery. By convention preoperative antibiotic prophylaxis may be indicated in cases in which surgery is prolonged (generally longer than 2 hours), in immunocompromised patients, when implants are employed, and in cases dealing with trauma. Again, because of a lack of any hard data, one can only theorize as to the reasons for each of these indications. Prolonged cases may subject the patient to increased risk of exogenous contamination from the operating suite. The immunocompromised patient may need the bolster that the antibiotic gives to the immune system. Implants have been shown to produce a localized area of immune compromise in their vicinity, and trauma has been shown to also cause an immune compromise. Some of the best data regarding surgical prophylaxis come from the literature on

open fractures. A marked decrease in the rate of operative infections was noted when class 3 open fractures received antibiotic prophylaxis prior to fixation.[80]

As stated in the first rule of prophylaxis, levels should be at their optimum as the tissues are exposed. For this reason, an intravenous antibiotic should be started about 20 minutes prior to the incision, and an intramuscular antibiotic closer to 1 hour prior. There is little evidence on the efficacy of oral antibiotic usage in this scenario. The antibiotic selected should be directed toward staphylococcus, the most frequent cause of postoperative infections in the lower extremity. The half-life of the drug should be prolonged so that fewer doses can be given, saving money. A first-generation cephalosporin such as cefazolin appears ideally suited for this task. If there is a high incidence of methicillin-resistant pathogens in the hospital prophylaxis with vancomycin may be indicated.

Trauma

Nowhere is the first rule breached more frequently than in the case of prophylaxis for trauma. Patients reporting to an office or emergency room with an uncomplicated puncture wound or laceration are frequently dosed with antibiotics. In fact there are few data to support this usage. Fitzgerald and Cowan found that in their study of 465 patients not given antibiotics following puncture wounds to the foot, only two required incision and drainage and one of those had a retained foreign body.[19] Likewise, Thrilby et al. found that in patients receiving suture closure of simple lacerations prophylactic antibiotics did not alter the rate of infection.[81]

Endocarditis Prophylaxis

Frequently, practitioners performing surgery on patients with histories of rheumatic heart disease, mitral valve prolapse, or valve replacement are faced with the question of endocarditis prophylaxis. Frequently the subject is broached by the patient used to taking penicillin each time a dentist works on his or her teeth. The principle behind this practice is to prevent the transient bacteremia caused by manipulation of heavily contaminated areas such as the oral cavity, the genitourinary tract, or the GI tract. Furthermore, attention is directed toward streptococcus, one of the most common causes of bacterial endocarditis and that organism found in these regions. Surgical procedures on the foot do not cause the same massive degree of bacteremia found in these other areas. Neither the American Heart Association nor the *Medical Letter* include clean elective bone surgery in their indications for prophylaxis.

REFERENCES

1. Vo NM, Watson S, Bryant LR: Infections of the lower extremities due to gas forming and non gas forming organisms. South Med J 79:1493, 1968
2. Suss SJ, Middleton DB: Cellulitis and related skin infections. Am Fam Practice 36:126, 1986
3. Stedman's Medical Dictionary. 24th Ed. Williams & Wilkins Co, Baltimore, 1987
4. Little JR, Kobayashs GE: Bacteriology and infection in the diabetic foot. p 97. In Levin ME, O'Neal LW (eds): The Diabetic Foot. St Louis, CV Mosby, 1977
5. Murphy PA: Temperature regulation and the pathogenesis of fever. In Mandell GL (ed): Principles and Practice of Infectious Diseases. 2nd Ed. Churchill Livingstone, New York, 1985
6. Dinerello CA, Wolff SM: Pathogenesis of fever in man. N Engl J Med 298:607, 1978
7. Stumacher RJ: Clinical Infectious Diseases. WB Saunders Company, Philadelphia, 1987
8. Harris RL, Musher DM, Bloom K et al: Manifestations of sepsis. Arch Intern Med 147:1895, 1987
9. Monson TP, Nelson CL: Microbiology for orthopedic surgeons: selected aspects. Clin Orthop Related Res 190:14, 1984
10. Mackowiak PA, Jones SR, Smith JW: Diagnostic value of sinus tract cultures in chronic osteomyelitis. JAMA 239:2772, 1978
11. Hook EW, Hooton TM, Horton CA et al: Microbiologic evaluation of cutaneous cellulitis in adults. Arch Intern Med 146:295, 1986
12. Epperly TO: The value of needle aspiration in the management of cellulitis. J Fam Pract 23:337, 1986
13. Johanson P: Pseudomonas infections of the foot following puncture wounds. JAMA 204:170, 1968
14. Swartz MN: Cellulitis and superficial infections. In Mandell GL (ed): Principles and Practice of Infec-

tious Diseases. 2nd Ed. Churchill Livingstone, New York, 1985
15. Downey MS, Yu GV: Post-saphenous phlebectomy donor leg cellulitis. J Am Podiatr Med Assoc 77:277, 1987
16. Abramson C, Steinmetz R: Antifungal activity of *Pseudomonas aeruginosa* in gram-negative athlete's foot. J Am Podiatry Assoc 73:227, 1983
17. Kosatsky T, Kleeman J: Superficial and systemic illness related to a hot tub. Am J Med 79:10, 1985
18. Eells LD, Mertz P, Piovanetti Y: Topical antibiotic treatment of impetigo with mupirocin. Arch Dermatol 122:1273, 1986
19. Fitzgerald R, Cowan J: Puncture wounds of the foot. Orthop Clin North Am 6:965, 1975
20. Houston A, Roy W, Faust R, Ewin DM: Tetanus prophylaxis in the treatment of puncture wounds of patients in the deep South. J Trauma 2:439, 1962
21. Chusid MJ, Jacobs WM, Sty JR: Pseudomonas arthritis following puncture wounds of the foot. J Pediatr 94:429, 1979
22. Miller E, Semian D: Gram-negative osteomyelitis following puncture wounds of the foot. J Bone Joint Surg 57A:535, 1975
23. Lang A, Peterson H: Osteomyelitis following puncture wounds of the foot in children. J Trauma 16:993, 1976
24. Joseph WS, LeFrock JL: Infections complicating puncture wounds of the foot. J Foot Surg 26:530, 1987
25. Siebert WT, Dewan S, Williams TW: Case report: Pseudomonas puncture wound osteomyelitis in adults. Am J Med Sci 283:83, 1982
26. Fritz R: Concerning the source of Pseudomonas osteomyelitis of the foot (letter). J Pediatr 91:161, 1977
27. Mahan KT, Kalish SR: Complications following puncture wounds of the foot. Am Podiatry Assoc 72:497, 1982
28. Minnefor AB, Olson MI, Carver DH: Pseudomonas osteomyelitis following puncture wounds of the foot. Pediatrics 47:598, 1971
29. Green N, Bruno J: Pseudomonas infections of the foot after puncture wounds. South Med J 73:146, 1980
30. Jacobs RF, Adelman L, Sack C, Wilson CB: Management of Pseudomonas osteochondritis complicating puncture wounds of the foot. Pediatrics 69:432, 1982
31. Coffey JA Jr., Harris RL, Rutledge ML: *Vibrio damsela:* another potentially virulent marine vibrio. J Infect Dis 153:800, 1986
32. Sanders WE: Other mycobacterium species. In Mandell GL (ed): Principles and Practice of Infec-

tious Diseases. 2nd Ed. Churchill Livingstone, New York, 1985

33. Bell ET: Atherosclerotic gangrene of the lower extremities in diabetic and non-diabetic persons. Am J Clin Pathol 28:27, 1957

34. Joseph WS, LeFrock JL: The pathogenesis of diabetic foot infections—immunopathy, angiopathy, and neuropathy. J Foot Surg 26:57, 1987

35. Ellenberg M, Bifkin H (eds): Diabetes Mellitus: Theory and Practice. p 734. McGraw-Hill, New York, 1970

36. Bates G, Weiss C: Delayed development of antibody to staphylococcus toxin in diabetic children. Am J Dis Child 62:346, 1941

37. Richardson R: Immunity in diabetes: influence of diabetes in the development of antibacterial properties in the blood. J Clin Invest 12:1143, 1933

38. Mowat AG, Baum J: Chemotaxis of polymorphonuclear leukocytes from patients with diabetes mellitus. N Engl J Med 284:621, 1971

39. Molenaar DM, Palumbo PJ, Wilson WR, Ritts RE, Jr.: Leukocyte chemotaxis in diabetic patients and their non-diabetic first degree relatives. Diabetes 25:880, 1976

40. MacCuish AC, Urbaniak SJ, Campbell CJ et al: Phytohaemagglutinin transformation and circulating lymphocyte subpopulation in insulin-dependent diabetic patients. Diabetes 23:708, 1974

41. Robertson WB, Strong JP: Atherosclerosis in patients with hypertension and diabetes mellitus. Lab Invest 18:538, 1968

42. Dinerstein C, Mason R, Giron F: Lower extremity complications of diabetes mellitus. Surg Rounds 7:26, 1984

43. LoGerfo FW, Coffman JD: Vascular and microvascular disease of the foot in diabetes. N Engl J Med 311:1615, 1984

44. Zatz A, Brenner BM: Pathogenesis of diabetic microangiopathy: the hemodynamic view. Am J Med 80:443, 1986

45. Rashkin P, Pietri AO, Unger R, Shannon WA: The effect of diabetic control on the width of skeletal-muscle capillary basement membrane in patients with type I diabetes mellitus. N Engl J Med 309:1546, 1983

46. Brown MJ, Asbury AK: Diabetic neuropathy. Ann Neurol 15:2, 1984

47. Greene DA, DeJesus PV, Winegrad AI: Effects of insulin and dietary myoinositol on impaired peripheral motor nerve conduction velocity in acute streptozotocin diabetes. J Clin Invest 55:1326, 1975

48. Greenwood AM: A study of the skin in 500 cases of diabetes. JAMA 89:774, 1927

49. Alteras I, Saryt E: Prevalence of pathogenic fungi in the toe-webs and toe-nails of diabetic patients. Mycopathologica 67:157, 1979

50. Huntley AC: The cutaneous manifestations of diabetes mellitus. J Am Acad Dermatol 7:427, 1982

51. LeFrock JL, Blais F, Schell RF et al: Cefoxitin in the treatment of diabetic patients with lower extremity infections. Infect Surg 2:361, 1983

52. Waldvogel FA, McDoff G, Swartz MN: Osteomyelitis: a review of clinical features, therapeutic considerations and unusual aspects. N Engl J Med 282:198, 1970

53. Sharp CS, Bessman AN, Wagner FW, Jr. et al: Microbiology of superficial and deep tissues in infected diabetic gangrene. Surg Gynecol Obstet 149:217, 1979

54. Sapico FA, Canwati HN, Witte JL et al: Quantitative aerobic and anaerobic bacteriology of the infected diabetic foot. J Clin Microbiol 12:413, 1980

55. Friedman SA, Gladstone JL: The bacterial flora of peripheral vascular ulcers. Arch Dermatol 100:29, 1969

56. Khan O, Wagnon W, Bessman AN: Mortality of diabetic patients treated surgically for lower limb infection and/or gangrene. Diabetes 23:287, 1974

57. Sapico EL, Witte JL, Canawati HN et al: The infected foot of the diabetic patient. Quant Microbiol 6(suppl 1):S171, 1984

58. Bessman AN, Sapico FL, Tabatabai M: Persistance of polymicrobial abscesses in the poorly controlled diabetic host. Diabetes 35:448, 1986

59. LeFrock JL, Blais F, Schell RF et al: Cefoxitin in the treatment of diabetic patients with lower extremity infections. Infect Surg 2:361, 1983

60. Calandra G, Raupp W, Brown K: Treatment of lower extremity skin and soft tissue infections in diabetics with imipenem/cilastatin. Abstract, 15th International Congress of Chemotherapy, Istanbul, Turkey, 1987

61. Smith N: Observations on the pathology and treatment of necrosis (reprinted). Rev Infect Dis 8:505, 1986

62. Chandrasekar PH, Narula AP: Bone and joint infections in intravenous drug abusers. Rev Infect Dis 8:904, 1986

63. Quie PG, Belani KK: Coagulase negative staphylococcal adherence and persistence. J Infect Dis 156:543, 1987

64. Cierny G, Mader JT, Penninck JJ: A clinical staging system for adult osteomyelitis. Contemp Orthop 10:17, 1985

65. Buckholz JM: The surgical management of osteo-

myelitis: with special reference to a surgical classification. J Foot Surg 26:517, 1987

66. Park HM, Wheat LJ, Siddiqui AR: Scintigraphic evaluation of diabetic osteomyelitis: concise communication. J Nucl Med 23:569, 1982

67. Park HM, Burt RW, Mock BH: Simultaneous 3-phase bone scan and In-111 WBC in the evaluation of neuropathic foot disease. (Abstract, 34 Annual meeting, The Society of Nuclear Medicine.) J Nucl Med 28:649, 1987

68. Roach JW: Early diagnosis and treatment of acute hematogenous osteomyelitis in children. Infect Surg 2:913, 1983

69. Ang-Fonte GZ, Rozbork MB, Thompson GR: Changes in nongonococcal septic arthritis: drug abuse and methicillin-resistant *Staphylococcus aureus*. Arthritis Rheum 23:889, 1980

70. Goldenberg DL, Cohen AS: Acute infectious arthritis. Am J Med 60:369, 1976

71. Rosenthal J, Giles GB, Robinson WD: Acute nongonococcal infectious arthritis. Arthritis Rheum 23:889, 1980

72. Goldenberg DL, Brant KD, Cohen AS: Treatment of septic arthritis. Arthritis Rheum 18:83, 1975

73. LeFrock JL, Kannangapa DW: Bacterial arthritis. In Kass E (ed): Current Therapy in Infectious Disease 1983–1984. BC Decker, Philadelphia, 1983

74. Black J, Hunt TL, Godley PJ: Oral antimicrobial therapy for adults with osteomyelitis or septic arthritis. J Infect Dis 155:968, 1987

75. Weinstein L, Dalton AC: Host determinants of response to antimicrobial agents. N Engl J Med 279:467, 1968

76. Safety of antimicrobial drugs in pregnancy. Med Lett 29:61, 1987

77. Moellering RC: Principles of anti-infective therapy. In Mandell GL (ed): Principles and Practice of Infectious Diseases. 2nd Ed. Churchill Livingstone, New York, 1985

78. Allgöwer M, Durig M, Wolff G: Infection and trauma. Surg Clin North Am 60:133, 1980

79. Nelson CL: The prevention of infection in total joint replacement surgery. Rev Infect Dis 9:613, 1987

80. Gustilo RB, Anderson JT: Prevention of infection in the treatment of one thousand and twenty five open fractures of long bones. J Bone Joint Surg [Am] 58:453, 1976

81. Thrilby RC, Blair AJ III, Thal ER: The value of prophylactic antibiotics for simple lacerations. Surg Gynecol Obstet 156:212, 1983

82. Scurran BL: Foot and Ankle Trauma. Churchill Livingstone, New York, 1989

Neoplasms That Involve the Skin, Soft Tissue, and Bone of the Foot — 14

Dennis Anderson, D.O., Cmdr. M.C., U.S.N.R.

Neoplasm, as defined in general pathology, refers to "new growth." This chapter deals with the most common neoplasms found on the skin of the foot, as well as those that involve soft tissue and bone. Berlin, in his article in the *Journal of American Podiatric Association*, presented a table that listed the 25 most common benign lesions.[1] Some of the lesions listed are not considered neoplasia, but rather result from fibrosis, degeneration, or in some cases a metabolic disorder. This chapter by definition then excludes these types of processes and concentrate solely on tumors.

Exhaustive lists for histologic classification of soft tissue tumors as well as bone and skin are easily found in the World Health Organization Histological Classification of Tumors or in specific Armed Forces Institute of Pathology Fascicles. In this chapter those lesions that are most commonly encountered are included, while the more esoteric or rare neoplastic processes are excluded. The histological classification used in this chapter is as follows:

I. Skin Neoplasms
  A. Benign neoplasms of surface epidermal origin
    1. Verruca plantaris
    2. Seborrheid keratosis
    3. Clear cell acanthoma
    4. Keratoacanthoma
  B. Premalignant neoplasms of surface epidermal origin
    1. Actinic keratosis
    2. Bowen's disease
  C. Malignant neoplasms of surface epidermal origin
    1. Basal cell carcinoma
    2. Squamous cell carcinoma
  D. Neoplasms of cutaneous appendages: eccrine
    1. Eccrine poroma
    2. Eccrine carcinoma
  E. Benign neoplasms of vascular origin
    1. Granuloma pyogenicum
    2. Angiokeratoma
    3. Glomus tumor
    4. Hemangiopericytoma
  F. Malignant neoplasms of vascular origin
    1. Kaposi sarcoma
    2. Angiosarcoma
  G. Benign pigmented neoplasms of melanocytic origin
    1. Lentio benigna
    2. Junctional nevus
    3. Intradermal nevus
    4. Compound nevus
    5. Blue nevus
  H. Malignant pigmented neoplasms of melanocytic origin
    1. Lentigo maligna

2. Superficial spreading melanoma in situ
3. Superficial spreading melanoma
4. Nodular melanoma
5. Malignant melanoma arising in compound nevus
I. Malignant neoplasms of lymphoid cell origin
   1. Lymphoma
   2. Mycosis fungoides
II. Neoplasms of soft tissue origin
  A. Fibrous tissue origin
    1. Dermatofibroma
    2. Giant cell tumor of tendon sheath
    3. Fibroma
    4. Fibrosarcoma
  B. Smooth muscle origin
    1. Leiomyoma
    2. Leiomyosarcoma
  C. Lipocyte origin
    1. Lipoma
    2. Liposarcoma
  D. Nerve tissue origin
    1. Neuroma
    2. Neurofibroma
    3. Neurolemmoma
III. Neoplasms that arise from bones of the foot
  A. Neoplasms that form bone—benign and malignant
    1. Osteoid osteoma
    2. Osteoblastoma
    3. Osteogenic sarcoma
    4. Juxtacortical osteogenic sarcoma
  B. Neoplasms that form cartilage—benign and malignant
    1. Osteochondroma
    2. Enchondroma
    3. Juxtacortical chondroma
    4. Chondroblastoma
    5. Chondromyxoid fibroma
    6. Chondrosarcoma
  C. Neoplasms of fibrous connective tissue origin—benign and malignant
    1. Desmoplastic fibroma
    2. Fibrosarcoma
  D. Neoplasms of histiocytic or fibrohistiocytic origin—benign and malignant
    1. Giant cell tumor
    2. Nonossifying fibroma
    3. Ewing's sarcoma
  E. Neoplasms of blood vessel origin—benign and malignant

1. Hemangioma
2. Malignant hemangioendothelioma
F. Neoplasms of lymphoid tissue origin
   1. Non-Hodgkin's lymphoma

If the reader desires more detailed information, a list of a number of excellent textbooks regarding skin, soft tissue, or bone neoplasms has been included at the end of this chapter.

SKIN NEOPLASMS

This section of the chapter deals with skin neoplasms. I have included a list of words and their definitions at the beginning of this section so that the reader may have a better understanding of certain key words used when describing the histologic patterns associated with each neoplasm.

Definition of Terms

Acantholysis—loss of the ability of two epithelial cells to stick tightly together

Acanthosis—the epidermis thickens mainly as a result of increased proliferation of the prickle layer (stratum malpighii)

Anaplasia—atypical appearance of nuclei found in malignant neoplastic cells. The atypical nuclei demonstrate pleomorphism, high nuclear-to-cytoplasmic ratio, and abnormal mitotic figures

Bulla—a cavity found within the epidermis or beneath it that is filled with fluid or plasma

Crust—fibrin, serum proteins, and cellular debris that are deposited upon the surface of the epidermis

Dendrite cells—melanocytes and Langerhans' cells

Dyskeratosis—epidermal cells that are prematurely keratinized

Excoriation—tearing away of the epidermis, which leaves a superficial ulcer

Hyperkeratosis—markedly thickened epidermis

Keratinocyte — a squamous epithelial cell found within the epidermis

Keratohyalin — irregularly shaped granules that are deeply basophilic; these are found in the basal layer of the epidermis

Melanocyte — a dendritic cell found in the basal layer of the epidermis

Melanophage — a macrophage or histiocyte that has ingested melanin granules

Papillomatosis — upward proliferation of the subdermal papillae, which causes the surface of the epidermis to appear wavy

Spongiosis — epidermal intercellular edema

Normal Skin

For comparative purposes, I would like to describe normal skin. Figure 14-1 demonstrates a section from normal skin. The skin is divided into an epidermis and dermis. The epidermis is composed of four layers: (1) the basal layer, (2) the squamous cell layer, (3) the granular layer, and (4) the horny layer. Within the dermis are certain adnexal structures that consist of eccrine glands, apocrine glands, and sebaceous glands. The dermis is rich in a connective tissue matrix and the adnexal

structures are found throughout the dermis, as well as vessels and nerve structures.

Benign Neoplasms of Surface Epidermal Origin

Verruca Plantaris[2-4]

This lesion, caused by a papillomavirus, produces a verrucous tumor (or wart). The most common serotype associated with verruca plantaris is human papillomavirus (HPV)-2 or HPV-4. The sole of the foot is frequently involved, but the lateral aspects or tips of the toes may also be affected. Grossly, the plantar warts are often covered by a thick callus and appear raised above the epidermal surface. When the thick callus is removed, the underlying wart is usually soft and white, and may occur in clusters or as so-called mosaic warts.

Figure 14-2 demonstrates the histology of a papillomatous epidermal wart with striking acanthosis as well as hyperkeratosis. Vacuolization of cells within the granular layer and upper portion of the malpighian layer is a common feature. Clumped keratohyaline granules are not as numerous when compared to verruca vulgaris. Occasionally, the verruca plantaris lesion demonstrates focal

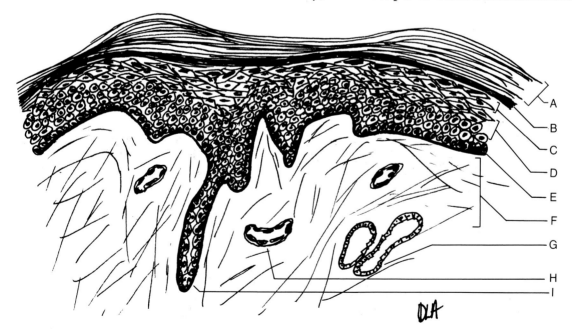

Fig. 14-1. Normal skin. **A,** horny layer; **B,** granular layer; **C,** Prickle cell layer; **D,** transition zone; **E,** basal layer; **F,** dermis; **G,** sweat gland; **H,** vessels, **I,** rete ridge.

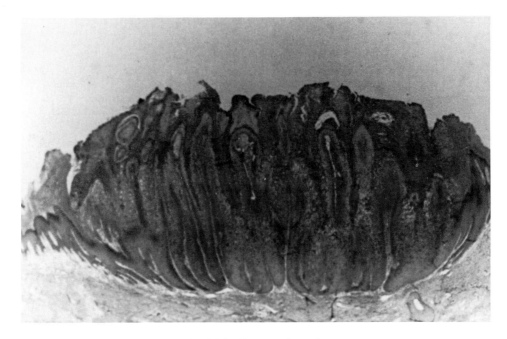

Fig. 14-2. Verruca plantaris.

heavy inflammation, composed mostly of lymphocytes as well as some neutrophils.

Seborrheic Keratosis[5,6]

These neoplasms, thought to be derived from the epidermal basal cell layer, usually appear during middle age. They are rarely seen on the sole of the foot, but may occur anywhere on the trunk, face, or extremities. Grossly, they appear as raised, sharply circumscribed lesions with a friable, verrucous-appearing surface. Often deeply pigmented, they appear gray-black because of melanin pigment within the keratinocytes. They vary in size from a few millimeters to several centimeters in diameter. Microscopically six histologic varieties are commonly found: acanthotic, hyperkeratotic, adenoid, clonal, irritated, and melanoacanthoma. For the sake of discussion we will deal almost exclusively with the acanthotic type.

The acanthotic type is one of the most common skin neoplasms observed in clinical practice. Figure 14-3 demonstrates the histology of a reticulated, acanthotic type of seborrheic keratosis. The acanthotic epidermis is raised above the adjacent, normal epidermis. Several "pseudohorn cysts," which represent hyperkeratotic invaginations, are seen. A few true horn cysts may also be present. Numerous small basaloid keratinocytes are noted, and melanin pigment is found in the keratinocytes. Some dermal melanophages are also found in the epidermal neoplasm. Although not difficult to diagnose microscopically, the lesions may present a problem clinically. Occasionally malignant melanoma is mistaken for seborrheic keratosis; however, on histologic section, seborrheic keratosis does not contain malignant nevus cells. Also, seborrheic keratosis is thought to represent squamous cell carcinoma of the verrucous pattern, but on histologic examination malignant keratinocytes are not present.

Clear Cell Acanthoma[7,8]

Clear cell acanthomas are neoplasms composed of large, glycogen-rich keratinocytes. These neoplasms, located on the lower extremities particularly near the ankle, appear as solitary, reddish nodules or plaques that are slow growing. Often covered by a thin crust, they exude some moisture. Microscopically (Fig. 14-4) these neoplasms demonstrate a prominent clear zone of epidermis that

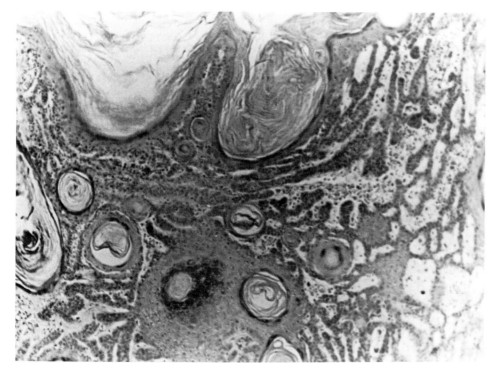

Fig. 14-3. Seborrheic keratosis.

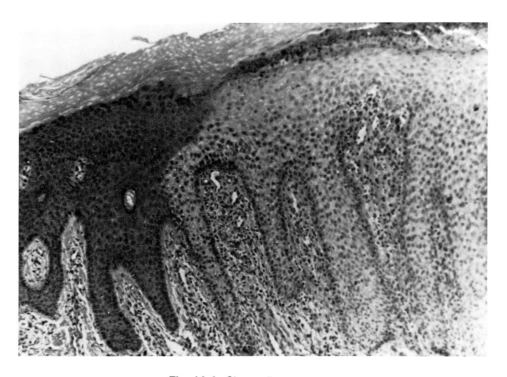

Fig. 14-4. Clear cell acanthoma.

reveals large keratinocytes. The keratinocytes contain a uniformly clear cytoplasm with benign nuclei. Parakeratosis is also seen. Decreased melanin is found in the affected area, and acanthosis, as well as elongation of the rete ridges, is seen. Capillaries are frequently found in the dermal papillae, and occasionally chronic inflammatory cells are located near the dermal-epidermal junction. Special stains for glycogen, which include periodic acid–Schiff (PAS; diastase positive), show large amounts of glycogen within the cells. Occasionally the neoplasm may demonstrate fragmented white blood cells sprinkled throughout the main lesion that appear as nuclear dust.

Keratoacanthoma[9,10]

Keratoacanthomas have not been reported on the soles of the feet, but may appear on any other sun-exposed surface, particularly the dorsal surface of the legs. Keratoacanthomas are thought to arise from a viral source, and are believed to start with hyperplasia of the infundibular epithelium of one or several adjoining hair follicles. Keratoacanthomas grossly appear as solitary lesions, but multiple lesions have been reported in a few cases. Typically, the lesions are large, dome-shaped, fleshy nodules with a crater that appears umbilicated. The crater is covered by a thickened layer of hyperkeratotic cells.

Microscopically (Fig. 14-5) a large keratin-filled crater is seen. The crater is surrounded by an irregular epidermal proliferation that extends up over the crater and lies against it in a buttress or shelflike manner. Many of the epithelial cells are larger than normal, and appear "glassy" due to partial keratinization. Parakeratosis is found within the central keratotic masses. Horny pearls, as well as dyskeratotic cells, may occasionally be seen. At the base of the lesion, young germinative cells, which show numerous mitoses, are noted. Some of the mitoses may also appear atypical. Dense inflammatory cell infiltrates are seen adjacent to the base of the lesion.

Distinguishing a well-differentiated squamous cell carcinoma from a keratoacanthoma may be

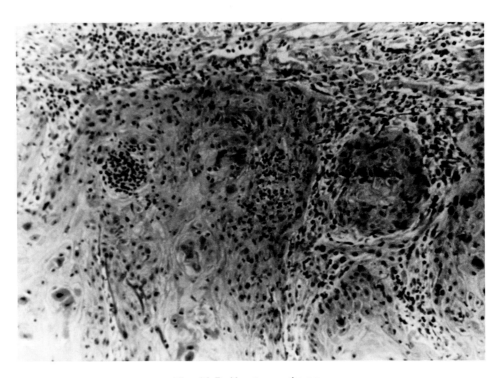

Fig. 14-5. Keratoacanthoma.

quite difficult, if not impossible. Structural features that lean more toward a benign keratoacanthoma include rapid growth, lack of significant nuclear atypia, and the presence of a button or collar surrounding the crater of the lesion.

Premalignant Neoplasms of Surface Epidermal Origin

Actinic Keratosis (Solar Keratosis)[11,12]

Actinic keratosis is a premalignant lesion of the surface epidermis that may undergo transformation into a squamous cell carcinoma. The culmulative effects of ultraviolet radiation are thought to induce the epidermal atypia associated with this condition. Actinic keratosis is most frequently seen in fair-skinned individuals who have a long history of sun exposure. All areas of the skin, including the lower extremity, have been reported as developing actinic keratosis. Grossly, erythema with focal scaling or hyperkeratosis is seen. Lesions are usually less than 1 cm in diameter. Occasionally, some ac-

tinic keratoses are pigmented and demonstrate peripheral spreading that closely mimics superficial spreading melanoma.

Five types of actinic keratosis may be recognized histologically, and are classified as hypertrophic, lichenoid, bowenoid, acantholytic, and atrophic. Figure 14-6 demonstrates the histology of the hypertrophic type of actinic keratosis. Varying degrees of hyperkeratosis, as well as parakeratosis, are seen. Careful examination of the lower portion of the epidermis demonstrates disorderly pleomorphic keratinocytes as well as several dyskeratotic cells. Nuclear atypia is frequently found in the keratinocytes, and on careful examination of the dermis solar degeneration, as well as solar elastosis and inflammation, are noted.

Squamous cell carcinoma is associated with actinic keratosis, and multiple microscopic sections may be necessary in order to prove the presence of squamous cell carcinoma. Radiation dermatitis may mimic actinic keratosis, but is separated from this entity by history and the absence of solar degeneration. Melanoma may also mimic actinic keratosis,

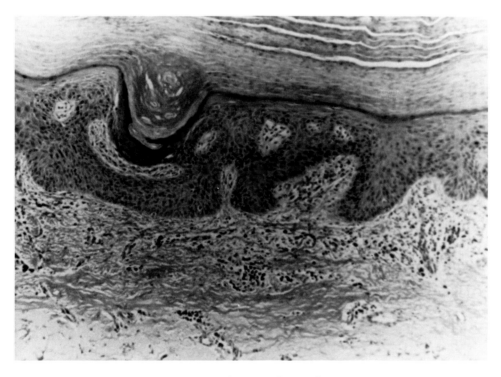

Fig. 14-6. Actinic keratosis.

but no malignant melanocytes are noted in the epidermis of the actinic keratotic lesion.

Bowen's Disease (Carcinoma In Situ)[13,14]

Bowen's disease is not related to sun exposure, and may be found in both sun- and non-sun-exposed areas. Electron microscopy of Bowen's disease demonstrates many dyskeratotic cells with no evidence of melanocytes or basaloid cells. Bowen's disease, like actinic keratosis, may undergo transformation into squamous cell carcinoma. The site of origin of Bowen's disease may be any sun-exposed, as well as non-sun-exposed, surface, including the foot. However, the sole is rarely involved by this process. Grossly, a slowly growing and enlarging erythematous patch or plaque is seen that has nodular, as well as focal, somewhat crusted areas. Little or no infiltration is seen, but a sharp irregular outline of the lesion is usually present.

Microscopically (Fig. 14-7) the epidermis is acanthotic, and the rete ridges are blunt to slightly rounded. Hyperkeratosis, as well as parakeratosis, may be present. Moderate to severe vacuolization of the epithelial cells is seen, and nuclear atypia is frequent with a high nucleus-to-cell (N : C) ratio as well as increased atypical mitotic activity. Lower levels of the epidermis demonstrate large hyperkeratotic nuclei. Large eosinophilic dyskeratotic cells are scattered throughout the lower portion of the epidermis. The dermis demonstrates a chronic inflammatory cell infiltrate that appears to be reactive to the neoplastic process.

Malignant Neoplasms of Surface Epidermal Origin

Basal Cell Carcinoma[15-17]

Two views are held regarding basal cell carcinoma. Lever believes that basal cell carcinomas are not true carcinomas but are nevoid tumors or hamartomas derived from primary epithelial germ cells.[15] Basal cell carcinomas would be neoplasms originating from incompletely differentiated immature cells and not from true anaplastic cells. However, other authors regard basal cell carcinomas as true carcinomas because of the similar

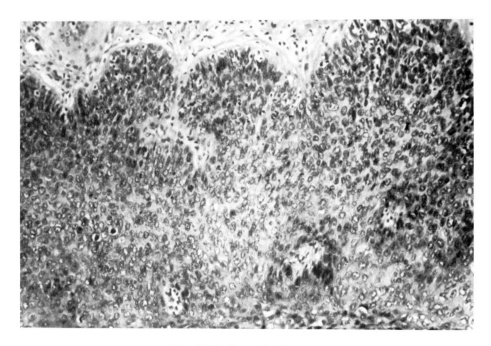

Fig. 14-7. Bowen's disease.

histogenesis of basal cell carcinomas and squamous cell carcinomas. Basal cell carcinomas usually develop during middle age or later life. Most commonly observed in areas of sun-damaged skin, the face and upper extremities are particularly prone to this condition. The condition is also noted in fair-skinned individuals with a history of long-term exposure to sunlight. Basal cell carcinomas have been reported on the sole as well as the dorsal surface of the foot. Basal cell carcinomas rarely metastasize, but have a tendency to ulcerate and invade underlying structures. If this condition is left unchecked in and around the nose and eyes, severe, extensive tissue damage and subsequent surgical reconstruction procedures may be necessary. On the foot, the condition can lead to large areas of scar after proper excision.

Grossly, five clinical types of basal cell carcinoma are noted: noduloulcerative, superficial, cystic, morphea-like, and pigmented. This section deals exclusively with the noduloulcerated basal cell carcinoma. Information on the other histologic types of basal cell carcinoma may be found in any of several dermatopathology textbooks included at the end of this chapter.

Basal cell carcinoma of the noduloulcerated type appears as transluscent, somewhat pearly nodules extending above the surface of the skin. Central ulceration is noted, but occasionally irregular ulceration occurs. Figure 14-8 demonstrates the microscopic appearance a typical noduloulcerated basal cell carcinoma. The epidermis is somewhat flattened and thin, while the dermis contains numerous uniform islands of tumor cells. A connection of the tumor cells to the superficial epidermis is often observed. The individual islands or nests of tumor cells are surrounded by a slightly loose or edematous stroma. Individual nests demonstrate two types of nuclei. The outer periphery of tumor cells demonstrates compact, hyperchromatic nuclei that tend to be cuboidal and arrange themselves in a picket fence manner. The more centrally located tumor cells are somewhat vesicular and haphazardly arranged. Chronic inflammatory cell infiltrates are commonly observed within the dermis.

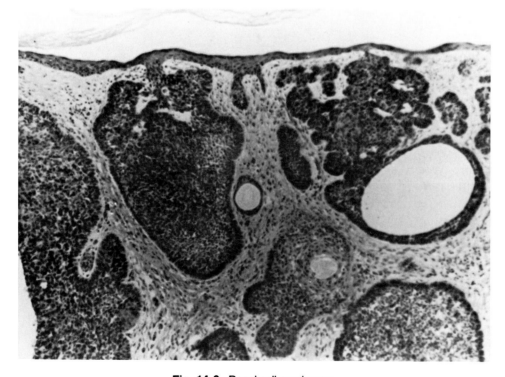

Fig. 14-8. Basal cell carcinoma.

Squamous Cell Carcinoma[18-21]

Squamous cell carcinoma is a malignant neoplasm derived from the epidermis. Although associated with premalignant conditions such as solar keratosis, Bowen's disease, premalignant leukoplakia, radiation keratosis, and arsenic keratosis, it may arise de novo. Squamous cell carcinoma may develop at the margins of chronic ulcers, as well as burn scars. Verrucous squamous cell carcinoma usually originates on the sole of the foot. The ulcers may be very large and show some raised margins. The surface of the neoplasm may be quite papillomatous or verrucous in appearance, resembling keratoacanthoma. Local tissue destruction is rather severe, but there is little tendency to produce regional metastasis. In one case that I personally examined, the patient had a long-standing history of unrecognized verrucous squamous cell carcinoma of the sole of the foot that metastasized to the inguinal lymph nodes. No other organs were involved by this process.

Microscopically (Fig. 14-9) verrucous squamous cell carcinoma shows striking hyperkeratosis, parakeratosis, acanthosis, and papillomatosis. The dermis is invaded by broad bands of malignant squamous cells composed of horn pearls, as well as dyskeratotic cells. In the case that I reviewed, several sections were required to confirm the diagnosis of verrucous cell carcinoma because many of the larger areas appeared completely benign.

Four grades are usually assigned when describing microscopic features of squamous cell carcinomas, and a reasonable attempt should be made to assign a grade to the carcinoma. Grade 1 is associated with a neoplasm in which 75 percent of the cells are quite differentiated and atypicality of the nuclei is very mild. In Grade 2 neoplasms, the number of well-differentiated cells drops to 50 to 75 percent. A definite increase in nuclear atypia occurs, and horn pearls, as well as dyskeratotic cells, are usually observed. In Grade 3 neoplasms, 25 to 50 percent of the cells are well differentiated, while the rest demonstrate high N:C ratios and atypia of the nuclei. In Grade 4 neoplasms, less than 25 percent of the cells are well differentiated, and nuclear atypia is severe. Spindle-like cells are noted, and intracellular bridges are very difficult to

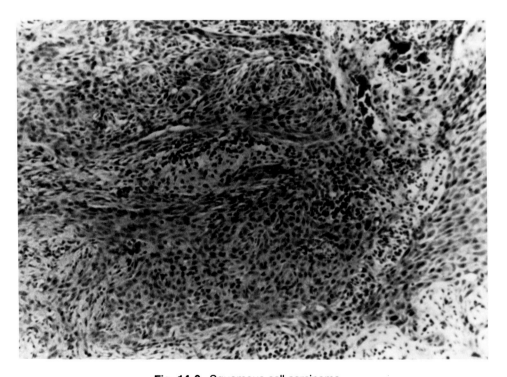

Fig. 14-9. Squamous cell carcinoma.

find. Most squamous cell carcinomas demonstrate large pleomorphic nuclei with prominent nucleoli.

Neoplasms of Cutaneous Appendages: Eccrine Differentiation

Eccrine Poroma

Eccrine poromas are thought to be derived from the outer layer of poral epithelial cells that are found lining the outer layer of the intraepidermal eccrine duct. They occur most often on the sole of the foot or the sides of the foot. However, they are frequently noted on the palms, neck, chest, and fingers. Eccrine poromas appear as somewhat pedunculated reddish-brown masses. They are rather firm in consistency, and are painless. Microscopically, tumor cells are fairly small and are quite uniform in appearance. No palisading at the periphery of the tumor occurs. Within the tumor, tubular structures resembling eccrine ducts are easily seen. The cells are strongly PAS positive, because of the heavy deposits of glycogen within individual cells. The tumor cells seldom appear as masses and may be entirely intradermal or entirely intraepidermal. The supporting stroma shows rich vascularization. Eccrine poromas can be differentiated from seborrheic keratosis simply because eccrine poromas grow downward and have tubular structures present. Pseudohorn cysts are absent. Eccrine poromas can be differentiated from basal cell carcinomas because they appear to have more cytoplasm and have distinct intercellular bridges as well as glycogen.

Malignant Eccrine Poroma

Malignant eccrine poromas may arise from a typical poroma. These lesions appear as nodules on the sole or sides of the foot, and may demonstrate some ulceration, particularly in the center of the lesion. Unfortunately, malignant eccrine poromas have a potential to produce widespread metastasis and death. Cutaneous metastasis is common, and the neoplasm may have a dermal or epidermal distribution. Histologically, malignant eccrine poromas demonstrate areas composed of normal eccrine cells that are completely benign with sudden demarcation into malignant zones showing anaplastic cells. The anaplastic or malignant cells are large and quite hyperchromatic, with irregularly shaped nuclei. The cells may be multinucleated, and are rich in glycogen.

Benign Neoplasms of Vascular Origin

Granuloma Pyogenicum[22]

Granuloma pyogenicum usually occurs as a single lesion. It most often is noted on the face and fingers, but some cases have been reported involving the foot, particularly the dorsal surface and near the toes. Grossly, granuloma pyogenicum are slightly pedunculated, dark red or reddish-brown, nodular lesions that show superficial ulceration and crusting. The lesions bleed quite easily when traumatized. Granuloma pyogenicum rarely grows beyond 0.5 cm in diameter. The cells of the granuloma pyogenicum are derived from endothelium that in essence shows endothelial proliferation and closely mimics a capillary hemangioma. Figure 14-10 demonstrates the microscopic appearance of a typical granuloma pyogenicum. The lesion is raised above the surface, and the epidermis appears quite thin with a somewhat acanthotic margin or so-called collarette. Within this zone is a circumscribed cluster of young capillaries lined by prominent endothelial cells. Some masses of endothelial cells are also noted with very little vascular lumen being identified. The endothelial cells as well as lumens are generally separated from each other by edema as well as loose connective tissue. Ulceration of the epidermis may be seen that is often secondarily inflamed.

Differential diagnosis would include Kaposi's sarcoma as well as a nodular malignant melanoma. In the case of Kaposi's sarcoma, fibroblastic proliferation, as well as vascular slits and hemorrhage, are seen. Granuloma pyogenicum does not demonstrate these features. Differentiation from a malignant melanoma, nodular type, is not difficult based on the presence of malignant melanocytes.

Angiokeratoma[23]

Five types of angiokeratoma occur. The discussion in this chapter concerns the Mibelli types. An-

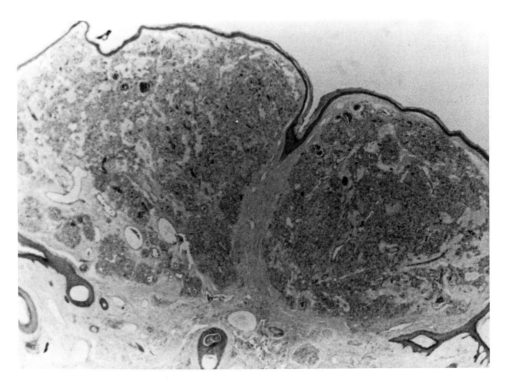

Fig. 14-10. Granuloma pyogenicum.

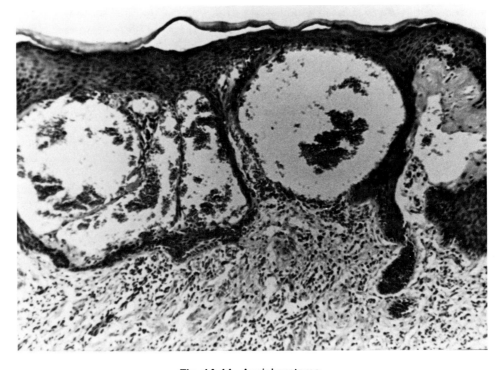

Fig. 14-11. Angiokeratoma.

giokeratoma of Mibelli usually develops in childhood or adolescence and is seen principally on the fingers and toes. The lesions are usually bilateral. Grossly, the lesions appear as hyperkeratotic, red papules on the dorsal surface of the skin. They average around 2 to 4 mm in diameter and may be soft or even compressible. Figure 14-11 demonstrates the microscopic appearance of a typical angiokeratoma. The epidermis shows hyperkeratosis, as well as papillomatosis and acanthosis. In the papillary dermis, numerous engorged, dilated capillaries are noted. The dilated capillaries impinge on the epidermis, and in some instances appear to be surrounded by the epidermis. Although referred to as "blood cysts," careful observation reveals no discernible endothelial lining.

Solitary Glomus Tumors[24]

Glomus cells are usually thought to be derived from vascular smooth muscle cells. Glomus tumors usually demonstrate a violaceous, slightly raised lesion commonly located on the distal part of the digits. The nodules are very tender, and sometimes give rise to extreme pain. They rarely exceed a few millimeters in diameter. Microscopically (Fig. 14-12) the glomus tumor lesions appear encapsulated. Numerous vessels lined by single layers of endothelial cells are noted. External to the endothelial cells are sheaths and nests of glomus cells. The glomus cells have faint cytoplasm and large round to oval nuclei. The glomus cells appear rather uniform. The stroma surrounding the cells is edematous, containing scattered fibroblasts as well as numerous mast cells. If Bodian stains are performed, several nerve fibers in the paravascular stroma are noted. Smooth muscle fibers are often also seen in the stroma.

Hemangiopericytoma[25,26]

Hemangiopericytomas are considered to be derived from pericytes, or cells that are found in the walls of capillaries and venules. Developing in skin and other tissues, the lesions are noted in somatic soft tissue, especially in the muscle, vascular, or subcutaneous tissue of the lower extremities. The subcutaneous lesions may be small and resemble

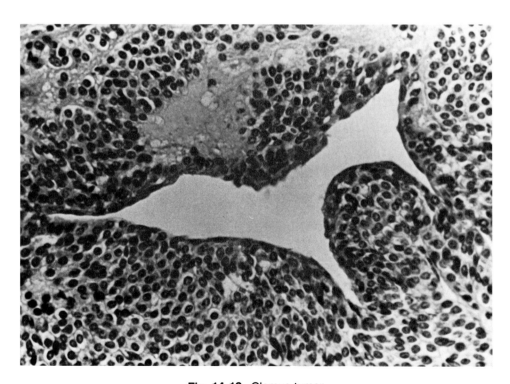

Fig. 14-12. Glomus tumor.

lipomas or epidermal inclusion cysts. However, they may reach considerable size and have been seen to invade underlying structures. Grossly, the cutaneous lesions appear as large indurated red plaques or nodules that are often invasive. Some authors consider hemangiopericytomas as neoplasms that represent low-grade soft tissue sarcomas. The frequency of metastasis is difficult to predict.

Microscopically, the vessels are lined by somewhat flattened endothelial cells. The lumen is surrounded by densely aggregated spindle-shaped pericytes. Nuclear atypia is noted in those cells with malignant potential, and there is a variation of mitotic activity noted from field to field. Special stains demonstrate a meshwork of reticulum fibers around the pericytes. Pseudocapsules are usually present. Glomus tumors can be differentiated from hemangiopericytomas principally by the presence of small glomus cells that are fairly homogeneous in size. Kaposi's sarcoma shows more conspicuous vascular proliferation, with prominent endothelial cells and always extravasation of erythrocytes into the stroma.

Malignant Neoplasms of Vascular Origin

Kaposi's Sarcoma[27–29]

A striking increase in Kaposi's sarcoma has occurred in the population of patients who are human immunodeficiency virus (HIV) positive. Kaposi's sarcoma was in the past noted in elderly, Caucasian males of Middle East descent. The lesions usually appeared as a single plaque or nodule. The classic form of Kaposi's sarcoma, not associated with the acquired immunodeficiency syndrome (AIDS) patient, tends to develop in the lower extremities or foot. The lesions are brownish-violet, and may appear as plaques or nodular configurations. However, verrucous-appearing and ulcerated forms of Kaposi's sarcoma are also noted. Multiple lesions of Kaposi's sarcoma may develop. Although lymph node and visceral involvement may occur, the lesions are thought to develop locally rather than metastasize. Patients with AIDS tend to develop Kaposi's sarcoma more rapidly than patients with the classic form of Kaposi's sarcoma, and usually

develop smaller, more numerous lesions. No predilection for the lower extremities appears to exist for Kaposi's sarcoma in AIDS patients; rather, the lesions may develop in any other area, particularly the upper extremities and face. Kaposi's sarcoma appears to be a slowly progressive disease that may cause death in 10 to 20 percent of those affected. Death is usually the result of hemorrhage caused by lesions in vital organs such as the gastrointestinal tract or lung.

Figure 14-13 demonstrates the microscopic appearance of a typical Kaposi's sarcoma. Kaposi's sarcoma is thought to be derived from mesenchymal cells that differentiate toward vascular tissue as well as fibroblasts. Two stages are noted, an *inflammatory stage* and a *proliferative stage*. The inflammatory stage is composed of the inflammatory cells related to a granulation-type tissue. The inflammatory stage demonstrates numerous dilated capillaries, as well as scattered infiltrates of histocytes, lymphocytes, and plasma cells. Some capillaries are lined by prominent endothelial cells with somewhat irregular vascular slits or lumens. Extravasated red blood cells and hemosiderin deposits are commonly present. The proliferative stage demonstrates vascular as well as fibroblastic proliferation. The vascular component demonstrates irregularly arranged lumina lined by single layers of endothelial cells. The endothelial cells form large, vascular slits or networks that are congested with red blood cells. Nuclear atypia may also be noted within the endothelial cells. The fibroblastic component demonstrates numerous spindle-shaped cells that appear as dense aggregates. Red blood cells are noted between the spindle-shaped cells. Atypia is noted in the fibroblastic cells, and mitotic figures are easily found. The stroma appears edematous, and hemosiderin is present. In long-standing lesions, collagenization due to the maturation of fibroblasts is noted. The fibroblastic component may be so predominant that it closely mimics fibrosarcoma.

Angiosarcoma[30,31]

Angiosarcomas, considered rare lesions, are often noted in elderly individuals. Angiosarcomas, referred to as malignant hemangioendotheliomas, appear as small, bruiselike patches that can develop into either plaques or hemorrhagic nodules.

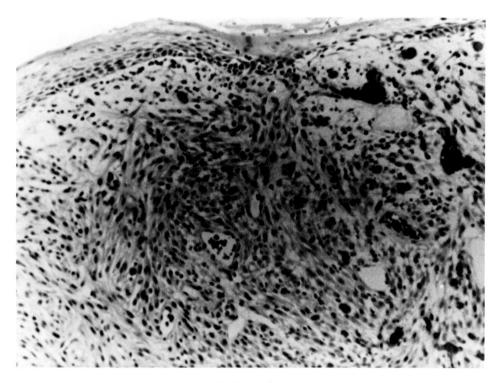

Fig. 14-13. Kaposi's sarcoma.

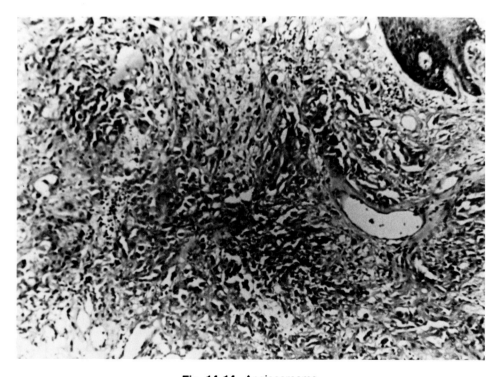

Fig. 14-14. Angiosarcoma.

They clinically resemble malignant melanoma. Hemorrhagic nodules can be observed in some cases. The nodules may be located more in the soft tissue rather than the skin. Local invasion is more commonly seen than distant metastasis. Microscopically (Fig. 14-14) the lesions demonstrate vascular lumina, lined by polyhedral, atypical-appearing endothelial cells that contain eosinophilic cytoplasm. Numerous atypical nuclei are noted. Occasional vascular clefts are seen, and in some cases the malignant endothelial cells can be seen to penetrate between collagen bundles. Some demonstrate anastomosing channels, whereas others show hyperproliferative cellular components with slit-like structures.

Benign Pigmented Neoplasms of Melanocytic Origin

Lentigo Benigna[32]

Lentigo benigna lesions are sometimes confused with ephelides or freckles. Freckles are hyperpigmented macules that are usually related to sun exposure. Freckles are not true neoplasms because an increase in basal layer melanization occurs but there is no genuine proliferation of melanocytes. Lentigo benigna lesions may occur anywhere on sun-exposed skin. Many times they are clinically indistinguishable from junctional nevi. Grossly, the lesions appear as brown macules and vary from one to several distributed over skin that has a long history of sun exposure. Microscopically (Fig. 14-15) elonated rete ridges are observed. In some instances areas of anastomoses are demonstrated. Typically, a diffuse proliferation of the basal melanocytes occurs. The lesions rarely develop into malignant melanoma. Examination of the dermis will usually demonstrate some sun or solar damage with solar degeneration of the collagen.

Junctional Nevus

A junctional nevus is a hyperpigmented, macular-appearing structure that may occur anywhere on the surface of the skin. It is not associated with sun exposure. Junctional nevi may be present at birth or appear at any age. Most appear solitary, and occur on the sole of the foot as well as between

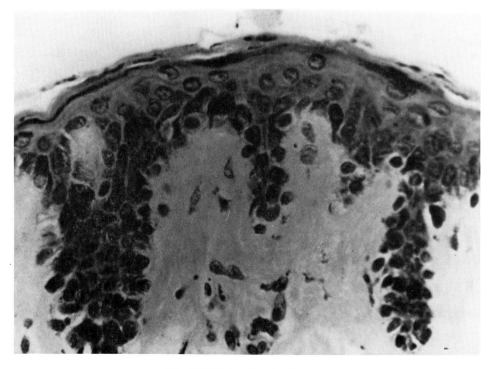

Fig. 14-15. Lentigo benigna.

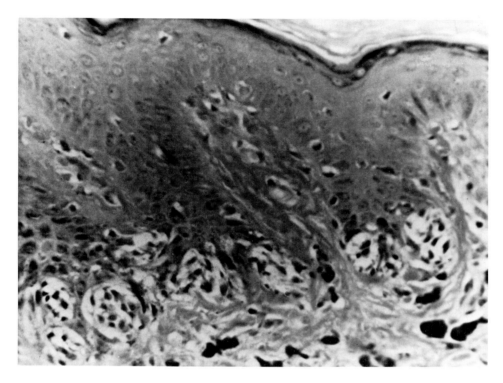

Fig. 14-16. Junctional nevus.

the digits. Microscopically, (Fig. 14-16) the nevus cells, which are benign melanocytes, are well circumscribed and appear in nests near the epidermal-dermal junction. They also may appear in the lower portion of the epidermis. Most nevus cells appear somewhat dendritic or bipolar; however, some may appear cuboid or spindle shaped with little or no melanization. Some junctional nevi show acanthosis with partial nesting of benign melanocytes. Occasionally some junctional nevi become active or "atypical" in appearance. The atypical junctional nevi demonstrate a moderate dermal infiltrate of chronic inflammatory cells and some melanophages. The presence or absence of nuclear atypia is helpful in discriminating between benign junctional nevus and lentigo maligna. Typical junctional nevi do not show abnormal or significant mitotic activity.

Intradermal Nevus

Intradermal nevi are raised, somewhat fleshy appearing lesions that demonstrate various degrees of pigmentation. Some lesions actually show no pigmentation. A few of the intradermal nevi are somewhat polyploid and contain hair, which is noted to project from the surface of the nevus. Microscopically (Fig. 14-17) intradermal nevi do not demonstrate junctional nevus cells. The nevus cells are arranged in nests, as well as cords and sometimes strands, within the dermis. The intradermal nevus are somewhat polyploid or papillomatous in appearance. At base of the nevus, fewer cells are noted, and the nevus cells appear to be mature and smaller. Melanization, which in some instances is rather pronounced, is usually located in the upper portion of the lesion. Occasionally inflammation in or around the nevus cells or nests is seen. A special concern is distinguishing benign intradermal nevus cells from malignant melanoma. An intradermal nevus will usually show maturation in the deeper dermis, whereas malignant melanoma will not show this process. Deep or scattered melanization is seen more in melanoma than in intradermal nevus.

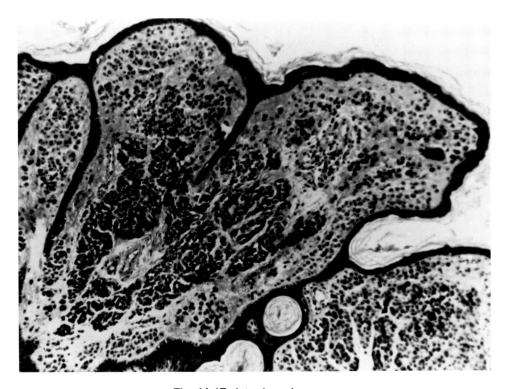

Fig. 14-17. Intradermal nevus.

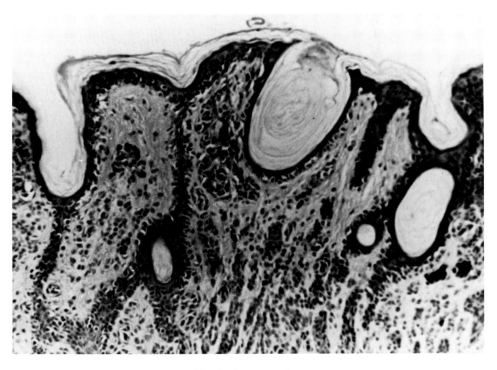

Fig. 14-18. Compound nevus.

Compound Nevus

A compound nevus is a somewhat large, raised hyperpigmented lesion and in many instances has a verrucous-appearing surface. In other instances, the compound nevus is somewhat hyperpigmented and nodular. Microscopically (Fig. 14-18) the compound nevus demonstrates both junctional and intradermal nevus cells. Both of these components are histologically similar to those previously described under junctional nevus and intradermal nevus. It is interesting to note that some acanthosis and/or papillomatosis may be seen near the overlying epidermis.

Blue Nevus[33,34]

Blue nevi are generally small lesions averaging less than 5 mm in diameter. Located on the head and neck, as well as dorsal surface of the foot and upper and lower extremities, the lesions appear as somewhat nodular or raised, deeply pigmented structures. The lesions are commonly mistaken for malignant melanoma. The color associated with the blue nevus is due to scattering of melanin pigment within the dermis. Two types of blue nevus are noted: common and cellular. The cellular blue nevus demonstrates numerous spindle cells that have little or no melanin. The common blue nevus contains cells that resemble normal melanocytes and some melanophages. Malignant transformation of a blue nevus into a malignant melanoma is rare. Microscopically (Fig. 14-19) the common blue nevus demonstrates large numbers of heavily melanized cells that occupy large areas of the mid- to lower dermis. Occasionally lesions may localize toward the epidermis, but there is no extension into the fat. In many cases the melanized cells are concentrated around blood vessels or other adnexal structures. Other varieties of the blue nevus show a lesion that has a fibrotic appearance. Cellular blue nevi tend to extend quite deeply but they do not invade other adjacent tissue or structures.

Malignant Pigmented Neoplasms of Melanocytic Origin[35-39]

Malignant melanomas represent changes that depart from the pattern of normal melanin-pigmented tumors. The departure may be mild to se-

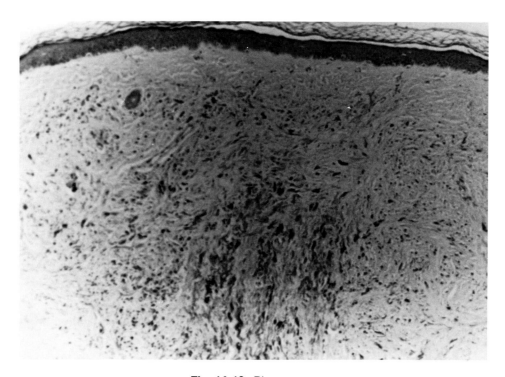

Fig. 14-19. Blue nevus.

Table 14-1. Various Classifications of Melanoma

Clark-McGovern classification
 Level I (melanoma in situ): Tumors cells are limited to the epidermis
 Level II: Tumor cells involve the papillary dermis
 Level III: Tumor cells fill the papillary dermis
 Level IV: Tumor cells involve the tricular dermis
 Level V: Tumor cells involve the subcutaneous fat
Breslow classification (depth of penetration)
 1. Less than 0.76 mm: Good pronosis, prophylactic lymph node dissection not indicated
 2. Between 0.76 and 1.5 mm: Value of prophylactic lymph node dissection uncertain
 3. More than 1.5 mm: Prophylactic lymph node dissection believed to improve prognosis
Bagley et al. classification
 Low risk: Less than 0.76 mm and Clark level II or III
 Moderate risk: Less than 0.76 mm but Clark level III
     Melanoma between 0.76 and 1.5 mm
     Melanoma more than 1.5 mm and Clark level III
 High risk: Melanoma more than 1.5 mm and Clark level IV or V

vere in nature and extent. The biologic potential of these malignant melanocytic neoplasms cannot always be determined with certainty from the microscopic morphology or the clinical history. In fact, minimal-deviation melanomas represent a category of malignant melanomas that demonstrates subtle histologic changes but do indeed represent melanomas. Many factors may influence the outcome or prognosis of melanoma.

There are three systems used to classify melanomas (Table 14-1). The Clark/McGovern system[37–39] is used by many pathologists. Another classification, proposed by Breslow,[36] is used in conjunction with Clark and McGovern's system. Bagley et al. have proposed a third classification.[40]

Lentigo Maligna

Lentigo maligna melanoma appears to be related to cumulative effects of solar damage to the skin. Lentigo maligna melanoma is believed to be preceded by an in situ phase or "Hutchinson's freckle," which may last for many months. The process then appears to spread laterally before frank invasive melanoma develops. The lesions usually develop in elderly patients, but may also be seen in middle age. Grossly the lesions show large macular areas somewhat mottled by a hyperpigmented zone. Indistinct margins are observed, and amelanotic zones found within the process may represent a regression of the whole process in that area. Clinically, the lesions have been mistaken for Bowen's disease. If the lentigo maligna melanoma develops frank foci of invasive melanoma, nodules or areas of induration and even ulceration may be seen.

Microscopically (Fig. 14-20) the abnormal proliferative basal melanocytes are haphazardly arranged with very little nesting. Nuclear atypia is commonly observed, and multinucleated giant cells may be present. A lymphocytic infiltrate is usually noted in the dermis. In other areas, the melanocytes may be quite atypical and spindle shaped. This process may involve and extend down to the outer root sheaths of hair follicles.

Lentigo Maligna Melanoma

Approximately 50 percent of the lentigo maligna will develop frankly invasive melanoma. The lesions are usually nodular and deeply pigmented and show areas of crusting, induration, and hemorrhage. Zones of hypopigmentation, thought to be due to tumor regression, may be seen. Microscopically, the malignant melanocytes extend downward from the dermal-epidermal junction and appear as groups or contiguous sheets. The epidermis, particularly the upper portion, does not show invasion. The tumor cells are often spindle shaped, and nuclear pleomorphism is quite prominent. The individual malignant melanocytes may appear heavily pigmented, but some groups of amelanotic cells are also noted. Fibrosis or desmoplasia of the dermis is also observed focally.

Superficial Spreading Melanoma In Situ

Superficial spreading melanoma is not limited to sun-exposed areas. Typically the superficial spreading melanoma appears as a flat, hyperpig-

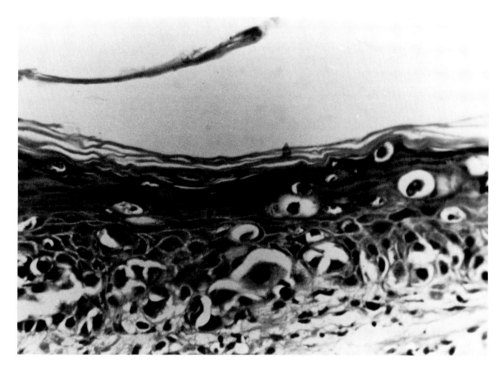

Fig. 14-20. Lentigo maligna.

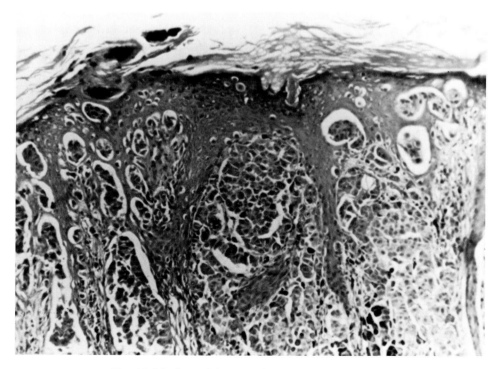

Fig. 14-21. Superficial spreading malignant melanoma.

mented lesion with irregular edges. It usually has a prolonged in situ phase, but then begins to spread laterally and vertically. The vertical invasion tends to be much earlier than that encountered in lentigo maligna melanoma. The prognosis is much worse in superficial spreading melanoma than in lentigo maligna melanoma. Of all the forms of malignant melanoma, superficial spreading melanoma is the most common, and can develop from preexisting benign nevi.

Microscopically, the thickness of the epidermis appears normal. The melanoma cells, cuboidal to pagetoid in appearance, show significant upward invasion into the epidermis. Nuclear pleomorphism is quite pronounced, and granules of melanin are often noted in the cytoplasm of the malignant melanocytes. Solar damage is usually not prominent, but a sprinkling of chronic inflammatory cells is usually noted in the upper portion of the dermis.

Superficial Spreading Melanoma

Superficial spreading melanomas are irregularly shaped and often have a coiled, somewhat irregular margin. The surface is also somewhat irregular, with numerous nodular components. The melanomas demonstrate different shades of black and blue pigmentation. Occasionally, a hypopigmented zone is noted that could represent regression. The lesions demonstrate satellitism, as well as some hyperpigmented halos around individual tumor nodules.

Microscopically, upward invasion, including the surface of the epidermis, is commonly seen (Fig. 14-21). Malignant cells show downward invasion that can include the papillary dermis as well as Clark/McGovern level III. Often the malignant melanoma cells appear pagetoid, and a chronic inflammatory cell infiltrate is noted in and around the malignant tumor cells. In other lesions, deep invasion, including the reticular dermis, may be present. The individual malignant nevus cells appear pagetoid and demonstrate a ground glass cytoplasm with prominent nuclei. Prominent nucleoli are seen within the individual nuclei, and pleomorphism is commonly observed throughout the tumor infiltrate.

Nodular Melanoma

Nodular melanomas appear as dome-shaped, rather large polypoid lesions that may arise de novo. Margins in and around the melanoma are sharp, but occasionally satellite lesions may develop. In nodular melanomas, the malignant nevus cells grow vertically from the time of inception. Nodular melanomas are most often found on the dorsal surface of the foot, whereas the superficial spreading malignant melanomas are found more often on the sole of the foot.

Microscopically, the malignant melanocytes demonstrate a rather striking downward growth. The tumor cells are somewhat compact and as a rule do not spread laterally. Invasion of the epidermis is seen. Occasionally a nodular melanoma, particularly the epithelial type, may mimic squamous cell carcinoma and be diagnosed as such. However, malignant melanomas do not demonstrate intercellular bridging or dyskeratosis. Squamous cell carcinomas do not demonstrate the presence of malignant nevus cells. Some nodular melanomas are amelanotic, and special staining may be necessary to rule out squamous cell carcinoma.

Malignant Melanoma Arising in Compound Nevus

Most malignant melanomas that develop from preexisting nevi usually arise from the junctional component. Malignant melanocytes are intermingled with benign nevus cells, and careful evaluation, as well as several histologic sections, may be necessary to confirm that the lesion represents a malignant melanoma.

Malignant Neoplasms of Lymphoid Cell Origin

Mycosis Fungoides[40-42]

Mycosis fungoides is thought to be a malignant neoplasm derived from T lymphoblasts. Mycosis fungoides primarily affects the skin, but various other visceral organs, as well as lymph nodes, may be affected. Mycosis fungoides, a slowly progressing lymphoma, usually has its onset in or after the fifth decade of life. Three stages are associated with the disease: premycotic stage, plaque stage, and tumor stage. Any stage may be associated with visceral involvement. The most common visceral organs affected include the spleen, liver, gastrointestinal tract, lung, bone marrow, and visceral lymph nodes. Sézary syndrome, a leukemic expression of mycosis fungoides, is associated with hepatosplenomegaly and lymphadenopathy, as well as exfoliative dermatitis and leukocytosis. Typical Sézary cells may be seen in the peripheral smear and appear as large T lymphoblasts with indentations or irregular nuclei. Intense pruritis is associated with any stage of mycosis fungoides but most often is reported in the premycotic stage, as is exfoliative dermatitis. The site of predilection includes any zone of skin, including the foot as well as lower extremities.

Grossly, the various stages differ in appearance. In the *premycotic stage,* the lesion resembles dermatitis or psoriasis and shows large plaques that may be mistaken for parapsoriasis or psoriasis. Diagnosis of mycosis fungoides in the premycotic stage is sometimes difficult and may require several biopsies over a long span of time in order to confirm the clinical suspicion. The *plaque stage* demonstrates large, erythematous, violaceous or brownish-tan plaques that show superficial scaling. Many of these lesions show a central clearing, giving the plaque a somewhat annular appearance. However, alterations in appearance are quite common in this stage. Finally, the *tumor stage* of mycosis fungoides shows very large, raised, violaceous or brownish-tan nodules. Umbilications or ulcerations are commonly observed on the surface of the tumor. Large confluent tumors may be associated with this stage.

Microscopically, the premycotic stage can be difficult or impossible to diagnose. However, the plaque stage, as well as tumor stage, show certain common histologic features. Examination of the epidermis demonstrates Pautrier microabscesses. The microabscesses are composed of malignant T lymphoblasts. The mycosis cell shows a convoluted, hyperchromatic nucleus. The superficial surface of the epidermis shows psoriaform changes closely resembling psoriasis. Elongation of the rete ridges and widening or thickening of the papillae are noted. Within the dermal papillae, a bandlike

infiltrate, as well as telangiectasia, are observed. In addition to the malignant T lymphoblasts, the bandlike infiltrate is composed of lymphocytes, histiocytes, plasma cells, and eosinophils. The tumor stage demonstrates a very thick plaque composed of an infiltrate of mycosis cells as well as the various other cells previously described. The infiltrate usually occupies a greater portion of the dermis in the tumor stage as compared to the other two stages. The premycotic stage shows very sparse to minimal numbers of mycosis cells, in addition to the lymphocytes, histiocytes, and occasional eosinophils and plasma cells.

NEOPLASMS OF SOFT TISSUE ORIGIN

Examination of the classification of soft tissue neoplasms presented at the beginning of this chapter will help in stressing those tumors most relevant to our discussion. Numerous textbooks on soft tissue neoplasms have been printed and are currently available for consultation. After examining any one of these textbooks, it will become quite apparent to the reader that there are numerous conditions and neoplasms derived from soft tissue. However, the main concern in this chapter is presenting those neoplasms that are most likely to be seen by the practicing clinician. Therefore, the discussion is restricted to those previously listed, the reader is left to explore in more detail other interesting or esoteric lesions discussed in those textbooks.

Fibrous Tissue Origin

Dermatofibroma[43]

Dermatofibromas are neoplasms derived from fibrous connective tissue. Dermatofibromas, also called histiocytomas, fibrohistiocytomas, and sclerosing hemangiomas, are solitary lesions commonly located on the lower legs. The overlying epidermis appears hyperpigmented and somewhat violaceous. Rarely found on the soles of the foot,

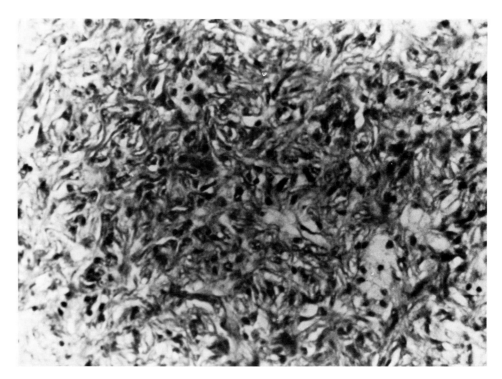

Fig. 14-22. Dermatofibroma.

they usually present as somewhat elevated, slightly protruding structures that tend to flatten with time.

Figure 14-22 shows the dermal portion that demonstrates a haphazardly arranged mass of fibrotic connective tissue that is poorly demarcated. However, a clear zone between the epidermis and the dermatofibroma structure exists. Newly formed collagen bundles are easily observed. Giant cells may be seen that may contain lipids and have the appearance of "Touton giant cells." The so-called histiocytoma, a variant of the fibrous type of dermatofibroma, demonstrates large numbers of histiocytes in the dermis, and some deposits of hemosiderin as well as occasional lipid droplets are also observed. In the hemangiomatous type, proliferative capillaries are present.

Giant Cell Tumor of Tendon Sheath[44]

A giant cell tumor of the tendon sheath, or localized nodular tendosynovitis, is a benign lesion that is not a true neoplasm. The lesions are usually solitary and may arise from either tendon sheaths, joints, or bursa of the large joints. Grossly, the lesion often appears as a subcutaneous mass that is quite painful. Microscopically (Fig. 14-23) a mixture of giant cells, fibroblasts, and lipid deposition is seen. The histiocytes are often spindle shaped, and foreign body types of giant cells, as well as mild fibrosis, are commonly observed.

Fibroma

Fibromas usually occur in the deep tissues. A fibroma appears as a somewhat circumscribed, firm, encapsulated tumor. Histologically, fibromas are composed of numerous bland fibroblasts. Fibromas may be mistaken for completely benign lesions, but may lead to localized infiltration and, in the case of some "benign fibromas," distant metastasis. The clinician is cautioned in regarding fibrous tissues or fibromas as just a benign proliferation of bland fibroblasts, when in fact they could represent low-grade fibrosarcomas.

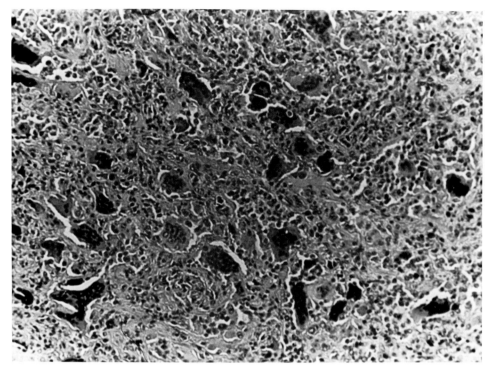

Fig. 14-23. Giant cell tumor of tendon sheath.

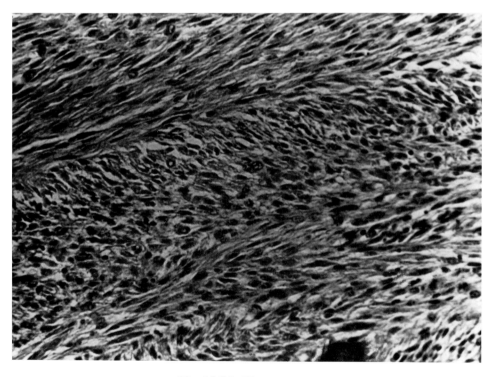

Fig. 14-24. Fibrosarcoma.

Fibrosarcoma[45]

Fibrosarcoma, a malignant neoplasm, is composed of anaplastic fibroblasts that appear epithelioid or in some areas stellate as well as spindle shaped. Epithelioid sarcomas are typically located on the palms and soles of the feet as well as the volar surfaces of the fingers and the forearms. These neoplasms usually spread along tendons or fascial planes, but nerves and blood vessels are also favorite routes of dissemination. They may metastasize to regional lymph nodes as well as pulmonary structures, and have a very high rate of recurrence.

Microscopically, (Fig. 14-24) malignant fibrous stroma, as well as epithelioid cells with multiple foci of necrosis, are seen. Some mucin is also present. Examination of the fascial planes as well as tendon sheaths demonstrates infiltration by this neoplasm, and the skin may show some erosion and infiltration. The appearance of malignant, spindle-shaped fibroblasts is similar to the so-called dermatofibrosarcoma protuberans. A definite area of palisading of the tumor cells around focal areas of necrosis is observed. Bizarre giant cells or Touton giant cells and osteoblasts are not normally seen.

Smooth Muscle Origin

Leiomyoma[46]

Four types of leiomyomas have been described in the literature: solitary cutaneous leiomyoma, multiple cutaneous leiomyoma, solitary genital leiomyoma, and solitary angioleiomyoma. The solitary cutaneous leiomyomas are usually reddish-brown nodules that may be rather large. The solitary angioleiomyomas are usually subcutaneous nodules located on the lower extremities. In this section attention is focused on the solitary cutaneous leiomyomas and angioleiomyomas.

The solitary leiomyomas as well as multiple cutaneous and solitary genital leiomyomas, have the same histologic features (Fig. 14-25). The tumor is not well demarcated, but is composed of anastomosing groups of elongated smooth muscle fibers intermingled with collagen. Individual nuclei are elongated, spindle shaped, and slightly hyperchromatic. The muscle fibers are slightly wavy and closely resemble nerve tissue. Special stains applied to the leiomyoma stain the smooth muscle red and the collagen blue. The special Mason

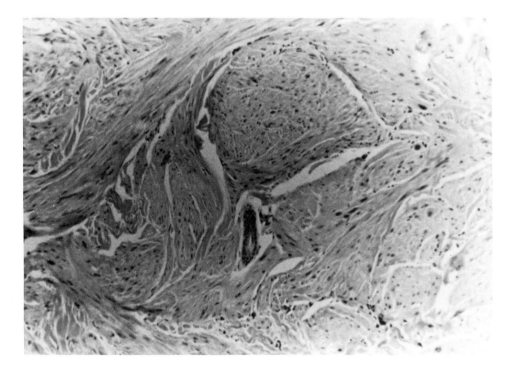

Fig. 14-25. Leiomyoma.

trichrome stain is necessary because immature collagen and nerve may appear quite similar to smooth muscle.

Histologically, the angioleiomyomas are solitary lesions that appear slightly encapsulated. Numerous vessels are seen that show thick smooth muscle in the walls. The lesions are usually tender. The smooth muscle found in the vessel walls often connects with smooth muscle fibers between vessels. The Mason trichrome stain is strikingly positive.

Leiomyosarcoma[47]

Leiomyosarcomas are very rare malignant tumors that may be seen in the subcutaneous tissue or dermis of the skin. Any area on the foot can develop this process, but it is more commonly observed on the dorsal surface. Nodules are large and associated with pain or tenderness. Cutaneous leiomyosarcomas have a better prognosis than the subcutaneous type, which are associated with increased incidence of metastasis and a reported high fatality rate.

Microscopically (Fig. 14-26) leiomyosarcomas do appear similar to benign cutaneous leiomyomas, but very careful histologic examination demonstrates nuclear atypia with definite increased numbers of mitotic figures. Focal areas of hemorrhage and necrosis may be seen, as well an occasional bizarre giant cell. A pseudocapsule may be noted at the edge of the neoplasm, and the muscle fibers are arranged quite haphazardly. Small vessels may also be seen within the tumor mass. Mason's trichrome stain is helpful in determining the presence of a smooth muscle tumor.

Lipocyte Origin

Lipoma[48]

Lipomas are tumors that are derived from benign lipocytes. They are usually solitary but may be multiple. They are soft, subcutaneous neoplasms with a lobulated appearance. Occasionally, a lipoma may become rather large in size. A subcutaneous lipoma is often slightly freely moveable. The deeper le-

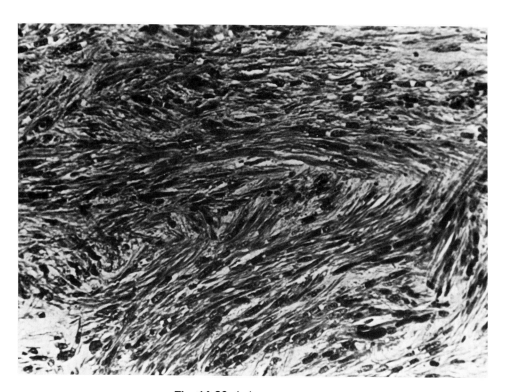

Fig. 14-26. Leiomyosarcoma.

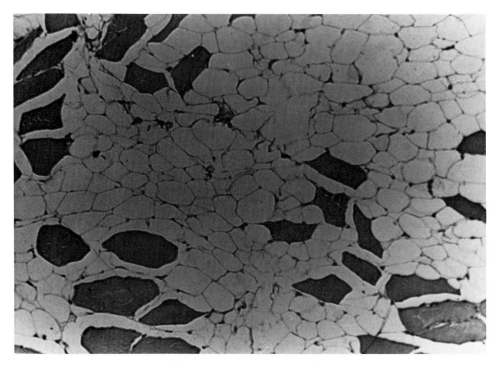

Fig. 14-27. Lipoma.

sions are usually fixed, but soft to palpation. Figure 14-27 demonstrates the microscopic appearance of a typical lipoma. A thin fibrous capsule may be present, and the tumor cells are composed of benign normal lipocytes.

Liposarcoma[49,50]

Liposarcomas are rare malignant neoplasms of lipocyte origin that arise from the deep subcutaneous tissue or fat. They are not derive from preexisting lipomas, and are seen in the fascial planes between muscles. They are locally invasive and do not readily metastasize. Microscopically (Fig. 14-28) liposarcomatous cells show lipocytes with eccentric nuclei. Each nucleus demonstrates a varying degree of nuclear atypia. As the malignant lipocytes become less differentiated, the nuclei often appear larger, are centrally placed, and have multiloculated cytoplasm with occasional bizarre multinucleated giant cells. Occasionally, poorly differentiated liposarcoma is found in the subcutaneous tissue, and special fat stains are necessary to determine that the neoplasm is of lipocyte origin.

Nerve Cell Origin

Neuroma[51,52]

Morton's neuroma is not a true neoplasm, but represents a regenerative response due to hypertrophy of the plantar nerve sheath through fibrosis. These pseudoneoplasms are generally found between the third and fourth metatarsal heads. Idiopathic neuroma (neuroma cutis), an extremely rare lesion, is most often localized in or around the oral mucosa. Traumatic neuromas also represent a regenerative response, and are often referred to as amputation neuromas. Microscopically (Fig. 14-29) idiopathic neuromas appear as enlarged nerve bundles composed of true Schwann cells. Myelinated as well as nonmyelinated nerve fibers are also observed. Traumatic neuromas, on the other hand, appear as a densely fibrous matrix with few Schwann cells.

Neurofibroma (Solitary Type)[53]

Neurofibromas occur as solitary cutaneous lesions. When multiple cutaneous lesions are noted, the condition known as von Recklinghausen's dis-

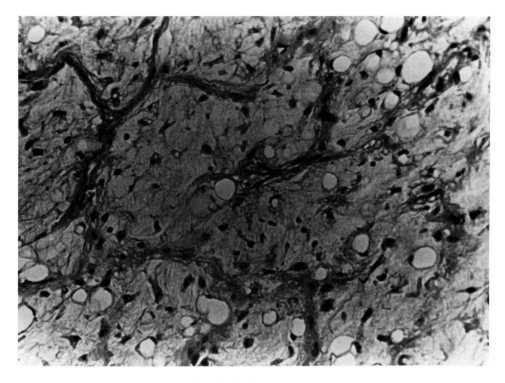

Fig. 14-28. Liposarcoma.

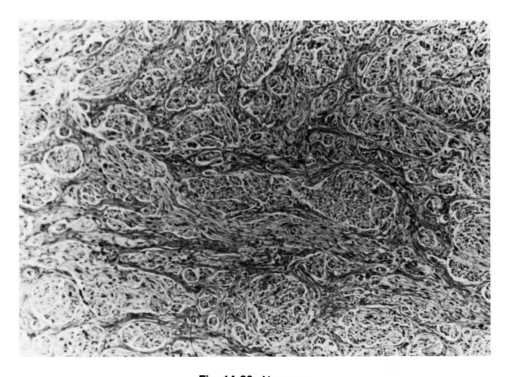

Fig. 14-29. Neuroma.

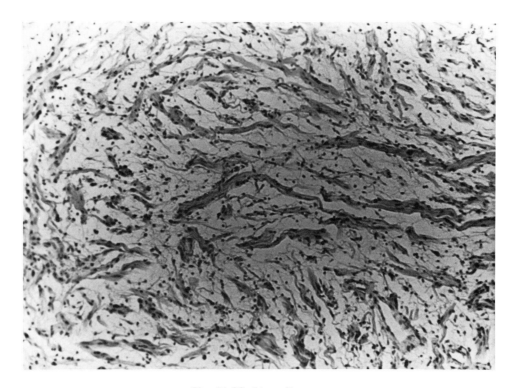

Fig. 14-30. Neurofibroma.

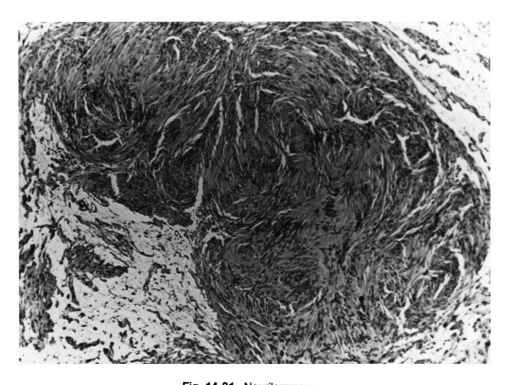

Fig. 14-31. Neurilemmoma.

ease may be present. However, this discussion deals only with the solitary type of neurofibroma. Usually the solitary type is rather soft in consistency. The lesions are flesh colored or violaceous, and are somewhat pedunculated in appearance. Histologically (Fig. 14-30) the neurofibromas are well-circumscribed lesions that may infiltrate the dermal connective tissue. The tumor is composed of thin, wavy fibers arranged loosely. The fibers extend in various directions. The nuclei are oval to spindle shaped and quite uniform in size. Most nuclei are arranged in parallel rows but a few develop a Verocay body, which is described under "Neurilemmoma." Mitotic figures are extremely scarce. Special nerve stains are usually positive and demonstrate long, thin nerve fibers admixed with thin, waxy connective tissue fibers.

Neurilemmoma[54]

Neurilemmomas are solitary soft lesions usually developing along the course of the digital nerve. Located within the subcutaneous tissue or interdermally, they are often painful and can reach rather large size. On sectioning a neurilemmoma, a well-defined capsule is observed. Malignant transformation is extremely rare. Microscopically (Fig. 14-31) the tumor appears well encapsulated, and rather dense masses of elongated spindle-shaped nuclei are seen to be embedded in a homogeneous collagenous matrix. The nuclei often palisade in their arrangement, and double palisading is what is referred to as Verocay bodies. Nerve fibers are few in number, but the lesion may have a very highly vascular stroma.

NEOPLASMS THAT ARISE FROM BONES OF THE FOOT

Neoplasms That Form Bone— Benign and Malignant

Osteoid Osteoma[55,56]

Osteoid osteoma, a benign osteoblastic lesion usually less than 1 cm in diameter, is surrounded by a zone of reactive bone formation. The nidus, or well-demarcated core, of osteoid osteoma is usually found in the cortex of the bone or the medulla.

Osteoid osteoma accounts for approximately 2 to 4 percent of all excised primary bone tumors found in the foot or ankle area. Most patients are children and young adults. Osteoid osteoma occurs twice as often in males as in females.

Clinically, the patient complains of pain that worsens at night and, if treated with aspirin, improves dramatically. The patient may limp, and in some instances, synovitis or tissue swelling may be noted in and around metatarsal and phalangeal structures. Occasionally, the pain is not localized within the bone, but referred pain in a nearby joint may be present. Radiographically, the nidus often appears radiolucent. If the nidus is located near the cortical structure, a radiopaque center is surrounded by a ringlike band of radiolucent halo. Variable degrees of periosteal sclerosis are also noted.

Grossly, the osteoid osteoma may appear entirely within the cortex, or it may lie on the inner surface of the cortex, or may be located completely within the spongiosa. The lesions may vary in appearance, but often are cherry red to yellow-white.

Histologically (Fig. 14-32) cartilage is never seen in an osteoid osteoma. A mixture of osteoid as well as newly formed bone is seen. The fibrovascular stroma demonstrates newly formed bone with minute amounts of osteoid. Osteoclastic activity is readily observed in the lesions, and the lesions are completely benign. The course of treatment involves local excision. Surgical intervention usually relieves the symptoms.

Several other conditions, including osteoblastoma, osteosarcoma, solitary endostosis, osteomyelitis, Ewing's tumor, metastasis, and eosinophilic granuloma, must be differentiated from osteoid osteoma. Osteoblastomas are large lesions usually greater than 2 cm in diameter that tend to expand the bone rather than have a small nidus. A small, thin border of reactive sclerosis is generally seen rather than the larger zones noted with osteoid osteoma.

Radiologically, cloudlike densities are noted within the osteosarcoma, and distinct histologic features are seen. Enostosis does not cause pain or reactive bone sclerosis and is composed of lamellar bone instead of the woven bone noted in osteoid osteoma. In cases of osteomyelitis, white blood

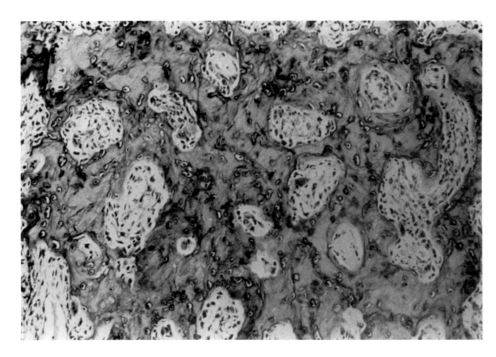

Fig. 14-32. Osteoid osteoma.

cells are seen, and reabsorbed bone and fragments are noted to occasionally lie within a central nidus. Ewing's tumor and eosinophilic granulomas are best diagnosed histologically. Biopsy materials, as well as imprints and special stains, are very useful in differentiating these conditions from osteoid osteoma. A metastasis will rarely involve the foot or ankle area, and the exact nature of the radiolucent area can be determined histologically.

Osteoblastoma[57,58]

Osteoblastoma is a rare, benign lesion composed primarily of osteoid and bone. Larger than an osteoid osteoma and sometimes painful, osteoblastomas show very little, if any reactive peripheral bone formation. Approximately 5 to 9 percent of osteoblastomas are located in the ankle and the phalangeal areas of the foot. More than 80 percent of the patients are younger than 30 years of age, with most patients between 10 and 20 years of age. The incidence of the disease is twice as great in males as in females. Patients usually complain of dull, aching, localized pain. Unlike osteoid osteoma, the pain is not nocturnal and salicylates do not offer much relief. Occasionally, slight local tenderness and swelling are seen in and around the phalanges and metatarsal structures.

Radiographically, the growth of the tumor demonstrates fusiform expansion. The lesions are usually well circumscribed and radiolucent. A thin shell of peripheral new bone is noted; however, abnormal periosteal reactions are uncommon. On gross examination, the tumor appears reddish brown, friable, and hemorrhagic. Some cystic degeneration, as well as central softening, is seen, and the lesion varies anywhere from 2 to 3 cm in diameter. On cut surface, a highly vascular, gritty, cystic lesion is observed.

Microscopically (Fig. 14-33) osteoblastomas closely resemble highly malignant osteogenic sarcomas. Careful examination shows the absence of cellular pleomorphism and increased or abundant amounts of osteoid tissues are seen. Areas where necrosis is observed show vascular channels as well as some fibroblastic tissue mixed with focal calcified woven bone. However, cartilage has not been reported in association with osteoblastoma.

Osteoblastomas must be differentiated from osteosarcomas, osteoid osteoma, and giant cell tumor

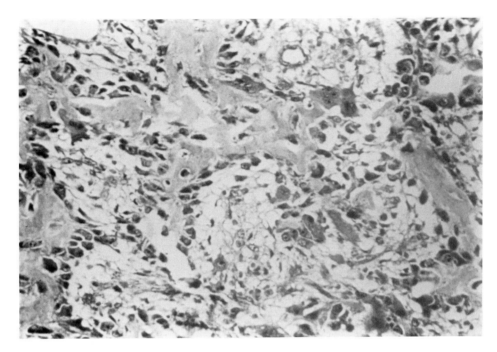

Fig. 14-33. Osteoblastoma.

with osteoid and woven bone production, as well as hyperparathyroidism. In the case of osteoblastoma versus osteogenic sarcoma, one does not normally see cartilage formation or calcified woven bone with little stroma and sparse vessels in osteoblastoma. In contrast to the giant cell tumor with osteoid production, the osteoblastoma does not produce areas of solidly packed giant cells and stroma cells. The course of an osteoblastoma is usually benign, and the treatment involves curettage and packing with bone chips. Recurrences are very unusual.

Osteogenic Sarcoma[59,60]

Osteogenic sarcoma is a malignant neoplasm of bone. The malignant stroma consist of proliferating spindle cells that directly product osteoid or immature bone. Individual stromal cells vary from mildly to frankly anaplastic-appearing structures. The tumors may produce malignant cartilage in addition to the malignant stroma. Less than 1 percent of primary osteogenic sarcomas involve the phalanges and talus bone. Osteogenic sarcoma of the foot and other bones can occur at any age, but most patients are afflicted before the age of 30 and there is a remarkable peak noted in the 10- to 20-year age group. Osteogenic sarcoma is seen more frequently in males than females.

Many patients are unaware of the neoplasm until a minor injury is sustained by the bone or articular structures of the foot. Slight to moderate pain is reported by the patient in addition to the swelling and some erythema around the articular structures of the foot. Occasionally, a pathologic fracture causes moderate stabbing pain in the lower leg or foot region.

Radiographically, osteogenic sarcoma appears as a large, bulky tumor that breaks through the cortex. Although osteogenic sarcomas are very dense, bone production results in a periostic reaction that closely resembles a cloudlike structure or "thermonuclear blast."

Close examination of the bone reveals a large, bulky, somewhat "hair-on-end" neoplasm eroding through the bone and cortex and lifting the periosteum. The tumor, if it involves the soft tissue, appears as a large, lobulated mass that may be extremely hard to soft. Hemorrhage is noted that

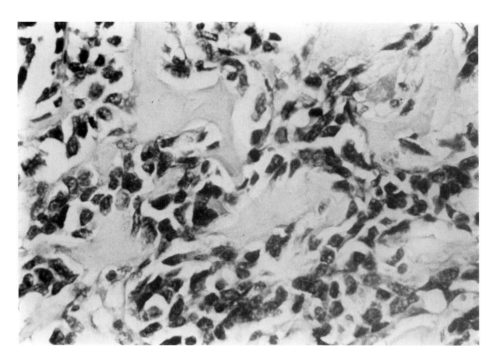

Fig. 14-34. Osteogenic sarcoma.

represents focal vascular proliferation. Osteosarcoma appears to be predominently lytic, explaining the vascular component noted in the hemorrhagic multicystic-appearing tumor stroma. Histologically (Fig. 14-34) definite anaplastic stromal cells demonstrating very atypical and bizarre nuclei can be observed. The nuclei are quite prominent, and mitotic figures are brisk. Osteoid is produced with or without woven bone. Other forms of osteogenic sarcomas may produce a fibrosarcomatous, chondrosarcomatous, or telangiectatic pattern.

Osteogenic sarcoma is one of the most malignant tumors known to man, and more than 80 percent of the patients die within 2 years of diagnosis in spite of amputation or radiation treatment. In other long bone involvement by osteogenic sarcoma, the metastases were most frequently noted in the lung. Primary osteogenic sarcoma of the foot is noted in less than 1 percent of all reported osteogenic sarcomas, and the exact nature of a primary osteogenic sarcoma of a foot is uncertain. Evaluation for tumor metastasis to local lymph nodes is necessary, and amputation should be considered.

Juxtacortical Osteogenic Sarcoma

Juxtacortical osteogenic sarcoma is a malignant bone tumor that arises from the periosteal surface of bone. Most patients are between 20 and 30 years of age. Less than 5 percent of all primary juxtacortical osteogenic sarcomas arise within bony structures or periosteum of the foot.

The patient usually complains of a mass with a dull aching pain over the periosteal surface of the foot bones. Radiographic examination shows the lesion to be a quite irregular, somewhat lobulated and densely radiopaque tumor. Grossly, most lesions are bulky and for the most part appear to encircle the cortex of the bone. On cut surface, the neoplasms appear grayish white.

Microscopically, three grades of tumor are noted: grade I (low grade), grade II (intermediate), and grade III (high grade). The grades are determined from the cellularity of the lesions as well as the amount of fibroblastic stroma and number of mitotic figures. Malignant osteoid as well as cartilage is seen in the high-grade tumors.

Treatment of the tumor consist of en bloc resection for grade I and grade II tumors. Grade III tumors require amputation as well as high-dose multidrug therapy.

Neoplasms That Form Cartilage — Benign and Malignant

Osteochondroma[61]

Osteochondromas is a cartilage-capped bony protrusion found on the external surface of a bone, and is considered to be derived from the epiphyseal plate. Osteochondromas are diagnosed in from 8 to 11 percent of biopsied primary bone tumors. However, in a series of several hundred solitary lesions, osteochondromas of the foot and ankle structures represented less than 1 percent. More than 60 percent of patients with osteochondromas were males, and most ranged from 10 to 30 years of age, with the highest incidence between the ages of 15 and 25.

The main complaints of patients with osteochondromas are related to the size of the tumor, and the most frequent complaint was that of a hard swelling of long duration. Bony protuberances, with or without pain, have also been recorded in the literature.

Radiographically, the bone appears as a projection composed of cortex that may appear pedunculated. Irregular zones of calcification, particularly in the cartilaginous cap, may be present. The cap is composed of benign cartilage. Extensive calcification of the cartilaginous cap should raise the question of malignant transformation. Grossly, the osteochondroma may appear either sessile or pedunculated. Many are somewhat cauliflower shaped with or without a stalk. On cut surface, the cortex of the bone is noted, and the periosteum covering the tumor's cortex is continuous with the uninvolved underlying bone.

Histologically (Fig. 14-35) an irregular, benign cartilage cap covers spongy and cortical bone and the bone may be lamellar or woven in appearance. Individual clusters of chrondrocytes and calcified foci of degenerate cartilage are commonly seen. Most osteochondromas are benign, and usually are cured by a complete excision. Recurrences occur in

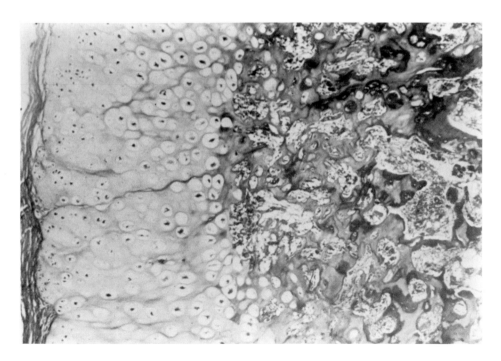

Fig. 14-35. Osteochondroma.

less than 2 percent of primary osteochondromas, and are usually the result of incomplete excision.

Enchondroma[62]

Solitary enchondroma is a benign neoplasm composed of either hyaline or fibrocartilaginous tissue that arises within the medullary portion of the bone. Enchondromas may either be solitary or multiple. Of the primary solitary enchondromas reported in the skeletal system, approximately 1 to 7 percent have been noted to involve the foot or ankle structures. Both sexes are about equally affected, but most patients involved are between 20 and 40 years of age, with 34 years of age reported as the average. The lesions develop slowly and are well established before the patient seeks medical attention for a painful area reported in the foot.

Radiographically, the lesions represent a well-circumscribed area of rarefaction that expands and may deform the particular bone. The lesion is usually confined to the medullary portion of the bone. No focal cortical erosion or bone expansion appears. Upon gross examination islands of glistening cartilage are observed. On cut surface calcified cartilage appears yellowish with some grittiness.

Microscopically (Fig. 14-36) benign cartilage is noted, but some enchondromas demonstrate islands of numerous binucleated chondrocytes. Plates of lamellar bone surround the lobules of cartilage. The lamellar bone may partially or completely surround individual islands of organized chondrocytes. Some enchondromas demonstrate bland islands of heavily calcified cartilage, which may appear mosaic-like or take on a jigsaw puzzle pattern.

The treatment of choice is surgical intervention with curettage. After adequate curettage, cancellous bone chips should be introduced into the medullary cavity. Prognosis of an enchondroma is usually good, and recurrence is extremely low even after curettage. If an enchondroma recurs, it may be necessary to resect the surrounding shell of bone and institute a graft procedure.

Chondroblastoma[63-65]

Chondroblastoma is a rare, benign bone tumor of immature cartilage localized in the epiphysis. Of several hundred primary chondroblastomas of bone, approximately 9 percent involve the bones of the foot. Sixty percent of patients with chondro-

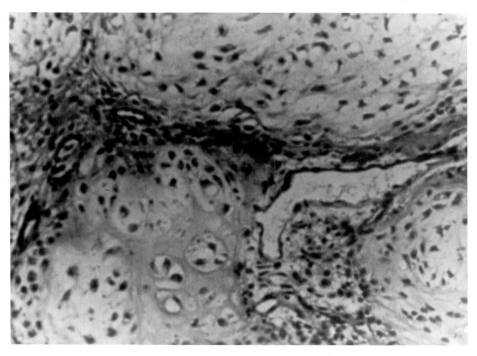

Fig. 14-36. Enchondroma.

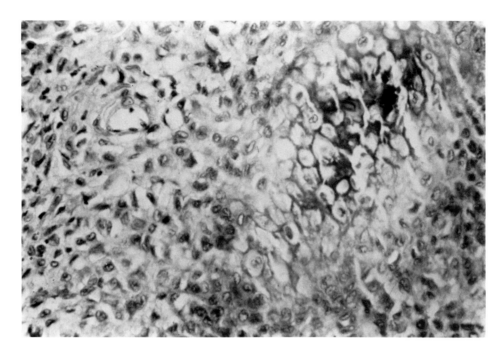

Fig. 14-37. Chondroblastoma.

blastomas are males. The vast majority of cases range in age from 10 to 20. Physical findings for a benign chondroblastoma are of little diagnostic value. Occasionally localized tenderness and nonspecific pain in the foot region is reported.

Radiographically, chondroblastomas demonstrate a central region of bone destruction that is sharply outlined from the surrounding normal bone. The lesion is well circumscribed with a thin, sclerotic boundary. Depending upon the presence and severity of calcification within the chrondroblastoma, mottled areas are noted within radiolucent zones. On gross examination, most chondroblastomas are small. A thin zone of sclerotic bone surrounds the tumor cells. The bulk of tumor may be grayish pink to pinkish tan and may contain focal zones of hemorrhage or necrosis. In a few cases, the matrix may mimic a chondroma.

Histologically (Fig. 14-37) the tumor demonstrates proliferating chondroblasts. The cells are usually uniform, polyhedral, and quite packed. Under low power the cells may be difficult to distinguish from plasma cells. Some giant cells may be interspersed among the chondroblasts. Scanty interstitial matrix separates individual chondro-

blasts. Whole areas of calcification may be easily detected. Some chondroblastomas are associated with secondary aneurysm of bone cyst formation.

Chondroblastomas demonstrate very low aggression. The best treatment for chondroblastoma is local curettage. Bone grafting may be necessary to repair a large surgical defect. Some patients receiving radiation therapy have developed sarcomas, and radiation treatment is now considered unnecessary.

Chondromyxoid Fibroma[66,67]

Chondromyxoid fibroma is a benign tumor of bone that produces fibrous, myxoid, and chondroid tissues in various proportions. The chondromyxoid fibroma may be mistaken for chondrosarcoma or myxoid chondrosarcoma. The disease appears more frequently in males than in females. An increased incidence of chondromyxoid fibroma occurs in patients ranging from 10 to 30 years of age. The symptom associated with chondromyxoid fibroma is pain of several years' duration, but many of the tumors may be asymptomatic.

Radiographically, the chondromyxoid fibroma is

a sharply outlined, somewhat eccentric structure that is seen to expand the bone. Foci of rarefaction are also noted. A few chondromyxoid fibromas show punctate calcifications. Upon gross examination, the tumor appears to represent typical fibrocartilage. A smooth, firm surface is usually noted that appears glistening and yellowish white. The lesion is well circumscribed and multilobulated. The tumor is usually small.

On multiple cut sections sharp delineation from the surrounding bone is seen. Careful examination reveals a thin, sclerotic zone of bone adjacent to the neoplasm. Histologically (Fig. 14-38) the tumor may be composed of myxomatous zones admixed with fibrous or chondroid zones of tissue. Nuclei of individual cells may be oval or spindle shaped, but occasional nuclei are round. Nuclear atypism may be noted. Globules of myxoid tissue separated from one another by cellular zones may be noted. Occasionally small calcified foci are seen. Stellate-appearing or spindle-shaped cells are usually seen within a myxoid background.

Block excision of the affected area is the treatment of choice because there is a high degree of recurrence if curettage is the only treatment used. Bone grafting may be necessary if the tumor is extensive. Occasionally amputation is required for cure.

Chondrosarcoma[68-70]

Chondrosarcoma is a malignant neoplasm composed of fully developed cartilage and lacking osteoid. Less than 1 percent of all primary bone neoplasms diagnosed as chondrosarcomas involve the foot. Approximately 60 percent of patients with chondrosarcomas are males. The incidence of chondrosarcoma varies, but the average for males is 40 and that for females is 43. Pain or minor discomfort and swelling may be noted in patients with primary chondrosarcoma of the bone of the foot. The characteristics of pain or swelling are not distinguishing, and do not aid in the differential diagnosis.

Radiographically, primary chondrosarcomas demonstrate osseous destruction with a mottled

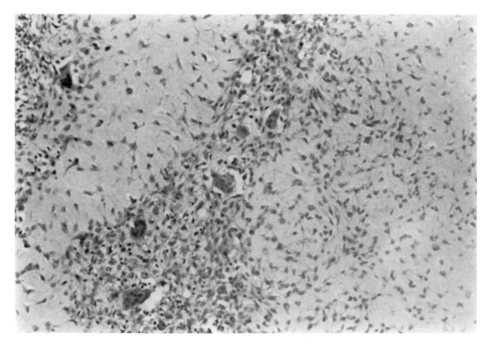

Fig. 14-38. Chondromyxoid fibroma.

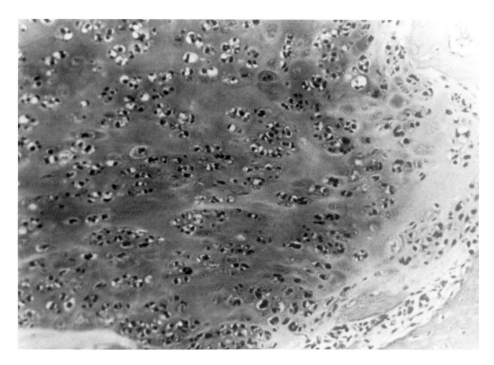

Fig. 14-39. Chondrosarcoma.

appearance, secondary to central calcification. Cortical destruction of the surrounding bone allows for extraosseous extension of the chondrosarcoma. Some chondrosarcomas may not involve the medullary cavity, and show little cortical destruction. The mass usually contains small foci of calcification. Chondrosarcomas are composed of lobules of cartilaginous tissues that coalesce. On cut surface, the lobules may demonstrate central necrotic, liquified, or cystic spaces. Small calcific zones, representing osseous masses, are also identified. A myxomatous quality noted in the firm hyalin cartilage is suggestive of malignancy, but histologic examination is needed to confirm the diagnosis. Metastasis to regional lymph nodes as well as other visceral organs is rare.

Histologically (Fig. 14-39) low-grade chondrosarcomas are difficult to distinguish from chondromas. Many of the histologic features are subtle and difficult to distinguish from benign cartilage-producing tumors. It is essential that the examining pathologist have access to the radiographs. Low-grade chondrosarcomas contain numerous carti-

lage cells that demonstrate binucleated forms and show definite variations in size and shape. A slight increase in the total number of cells is observed. Giant cartilage cells with numerous pleomorphic or bizarre forms may be noted. As the chondrosarcoma takes on a higher grade, a marked increase in the number of cartilage cells and pleomorphism of the individual nuclei occurs. The highest grade chondrosarcoma shows numerous spindle cells and a frank, marked increase in cellularity. Some areas of myxomatous changes are clearly noted. In order to reach the correct diagnostic decision, various criteria should be taken into account. The criteria depend on histologic and radiographic features as well as size, pain, invasiveness, extraosseous extension, and rapid growth.

Surgery is the treatment of choice. Chondrosarcoma appears to be quite radiotherapy resistant. Chondrosarcomas are noted to recur 5 to 10 years after surgical resection. The patient must be followed over long periods of time to determine if recurrence or metastasis to the lung or other internal parenchymal organs has taken place.

Neoplasms of Fibrous Connective Tissue Origin — Benign and Malignant

Desmoplastic Fibroma[71]

Desmoplastic fibromas are rare, benign tumors of fibrous connective tissue origin, characterized by an overwhelming amount of collagen formation with sparse numbers of oval or disk-shaped fibroblasts. Microscopic evidence of pleomorphism, abnormal or increased mitotic activity, and increased cellularity indicates a counterpart to this lesion, namely a malignant fibrosarcoma. Desmoplastic fibromas have been reported in the foot, and of the two noted in the literature, the calcaneus and the distal end of the femur were involved. These neoplasms are most often seen in patients between 10 and 20 years of age. The lesions fail to present distinguishable symptoms and signs. Pain is usually a late manifestation of this neoplasm, and the painful area appears to be located near a joint space.

Radiographically, the lesion appears well demarcated and is considered to be osteolytic. An expanded radiolucency with a very thin overlying cortex is observed. However, very little, if any, periosteal reaction is seen. Grossly, the tumor is somewhat whitish gray and rubbery-firm. Occasional ossification and calcification are noted. Many of the lesions appear to be pseudoencapsulated.

Histologically (Fig. 14-40) the lesions are somewhat devoid of cells and exhibit a heavy band of collagen fibers. In other areas, increased numbers of fibrous connective tissue may be admixed with mature fibroblasts. The nuclei of the individual fibroblasts appear spindly and mitotic figures are extremely scarce or absent. The separation of a low-grade malignant fibrosarcoma in some instances is extremely difficult. Low-grade fibrosarcomas usually demonstrate plump, hyperchromatic nuclei with an occasional mitotic figure. The usual treatment of these neoplasms is wide resection and thorough curettage with some bone grafting.

Fibrosarcoma[72,73]

Fibrosarcoma of the bone is a malignant tumor composed of anaplastic, fibroblastic tissue admixed with varying amounts of collagen material but with no evidence of osteoid, or cartilage. The lesions

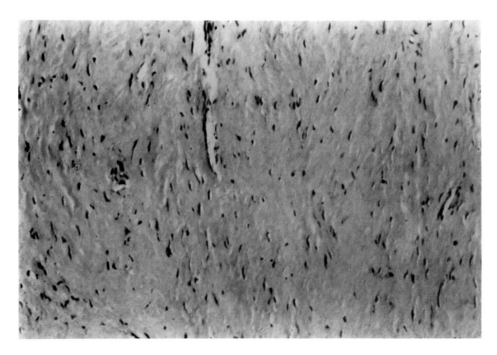

Fig. 14-40. Desmoplastic fibroma.

may develop in periosteal or intermedullary locations, and the majority of cases found in the foot develop from medullary sources. Most medullary types of primary fibrosarcoma develop in persons age 10 through 19 years and 30 through 50 years, with an average age of approximately 40. Medullary lesions present as a painful swelling, while the periosteal tumors present as more of a subcutaneous mass.

Radiographically, medullary fibrosarcoma presents as a lytic lesion noted within the bone with thinning and widening of the overlying cortex. Grossly, fibrosarcomas are usually located near the ends of the long bones or close to metaphyseal areas. The tumor is usually grayish white and somewhat rubbery-firm with focal hemorrhage or necrotic zones located in larger lesions.

Note that fibrosarcoma of bone is identical to soft tissue fibrosarcomas. In the well-differentiated or low-grade tumor, ample collagen deposition with interdigitating fascicles of malignant fibroblasts and a "herringbone arrangement" are seen. Mitoses are present but not numerous. However, in the more undifferentiated types of fibrosarcoma, a definite increase in cellularity with abnormal numbers of mitoses is seen. Large tumor cells are haphazardly arranged in the malignant fibrous matrix throughout the tumor. Treatment consists of amputation or disarticulation of the foot.

Tumors of Histocytic or Fibrohistocytic Origin — Benign and Malignant

Giant Cell Tumor[74,75]

Giant cell tumor of bone is considered to be an aggressive lesion of fibrohistocytic origin. Of the 265 cases reported in one series, 13 of them involved the lower portion of the femur or tibia, as well as various bones of the foot. Clinically, the patients complain of intermittent aching pain with some local swelling, tenderness, and limited movement in or around the foot. Twenty- to 29-year-old patients are the most common age group affected by this neoplasm, with an average patient age of approximately 33 years.

Radiographically, giant cell tumors of bone demonstrate expanded central areas of radiolucency. In some areas, a slight suggestion of fine trabeculation is noted. The center of the neoplasm is more lucent, with a gradual increase in density noted toward the periphery. Grossly, the tumor appears fleshy and somewhat grayish white, and hemorrhage as well as focal cystic areas are seen. Some zones of fibrosis are also apparent. Histologically, a benign giant cell tumor of bone is identical to a giant cell tumor of the tendon sheath.

When the examiner is satisfied that the radiographic and clinical data support the diagnosis of giant cell tumor, it is appropriate to make this diagnosis. The presence of giant cells alone is not specific for giant cell tumor because bone cysts as well as fibromas, chondroblastomas, and granulomas may also contain sparse to many giant cells. However, in this case the numerous giant cells are separated by a scanty amount of intercellular, irregular stroma that appears somewhat spindle shaped, and the giant cells contain numerous nuclei.

The prediction of the potential for malignancy of giant cell tumors is based upon a Grade 1 through Grade 3 classification. In Grade 1, the giant cell tumor is relatively benign, and numerous giant cells are seen with little stroma found between individual giant cells. The borderline lesions are Grade 2, and demonstrate more stroma with fewer giant cells. The stromal cells are somewhat spindly and elongated. The cellular components also demonstrate atypia of the stromal cells with moderate numbers of mitotic figures. However, the cytologic features still do not represent frank anaplasia or malignancy. In Grade 3, or the fully malignant giant cell tumor, the spindle cell component is sarcomatous in appearance and giant cells are sparse. There is a potential for metastasis to various organs from a malignant cell tumor of bone. The literature contains numerous reports of "benign" giant cell tumors of bone that have metastasized to the lungs, probably representing more of an iatrogenic seeding of blood vessels rather than true metastasis. However, malignant giant cell tumors of bone can metastasize to local as well as distant organs. There are numerous reports of recurrence of the tumor as a result of insufficient or inadequate excision. Treatment consists of resection and bone grafting.

Nonossifying Fibroma[76]

Nonossifying fibromas are well-delineated lytic lesions that appear near the metaphyseal region of the long bones. Most of the cases of nonossifying fibroma are seen in children from the ages of 4 to 8 years. The tumors are rarely seen after puberty. Clinically, the lesions seldom cause complaint and are frequently observed on x-rays taken for entirely unrelated causes. Radiographically, the lesions appear as multiple "eccentric bubbles" that are lined by a thin, sclerotic rim of bone. Grossly, the neoplasms appear yellow to dark brown, and there appears to be no disruption of the overlying cortex.

Histologically (Fig. 14-41) these lesions are composed of numerous or quite compact spindly fibroblastic cells that arrange themselves in whirls or storiform patterns. Multinucleated giant cells are seen admixed with the storiform fibroblastic cells. Hemosiderin pigment may be deposited within the individual multinucleated giant cells or within some of the spindly stromal cells. Collagen formation is usually absent. The lesions are usually treated by curettage or block excision if they become large enough to cause localized fractures or pathologic fractures and instability.

Ewing's Sarcoma[77,78]

Ewing's sarcoma is thought to be a primitive malignant tumor derived from the connective tissue framework found in the bone marrow. In one series, seven cases were noted in which Ewing's sarcoma involved various bones of the foot. Most patients afflicted by Ewing's sarcoma are under the age of 30, and most cases occur within the first two decades of life. Clinically, patients complain of fever, and anemia, leukocytosis, and an undefined increase in sedimentation rate are noted. Pain and swelling are seen in and around the involved bone, and the pain will eventually become persistent, dull to severe in intensity.

Radiographically, Ewing's sarcoma bone presents a somewhat onion peel or "cracked ice" appearance. Many zones of patchy mottled medullary bone destruction are seen. Grossly, the tumor, which is located within interosseous bone, presents

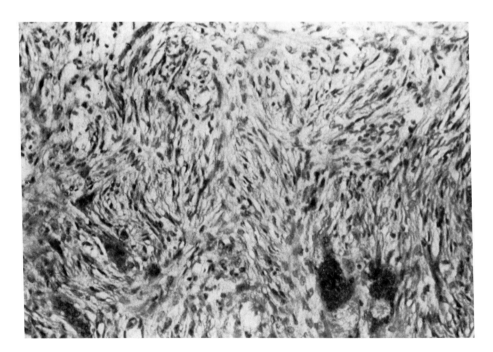

Fig. 14-41. Nonossifying fibroma.

as a somewhat firm, white neoplasm. However, if the neoplasm breaks through the cortex, the tissue becomes soft, hemorrhagic, and very friable. Unfortunately, metastatic spread of Ewing's sarcoma to other organs frequently occurs, and the lungs and regional lymph nodes are most often involved by this process.

Histologically (Fig. 14-42) large clusters of compact, round nests of tumor cells lacking any true rosette formation are seen. Special stains demonstrate fibrous septa surrounding tumor cells. Close examination of individual tumor cells reveals a moderately enlarged nucleus with a very thin or poorly defined cystoplasmic rim.

Treatment of Ewing's sarcoma has included both multidrug chemotherapy and radiation. However, the 5-year survival rate is only approximately 50 percent. The poor survival rate is in part due to diffuse osseous involvement, as well as soft tissue infiltration, and extension as well as metastasis. It is hoped that new chemotherapeutic agents will improve the survival rate.

Neoplasms of Blood Vessel Origin —Benign and Malignant

Hemangioma[79,80]

Hemangiomas of bone are considered to be benign lesions composed of capillary or venous blood vessels. Hemangiomas can be found in fairly young patients, but are more frequently observed in middle-aged to older-aged adults, with the incidence increasing with age. Clinically, hemangiomas of bone rarely present clinical symptoms or signs. If any symptom is present, it is usually vague and somewhat insidious in nature and consists of pain in and around the affected bone of the foot.

Radiographically, hemangiomas of bone demonstrate linear reactive ossifications. The radiographs reveal finely mottled osteoporosis with large zones that produce a "sunburst" appearance. On gross examination, the neoplasm is usually reddish-brown and quite hemorrhagic. Microscopically (Fig. 14-43) the individual bony tissue is separated

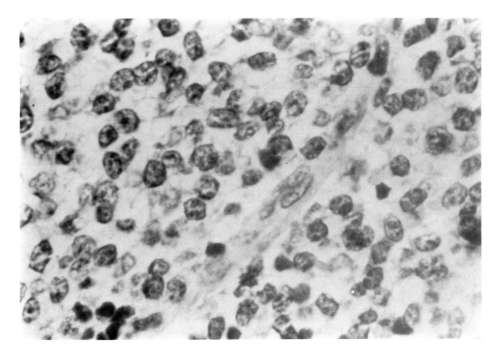

Fig. 14-42. Ewing's sarcoma.

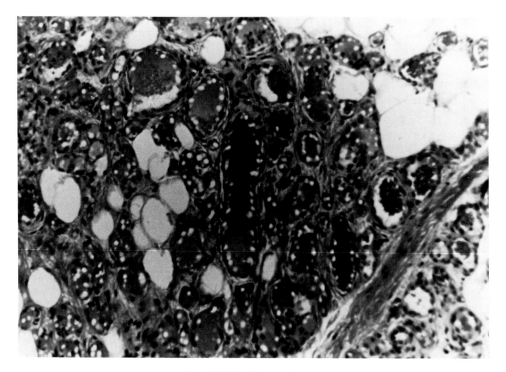

Fig. 14-43. Hemangioma.

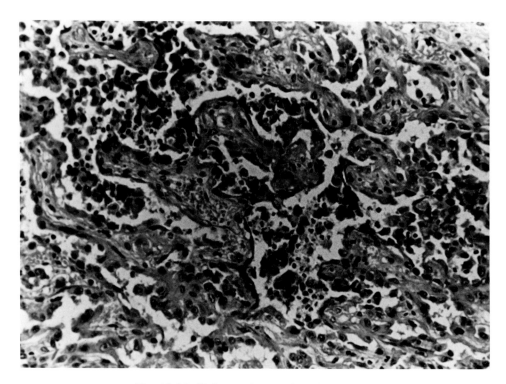

Fig. 14-44. Malignant hemangioendothelioma.

by fat tissue, numerous lobules of capillary tissue, and larger feeding vessels. The epithelium and endothelial cells lining the individual vessels are somewhat flat, small, and uniform. Mitotic figures are not easily found. In some cases, the capillary proliferation is rather diffuse, and the patient may go on to form the so-called cavernous type of hemangioma composed of numerous, multiple, large, thin-walled blood vessels, as well as very flattened slitlike spaces lined by thin, flat endothelial cells.

Malignant Hemangioendothelioma of Bone (Angiosarcoma)[81]

Malignant hemangioendothelioma of bone is a neoplasm composed of frankly malignant, atypical endothelial cells, which are immature in appearance. This neoplasm is rather rare, and only a few cases have been found that involve the foot. Clinically, the patient usually complains of a dull, well localized pain with some tenderness and swelling. The duration of the symptoms may be from several weeks to months.

Radiographically, these malignant neoplasms are generally localized near the metaphyseal plates. The tumors appear quite osteolytic and expansive, demonstrating minimal periosteal reaction. The overlying cortex is partially to totally eroded, and a small zone of sclerosis may be observed. Grossly, the lesions appear soft, fleshy, reddish tan, and highly vascular. Many appear to represent more of a blood clot than a true neoplasm.

Microscopically (Fig. 14-44) under low power the neoplasm demonstrates numerous proliferating vascular channels arranged haphazardly and separated by a hypocellular, somewhat eosinophilic matrix. Under low power, the neoplasms appear entirely benign. However, under high power profound vascular proliferation with prominent and quite atypical-appearing endothelial cells are observed. Mitotic figures are also observed.

Treatment of these malignant neoplasms includes major amputation or total resection of the tumor. Prognosis for these patients appears to remain dismal, with only approximately 20 percent surviving 5 years.

Neoplasms of Lymphoid Tissue Origin

Non-Hodgkins Lymphoma[82–86]

Primary lymphoma of bone, non-Hodgkins type, is considered a very rare, extranodal malignant lymphoproliferative disorder, arising in soft tissues and bone. Table 14-2 demonstrates the various types of classification of lymphoma as proposed by Rappaport[85] and a variation of the chart as proposed by Lukes and Collins.[84]

Primary lymphoma of the bone is most commonly observed in the second decade of life and is extremely rare in young children. The mean age of males affected by this neoplasm is approximately 35 years, and that for females is 46 years.

Radiographically, no definitive findings are noted. Occasionally, patients will present with a lytic, somewhat mottled type of destruction of the cortex bone. Grossly, the neoplasm is whitish and

Table 14-2. Non-Hodgkins Lymphoma Classification

Rappaport		Lukes and Collins	
I.	Nodular	I.	
	A. Poorly differentiated lymphocytic		A. Small and large cell–cleaved
	B. Mixed cellularity		B. Large cell–cleaved and noncleaved
	C. Histiocytic		C. Large cell–cleaved and noncleaved
II.	Diffuse	II.	
	A. Well-differentiated lymphocytic		A. Small lymphocytic, plasmary—bid
	B. Poorly differentiated lymphocytic		B. Usual small cleaved
	C. Histiocytic		C. Large cleaved and noncleaved
III.	Lymphoblastic	III.	
	A. Convoluted		A. Convoluted
	B. Nonconvoluted		B. Nonconvoluted
IV.	Burkitt's	IV.	Small noncleaved
V.	Undifferentiated (non-Burkitt's)	V.	Small noncleaved

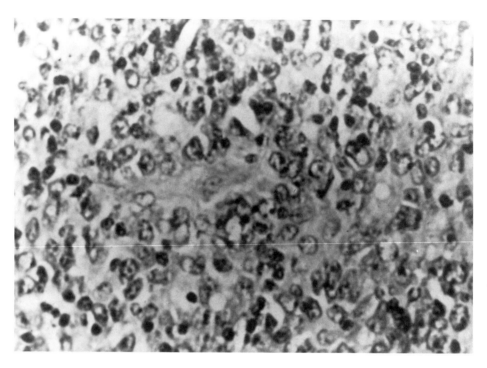

Fig. 14-45. Non-Hodgkins lymphoma.

slightly firm to friable. Figure 14-45 represents a reticulum cell sarcoma (a variant of lymphoma) that demonstrates a large nucleus with well-demarcated borders. The cytoplasm is pale and abundant, and the intercellular reticulum fibers completely surround individual cells. The nuclei often are oval and indented. Other types of lymphoma may present large or small cells that may be cleaved or noncleaved.

Treatment of lymphomas involving bone is radiation. However, the prognosis for non-Hodgkins type lymphoma remains guarded, with 50 percent of the patients surviving 5 years.

REFERENCES

1. Berlin A: J Am Podiatr Assoc in press, 1989
2. Becker S: The pigmentary form of verruca plantaris. Arch Dermatol Syph 34:265, 1936
3. Chapman CB, Drusin LM, Todd JE: Fine structure of the human wart. Am J Pathol 42:619, 1963
4. Berman A, Winkelmann RK: Flat warts undergoing involution. Histological findings. Arch Dermatol 113:1219, 1977
5. Headington J: Tumors of the hair follicle: a review. Am J Pathol 85:480, 1976
6. Reichis A: Seborrheic keratosis. Arch Dermatol Syph 65:596, 1952
7. Brownstein M: The benign acanthomas. J Cutan Pathol 12:172, 1985
8. Brownstein M, Fernando S, Shapiro L: Clear-cell ancanthoma: clinicopathologic analysis of thirty seven new cases. Am J Clin Pathol 59:306, 1973
9. Ade T, Acherman A: The many faces of kerato-acanthoma. J Dermatol Surg Oncol 4:498, 1978
10. Ghadially F, Barton B, Kerridge D: The etiology of keratoacanthoma. Cancer 16:603, 1963
11. Brownstein M, Rabinowitz A: The precursors of cutaneous squamous cell carcinoma. Int J Dermatol 18:1, 1979
12. Ravits H: Precancerous lesions of the skin and mucous membranes. Geriatrics 17:367, 1962
13. Collen J, Herdington J: Bowen's and non-Bowen's squamous intraepidermal neoplasia of the skin. Arch Dermatol 116:422, 1980

14. McGovern V: Bowen's disease. Australas J Dermatol 8:48, 1965
15. Lever W: Pathogenesis of benign tumors of cutaneous appendages and of basal cell epithelioma. II Basal cell epithelioma. Arch Dermatol Syph 57:709, 1948
16. Lewis H, Stensans C, Okun M: Basal cell epithelioma of the sole. Arch Dermatol 91:623, 1965
17. Mehregan A, Pinkus H: Intraepidermal epithelioma: a critical study. Cancer 17:609, 1964
18. Brodin M, Mehregan A: Verrucous carcinoma. Arch Dermatol 116:987, 1980
19. Glass R, Spratt J Jr., Perez-Mesa C: Epidermoid carcinomas of the lower extremities: an analysis of 35 cases. Arch Surg 89:955, 1964
20. Reingold I, Smith B, Graham J: Epithelioma cuniculatum pedis: a variant of squamous cell carcinoma. Am J Clin Pathol 69:561, 1978
21. Seehafer J et al: Bilateral verrucous carcinoma of the feet. Arch Dermatol 115:1222, 1979
22. Rowe L: Granuloma pyogenicum: differential diagnosis. Arch Dermatol 78:341, 1958
23. Imperial R, Helwig E: Angiokeratoma. Arch Dermatol 95:166, 1967
24. Tsureyashi M, Enjoji M: Glomus tumor: a clinicopathologic and electron microscopic study. Cancer 50:1601, 1982
25. Bachwinkel K, Diddams J: Hemangiopericytoma. Cancer 25:296, 1970
26. Enzinger F, Smith B: Hemangiopericytoma: an analysis of 106 cases. Hum Pathol 7:61, 1976
27. Bhiefarb S: Kaposi's Sarcoma. Charles C Thomas, Springfield, IL, 1957
28. Blumenfeld W, Egbert B, Sagebiel R: Differential diagnosis of Kaposi's sarcoma. Arch Pathol Lab Med 109:123, 1985
29. Mali J, Kuper J, Hamers F: Acroangiodermatitis of the foot. Arch Dermatol 92:515, 1965
30. Girard C, Johnson W, Graham J: Cutaneous angiosarcoma. Cancer 26:868, 1970
31. Maddox J, Evans H: Angiosarcoma of skin and soft tissue. Cancer 48:1907, 1981
32. Mehregan AH: Lentigo senilis and its evolution. J Invest Dermatol 65:429, 1975
33. Keioikdm JG, Richards DB: The interrelationship of blue and common nevi. J Pathol 95:37 1968
34. Mishiwa Y: Cellular blue nevus. Melanogenic activity and malignant transformation. Arch Dermatol 101:104, 1970
35. Arrington JR III, Reed RJ, Ichinase H et al: Plantar lentiginous melanoma. Am J Surg 1:131, 1977
36. Breslow A: Thickness, cross-sectional areas and depth of invasion in the prognosis of cutaneous melanoma. Ann Surg 172:902, 1970
37. Clark WH. Jr: A classification of malignant melanoma in man correlated with histogenesis and biological behavior. pp. 621–647. In Montogna W, Hu F (eds): Advances in Biology of the Skin. Vol. 8. The Pigmentary System. Pergamon Press, New York, 1964
38. McGovern VJ: The classification of melanoma and its relationship with prognosis. Pathology 2:85, 1970
39. McGovern VJ, Mikm MC Jr., Bailly C et al: The classification of malignant melanoma and its histologic reporting. Cancer 32:1446, 1973
40. Ackerman A, Flaxman B: Granulomatous mycosis fungoides. Br J Dermatol 82:397, 1970
41. Epstein E et al: Mycosis fungoides. Medicine 51:61, 1972
42. Norris D: The pathogenesis of mycosis fungoides. Clin Exp Dermatol 6:77, 1981
43. Vilanova J, Flint A: The morphological variations of fibrous histiocytomas. J Cutan Pathol 1:155, 1974
44. Carsteus PHB: Giant cell tumors of tendon sheath. Arch Pathol 102:99, 1978
45. Pritchard DJ, Soule EH, Toybi WF et al: Fibrosarcoma, a clinicopathological and statistical study of 199 tumors of the soft tissues of the extremities and trunk. Cancer 33:808, 1974
46. Fisher W, Helwig E: Leiomyomas of the skin. Arch Dermatol 88:510, 1963
47. Chavers E et al: Leiomyosarcoma in the skin. Acta Derm Venereol (Stockh) 52:288, 1972
48. Sahl W Jr.: Mobile encapsulated lipomas. Arch Dermatol 114:1684, 1978
49. Enterline H et al: Liposarcoma: a clinical and pathological study of 53 cases. Cancer 13:932, 1960
50. Reszel P, Soule E, Coventry M: Liposarcoma of the extremities and limb girdles: a study of 222 cases. J Bone Joint Surg [Am] 48:229, 1966
51. Graham W, Johnston C: Plantar digital neuroma. Lancet 273:470, 1957
52. Kite H: Morton's toe neuroma. Southern Med J 59:21, 1966
53. Owen D: Pacinian neurofibroma. Arch Pathol Lab Med 103:99, 1979
54. Das Guptas T et al: Benign solitary schwannoma (neurilemmoma). Cancer 24:355, 1969
55. Wilkinson RH: Osteoid osteoma. Postgrad Med 49:61, 1971
56. Dahlin DC, Johnson EW: Giant osteoid osteoma. J Bone Joint Surg 36:559, 1954
57. Giannestras NJ, Diamond JR: Benign osteoblastoma of the talus. J Bone Joint Surg 40:469, 1958
58. Maar D, Dornetzhuber V: Benign osteoblastoma ossis tali resembling tuberculosa. Acta Chir Orthop Traumatol Cech 41:362, 1974

59. Coventry MB, Dahlin DC: Osteogenic sarcoma. A critical analysis of 430 cases. J Bone Joint Surg 39:741, 1957
60. Dahlin DC, Coventry MB: Osteogenic sarcoma. A study of 600 cases. J Bone Joint Surg 49:101, 1967
61. Harsha WN: The natural history of osteocartilaginous exostoses (osteochondroma). Am Surg 20:65, 1954
62. Jaffe HL, Lichtenstein L: Solitary benign enchondroma of bone. Arch Surg 46:480, 1943
63. Breck CW, Emmett JE: Chondroblastoma of the talus, a case report. Clin Orthop 7:132, 1956
64. Dahlin DC, Ivnis JC: Benign chondroblastoma. A study of 125 cases. Cancer 30:201, 1972
65. Moore TM, Roe JB, Harvey JP Jr.: Chondroblastoma of the talus. A case report. J Bone Joint Surg 59:830, 1977
66. Gacyk W, Pikiel L, Bilczuh B et al: Chondro-myxoid fibroma of the calcaneus. Chir Maryaclow Ruchu Ortop Pol 36:127, 1971
67. Rahiani A, Beabout JW, Ivnis JC et al: Chondromyxoid fibroma: a clinicopathologic study of 76 cases. Cancer 30:726, 1972
68. Barnes R, Etto M: Chondrosarcoma of bone. J Bone Joint Surg [Br] 48:729, 1966
69. Dahlin DC, Salvador AH: Chondrosarcomas of bones of the hands and feet—a study of 30 cases. Cancer 34:755, 1974
70. Sairerkin NG, Gallagher P: A review of the behavior of chondrosarcoma of bone. J Bone Joint Surg [Br] 61:395, 1979
71. Rabhan WN, Rasai J: Desmoplastic fibroma. Report of 10 cases and review of the literature. J Bone Joint Surg [Am] 50:487, 1968
72. Chen V, Lennortz KJ: A case of sarcoma of the talus giving the radiographic appearance of a "cyst." Z Orthop 113:1027, 1975
73. Dahlin DC, Ivins JC: Fibrosarcoma of bone. A study of 114 cases. Cancer 23:35, 1969
74. Barnes R: Giant-cell tumor of bone. J Bone Joint Surg [Br] 54:213, 1972
75. Goldenberg, RR, Campbell CJ, Bonfiglio M: Giant-cell tumor of bone. An analysis of 218 cases. J Bone Joint Surg [Am] 52:619, 1970
76. Compere CL, Coleman SS: Non-osteogenic fibroma of bone. Surg Gynecol Obstet 105:958, 1957
77. Dahlin DC, Coventry MB, Scanlon PW, Ewing's sarcoma. A critical analysis of 165 cases. J Bone Joint Surg [Am] 43:105, 1961
78. Nouri MM, Hashemian H: Ewing's tumor. Review of 73 cases. Int Surg 60:478, 1975
79. Dorfman HD, Steiner GC, Jaffe HL: Vascular tumors of bone. Hum Pathol 2:349, 1971
80. Lidholm SV, Lindbom A, Spjut HJ: Multiple capillary hemangiomas of bones of the foot. Acta Pathol Microbiol Scand 51:9, 1961
81. Bundeus WD Jr., Brighton CT: Malignant hemangioendotheliomas of bone. Report of two cases and review of the literature. J Bone Joint Surg [Am] 47:762, 1965
82. Desai P, Meher-Homji D, Paysraster J: Malignant lymphoma. Cancer 18:25, 1965
83. Lukes R, Collins R: A functional approach to the classification of malignant lymphoma: recent results. Cancer Res 46:18, 1974
84. Rappaport H: Atlas of Tumor Pathology: Section 3, Tumors of the Hematopoietic System. Fascicle 8. Armed Forces Institute of Pathology, Washington, DC, 1966
85. Boston HC Jr., Dahlin DC, Ivins JC et al: Malignant lymphoma (so-called reticulum cell sarcoma) of bone. Cancer 34:1131, 1974
86. Short JH: Malignant lymphoma (reticulum cell sarcoma) of bone. Radiography 43:139, 1977

BIBLIOGRAPHY

Dermatopathology

Lever WF, Shaumburg-Lever G: Histopathology of the Skin, 6 ed. JB Lippincott, Philadelphia, 1983

Mehregan AH: Pinkus' Guide to Dermatohistopathology, 4 ed. Appleton-Century-Crofts, East Norwalk, CT, 1986

Okun MR, Edelstein LM, Fisher BK: Gross and Microscopic Pathology of the Skin, 2 ed. Dermatopathology Foundation Press Inc., Canton, MA

Soft Tissue

Enzinger FM, Weiss A, Sharon W: Soft Tissue Tumors. CV Mosby Company, St. Louis, 1983

Stout AP, Lattes R: Tumors of the Soft Tissues. Atlas of Tumor Pathology. Fascicle 1, Armed Forces Institute of Pathology, Washington, DC, 1967

Bone Pathology

Mirra JM, Gold RH, Marcove RC: Bone Tumors Diagnosis and Treatment, 3 ed. JB Lippincott, Philadelphia, 1980

Dahlin DC: Bone Tumors, Charles C Thomas, Springfield, Ill, 1978

Ackerman LV, et al: Tumors of Bone and Cartilage, Atlas of Tumor Pathology. Fascicle 5, Armed Forces Institutes of Pathology, Washington, DC, 1967

Arthritis

15

Leonard A. Levy, D.P.M., M.P.H

This chapter focuses on the more common rheumatic diseases, with emphasis on their manifestations in the foot and contiguous structures, and to a lesser extent on uncommon rheumatic disorders that have significant involvement in the lower extremity. These include the following:

Diffuse connective tissue disease
   Rheumatic arthritis
   Systemic lupus erythematosus
   Progressive systemic sclerosis
Ankylosing spondylitis, Reiter's syndrome, and psoriatic arthritis
Degenerative joint disease
Gout and pseudogout
Nonarticular rheumatism
   Fibrositis
   Tendinitis and Bursitis
   Fasciitis
   Miscellaneous pain syndromes
Reflex sympathetic dystrophy and related causalgic states

Other texts provide detailed discussions of all types of rheumatic diseases and related entities that are beyond the scope of this chapter.

RHEUMATOID ARTHRITIS

With respect to the early symptoms of rheumatoid arthritis, foot problems outrank in frequency those of the hand and are second only to those of the knee, according to Calabro.[1] However, 90 percent of rheumatoid arthritis patients find that their feet become affected (Table 15-1). Major disability occurs in many individuals as a result.[2]

Typically, the first areas to become involved are the metatarsophalangeal joints. Light pressure to these joints, compression, and active as well as passive movement, especially plantar flexion, cause pain or tenderness. Not infrequently the heel may be painful as a result of plantar fasciitis, Achilles tendinitis, or bursitis.[1] As the disease process continues, the inflammation may eventually lead to contractures of ligamentous structures, resulting in sometimes severe hallux valgus, fibular or lateral deviation (analogous to ulnar deviation), and hammering of the toes. Associated subluxation of the metatarsophalangeal joints is another common finding in the foot.

These deformities are most typically associated with the buildup of hyperkeratotic tissue as a result

Table 15-1. Results and Causes of Foot Deformities or Problems in Rheumatoid Arthritis

Deformity or Problem	Cause or Result
Muscle spasm ↓	Flexion deformity results, since this is the least painful position for the joint.
Muscle atrophy ↓	Causes decreased muscle strength.
Subluxation and dislocation ↓	Due to stretched joint capsules and ligaments. Leads to cocked-up toes and clawlike appearance.
Capsular and ligamentous contracture ↓	Due to fibrosis.
Rupture of tendons	

of the pressure and rubbing of shoes and the excessive weightbearing on the heads of one or more subluxed metatarsophalangeal joints. Thus, while the joints themselves are inflamed during the active stage of the disease, the burden of weightbearing and the compression of shoes increase the pain greatly. This in itself can lead to limitation of motion if not disability. Pain is often markedly increased by the addition of considerable and even small amounts of hyperkeratotic tissue on the plantar surfaces of the feet overlying the metatarsal heads, the tibial border of the first metatarsophalangeal joint, and the dorsal and distal aspects of the toes.

Additional problems in the foot may result from vascular lesions accompanying the disease. Proliferation of the intima of small vessels can affect digital areas. Such an arteritis can lead to sensorimotor neuropathy, ulceration, necrosis of the skin, and even gangrene of the digit in rare situations. The periungual areas and the digital pulp may present with brown spots due to ischemia. There are also reports of malleolar ischemic ulcerations. Patients with the vasculitis of rheumatoid arthritis usually have a high titer of serum rheumatoid factor.[3,4]

Neuropathy

Abnormalities of the peripheral nerves can occur in rheumatoid arthritis. Foot-drop, for example, as well as a patchy loss of sensation may occur in either or both feet as a manifestation of vasculitis.

There may be a mild, symmetric and distally located neuropathy, which does not appear to be related to vasculitis and has a better prognosis. This is found more often in elderly victims of the disease.

As a result of entrapment neuropathy, anterior tibial nerve palsy resulting in foot-drop may occur. As in tarsal tunnel syndrome from other causes, the syndrome when caused by rheumatoid arthritis may also result in pain and paresthesia in the heel and the medial aspect of the foot.[5,6]

Felty's Syndrome

Since splenomegaly occurs in about 10 percent of patients with rheumatoid arthritis, it is important to mention Felty's syndrome. This is a form of rheumatoid arthritis with both splenomegaly and leukopenia; there may be associated leg ulcers as well as hyperpigmented skin.

Since rheumatoid arthritis can affect any diarthrodial joint, it is not surprising that the small joints of the feet are so commonly involved. At the onset there may be any pattern of joint involvement; thus, in some instances the initial and only symptoms may be in the foot. Usually, however, the condition is bilateral, symmetric, and polyarticular. Typically after being present in the small joints of the feet during the early part of the disease, as the condition becomes established it may spread to the subtalar joints and the ankles.[7]

Limitations of both flexion and extension of the foot may occur, along with pain due to involvement of the ankle mortise joint. The calcaneus may become inflamed; the result is considerable pain on weightbearing when the plantar surface is involved. When the bursa under the insertion of the Achilles tendon becomes inflamed in rheumatoid arthritis, pain also results and is more pronounced on walking. It is not typical for patients with rheumatoid arthritis to have interphalangeal joint synovitis. More commonly the metatarsophalangeal joints are involved. Inversion and eversion produce symptoms when there is subtalar joint involvement.

Although morning stiffness is most commonly discussed with regard to the fingers and hands, its presence in the feet and toes must not be left unrecognized. This sensation of stiffness is thought to be due to congestion in the synovium as well as joint capsule thickening. There may also be an increase in the volume of synovial fluid (effusion), creating stiffness.[8]

Radiology

Although there are no diagnostic features specific to rheumatoid arthritis, it is differentiated from degenerative arthritis and other inflammatory arthritides by the fact that typical rheumatoid arthritis in the feet is symmetric when it is well established and has a predilection for the metatarsophalangeal joints. In addition, there is a relative lack of bone formation when there is advanced joint destruction.

Initially one sees soft tissue swelling, which may be fusiform in nature in the toes. Bone atrophy is an early finding, often in juxta-articular areas. As a result of articular cartilage loss, there is a uniform narrowing of the interosseous joint space. This is irreversible, usually preceding or coinciding with bone erosion. In rare instances, there is slight widening of the joint space probably as a result of ligamentous laxity and joint effusion.

Lack of new bone formation is characteristic of rheumatoid arthritis. The presence of exuberant bone is enough evidence to make one look for another diagnosis.

Bone erosions in the feet are frequent, occurring near the attachments of the joint capsule, especially on the medial aspects of the metatarsal heads. However, erosion of the fifth metatarsal most frequently occurs on the lateral aspect.

There may also be erosion seen on radiography at the calcaneus next to the retrocalcaneal bursa, as well as spur formation at the attachment of the plantar fascia. Pseudocysts, which are really marginated cystlike erosions in the subchondral bone, may appear to be unconnected to the joint. These pseudocysts only occasionally occur in the small joints of the feet. Bone never returns to normal at the location of erosions.

Bone ankylosis may be seen at the tarsal joints, less commonly at the interphalangeal joints, and rarely in the metatarsophalangeal joints. Secondary osteoarthritis may occur in rheumatoid arthritic patients, especially in weight-bearing joints

as a result of impairment of mechanical function. However, the osteophytes seen are usually small and poorly developed, with minimal subchondral sclerosis, compared to the osteophytes one sees in osteoarthritis.

In juvenile rheumatoid arthritis the ankles are commonly affected, and during the early years the feet are usually spared. New bone is easily stimulated, especially in the metatarsals. It is more common than in adults probably because in children there is linear subperiosteal bone apposition adjacent to involved joints. Bony ankylosis is also more common in juvenile rheumatoid arthritis.[9]

Patient Management

In rheumatoid arthritis and perhaps most multisystem arthritides, often the most important aspect of patient management, especially early in the disease, is the establishment of a specific diagnosis. In many instances the patient with joint symptoms in the feet may go directly to the podiatric physician, and a clinical diagnosis may be made at that time. Very frequently, however, the spectrum of problems and findings requires the intervention of the rheumatologist to establish a specific diagnosis.

A team approach to the management of these patients is essential not only to ensure that as specific a diagnosis as possible has been made, but also to develop a therapeutic plan that is comprehensive and coordinated rather than fragmented. Working in this multidisciplinary context provides the patient with the benefit of a maximum degree of medical and surgical input, involving those physicians with extensive knowledge of applied immunology, clinical pharmacology, and the natural history of rheumatologic conditions. It also provides those from podiatric medicine and other disciplines with surgical experience, biomechanical skills, and other effective local and generalized rehabilitative approaches.

The role of the podiatric physician may include a major contribution to the relief of pain and restoration of function. This not only leads to reduction in disability and in impairment of locomotion but also contributes to the psychological and social well-being of the patient by increasing independence and the ability to engage in occupational and recre-

Table 15-2. Therapeutic Modalities Employed in the Management of Rheumatoid Arthritis

Biomechanical therapy
  Orthotic devices
  Protective padding and shoe inserts
  Advice about shoes
  Specially molded shoes
  Immobilization
Drug therapy
  Aspirin
  Nonsalicylate analgesics and other nonsteroidal anti-
    inflammatory drugs
  Local injection of anesthetics into trigger points or
    periarticularly
  Intra-articular injection therapy
  Corticosteroids systemically
Physical therapy
  Canes, walkers
  Exercise in warm water (e.g., warm swimming pool)
  Wet heat (e.g., wet towels, whirlpool)
  Paraffin bath
  Other modalities
Surgical intervention
  Tendon release or lengthening
  Correction of single or multiple hammer toes or other
    lesser deformities
  Hallux valgus correction
  Joint implants
  Total-foot rehabilitative surgery
Education and counseling
  Patient
  Family of patient
  Health care providers
Combinations of any of the above.

ational activities that are as normal as possible. Accomplishing the goals of pain relief and functional improvement may include the use of the modalities listed in Table 15-2.

The details of these therapeutic approaches are covered, often extensively, elsewhere in this text.

SYSTEMIC LUPUS ERYTHEMATOSUS

Another chronic inflammatory disease that may affect the foot and may be extremely difficult for even the rheumatologist to differentiate from rheumatoid arthritis is systemic lupus erythematosus (SLE). The most common manifestation of SLE is joint involvement.[11] Joint pain and swelling may precede the onset of multisystem disease by many years. At the time of diagnosis in 75 percent of SLE patients, arthritis is present with objective evidence of pain on motion, tenderness, or effusion. However, arthralgia is present in 95 percent of SLE patients.[12]

Among the joints most commonly involved are the proximal interphalangeal joints. Involvement is most often symmetrical, with 80 percent of patients having morning stiffness. Nodules occur in SLE in 7 percent of patients. These are histologically similar to those occurring in rheumatoid arthritis. Palpable purpuric lesions may be found on the legs. Vasculitic lesions may occur on the toes as tender erythematous nodules. Periungual erythema is noted in about 10 percent of SLE patients, as well as splinter hemorrhages.[13]

Very common in SLE patients who have active systemic disease is livedo reticularis. This can precede the occurrence of gangrene. In some patients, ulcers over the malleoli, ecchymoses, petechiae, gangrene of the toes, and dystrophic nail changes may be seen. Raynaud's phenomenon occurs in as many as 15 percent of patients.[12]

Drug-related lupus-like syndromes have been reported, but often the evidence is highly circumstantial. Those drugs most firmly established as capable of producing an SLE-like state are hydralazine (which is no longer widely used in treating hypertension), procainamide, and anti-seizure medications. Procainamide is the most common agent implicated. Upon withdrawal of this drug the clinical syndrome and antinuclear antibodies in the serum disappear.[14]

Many features of rheumatoid arthritis and SLE overlap, and it is difficult to distinguish one from the other early in the course of their natural history. Articular involvement in SLE resembles that of rheumatoid arthritis. As many as 20 percent of SLE patients test positively for rheumatoid factor, and two-thirds of rheumatoid arthritis patients have antinuclear antibodies present. Rheumatoid arthritis patients may also have a positive LE cell reaction in 15 to 20 percent of cases.[12]

Radiology

In about 15 percent of patients who have SLE, deforming arthritis is seen after 4 years without radiographic evidence of erosions. Swan-neck deformities may be seen, but these are largely reducible, unlike those of rheumatoid arthritis.[12]

Patient Management

The approach to managing the SLE patient employs most of the principles established for the rheumatoid arthritic. These include adequate diagnosis, development of an individualized program of treatment, and patient education. Although the systemic care of this disease may be managed by a rheumatologist, general internist, or family practice physician, the podiatric physician often has a pivotal responsibility. The podiatrist may be the patient's initial contact because of joint, nail, or skin manifestations in the foot. These findings may be recognized as being highly suspicious for SLE, or at least SLE is included in the differential diagnosis. In addition, the podiatric physician can make a major contribution by participating in the care of the foot problems that may be present and may be the focus of pain and disability. To the degree possible, the podiatric physician's contribution should be as part of a team effort, consisting at least of interdisciplinary communication, so that the total care the patient receives is not only comprehensive but coordinated. Failure to establish such communication leads to fragmented care, with a greater risk for the development of iatrogenic complications.

PROGRESSIVE SYSTEMIC SCLEROSIS

Progressive systemic sclerosis (PSS), previously labeled scleroderma, is a generalized connective tissue disorder consisting of fibrotic and degenerative changes not only in the skin, but also in the synovium, the digital arteries, and the small arteries of the esophagus, intestines, heart, lungs, kidney, and thyroid. It may occur in a form characterized by diffuse scleroderma and early involvement of the internal organs. A severe form of the disease in which several decades may pass before there is involvement of the visceral organs, and in which only the distal portions of the extremities are affected, is called CREST syndrome. This syndrome includes calcinosis cutis (C), Raynaud's phenomenon (R), esophageal dysfunction (E), sclerodactyly (S), and telangiectasia (T), as well as the

much later presenting internal manifestations. Fibrosis of the skin and internal organs in PSS is due to overproduction of collagen.

PSS affects women three to four times more frequently than men, and occurs most often in persons aged 30 to 60 years. Swelling of the feet may be the initial complaint. Joint pain and stiffness in the feet may also be initial symptoms. The early edema tends to be painless, symmetric, and pitting. This lasts a few weeks or several and is followed by thickening, tightening, and hardening of the skin. As the disease progresses, the skin becomes taut and shiny. Subcutaneous calcifications may appear at the tips of the toes (calcinosis circumscripta). These may be punctate in nature. In about 98 percent of patients with PSS, Raynaud's phenomenon occurs. This symptom may precede other evidence of PSS by many years. As a result of joint stiffness and synovial fibrosis, severe flexion contractures may occur.[15]

Morphea and Linear Scleroderma

Morphea and linear scleroderma are localized forms of scleroderma. Morphea may present with one or more erythematous or violaceous areas on the skin. These areas may be small or large plaques or sometimes droplike spots called guttate morphea. The lesions may become waxy or ivory-colored. After a period of months or years, the skin may soften spontaneously. Morphea can occur at any age.

Linear scleroderma usually develops in childhood and is characterized by a linear streak or band of sclerosis on the lower extremities, sometimes involving its entire length. Overlap between morphea and linear scleroderma can occur, with patches of morphea found in linear scleroderma patients.[16]

Radiology

Absorption of the tufts of the terminal phalanges is frequently seen, often with atrophy of the soft tissue and subcutaneous calcinosis. Patients with CREST syndrome may have severe bone erosion leading occasionally to complete dissolution of the terminal and infrequently the middle phalanx. Patients with linear scleroderma may also have melorheostosis, a linear fibrotic hyperostosis of bone.[12]

Patient Management

Like most rheumatologic disorders, PSS requires the involvement of a health care team in spite of the many gaps that exist in its treatment. Although corticosteroids, colchicine, and D-penicillamine are being used, no single drug has proven to be effective in adequately controlled studies. D-Penicillamine interferes with the intermolecular cross linking of collagen. Colchicine reduces the accumulation of collagen by blocking the conversion of procollagen to collagen.

The podiatric role in patient management, like much of the therapy for the PSS patient, is supportive in nature. Advising the patient to avoid exposure to cold to reduce the symptoms of Raynaud's phenomenon is seemingly simple but essential. The podiatric physician can also help the patient avoid using tobacco because of its vasoconstricting properties. Although a number of vasodilating drugs have been used, the results are disappointing. Similarly disappointing is the treatment of calcinosis seen in PSS with such regimens as probenecid, which causes hypophosphatemia, and a low-calcium diet.

ANKYLOSING SPONDYLITIS

Ankylosing spondylitis is one of the seronegative arthropathies interrelated with psoriatic arthropathy, Reiter's syndrome, and other arthropathies. They are associated with HLA-B27.[17,18] There is an absence of serum rheumatoid factor, and rheumatoid nodules are not found. In these conditions inflammation develops at the site of ligamentous insertions into bone (enthesopathic).[19] Ankylosing spondylitis affects both sexes, although males more frequently, and males have more symptomatic disease. Although the term is derived from Greek roots meaning "crooked vertebra," there are significant findings in the foot. At presentation 20 percent of patients have asymmetric peripheral arthropathy of the lower limb. Other findings include peripheral joint involvement and plantar fasciitis. Joint involvement is more frequent in the lower limb than in the upper extremity. Other extraspinal symptoms are dactylitis, calcaneal periostitis at the site of the Achilles tendon insertion, and plantar spurs.

Radiology

Findings in the foot are related to the enthesopathic pathology of the disease, resulting in new bone formation in some instances, such as heel spurs. In addition, calcaneal periostitis is seen at the insertion of the Achilles tendon. Destructive arthritis of the feet, however, with bone erosion demonstrable on radiography, is relatively uncommon in ankylosing spondylitis except for calcaneal erosions. This is usually a late occurrence.[12,23]

Patient Management

As with many other rheumatologic disorders, ankylosing spondylitis is best managed in a multidisciplinary manner. The nonpodiatric aspects of the condition are usually approached by the administration of nonsteroidal anti-inflammatory agents along with an active exercise program and physical therapeutic modalities. Occasionally surgical intervention is indicated, including wedge osteotomy of the vertebral areas affected.

Podiatric involvement is essentially supportive, but there is potentially the capability to reduce morbidity and allow patients to engage more comfortably in their occupational and social activities. This may be achieved by accomodative and weight-dispersing orthotic devices, as well as by local physical therapeutic modalities.

REITER'S SYNDROME

In the United States and Canada, as in the United Kingdom, most cases of Reiter's syndrome follow venereal exposure. A postdysenteric type appears in Europe, Africa, and Asia. The disease is characterized by urethritis, conjunctivitis, arthritis, and a cutaneous manifestation on the soles (and sometimes on the palms) called keratoderma blennorrhagica.[20]

The lesions of keratoderma blennorrhagica appear about 4 to 6 weeks after urethritis and may be indistinguishable from psoriasis. In fact, they are histologically identical to pustular psoriasis. Some feel that there is an association between psoriasis and keratoderma blennorrhagica because the lesions sometimes progress to form frank psoriasis. This dermatologic manifestation of Reiter's syndrome has been reported in from 10 to 30 percent of patients. It first presents with small red to yellowish-brown vesicles or papules, which are firm but not tender. Sometimes these lesions become confluent. Patients with the postdysenteric form of the disease are less frequently affected with keratoderma blennorrhagica.

Weight-bearing joints such as the ankles and knees are commonly affected. Few joints are typically involved in the nonsymmetric arthritis that characteristically occurs. In rare instances only a single joint is involved. Acute inflammation and swelling are seen with joint effusion along with wasting of muscles in the affected areas. Achilles tenosynovitis is not a rare manifestation of the disease. After complete remission, multiple recurrences are frequent, with the development of residual joint damage especially at the heads of the metatarsals. Involvement of the calcaneus at its inferior and posterior aspects may result from periostitis. The painful condition that can result is sometimes called "lover's heel" and is classically accompanied by calcaneal spurs.[12]

Radiology

Reiter's syndrome and psoriatic arthritis are difficult to distinguish. There is a predilection for the joints of the lower extremities, especially the metatarsophalangeal joints. Like psoriatic arthritis, Reiter's syndrome has a predilection for the interphalangeal joint of the great toe as well as the heels. Characteristically there are erosions of the calcaneus at the posterior superior and posterior inferior aspects, as is also the case in psoriatic arthritis. This is especially associated with reactive bone formation. At the metatarsophalangeal joints in par-

ticular, severe bone destruction can occur. There does not seem to be a predilection for joints of a single ray or for the terminal interphalangeal joints of the hand.[21,22]

Nail deformities similar to those seen in psoriasis may be present. There is hyperkeratosis with extensive buildup of cornified material under the nail, and this can result in loss of the nail.[12]

Patient Management

Symptomatic treatment is the approach to the patient with Reiter's syndrome. This is best provided through the use of the team approach. Nonsteroidal anti-inflammatory drugs are widely used for the arthritis along with physical therapeutic modalities. Injection of corticosteroids around the Achilles tendon and in the plantar fascia has proven to be helpful in patients with Reiter's syndrome affecting these areas.

PSORIATIC ARTHRITIS

The distal interphalangeal joints are typically involved in psoriatic arthritis. There is frequent metatarsophalangeal joint involvement as well. Except for the less common arthritis mutilans that may occur, psoriatic arthritis is usually not as painful and disabling as rheumatoid arthritis. Some patients with psoriatic arthritis have asymmetric involvement of two or three joints, whereas others have a symmetrical polyarthritis indistinguishable clinically from rheumatoid arthritis.

Nail involvement is seen in 80 percent of patients with psoriatic arthritis. Those patients with psoriasis without arthritis have nail involvement only 30 percent of the time. The toes with nail involvement tend to be those that have distal interphalangeal joint arthritis.

Except for the fact that fibrosis is more prominent in psoriatic arthritis, the synovitis that occurs is similar to what is seen in rheumatoid arthritis histologically. In psoriasis patients with bilaterally symmetric arthritis, joint involvement typically does not differ to any extent from that seen in rheumatoid arthritis patients. An exception to this is the involvement of the distal interphalangeal joints classically seen in the patient with psoriatic arthritis.[12]

Radiology

Although the radiologic picture of psoriatic arthritis is similar to that of rheumatoid arthritis, there is a predilection for the terminal interphalangeal joints, and involvement of joints of a single ray is typically seen. There also is a predilection for the interphalangeal joint of the hallux along with more severe involvement of the feet than of the hands. Reabsorption of the terminal tuft of the great toe may be seen along with sclerotic changes in the terminal phalanx. Despite sometimes extensive joint destruction, osteoporosis is frequently absent. The bone may taper to appear like a pencil in a cup as a result of the erosion of bone along the diaphysis of the metatarsal beyond its capsular attachment. At the posterior superior and posterior plantar aspects of the calcaneus, erosions are common with new bone apposition.

Patient Management

Aspirin and other nonsteroidal anti-inflammatory drugs are used in the care of psoriatic arthritis. Intra-articular corticosteroids also provide temporary relief, as do physical therapeutic modalities. Corticosteroid therapy usually is quite effective for both joint and skin symptoms, but requires large doses in most instances, predisposing patients to the side effects of these drugs. As with the other arthritides, a multidisciplinary approach to managing patients with psoriatic arthritis is to be encouraged.

OSTEOARTHRITIS

The most common disease of the peripheral diarthrodial joints is osteoarthritis. This disease is characterized by progressive deterioration and loss of articular cartilage. Reactive changes occur at the margins of the joints and in subchondral bone. Pa-

tients experience slowly developing pain in the joints, stiffness, and enlargement of the joints with limitation of motion. Synovitis may occur secondarily.

Early in the course of the disease, pain occurs after joint use and is relieved by rest. As the disease progresses, pain occurs even with minimal motion or at rest and may even be present at night. Crepitus, a feeling of crackling or grating when a joint is moved, is often present along with pain on passive motion. Synovitis causes enlargement of joints as do increased amounts of synovial fluid or proliferative changes of cartilage and bone.

Spur formation at the dorsolateral and medial aspects of the distal interphalangeal joints of the toes is the counterpart of what is seen in the fingers, where it is referred to as Heberden's nodes. When seen at the proximal interphalangeal joints these are called Bouchard's nodes. Flexor and lateral deviations of the distal phalanx are also seen. Mucoid cysts, which are gelatinous filled cysts similar to a ganglion, may be precursors of Heberden's nodes.

Tight shoes may aggravate osteoarthritis of the first metatarsophalangeal joint. One can usually palpate irregularities in joint contour. Tenderness is common, especially when the bursa over the first metatarsophalangeal joint is secondarily inflamed at the medial aspect.

In most patients, laboratory findings such as the erythrocyte sedimentation rate (ESR) and synovial fluid are normal. The ESR may be slightly elevated in patients with erosive inflammatory or generalized forms of the disease. In many osteoarthritic joints with effusion there may be crystals of calcium pyrophosphate dehydrate and/or apatite.

Patients with involvement of weight-bearing joints are more likely than others to have some disability resulting from the disease. Because there is often distal interphalangeal joint involvement, it may be difficult to differentiate osteoarthritis from Reiter's syndrome, psoriasis, and the arthritis of chronic ulcerative colitis. In addition, seronegative rheumatoid arthritis must be differentiated from osteoarthritis.[12]

Radiology

Primary osteoarthritis has a predilection for weight-bearing joints, especially in the foot at the first metatarsophalangeal joint. Involvement of the tarsal joints is not typical as it is in rheumatoid arthritis. The tibiotalar joint also is rarely involved, but when it is one should consider that the condition may be secondary osteoarthritis. Radiographic changes develop gradually over years. Except for erosive osteoarthritis, which shows changes over months, rapidly developing major x-ray changes are a clue that the patient may have a disease other than osteoarthritis. It is not usual for the cartilages in the medial and lateral compartments of the same joint to be affected simultaneously. As cartilage degenerates, a characteristic sclerosis of the subchondral cortex occurs as a result of excessive mechanical stress. Osteophytes develop due to cartilage hyperplasia as a result of endochondral bone formation. This subchondral sclerosis (eburnation) and osteophyte formation indicate that there are degenerative changes in the adjacent articular cartilage. Metaplastic, cartilaginous, and osseous bodies within the joint are called "mice" and may be found in the advanced stages of the disease.

Cystlike rarefactions in the subchondral bone may be seen in osteoarthritis. They may collapse, causing marked joint deformity. Whereas osteoporosis, soft tissue atrophy, and subluxation are features of rheumatoid arthritis, they are not seen in osteoarthritis. However, minimal or moderate malalignment due to intra-articular and para-articular bone production may frequently occur. Therefore, one may see hallux valgus, but ulnar deviation is not usually present. The metatarsophalangeal joints are not usually affected as they are in rheumatoid arthritis. However, uniform narrowing of the interosseous spaces may occur at the metatarsophalangeal joints without marginal bone erosions. Ankylosis is common at the interphalangeal joints only in cases of osteoarthritis of the erosive type.[23,24]

Patient Management

Protecting the involved joints of the feet from overuse or abnormal weightbearing, which is probably a major contributing cause, is essential. Shifting of weight from the painful lower extremity to the opposite limb places three to four times the amount of force on that extremity. Weight reduction should be encouraged in obese patients. Physical therapy is useful, sometimes relieving spasm and associated pain. Often simple application of warm wet packs or warm soaks is helpful. Periarticular injections of local anesthetics are often very effective at the metatarsophalangeal joints by reducing spasm and dilating small vessels supplied by the autonomic nerves in the area. Injection of about 0.75 ml of a local anesthetic in the first and third interspaces around the metatarsophalangeal joints of a patient with marked spasm and pain in the forefoot often brings dramatic relief for several hours or days initially and more prolonged relief when repeated weekly. This regimen can often be reduced to every other week, then monthly, and often even longer intervals. This therapy also permits the patient to maintain muscle function and strength through walking, which is less painful because of the reduction of spasm, which frequently persists long after the local anesthetic has been metabolized (MD Steinberg, personal communication).

Aspirin and other nonsteroidal agents are helpful in many patients. The drug of choice still is aspirin, because of its analgesic and anti-inflammatory properties as well as its low cost. Oral or parenteral adrenocorticosteroid therapy is contraindicated. However, injecting osteoarthritic areas with corticosteroids can be helpful in acute situations. Intraarticular corticosteroid injections should be given with great caution in weight-bearing areas. If given too frequently, they could accelerate joint deterioration by masking pain and leading to overuse of the joint. Pericapsular and ligamentous injection of a local anesthetic around involved joints as described above may provide considerable relief without nearly as much hazard.

Sometimes surgical procedures are indicated when conservative measures prove inadequate. Surgery can include arthroplasty, osteotomy, fusion, and partial or total prosthetic replacement. Some of these procedures also help to bring nondiseased articular cartilage into a more functional position.

GOUT

An ancient disease, gout presents with recurrent paroxysms of violent articular inflammation, provoked by the precipitation of monosodium urate monohydrate in the joint cavity. If the condition is neglected or if therapy is not adequate, gross deposits of sodium urate called tophi may be found in and around the joints and in the kidneys.

The arthritis of gout is a complication of prolonged hyperuricemia. In adults, normal serum urate concentration is 4.0 ± 1.0 mg/dl in women and 5.1 ± 1.0 mg/dl in men. After menopause, female serum uric acid levels rise to approach the level found normally in males. In children of both sexes the level is 3.5 to 4.0 mg/dl until puberty, when it rises to the levels found in adults.[12]

Although 5 percent of adults have been found to have hyperuricemia, only a small proportion of these develop gouty arthritis. In 10 to 15 percent of these patients gouty arthritis is preceded by nephrolithiasis (kidney stones).[25]

Hyperuricemia is classified as either primary or secondary. Primary hyperuricemia is associated with specific enzyme defects, which ultimately result in the overproduction of uric acid, or is due to some undefined molecular defects leading to overproduction or underexcretion of uric acid. Some cases of primary gout have a genetic basis, but others do not. In secondary hyperuricemia, patients develop the condition as part of the course of some other disease or because of certain drugs.

Secondary gout due to overproduction of uric acid is most frequently caused by an increased turnover of nucleic acids. Some of the many conditions that may cause this are the myeloproliferative and lymphoproliferative disorders, multiple myeloma, secondary polycythemia, pernicious anemia, certain hemoglobinopathies, thalassemia, other hemolytic anemias, infectious mononucleosis, and certain carcinomas. Renal causes of secondary hyperuricemia include renal insufficiency, most of the diuretics, chronic lead intoxication, low doses of aspirin (large doses elevate uric acid levels), pyrazinamide, ethambutol, ethanol, and organic acidosis. Fasting may also cause hyperuricemia by increasing plasma levels of acetoacetic and β-hydroxybutyric acids.[12]

One-fourth of gouty patients give a family history of the disease. Males constitute 80 to 85 percent of patients affected and are mainly middleaged and older. Postmenopausal women also are not infrequent victims. In men past 40 years of age,

gout is the most common inflammatory joint disease. The peak period for gouty arthritis is between 40 and 60 years of age.[26]

A typical attack is monoarticular, although rarely a few other joints may also be involved. The lower limbs, especially the first metatarsophalangeal joints, are involved initially (in 75 percent or more of all patients). The tarsal joints, ankles, and knees also are not infrequently the site of an attack. Typical cases have an acute onset, often at night, with exquisite pain and swelling as well as erythema. These features often make gout hard to distinguish clinically from cellulitis or thrombophlebitis. Mild attacks may last several days if not treated, whereas severe conditions may last for weeks. When the inflammation subsides, desquamation of the skin in the area is often seen, and the joint returns to its normal state. Between attacks no abnormalities may be present and the patient may be symptom free.[12]

Clinically or radiologically detectable tophi may be found, especially in longstanding cases that have not been treated with hypouricemic agents. Common areas where tophi are found in the lower extremity are the synovium, subchondral bone, the infrapatellar tendon, and the Achilles tendon.

Chronic gouty arthritis may result in joint deformity, especially in patients with tophi, who tend to have more severe and frequent attacks. This deformity is caused by erosion of cartilage and subchondral bone due to inflammatory reaction to tophaceous material in the joints. Joint cartilage destruction in chronic gout can lead to secondary osteoarthritis with or without chondrocalcinosis.

The metatarsophalangeal joint may be the most frequent target of an attack of acute gouty arthritis because of the relatively low temperature in that part of the body and the fact that this joint bears more weight per square centimeter than any other joint in the body. The low temperature causes the precipitation of the supersaturated solution of uric acid, as does the local joint trauma due to weightbearing. As urates precipitate out of solution, their sharp crystals irritate the joint, start the process of inflammation, and decrease the pH. A low pH also perturbs a supersaturated solution and contributes further to crystallization.[27]

A history of uric acid kidney stones and hyperuricemia and a family history of gout strengthen the evidence needed to diagnose the condition, but none of these is pathognomonic for the disease. One may have hyperuricemia without gout, and one may have gout without demonstrable hyperuricemia because uric acid levels may have been artificially reduced by large doses of aspirin, phenylbutazone, corticosteroids, or other anti-inflammatory agents.

A definitive diagnosis is made by aspiration of monosodium urate monohydrate crystals from an inflamed or even a symptomatic joint. Demonstration of such crystals in aspirates or tissue secretions of tophaceous deposits also is evidence for a definitive diagnosis of gout. A small amount of synovia obtained from the first metatarsophalangeal joint is all that is needed.[28]

Radiology

Joint effusion is frequently seen in acute gout as well as in the chronic tophaceous state of the disease. Tophi are seen as nodules or as lobulated masses near joints or sometimes adjacent to the diaphysis. When they occur, tophi are most common on the dorsum of the foot and ankle and on the Achilles tendon. Bone erosions often develop near tophi. They may be intra-articular or para-articular. There is only a little interosseous space narrowing early in the disease, with narrowing commonly found later in the disorder.

Gout can be mistaken on radiography for rheumatoid arthritis because of the presence of bone erosions, but in gout there is an overhanging margin, which is a segment of eroded cortex extending over the cortex and displaced from the normal bone contour. This appears as a punched-out area, which helps to distinguish it from the erosions of rheumatoid arthritis.[29]

Subperiosteal bone apposition is occasionally present in the metatarsals. Occasionally joint ankylosis is seen. Osteoporosis and soft tissue atrophy, present in rheumatoid arthritis, are not found in gout. However, when chronic arthritis develops in gouty patients, regional osteoporosis may be seen.

The characteristic malalignments or subluxations seen in rheumatoid arthritis are not seen in gout. However, at the site of large intra-articular tophi and ligamentous and bone destruction there may be gross deformity. Secondary osteoarthritis caused by gout may result in minimal malalignment. Bone erosion and tophi are radiologically evident only after years of attacks.

Patient Management

The metabolic nature of gout is such that interdisciplinary cooperative efforts make for the best management plan. The podiatric physician may be the first member of the health care team to see the patient, especially if an acute gouty attack prompts the visit. The care of the acute attack usually has little effect on the hyperuricemia itself (except when phenylbutazone is used). Because of the toxic effects (nausea and diarrhea) that patients experience with colchicine, this ancient drug is often not given, and nonsteroidal anti-inflammatory agents, which are at least as effective, may be prescribed. Indomethacin (Indocin) has been found to be very effective in doses of 50 mg three or four times daily for 4 to 7 days, with little problem of toxicity. Some patients may experience gastrointestinal symptoms, headaches, and other toxic effects, requiring the use of another drug. Ibuprofen, fenoprofen, naproxen, tolmetin sodium, sulindac, and piroxicam have also been shown to be effective against acute attacks of gout. It is advisable to use the maximal recommended dose early in the attack and then to reduce the dose gradually when the symptoms have resolved. Phenylbutazone and oxyphenbutazone are very effective, but great caution is recommended because of their potential for causing bone marrow suppression. The availability of other effective nonsteroidal agents makes the use of these drugs not as essential.

Colchicine, although more specific than the anti-inflammatory agents against gout, is no more effective. However, if it is prescribed for a patient in a full-blown acute attack, one 0.6-mg tablet should be taken every hour until pain is relieved or nausea or diarrhea occurs. A total of no more than 12 tablets should be given in any 24-hour period. About 75 percent of patients respond to colchicine during an acute attack. The earlier in the attack the colchicine is started, the more likely it is that the patient will respond. Patients frequently fail to respond because of a delay in initiating this therapy.

Since most patients respond so rapidly (within 48 hours) to colchicine therapy, it is often also of diagnostic value. Occasionally, however, one may get a response to colchicine in patients with pseudogout, apatite deposition disease, or sarcoid arthritis. Although the mechanism of action of colchicine is still under investigation, it is believed that it acts by interfering with polymorphonuclear leukocyte function.

Between attacks, or to avoid an attack, it is important to eliminate the hyperuricemic body pools of gouty patients. This is best managed by a physician who has much experience in the treatment of patients with hyperuricemia; this may be the rheumatologist, the internist, or in some instances the family practice physician. Treatment may involve the use of uricosuric agents such as probenecid or, when that fails, sulfinpyrazone. Uricosuric agents are started in low doses and gradually increased over 7 to 10 days to avoid precipitating an acute attack. Probenecid 1 to 3 grams daily is given in divided doses, since its half-life is 6 to 12 hours. A mean fall of the serum urate concentration by one-third results. Sulfinpyrazone is used with phenylbutane is toxic or ineffective. It is given in doses that attempt to reach the desired serum urate concentrates. This should not exceed 800 mg/day in divided doses. Salicylates should not be taken when these drugs are used, since they nullify the uricosuric effect. However, acetaminophen can be used without such problems in patients requiring an analgesic or antipyretic agent when they are taking a uricosuric drug. Allopurinol is now frequently used instead of uricosuric agents. It inhibits uric acid production by blocking the conversion of hypoxanthine to xanthine and xanthine to uric acid via the inhibition of the enzyme xanthine oxidase. It is administered in doses of 300 to 800 mg/day. Most patients are able to take the drug without side effects, and rarely have the side effects that sometimes occur been serious. They include rashes, transient liver function problems, and transient leukopenia. Like the uricosurics, allopurinol is started in small doses and gradually increased to avoid precipitating an attack of gouty arthritis.

No rationale is provided to treat asymptomatic hyperuricemia. However, it should be pointed out that the risk of developing acute gouty arthritis increases as the serum urate concentration does. Patients with concentrations greater than 9 mg/dl have a very high risk of developing clinical symptoms of gout.[12]

Patients with tophi on weight-bearing areas or at sites of excessive pressure as well as those who have tophi that drain would benefit from excision of these lesions. Joints that are severely deformed and are compromising motion or weightbearing may benefit from an arthroplasty. However, serum uric acid should be controlled before surgical intervention for tophi or deformed joints is undertaken. This is best done through the cooperative efforts of the foot surgeon and the physician responsible for control of the metabolic defect.

NONARTICULAR RHEUMATISM

Fibrositis

Fibrositis affecting the foot and ankle area is characterized by tenderness without, in most cases, any objective findings. There may be several points of tenderness in other parts of the body as well, or the tenderness may be limited to one area such as the foot. Primary fibrositis patients have no associated disease, whereas in the secondary type some other disease state is related to the condition.

Symptoms include pain, tenderness, and stiffness. The pain when present is sometimes aggravated by fatigue or chilling. Stiffness may result in varying degrees of disability. Most patients with this problem are female. Sometimes tender areas do not involve muscles. Pain may disappear after injections of a local anesthetic.

Salicylates in low doses are often helpful, as are heat, massage, electrical stimulation, and injections into "trigger points." Orthotic devices to place the feet in a more biomechanically sound position may be helpful, as is exercise therapy.[30,31]

Tendinitis, Bursitis, and Fasciitis

Tendinitis, bursitis, and fasciitis are painful conditions which in the foot and ankle area can result in considerable reduction in mobility, which is aggravated by weightbearing and pressure. These conditions most frequently are the result of trauma, which very frequently is a result of biomechanical abnormality, and are aggravated by activities that may range from normal walking to physical fitness activities or sports. Improperly fitted shoes, obesity, and certain occupational activities may be primary or secondary causes of these conditions.

Injection of corticosteroid agents into or around an affected tendon sheath, or intrabursally after aspiration in the case of bursitis, can often be helpful. This can coincide with protective measures to avoid pressure over bursal areas such as felt or foam rubber aperture pads; open, cutout, or special shoes; or orthotic devices. Occasionally surgical treatment is necessary to remove a bursa and correct an underlying bony deformity, which often may be the major direct cause of the problem. Sometimes when tendinitis is present it is necessary to put an area at rest by means of a cast, splint, or other form of temporary immobilization, to avoid using the involved tendon. Physical therapeutic measures, ranging from exercise programs to the use of heat in the form of baths, whirlpool, wet towels, or paraffin, may sometimes be helpful. Diathermy and ultrasound therapy are also used in treating these conditions.[32]

REFLEX SYMPATHETIC DYSTROPHY

Reflex sympathetic dystrophy is classified among the rheumatic diseases as a neuropathic disorder. It is discussed in detail elsewhere in this text. These syndromes are characterized by causalgia, which is a distinctive, nonsegmental pain in one or more extremities. Accompanying the causalgic state are trophic skin changes, vasomotor instability, and increased local blood flow. It may be precipitated by trauma of even a minor nature, immobilization, and personality type. As many as one-third of all patients have no etiologic event that can be identified. When the lower extremity is involved, the whole foot is usually affected, although sometimes only one ray is involved. Tenderness and swelling are accentuated around joints.

Patchy osteoporosis of the feet is sometimes seen in radiographs of patients with reflex sympathetic dystrophy and is called Sudeck's atrophy. Crumbling erosions similar to what is seen in rheumatoid arthritis are often seen on the radiographs. On average, one-third of the bone mineral in the affected extremity is lost. After the initial acute stage, trophic changes are often seen in the skin. A final stage, called the atrophic stage, is characterized by thinning of the skin, subcutaneous tissue, and muscle, and eventually leading to contractures in some cases.

A combination of analgesics with exercise therapy has been used. Sometimes nonsteroidal anti-inflammatory agents are effective. Corticosteroids have also been employed, as have frequent sympathetic blocks with local anesthetics. In some severe cases surgical sympathectomy is performed, provided that local sympathetic blocks have been shown to produce some relief.[12]

REFERENCES

1. Calabro JJ: A critical evaluation of the diagnostic features of the feet in rheumatoid arthritis. Arthritis Rheum 5:19, 1962
2. Rodnan GP, Schumacher HR, Zraifler NJ: Primer on the Rheumatic Diseases. 8th Ed. p 163. Arthritis Foundation, Atlanta, 1983
3. Schmid FR, et al: Arteritis in rheumatoid arthritis. Am J Med 30:56, 1961
4. Mongan EL, Cass RM, Jacox RF, et al: A study of the relation of seronegative and seropositive rheumatoid arthritis to each other and to necrotizing vasculitis. Am J Med 47:23, 1969
5. Pallis CA, Scott JT: Peripheral neuropathy in rheumatoid arthritis. Br Med J 1:1141, 1965
6. Chamberlain MA, Bruckner FE: Rheumatoid neuropathy: clinical and electrophysiological features. Ann Rheum Dis 19:609, 1970
7. Hurd ER: Extraarticular manifestations of rheumatoid arthritis. Semin Arthritis Rheumatol 8:151, 1979
8. Spivak JL: Felty's syndrome: an analytic review. Johns Hopkins Med J 141:156, 1977

9. Martel W: Radiologic manifestations of rheumatoid arthritis with particular reference to the hand, wrist and foot. Med Clin Am 52:655, 1968

10. Martel W: Roentgenographic features of the rheumatic diseases. p 74. In Rodnan GP, Schumacher HR, Zraifer NJ: Primer on the Rheumatic Diseases. 8th Ed. Arthritis Foundation, Atlanta, 1983

11. Rothfield NF: Systemic lupus erythematosus: clinical and laboratory aspects. In McCarty DJ (ed): Arthritis and Allied Conditions. 9th Ed. Lea & Febiger, Philadelphia, 1979

12. Rodnan GP, Schumacher HR, Zraifler NJ: Primer on the Rheumatic Diseases. 8th Ed. pp 52, 63, 177–179, 89–92, 180–181, 104–107, 120–127, 165–167. Arthritis Foundation, Atlanta, 1982

13. Hahn BH, Yardley JH, Stevens MB: Rheumatoid nodules in system lupus erythematosus. Ann Intern Med 72:49, 1970

14. Blomgren SE, Condemi JJ, Vaughan JH: Procainamide-induced lupus erythematosus. Am J Med 5:338, 1972

15. LeRoy EC: Scleroderma (systemic sclerosis). p 1211. In Kelley WN, Harns ED Jr, Ruddy S, Sledge CB (eds): Textbook of Rheumatology. WB Saunders, Philadelphia, 1981

16. Jablonska S, Rodnan GP: Localized forms of scleroderma. Clin Rheumatol Disorders 5:215, 1979

17. Wright V, Moll JMH: Seronegative Polyarthritis. Amsterdam, North-Holland, 1976

18. Editorial: HLA-B27 and the risk of ankylosing spondylitis. Br Med J 2:650, 1978

19. Ball J: Enthesopathy of rheumatoid and ankylosing spondylitis. Ann Rheum Dis 30:213, 1971

20. Ford DK: Reiter's syndrome. Bull Rheum Dis 20:588, 1970

21. Martel W, Braunstein EM, Borlaza G, et al: Radiologic features of Reiter's disease. Radiology 132:1, 1979

22. Martel W: Radiological manifestations of Reiter's syndrome. Ann Rheum Dis, 38:suppl. 12, 23, 1979

23. Kidd KL, Peter JB: Erosive osteoarthritis. Radiology 86:640, 1966

24. Sokoloff L: Osteoarthritis. p 110. In Ackerman LV, Spjut HJ, Abell MR (eds): Bones and Joints. Williams & Wilkins, Baltimore, 1976

25. Hall AP, Barry PE, Dawber TR, McNamara PM: Epidemiology of gout and hyperuricemia: a long term population study. Am J Med 42:27, 1967

26. Becker MA, Seegmiller JE: Genetic aspects of gout. Annu Rev Med 25:15, 1974

27. Levy LA: A rationale for gouty arthritis affecting the first metatarsophalangeal joint. J Am Podiatr Med Assoc 77:643, 1987

28. Wallace SL, Robinson H, Masi AT, et al: Preliminary criteria for the classification of the acute arthritis of primary gout. Arthritis Rheum 20:895, 1977

29. Martel W: The overhanging margin of bone: a roentgenologic manifestation of gout. Radiology 91:755, 1968

30. Smythe HA: Nonarticular rheumatism and the fibrositis syndrome. p 881. In McCarty DJ Jr (ed): Arthritis and Allied Conditions, 9th Ed. Lea & Febiger, Philadelphia, 1979

31. Smythe HA: Fibrositis syndrome. p 706. In Conn HF (ed): Current Therapy. 27th Ed. WB Saunders, Philadelphia, 1975

32. Hench PK: Nonarticular rheumatism. In Katz WA (ed): Rheumatic Diseases: Diagnosis and Management. JB Lippincott, Philadelphia, 1977

Peripheral Nerve Disorders

16

Mark E. Landry, D.P.M.

As recently as 1981, 40 percent of patients with a general history of chronic peripheral neuropathy who entered a hospital did not obtain a definitive diagnosis or etiology of their neuropathy.[1] In the same year, however, improved diagnoses with more aggressive evaluations were reported at a major medical center.[2] In spite of the complexity of peripheral nerve disease, advances have been significant in the past decade. Confusing terminology and eponyms are being avoided. Simplified classification schemes based on anatomic sites of origin and genetic groups have been developed.[3-6] Computed tomography and magnetic resonance imaging (MRI) are rapidly outdating myelography with its inherent risks.[7] Clinical electrophysiology and nerve biopsy have added dimensions to our knowledge of neuropathy. As a testament to the recent advances, consider the tarsal tunnel syndrome: first described and accepted as a clinical entity by Keck[8] in 1962, it was recently the subject of a bibliography including over 100 references.[9]

CLASSIFICATION OF PERIPHERAL NEUROPATHY

Peripheral neuropathy can affect the myelin sheaths, the axon, or the centrally located cell body. The nerves encountered peripherally are merely cytoplasmic extensions of the cell body, supported by connective tissue, and of specialized myelin-producing Schwann cells. Injure the cell at the spinal cord, and the cell and its long axon will die. Injure the axon or myelin sheath, and a repair process may restore what otherwise would be a temporary motor and/or sensory loss. A severe crush of complete laceration to the axon results in distal axonal (Wallerian) degeneration. Finally, many systemic diseases affect the peripheral nerves and must also be considered.

Peripheral neuropathy is divided into two broad categories. It is either symmetric, involving many nerves (polyneuropathy), or asymmetric and local-

377

ized, involving one or several branches of a nerve trunk (mononeuropathy or focal neuropathy). When more than one site is involved the term *multifocal neuropathy* is used.

Polyneuropathy

There are several classifications of polyneuropathies (see Tables 16-1 through 16-7). Polyneuropathy is seen in metabolic, toxic, infective (and postinfective), and hereditary diseases. Common examples of each of these include diabetes mellitus, lead poisoning (plumbism), leprosy, (Guillain-Barré syndrome is a postinfectious autoimmune response), and hereditary motor and sensory neuropathy type I (HMSN type I), respectively. HMSN type I is also known as the hypertrophic type of Charcot-Marie-Tooth disease.

Polyneuropathy can also be classified anatomically, stressing the site of initial pathology. For example, patients with uremia present with neuropathy involving demyelination (as commonly measured by slower nerve conduction studies); however, it has been shown that this neuropathy was secondary to an initial axonal degeneration.[6] Polyneuropathy can also be classified by its clinical onset and, finally, by its involvement of the sensory, motor, or autonomic systems or combinations thereof.

Distal axonopathy occurs most commonly in toxic neuropathies and probably accounts for many metabolic and hereditary neuropathies, in addition to the more obvious segmental demyelination.[6] Degeneration of the nerve begins distally and progresses proximally ("dying back").[10,11] The long axons to the lower extremity are affected first, followed later by involvement of the hands.

Polyneuropathy may primarily affect the myelin as seen in Guillain-Barré syndrome and in diphtheria, among other diseases (Table 16-1). Less frequently the neuropathy starts at the cell body, as in mercury toxicity and pyridoxine megavitaminosis.[6]

Polyneuropathy is commonly described according to its clinical onset (Table 16-2).[12] Examples of acute onset include the ascending paralysis of Guillain-Barré syndrome, diphtheria, acute intermittent porphyria, and paralysis from toxins including arsenic, thallium, hexacarbons, dapsone, and nitrofurantoin. Subacute clinical patterns are seen with metabolic diseases such as diabetes and uremia, nutritional deficiencies, inflammatory diseases such as systemic lupus erythematosus and rheuma-

Table 16-1. Anatomic Classification of Peripheral Neuropathy

Two overall types —	1. Symmetrical generalized
	2. Focal and multifocal

1. Symmetrical generalized neuropathies (polyneuropathies)

Distal axonopathies	Toxic — many drugs, industrial and environmental chemicals
	Metabolic — uremia, diabetes, porphyria, endocrine
	Deficiency — thiamine, pyridoxine
	Genetic — HMSN II
	Malignancy-associated — oat-cell carcinoma, multiple myeloma
Myelinopathies	Toxic — diphtheria, buckthorn
	Immunologic — acute inflammatory polyneuropathy (Guillain-Barré) chronic inflammatory polyneuropathy
	Genetic — Refsum disease, metachromatic leukodystrophy
Neuronopathies	
somatic motor	Undetermined — amyotropic lateral sclerosis
	Genetic — hereditary motor neuronopathies
somatic sensory	Infectious — herpes zoster neuronitis
	Malignancy-associated — sensory neuronopathy syndrome
	Toxic — pyridoxine sensory neuronopathy
	Undetermined — subacute sensory neuronopathy syndrome
autonomic	Genetic — hereditary dysautonomia (HSN IV)

2. Focal (mononeuropathy) and multifocal (multiple mononeuropathy) neuropathies
   Ischemia — polyarteritis, diabetes, rheumatoid arthritis
   Infiltration — leukemia, lymphoma, granuloma, schwannoma, amyloid
   Physical injuries — severance, focal crush, compression, stretch and traction, entrapment.
   Immunologic — brachial and lumbar plexopathy

(From Schaumburg, et al.,[6] with permission.)

toid arthritis, paraneoplastic disease, and toxins, including disulfiram (Antabuse), nitrous oxide, and other metallic and industrial toxins. Chronic clinical patterns include the hereditary motor and sensory polyneuropathies (Tables 16-2, 16-3, 16-4, 16-5, and 16-6).

In addition, polyneuropathy can involve the sensory, motor, and autonomic nerves to varying degrees (Tables 16-3 and 16-4). Charcot-Marie-Tooth (HMSN type I) disease and Guillain-Barré syndrome affect the motor nerves more, whereas diabetes and leprosy more commonly affect the sensory nerves. Moreover, autonomic neuropathy is encountered in insulin-dependent (type 1) diabetics.

Whereas complications of diabetic polyneuropathy are commonly treated by American po-diatrists, up to 20 million people worldwide are affected with the most commonly treatable neuropathy, that arising from leprosy, uncommon though the disease is to the Western world.[6]

Symptoms more often start with numbness, although a deep aching with tingling and an urge to move the legs ("restless legs") are seen not infrequently.[12] An intense, burning foot pain occurs less often but is of more obvious concern to the patient. Polyneuropathies involve varying degrees of mixed sensory, autonomic, and motor dysfunction. Therefore, weakness and fatigue are seen in the sensory polyneuropathies as well.

Signs of autonomic dysfunction include anhidrosis and orthostatic edema. Extreme vascular fluctuation in Guillain-Barré syndrome can bring about a life-threatening hypertensive crisis.

Table 16-2. Classification of Polyneuropathies Based on Clinical Pattern

Clinical Type	Manifestations	Causes
Acute fulminant	Ascending or descending symmetrical paralysis, usually predominantly motor; may involve cranial nerves and/or respiratory muscles	Landry-Guillain-Barré Diphtheria Acute intermittent porphyria Toxins: nitrofurantoin, dapsone, thallium, hexacarbons, arsenic
Subacute	Distal symmetrical; mixed motor and sensory loss; legs affected more than arms	Metabolic: diabetes, uremia Nutritional: vitamin deficiency (*e.g.*, thiamine), but all of B complex Inflammatory: systemic lupus erythematosus, rheumatoid arthritis Paraneoplastic: carcinomas, lymphomas, myeloma Toxins: general drugs—Antabuse, ethylene oxide, isoniazid, lithium, nitrofurantoin, nitrous oxide, thalidomide Toxins: anticancer drugs—Adriamycin, Ara-C, 5-azacytidine, cis-platinum, hexamethylmelamine, m-AmSA, methyl GAG, mizonidazole, procarbazine, vincristine, VP-16-213 Toxins: metals—arsenic, lead, mercury, thallium Toxins: industrial—acrylamide, carbon disulfide, chlordecone, clioquinalone, 2,4-dichlorophenoxyacetic acid, dimethylaminopropionitrile, methylbromide, methylbutylketone, *n*-hexane, organophosphates, trichloroethylene, triorthocresyl phosphate, styrene
Chronic, slowly progressing	Distal symmetrical; mixed motor and sensory loss	Hereditary motor and sensory neuropathies, types I to IV Hereditary sensory neuropathy, types I to IV Chronic inflammatory polyneuropathy Tangier disease Amyloidosis Leprosy°
Chronic relapsing	Distal symmetrical; mixed motor and sensory loss	Probably a variant of Landry-Guillain-Barré

° Usually patchy, not distal symmetrical; may involve face.
(From Swanson,[12] with permission.)

Table 16.3 Predominantly Motor Neuropathies

Landry-Guillain-Barré syndrome
Acute intermittent porphyria
Diabetic amyotrophy
HMSN type I°
HMSN type II°
Nitrofurantoin
Dapsone
Lead
Mercury
Subacute motor neuronopathy†

° HMSN is the abbreviation for hereditary motor and sensory neuropathy (Dyck, Thomas). Types I and II correspond to neuropathies that are also referred to as Charcot-Marie-Tooth disease, peroneal muscular atrophy, or Roussy-Lévy syndrome.
† This is a paraneoplastic neuropathy that may be seen as a complication of lymphoproliferative disorders.
(From Swanson,[12] with permission.)

Mononeuropathy

Mononeuropathy, or focal neuropathy, is most commonly caused by trauma, although many systemic diseases may predispose the patient. Carpal and possibly tarsal tunnel syndrome is seen in numerous conditions, including diabetes, pregnancy, and rheumatoid arthritis.[13] Other causes of mono-

Table 16-4. Predominantly Sensory Neuropathies

Diabetic distal sensory neuropathy
Alcoholic (vitamin-nutritional deficiency) (some cases)
Amyloidosis (some cases)°
Tangier disease (high-density lipoprotein deficiency)°
Pyridoxine excess
HSN I (hereditary sensory neuropathy of Denny-Brown)†
HSN II (congenital sensory neuropathy, Morvan's disease)†
HSN III (familial dysautonomia, Riley-Day syndrome)†
HSN IV (congenital insensitivity to pain)†
Subacute sensory neuropathy (paraneoplastic dorsal root ganglionitis)
Chronic neuropathy of rheumatoid arthritis
Leprosy
Chloramphenicol
Ethionamide
Glutethimide
Metronidazole/misonidazole
Nitrous oxide
Cis-platinum
Chronic arsenic intoxication
Thallium intoxication

° Pain and temperature losses may predominate in these neuropathies.
† HSN is the abbreviation for hereditary sensory neuropathy (Schaumburg).
(From Swanson,[12] with permission.)

neuropathy include thermal, electrical, and radiation injury; vascular lesions; neoplastic or granulomatous lesions; and peripheral nerve tumors and pseudotumors (e.g., Morton's neuroma).

Direct laceration, missile wounds, fractures, and severe contusions cause varying degrees of nerve injury (see classification below). Indirect injury such as soft tissue compression with an improperly applied tourniquet can cause temporary or even permanent nerve damage. Not uncommonly, one might cross one's legs routinely and develop distal paresthesias and even a palsy of the dorsiflexors from chronic compression of the common peroneal nerve as it courses around the fibular neck. The peroneal nerve and its more proximal portion in the sciatic nerve are readily susceptible to compressive injuries.

The surgeon must be wary of prolonged lateral recumbent positioning of the patient on the operating table. A long sleep in which the patient lies on one arm, often after ethanol intoxication, may lead to a "Saturday night palsy." Fortunately, these neuropathies are usually reversible (class 1 neuropraxia). Radiculopathy of L4, L5, and S1 must be ruled out as well (see Ch. 8).

Entrapment is a form of compression.[7] The nerve is restricted and compressed by abnormal adjacent soft tissue and/or bone, often near a joint.[14] The nerve becomes constricted and narrowed at the entrapment and edematous proximally. Myelin distortion and demyelination take place. Electrophysiologic nerve conduction studies are delayed in velocity because of the demyelination. This is especially true of the orthodromic sensory nerve action potential (SNAP) studies. The tarsal tunnel syndrome is the most commonly acknowledged nerve entrapment of the foot.

Acute compression occurs in the compartment syndromes. The anterior compartment syndrome of the lower leg is an emergency situation in which both neurologic and vascular status are in jeopardy of permanent damage. Exercise can lead to the intense increase in interstitial fluids confined to the unyielding anterior compartment. Fasciotomy of the compartment may be required.[7]

Morton's neuroma is the most common focal neuropathy of the foot.[15] It has been considered by some authors to be an entrapment.[14-17] As discussed below, the etiology of Morton's neuroma is not fully understood; however, more often it is considered a traumatic lesion resulting from repeated compression. It is actually a neural fibrosis and not a true neuroma.

Tumors are a relatively rare cause of mononeuropathy. The most common tumor seen is the benign schwannoma.[5] Peripherally, no age or sex distribution can be appreciated. Schwannomas can be observed in larger peripheral nerves on flexor surfaces, but generally not in the smaller cutaneous branches.[18] Neurofibromas are seen subcutaneously in Von Recklinghausen's disease. Isolated cases have been observed in the foot.[19] Malignant nerve tumors are extremely rare in the foot. These tumors (malignant schwannoma and sarcomatous change of neurofibromatosis) may occur in patients with Von Recklinghausen's disease.[20]

Traumatic neuromata are seen following laceration or surgery. An amputation neuroma is a fibrous terminal bulb, occasionally symptomatic at healed amputated sites. Neuroma-in-continuity is simply an undesired and proliferated repair of a partially divided nerve.[21]

THE PERIPHERAL NERVE

The peripheral nerves are bundles of nerve fibers or fascicles partly enveloped by myelin and supported by connective tissue: the epineurium, perineurium, and endoneurium.[22] As the more proximal nerve trunk undergoes distal division, the terms for the connective tissue covering change: the perineurium becomes epineurium, and the endoneurium becomes perineurium. At the level of the foot, the smaller sensory nerves may be composed of 4 to 14 bundles of nerve fascicles separated by perineurium and covered by an epineurium (Fig. 16-1).

Non-weight-bearing nerve branches such as the sural nerve show well-spaced myelinated axons on cross section. In contrast, the plantar interdigital nerves are not as rounded in shape, demonstrate degeneration of and a decrease in the total number of myelinated axons, and exhibit a thickened epineurium (Figs. 16-2 and 16-3).

Unmyelinated fibers are just as numerous as myelinated fibers, but they are not as visible on routine microscopy. A thin myelinated sheath is seen in association with several "unmyelinated" fibers. Nerve conduction studies are done on the faster (by saltatory conduction) myelinated fibers. In many kinds of neuropathy, demyelination and a reparative remyelination of the larger fibers are appreciated in both biopsy and electrophysiologic testing.

A myelinated nerve fiber is enveloped in multiple layers of myelin produced from one single Schwann cell juxtaposed between nodes of Ranvier. Ordinarily, the distance between two nodes (called a segment) is at least 1,000 μm.[23]

Myelin is dependent on both the Schwann cell and the adjacent axon for its continued existence.[6] Distal axonopathies lead to segmental demyelination with preservation of the Schwann cells. However, a primary loss of myelin does not disrupt the axon, although it does significantly slow conduction. Schwann cell division permits alignment of the Schwann cells along the denuded axon to remyelinate the fiber, but with shorter internodal lengths of perhaps 300 μm.[23] However, this intercalation of the remyelinated segments, once fully restored, only slightly decreases the nerve conduction velocity.

If the cell body is destroyed at the level of the spinal cord, the entire nerve dies as well. In cases where the nerve is completely lacerated or suffers a severe crush injury, or even in chronic compression syndromes such as Morton's neuroma, distal degeneration of the axon and myelin results (Wallerian degeneration).

CLASSIFICATION OF NERVE INJURY

Trauma from compression, or direct injury, is the most common cause of isolated focal neuropathy. Seddon[14] outlined three classes of peripheral nerve injury. Sunderland[22] further classified these injuries into five categories. However, Seddon's classification, which follows, has been used since World

Table 16-5. The Principal Hereditary Sensory Neuropathies (HSN)

Mayo Nomenclature	Alternative Names	Inheritance	Clinical and Electrophysiologic Features	Pathology	Pathogenetic Hypothesis	Comments
HSN type I	Dominantly inherited sensory neuropathy. Hereditary sensory neuropathy of Denny-Brown.	Autosomal dominant	Rare. Onset in second decade. Progressive distal extremity sensory loss. Mutilation of feet. Pain and temperature sense more affected than touch-pressure. Occasional lancinating pain. Sweating impaired in distal extremities. Motor nerve conduction normal. Preserved sensory action potentials (A-alpha component) in earlier stages with abnormal A-delta and C-fiber potentials. Proximal tendon reflexes and autonomic function spared (except sweating). Life expectancy normal with good foot care.	Proximal-to-distal gradient of fiber loss. Unmyelinated and small myelinated fibers more depleted than myelinated large fibers.	Pathology and clinical data support hypothesis of slowly progressive sensory distal axonopathy.	Firm correlation of sensory deficit with fiber-type loss on morphologic and electrophysiologic studies. Sparing of proximal autonomic function helpful in differentiating from amyloid neuropathy. Increased synthesis of immunoglobulin A in one kinship.
HSN type II	Congenital sensory neuropathy. Recessive hereditary sensory neuropathy. Morvan's disease.	Autosomal recessive	Rare. Onset in early childhood or at birth. Progression poorly documented. Hands and feet mutilated, pathologic fracture common. Distal touch-pressure may be affected earlier; eventually all modalities involved. Sensory loss not confined to extremities. All tendon reflexes lost. Distal sensory conduction profoundly affected. Motor nerve conduction near normal. Prognosis not known.	Mild proximal-to-distal gradient of fiber loss. Myelinated fibers severely depleted, unmyelinated fibers less so. Occasional degenerating fiber present on biopsy. Some distal segmental demyelination and remyelination.	Morphologic evidence somewhat supports hypothesis similar to HSN type I. Xenograft studies indicate no disorder of Schwann cells.	Morphology supports notion of a progressive, degenerative condition; clinical state often seems static.

| HSN type III | Riley-Day syndrome. Familial dysautonomia. | Autosomal recessive. Predominantly in Jewish families. | Rare. Onset in infancy. Autonomic dysfunction prominent: absent lachrymation, labile sweating, blood pressure, and temperature. Loss of taste. Generalized diminution of pain-temperature sensation. Preserved touch sensation. Short stature, scoliosis. Hyporeflexia. Decreased amplitude of sensory action potentials, mild slowing of motor conduction. Mutilation unusual. Decreased life expectancy. | Sural nerve has near-total absence of unmyelinated axons and reduced numbers of myelinated axons. Slow progression with age. Reduced number of neurons in sympathetic, dorsal root, gasserian, and spheno-palatine ganglia. Ciliary ganglia normal. No CNS change aside from progressive dorsal column degeneration, and depletion of preganglionic sympathetic neurons. | Congenital absence of autonomic and sensory ganglia and peripheral processes indicates disorder of embryogenesis, with mild progressive degenerative disease of neurons. Role for diminished nerve growth factor in embryo and postnatal period has been postulated. | Relationship of abnormal levels of catecholamine metabolites and low serum dopamine β-hydroxylase to the labile autonomic clinical phenomena unclear. Diagnosis usually established shortly after birth; may be initially misdiagnosed as HSN type IV. |
| HSN type IV | Congenital insensitivity to pain. Congenital sensory neuropathy with anhidrosis. | Autosomal recessive | Very rare. Onset in infancy. Widespread absence of pain-temperature sensation. Strength normal. Episodic fever. Absent sweating. Mental retardation. Mutilation usual. Short stature. | PNS incompletely studied. Reduced number of smaller neurons in dorsal root ganglia. | Pathogenesis may resemble that of HSN type III, but insufficient data to support this notion firmly. | Mental retardation and lack of sweating help distinguish from HSN type III. More clinical, pathologic and basic studies needed. |

(From Schaumburg et al.,[6] with permission.)

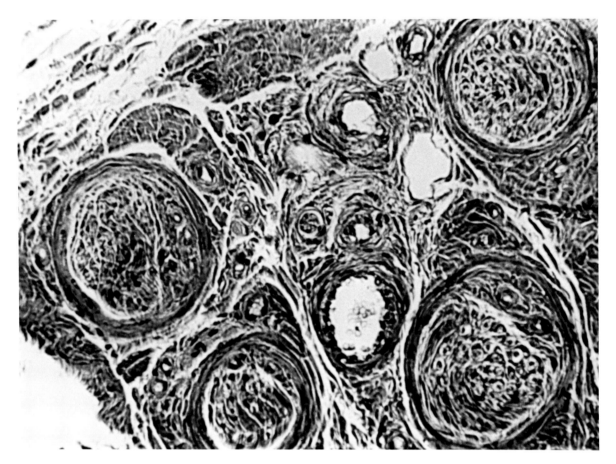

Fig. 16-1. A grouping of four nerve fascicles from a cadaveric sural nerve. (Magnification ×40.)

War II and is practical for evaluating the prognoses of different nerve lesions.

Class 1 (Neuropraxia). Compressive injuries (from tourniquets and casts) result in a transient loss of sensation and/or function lasting from several days to several weeks. Paranodal demyelination occurs, followed by remyelination. A nerve conduction study would exhibit slower velocities (distal latencies) until remyelination takes place.

Class 2 (Axonotmesis). A crush or severe compressive injury involved degeneration of the axon as well. The connective tissue, including the basal lamina of the Schwann cell, remains intact. Wallerian degeneration occurs distally. However, with Schwann cell division and alignment along the endoneural tube, axonal regeneration begins shortly after the injury. The prognosis is good for restoration of function, although it may take weeks.

As remyelination takes place, the internodal lengths become shorter along the restored nerve; hence, nerve conduction may be slightly delayed. A partial injury or laceration in which some of the fascicles are preserved will present a normal conduction velocity, but with a decreased amplitude of the action potential, which directly correlates with the number of participating fibers.

Class 3 (Neurotmesis). The axon and the connective tissue are lacerated and the ends are not realigned. Wallerian degeneration takes place. Sprouting of the proximal nerve end occurs to no avail. Amputation neuromata and aberrant regeneration are seen. No nerve action potentials are recorded with a complete laceration.

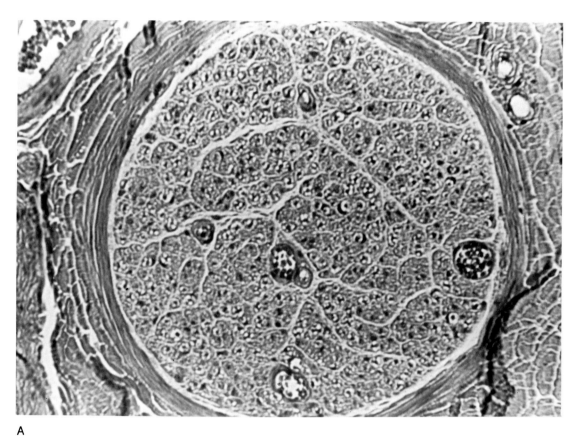

A

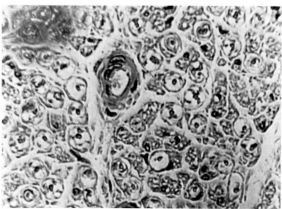

B

Fig. 16-2. (A) Cross section of one fascicle of a sural nerve. Note the numerous myelinated axons (darkened centers of what appear to be empty ovoid discs). (Magnification × 100.) **(B)** Higher magnification. In routine hematoxylin-eosin stain the myelin (clear area about the central axons) does not take up the stain. (Magnification × 400.)

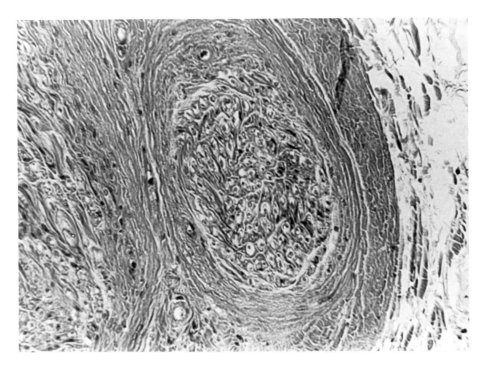

Fig. 16-3. Individual fascicle of a control interdigital plantar nerve. Note the more flattened appearance, the irregular shapes of the myelinated axons, and the thickened epineurium. (Magnification ×100.)

DIAGNOSTIC CONSIDERATIONS

As with any disease or injury, a thorough history and examination are prerequisites. A more complete neurologic examination should be performed when neuropathy is suspected. The entire course of the affected nerve should be examined in focal neuropathy. The body should be inspected for cutaneous abnormalities including neurofibromas, café-au-lait spots, and depigmented and anesthetic patches. These may point to a diagnosis of neurofibromatosis or leprosy. In making the latter diagnosis, the geographic origin of the patient would also be considered.

Amyotrophic lateral sclerosis and syringomyelia are just two examples of diagnoses that might be overlooked unless a complete physical is performed. The physician must be thoroughly cognizant of the signs and symptoms of peripheral vascular disease. Often, the patient with peripheral neuropathy may complain of "poor circulation," when in fact the "pins and needles" sensation he or she is experiencing may be distal paresthesias.

Warmth, erythema, and pain along the course of a vein should lead the examiner to consider superficial phlebitis. Appropriate laboratory blood work should be ordered to rule out infectious or inflammatory processes and to screen for any metabolic disorders. Hypokalemia must always be ruled out when weakness is a presenting symptom.

How long have the symptoms been present? What was the nature of the onset? Are the symptoms increasing in intensity? in frequency? in duration? Are they intermittent?

Symptoms of Guillain-Barré, vascular lesions affecting a nerve, and radiculopathy can begin abruptly. Ingestion or exposure to toxins can bring on a polyneuropathy in a period of weeks; intense foot pain may ensue. Many of the metabolic and hereditary neuropathies present insidiously over a period of months or years. The diabetic patient might initially relate deep, aching cramps and/or a burning foot pain. In other polyneuropathies, deformity and ataxia may be the presenting symptoms. Younger patients may present with genetic polyneuropathy, whereas malignancy and associated vascular lesions are considered more likely in older individuals.

Of course, the family history is important, as both motor and sensory neuropathies can be inherited. Connective tissue disorders affecting the peripheral nerves can likewise be inherited. A previous history of hip, back, or pelvic surgery, including pregnancy and delivery, or trauma may be a significant factor in a resultant mononeuropathy or multifocal neuropathy.

When evaluating suspected motor weakness, myopathy should be ruled out by its proximal involvement and by a check of the serum creatine kinase. Polyneuropathies usually start distally in the feet, fade proximally, and then progress into the hands in a "glove and stocking" distribution. However, neuropathy in diabetes can present proximally in what is usually an asymmetric painful weakness of the anterior thigh muscles (diabetic amyotrophy). Upper motor neuron lesions can usually be recognized (Ch. 8). Hysterical neuropathy is revealed by the patient's bizarre and conflicting signs. To unmask a false radiculopathy, a straight leg raise can be simulated with the patient sitting; the foot is suddenly dorsiflexed on an extended knee. If the patient shows a complete loss of pain and touch without loss of temperature, position, or vibration sense, suspect spurious symptoms and/or hysteria.

Leg and Back Pain

Some of the more common lesions of the low back and hip that can present with foot and leg pain (see Ch. 8 and refs. 7, 12, 24, 25, and 26) are neurogenic stenosis, lumbar disc pain from either a herniated disc or a bony root entrapment (spondylosis), cauda equina syndromes, the piriformis syndrome, and other causes of sciatica.

The patient with neurogenic stenosis presents symptoms similar to intermittent vascular claudication. Calf and foot pain are brought on with activity such as walking. In contrast to radiculopathy from a herniated disc, pain will not be noticed with straining, coughing, or sneezing, nor will there be muscle spasm. The patient is usually at least middle-aged without any significant previous history of back pain, although geriatric patients with chronic degenerative spondylosis may present with a combination of lesions including stenosis. Neurogenic stenosis is seen in cauda equina claudication. The diagnosis is usually clinched by a myelogram and other radiographic studies (see "Radiologic Tests" below). The anteroposterior diameter of the spinal canal is measured to appreciate the stenosis.

Lumbar disc pain may be present with only the symptom of foot pain or leg pain. The pain may be brought on when the patient is lying prone. Curling up on the side may relieve the symptoms. The dermatomes and myotomes as well as the reflexes should be checked to detect the approximate level of the radiculopathy. This is reviewed in Chapter 6.

In gait, the patient with a lumbar nerve root pain will list away from the compressed side and will characteristically stand with a rolled pelvis and flattened lumbar spine. Paravertebral muscle spasm may be observed and palpated. If the straight leg raise is positive, electromyography, appropriate radiographic studies, and consultation are in order.

Cauda equina syndromes include neurogenic claudication, primary tumors of the cauda equina, central disc herniation, malignant disease, and spinal arachnoiditis.[7] Pain and paresthesias can be present from the thigh to the sole of the foot. The patient may walk with an odd gait due to unilateral hamstring spasm. Straight leg raise can be exquisitely sensitive. Tumors such as ependymomas and neurofibromas may affect the younger patient as well. The mother may think the child has a foot problem because of the gait disturbance. If the tumor is high enough (approaching L5), Babinski's sign can be present. These patients also lose control of the sphincter. Metastasis, especially from breast and prostate cancer, must be considered.

Spinal arachnoiditis, which can occur anywhere, commonly occurs in the lumbosacral region. The arachnoid becomes scarred and thickened, bonding to the pia and the dura. The local circulation is jeopardized. This scar tissue unfortunately occurs after lumbar surgery and after the injection of oil-based contrast dyes used in myelography.

Disorders of the lumbosacral plexus must also be considered in the differential diagnosis of leg pain. Adjacent soft tissue tumors and retroperitoneal hemorrhage present with subacute pain radiating from the low back to the leg. Paresthesias and motor weakness follow. The tumors are often more insidious and may preclude venous and/or lymphatic return, leading to often unilateral pedal edema. A warm, dry foot may be observed when the sympathetic trunk is involved.[23]

Diabetics may have a lumbar plexopathy (amyotrophy), often in association with distal polyneuropathy. In the proximal neuropathy, severe pain is present mostly in the back, hips, and proximal thighs. Weakness is present mostly about the pelvic girdle.

Piriformis syndrome is a controversial entity. It is a focal neuropathy of the sciatic nerve. The piriformis muscle, an external hip rotator, is thought to compress the sciatic nerve. Pain is localized about the thigh and buttocks. To check for this, the patient lies prone and with the knee flexed, and the thigh is internally rotated to elicit pain.

Finally, other causes of sciatica should be considered. Patients on anticoagulant therapy may have hemorrhage in the posterior thigh, thus contributing to a focal sciatic neuropathy. Short-legged obese patients may develop sciatica from sitting on the edges of chairs.

The Physical Examination

The motor system should be evaluated first by observing the gait and stance. This can be included with a routine biomechanical and gait analysis. Pes cavus or any other unusual foot or gait disorder is observed. Weakness of specific myotomes along with absence of reflexes is a more accurate and reliable guide to diagnosis than the paresthesias and hypesthesias observed in the dermatomes. Gross muscle atrophy with muscle fasciculations may be observed in the patient with mononeuropathy. Peroneal atrophy is seen in hereditary polyneuropathy.

Loss of muscle mass, however, is not seen as frequently in focal neuropathies within the foot. Muscle testing is graded from zero to five as reviewed in Chapter 8. The muscle flexors in the foot can be checked and compared to each other. This is done by asking the patient to flex the toes 5 to 10 times against the examiner's resistance.

Very simply, and with caution to remember individual variations of innervation, the following myotomes should be kept in mind: The patient should be able to raise the great toe in gait; this tests the L5 root. To further evaluate an L5 radiculopathy, manual testing and an electromyogram of the gluteals and the posterior tibial muscle would help differentiate a foot-drop secondary to a lesion affecting only the common peroneal nerve.

The anterior tibial muscle is innervated by a preponderance of fibers from L4, although in a minority of cases it may be supplied more with fibers from L5.[25] To further evaluate an L4 lesion, the patient is asked to do partial knee-bends to check the quadriceps.

The flexor hallucis and flexor digitorum longus and gastrocnemius muscles all adequately reflect S1 and S2 function. Hamstring strength testing permits discrimination between the medial tibial and lateral peroneal components of the sciatic nerve. Testing the biceps femoris is more specific for the peroneal side of the sciatic nerve (L4, L5, S1, S2). The remainder of the hamstrings are innervated by the tibial side of the sciatic nerve (L4, L5, S1–S3). The peroneal side of the sciatic nerve is composed mostly of fibers from L5, whereas the tibial side has more fibers from S1.

Radiculopathy and other more distal focal neuropathies do not always present with a clearly defined area of anesthesia. Rather, a patchy distribution of paresthesias and sensory loss will often be observed. Severe demyelination or complete interruption of the axon will result in a distal radiating area of anesthesia. However, the "signature area" will vary considerably because of variability in branching and because of anastomosing between the branches. Nevertheless, the classic means of testing the dermatomes on the foot is by running a sewing wheel from medial to lateral to check, respectively, L4, L5, and S1.

Sensory changes seen in polyneuropathy might include a loss of pain and temperature sensation (small-fiber involvement). Sharp and dull touch are checked with a cotton-tipped wooden applicator.

To check loss of temperature, a wooden dowel can be warmed and placed next to the patient's skin, followed by a cold coin. This small-fiber loss of sensation is frequently seen in the stocking and later the glove distribution.

Large-fiber loss includes a loss of vibration sense and proprioception, resulting in ataxia. This is seen in Friedreich's ataxia and in uremic neuropathy. Often vibration loss is one of the first signs observed in polyneuropathy. The tuning fork should be set at 128 Hz. The deep tendon reflex of the Achilles tendon is also an earlier-lost sensation, except amyloidosis where it may be seen late.[12] Diabetics often show a pattern of mixed large- and small-fiber neuropathy, much of which is not subjectively appreciated. Vibration and temperature thresholds have been found to be elevated in asymptomatic type 1 diabetics.[27]

In tabes dorsalis and in less common types of diabetic neuropathy, lightning-like pains shoot through the legs. In this type of neuropathy, not uncommonly seen by podiatrists, the foot should be inspected for ulcers and felt for any unusual warmth about the midtarsal joints, where arthropathy occurs (Fig. 16-4).

Fasciculations and cramps may occur in the patient with metabolic polyneuropathy. Diabetics and alcoholics may experience cramps in their feet or calves in the morning or at any time upon stretching. Squeezing the calf or foot may elicit undue pain and discomfort deep within the muscle.

Autonomic innervation parallels the sensory dermatomes. Autonomic neuropathy is seen in diabetics. The patient should be observed for orthostatic edema and vascular discoloration. The nails are often thick, brittle, and friable. The skin may be shiny and appear thin. To further test the autonomic system, check for the presence of sweating. Scratch the skin and look for the hyperemic response. Autonomic neuropathy is particularly evident in reflex sympathetic dystrophy (causalgia).

When one is evaluating a focal neuropathy, the entire course of the nerve and other muscles innervated by the trunk nerve from the back to the foot should be examined. Multifocal neuropathies should always be considered. Tinel's sign may be present as well as a palpable lesion. The peripheral nerves may be relatively thickened as a result of chronic demyelination and reparative remyelina-

tion and intraneural scarring. The auricular nerve below the ear may be visible in Charcot-Marie-Tooth disease as well as other peripheral nerves of the foot.

The examiner should readily identify the intermediate dorsal cutaneous branch of the superficial peroneal nerve (Lemont's nerve), which has been reported to undergo tension injury in the common inversion sprain.[28] Occasionally the intermediate, medial, and proximal superficial peroneal nerve can be seen, especially when supinating the foot.

Entrapment of the superficial nerve has been reported.[29] Marked tenderness was localized 10 cm above the lateral malleolus, with distal pain radiating dorsally onto the foot. Surgical release of the entrapment may be required.

The sural nerve may sometimes stand out and be visible. The larger tibial nerve can be palpated behind the medial malleolus immediately posterior to the posterior tibial artery. Finally, the common peroneal nerve can also sometimes be palpated by the head of the fibula. Most nerves in the foot come from the sciatic root, the exception being the saphenous nerve on the dorsomedial part of the foot. Figure 16-5 shows the course of the sciatic nerve and its distal branches. These are the fibers more commonly involved in traumatic mononeuropathies of the limb and foot.

Radiologic Tests

Once neuropathy is suspected and/or referral is made to the neurologist, a myelogram may be ordered to evaluate the spinal cord and any herniation or bony impingements on the nerve root. Stenosis of the canal can sometimes be appreciated.

Computed tomography (CT) scanning is supplementing myelography. Myelography views the entire length of the spinal cord whereas CT provides transverse slices. Magnetic resonance imaging (MRI) enhances soft tissue abnormalities in association with bone (Fig. 16-6).[29] MRI provides more accurate structural information. Radiopaque dyes can be used to inject bursae and/or tendon sheets that may be impinging upon an adjacent nerve (Fig. 16-7).

Xeroradiography has been used with limited success to evaluate neuromas in the foot.[30] Sullivan's

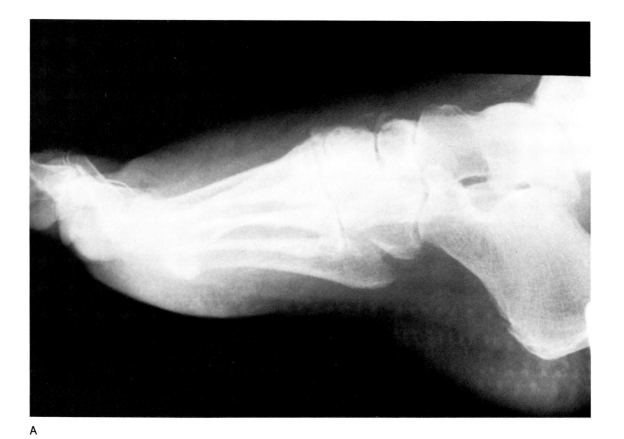

A

B

Fig. 16-4. (A) Early Charcot joint in a diabetic. **(B)** Three months later, extensive destruction takes place at the more commonly occurring Lisfranc and Chopart joint levels.

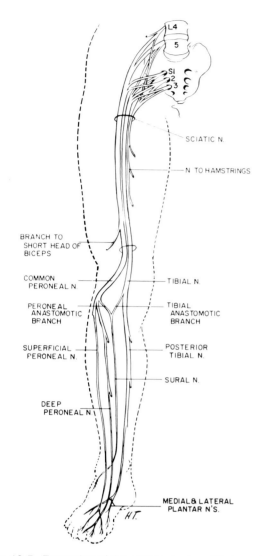

Fig. 16-5. Formation of the sciatic nerve and its branches. (From Liverson and Speilholz,[26] with permission.)

sign[31] on a standard radiograph is seen in some cases of Morton's neuroma or interdigital cyst at either the third or the second interspace. Of course, previous fractures or bony exostoses may cause impingement on adjacent nerve structures as well. Routine radiographs may show this.[32]

Electrodiagnostic Testing

There are two general types of electrodiagnostic study employed by podiatrists when evaluating focal neuropathy of the foot: nerve conduction studies including distal latency times, and electromyography (EMG). Nerve conduction studies can evaluate either motor or sensory activity. The resultant compound action potential can then be recorded at a distal or a proximal site.

Historically, nerve conduction studies have involved proximal stimulation of a motor nerve with observation of a distal response. For example, the tibial nerve would be excited above the ankle and a distal compound motor action potential (CMAP) would be recorded at either the abductor hallucis or the abductor digiti quinti muscle. The resting nerve potential is about 70 μV and relatively negative on the inside of the axolemma. During depolarization of the nerve, the exchange of sodium and potassium ions brings about an action potential of 50 μV inside the nerve. Sodium flows out, potassium returns, and repolarization of the nerve takes place.

Conduction is carried by saltatory motion between the nodes on the larger myelinated fibers at speeds of about 50 m/sec. Unmyelinated fibers may conduct at rates as slow as 12 m/sec.[7]

The aggregation of numerous depolarizing and repolarizing fibers contributes to the resultant compound action potential. Muscle depolarization is summated into characteristic amplitudes, whereas nerve action potentials are polyphasic.

Compound sensory action potentials (CSAP) are now commonly being recorded. This is done by placing a surface electrode over a superficial sensory nerve in the foot, applying a stimulus, and recording the proximal action potential. Ring electrodes on the digits are also in popular use. This type of sensory nerves measurement is also sometimes referred to as sensory nerve action potential (SNAP) testing. These potentials appear to be of greatest value in diagnosing tarsal tunnel syndrome. Unfortunately, they are of questionable value in diagnosing Morton's neuroma.

The period from the proximal stimulation to the recorded CMAP is referred to as the distal latency time. It is usually on the order of 5 to 6 msecs in the tibial nerve in tarsal tunnel syndrome. The velocity is usually in the range of 50 m/sec.

The recorded CMAP amplitude is proportional to the number of units (fibers) depolarizing. The CMAP duration reflects the relative grouping or

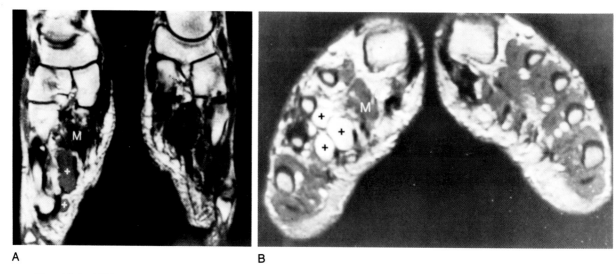

A   B

Fig. 16-6. MRI scan demonstrating soft tissue neuromas and adjacent bursae (+). (Courtesy of Dr. David Sartoris.)

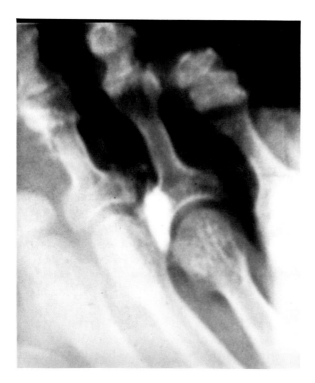

Fig. 16-7. Radiopaque dye can be used to determine the presence and size of an intermetatarsal bursa that may be impinging upon the interdigital nerve.

uniformity of the depolarizing motor units. If the nerve fibers are in part demyelinated, and conduction is slower, the depolarization of the muscle units will occur in a more dispersed manner. Hence the CMAP will be prolonged in demyelinated neuropathy. Its amplitude will be less if the number of motor units firing at any one time is less. Figure 16-8 shows normal and abnormal nerve conduction studies and EMG recordings as might be seen in tarsal tunnel syndrome.

CSAP can be stimulated distally and recorded proximally. When studying a sensory nerve, the velocity is measured from two different proximal locations. As with the CMAP measurement, the amplitude reflects the number of firing nerve fibers, and the duration of the CSAP measures the uniformity of the conductions (Fig. 16-8).

Finally, mixed nerve motor and sensory nerves are stimulated at one point, and depolarization occurs both distally and proximally. The motor fibers cause an antidromic or distal muscular response. The sensory axons depolarize proximally in the orthodromic direction. Moreover, the proximal depolarization to the spinal cord causes activation of the anterior horn cells, resulting in a secondary antidromic action potential occurring a few milliseconds after the initial CMAP. This smaller sec-

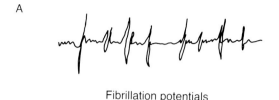

Fibrillation potentials

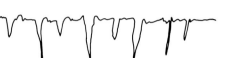

Positive sharp waves 100 ms

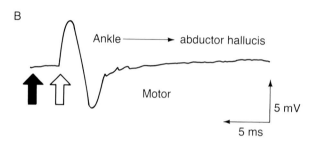

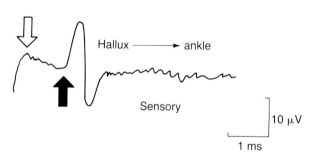

A

B

Ankle ⟶ abductor hallucis

Motor

5 mV

5 ms

Hallux ⟶ ankle

Sensory

10 μV

1 ms

Fig. 16-8. Electrodiagnostic recordings. **(A)** Abnormal muscle recordings of EMG. **(B)** Antidromic motor and orthodromic sensory nerve conduction studies.

ondary action potential is known as an **F-wave.** It is useful to measure this potential when radiculopathy or plexopathy is being considered.

The H-reflex is similar to the F-wave except that the motor response seen with the contraction of the muscle groups supplied by the sciatic nerve is the deep tendon reflex (i.e., the Achilles reflex). However, clinical testing of the deep tendon reflexes

resulting in an α motor neuron response of the gastrocnemius is similarly reliable, thus precluding any practical need of the H-reflex.[7]

The relative value of SNAP in both tarsal tunnel and Morton's neuroma is discussed later in this chapter, and an order of hierarchy reflecting the relative validity of electrodiagnostic tests is presented as well.

EMG is directly useful to the podiatrist to confirm any aberrant activity of the intrinsic muscles of the sole of the foot. A neurologist would more often use EMG to confirm any clinical suspicions of weak muscle groups seen in nerve root lesions. The EMG would help confirm the level of nerve root damaged.

Normally, there should be an absence of electrical activity in the resting muscle. Positive sharp waves and fibrillation potentials are seen when the muscle innervation has undergone Wallerian degeneration (axonopathy). These usually appear in about 10 to 20 days following a complete laceration of the nerve to the muscle[7] (Fig. 16-8A).

The abnormal EMG responses seen in focal neuropathies, including fibrillation potentials and positive sharp waves, are not specific to neuropathy. This muscle activity is seen in myopathy and muscular dystrophy as well.

During voluntary muscle contraction the motor unit potentials are summated and present a characteristic amplitude and wave shape. Neurogenic motor unit potentials have larger amplitudes and a polyphasic configuration. If, following an injury, the axon is preserved, detectable motor unit potentials will be preserved and revealed by EMG. In class 2 and 3 nerve injuries no EMG activity will be recorded at first. After a month, either aberrant activity or evidence of regeneration demonstrating the nerve injury to be either class 2 or class 3 will be seen. If there has been axonal degeneration of a number of fascicles, the amplitude of a motor unit potential will be reduced. Focal demyelination and remyelination will disperse the CMAPs.

EMG and nerve conduction studies test the integrity of the larger myelinated nerves. They do not test the smaller unmyelinated fibers. Unmyelinated fibers of the autonomic system can be tested by inducing sweating and observing the respective dermatomes.

DISEASES INVOLVING POLYNEUROPATHY

Sir William Osler said, "He who knows syphilis knows medicine." Fortunately, little syphilis is seen today. In its place, however, one might attempt to know and appreciate the many diseases that can present as some form of polyneuropathy. Therefore, to update Osler's now-outdated dictum, to know peripheral neuropathy is to know medicine.

The polyneuropathies reviewed here are the more common ones, especially those commonly seen by podiatrists, including diabetic neuropathy and hereditary motor and sensory disorders (Table 16-6).

Diabetic Neuropathy

Diabetic neuropathy is probably the polyneuropathy most frequently seen by clinicians in the United States. Diabetic patients can have a wide range of peripheral nerve disorders, including polyneuropathies and mononeuropathies and mixtures of the two. The polyneuropathy can be either a distal sensory neuropathy or an autonomic neuropathy. A rapidly reversible neuropathy is also seen in patients with uncontrolled hyperglycemia.

Diabetic polyneuropathy affects males and females equally. There is a prevalence of distal polyneuropathy of about 50 percent among diabetics of 25 years' duration.

Focal neuropathies are also commonly seen in diabetics. A patient may have a mixed pattern of involvement consisting of proximal thigh paresthesias and weakness (amyotrophy), carpal tunnel syndrome, and symmetric burning feet.

The sensory neuropathy is symmetric and usually starts with an imperceptible degree of numbness. Early increases in the threshold of the vibratory and temperature responses have also been shown.[33] Both large and small nerve fibers undergo selective segmental demyelination and possibly axonopathy. The sensory neuropathic patient may have muscular pain and cramps, burning feet, or distal paresthesias. Hypesthesia may commonly be present in the feet, followed later by the hands in a stocking-and-glove distribution.

Diabetics may also have autonomic neuropathy, which may affect other bodily functions including the genitourinary, gastrointestinal, and reproductive systems. The vascular tone may be jeopardized, leading to orthostatic edema and other trophic changes. These changes might be thin, shiny skin, hair loss, and thickened nails. The jeopardized vascularity may serve to shunt vital blood supply to inflamed areas of the foot and cause rarefaction of bone.[34,35] This further increases the gravity of minor infections in the diabetic foot.

The diabetic patient may have hyperpathic signs (e.g., burning feet), numb feet in the stocking distribution, or the less commonly seen (but with greater complications) pseudotabetic pattern. Selective fiber involvement has been suspected.[33,34,36]

The pseudotabetic pattern in diabetes is similar to tabes dorsalis in that the dorsal column of fibers (proprioception and vibration) is affected. In more advanced cases, the patient may have to walk with a wide stance and look at the floor as the feet are placed in an almost slapping manner. The patient may have lightning-like pain shooting through the feet and legs. Both tabetic patients and diabetics

Table 16-6. Classification of Polyneuropathies

Metabolic	Hereditary	Toxic	Ischemic	Inflammatory	Other
Diabetes	Hereditary motor and	Ethanol abuse	Necrotizing angiitis	Guillain-Barré	Carcinoma
Nutritional	sensory	Pharmaceutical	Rheumatoid arthritis	syndrome	Lymphoma
Porphyria	neuropathies (e.g.,	Environmental	Polyarteritis nodosa		Multiple myeloma
Uremia	Charcot-Marie-	Biologic	Systemic lupus		Dysproteinemia
Hypothyroidism	Tooth disease)		erythematosus		Amyloidosis
	Hereditary amyloidosis				Leprosy
	Hereditary lipid				Diphtheria
	disorders				Herpes zoster
					Sarcoidosis
					Tabes dorsalis

can develop neuropathic ulcers (e.g., malperforans) and severe arthropathy. In this pattern, Romberg's sign is present and deep tendon reflexes are diminished or absent. The radiographic and clinical signs will not correlate with the minimal symptoms the patient may have. The foot will be warm, swollen, and sometimes erythematous. Osteomyelitis must be ruled out.

Ground bone chips can be seen in the early radiographs. Figure 16-4 shows the marked destruction that can occur in a neuropathic joint. Autonomic disorders including impotence, bladder atony, and pupillary abnormalities are also more commonly associated with this pattern. Arthropathy is generally treated conservatively with bracing or casting.

The pathomechanism of distal polyneuropathy is unclear. In chronic cases both segmental demyelination and axonopathy are seen. No longer is the vasa nervorum implicated as the cause of distal polyneuropathy. The relative degree of neuropathy does not correlate with the thickening of the walls of the endoneural capillaries. Accumulation of nerve sorbital has been proposed.[10]

In contrast to diabetic polyneuropathy, mononeuropathy in diabetics is believed to have a vascular basis. Mononeuropathies are seen in the elderly and may have a more abrupt onset. They may improve spontaneously.

Differential diagnosis of the distal sensory polyneuropathy seen in diabetics should include paraneoplastic sensory neuropathy, nutritional deficiency, and polyarteritis nodosa. Leprosy can also mimic sensory neuropathy and should be ruled out by those treating susceptible populations.

Paraneoplastic sensory neuropathy involves a similar loss of sensation; however, signs of upper motor lesions may lead the clinician to suspect occult carcinoma or lymphoma.

Nutritional deficiency states, including those associated with chronic alcoholism, should be considered. A higher incidence of neuropathic ulcers is seen with the mixed abuse of alcohol, poor nutrition, and uncontrolled diabetes. Vitamin B_{12} deficiency affects the large-fiber pattern of sensory loss and loss of ankle jerks. Anemia might suggest vitamin B_{12} deficiency.

Polyarteritis nodosa is seen more in the younger individual. Usually more systemic illness is seen with this, including fever and an elevated erythrocyte sedimentation rate and blood urea nitrogen. Nerve biopsy is diagnostic.

Treatment of the sensory neuropathy must include strict control of hyperglycemia. Protective shoes and caution in using hot water as well as daily inspection of the feet for blisters or fissures help to prevent more serious and complicating infections. Malodorous ulcers should lead the clinician to suspect mixed bacterial infections and anaerobic bacteria. More salient features of the diabetic foot are reviewed in Chapter 20.

In summary, diabetics may show one of three patterns of distal polyneuropathy. Large-fiber involvement presents with absent ankle jerks and loss of light touch and vibratory sense. In severe cases proprioception is impaired. Less frequently seen is the small-fiber pattern, which is associated with pain and burning soles. The pseudotabetic pattern is seen where neuropathic ulcerations lead to severe infections, sometimes requiring amputation. Neuropathic arthropathy is the other hallmark of this pattern. Recent fiber studies have revealed selective large- and small-fiber demyelination and early autonomic involvement.[33,34,36]

Nutritional Polyneuropathy

Selective vitamin B_6 and B_{12} deficiencies are now rare in Europe and North America. Instead, combined vitamin B deficiency is commonly associated with alcoholism. Although alcohol by itself is considered a neurotoxin, more often chronic alcoholics fail to be well nourished. Among other nutrients, thiamine deficiency is thought to have a major role because of the excessive carbohydrate ingestion and resultant increased need for thiamine.[35]

Nutritional deficiencies appear to first affect the distal axons of the feet and secondarily affect the myelin.[35] Many of the sensory symptoms affecting small and large fibers are frequently seen in the feet. Cramps in the calves and painful soles are frequently seen. Weakness follows. The full burning foot syndrome may ensue. Alcoholics with poorly controlled diabetes are seen with regularity in podiatric clinics in the larger U.S. cities.

Malabsorption syndromes can bring about a vitamin B_{12} deficiency. Neurologic symptoms include optic neuropathy, myelopathy, and peripheral sensory neuropathy.

Guillain-Barré Neuropathy

Guillain-Barré syndrome is a more rapidly evolving polyneuropathy. Extensive demyelination of the motor nerves occurs. It may sometimes be referred to as Landry's paralysis or Landry-Guillain-Barré syndrome. Many times it follows a nonspecific viral infection. Immunization with the vaccine for A/New Jersey influenza (swine flu) caused an outbreak in the early 1980s. However, the condition is present worldwide. It is a leading cause of paralysis in young adults, with an incidence of 9.5 cases per million in the United States.[6] It is also seen in an older age group between the fourth and sixth decades.

Although the precise etiology is not known, Guillain-Barré syndrome is generally believed to be an autoimmune response with delayed hypersensitivity primarily confined to the peripheral nervous system. In 60 percent of cases a preexisting upper respiratory or gastrointestinal illness was revealed in the history.[6]

Progressive symmetric weakness starting in the feet and legs, with hyporeflexia is commonly seen. Difficulty walking is frequently an early complaint. The weakness then ascends over the entire body. Although full recovery takes place in most cases by 6 months, life-threatening breathing paralysis may occur. These patients must be admitted to a hospital to prevent and guard against any pulmonary complications. There is a 5 percent mortality rate. Rarely, recurring inflammatory polyneuropathy is seen.

Toxic Polyneuropathy

Many drugs and environmental chemicals are thought to contribute to the semiology of distal axonopathy. Fewer are actually understood to cause neuropathy. Many new drugs are being reported to have peripheral neuropathy as a possible side effect. Regrettably, many industrial chemicals, fertilizers, and pesticides have been found to be neurotoxic after widespread use. Thallium, the hexacarbons, the monomer of acrylamide, and organophosphates are chemical groups known to be neurotoxic. Two well-known neurotoxic drugs are

isoniazid (INH) and vincristine (Oncovin, used in leukemia and lymphoma). (For more information on the numerous toxins contributing to polyneuropathy, see refs. 1, 5, 6, 10, and 12).

Well-nourished alcoholics are seen with neuropathy; here alcohol is directly associated with neuropathy and considered a toxin. Distal axonopathy presents with numbness and pins and needles in the tips of the digits (acroparesthesia). An unsteady gait may also be noticed. Signs of diminished temperature sensation, painful cramping, and loss of proprioception are observed.

An example of a biologic toxin is the exotoxin released by *Corynebacterium diphtheriae* in the acute infection of diphtheria. A polyradiculopathy occurs in 20 percent of cases 8 to 12 weeks after the acute infection. The toxin appears to inhibit myelin synthesis in the Schwann cell.[6] Fortunately, it is not seen in the United States but is still present in countries where vaccinations are not required.

Ischemic Polyneuropathy

Diffuse small-vessel disease, with necrotizing angiitis and ischemia, contributes to a generalized polyneuropathy seen in a number of arthritic disorders including rheumatoid arthritis, polyarteritis nodosa, and systemic lupus erythematosus (SLE). On biopsy, the epineural vessels are thickened, and axonal degeneration is seen. The symptoms of polyneuropathy are noticed less in light of other soft tissue and joint problems.

Patients with longstanding rheumatoid arthritis develop a mild distal sensory neuropathy. All senses are diminished equally, unlike the selective loss seen in diabetics. Occasionally some pain related to the neuropathy may occur. One should look for bilateral muscle soreness and cramping.

Two-thirds of patients with polyarteritis nodosa exhibit neuropathy at some time. Multiple focal neuropathy is common. The onset is often abrupt and painful, with anesthesia along the course of the affected nerve a classic feature. Total motor and sensory loss can follow in a few days. The arms may be affected as well as the legs. This condition is seen in elderly patients and the prognosis is poor.

About 10 percent of patients with SLE develop one of three neuropathic patterns: a Guillain-Barré type, diffuse distal sensory and/or motor neuropathy, or multiple focal neuropathies.

Infectious Polyneuropathy

Although leprosy (Hansen's disease) is the leading cause of peripheral neuropathy in the world, it is rare in the United States. There are special centers in America that treat patients with Hansen's disease; fortunately these patients receive podiatric care.[37] Neuropathic ulcers and arthropathy are seen. Hansen's bacillus *(Mycobacterium leprae)* specifically attacks the peripheral nerves. Therefore, all lepers have peripheral neuropathy.

Herpes zoster is caused by the varicella-zoster virus. It, too, specifically infects the peripheral nerves. Although the thoracic spinal roots are involved more in the common shingles, the lumbar roots can be affected in up to 15 percent of cases.[12] Skin vesicles are seen 1 to 3 weeks following the onset of rather severe pain in the respective dermatome. Segmental paralysis can occur, but in general the prognosis is good.

End-stage or tertiary syphilis including tabes dorsalis is not seen today in such numbers as before the advent of penicillin. The symptoms of tabes dorsalis are comparable to a severe form of diabetic polyneuropathy. Lancinating pain occurs, along with neuropathic ulcers and joint destruction from sensory loss. Arthropathy is more common in the knee in tabes dorsalis, and more common in the midtarsal joints in diabetes.

Sarcoidosis is a granulomatous disease of unknown etiology affecting multiple systems. Therefore, other medical signs and symptoms are present, including pulmonary infiltration, lymphadenopathy, and skin lesions.

Peripheral polyneuropathy is seen in only 5 percent of cases.[6]

OTHER METABOLIC POLYNEUROPATHIES

Hypothyroidism

Mononeuropathy from swollen adjacent soft tissue is more closely associated with hypothyroidism, especially carpal tunnel syndrome. When carpal or tarsal tunnel syndrome is seen in a patient, hypothyroidism should be suspected and ruled out. Polyneuropathy is rare. It is common to see it first in the feet and then in the hands. The patient's feet are tired and weak and the patient has an unsteady gait. Paresthesias, cramping, and numbness may also occur. The pathomechanism appears to involve both the axon and concomitant Schwann cell dysfunction. With proper hormonal therapy, signs of polyneuropathy usually disappear within 6 months.[6]

Porphyria

Three of six relatively rare types of porphyria have an associated polyneuropathy. The most common and, hence, most studied is acute intermittent porphyria (AIP). Less is known about variegated porphyria and hereditary coproporphyria.

In porphyria, there is a deficiency in essential enzymes normally used for the production of the heme molecule. Porphyria can be a serious, life-threatening disease. Motor weakness predominates as in Guillain-Barré syndrome. The upper and proximal extremities are more often involved than the legs and feet.

Acute exacerbations are brought on with certain drugs, including barbiturates and griseofulvin. Special precautions must be taken with any anesthesia given to patients with a past history of porphyria. Recovery usually takes place within 2 months after the acute symptoms appear, but recurrent episodes may occur at any time. It may take more than a year for the distal nerves in the feet and hands to fully reinnervate.[5-7]

Uremic Neuropathy

When the kidney cannot excrete metabolites, they play havoc on the peripheral nerves as well as on other systems. Hence, these patients are usually very sick and not first seen with complaints of peripheral neuropathy. Approximately half of all patients on renal dialysis have neuropathy. It is often observed to be reversible following dialysis. Paresthesias commonly occur in the feet. Today's therapy, including increasingly successful renal transplantation, has largely controlled the associated polyneuropathy seen in uremia. The myelin break-

Table 16-7. The Principal Hereditary Motor and Sensory Neuropathies (HMSN)

Mayo Nomenclature	Alternative Names	Inheritance	Clinical and Electrophysiologic Features	Pathology	Pathogenetic Hypothesis	Comments
HMSN type I	Hypertrophic form of peroneal muscular atrophy (PMA). Hypertrophic form of Charcot-Marie-Tooth (CMT) disease. Roussy-Lévy syndrome (some cases).	Usually autosomal dominant (linked to Duffy locus on chromosome 1), rarely autosomal recessive. Recessive cases are more severely affected. Marriage of two affected individuals has produced children resembling recessively inherited HMSN type I.	Not an uncommon condition. Many mild, asymptomatic cases. Onset in childhood, adolescence or later. Slowly progressive distal atrophy and weakness. Little sensory loss. Nerves often enlarged. Pes cavus common, scoliosis unusual. Essential tremor in some individuals. Sensory and motor conduction diffusely affected, motor may be extremely slow. Abnormal visual and auditory evoked potentials indicate optic and acoustic nerve involvement in some cases. Normal active life span common.	Distal segmental demyelination, remyelination and onion bulbs. Fewer myelinated axons of large diameter in distal nerves. CNS normal except for dorsal columns.	Pathology and morphometry suggest primary axonal disorder (distal axonopathy). Xenograft studies and abnormal axonal transport of dopamine β-hydroxylase support this hypothesis.	The "classic" form of CMT disease or PMA. Mild cases widely misdiagnosed as orthopedic foot disorders. Rare variants associated with optic atrophy, deafness, or spastic paraplegia.
HMSN type II	Neuronal form of PMA. Neuronal form of CMT disease.	Usually autosomal dominant, rarely autosomal recessive; recessive cases more severely affected.	Less common than HMSN type I. Onset most often in 2nd decade. Progressive distal weakness and atrophy similar to HMSN type I. Sensory and motor nerve conduction only mildly abnormal.	Nerves not enlarged. Fewer myelinated axons of large diameter in distal nerves. Rare demyelination, few onion bulbs. No reliable autopsy report.	Generally held to represent disease of motor and sensory neurons. Not a variant of spinal muscular atrophy (SMA), although a distal form of SMA with features resembling other types of CMT disease but without sensory involvement exists.	Often clinically indistinguishable from HMSN type I. Nerve conduction study usually essential for differential diagnosis. Intermediate forms between types I and II proposed but not established.

HMSN type III				
Dejerine-Sottas disease. Hypertrophic neuropathy of infancy. Congenital hypomyelination neuropathy.	Autosomal recessive. Probably genetically heterogeneous.	Rare. Onset in infancy, or from birth. Slowly progressive motor and sensory loss, and ataxia. Scoliosis and pes cavus frequent. Enlarged nerves. Short stature. Patients often severely disabled in adult life. Occasional pupillary abnormality. Motor nerve conduction velocity severely reduced, sensory action potentials unrecordable.	Enlarged nerves. Hypomyelination. Long demyelinated axon segments and many onion bulbs.	One case with decreased nerve cerebroside and increased liver ceramide monohexoside sulfate. Primary Schwann-cell disorder possible.	Need for confirmation of disordered lipid metabolism.

(From Schaumburg et al.,[6] with permission.)

down in uremic polyneuropathy is now known to be largely secondary to the distal axonopathy.[6]

Acromegaly

Acromegalic patients can develop distal paresthesias and numbness. Segmental demyelination takes place. Mononeuropathy is also seen in this endocrine disorder.

HEREDITARY DISORDERS

A number of hereditary metabolic disorders affect the peripheral nervous system. Hereditary amyloidosis deposits fibrous protein within the nerve. There are several lipid disorders that generally will be detected at a young age because of their other symptoms. These disorders are due to a defect in an enzyme used in breaking down fats or in producing lipoproteins. Sulfatide lipidosis, Krabbe's disease, Tangier disease (high-density lipoprotein deficiency), and Fabry's disease are examples. They are, however, quite rare. Peripheral limb weakness and clumsiness are seen later in these diseases and not particularly at the onset.

Another rare group of hereditary diseases are the hereditary sensory neuropathies. There are four types as classified by the Mayo Clinic.[5,6] All are very rare. In all except type 1 the onset is in infancy; type 1 is seen in the second decade. The feet are insensate and become mutilated with ulcers and arthropathy early on. Care of the feet is mandatory (Table 16-5).

Charcot-Marie-Tooth Disease

A more common hereditary disease that frequently goes undiagnosed is Charcot-Marie-Tooth disease (HMSN type I). The telltale signs are pes cavus and peroneal atrophy. A Norwegian study reported a prevalence of 41 per 100,000. The dominant form, HMSN type I, occurred at a rate of 36 per 100,000; an X-linked recessive form, HMSN type II, occurred at a rate of 3.6 per 100,000; and an autosomal recessive form, HMSN type III had a prevalence of 1.4 per 100,000.[38]

Table 16-7 summarizes the pertinent facts of all three types. The podiatric clinician should be familiar especially with types I and II, as both may likely have foot deformity as the presenting complaint.

Charcot-Marie-Tooth disease has commonly been classified into a dominant and a recessive form. The more common dominant form, HMSN type I, exhibits slowing of the nerve conduction velocities, a hypertrophic "onion bulb" appearance of the peripheral nerves, and the characteristic "inverted champagne bottle" leg deformity. The recessive form exhibits the same characteristics; however, the nerve conduction velocity is less attenuated.[2-5]

Since Charcot-Marie-Tooth disease is universally recognized as a genetic, autosomal dominant syndrome, it is important to ascertain the patient's history. Geneticists are attempting to find the unifying factor that links the disease within families. It was hypothesized that its etiology was due to one unit trait (i.e., conditioned by a single defective gene). Patterns of inheritance may be dominant, recessive, or sex-linked, but in each family a distinctive pattern is preserved.

Dyck and Lambert classified Charcot-Marie-Tooth disease into HMSN type I (dominantly inherited hypertrophic neuropathy) and HMSN type II (neural-type peroneal muscle atrophy).[3-5] These types are similar to the dominant and recessive forms already discussed. The cardinal features of HMSN type I include autosomal dominant inheritance with symptomatic onset in the 20- to 40-year age group.[3] A slow progression of cavus foot deformity, abnormal gait, weakness of the small muscles of the hands and feet, decreased deep tendon reflexes, mild loss of sensation, and enlargement of the peripheral nerves are observed. Sometimes patients with HMSN type I become accommodated to their disability and do not notice the slow progression of deformity and weakness. These patients also have decreased motor and sensory nerve conduction velocities in the limbs and other isolated peripheral nerves. Evidence of axonal atrophy with segmental demyelination and remyelination (onion bulb formation) of the nerves in the limbs is found.

Lambert and Dyck's HMSN type II exhibits large motor unit potentials and fasciculations in the presence of normal conduction velocities.[4] The clinical characteristics of this group are much the same as in HMSN type I; however, type II has a later onset of symptoms. The peripheral nerves are not palpably enlarged, weakness of the hand muscles is less severe, and weakness of the ankle plantar flexor group is more severe in HMSN type II.

The neuronal degeneration that occurs in type II affects the proximal and distal portions of motor and sensory nerves. Enough neurons remain unaffected so that nerve conduction velocities are not appreciably slowed. The specific population of peripheral neurons most affected in HMSN type II consists of those supplying the lower limbs.

Dyck and others[5] stated that certain HMSN type I patients exhibited the same locus for the Duffy blood group on chromosome 1. Of two kinships that were studied in this work, one displayed this finding, and the other exhibited no similarity in genetic pattern. The authors concluded that genetic heterogeneity among kinships with Charcot-Marie-Tooth disease was the more probable finding.

In contradiction of earlier work, Dyck and Lambert in 1968 concluded that slow nerve conduction velocities did not necessarily correlate with the severity of sensory loss in foot deformity, thus calling into question the use of the HMSN type I and II categories for Charcot-Marie-Tooth disease.[5] This conclusion was later supported by Brust, Lovelace, and Devi,[39] who attempted to categorize Charcot-Marie-Tooth patients by nerve conduction velocity studies. They concluded that Dyck and Lambert's classification was artificial and proposed that clinical and electrodiagnostic criteria were not sufficient to grade categories of Charcot-Marie-Tooth disease.

In support of this opinion, Humberstone[40] reported on the university of nerve conduction velocity abnormalities in patients with Charcot-Marie-Tooth disease. Jones et al.[41] believed that sensory nerve conduction velocity could vary by as much as 10 m/sec between the right and left arms of the same patient. This negates the use of sensory nerve conduction velocity measurements as a classification tool, as does the finding by Jones that these velocities can also vary from segment to segment along the same nerve in a majority of patients.

Jones also discussed the phenomenon of axonal degeneration followed by secondary remyelination, which commonly occurs in Charcot-Marie-Tooth disease. He proposed that ultimately this process leads to a decrease in nerve conduction velocity, but depending on what stage in the process a patient is in, the patient could be classified into either HMSN type I or type II.

However, studies by Buchthal and Behse support Dyck and Lambert's classification.[42] On the basis of peripheral nerve biopsies and nerve conduction velocity studies, these authors felt that HMSN types I and II were two distinct diseases that may be difficult to differentiate by purely clinical findings. Dyck and Lambert's classification was also supported by Bradley et al.[43] In addition to HMSN types I and II, they described an intermediate group of patients. Segmental demyelination and onion bulb formation was observed in this group, as in HMSN type I, but nerve hypertrophy was not observed, as in HMSN type II.

Sabir and Lyttle[44] utilized muscular aspects of Charcot-Marie-Tooth disease to classify the pes cavus deformity. Their category I consisted of flexible, correctable cavus foot deformities. Category II cavus feet displayed equinus with first ray pronation and clawing of the great toe, which was nonreducible. Category III presented equinus of the forefoot, a varus calcaneus, and no structural abnormalities on radiographic examination. Category IV displayed structural abnormalities with some tarsal movement present. Category V cavus foot was rigidly fixed, with pronounced structural changes, dorsal dislocation of digits, and plantar keratoses. This categorization of pes cavus helped to clarify muscle involvement and treatment planning for Charcot-Marie-Tooth patients.

Muscle Pathology

Although the disease has been characterized as a peroneal muscular atrophy, the peroneal muscle group is not generally involved in the initial stage of Charcot-Marie-Tooth disease. Rather, the intrinsic muscle groups of the foot are most commonly affected first. Sabir and Lyttle[44] argue that because Charcot-Marie-Tooth disease is a process of centrifugal degeneration of long axons, the degeneration pattern proceeds in a predictable fashion. The muscles supplied by the longest axons of the sciatic nerve are affected first, followed by muscles with smaller bulk, followed by muscles with larger mass. Thus, the specific order of denervation of lower limb musculature would proceed from the foot intrinsics, to the long and short digital flexors, to the peroneal groups, and, finally, to the gastrocsoleus complex.

The intrinsic muscles function similarly as a group. The interossei muscles produce abduction or adduction of the digits, flexion of the proximal phalanges, and extension of the middle and distal phalanges. Flexion of the proximal phalanx is very important. With loss of interossei power, the proximal phalanx extends, with increased flexion of the middle and distal phalanges, thereby producing severe hammering at the proximal interphalangeal joint. With increased rigidity of this condition, constant trauma can eventually produce discomforting corns and possible ulceration.

The flexor digitorum longus muscle originates from the posterior aspect of the tibia; its tendon passes behind the medial malleolus and then inserts into the lateral four distal phalanges. This muscle flexes the distal phalanges; however, Duchenne[45] believed that some weak plantar flexion of the proximal phalanges was also produced. The flexor digitorum brevis muscle flexes the middle phalanges and also weakly flexes the proximal phalanges. The distal phalanges also appear to flex with contraction of this muscle, according to Duchenne, but no resistance to extension is produced.

The extensor digitorum longus muscle extends the lateral four proximal phalanges fully on their metatarsals. When the foot is dorsiflexed, the two distal phalanges of each toe flex, and the proximal phalanges extend even further. As the intrinsic muscles are lost in Charcot-Marie-Tooth disease, the long extensors become maintainers of hammer digit deformity. A gentle flexion deformity of the digits could be corrected with extensor tenotomies, but as the deformity is maintained over time, bony adaptation occurs. An arthroplasty of the proximal interphalangeal joint, combined with a long extensor tenotomy and metatarsophalangeal joint capsulotomy, may be required.

As the short plantar muscles undergo denervation and atrophy in Charcot-Marie-Tooth syndrome, shortening occurs. This causes the rearfoot and forefoot to be drawn closer together, raising the height of the longitudinal arch. With shortening of these muscles and weakening of the interossei, the relative force of muscle groups that extend the proximal phalanges and flex the middle and distal phalanges increases. The bases of the proximal phalanges progressively depress the heads of the metatarsals, and the plantar fascia contracts.

The actions of the peroneus longus muscle are to plantarflex the first metatarsal head and to plantarflex and pronate the foot. In Charcot-Marie-Tooth disease, the foot supinators will be unopposed with peroneal atrophy, thereby producing a cavus foot deformity.

Treatment

In the past, a triple arthrodesis was performed on most Charcot-Marie-Tooth patients. The primary concerns of the patient and the surgeon are most often those of a plantigrade foot, with adequate midfoot-hindfoot motion and increased forefoot stability. The triple arthrodesis, therefore, does not adequately address the true disability. Alternate procedures have been proposed and include proximally placed dorsally closing wedge osteotomies to reduce forefoot cavus; the Dwyer closing wedge osteotomy to reduce heel inversion; plantar fasciotomies; and digital arthroplasties with long extensor tenotomies.[46]

Surgery in Charcot-Marie-Tooth victims has not always been reported to be successful, and this fact underlines the importance of complete patient evaluation before such intervention. Every muscle should be evaluated and each deformity fully assessed.

FOCAL NEUROPATHIES OF THE FOOT AND LEG

Proximal lesions to the sciatic nerve and to a much lesser extent the femoral nerve and to their respective roots must be considered in cases of distal neuropathy in the lower leg. Virtually all focal neuropathies including motor deficiencies of the lower leg and foot are in regions supplied by the sciatic nerve (Fig. 16-5). Very few lesions are seen in the saphenous nerve, which is supplied by the femoral nerve.

If the patient presents with a peroneal foot-drop,

can he or she invert the foot? Lack of inversion points to a lesion higher than the common peroneal nerve (see below and Ch. 8). The course of the nerve should also be palpated for any proximal tenderness. An endogenous lesion in the thigh of the patient may be pressing on the tibial component of the sciatic. Notably, there will be weakness in muscles not supplied by the common peroneal (e.g., the posterior tibial muscle). If an L5 root lesion were the problem, the gluteal muscles would be weak as well.

Most commonly, focal neuropathies in the foot and leg are caused by external trauma. Internal causes include tumors (although these are rare, the schwannoma is the most common),[21] ischemia (multifocal neuropathies are seen in rheumatoid arthritis and polyarteritis nodosa), hemorrhage (especially proximally by the sciatic trunk in elderly or otherwise predisposed individuals),[7] and anatomic variations that might predispose the patient to nerve entrapment syndromes.

Saphenous Nerve

The saphenous nerve is the continuation of the femoral nerve on the medial side of the leg. It is seldom injured except by laceration.[47-51] Operation on the saphenous vein may damage the nerve, resulting in distal paresthesias.[47,50,51] The infrapatellar branch is occasionally lacerated in knee operations, giving rise to "gonyalgia paresthetica."[48,51]

The saphenous nerve has been alleged to be entrapped just as it exits the subsartorial (Hunter's) canal proximal to the knee.[52] More recently, the existence of this type of entrapment has been questioned.[7] Malay provides a more detailed description of this possible entrapment.[50]

Paresthesia along the distal course of the saphenous nerve onto the dorsomedial aspect of the foot will be seen. Usually the cause is obvious from the history and the presence of a scar on examination. A neuroma-in-continuity (see above) may be palpable. Because its innervation is from L3-L4, proximal L4 radiculopathy and partial femoral neuropathy must be ruled out. Testing the strength of the quadriceps can help rule out proximal involvement.

Common Peroneal Nerve

The common peroneal nerve is one of the most vulnerable to external compression injuries.[7,54] Injury results quite commonly from crossing the legs. The patient may complain of numbness down the lateral side of the leg, and the examiner may discover some weakness in dorsiflexion. Upon questioning, the patient may admit to the habit of constantly crossing one leg over the other.

Certain occupations may predispose the patient to common peroneal nerve injury, as was the case in a group of workers picking strawberries in a squatting position.[52] Of direct concern to the clinician is the danger of prolonged positioning of the patient on the operating table or injudicious casting, which can lead to a neuropraxic injury.[53] It may take weeks of encouragement for the patient to recover from an iatrogenic foot-drop.

Blunt trauma is a common cause of peroneal neuropathy. As already mentioned, the peroneal component of the sciatic nerve is susceptible to trauma as well. Therefore it is critical to evaluate the entire course of the nerve and perform a straight leg raise test to rule out any proximal radiculopathy.

Entrapment of the common peroneal nerve may be seen with less frequency.[50,53] This condition has been confirmed surgically.[7] Constriction (with demyelination) was observed at the fibrous fibular tunnel by the origin of the peroneus longus. After wrapping around the fibular neck, the nerve then pierces this origin. Proximal swelling of the nerve was also noted.[54]

The common inversion ankle sprain can affect the proximal part of the common peroneal nerve. In a prospective series of 66 ankle sprains, EMG and nerve conduction studies showed damage to the peroneal nerve in 17 percent of the patients.[55]

One must consider single or multiple focal neuropathies in patients with diabetes and rheumatoid arthritis. In one study, up to one-third of the diabetics had mononeuropathy of the common peroneal nerve.[56] Thrombosis and embolism of the femoral or popliteal artery can cause a peroneal neuropathy, presumably as a result of ischemia.[57] Steppage gait may precede a palpable lesion by several days.[58] Ganglions, lipomas, giant cell cysts, and schwannomas all contribute to a peroneal palsy.[59]

Finally, idiopathic cases of lateral dysesthesia and/or motor weakness will be seen. Often, the patient may not recollect any blunt trauma, or the peroneal neuropathy may have even resulted from pressure during sleep.[7]

To differentiate common peroneal neuropathy from proximal lesions, look for weakness in muscles supplied by the medial trunk of the sciatic nerve. This would include weakness in the posterior tibial and gastrocnemius muscles. Radiculopathy of L5 would produce EMG aberrations in the gluteal and paraspinal muscle groups. Finally, an EMG of the biceps femoris would indicate involvement of the more proximal lateral (peroneal component) trunk of the sciatic nerve.

Temporary foot-drop should be managed with braces and regular physical therapy. Permanent peroneal neuropathy may require surgery to check the foot-drop. Posterior bony ankle blocks or tendon transfers may be done.[7,50]

Sural Nerve

Sural neuropathies commonly occur at the ankle, affecting only sensation on the lateral side of the foot. Surgical removal of Haglund's deformity, or os trigonum, and peroneal tendon work can all leave the surgeon with a disgruntled patient.

The sural nerve may be injured from ankle sprains and from fibrosis about the peroneal tendons.[7] Entrapment neuropathy has been reported recently in two cases.[60] One patient had a history of an ankle sprain several years earlier. The other patient had a palpable ganglion. Both patients had a positive Tinel's sign. Surgery brought improvement in both cases. No actual nerve constriction or proximal swelling was reported in the surgical findings, thus raising the question of possible entrapment rather than compression.[60]

The sural nerve is composed of anywhere from 8 to 14 fascicles that disseminate not only to the lateral fifth toe, but also to the skin and soft tissue above the base of the fourth metatarsal (see Fig. 16-1).[23] This medial branch is usually larger than the one going to the fifth toe and communicates with the intermediate cutaneous branch of the superficial peroneal nerve. The sural nerve also provides branches to the tarsal joints. Localized pares-

thesias may only be present on the dorsolateral aspect of the foot, sparing the fascicles to the fifth digit. An accessory deep peroneal nerve branch may also innervate the extensor digitorum brevis and may be involved in paresthesias here.

The sural nerve is commonly the nerve of choice for biopsies. Discomforting pins-and-needles sensations may be felt afterward for up to 2 years.[5]

The sural nerve has medial and lateral proximal branches: one from the common peroneal nerve and one from the tibial nerve. They join just below the knee, and not until the nerve reaches the lower third of the leg does it veer off toward the lateral malleolus. Proximal calf injuries and neoplasms should be ruled out.

Anterior Tarsal Tunnel Syndrome

Anterior tarsal tunnel syndrome was first described by Kopel and Thompson in 1960 and has been reported on by others since.[61-65] The deep peroneal nerve becomes traumatized somewhere along its course in front of the ankle. The nerve does flatten somewhat as it courses under the extensor retinaculum, but this has not been appreciated.[7,51,66] Tarsal spurs have been said to contribute to the syndrome.[64] Rigid pes cavus feet with forefoot valgus may also be contributory.[65] Tight or ill-fitting shoes have been implicated as well.[66] In a series of 20 cadavers, Borges et al.[65] showed the maximum point of contact to be at the dorsal talonavicular joint. The evidence for any precise and consistent site of entrapment of the deep peroneal nerve remains elusive.[7]

However, the symptoms of deep peroneal focal neuropathy are unequivocal.[50,51,61-66] The patient will complain of paresthesias on the top of the foot and numbness at the dorsal aspect of the first interspace.[65] Nocturnal pain is commonly relieved by movement of the foot. Extension and eversion appear to relax undue tension on the nerve.[51] Lying in bed with the foot supinated appears to bring about paresthesia.

Tinel's sign may be elicited at the anterior ankle. One should attempt to palpate the nerve just medial to the dorsalis pedis artery. The deep peroneal nerve sends innervation to the extensor digitorum brevis. This muscle should be palpated for any atrophy and compared to the opposite foot. The deep peroneal nerve also innervates the first interosseous muscle.

Distal motor latencies have been increased in electrodiagnostic testing,[65] above 7 msec compared to a more normal 5 msec.

Orthotics with valgus posting have brought relief.[66] Injections of corticosteroids may bring relief. Although some have recommended neurolysis for recalcitrant cases,[50] all efforts should be made to free any nerve entrapment or compression from articular exostoses.[51]

Superficial Peroneal Nerve

The intermediate cutaneous branch of the superficial peroneal nerve (Lemont's nerve) is precariously located, crossing just medial to the sinus tarsi. It can be stretched in severe ankle sprains and fractures.[28] Moreover, its superficial location lends it and its sister medial branch to direct compression injuries. Tinel's sign is not always present. A gentle stroking of the nerve can elicit a symptomatic response. The distal branches are almost routinely encountered in much podiatric surgery, as is further discussed below.

Tibial Nerve

The laciniate ligament or flexor retinaculum has been implicated as the cause of tarsal tunnel pain since 1962.[8,67] Commonly, paresthesias extend out the great toe.[68] The onset is usually insidious, although trauma can bring about symptoms more acutely. Gauthier et al.[69] described two different clinical patterns: (1) heel and arch pain that is increased during the day in walking and in standing, and (2) pain that is more discomforting at night or with rest. Generally, one does tend to associate rest or nocturnal pain with tarsal tunnel syndrome.

Tinel's sign is fairly reliable in revealing tarsal tunnel syndrome.[70] In a series of 21 feet with symptoms consistent with tarsal tunnel entrapment, Tinel's sign was present in 19, or 90 percent of the cases that underwent surgical release of the flexor retinaculum. In this same study in 1979, sensory nerve action potentials were tested and found to be significantly affected also in 19, or 90 percent

of the cases. In contrast, only 11 of the 21 cases demonstrated slowed motor conduction velocities. Specific deficits in the SNAPs included slowed velocities, decreased amplitudes, and even absent potentials.[70] Others have since supported the use of sensory nerve studies to more accurately diagnose tarsal tunnel syndrome.[71–73]

A true entrapment would constrict the nerve at the tarsal tunnel. Constriction with demyelination would occur directly under the ligament, as has been witnessed in the more familiar carpal tunnel syndrome. Moreover, proximal enlargement of the nerve should be observed. The axoplasm, impeded by the entrapment, accumulates proximal to the ligament. An increased vascular response would also be observed. This classic appearance of an entrapment as observed in tarsal tunnel syndrome has been infrequently reported.[74]

As noted, motor conduction studies have failed to consistently demonstrate significantly slowed velocities, as would be expected with demyelination, and as demonstrated rather reliably in carpal tunnel studies. Nor do we commonly see atrophy of the intrinsic musculature as in the hand. Do we see the patients with symptomatic feet before any motor deficit occurs? Is there an entrapment at the flexor retinaculum? Or, more often, is the entrapment distal? Does the preponderance of distal axonal polyneuropathy complicate the clinical picture of tarsal tunnel syndrome?

Significant entrapment should produce some hypesthesia along the medial or lateral plantar nerve signature areas, although this is not a consistent finding.[75] Pain is more often present in the arch and heel, with distal radiation occurring possibly out to the end of the great toe. Tinel's sign should be positive on percussion, or in some cases by rolling and massaging the nerve. Valleix's sign of proximal radiation with percussion at the laciniate ligament may be observed.

All of these signs may be located at a site distal (or rarely proximal) to the flexor retinaculum. A tourniquet can be inflated above the ankle to help rule out an adjacent imposing varicosity of the venae comitantes or ischemia.[76] Whether or not a dilated vein does in fact entrap the tibial nerve within the confined tunnel remains a matter of controversy.[7]

The abductor hallucis and other intrinsic muscles of the foot may appear atrophied or weak upon repeated flexion. Counterresistance should be given at the proximal bases of the digits to minimize the pull of the long flexors. Again, atrophy has not been observed in the foot as it has in the hands of patients with carpal tunnel syndrome. Isolated lesions along the course of the nerve should be ruled out by direct and careful palpation.

Pronation appears to be contributory. Empirically, orthoses bring relief, especially in patients with a short history. Pronating the hindfoot may help to elicit a Tinel's sign. Steroid anti-inflammatory injections can likewise bring relief in a small percentage of patients. For persistent cases resistant to conservative measures, nerve conduction and EMG studies should be ordered. Surgical intervention may be anticipated. The extent of any detectable mass should fully evaluated, possibly with MRI.

If motor velocity is tested, it is important to have the latencies sufficiently distal to the tarsal tunnel.[77] This maneuver will more effectively reveal any distal entrapment. The relative contribution of each electrodiagnostic test has been outlined by Johnson[78] (Table 16-8).

The flexor retinaculum has been noted in surgery to be unduly thickened at the "malleolar calcaneal axis," and more recently the more distal tunnels of each of the respective nerve and artery divisions (of the posterior tibial nerve and artery)

have been implicated. The transverse interfascicular lamina separating the more superior medial plantar vessels from the more inferior lateral plantar nerve and artery has been considered.[76,78] This division occurs approximately at the origin of the abductor hallucis, the porta pedis hiatus. Surgical exploration should be carried through to these distal tunnels to be sure no entrapment exists, especially about the medial plantar nerve (Fig. 16-9). The medial plantar nerve then exits the canal and courses next over the master knot of Henry, where the tendons of the flexor hallucis longus and the flexor digitorum longus cross. Tension in this area has been thought to contribute to entrapment of the medial plantar nerve.

The lateral plantar nerve courses obliquely and distally across the sole of the foot directly under the quadratus plantae. Nerve entrapment here has rarely been reported.

In Figure 16-10, multiple ganglia were removed from the inferior tarsometatarsal joints in a 27-year-old building contractor. A year of increasing paresthesia and numbness along the lateral side of his foot preceded his seeking definitive care. Return of normal sensation occurred within 6 weeks after surgery.

Beyond the master knot of Henry, the medial plantar nerve undergoes its first division just proximal to the midfoot. Here one branch continues medially under the abductor hallucis to become the medial plantar digital proper nerve (see discussion of Joplin's neuroma below). The lateral division of the medial plantar nerve courses distally between the abductor hallucis and the flexor digitorum brevis (Fig. 16-6). Ultimately it innervates the plantar surfaces of the first and second interspaces.

At this first division of the medial plantar nerve the intrinsic muscles may stretch the underlying nerve. A recent case of the author's involved distal paresthesia and plantar anesthesia along the course of the lateral division of the medial plantar nerve. Moreover, the point of tenderness was at the division. Localized entrapment was assumed to exist, although no appreciable constriction of the nerve was noted. The division of the medial plantar nerve inferior to the abductor hallucis acts like a sling. The exerting abductor hallucis constrains and places tension on the underlying divided medial plantar nerve (Fig. 16-11). Palpable and sympto-

Table 16-8. Hierarchy of Relative Value of Electrodiagnostic Tests for Tarsal Tunnel Syndrome[78]

Study	Abnormality in Tarsal Tunnel Syndrome
Sensory nerve conduction velocity	Decreased
Sensory nerve action potential (SNAP) or compound nerve action potential	Decreased
SNAP dispersion (duration) phenomenon	Increased
Motor potential amplitude	Decreased
Motor potential duration	Increased
Motor distal latency°	Increased
Motor conduction velocity	Decreased
Sensory latency (?)	Increased
Electromyography°	Fibrillations
	Positive sharp waves
	Complex discharges

° As tested for the abductor hallucis and abductor digiti minimi muscles. All other tests were done on the medial and lateral plantar nerves.

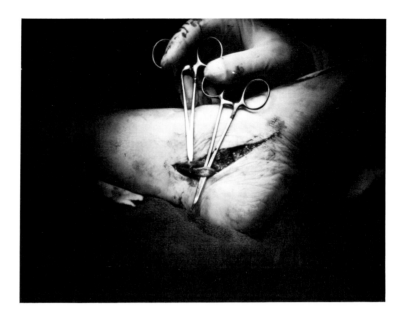

Fig. 16-9. During tarsal tunnel release both medial and plantar nerves are identified and followed as far distally as possible. The fan-shaped flexor retinaculum (laciniate ligament) becomes thicker distally.

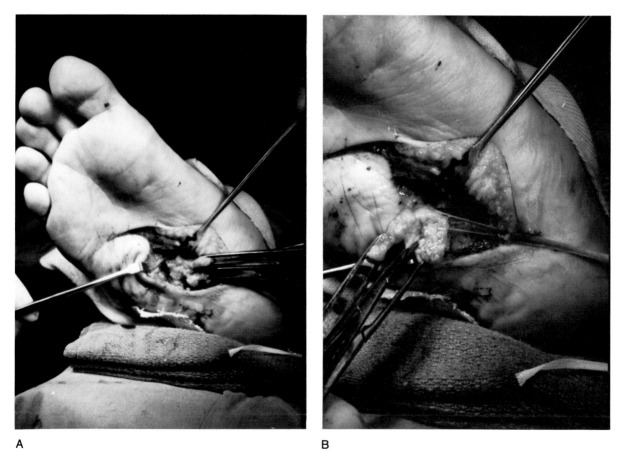

A

B

Fig. 16-10. Adjacent ganglia causing focal neuropathy of the lateral plantar nerve. Return of sensation along the lateral sole occurred within 6 weeks after surgery.

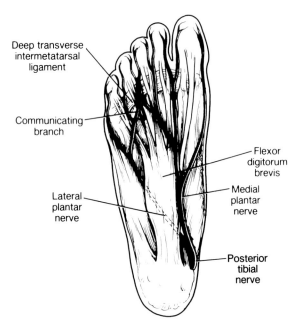

Fig. 16-11. Anatomy of the plantar nerves. (From Miller SJ: Surgical technique for resection of Morton's neuroma. J Am Podiatr Assoc 71:181, 1981, with permission.)

matic pain was localized at the beginning of the lateral branch of the medial plantar nerve.

Surgical separation of the muscle away from this branch brought prompt relief in this case. Some hypesthesia persisted 4 months postoperatively, but the patient's pain had diminished and she returned to her standing job by the sixth postoperative week.

MISCELLANEOUS FOCAL NEUROPATHIES OF THE FOOT

Several other focal neuropathies of the foot are less commonly seen. These include incisional neuromas, Joplin's neuroma, and miscellaneous entrapment and compression neuropathies about the more vulnerable medial and lateral sides of the foot. These are chronic fibrotic mononeuropathies, loosely termed neuromas and in some cases entrapments.[79–86]

Incisional neuromas are not infrequently seen.[79] As DuVries[32] stressed, incisions on the top of the foot should, in general, parallel the distribution of the sensory nerves. Kenzora[79] reviewed 55 sensory neuromas in 37 patients over a 4-year period. The medial and intermediate branches of the superficial and deep peroneal nerves were most frequently involved. In surgery these nerves must be mobilized about the sinus tarsus and frequently when removing exostoses from the dorsal tarsal bones. The sural nerve or an occasional accessory deep peroneal nerve may complicate an otherwise fairly simple elective surgery for os trigonum or Haglund's deformity.

In the past, the medial bunionectomy and implant arthroplasties were done through incisions with the ends plantarward. This, however, risks transection of the medial plantar digital proper nerve.[80] Dale Austin's routine approach for the medial incision followed Keller's incision: the ends were upward in the so-called "smile" incision. This incision avoids the plantar digital proper nerve, but the dorsal flap must be handled with care to avoid trauma to the more superomedial branch from both the medial dorsal cutaneous and the saphenous nerves. Careful medial dissection must be done when the more common dorsal incision for a bunionectomy is done. The medial plantar digital proper nerve has been reported in compressive and entrapped neuropathies.[80,81,83,84]

Incisional neuropathy can lead to failed surgery, including a brush with reflex sympathetic dystrophy (RSD). With determination, the surgeon should be able to turn about a potential RSD. Early signs include a reluctance of the patient to use the foot following surgery. The patient prefers to remain on crutches or in a wheelchair. The foot becomes edematous, discolored, and dyshydrotic. It is very sensitive on manual examination to the point where examination is almost impossible.

An overactive sympathetic nervous system is in play. It is crucial that the surgeon recognize these signs to thwart any further progress toward a fully developed RSD. Subsequent trophic changes lead to bony demineralization, contractures of the digits, unrelenting pain, and skin and nail friability.[82]

During one's surgical training, an appreciation of the general anatomy, the size of the respective nerves, and the whiter color of the nerve as it first appears directly under the superficial fascia should be developed through keen observation. Incisional neuromas can largely be avoided with proper care and respect for the usual and variant anatomic distributions of the distal sensory nerves of the foot.

Joplin's Neuroma

Joplin's neural fibrosis is much like the traumatic pathology seen in Morton's neuroma, but not always to the same degree. Although some authors have recommended excision, this must be done with discrimination. A merely entrapped medial plantar digital proper nerve may require only a release of entangled fibrotic tissue.[80,81]

The signs and symptoms of Joplin's neuroma are similar to those of other distal focal neuropathies: paresthesias with pain at the point of compression or entrapment are observed. The nerve may be subject to an overriding bunion condition. The nerve may roll under digital palpation. It is often symptomatic directly inferomedial to the first metatarsophalangeal joint, although more distal involvement has been reported.[81] Demyelination and intraneural fibrosis would be expected.

Case Study. A 33-year-old woman presented with tingling and pain directly inferomedial to the first metatarsophalangeal joint, having lasted for 6 months. She also had a moderate bunion and hyperpronation. No history of trauma was revealed except that as a child she may have hurt her foot when jumping from a swing. As a child she was a hemophiliac with HTP (hemophilia, thrombocytopenia, and purpura). She underwent a splenectomy at 12 years old. In 1980 she had a recurrent episode of thrombocytopenia.

A palpable nerve elicited a Tinel's sign with direct pain at the metatarsophalangeal joint. The diagnosis of entrapment was considered. An injection of prednisolone tebutate and bupivicaine was given at the first visit. This completely relieved her symptoms for about 2 days. A dancer's pad also helped. After several months of recurring pain, the patient elected to undergo surgical correction of the possible entrapment and bunion. Release of an apparent nerve entrapment and an Austin bunion-ectomy were achieved through a medial "smile" incision.

The medial plantar digital proper nerve was readily identified along the inferior half of the first metatarsophalangeal joint and was enlarged distally in a fusiform shape to almost twice the usual size (2 to 3 mm). At the central capsule the nerve was inflected 90 degrees cephalad. The nerve was bound at this inflection. Release of fibrous capsular tissue left a straight and slackened nerve. The bunionectomy was then done.

The post-operative course was uneventful. The neuropraxia of the medial digital proper nerve resolved in 3 months. No further complications have been encountered in 1 year's time. The patient's previous uncontrolled hemophilia may have contributed to scar formation at the first metatarsophalangeal joint.

Calcaneal Neuropathies of the Foot

Runners are often seen with irritation to the medial calcaneal nerve branch. A medial arch "cookie" or self-made arch support might be directly aggravating the nerve. The runner's shoes must be checked, and sources of irritations, including self-made arch supports, must be removed. Dexamethasone phosphate 4 mg can be used therapeutically. Taping or custom orthoses can be used to help prevent pronation of the heel if this persists.

If the lesion is chronic (present for at least 6 months), surgical intervention may be necessary. The medial calcaneal nerve is often superficial and thin and is quickly dispersed into branches and lost in the fat inferior to the heel. Although medial calcaneal neuritis does appear to be a true syndrome, earlier reports of a "lamp cord" sign were misleading and were confused with a local bursitis.[88] This author has never observed a medial calcaneal nerve the size of an interdigital "neuroma" causing a palpable click under the heel. Surgical interventions over 15 years, 13 of which have been spent looking for the heel neuroma, have failed to reveal any enlarged lesion. Thickened bursae have, in fact, been present when a lamp cord sign was observed. The calcaneal branch has been consistently observed to be relatively small in size (Figure 16-12), dispersing itself in about three branches into the fat and

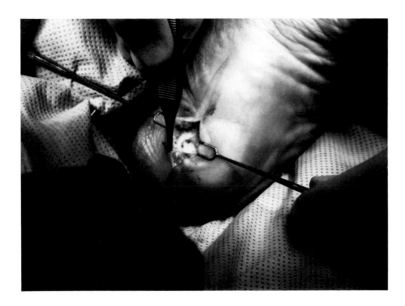

Fig. 16-12. Branches of the medial calcaneal nerve are commonly encountered during heel spur surgery. The chronically inflamed bursa will feel like a lamp cord transversely situated under the calcaneus.

bursae. Nevertheless, the smaller branches can become chronically inflamed, and, as Jones observed, the histologic picture of the nerves shows internal fibrosis occurring.

Jones and Przylucki[87] have introduced new concepts in the diagnosis and treatment of entrapment and compression neuropathy of the foot and ankle. Jones has used a diagnostic technique of local anesthesia to discriminate the level of the lesion between the tarsal tunnel and its distal branches. The aberrant branch of the lateral plantar nerve has been implicated in heel pain. Jones has supported this with pathologic finding of the nerve as it courses underneath the calcaneus, inserting into the abductor digit quinti. The nerve is both a sensory and a motor nerve. Symptoms include inferolateral heel pain accompanied by nocturnal rest pain. Jones also elaborated on the involvement of the medial calcaneal branch and the more distal nerves, as they may be involved in the etiology of heel and arch pain.

Generally, inferior heel pain has been described as being more symptomatic on first arising in the morning and after sitting for a period of time. An initial antalgic gait soon works itself out to the point where the pain somewhat diminishes and the patient can resume a normal gait. Although this is a more typical history, the nagging pain may be present regardless of the activity. Jones uses local anesthetic blocks to determine the level of nerve involvement. One to two milliliters of local anesthetic can be injected subcutaneously between the medial malleolus, the posterior superior malleolus, and the posterior superior calcaneus. This would help rule out trauma to the medial calcaneal branch if relief were obtained.

Like the calcaneal branch, the aberrant lateral branch coming off the lateral plantar nerve can become irritated. Again, the nerve does not appreciably enlarge but rather shows evidence of perineural fibrosis that thickens, more so internally. Here, too, in chronic cases, the symptoms of inferior or lateral heel pain may be relieved by local injection to help diagnose the condition.

In neuritis of the lateral branches, a decrease in motor activity to the abductor digiti quintus is also observed. The patient cannot abduct the fifth toe away from the fourth. This is a common finding in pes cavus and adductus feet.

MORTON'S NEUROMA

Morton's "neuroma" as it is known to most American clinicians, is likely the most common intrinsic nerve disorder of the foot. In Great Britain,

Table 16-9. Comparative Studies of Morton's Neuroma

Author and Reference	No. of Patients	No. of Procedures	Unilateral (Multisites)	Bilateral	Interspace Third	Interspace Second	No. Female	Average Age	Average Follow-up	Percentage Successful	Comment
Gauthier[105]	206	304	128(70)	106	233(77%)	38(13%)	187(90.8%)	54	21 mos.	83%	Released ligament only, related to pes cavus and hallux valgus, considered entrapment.
Lassmann[116]	133	145	121(24)	n.s.	65(45%)	76(52%)	°	°	n.s.	°	°Seen more in women 40 to 60; surgery provides "lasting relief . . . with no recurrences." Review histopathology.
Bartolomei and Wertheimer[90]	97	114	81(8)	24	72(64%)	33(29%)	78(80%)	47	n.s.	n.s.	Correlated with obesity.
Mann and Reynolds[114]	56	76	46(n.s.)	15	46(46%)	53(53%)	53(95%)	55	22 mos.	80%	Disputed traction theory to third interspace; no abnormal foot types noted. States ligament repairs itself.
Gudas and Mattana[115]	43	59	27(5)	11	51(86%)	3(5%)	36(84%)	43.5	51 mos.	79%	Denies entrapment theory, leaves ligament intact.

n.s., not stated.

the disorder is more frequently referred to as Morton's metatarsalgia. Synonyms are numerous and discussed further below. A more complete list of terms has been provided by Miller.[89]

Signs and Symptoms

Symptoms are paroxysmal and intermittent, most often occurring at the third interdigital cleft. Paresthesias may radiate into the third or the fourth digit as well as proximally. The attacks often occur while the patient is shod and walking, prompting removal of the shoe for relief. Manipulation of the toes and foot seems to help.[89-94] Intermetatarsal mononeuropathy may also occur at the second and less frequently at the first interdigital clefts. It rarely occurs in the fourth interspace. Women are seen with this condition more often than men, presumably because of shoe aggravation. The disorder generally affects middle-aged persons (Table 16-9).

Mulder's[95] click has been modified to include lateral compression.[94] The examiner palpates plantar and distal to the intermetatarsal ligament with one index finger. The other hand simultaneously applies lateral compression to click the neuroma in and out of the space between the metatarsal heads. (Of course, this must be done cautiously in the symptomatic patient.) Other signs seen less often include hypesthesia within the digital cleft. This can be tested with a cotton-tip applicator. A sewing wheel can be used at the tips of the toes.

Etiology

Among the numerous etiologies suggested in the past, ischemia has largely been discredited.[96,97] Plantar neuromas are frequently associated with repeated microtrauma during weightbearing or with direct pressure. Whether or not an impending bursa,[98-104] ligament,[105] or phalanx[32] plays an associated role is for the surgeon to determine when surgical correction is considered. (Figs. 16-13 and 16-14).

Recent studies indicate that the intermetatarsal bursae may contribute to excessive pressure on the nerve,[98-104] as Mulder[95] first suspected. This theory is still being explored and may be included among numerous other previously proposed etiologies.[89,93,96,97,105-110]

Histologic Appearance

Histologically the nerve shows evidence of trauma, with endo- and perineural fibrosis and endoneural edema to a varying degree. Demyelination is seen early with edema, mucinous degen-

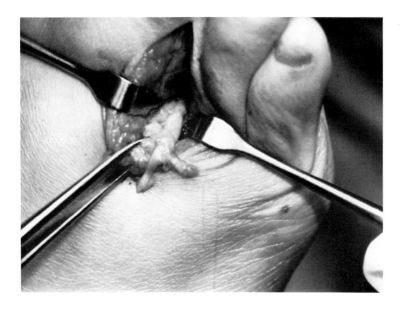

Fig. 16-13. Perineural fibrosis (Morton's neuroma) reflected proximally after incising the distal branches to the adjacent third and fourth toes.

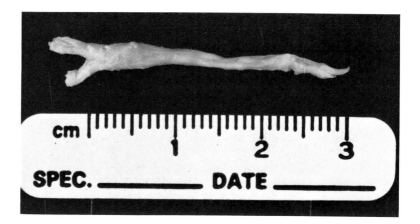

Fig. 16-14. Once the lesion is excised and denuded of adjacent fat and synovial tissue, its overall size may be unimpressive. Note the thickening of the nerve just proximal to its digital branches. This nerve was from the second interspace of a relatively small woman.

eration, and fibrosis (Figs. 16-15 to 16-17). Distal Wallerian degeneration of the axons can take place in more chronic neuromas. Ultimately, axonal loss is seen, with resultant sclerosis, hyalinization, and a generalized increased collagenation of the nerve. Less commonly seen in the plantar neuroma is sufficient remyelination and restoration of nerve fascicles.[111] Electron microscopic studies were done by Goldman,[111] who found (1) demyelination and remyelination of the large fibers, (2) resprouting of the axon, and (3) phagocytosis of myelin débris by the perineural epithelial cells.

Treatment

Conservative therapy is not without merit.[112] A Fay metatarsal bar can be used to eliminate most of the pressure on the forefoot and the associated pain seen with Morton's neuroma. A pad or raise in an orthotic can similarly relieve the symptoms. A 1 ×

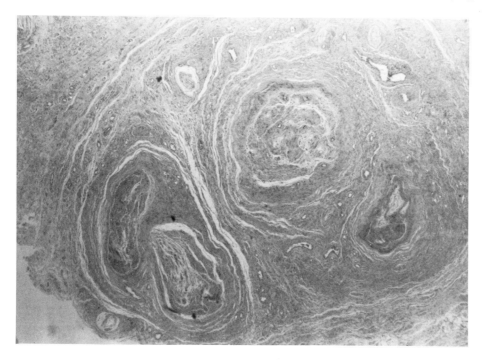

Fig. 16-15. The fascicles of a Morton's neuroma, deformed in their ovoid shape, show a significant loss of myelinated fibers and exhibit endo- and perineural fibrosis. (Magnification ×40.)

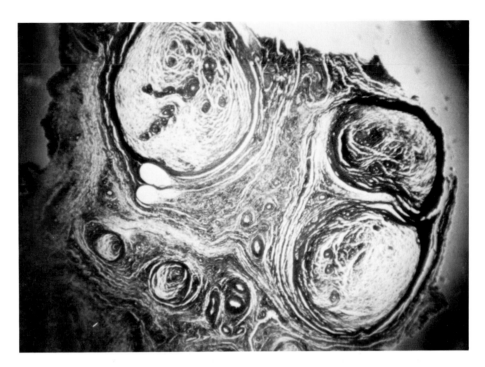

Fig. 16-16. A more recent neuroma less than 6 months in duration from the second interspace shows marked endoneural edema and significant demyelination. (Magnification ×40.)

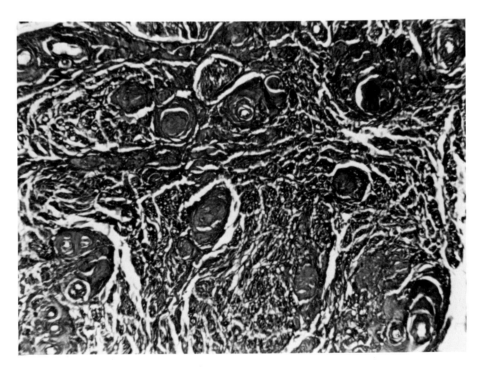

Fig. 16-17. Higher magnification (×400) with a special myelin stain (luxol-fast blue) shows a significant loss of myelinated axons in this Morton's neuroma.

1 × ⅛ inch foam pad can be placed with just one corner lifting and spreading the interspace between the metatarsal heads. The bulk of the square is placed proximal to the metatarsal heads.[112] This affords temporary relief. The use of injectable, steroidal, anti-inflammatory drugs should be considered.[112,113] Generally, conservative therapy should be rigorously attempted, especially if the patient has had symptoms for less than 6 months.

Surgical excision of the traumatized nerve is now performed in patients with a history of chronic and unrelenting pain and discomfort. The common interdigital nerve is excised just inferior, posterior, and anterior to the intermetatarsal ligament. This provides permanent relief in about 80 percent of patients (Table 16-9).

Surgical removal of the interdigital nerve and its common branch must be done far enough proximal to the intermetatarsal ligament to prevent an amputation or stump neuroma from forming in the scar. Gentle traction on the nerve before incising it permits the nerve to recede into the fascial planes, lessening the chance of a stump neuroma. Recurrent stump neuromas are readily removed through a plantar incision between the weight-bearing metatarsal heads. The close proximity of the second and third metatarsals sometimes leads the surgeon to consider the plantar or European approach.

Gauthier[105] has successively treated interdigital neuroma by releasing the intermetatarsal ligament. He considers the mononeuropathy a result of entrapment. Using a dorsal approach, he may have obliterated the superiorly located intermetatarsophalangeal bursae. The majority (77 percent) of his cases involved the third interspace (Table 16-9). He also observed an association with pes cavus, but with no criteria defined. Wachter et al.[108] did show how pes cavus may contribute to excess tension on the plantar nerve. However, others still discredit any associated foot type and any traction theory.[114]

In contrast to proximal swelling and narrowing of the nerve in carpal tunnel entrapment, Morton's neuroma is thickened at the distal edge of the ligament.[105] Moreover, no significant constriction (caused by demyelination) of the common trunk under the ligament is commonly observed.

Bartolomei and Wertheimer[90] reviewed hospital charts and correlated incidence of the neuroma with obesity. Like the majority of current studies, they support surgical excision of the nerve. Gudas and Mattana[115] also support surgical excision following trials of conservative therapy. Although they reported satisfactory results in 79 percent of cases, they further improved their results with an additional postoperative injection of steroids in patients who continued to have symptoms. Interestingly, they surgically repair the intermetatarsal ligament or leave it intact.

It is difficult to argue against the more common dorsal incision when excising a neuroma from the third interspace. Here the metatarsals are more mobile, permitting the use of a baby laminar spreader to effectively expose the intermetatarsal ligament and the underlying nerve.

Historical Review

European and historical accounts commonly referred to the disorder as Morton's metatarsalgia.[98,100,105,107,116–123] More recently Morton's neuralgia[93,94] and interdigital neuropathy[125] have been used. Other historically used terms include Morton's disease[121] and Morton's toe[123] (not to be confused with Dudley Morton's[118] short first metatarsal and hallux).

The more often described Morton's metatarsalgia gives proper credit to Thomas Morton,[106,128] who in 1876 described the "peculiar and painful affliction of the fourth metatarsophalangeal articulation." His suspected etiology was a pinched interdigital nerve between the fourth and fifth metatarsals. Removal of the head and base of the fourth metatarsophalangeal joint prompted a cure along with a shortened toe.[106]

A generation before Morton's[106] report of surgical correction, Durlacher[109] accurately described the "neuralgic affection" that "occasionally attacks the plantar nerve on the sole of the foot, between the third and fourth metatarsal bones. . . ." The pain can be reproduced by the "mere pressure of the finger" at the plantar aspect. The symptoms also become "very severe while walking, or whenever the foot is on the ground.[11,109] Durlacher believed that spreading of the metatarsals in hypermobile feet exposed the nerve to injury. His conservative treatment included strapping the metatarsals closer together.

Morton[106] believed that hypermobility of the fifth metatarsal contributed to the pinching of the nerve. He did not excise or report on any involved pathology of the interdigital nerves, bursae, or joint capsules. Hoadley,[126] in the *Chicago Medical Record* in 1893, discredited Morton's[106] suspected etiology. Hoadley reported six cases in which the nerve was plantar to the intermetatarsal ligament, and he questioned its being pinched or trapped between the metatarsal bones. He was also the first surgeon to remove only the nerve. Tubby,[127] in a less radical manner than Morton, removed only the metatarsal head of the fourth metatarsophalangeal joint. Although he practiced this technique through 1912, he observed visible nodular masses on the interdigital nerves. In spite of this observation, resection of the fourth metatarsal head was the surgical procedure of choice through the late 1920s.[128]

Schuster[128] noted that there was a widespread belief that Morton's neuralgia was an unusual symptom of a depressed fourth metatarsal. Nutt,[119] for example, stated in his 1925 text that ". . . neuritis (was) caused by nerve pressure by the head of the fourth metatarsal." However, in 1927, Schuster's text from the First Institute of Podiatry rebuked this common belief and stated that "finding was . . . incidental and does not exist in the majority of cases."[128]

To his credit, Nutt[119] did precede Betts[107] in observing the communion of nerve branches between the medial and plantar nerves. There "may be pressure on one of the larger branches of the external plantar nerve or on the nerve formed by the communicating branches (between the lateral and medial plantar nerves).[119] In 1927, Schuster[128] recommended paddings to the fourth metatarsal head. He went on to state, ". . . until recently it was quite common to [excise the fourth metatarsal]" and "such procedure is hardly ever adopted . . . except . . . as a last resort."

In Foote's *Textbook of Minor Surgery*,[129] also published in 1927, surgery for Morton's toe was not recommended. Instead exercise, manipulation, and a support under the fourth metatarsal head were prescribed. There appeared to have been a drift away from the bone resection procedure for neuroma. Contemporary accounts indicate that it is still being done, but only rarely.

Little more appeared in the literature until the 1940s. Betts[107] from Australia boldly excised the interdigital "neuroma" through a plantar incision. Not one of 19 patients had any significant postoperative problems, including a dreaded plantar scar.

In 1943, the American surgeon McElvenny[124] shortly followed Betts in reporting excision of the "neurofibroma." He did this cautiously through the web space, avoiding a potentially problematic scar. In 1948, the British orthopedist Nissen[97] reported on his series of 33 cases. His findings of obliterated interdigital arteries led him to propose an ischemic etiology.[98] However, by 1949, and in subsequent studies, "control" interdigital arteries from cadavers were commonly obliterated in aged persons.[120–123,130]

By 1951, McKeever[117] of Houston, Texas, had published his dorsal approach for "interdigital neuroma." Interestingly, in 1941, when through a dorsal approach he was going to remove the metatarsal head and base of the proximal phalanx, he discovered with pressure on the sole a "large mass" presenting itself. From that point on he removed only the apparent neuroma, affording the patient "complete relief." McKeever had completed 73 procedures when he published his dorsal approach, the most common approach today in America. His procedure was "simple . . . done through a one inch dorsal incision . . . and took less than five minutes." In conclusion, he argued against the prolonged convalescence required with a plantar incision.[117]

Pathologic reports also appeared in the 1940s. King[130] noted increased connective tissue within the specimen. He referred to this as a "sclerosing neuroma" to differentiate it from the multiple sworls seen in amputation neuromas. Others noted the degeneration and reactive fibrosis as well as the presence of obliterated arteries and of an adjacent bursa.[94–103,111,116,120–123]

Recent Studies

Bossley and Cairney[100] have more recently implicated the intermetatarsophalangeal bursae as a possible cause of Morton's metatarsalgia. The presence of these bursae between the metatarsophalangeal joints and above the intermetatarsal ligaments was first described by Spatteholz.[103] Unfortunately this information is conspicuously absent in currently available textbooks.

Bossley and Cairney[100] injected radiopaque heated gelatin into the interdigital bursae of cadavers. It was found that the bursae were oval and about 2 to 3 cm in length, and that the center was directly over the intermetatarsal ligament (Fig. 16-7). The interdigital neurovascular bundle was directly inferior to the ligament. Compression of the foot expressed the bursae forward, presumably stressing the interdigital nerve. The bursa was often absent in the fourth interspace, and this might explain the rarity of neuromas located here.[100]

Although Mulder[95] credited his palpable click to the nerve, he noted the consistent finding of a more superiorly located bursa adherent to the nerve. He was unable to remove the nerve (from the plantar approach) without cutting part of the bursa.[95]

Earlier authors had suggested that bursitis led to the neurofibrosis. Reed and Bliss[120] reported in 1973, a "thickened bursal wall with hyalinized fronds projecting into the lumen." Vanio[104] and later others[98] stressed the possibility of early rheumatoid arthritis presenting symptoms of interdigital bursitis with symptoms of neuritis.

Nevertheless, injection of the intermetatarsophalangeal bursae with cortisone derivatives has met with limited success.[100,113] One cannot help but question the accuracy of the diagnosis; an inflamed bursal cyst would be expected to respond to cortisone injections, whereas chronically irritated nerves may continue to be irritated if not irreversibly damaged. As the diagnosis of neuroma improves with nerve conduction studies and other modalities (e.g., MRI), there may be more uniform consensus regarding treatment.

Other etiologies for Morton's mononeuropathy have been suggested. Excess pronation or supination has been postulated to stress the individual branches to the third or the fourth digit.[93] Empirically, orthotic devices used to control pronation have not entered common use.

In summary, Morton's neuroma is a reactive fibrosis of the common digital nerve, seen more commonly in middle-aged women. Surgical excision appears to still be a worthwhile procedure if conservative treatment is unrewarding. However, with surgical results unsatisfactory in one-fifth of cases, and as Milgram[112] cautioned, every effort should be made to (1) adequately inform the patient of the neuroma as well as other possibilities, (2) provide a fair attempt at conservative treatment, and (3) prepare the patient for the possibility of continued pain that might require postoperative therapy in one-fifth of the cases.

REFERENCES

1. Adam RD, Victor M: Principles of Neurology. 2nd Ed. McGraw-Hill, New York, 1981
2. Dyck PJ, Oviatt KF, Lambert EH: Intensive evaluation of unclassified neuropathies yields improved diagnosis. Ann Neurol 10:222, 1981
3. Dyck PJ, Lambert EH: Lower motor and primary sensory neuron diseases with peroneal muscular atrophy. I. Neurologic; Genetic and electrophysiology findings in various neuronal degenerations. Arch Neurol 18:603, 1968
4. Dyck PJ, Lambert EH: Lower motor and primary sensory neuron diseases with peroneal muscular atrophy. II. Neurologic; genetic and electrophysiologic findings in various neuronal degenerations. Arch Neurol 18:619, 1968
5. Dyck PJ, Thomas PK, Lambert EH, Bunge R: Peripheral Neuropathy. 2nd Ed. WB Saunders, Philadelphia, 1984
6. Schaumburg HH, Spencer PS, Peter S, Thomas PK: Disorders of Peripheral Nerves. FA Davis, Philadelphia, 1983
7. Stewart JD: Focal Peripheral Neuropathies. Elsevier, New York, 1987
8. Keck C: The tarsal-tunnel syndrome. J Bone Joint Surg 44A:180, 1962
9. Johnson M: Comprehensive anterior/posterior tarsal tunnel bibliography. Curr Podiatry 37(6):32, 1988
10. Schaumburg HH, Spencer PS: Clinical and experimental studies of distal axonopathy: a frequent form of nerve and brain damage produced by chemical hazards. Ann NY Acad Sci 329:14, 1979
11. Spencer PS, Sabori: MI, Schaumburg HH, Moore CL: Does a defect in the energy metabolism in the nerve fiber underlie axon degeneration in polyneuropathies? Ann Neurol 5:501, 1979

12. Swanson PD: Signs and Symptoms in Neurology. JB Lippincott, Philadelphia, 1984

13. Oloff JM, Jacobs AM, Jaffe S: Tarsal tunnel syndrome: a manifestation of systemic disease. J Foot Surg 22:302, 1983

14. Seddon H: Surgical Disorders of Peripheral Nerves. 2nd Ed. Churchill Livingstone, Edinburgh, 1975

15. Carrier PA, Janigan JD, Smith SD, Weil LS: Morton's Neuralgia: a possible contributing etiology. J Am Podiatry Assoc 65(4):313, 1975

16. Gauthier G: Thomas Morton's disease: a nerve entrapment syndrome. Clin Orthop Rel Res 142:90, 1979

17. Graham CE, Graham DM: Morton's neuroma: a microscopic evaluation. Foot Ankle 5(2):150, 1984

18. Eaton RG: Painful neuromas. p 196. In Omer GE, Spinner M (eds): Management of Peripheral Nerve Problems. WB Saunders, Philadelphia, 1980

19. Berlin SJ, Donick II, Block LD, Costa AJ: Nerve tumors of the foot. J Am Podiatry Assoc 65(2):157, 1975

20. Livingston KE, Huskings W: Tumors of the peripheral nerves. Surg Clin North Am 27:554, 1947

21. Harkin JC: Differential diagnosis of peripheral nerve tumors: p 658. In Omer GE, Spinner M (eds): Management of Peripheral Nerve Problems. WB Saunders, Philadelphia. 1980

22. Sunderland S: Nerves and Nerve Injuries. 2nd Ed. Churchill Livingstone, Edinburgh, 1978

23. Weller R: Color Atlas of Neuropathology. Oxford University Press, New York, 1984

24. Evans RJ, Watson CPN: Lumbosacral plexopathy in cancer patients. Neurology 35:1392, 1985

25. Thange D: The myotomes, L2-S2 in man. Acta Neurol Scand, 41: suppl. 13, 241, 1965

26. Liverson JA, Speilholz NI: Peripheral Neurology: Case Studies in Electrodiagnosis. FA Davis, Philadelphia, 1979

27. Heimans JJ, Bertelsmann FW, and Van Rooy JCGM: Large and small nerve fiber function in a painful diabetic neuropathy. J Neurol Sci 74:1, 1986

28. Lemont H: The branches of the superficial peroneal nerve and their clinical significance. J Am Podiatry Assoc 65(4):310, 1975

29. Sartoris DJ, Resnick D: Magnetic resonance imaging of podiatric disorders: a pictorial essay. J Foot Surg 26(4):336, 1987

30. Pagliano JD, Wexler CE: Xeroradiography for detection of neuromas in podiatry. J Am Podiatry Assoc 68(1):38, 1978

31. Sullivan JD: Neuroma diagnosis by means of x-ray evaluation. J Foot Surg 6:45, 1967

32. DuVries HL: Surgery of the Foot. 3rd Ed. CV Mosby, St Louis, 1973

33. Gabbay KH: The sorbital pathway and the complication of diabetes. N Engl J Med 288:831, 1973

34. Edmond ME, Roberts VC, Watkins PJ: Blood flow in the diabetic foot. Diabetologia 22:9, 1982

35. Behse F, Buchthal F: Alcoholic neuropathy: clinical, electrophysiological and biopsy findings. Ann Neurol 2:95, 1977

36. Watkins PJ, Edmonds ME: Sympathetic nerve failure in diabetes. Diabetologia 25:73, 1983

37. Cooper CT Jr: Hansen's disease: a podiatrist's experience. J Am Podiatry Assoc 65(4):300, 1975

38. Skre H: Genetic and clinical aspects of Charcot-Marie-Tooth's disease. Clin Genet 6:98, 1974

39. Brust JCM, Lovelace RE, Devi S: Clinical and electrodiagnostic features of Charcot-Marie-Tooth syndrome. Acta Neurol Scand, 58:suppl. 1, 1978

40. Humberstone PM: Nerve conduction studies in Charcot-Marie-Tooth disease. Acta Neurol Scand 48:176, 1972

41. Jones SJ, Carroll and Halliday AM: Peripheral and central sensory nerve conduction in Charcot-Marie-Tooth disease and comparison with Friederich's ataxia. J Neurol Sci 61:135, 1983

42. Buchthal F, Behse F: Peroneal muscular atrophy and related disorders. Part I. Clinical manifestations as related to biopsy findings, nerve conduction and electromyography. Brain 100:41, 1977

43. Bradley WG, Madrid R, Davis CJF: The peroneal muscular atrophy syndrome. J Neurol Sci 32:91, 1977

44. Sabir M, Lyttle D: Pathogenesis of Charcot-Marie-Tooth disease. Gait analysis and electrophysiologic, genetic, histopathologic and enzyme studies in a kinship. Clin Orthop 184:223, 1984

45. Duchenne DBA: Physiology of Motion, Demonstrated by Means of Electrical Stimulation and Clinical Observation and Applied to Study of Paralysis and Deformities (translated and edited by EB Kaplan) JB Lippincott, Philadelphia, 1949

46. Fenton CF, Schlefman BS, McGlamrey SD: Surgical considerations in the presence of Charcot-Marie-Tooth disease. J Am Podiatry Assoc 74(10):490, 1984

47. Garnjobst W: Injuries to the saphenous nerve following operations for varicose veins. Surg Gynecol Obstet 119:359, 1964

48. Wartenberg R: Digitalgia paresthetica and gonyalgia paresthetica. Neurology 4:106, 1954

49. Mozes M, Ouaknine G, Nathan H: Saphenous nerve entrapment simulating vascular disorder. Surgery 77:299, 1975

50. Malay DS, Dalton ED, Nava CA: Entrapment neuropathies of the lower extremities. In McGlamry ED (ed): Comprehensive Textbook of Foot Surgery. Williams & Wilkins, Baltimore, 1987

51. Dawson DM, Hallet M, Millender LH: Entrapment Neuropathies. Little, Brown, Boston, 1983

52. Seppalainen AM, Aho K, Unsitupa M: Strawberry picker's foot drop. Br Med J 2:767, 1977

53. Berry H, Richardson PM: Common peroneal nerve palsy: a clinical and electrophysiological review. J Neurol Neurosurg Psychiatry 39:1162, 1976

54. Maudsley RH: Fibular tunnel syndrome. J Bone Joint Surg 49B:384, 1967

55. Nitz AJ, Dobner JJ, Kersey D: Nerve injury and grades II and III ankle sprains. Am J Sports Med 13:177, 1985

56. Fraser DM, Campbell IW, Ewing J, et al: Mononeuropathy in diabetes mellitus. Diabetes 28:96, 1979

57. Ferguson FR, Liversedge LA: Ischemic lateral popliteal nerve palsy. Br Med J 2:333, 1954

58. Roffman M, Meades DG, Ullman G: Peroneal intraneural ganglion. Orthopedics 7(5):872, 1984

59. Barber KW, Bianco AJ, Soule EH, MacCarty CS: Benign extraneural soft tissue tumors of the extremities causing compression of the nerves. J Bone Joint Surg 44A(1):98, 1962

60. Raynor KJ, Raczka EK, Stone PA, et al: Entrapment of the sural nerve. J Am Podiatry Assoc 76(7):407, 1986

61. Kopell HP, Thompson WAL: Peripheral entrapment neuropathies of the lower extremity. N Engl J Med 262:56, 1960

62. Kuritz HM: Anterior entrapment syndromes. J Foot Surg 15(4)143, 1976

63. Ort L: Deep peroneal nerve entrapment: a case report. J Foot Surg 12:20, 1973

64. Subotnick S, McGlamry ED: Anterior impingement exostosis of the ankle. J Am Podiatry Assoc 66(12):958, 1976

65. Borges LF, Hallet M, Selkoe DJ, Welch K: The anterior tarsal tunnel syndrome: a report of two cases. J Neurosurg 54:89, 1981

66. Cangialosi CP, Schnall SJ: The biomechanical aspects of anterior tarsal tunnel syndrome. J Am Podiatry Assoc 70:291, 1980

67. Lam STS: A tarsal tunnel syndrome. Lancet 2:1354, 1962

68. Kushner S, Reid DC: Medial tarsal tunnel syndrome: a review. J Orthop Sports Phys Ther 6:39, 1984

69. Gauthier JC, Bruyn GW, Van Der Meer WK: The medial tarsal tunnel syndrome. J Neurol Neurosurg Psychiatry 33:97, 1970

70. Oh SJ, Sarala PK, Kuba T, Elmore RS: Tarsal tunnel syndrome: electrophysiological study. Ann Neurol 5:327, 1979

71. Guiloff RJ, Sherratt RM: Sensory nerve conduction in medial plantar nerve. J Neurol Neurosurg Psychiatry 40:1168, 1977

72. Iyer KS, Kaplan E, Goodgold J: Sensory nerve action potentials of the medial and lateral plantar nerve. Arch Phys Med Rehabil 65:529, 1984

73. Oh SJ, Kim HS, Ahmad BA: The near nerve sensory nerve conduction in tarsal tunnel syndrome. J Neurol Neurosurg Psychiatry 48:999, 1985

74. DeLisa JA, Saeed MA: The tarsal tunnel syndrome. Muscle Nerve 6:664, 1983

75. Kaplan PE, Kernahan WT: Tarsal tunnel syndrome: an electrodiagnostic and surgical correlation. J Bone Joint Surg 63:96, 1981

76. Srinivasan R, Rhodes J, Seidel MR: The tarsal tunnel. Mt Sinai J Med 47:17, 1980

77. Goodman CR, Kehr LE: Bilateral tarsal tunnel syndrome: a correlative perspective J Am Podiatr Med Assoc 78(6):292, 1988

78. Johnson M: Anatomy and electrodiagnosis of tarsal tunnel syndrome. Curr Podiatry 38(1):8, 1989

79. Kenzora JE: Sensory nerve neuromas—leading to failed foot surgery. Foot Ankle 7:110, 1986

80. Joplin RJ: The proper digital nerve, vitallium stem arthroplasty, and some thoughts about foot surgery in general. Clin Orthop 76:199, 1971

81. Merritt GN, Subotnick SI: Medial plantar digital proper nerve syndrome (Joplin's neuroma): typical presentation. J Foot Surg 21(3):166, 1982

82. Turf RM, Bacard BE: Causalgia classifications in terminology and a case presentation. J Foot Surg 25:284, 1986

83. Chioros PG, Frankel SL, Sidlow CJ: Sesamoid pain secondary to plantar neuroma. J Foot Surg 26(4):296, 1987

84. Lee B, Crowhurst JA: Entrapment neuropathy of the first metatarsophalangeal joint. J Am Podiatr Med Assoc 77(12):657, 1987

85. Fabrikant J, Califano PJ: Atypical neuroma of the lateral fifth metatarsal head. J Foot Surg 20(1):35, 1981

86. Thul JR, Hoffman SJ: Neuromas associated with tailor's bunion. J Foot Surg 24:342, 1985

87. Przylucki H, Jones CL: Entrapment neuropathy of

muscle branch of lateral plantar nerve: a cause of heel pain. J Am Podiatry Assoc 71:119, 1981

88. Davidson M: Clinical discourse: the medial calcaneal neuroma. Arch Podiatr Med Foot Surg 1:49, 1978

89. Miller S: Morton's neuroma: a syndrome. In McGlamry ED (ed): Comprehensive Textbook of Foot Surgery. Williams & Wilkins, Baltimore, 1987

90. Bartolomei FJ, Wertheimer SJ: Intermetatarsal neuromas: distribution and etiologic factors. J Foot Surg 22(4):279, 1983

91. Berlin SJ, Donick II, Black LD, Costa AJ: Nerve tumors of the foot: diagnosis and treatment. J Am Podiatr Assoc 65(2):157, 1975

92. Bratkowski B: Differential diagnosis of plantar neuromas. J Foot Surg 17(3)99, 1978

93. Carrier PA, Janigan JD, Smith SD, Weil LS: Morton's neuralgia: a possible contributing etiology. J Am Podiatry Assoc 65(4):315, 1975

94. Nissen KI: An exploration of Morton's neuralgia. Practitioner 227:1179, 1983

95. Mulder JD: The causative mechanism in Morton's metatarsalgia. J Bone Joint Surg 33B:94, 1951

96. Nissen KI: The etiology of Morton's metatarsalgia. J Bone Joint Surg 33B:293, 1951

97. Nissen KI: Plantar digital neuritis. Morton's metatarsalgia. J Bone Joint Surg 30B:84, 1948

98. Awerbuch M, Shephard E, Vernon-Roberts B: Morton's metatarsalgia due to intermetatarsophalangeal bursitis as an early manifestation of rheumatoid arthritis. Clin Orthop 167:214, 1982

99. Barziano I: The place of the intermetatarsal bursitis in the pathology of the interdigital web space. Proc Israeli Orthop Soc 10:112, 1986

100. Bossley CJ, Cairney C: The intermetatarsophalangeal bursa—its significance in Morton's metatarsalgia. J Bone Joint Surg 62B(2):184, 1980

101. Roberts PM: Fifty cases of bursitis of the foot. J Bone Joint Surg 1929

102. Shepard E: Intermetatarsophalangeal bursitis in the causation of Morton's metatarsalgia. J Bone Joint Surg 57B(1):115, 1975

103. Spalteholz W: In Barker LF (trans): Hand Atlas of Human Anatomy, 7th ed. p 381. JB Lippincott, Philadelphia, 1943

104. Vanio K: Morton's metatarsalgia in rheumatoid arthritis. Clin Orthop 142:85, 1979

105. Gauthier G: Thomas Morton's disease: a nerve entrapment syndrome. Clin Orthop 142:90, 1979

106. Morton TG: A peculiar and painful affliction of the fourth metatarsophalangeal articulation. Am J Med Sci 71:35, 1876

107. Betts LO: Morton's metatarsalgia: neuritis of the fourth digital nerve. Med J Aust 1:514, 1940

108. Wachter SD, Nilson RZ, Thul JR: The relationship between foot structure and intermetatarsal neuromas. J Foot Surg 23(6):436, 1984

109. Durlacher L: A Treatise on Corns, Bunions, the Diseases of Nails and the General Management of the Feet. Simkin Marshall, London, 1845

110. Graham CE, Graham DM: Morton's neuroma: a microscopic evaluation. Foot Ankle 5(2):150, 1984

111. Goldman F: Intermetatarsal neuromas, light and electron microscope observation. J Am Podiatr Med Assoc 76(6):265, 1980

112. Milgram JE: Morton's neuritis and management of post-neurectomy pain. In Omer GE, Spinner M (eds): Management of Peripheral Nerve Problems. WB Saunders, Philadelphia, 1980

113. Greenfield J, Rea J, Ilfeld F: Morton's interdigital neuroma: indications for treatment by local injections versus surgery. Clin Orthop 185:142, 1984

114. Mann RA, Reynolds JC: Interdigital neuroma—a critical analysis. Foot Ankle 3(4):238, 1983

115. Gudas CJ, Mattana GM: Retrospective analysis of intermetatarsal neuroma excision with preservation of the transverse ligament. J Foot Surg 52(6):459, 1986

116. Lassmann G: Morton's toe: clinical, light and electron microscopic investigation in 133 cases. Clin Orthop 142:73, 1979

117. McKeever DC: Surgical approach for neuroma of plantar digital nerve (Morton's metatarsalgia). J Bone Joint Surg 34A(2):490, 1952

118. Morton DJ: The Human Foot. Columbia University Press, New York, 1935

119. Nutt JJ: Diseases and Deformities of the Foot. p. 252. EB Treat, New York, 1925

120. Reed RJ, Bliss BO: Morton's neuroma. Arch Pathol 95:123, 1973

121. Ringertz N, Unander-Scharin ML: Morton's disease: a clinical and pathoanatomical study. Acta Orthop Scand 19:327, 1950

122. Winkler H, Feltner JB, Kimmestiel P: Morton's metatarsalgia. J Bone Joint Surg 30A:496, 1948

123. Scotti TM: The lesion of Morton's metatarsalgia (Morton's toe). Arch Pathol Lab Med 63:91, 1957

124. McElvenny RT: The etiology and surgical treatment of intractable pain about the fourth metatarsophalangeal joint (Morton's toe). J Bone Joint Surg 25:675, 1943

125. Oh SJ, Kim HS: Electrophysiological diagnosis of interdigital neuropathy of the foot. Muscle Nerve 7:218, 1984

126. Hoadley AE: Six cases of metatarsalgia. Chicago Med Rec 5:32, 1893

127. Tubby AH: Deformities Including Diseases of Bone and Joint. 2nd Ed. Vol 1. Macmillan, London, 1912

128. Schuster O: In Lewi MJ (ed): Foot Orthopedics. p 324. First Institute of Podiatry, New York, 1927

129. Foote EM: A Textbook of Minor Surgery. p 560. D Appleton and Co, New York, 1927

130. King LS: Note on the pathology of Morton's metatarsalgia. Am J Clin Pathol 16:124, 1946

Vascular Disorders

17

Anthony S. Kidawa, D.P.M.

The lower extremities, including the feet, have a predilection for development of organic vessel disease in the mature population and autonomic dysfunction in the young adult. Since this system is the primary cause of limb loss, appropriate diagnosis and treatment is imperative. In addition, since the surgical candidate must have adequate circulation to ensure uncomplicated recovery, the presurgical vascular assessment must be thoroughly understood and completed.

The assessment of the peripheral vasculature necessitates investigation of its three components: arterial, venous, and lymphatic vessels. The diagnosis of impaired circulation can, in most instances, be readily made through the use of simple clinical tests performed in the office. Various techniques are presented with a discussion of their applications and limitations.

Understanding the pathophysiology and diagnosis as it applies to the tissues of the lower extremities is important to the practitioner entrusted to treat the feet. All three forms of vessels comprising the peripheral vasculature are presented, with emphasis on local care and discussion of sophisticated procedures performed by the vascular surgeon or radiologist.

ARTERIAL PHYSICAL EXAMINATION

Inspection

Nutritional Disturbances

Examination will reveal the vascular status of the cutaneous and subcutaneous tissue. Presence of amputated digits, healed ulcers, open or infected ulcers, or depressed scars is adequate cause for suspicion of inadequate cutaneous flow when the common systemic causes of such findings have been ruled out.

Particular attention should be given to the texture of the skin. In cases of loose skin over joints, moderate arterial insufficiency is suspect, and chronic marked insufficiency is characterized by thinning (onion skin) over most surfaces of the feet and legs. Scaliness of the periungual and digital tissue also suggests inadequate flow.

Alterations in Nail Structure

Hypertrophic nails may result from trauma when this is indicated by history. Bilateral thickening of symmetric nails of the longest toes is associated

423

with chronic microtrauma from the toe box of shoes as a result of a short fit. Hypertrophy may also result from impaired arterial flow to the matrix and nail bed and involves many nails of one or both feet without discoloration (or with discoloration secondary to mycotic infection). With organic arterial insufficiency, a thickening, ridging, or brittleness is observed with a history of slow nail growth. In vasospastic disorders, thinning of the epinychium and merging with the posterior nail fold is observed.

Alterations in Hair Growth

Since hair is an appendage of skin, its growth is directly affected by the cutaneous circulation. Marked and chronic disturbances in arterial flow cause cessation in growth from distal to proximal. Consideration must be given for absence of hair as a result of chronic friction from clothing, shaving, or use of depilatories.

Skin Coloration

Interpretation of skin coloration is dependent upon the color acuity of the examiner and the natural spectrum of the source of illumination: incandescent (red), fluorescent (blue), or natural sunlight. Full-spectrum fluorescent tubes are marketed for office use and provide the best illumination.

The color of skin is dependent upon the oxygen saturation of the hemoglobin in the subpapillary venous plexus as transmitted to the surface through the relatively translucent epidermis. Since roughly 25 percent of the oxyhemoglobin is reduced in the cutaneous circuit, the oxygen saturation of the blood remains high and allows for perception of a normal pink color. This may be observed in most patients except for those with extremely deep pigmentation. With slight retardation of flow, the oxygen saturation is lower and rubor is evident, whereas in marked stagnation of flow, further oxygen consumption yields cyanosis. Finally, vascular standstill fully depletes the blood of oxygen, causing black coloration seen in gangrene, ecchymosis, and hematoma.

Palpation

Alterations in Skin Temperature

Decrease in skin temperature from proximal to distal is anticipated as a result of increasing sympathetic fibers and activity when the gradation is gradual and observed bilaterally. However, when the temperature decrease is marked and apparent in a short distance, it is pathognomonic of arterial disease. This may be assessed by manual testing with the back of the examiner's hand stroking all exposed nonsupportive surfaces from proximal on distally to the toes. Comparison is always made between bilateral symmetric sites. This technique allows for the following gradation: hot, warm, tepid (matching examiner's hand temperature), cool, or cold. A more objective assessment is possible with instrumentation discussed later in this chapter. Interpretation must allow for temperature variations due to season and clothing or local exposure to heat or air condition ducts.

Peripheral Pulses

When palpating the vessels in the lower extremities, the examiner should be comfortably positioned. The pressure applied is dependent upon the known depth and size of each artery. The fingers should be slightly spaced apart to preclude feeling one's own digital pulsations. If the amplitude of the pulse is feeble, the examiner can ensure that the palpated pulse is the patient's by simultaneously palpating another more prominent patient's pulse or the examiner's own radial pulse. The examiner may also squat down, bringing his or her own heart to a lower level than the pulse being palpated.

All pulses should be examined with regard to force, rate, and rhythm. Amplitudes are rated as follows:

$+\frac{1}{4}$ = Weak
$+\frac{2}{4}$ = Normal
$+\frac{3}{4}$ = Full
$+\frac{4}{4}$ = Bounding

Whenever noninstrumental evaluation is made, the notation is a fractional expression with the numerator representing the value ascribed and the denominator the maximum in the arbitrary scale utilized.

A natural progression for palpation is from the pedal vessels on proximally until normal pulses are identified. This may cause the examination to proceed to the iliac arteries and even the abdominal aorta. Supplemental evaluation of any of the arteries in the upper extremity is indicated to rule out Takayasu's pulseless disease or generalized arteriosclerosis.

Extrinsic Factors Affecting Pulsations. The parameters in the examination of peripheral pulses may be affected by factors other than the local arterial status. Since the heart is the prime mover of blood throughout the arterial system, pathologies that affect it are reflected in the distal arteries. Constrictive pericarditis diminishes pulse amplitude, as does congestive heart failure. Atrial fibrillation affects the apparent rhythm, and ectopic beats affect rhythm and amplitude. Other conditions that have an impact on the peripheral pulses include congestive heart failure, hypothyroidism, coarctation or calcification of the aorta, abdominal dissecting aneurysm, or stenosis due to expansive visceral or pelvic neoplasms.

Intrinsic Factors Affecting Pulsations. Organic changes of the vessels responsible for decreased pulse amplitudes include atherosclerosis, arteriosclerosis, and thromboangiitis obliterans. Dampening occurs in Mönckeberg's arteriosclerosis as a result of calcium deposits in the tunica media. Vasospastic conditions will also diminish pedal pulses, and erythromyalgia causes bounding pulses.

Auscultation

Vessels of ample size and pulsation that are available to palpation may also be studied by stethoscopic auscultation. Two distinct sounds are audible consistent with the systolic and diastolic components of cardiac activity. The first (systolic) signal is louder than the second (diastolic) signal. The sounds are distinctly clear and crisp. Their amplitudes are dependent on the pressure within the vessel, the size of the lumen, and the amount of interposed soft tissue that may dampen the transmission to the surface.

When the normal laminar flow is disturbed as a result of abrupt changes in the luminal dimension (e.g., poststenotic dilation or at a site of an aneurysm), eddy currents develop, with the turbulent flow being audible as a bruit. This characteristic change in sound may be heard during the systolic or diastolic component depending on the net change in pressure as a result of the stenosis. The bruit may be systolic or diastolic at a point of an enlarged chronic post-traumatic arteriovenous (A-V) fistula. The pitch is usually higher than normal. If significant disturbance of laminar flow occurs, this vortex may also be palpated as a thrill.

Flat surfaces over arteries are auscultated with the diaphragm of the stethoscope, whereas concave surfaces (e.g., posterior tibial artery) are best evaluated with the bell. Auscultation requires a quiet environment, particularly for the faint distal vessels. Auscultory evaluation of still smaller distal vessels requires a Doppler flow meter (described later).

Functional Studies

Considerable information of value may be obtained by studying the skin color of the lower extremities when stressed in the elevated and dependent positions.

Horizontal (Phlebostatic) Position

With the patient lying supine on the examination table, inspection of the lower extremities normally reveals a pink flush to the skin. If rubor or cyanosis is evident, it is a sign of advanced arterial involvement, if systemic conditions that would cause hypo-oxygenation of blood have been ruled out.

Elevated Position

With the lower extremities in the elevated position, normally some loss of pink flush is anticipated as a result of loss of hydrostatic pressure of gravity. In cases of arterial stenosis, a marked blanching occurs within 1 minute. To facilitate this study, the patient is requested to wiggle the toes or feet, thereby draining part of the venous blood. This elevational pallor test, also known as Samuel's test, may be graded as mild, moderate, or severe. In the advanced states of blanching, accentuation of the plantar skin creases is observed as a result of atrophy of connective tissue.

If one of the pedal vessels is not palpable and is thought to be stenosed, an extension of this basic maneuver can be performed. With the extremity still elevated, the palpable pulse is fully compressed with sufficient digital pressure to temporarily occlude this vessel. If the nonpalpable artery is truly occluded, no flow can enter the foot, resulting in pallor of the sole. This Allen test, therefore, discriminates patent from occluded nonpalpable distal vessels, and requires a Doppler flow meter (described later).

Venous Filling Time

When the lower extremities are returned to the dependent position, refilling of the veins occurs within a few seconds. The superficial veins constituting the dorsal venous arcade refill from distal to proximal within 10 to 20 seconds as the blood courses from the arteries to the previously collapsed veins. If refilling occurs from proximal to distal and almost immediately, retrograde flow due to incompetent valves is identified. Therefore, this test is not reliable if venous insufficiency exists. The longer the refill after 20 seconds, the greater is the degree of arterial compromise.

Dependent Rubor. With continued dependency in the presence of impaired arterial flow, the skin color proceeds to a deep rubor. This state is positive with arterial insufficiency and is observed to involve more of the pedal skin as the condition worsens. With moderate proximal stenosis, the rubor is noted at the plantar surface of the toes and metatarsal area; as the stenosis advances, the rubor extends to the heel and dorsum of the foot. If the stenosis is distal, the rubor occurs in a stocking distribution, that is, beginning on all surfaces of the toes and progressing proximally to the forefoot, midfoot, and finally the rearfoot. This phenomenon is a result of pooling of blood in the subpapillary plexus with concurrent dilation to retain the rationed volume of blood perfusing slowly per unit of time.

Subpapillary Venous Plexus Filling Time

A simple test to evaluate the arterial inflow is application of pressure to the skin at any site of the lower extremity or to compress the nail plate against the underlying nail bed. This naturally causes blanching as the blood is expressed from the microvasculature. Release of pressure with the limb in the supine position allows an immediate return of color. A delay of from 2 to 5 seconds occurs depending on the degree of arterial compromise. This same procedure with the limb elevated causes a commensurate delay in filling time by about 2 seconds since the flow is upgrade against gravity.

This test can predict the viability of tissue. A return of color in a ruborous foot connotes adequate collateral flow, whereas no return of color suggests that the tissue will proceed to undergo gangrenous changes.

VENOUS PHYSICAL EXAMINATION

Inspection

Nutritional Disturbances

Inspection of the skin will reveal the status of the deep and superficial venous systems. The presence of pretibial pitting edema, ruborous or brawny dermatitis, or ulceration of the medial portion of the leg suggest inadequate venous return.

Particular attention is given to skin when induration is noted to exclude the possibility of thyroid dysfunction or scar formation as a result of trauma, infection, or surgery. Deep pigmentation and induration are the sequelae of deep thrombophlebitis and have acquired the characterization of postphlebitic syndrome.

Alterations in Venous Structure

Normally the superficial veins are not apparent except when carefully examined in the Caucasian; they are nearly never apparent in darker pigmented skin. When they are easily identifiable but maintain normal distribution, they are considered merely superficial. This is observed commonly in slender individuals with minimal subcutaneous adipose tissue for protective covering. With overt valvular incompetency, the substantial hydrostatic pressure head expands the veins, thereby increasing their capacitance. With time the dilation in the transverse plane causes varices while the dilation in the longitudinal axis yields tortuosity. Weakening of the venous wall is also a natural result, with risk of rupturing. Continuous retrograde pressure on the venioles may cause dilation of these structures in the dermis to a point of clinical recognition as spider nevi or telangiectasia.

Functionally, the deep system consisting of the vena communicantes conducts over 80 percent of the blood from the leg to the heart. It receives blood from the leg muscles as well as the perforating veins from the superficial system. When valvular incompetency occurs within the deep system, there is regurgitation of blood to the superficial system via the perforators. These vessels must also dilate to accept an unnatural higher volume of blood, thus precluding valvular coaptation and allowing reversal of flow. These perforating veins, numbering about four, are spaced about 3 cm apart as they anastomose with the long saphenous vein. At the point of anastamosis of the lowest perforator, dilation occurs in the long saphenous vein above the medial malleolus. Attendent with this phenomenon is diapedesis of the blood cells, pushed by the higher than normal head of pressure, into the extravascular soft tissue compartments. The hemoglobin is biodegraded to hemosiderin, whose iron content is permanently deposited in the skin. This results in hyperpigmentation with attendant hardening as a result of scarring from the inflammatory response to the extravascular blood cells. The plasma similarly accumulates in the intercellular spaces as a result of the tremendous intraluminal pressure head of retrograde flow at the veniole end of the capillaries, and is clinically manifested as pitting edema.

When edema is evident, its level of presentation must be identified as well as its character for pitting or nonpitting. To identify its nature, digital compression is applied for 15 to 30 seconds over any osseous prominance. After release of pressure, a pit remains in pitting edema whereas none remains in nonpitting edema. Pitting edema is graded on an arbitrary scale. The broader the scale, the more defined is the notation of subtle differences. A recommended scale is as follows:

$$+\tfrac{1}{7} = \ 5 \text{ mm deep}$$
$$+\tfrac{2}{7} = 10 \text{ mm deep}$$
$$+\tfrac{3}{7} = 15 \text{ mm deep}$$
$$+\tfrac{4}{7} = 20 \text{ mm deep}$$
$$+\tfrac{5}{7} = 25 \text{ mm deep}$$
$$+\tfrac{6}{7} = 30 \text{ mm deep}$$
$$+\tfrac{7}{7} = 35 \text{ mm deep}$$

Edema of systemic origin (i.e., cardiac or renal failure) is pitting and progresses to the bases of the toes, whereas venous edema is also pitting but is limited to the ankle. Lymphatic edema is nonpitting and extends to and involving the toes.

Palpation

Alteration in Skin Temperature

Valvular incompetency leads to venous insufficiency, whether of the deep, perforating, superficial, or communicating veins. This state of itself does not cause any skin temperature alteration; however, when the vessels are inflamed as a result of trauma or stasis, as in superficial phlebitis or deep thrombophlebitis, an increase in the skin temperature is readily palpated. The demarcation is acutely circumscribed in superficial or regional phlebitis, whereas in deep phlebitis the increase in temperature is more widespread.

Superficial Veins

Examination of the venous system is indicated when clinical varicosities are evident and when symptoms presented are of venous origin. The superficial and communicating veins may be palpated clinically whereas the perforating and deep can only be studied directly with use of instrumentation.

Extrinsic Factors Affecting Veins. The clinical evidence of varicose veins may be attributed to factors other than venous dysfunction. Since venous blood is directed toward the heart, pathologies that involve the heart or organs between the lower limbs and the heart may affect the venous status. With right-sided backward failure, cor pulmonale, hepatic cirrhosis, portal hypertension, intra-abdominal neoplasms, pregnancy, trauma involving the inferior vena cava, or venous hypertension, pooling of blood may occur, leading to greater hydrostatic pressure and eventual varicose development.

Intrinsic Factors Affecting Veins. Should interview or examination rule out any extrinsic factors as the etiology for varicosities, the probability of local factors must be considered. Congenital weakness of walls has been identified and should be ruled out when there exists a positive familial history and when onset was during the adolescent years. The possibility of venous or valvular damage as a result of trauma must also be considered. Women with softer skin have somewhat lesser support for the veins and are more likely to develop varices.

Functional Studies

Valuable information regarding the location of incompetent segments or thrombosis of the deep veins may be obtained from studying the drainage or lack of it with the limbs in elevated or dependent positions.

Elevational Test

If the feet are ruborous or cyanotic on dependency, and following elevation the normal color returns, venous hypertension or insufficiency is the etiology. This is a result of excessive retrograde hydrostatic pressure on the subpapillary venous plexus, with arterial blood being shunted via the normal A-V anatamosis to the venous channels while not perfusing the cutaneous plexus.

Percussion Test

Percussion of the great saphenous vein identifies valvular incompetence. With the patient standing and the veins fully distended, a vein is struck above the level of the knee with one hand while the other hand palpates a segment of the vein in the leg. Perception of an impulse distal to the area struck indicates incompetence of the intervening valves.

Brodie-Trendelenburg Test

This test demonstrates valvular competency in the great saphenous vein and the branches communicating with the deep femoral vein. The lower extremity is elevated vertically until drained of venous blood. A tourniquet is applied at midthigh to a pressure of about 70 mm Hg, and the patient stands upright. The tourniquet is removed in 60 seconds. Normally arterial flow from below refills the veins in about 35 seconds. With the tourniquet applied, faster filling indicates incompetence of the communicating veins. Normally when the tourniquet is released, no further increment of blood is added from above; any additional flow indicates saphenous valve incompetence.

Perthes' Test

This tests valvular competence in the deep femoral vein and its communications. A tourniquet is applied at midthigh to 70 mm Hg pressure with the patient standing, and the veins are distended with blood. The patient is required to walk for 5 minutes with the tourniquet in place. With normal competent valves and patent lumens in the deep veins, the size of the superficial veins is reduced with exercise.

Homan's Sign

This test is beneficial in the diagnosis of deep thrombophlebitis. The calf at its widest upper portion is manually compressed. If pain is elicited the test is positive. If there is no response, the procedure may be augmented by dorsiflexing the foot, thereby stretching the deep veins and further limiting the lumen of the thrombosed vein. The rapid evacuation of blood from the gastrosoleal veins will produce pain because of the inability of the thrombosed deep veins to accept and propagate the bolus of blood to more proximal vessels. A more precise knowledge of the amount of compression required to elicit pain can be determined by applying of a pressure cuff and noting the amount of compression required to reach the pain threshold. This can then be compared accurately at time of future readings.

Since unrelated conditions in the same location can be a source of pain, these conditions must be eliminated from the differential diagnosis. False-positive diagnoses can occur if any of the following are the etiology of pain: acute or chronic cellulitis, myositis, dermatitis, local hemorrhage, rupture or contusion of muscle, or superficial phlebitis.

LYMPHATIC PHYSICAL EXAMINATION

Inspection

Alterations in Skin Texture

Lymphatic disease may present with a spectrum of skin changes, including dryness, nodules, tumors, and even verrucoid dermatoses. The most important clinical finding in long-standing lymphatic dysfunction is thickening of the dermis (Fig. 17-1). The hyperplasia that develops is a physio-logic response to the tremendous pressure as a result of chronic increasing edema.

In the early stages, dryness is apparent with associated thickening of stratum corneum and dermal hyperplasia. This process continues until the hypertrophied dermis is readily palpated by grasping it between two fingers. It has been demonstrated that this hyperplastic activity may produce a dermis over 1 inch thick. At this terminal stage hypertrophied papilla that originally gave the appearance of "pigskin" progress to large verrucoid nodules and skinfolds. This state is commonly termed *elephantiasis*.

Alterations in Fluid Dynamics

Because of lymphatic dysfunction, proteins of high molecular weight saturate the fluids that are normally transported via the lymphatic conduits. The fluids accumulate in the intercellular compartments as well as intracellularly. This results in edema that is nonpitting and extending from the toes proximally to a level of normal lymphatic function. If hypoplasia of lymphatic channels is the underlying factor, the lymphedema may involve the entire lower extremities. Unlike edema of venous or systemic origin, which resolves after elevation or a night's rest, lymphedema responds much more slowly to elevation, and, depending on the chronicity, it may not resolve at all.

Palpation

Alteration in Contour

The lymphatic channels and nodes are not normally evident to inspection or palpation. However, if an infection is not localized to the foot, but begins to extend to adjacent tissue, it will invade the lymphatic channels, and inflammation of these vessels will occur. This lymphangiitis is evident clinically by its red streaks and may be palpated as being hyperthermic.

If the infection migrates into the lymph channels and is not controlled, the lymphatic nodes will attempt to thwart further dissemination of the infection by accumulating the organisms and toxins. This results in distention of these nodes, known as lymphadenopathy. These nodes now may be pal-

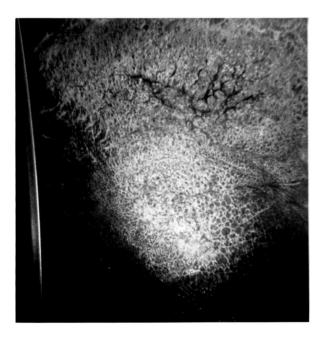

Fig. 17-1. Lymphatic blockage leads to fibrous tissue accumulation in the subcutis, resulting in thickening of the stratum corneum and hypertrophy of the dermal papilla causing a "pigskin" appearance.

pated in the popliteal fossa (popliteal lymphade-nopathy) or more commonly in the groin (inguinal lymphadenopathy). These nodes are also functional in attempting to curb metastasis of neoplasms.

Systemic lymphadenopathy of Hodgkin's disease would present in these nodes as well as in the axilla and infra-auricular, submandibular, and submaxillary areas.

NONINVASIVE VASCULAR EXAMINATION

The clinical examination provides the experienced practitioner most of the information necessary for establishing a working diagnosis. The addition of instrumental examination aids in the definition of the pathology as well as its qualitative and quantitative parameters. Therefore, the noninvasive instrumental examination characterizes the vasculopathies involving the arterial and venous components of the peripheral circulation. Since the lymphatic system does not possess similar active dynamics, it is not evaluable by noninvasive techniques.

Diascopy

When concentrations of blood at the skin level exceed that normally present in the rete pegs, the areas are clinically evident as red or blue discolorations. The presentation may be linear, patchy, or spotty. It is desireous to differentiate whether the blood is intra- or extravascular.

Superficial microcirculatory vessels may be distended and can be identified on inspection. Typical ectatic arterial lesions are classified as *angiomas,* which are congenital, whereas dilated venioles are termed *telangiectasia* and are principally acquired. Angiomas are patchy whereas telangiectasia are linear in distribution.

Lesions that are spotty and discolored represent extravasation of blood from capillaries, arterioles, or venules into the adjacent extravascular tissue. These may be present as petechiae, which result from vessel wall weakness and breakage or from increased permeability. They usually appear in areas of the skin that are subject to pressure, such as the heels, and are characteristically observed in patients with thrombocytopenia. The simple procedure of determining blood pressure may cause petechiae to develop in the segment distal to the occluding cuff. Suspicion of this tendency may be confirmed by the tourniquet test with the cuff applied to as distal a segment as possible, preferably the ankle or wrist. The petechiometer is a specialized instrument that employs the suction principle to apply negative pressure to a small surface area of the skin. If capillary fragility causes petechia formation, it is limited to a small area, and, with a built-in magnification lens, the character and count of the lesions can be determined. These lesions may also be evident in the posterior thigh, are perifollicular, and are associated with scurvy. Splinter hemorrhages present typically as linear streaks due to microemboli that lodge in the cutaneous vessels and secondary rupture of vessel wall. These lesions are characteristic of infective endocarditis.

Any transparent rigid material may be employed as a diascope. Glass slides or even reading glasses may be used. The lesion to be differentiated is compressed with the diascope, and the persistence or disappearance of the discoloration is noted. Lesions with extravasated and coagulated blood will not disappear whereas those with dilated vessels will disappear as the pressure on the skin exceeds that of the vessel, causing its collapse.

Oscillometry

The oscillometer objectively evaluates the arterial pulsations. With each pulsation there is arterial expansion that displaces all soft tissue, including skin. The air contained within the pneumatic cuff is also displaced through tubing, past a valve to a sensitive aneroid that depicts this displacement on a scale. Since this technique is a gross demonstration of volume displacement, the scale is interpreted in units of millimeters. A recommended notation of the study results is:

Oscillometric Index

$$= \frac{\text{mm maximum excursion}}{\text{mm least pressure}}$$

whereby the denominator of this fraction represents the least pressure it takes to attain the greatest excursion. This recording is an index that allows for comparison of one extremity level to other levels on the ipsi- and contralateral sides. The studies are performed sequentially at the pedal, ankle, below-knee, above-knee, and groin levels.

Since the pulse of an artery is reflected to the surface through intervening soft tissue, the cuff should be applied to the limb with its most sensitive portion (i.e., the bladder section with tubing) directly over the vessel studied. Decreased pulsations due to stenotically reduced pressures yield decreased excursions. At a level just proximal to a stenosis or occlusion, lateralization of the forward head of arterial pressure yields a higher reading than at the same level of the pathology-free companion limb.

Oscillometric readings inconsistent with other clinical findings are observed as a result of improper application of the cuff over the artery. Higher than normal readings may be observed if the patient is slender, hypertensive, or hyperthyroid, or has decreased vasomotor tone as in erythromelalgia. Lower readings are observed in obese, muscular, hypotensive, and hypothyroid patients, as well as those with constrictive pericarditis, coarctation of the aorta, congestive heart failure with or without peripheral edema, dissecting aneurysm, peripheral edema, or neoplasms compressing vessels in the thorax, abdomen, or pelvis. Other compressive forces against the peripheral arteries would similarly decrease the oscillometric index (e.g., fractures, dislocations, and extensive effusion). Figure 17-2 summarizes normal and abnormal results obtained by this and other diagnostic techniques.

Temperature Gradients

The temperature of a part is dependent principally on the volume of blood perfusing it, assuming that the body is normothermic. The quantity of perfusing blood is governed by the state of tonicity of the microvasculature. This in turn is controlled by the smooth muscles in the vessel walls that are influenced by metabolites, hormones (thyroid, adrenal, and pituitary), and the autonomic nervous system. The sympathetic component exerts the most influence while activating constriction or yielding dilation. The greatest concentration of the sympathetic fibers is at the distal anatomic segments, including the toes.

Thermometry

Any thermocouple or skin thermometer may be employed in determining the skin temperature of a part. Electronic devices usually indicate temperatures to within one-tenth of a degree Fahrenheit. This instrument objectively quantitates the temperature, which is preferable to subjective and only qualitative palpation.

The probe is usually placed at multiple symmetric sites from proximal to distal. Relatively avascular bony prominances are avoided. Typical points of interrogation for temperatures would include the pulp of any toe, the dorsum of the foot, lateral leg, and anterior thigh. The temperatures should be observed to gradually decrease from proximal to distal in decrements of about 6 to 8°F. Any segmental decrease in excess of this range warrants scrutiny.

Thermography

This instrument translates ranges of temperatures into a visual form of colors or shades of gray. Two formats exist that provide the same information. The electronic variant employs an infrared camera-like sensor that detects varying amounts of heat or infrared radiation emitted from any source. This information is electronically processed and is projected on a monitor screen in various shades of color or gray. By selection of sensitivity and discrimination of temperature ranges, the unit projects a color image outline of anything in its field of view, with colors ascribed to each programmed difference in temperature.

The contact form of thermography has cholesterol crystals that are suspended in a medium that is applied over rubber dam material. This sheet of crystals is applied to the anatomic surface. The heat is conducted to the crystals, causing varying amounts of expansion that refracts light into a spectrum of colors. Hence areas of one temperature are visualized in one color while other areas of other temperatures are seen in different colors.

Either of these formats have a distinct advantage over manual palpation for temperature or even

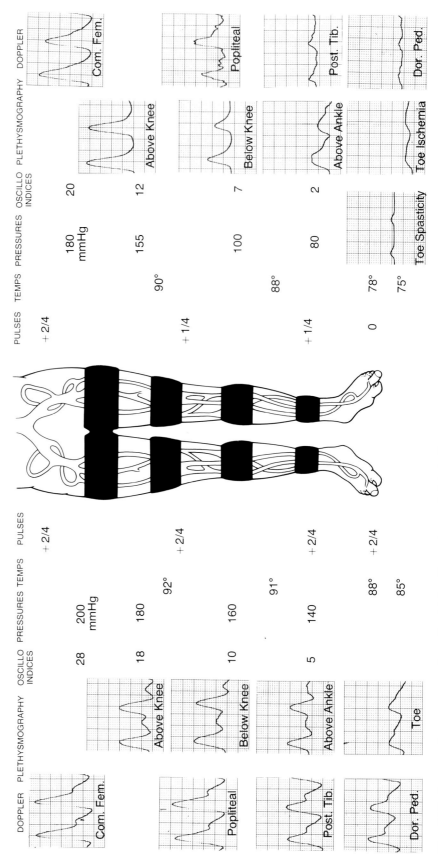

Fig. 17-2. Comparative summary of results obtained by various arterial studies.

thermometry since they provide a visual form of temperature variations over a broad area and in small increments. Fine temperature detail, such as coolness over a superficial vein or hyperemia of a psoriatic lesion, may be appreciated. The vascular applications include localization of A-V fistulas, and early detection of thrombophlebitis, vasospastic or vasodilatory crises, and neurovascular deficits.

Segmental Systolic Pressures

Groin to Ankle Levels

Systolic pressures are typically determined at the groin, the above- and below-knee levels, and the ankles. The cuff for each of these levels should have a width approximately the same as the diameter of the part examined. Straight cuffs are usually employed, although contour cuffs for the thighs are commercially available to better fit the conical shape at these levels.

The principle is the same as that for determination of systemic blood pressure at the brachial artery. However, instead of a stethoscope, a Doppler probe is used to auscultate the vessels. For determination of thigh pressures, the Doppler probe may be applied at the popliteal artery or either the dorsalis pedis or posterior tibial artery. The latter two vessels are auscultated sequentially for pressure determinations of the below-knee and ankle levels. Another technique for determination of these same pressures is a photocell plethysmographic probe applied to any digit. However, this approach only yields the segmental pressure of the tibial vessel that has the higher pressure, whereas the Doppler probe allows the examiner to evaluate more discriminately the pressure in each vessel at all sites.

The arterial pressure decreases negligibly from the heart through the major vessels. It is at the level of the medium-sized arteries, especially at the end arteries, called pressor vessels, that the pressure drops precipitously. This is a result of increasing number of smooth circular muscles in the periphery as well as increased numbers of sympathetic fibers regulating the vasomotor tone. The natural pressure decrease from proximal to distal in either upper or lower extremities, therefore, is due to

decreasing volume of soft tissue to dampen the cuff pressure from occluding the vessel.

The segmental pressures naturally decrease from proximal to distal by decrements not to exceed 20 mmHg from one level to the next. A decrease in excess of this indicates a stenotic lesion that has intra-arterially dampened the forward head of pressure between the two cuff sites. The pressures are also compared to the contralateral limb at the same level. This comparison should yield readings within 10 mmHg, allowing for minor variations in anatomic development or in examination technique. Distal pressures that seem higher than more proximal levels are due to a greater volume of tissue that is dampening the pressure from compressing the vessel (e.g., increased muscle mass, edema, or fat). This may also be observed when arterial sclerosis of the distal vessel is precluding the artery from being compressed.

Digital Pressures

Special small cuffs of various sizes with Velcro attachments are available to be applied to the base of a toe. Usually the hallux is chosen to be studied, and it serves as an index of the most acral pressures to the other toes. Since only the glomus of anastomotic small vessels exists at the digital pulp, a photocell plethysmographic probe is utilized rather than a Doppler probe. The point of return of plethysmographic waves as the pressure within the digital cuff is decreased indicates the digital systolic pressure. Any digital pressure in excess of the ankle pressure is indicative of sclerosis of the microvasculature and is termed *arteriolosclerosis.*[1]

Ischemic Indices

It has been determined that the arm and ankle have typically the same girth, and hence segmental pressure, although the ankle pressure may be slightly higher because of a lifelong erect posture exerting both systolic and hydrostatic pressure of gravity. Hence this relationship has evolved to a universally accepted Ankle/Arm Index with a normal value of 1.00 to 1.20. If any stenotic lesion in the lower extremity lowers the ankle pressure, the resultant index decreases proportionally. Indices of 0.90 to 0.70 are usually associated with claudication; indices between 0.70 and 0.50 are associated with nocturnal cramping and pain on elevation; indices below 0.50 are consistent with intermittent or near-constant rest pain. This relationship only defines the ability of the arteries to transmit a head of pressure to the level of the ankle and does not indicate the status of the pressure at the pedal or digital levels. The Toe/Ankle Index indicates this distal circulation and has a normal value of 0.80 to 1.00. For the diabetic, these values are usually 0.10 to 0.20 higher as a result of accepted complications of arteriosclerosis.

The indices are also useful in assessing the level of vascularity in the lower extremities as well as in the digits. Various observers have studied these values and reported differing views on anticipated healing and limb salvage. The results have varied based on the skill of the surgeon, choice of procedure, and assessment of the hemodynamics of flow prior to surgical intervention or revascularization.

Doppler Evaluation

Doppler ultrasound or flow meter works on the principle that any moving object in the path of the sound beam shifts the frequency of the transmitted signal. Thus the emitting ultrasound beam of constant frequency penetrates all intervening soft tissue layers until striking a moving column of blood. The velocity of blood flow alters the frequency reflected back through the same soft tissue to a receiving crystal. This is termed the *Doppler shift*, with greater velocity yielding higher frequency and slower velocity yielding lower frequency.

The reflected signal is electronically processed and amplified to be heard through a speaker for audible interpretation of frequency shift. Recognizable patterns exist for normal and disease states. A visual interpretation also is possible through spectral sound analysis. Strip chart–recorded analog tracings of the signal serve as a permanent record of the Doppler study. Some instruments also have the capacity of recording forward and reverse flow.

Arterial Examination

The vessels that are typically insonated with the Doppler probe are the common femoral, popliteal, dorsalis pedis, and posterior tibial. The probe is positioned over the artery and held steady at a 45-degree angle facing the direction of oncoming flow. The audible signal is evaluated for amplitude, pitch, phasicity, and character. A 7- to 9-MHz crystal is suitable for arterial studies.

The normal arterial signal has an amplitude and pitch appropriate for the vessel size, velocity, and pressure. The character is usually crisp. The phasicity varies from two to four audible components for each pulse. The first signal represents the forward flow in relative time to left ventricular systole. The second signal is somewhat lesser in amplitude and represents the reversal of flow due to vessel wall recoil at early diastole. The third component is of still lesser amplitude and represents the continued forward flow of blood to the next segment of the artery. Its timing is at late diastole and it may not be heard because of low systemic and pulse pressure or decreased volume in smaller caliber vessels. The fourth signal is only heard with the extremity elevated and represents a second reversal of flow when the end-diastolic pressure is overcome by the hydrostatic pressure of gravity and when the heart rate is lesser than 60 beats per minute.

The analog tracings in bidirectional systems accurately scribe the direction of flow at various phases of the cardiac or pulse cycle. Forward flow is graphed above the baseline and reverse or negative flow below the baseline. Since each successive signal is quieter as a result of redirection of flow, the waves are scribed sequentially with lesser amplitudes. Disappearance of component signals is always from the last or quietest to the first.

The hemodynamics of flow are altered at the site of stenosis. The loss of vessel wall recoil in atherosclerosis results in monophasic signals with a knocking character as the blood strikes the projecting plaque. The signal from the narrowed lumen at midplaque level is high in pitch because of the jettisoning of blood flow, while the amplitude is proportionally decreased as a result of lesser volume of flow. The signal at this level also remains monophasic. The poststenotic region is characterized by roughness of signal as a result of turbulence of eddy currents as the vessel diameter increases. By stethoscopic auscultation, this lesion site would generate a bruit, and a thrill would be palpable. If the lesion is of significant length and occlusive depth, the signal also remains monophasic. Should a collateral vessel of adequate luminal diameter provide a sufficient volume of blood poststenotically, the biphasicity of signal may return at more distal levels.

More peripheral arteriosclerosis without plaque formation also presents with alteration of flow hemodynamics. As the vessel hardens as a result of intimal and some medial coat sclerosis, the recoil of elasticity is lost, and the second and subsequent phases of the signal disappear.

Venous Examination

Until the refinement of the Doppler instrument, the venous system was evaluable indirectly by the tourniquet tests previously described or by invasive venography. The latter technique oftentimes initiated thrombophlebitis as a result of injury of the venous wall by venipuncture and the injection of the dye into a vessel with a slow rate of flow, causing chemical damage to the walls near the site of injection. Allergic reactions as well as anaphylaxis were periodic complications.

Doppler evaluation of the deep and nonpulsatile veins is now a valuable adjunct to chairside assessment of these structures. Its limitations are the evaluation of the vein only at the site insonated and the operator's knowledge of the venous anatomy.

Since the venous flow is slower and the veins are more superficial than the arteries, a probe of 2 to 4 MHz is preferable. The veins are evaluated for patency, spontaneity, augmentability, and rhythmicity of flow, as well as for valvular competency. The deep veins that are usually studied include the femoral, popliteal, and posterior tibial. Although the superficial veins usually are evaluable by inspection, the short and great saphenous may also be insonated.

With the patient in a phlebostatic supine position, the probe is placed over any of the vein sites. If spontaneity of flow is not prominent, the examiner may experience difficulty in locating the vein. Isolation of the vein may be accomplished by locating the artery, which pulsates, and moving the probe to the adjacent vein. In patients with associated arterial compromise where the arterial pulsations are not evident, the examiner must mildly compress the distal tissue to augment venous outflow past the probe site. Excessive compression necessitates a 10- to 20-second pause before the next compressive maneuver to allow the vein a normal refilling.

Once the vein is located, the casual "blowing wind" sound of passive venous flow is evaluated. This is more prominent in the proximal veins but may also be heard in the distal posterior tibial vein. If spontaneity is identified, the signal is monitored for 5 to 10 seconds and identified as to rhythmicity. (For example, the flow may be apparent during pulmonary expiration and ceases momentarily during inspiration). This is as a result of diaphragmatic descent during inspiration, which increases intra-abdominal pressure and precludes venous emptying from the extremity to the inferior area cava.

With the probe in continued position, the distal tissue is fully compressed and augmentability of flow is identified as a sudden increase in signal amplitude. On release of manual pressure, normally no signal is audible because valvular coaptation precludes reflux. In cases of valvular incompetency resulting from scarring, tearing, or separation with widening of the vessel as in a varicosity, the leaflets do not close and allow regurgitation past the probe to the distal vein. The anatomic segment proximal to the probe is then compressed. Normally no signal is audible because of valvular closure; incompetency of the valve leaflets allows reversal of flow and an audible flow signal. Having emptied the venous segment above the probe with full compression, the vein has no volume to exert any pressure while the distal, momentarily engorged venous site has significant pressure that must be relieved. On proximal decompression, this volume and pressure is released to the previously emptied level, and a rush of venous outflow past the probe is heard. With valvular incompetency the valves do not engage, allowing reversal of flow past the probe on proximal compression as well as forward flow on decompression. In summary, there exists to-and-fro flow with valvular insufficiency, and flow signals are heard with manual compression and decompression at levels distal and proximal to the probe sites.

Plethysmographic Evaluation

Plethysmography is the scribed recording generated by a device capable of detecting changes in volume of an anatomic segment that are usually due to blood flow. Various instruments have been developed to measure such volumetric changes. Electrical conductivity and its resistance have been employed in strain gauge and impedance plethysmographs, whereas infrared or incandescent light passed into tissue and reflected back is measured by a photocell. The pneumatic plethysmograph measures the amount of fluid, air or liquid, that is displaced in a container when the volume changes occur with blood flow variations. For ease of clinical application, current pneumatic systems employ an air-containing cuff that envelopes a limb segment.

Arterial Examination

Segmental Plethysmography. In examination of the peripheral pulses, the examiner applies varying pressures at different arterial sites. Excessive or inadequate pressure yields lesser pulse amplitudes than does intermediate pressure. Maximal pulse excursions are palpable at the vessel's mean pressure, which is midway between systolic and diastolic pressures. The palpating digital pressure is readily adjusted by the examiner until the maximal excursion is realized. In evaluating the peripheral pulse by oscillometry, the mean pulse pressure is unknown, forcing the examiner to seek the maximal deflection by initiating the study at a high pressure and decreasing the cuff pressure in 10-mm Hg decrements until the maximal deflection is attained. Continued lowering of the cuff pressure decreases the oscillations until no readings are evident at the lowest pressures. This is akin to no palpable pulse excursion with just the laying of fingers over a pulse site.

Segmental pneumatic plethysmography is in actuality recording oscillometry. Instead of reading the oscillometric excursions of the needle, the stylus scribes the same deflective pattern as a graph recording. The morphology of the scribed plethysmographic waves is consistent with the pulse contour, which may be palpated and differentiated only by a very experienced clinician.

The normal arterial pulse wave is scribed at the universal chart speed of 25 mm/sec. Its morphology consists of an upswing from the baseline, termed the *anacrotic limb,* and a downswing from the peak, termed the *catacrotic limb.* Along the length of the catacrotic limb is a depression known as the *dicrotic notch.* The crest of the wave is normally attained within the first one-third or 35 percent of the wave length, and its peak is sharp. The anacrotic limb is a reflection of the expanding vessel as it accepts the pulsatile volume in time with left ventricular systole. The dicrotic notch is reflective of the arterial wall recoil due to normal rebound of the elastic fibers and occurs at early left ventricular diastole. This notch in vessels most proximal to the heart is indicative of aortic valvular function.

The sclerotic vessel resists dilation with prolonged crest times (approaching 50 to 75 percent in advanced cases of atherosclerosis), various degrees of rounding of peaks, absence of dicrotic notching consistent with marked decrease or absence of recoil, and decrease of amplitudes consistent with lessened wall excursions.

Digital Plethysmography. Evaluation of the digital arterial pulsations, and hence perfusion of the cutaneous circuit that comprises the highest percentage of vascularized tissue, is based on the same principle as segmental plethysmography. The digital arteries, possessing vasomotion characteristics identical to those of more proximal vessels, demonstrate the same scribed morphologic features.

The pneumatic plethysmograph may employ small digital cuffs or a rigid plastic cup that is sealed at its base to preclude an air leak and that has a port with tubing conveying the displaced air to a sensor in the body of the instrument. The cupped format of this device has the advantage of ensuring analysis of a consistent volume of digital tissue as well as volume standardization.

The photocell plethysmograph utilizes a light source with an incandescent bulb or an infrared diode and an appropriate light spectrum – matched photocell sensor. The light passed through the tissue is reflected back with different intensity depending on the volume of red cells carried into the glomus of a digit with each pulsation. Its advantages are feasibility of application to all digits and detection of minor volume changes.

These forms of plethysmography have the advantage of defining the pulsations at the most acral limits of the arterial tree where the end arteries have a predilection for vasospasticity and small vessel disease.

Venous Examination

The deep venous system transfers approximately 85 percent of the venous blood from the lower extremities back to the heart. Its flow is dependent on some residual pressure from the arterial side but mostly from muscular contractions. Since the rate of flow is slow and passive, on insult a cascading set of events leads to thrombosis. This results in damming of venous blood that is identified by associated signs and symptoms. Evaluation of this entity is nonspecific by Homan's sign or venous Doppler probe and necessitates the sensitivity of venous plethysmography.

This instrument may be of the strain gauge, pneumatic, impedance, or direct current–coupled photocell design. Each type is capable of detecting the slow change in limb volume associated with retarded outflow. The studies determine the capacitance and maximum venous outflow when the veins are temporarily cuff-occluded at the thigh level.[2,3]

A sensing device is placed at the calf level whose character depends on the design — expansive metallic tube (strain gauage), two separate metallic ribbons (impedance), photocell, or air bladder (pneumatic). In the normal extremity, venous occlusion of the venous system is accomplished by inflating the thigh cuff to 70 mm Hg. This is below arterial pressure, thereby allowing inflow past the cuff but ceasing venous outflow. The resultant tourniquet effect causes a slow but measurable distention of the peripheral veins until their natural capacitance is reached. The venous plethysmograph records this change in leg volume with a slow staircase rise of the stylus until a plateau is reached. On rapid full deflation of the thigh cuff the engorged veins, with a high-pressure gradient, evacuate the surplus of blood, termed the *maximal venous outflow*, within 3 seconds.

In deep thrombophlebitis the distal veins are already partially engorged, so that the thigh tourniquet succeeds in only trapping some additional venous blood; therefore, the measurable venous

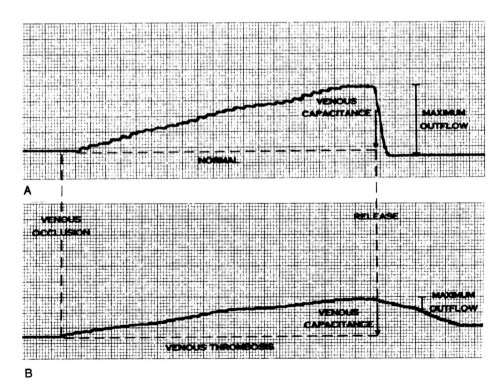

Fig. 17-3. Top. Normal venous patency demonstrates considerable capacitance, with maximal outflow occurring within 3 seconds. **Bottom.** Venous thrombosis of the deep veins exhibits decreased additional capacitance and lesser and retarded maximal outflow.

capacitance is less than normal. On deflation of the thigh cuff, the fully engorged deep veins are relieved of the increased pressure gradient although at a slower rate because of the obstructing thrombus; hence, the maximum venous outflow is longer than 3 seconds (Fig. 17-3).

Doppler Ultrasonic Imaging

The basic application of Doppler ultrasound in auscultating the velocity and other characteristics of flow has been extended to the imaging of vessels and other structures. This procedure allows the visualization of vessel morphology without the time, discomfort, and expense associated with contrast studies.

The Doppler's transducing handpiece may be held parallel and over the vessel's long axis and display a longitudinal view, or perpendicular to the vessel axis and presenting a transverse image of the lumen and wall. Where anatomically feasible, a vessel may be longitudinally imaged in the frontal or sagittal plane, thereby ensuring visualization of all wall surfaces for luminal defects. Any motion or activity of thrombi during systole and diastole is also identifiable.

Since the Doppler is sensitive to movement, the column of blood in its laminar and vessel-expansive flow is projected as a darkened area. The vessel wall, and any atheromatous plaque formation, which is nonmobile, reflect the signal at the same frequency as emitted and are visualized as whitened structures. Thus the morphologic presentation of the vessel wall as well as the plaque, including the relative density, are assessed. The degree of whiteness is directly proportional to the varying densities of the plaque or wall as defined by presence or absence of attendant calcification or fibrin-entrapped blood cell elements. Softer cholesterol plaques that are free-standing or mixed with hardened plaques thus may be differentiated.[4]

Doppler Spectral Analysis

Insonation of a vessel yields a reflected signal that has a character consistent with the hemodynamics of flow. This is a near constant for each named vessel. As the normal laminar flow is disturbed, the altered flow yields reflected signals that may be harsh or roughened and of altered pitch. The trained examiner can usually detect the obvious character changes of the Doppler-reflected signals but can only scribe their analog form.

By Doppler spectral analysis, the audible signal is presented in visual form with a segregation of the various pitches that constitute it. The reflected signal frequency is displayed along the x axis and wavelength consistent with time is visualized on the y axis. The number of signals for each pulse is also reflected in the general outline of the spectral plot.

The normal arterial signal is characterized by a crisp multiphasic sound of near-common frequency pitch as a result of a constant rate of flow along the entire width of the vessel's lumen. Such a signal's spectral analysis displays a concentration of pitches in a small frequency range with an overall multiphasic wave outline (Fig. 17-4A). The stenotic arterial signal is heard as a high-pitched sound that is monophasic. This signal is reflected by spectral analysis as a concentration of higher pitched sounds on the x axis that may be monophasic in spectral outline. The signal from a poststenotic area having characteristic eddy currents is audible as a roughened monophasic sound. Its spectral analysis is identified to be of broadened frequency as a result of the combination of varying velocities along the width of the vessel site, and of a singular monophasic outline.[5]

Duplex Imaging

Although Doppler ultrasound angiography and spectral analysis contribute significantly to the noninvasive evaluation of the peripheral vasculature by visualization of the morphology and the reflected signal, the examiner is forced to combine the results in establishing the diagnosis. These sequential studies force the examiner to address exactly the same location in categorizing the flow deficit.

The combination of ultrasound imaging and spectral analysis is known as a duplex system. Its obvious advantage is the simultaneous assessment

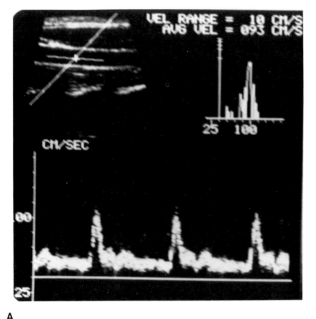
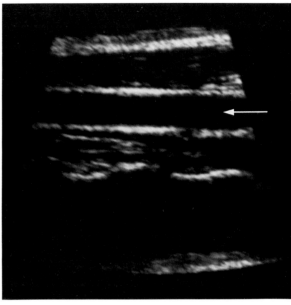

A   B

Fig. 17-4. (A) Doppler spectral analysis of an arterial signal demonstrating normal hemodynamic flow characteristics. The frequencies are not broadened and a biphasic contour is recognized. This, coupled with real-time imaging, constitutes a duplex study. **(B)** Real-time B-mode ultrasound image of a patent artery demonstrated by a blackened area of high-velocity flow and high-frequency signals. The lighter adjacent structures demonstrate visible detection of low-frequency reflected signals.

of a particular vessel segment by both techniques. Since the Doppler ultrasound component is of a pulsed format, its depth of focus can be electronically controlled. The examiner, therefore, has the ability to evaluate the hemodynamics of flow at any observed point in the lumen. The varying flow characteristics can be assessed at the pre-, intra-, and poststenotic areas in the immediate proximity of the plaque, as well as those on the other side of the wall free of plaque formation. In summary, the anatomic morphology (Fig. 17-4B) as well as the laminar flow or its alteration in any vessel can be studied at the near and far wall or any point in between, as well as other points of interest, including bifurcation levels, collateral vessels, aneurysms, or fistulas.[6]

This form of instrumentation has significant computer capability, allowing for postprocessing of raw data. Therefore, the velocity of flow at any point 1.50 mm or larger can be determined as well as degree of stenosis by area or diameter. Newer

models have even added color to designate the directionality and velocity of flow.

Magnetic Resonance Imaging

Following the development of sound to evaluate the peripheral circulation, magnetic energy was introduced, which has the potential to produce an image of good resolution. Since all nuclei have a native resonating frequency proportional to the local magnetic field, an imposed magnetic gradient changes that frequency and is detected by a spectrometer. Proton migrations are identified after repetitive applications of pulsed magnetic fields, yielding an image of stationary tissue. Because of the motion of blood, only the internal structures of vessels, including thrombi, are delineated. Since the sensor may be positioned in any direction, triplane studies of vascular structures are possible. Also, since ischemic tissue reacts differently than normal viable tissue, evaluation of the effects of embolic crises is feasible.[7]

INVASIVE VASCULAR EXAMINATION

The traditional evaluation of the peripheral vasculature has been by radiography with injection of an opaque dye. The resultant arteriogram, venogram, or lymphangiogram remains the gold standard by which all less invasive or noninvasive techniques are judged as to sensitivity and specificity. Other less invasive procedures have developed with advancement of computer science, including scanning for radioactive deposits and digital subtraction angiography.

Arteriography

Identification of the anatomic distribution of the peripheral arteries or any associated morphologic changes requires an opaque dye that is carried by the blood to all distal tributaries. The dye is conventionally injected directly into the aorta at or below the renal arteries, and the resulting image is termed an *aortogram*. In the retrograde aortographic technique, a catheter is fed through the common femoral artery up to the aorta above the bifurcation level, and the dye is injected. The usual volume of injected dye is 350 to 500 ml, and it is administered as a bolus. Given the chemical nature of the dye, it causes pain locally on injection as well as distally during its distribution through all peripheral arteries.

Since the dye is mobilized and diluted downstream by the blood, a series of radiographic flat plates are prepositioned in the examination table. The first flat plate is exposed at the aortic level, followed by serial plates in a distal sequence with slight overlap. The arteriogram thus demonstrates the anatomic distribution of all patent arteries with some retrograde filling of arteries distal to occluding thrombi from anastomotic vessels. The dilation of collateral vessels is also clearly identified. Areas along the distribution of an artery that are occluded are not evident because of lack of dye flow through the segment. Recently developed aneurysms are visualized as an expected dilated defect, whereas older aneurysms may be missed because of filling of the expanded defect by thrombus, leaving a usable lumen the size of the vessel before the aneurysm. Near and far wall thrombi may also be missed since the dye appears to fill the entire width of a vessel. Ulcerating thrombi demonstrate dye penetration into the defect, as do intimal tears. Some smaller anastomotic vessels may not be visualized because of lack of diversion of the dye-carrying blood during the time of study, while the most acral vessels may carry blood with excessively diluted dye for imaging.

This technique is considered anatomic and serves the surgeon as a map for incisional approach. It also may provide the vascular surgeon a basis for choice of surgical procedure, including incisional thrombectomy, enarterectomy, synthetic or autogenous saphenous bypass graft, in situ saphenous bypass, or such less invasive procedures as laser thrombectomy, percutaneous angioplasty, or enzymatic thrombolysis.

Digital Subtraction Angiography

With the advancement of computer science, traditional arteriography has been modified. This lesser invasive procedure requires about 1/10th the original dose of the dye and reduces the risk of allergic reactions and chemogenic thrombosis.

In this procedure, baseline radiographs are taken and the information stored in a computer. With no patient movement, 50 ml of dye is injected into an artery as previously described. As the dye is carried via the bloodstream into more distal vessels, serial radiographic views are again taken. The additional information on these secondary plates is the result of appearance of the arteries as they fill with the injected dye. This information is again entered into the computer. The computer then digitally subtracts the baseline information, including osseous and soft tissue structures, leaving an image of only the injected arteries. Since the dose of the dye was low, the resultant image is of decreased contrast.

By computer enhancement, the vessel images are improved to be readily identified. Since the image may be reversed, the final arteriogram may be presented in a negative or positive format.

Venography

As in conventional arteriography, identification of the anatomic configuration of the deep, communicating, perforating, and even superficial veins is accomplished by injection of a dye suspension. Besides the anatomic placement of veins, dilations of deep varices and thrombi may be visualized as well as valvular structures.

Venography is primarily employed for the identification of deep thrombophlebitis; however, the procedure itself is known to cause this very condition. This is because of injury of the endothelium with needle penetration and the high concentration of the dye, which is particularly caustic to the endothelium since it lingers longer in the injected vein as a result of slower and passive venous flow.

The technique involves injection of the radiopaque dye into an identifiable superficial vein, usually at the pedal dorsal venous arcade. Since the superficial veins anastomose with each other by communicating veins and penetrate via the perforators into the deep system, all four types of veins are visualized. Because the superficial dorsal arcade veins are small, the injection technique is slower than in arteriography and lasts for a longer period of time. If care is not exercised, extravasation of the dye to adjacent structures results in spreading of the dye along a plane beneath the skin. This leads to tissue reaction to the concentrated dye and eventual sloughage of the skin (Fig. 17-5).

Lymphangiography

Because of the colorless plasma that the lymphatic channels convey, these structures were the last component of the circulatory system to be discovered. The lymphatic flow is also pulseless and moves at the same rate as that of the veins, with valves to prevent regurgitation. Furthermore, the lymphatic channels accompany the deep and superficial veins and respectively drain the intermuscular fluids and the interstitial cutaneous fluids.

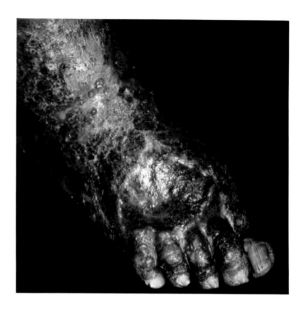

Fig. 17-5. Sloughage of the dorsum of the foot and proximal skin of all the toes secondary to extravasation from a dorsal vein of opaque dye used for venography to rule out deep thrombosis.

Evaluation of these channels is necessary to identify ectasia, insufficient development, or blockage due to compression, inflammation, infection, adjacent expansile lesions, fracture impingement, or iatrogenic surgical damage.

Since these channels are not evident on clinical examination, no vessels may be directly approached. Methylene blue dye, therefore, is slowly injected subcutaneously or intradermally at the distal pedal level of the toe web. This extravascular injected dye is conveyed to the open-ended lymphatic capillaries and carried to small channels that receive the same dye from other tributaries. This confluency of small lymphatics concentrates the dye into larger vessels until a discrete channel is identified bearing a blue color. The lymph channel is then injected with 10 to 12 ml of a non-water-soluble radiopaque dye at a slow gravity-feed rate because of its small caliber and venous-equivalent rate of flow.

Immediately after injection, a flat plate radiograph is taken that demonstrates the lymphatic channels. A repeat radiograph may be taken in 24 hours to visualize the popliteal and inguinal nodes, which retain the dye for longer periods of time.

Radionuclide Venography

In recent years isotopes have been used increasingly in the study of venous disease. These have been considered less invasive and have developed into routine clinical tests. Two well-established scintiscanning techniques employ the injection of radiopharmaceutical materials containing iodine-125 or technetium-99m.

The ^{125}I fibrinogen test is based on the observation that when injected, it is incorporated into the developing thrombus and is detected by an external scintillation meter. Since multiple passes are required before a measurable amount of this preparation has adhered to the thrombus, the diagnosis cannot be established until 24 to 48 hours after injection. This serves as a major drawback since therapy can be withheld pending results of study.[8]

The ^{99m}Tc plasmin test incorporates porcine plasmin (a mixture of plasminogen and streptokinase) labeled with technetium. This preparation remains stable for at least 29 hours and rapidly accumulates in thrombi. After a dorsal intravenous administration, the radioactivity is measured at 5- and 30-minute intervals along several thigh and calf levels. Each point's radioactivity is measured for 10 minutes. Counts vary between 2,000 and 5,000 at each leg point. By calculation of point and time difference in values, the diagnosis is established.[9]

These studies with iodinated and technetium isotope contrast agents can diagnose deep thrombophlebitis with very reliable sensitivity; however, the specificity, with false positives, remains a concern to clinicians.

ANOMALIES OF BLOOD SUPPLY TO THE LOWER LIMB

The development of the many branches and anastomoses of the blood vessels leads to a standard anatomic pattern that is surprisingly common. However, certain aberrations from the classic pattern are not unanticipated. Duplication of arteries can be of benefit in cases of trauma or disease, whereas congenital absence is not. Sometimes vessels branch and pass too close to osseous or musculotendinous structures and are impinged upon during extreme ranges of motion.

The arteries of the lower limbs derive from the fifth lumbar artery, with the original branches being the sciatic, saphenous, and external iliac. As the typical named arteries develop, these precursor vessels regress, although in rare instances they can persist.[10]

Popliteal Artery Entrapment Syndrome

This syndrome was first described by a medical student at the University of Edinburgh and has since been identified by others to be unusual but not rare. Instead of the popliteal artery passing from the hiatus of the adductor magnus to the center of the popliteal space between the head of the gastrocnemius muscle, it courses almost vertically downward. In so doing it is compressed frequently by the medial head of the gastrocnemius muscle and sometimes by the plantaris and semimembranosus.

Four variants of entrapment are classically recognized. Type 1 has the artery looping medially and under the normally placed medial head of the gastrocnemius. Type 2 shows less looping as the artery follows the same course but the medial gastrocnemius head originates more laterally. Type 3 demonstrates a varying-width accessory head of the medial head of the gastrocnemius that arises from the femur more laterally, with the artery impinged beneath the accessory head. Type 4 characterizes the artery as entrapped while passing beneath the popliteus muscle. In some instances, the accompanying popliteal vein is also entrapped, and the anomaly can occur bilaterally.

Entrapment of this artery, if sufficiently constrictive, can lead to fibrosis and thrombosis that may be partially or totally occlusive. Poststenotic dilation can occur that may lead to an aneurysmal defect as a result of frequent flexure at the knee joint. Any thrombosis that develops may embolize as a result of repetitive compression of the stenotic lesion and lead to peripheral ischemic symptoms.

Diagnosis of popliteal artery entrapment may

present a challenge. Although claudication is the presenting concern, it may not always be typically described. The type of entrapment and the degree of stenosis may allow the patient to be symptom free when jogging or running because the knee joint is not fully extended to compress the artery, whereas walking will incite claudication with knee extension and foot dorsiflexion. Any palpable bounding of the popliteal pulse indicates an aneurysmal formation of the popliteal artery, which may be de novo or as a complication of the entrapment syndrome. Loss or decrease of the popliteal or other peripheral pulses with the knee fully extended is diagnostic of this syndrome. Relief of leg or pedal ischemic rest pain with the knee flexed is also corroborative information.

Stethoscopic auscultation may yield an audible bruit, and Doppler insonation demonstrates a high-pitched jettisoned flow in knee extension, or monophasicity and roughness of character with the knee extended when the lumen is compromised by a thrombosis.

Operative release of the artery is indicated when symptomatic regardless of the presence or absence of an occlusion. Simultaneous contralateral musculotendinous sectioning is recommended prophylactically to preclude eventual occlusion. If a thrombosis is also present, it must be resected.

Absence of Dorsalis Pedis Artery

The dorsalis pedis artery classically lies lateral to the extensor hallucis longus tendon; however, it may course more laterally and be located over the second, third, or fourth metatarsal bases. In approximately 10 percent of the population, the dorsalis pedis artery is absent or so small as not to be palpable. This is of no clinical concern since the perforating peroneal artery is usually noted to be the alternate source of blood supply to the dorsum of the foot. If the posterior tibial artery is absent, the peroneal forms the plantar arteries. In essence, the peroneal artery may be viewed as the main source of blood supply to the lower leg and foot because it is the most consistently encountered artery. The perforating peroneal is located further laterally than the dorsalis pedis and may be found

to be just as full in its pulse amplitude. It should be sought in the absence of the dorsalis pedis artery.

Variations of the First Dorsal Metatarsal Artery

Three types of branchings have been identified for the first dorsal metatarsal artery. This vessel may take origin dorsally from the terminal portion of the dorsalis pedis artery, from the midportion of the deep branch in the first intermetatarsal space, or from a more plantar portion of the same deep branch. Irrespective of its origin, the first metatarsal blood supply is satisfied by its anastomosis with the first plantar metatarsal artery. Of clinical significance is its variations in origin, which are close to the surgical site for Akin bunionectomies, fibular sesamoidectomies, and adductor releases. Its integrity ideally should be preserved.[11]

Variations of the Plantar Arch

The plantar arch is formed typically by the lateral plantar artery and the deep plantar branch of the distal dorsalis pedis artery. Sometimes the plantar arteries are primarily derived as extensions of the deep plantar artery from the dorsalis pedis, and they may be the source of blood to the second through fifth metatarsal areas as well as the respective digits. The rarest formation has all the metatarsal arteries solely derived from the deep plantar branch without any contribution from the lateral plantar artery.

Common Vessel Wall Shared by Inferior Vena Cava and Abdominal Aorta

All arteries and veins have walls that are distinct to the respective vessels. On occasion, however, during the development of the vessels in the pelvic area, a common wall is shared by the distal abdominal aorta and the posterior portion of the proximal common iliac arteries with the inferior vena cava and its communicating common iliac veins.

The inferior vena cava lies in the midline of the abdominal cavity, whereas the abdominal aorta is to the left of midline. Both vessels have two common iliac branches, and therefore the left common iliac vein is crossed over by the right common iliac artery. Since the arterial wall expands during systole and since it carries blood under a high head of pressure, the venous lumen on the other side of the shared wall is subject to pulsatile compression. Over many years, the constancy of repetitive compression and small reflux in the left common iliac vein causes a distention of that vessel that results in relative venous hypertension. As a result, varicosities develop preferentially in the left lower extremity in most cases.

No treatment is rendered unless the venous hypertension is significant in its etiology of extensive varices. The vessels may be separated and a patch graft positioned over the defect, or a synthetic bifurcating graft may be implanted.

Arteriovenous Fistulas

Abnormal connections between arteries and veins may exist as variations in development. These are most common in the pulmonary circulation but are without any hemodynamic significance. When present in the lower extremity, the A-V fistulas short-circuit blood prematurely to the venous side, placing a burden on the right side of the heart and predisposing to heart failure. Any significant size of this malformation causes retardation of venous outflow from veins distal to the fistula, resulting in venous distention and varicose formation. Should local tortuosity become significant, the apparent aneurysm is termed a *cirsoid aneurysm*. This lesion has significant alteration of hemodynamics and may be readily auscultated as a bruit or palpated as a thrill. Its treatment is surgical dissection and separation.

Although not of congenital origin, the glomus tumor of a digit is an abnormal connection of multiple arterioles and venioles in a nail bed as a result of blunt trauma. Pulsations at this abnormal formation between nonyielding phalanx and toenail are extremely painful and throbbing in nature. Surgical extirpation is the only treatment.

VASOSPASTIC DISORDERS AFFECTING THE FOOT

The tonicity of the peripheral vasculature is controlled by endocrine and chemical substrates as well as by the autonomic nervous system. Intermittent periods of constriction or dilation are necessary to limit the volume of blood flow to the periphery, thus maintaining sufficient supply for other anatomic beds or to preserve life itself by moderating the body's heat balance.

The hypothalamus, as the heat regulator of the body, controls the distribution of blood via hormones and neural influence. Humoral substances (mainly polypeptides), secreted by the hypothalamic neurons, are conveyed by veins to the anterior pituitary, thus exciting adrenocorticotropic and thryrotropic hormonal secretion. In general, the anterior hypothalamus is concerned with parasympathetic activity and control of the pituitary gland. The posterior hypothalamus secretes vasopressin and influences sympathetic activity.

The chemical control by the pituitary gland is indirect since it releases thyroid-stimulating hormone to activate the thyroid. In turn, the released thyroid hormone increases the oxidative processes, transformation of glycogen to glucose, and the onset of shivering. Thyroid hormone also augments the β-adrenergic agonists of the adrenal medulla, whose function is controlled by the sympathetic nervous system. Therefore, adrenalin and thyroid hormone function synergistically in producing effects such as caridioacceleration, perspiration, tremulousness, and anxiety.

The sympathetic component of the autonomic nervous system has significant control over the peripheral vessels, the sweat glands, and the erector muscles of the hairs, whose effect is most pronounced when the body is suddenly chilled and "goose bumps" appear. Preganglionic medullated sympathetic fibers originate in the most lateral midportion of the spinal gray matter of spinal segments between the first thoracic and the second lumbar levels. These fibers pass laterally to the sympathetic chain to meet corresponding ganglia.

From these ganglia nonmedullated postganglionic fibers join the corresponding somatic nerve and are distributed to the blood vessels and skin of the appropriate dermatome. The fibers in the chain also extend downward to the fifth lumbar ganglionic level.

The somatic nerve that carries the sympathetic fibers to the foot is predominantly the posterior tibial nerve. The sympathetic fibers continue to divide and are most numerous in the acral part of the foot, particularly the toes. It is at this level that excessive sympathetic activity is most commonly seen.

Normal activity of the efferent sympathetics may be simply a reflex arc working in concert with the afferent sensory fibers, such as when the skin is scratched. The well-known triple response of Lewis is noted, with immediate blanching as a result of capillary injury followed by a flare of vasodilation from the axon reflex. The final wheal is not neurogenically related since it is caused by local histamine release. If the sensory fibers are damaged, the flare response does not occur, nor would dilation following cooling of a digit.

The sympathetics also assist in controlling the volume of blood that enters the lower extremities after rising from a sitting or recumbent position. By doing so, excessive blood entering the lower extremities with the greater hydrostatic pressure is prevented, thereby maintaining a sufficient volume to perfuse the cerebral tissue. Central sympathetic denervation allows excessive blood to enter the lower limbs, resulting in lowered pressure and postural hypotension with resultant vertigo.[12] Reflex vasomotor paralysis may also be confirmed by verifying the integrity of vagal activity. When challenged by holding the breath, reflex slowing of the heart and decreased cutaneous arterial pulsations are abolished.[13]

Raynaud's Syndrome and Disease

Raynaud described a phenomenon that is characterized by paroxysmal bilateral digital ischemia. The condition is attributed to excessive sympathetic activity. *Raynaud's syndrome* is the repetitive occurrence of the phenomenon induced by cold or emotional stimuli that is relieved by heat and is secondary to an underlying cause. *Raynaud's disease* is diagnosed 2 years after no etiology has been determined.

The syndrome is usually identified between the ages of puberty and 40 years, predominantly in women. It may be associated with occlusive arterial disease, either primary or secondary to nerve compression, such as in thoracic outlet or tarsal tunnel syndrome. Its underlying cause may also include collagen disease, blood dyscrasia, repetitive microtrauma, or exposure to chemicals any of which may be irritative to the sympathetic nerves, alter the arterioles, or generally cause sludging or rouleau formation.

The phenomenon is characterized by a trilogy of color changes progressing from white to blue to red. The initial stage of pallor is associated with constriction of the metarterioles and arterioles near the skin surface with reduced blood perfusion. The secondary cyanotic stage is associated with an extension of the spasticity to involve the venules in the subpapillary venous plexus, which retains what little arterial blood enters the cutaneous circuit and significantly reduces the oxygen tension of the sludged erythrocytes. The final stage of rubor is associated with a postocclusive reactive hyperemia that occurs to repay the metabolic debt caused by the occlusion while reestablishing the normal cellular oxygen and nutrient economy. At this stage the humoral influence of the local lactic acidotic millieu overcomes the sympathetic influence and the constricted smooth circular muscles, including all precapillary sphincters, relax to a dilated state.

Patients with this phenomenon have lesser native digital blood flow that is fully arrested during the crisis. Since the smooth circular muscles run a somewhat spiral course, constriction is predominantly in the transverse axis, although some longitudial shortening occurs as well. In the pure form of spasticity without intimal thickening, constriction leaves a patent lumen allowing for continued flow. With time, hypertrophy of the arteriole intima and muscular media occurs. This further retards the flow of blood, eventuating in rouleau formation, arteriole thrombosis, and digital gangrene since mild constriction markedly reduces the lumen as a result of increased wall thickness. If the end stage is not reached, the condition is characterized by greater frequency of attacks, particularly in the cold months. Chronic episodes have a cumulative effect of trophic changes with shiny, taut skin and tapering fingers resembling sclerodactylic digits. When the underlying cause is rheumatoid arthritis or scleroderma, severe digital deformities are a common complication. The cyanosis may be pronounced for longer periods of time over the years until a near-permanent discoloration is noted.

The phenomenon is identified clinically by the change in colors, which is bilaterally symmetric while involving the same digits to the same interphalangeal or metatarsal-phalangeal level. The crisis occurs when the digits are exposed to cold air or water and is associated with paresthesias that may advance to a numbing pain. Clinical onset of the phenomenon may be provoked by immersion of the part in cold water. Any emotional crisis aggravated by cold exposure may provoke an attack. During the reactive hyperemic phase, the profound dilation causes throbbing pain and a burning sensation.

Management of the syndrome is directed toward the underlying cause. Symptomatic relief for the syndrome or disease is directed at control of the emotional state, by medication if necessary, or at the vasoconstrictive tendency with vasodilators. Rauwolfia products as well as β-blocking agents have been used.[14] The calcium channel blocker family of compounds inhibit potential-dependent calcium channels, thereby reducing the increased contractile force exhibited in Raynaud's disease. Of paramount importance is the prophylaxis against exposure to cold.[15]

Acrocyanosis

Acrocyanosis is a symmetric, persistent cyanosis of the distal parts of the extremities, including feet and hands as well as the digits. Symptoms are limited to coldness and paresthesias, and there are no complications.

The condition is attributable to excessive sympathetic activity that constantly constricts the distal cutaneous arterioles. Excessive arteriolar tone is noted even at normal temperatures, although the discoloration may be more prominent in the

winter. The hypertonicity results in retarded passage of blood through the cutaneous microcirculation, with pronounced reduction of the hemoglobin yielding the blue discoloration. The cyanosis is manifest to the levels of the ankles and wrists, unlike Raynaud's syndrome, which presents with a trilogy of colors limited to the digits. The condition is more prevalent in women, who naturally have cooler acral segments and a higher core temperature as required for fetal nourishment in pregnancy.

Although trophic changes are rare, edema is sometimes an associated finding. The discoloration does not resolve on elevation of the extremity as in cases of venous congestion. It is also differentiated from cyanosis on dependency in advanced stages of arterial stenosis by normally palpable distal pulses. The cyanosis possibly may resolve on warming or change to a red color in the summer months, indicative of an intermediate level of erythrocyte oxygen saturation. The color does return to normal during sleep. This phenomenon suggests an emotional component to the etiology.

Treatment is usually unnecessary. Maintenance of a positive heat balance with protective covering of the extremities and head area are paramount measures for prophylaxis against the reflex sympathetic vasoconstriction. Vasodilators may be of benefit in the early stages, and sympathectomy may be considered for the chronic condition. Although the discoloration may persist for life, some improvement may be noted in later years.

Livedo Reticularis

Livedo reticularis is another rare vasospastic disorder that presents with red and blue blotchy discoloration of the skin, particularly in the lower extremities. The distribution is lacy and irregular, with central areas of normal skin appearance.

Three variants of the condition are clinically recognized. Cutis marmorata has mottling of skin on exposure to cold that disappears in a warm environment. This form seems to be a persistence of excessive dynamics of the cutaneous microvasculature from infancy, at which stage a cutaneous reticular discoloration is observed while bathing as a result of arteriolar constriction in the skin with loss of heat via evaporation from wetted skin. Livedo reticularis idiopathica also presents the same skin pattern in the extremities, which persists during cold and warm weather. Livedo reticularis symptomatica persists in warm weather and is associated with symptoms of coldness, pruritis, paresthesias, and sometimes pain. Cutaneous ulcerations may also be noted in the winter months.

All forms of livedo reticularis are seen predominantly in women up to the second or third decades of life. No etiology is known, although the symptomatic variant is associated with periarteritis nodosa and other occlusive arterial diseases. There is no racial predilection; however, this abnormality is common in patients with nervous instability.

The mechanisms responsible for the cutaneous discoloration is sympathetic mediated constriction of the arterioles and metarterioles with concurrent atony of the venules. The varying stages of constriction in different local arteriole-capillary beds defines the rate of blood flow and resultant coloration. Moderate rate of flow yields a reddish appearance with intermediate hemoglobin oxygen tension, whereas sluggish flow results in a cyanotic discoloration with marked reduction of the hemoglobin. Central areas of normal color have rapid flow, normal vessel tonicity, and normal 20 to 25 percent reduction of oxyhemoglobin. Therefore, central areas of normal color have normal arteriolar tone in the vessels that surface to the level of the cutaneous rete pegs. The peripheral discolored and mottled areas have hypertonic piercing arterioles and atonic venules in the subpapillary venous plexus. The symptomatic variant associated with organic vessel disease may have intimal and medial layer proliferation.

All forms of the condition have exaggeration of the livid network on exposure to cold. Elevation of the extremity does not resolve the discoloration, whereas warming does. The cutaneous ulcers in the symptomatic form usually resolve in the summer months with no sequelae. A feeling of coldness is usually associated with paresthesias in the discolored segments.

No treatment is usually required in the marmoratic form, and protection from cold exposure and vasodilators will control the more advanced lividic variants. The symptomatic type may require a sympathectomy if seasonal ulcerations are persistent.

In all cases, the use of tobacco in any form should be discouraged.

Unspecific Vasospasticity

Vasospasm of the manual and pedal arteries, particularly those of the digits, has been identified that does not present with the classic pattern of labeled disorders. This functional abnormality is more prevalent in women and anxious individuals.

This generic form of vasospasticity has excessive sympthetic activity and may, therefore, be termed *neurogenic vasospasticity.* As a consequence of the sympathetic overactivity, excessive sweat production is noted and vasoconstriction limits the amount of warm blood surfacing to the skin, leading to coldness by sensation and palpation. The combined effects allow the extremity to the described as cold and clammy.

Unspecified vasospasticity is noted in emotional or anxious individuals, including children, whose social or environmental stimuli must be explored, discussed, and accepted or removed before the signs and symptoms abate. Periods of normal skin perfusion are interrupted during periods of stress, with mentation invoking sympathetic and adrenal crises resulting in increased cardiac rate and pressure as well as reduced skin perfusion and hyperhidrosis. This fight-or-flight reaction diverts blood from the skin, which requires only basal volumes to remain viable, to the liver for glycolysis and energy to effect a decision, to the muscle to enact the decision, and to the brain to make and direct the decision. Therefore, stoic individuals rarely experience this syndrome. This form of vasospasticity may also be the chronic sequel to a remote history of cold injury. Finally, the syndrome may be associated with disuse atrophy of prolonged immobilization and with concurrent edema.

The diagnosis is one of excluding the named vasospastic disorders. Confirmation of this and all other vasospastic disorders is by thermography or thermometry, which registers the decreased skin temperature. Digital plethysmography records reduced pulsations due to hypertonicity of the smooth circular muscles while other morphologic analog wave features remain normal. Evaluation for additional constrictive capacity is accomplished by the vasovagal test, and reversibility for potential treatment is assessed by the postocclusive reactive hyperemia test. Additional dilatory maneuvers include consumption of an alcoholic beverage, interruption of sympathetic innervation by a posterior tibial nerve block, warming of the feet by insulation or a heating blanket, or warming of the abdominal splanchnic vasculature, as in the Landis-Gibbons reflex.

Treatment is directed toward direct relaxation of the arterial wall's smooth muscles with vasodilators taken day or night, or an alcoholic beverage at bedtime for vasodilation of the feet and toes at a time of most concern or observation. The vasodilators, in most instances, need only be taken during the winter months. β-Blocking and calcium channel blocking agents may also be considered. Individuals employed in cold or cool environments, such as butchers or secretaries in cool, air-conditioned offices, may need to take the medication routinely. Abstinence from tobacco is useful, and prophylactic protection from cold and moisture, as in skiing, is a necessity.

Erythromelalgia (Erythermalgia)

Although always discussed under the vasospatic disorders, erythromelalgia is a rare syndrome of paroxismal bilateral dilation of the pedal arteries, and less often the arteries of the hands. It is associated with redness, increased skin temperature, and burning pain akin to postocclusive reactive hyperemia; hence, the term *erythermalgia* encompasses all components of this syndrome.

The condition is classified as primary or idiopathic and secondary. The primary form occurs in otherwise healthy individuals, whereas the secondary form is associated with organic occlusive arterial disease, diabetes, and venous insufficiency. These conditions have a common basis of arteriole, capillary, and venule distention. Dependent rubor in arterial occlusive states is associated with arteriole dilation to preclude passage of blood to the venule side while its rate and volume is rationed from above per unit of time. Diabetes is complicated oftentimes by autonomic neuropathy, with a near-constant state of dilation in the end circulation. Venous insufficiency yields hypertension on the venular end of the microcirculation, with distention, decreased resorption, and progressive edema. Since the venous column is higher in the lower extremities, this condition is more prevalent in the feet than the hands.

In primary erythermalgia, increased heat is the predominant feature that incites pain. As the ambient temperature rises, a critical point is reached that triggers the vasodilative reaction and the symptom complex. It appears that heat is the stimulus rather than hypertension, since cuff occlusion of more proximal vessels does not offer relief when there is vascular standstill. Digital photocell plethysmographic studies have demonstrated that no increase in pulsations occurs when symptoms are present. Venous hypertension also contributes to the distress since venous occlusive tourniquets also incite crises.

Primary erythermalgia is bilateral and may begin during the adolescent years, whereas the secondary form tends to be unilateral and begins in middle age. It has occurred as a hereditary affliction affecting men more often than women. As the temperatures rise past an individual's critical point, the symptom complex becomes manifest. Warm weather and baths trigger a reaction, as does warming of feet by insulation under a blanket; therefore, individuals sleep with the feet uncovered and cooled by fan or air conditioning. Relief of pain during symptomatic episodes is usually attained by immersion of the feet into cold or iced water. Puffiness may be noted in areas of increased perfusion, although trophic changes are not observed unless associated with the attendant occlusive disease. Diagnosis is made by the direct observation of peripheral redness and tissue warming following provocation of an attack by heating or cuff applications. The ruborous appearance must be differentiated from that associated with occlusive disease where the cutaneous temperature is cool.

No complications are known to occur except for the mental distress of the burning pain. Prophylaxis against attacks includes use of well-ventilating footwear, such as sandles, while avoiding heat-retentive shoegear, including rubber soles, patent leather, synthetic materials, and boots, especially in the summer months. Treatment includes elevation of the bared lower extremities to assist venous outflow and to ventilate the skin in the primary form. Aspirin also ameliorates the symptoms, as do vasoconstictor agents.

OCCLUSIVE ARTERIAL DISEASES

The arterial system undergoes an aging process that leads to hardening of the walls and even plaque formation. Hence the vessels' capacity to function as elastic conduits is disturbed, and tissue perfusion is diminished, leading to various degrees of ischemia.

The most common organic disease class is arteriosclerosis. In its general form there is hardening of the vessel wall with some thickening. A specific entity, atherosclerosis, is distinguished for its lipid-rich deposits in thrombi that adhere to the vessel wall and frankly decrease the lumenal area. Collectively, these are the leading causes of arterial disease leading to significant morbidity. Finally, Mönckeberg's medial calcific arteriosclerosis is characterized by calcification of the media of extremity arteries.

Arteriosclerosis

Arteriosclerosis literally means hardening of the arteries. This is a diffuse process that involves all arteries and continues to advance at varying rates throughout life. There is intimal thickening, loss of elasticity, and calcium deposition, all of which contribute to the hardening process. In its terminal stages, after the age of 50, complete stenosis of the lumen occurs and is identified as arteriosclerosis obliterans.

The aging process of arteries is insidious but is known to be accelerated under certain conditions. Cigarette smoking has been demonstrated to contribute to intimal thickening as a result of injury from exposure to higher concentrations of carboxyhemoglobin at the vessel wall where the laminar flow is the slowest, and platelet dysfunction.

There is universal agreement that hypertension contributes significantly to the earlier development of arteriosclerosis, with the black population at greater risk. The intima is subject to greater shear forces, causing injury after prolonged periods. The vasa vasorum may also decrease the perfusion to the medial coat when constantly overcompressed during the significant expansion of the vessel wall while accepting the pulse volume during systole. This chronic repetitive hypoperfusion may lead to a cascading series of events eventuating in arterial wall sclerosis. It has also been well recognized that elevated blood pressure of hypertension is characterized by increased peripheral resistance. Since the contractile state of vascular smooth muscle is a function of intracellular calcium deposits, a decreased number of calcium binding sites in the muscular plasma membrane lead to hyperexitability. This in turn causes excessive contraction with increased resistance and hypertension. In summary, hypertension leads to arteriosclerosis and increased peripheral resistance, and these in turn beget hypertension to propagate the blood through rigid conduits to the peripheral tissue.

Diabetes also leads to accelerated arteriosclerosis, particularly in the tibial and pedal vessels. Calcification is also a concomitant finding. Coagulopathies with impaired platelet function have a thrombotic tendency, leading to diffuse intimal aggregation of blood cells.

The arteriosclerotic process involves all the major vessels of the lower extremities, although symptoms usually arise when the large and muscular vessels are involved. However, these vessels are usually associated with an atheromatous plaque and the diagnosis more correctly in these instances is atherosclerosis. The more distal tibial and pedal arteries rarely show lipid deposits and are more consistently identified as pure arteriosclerosis. The most distal vessels (i.e., the arterioles) are considered separately and termed *arteriolosclerosis*.

Claudication is usually the first symptom that arises with arteriosclerosis, since the major vessels such as the iliacs and femorals as well as the muscular nutrient arteries are involved. Dependent rubor is not noted since collateral flow is attained through available anastomotic or other nutrient arteries. When arteriosclerosis involves the tibial and pedal vessels, dependent rubor is identified since relatively no collateral flow is possible. The ruborous distribution is classic because all surfaces of the toes and forefoot are involved in a stocking distribution. If the intimal proliferative process continues to stenose the vessel, then the state of total or subtotal arteriosclerosis obliterans is reached. However, the diagnosis may be totally missed if the obliterative stage is not reached and the ankle pressures and ischemic indices are falsely or exceedingly high because of concurrent vessel wall calcification.

Treatment is dependent on the stage of the disease and the impairment it produces. Early stages may require no treatment because the process may remain stable for years. As the claudication distance decreases or nocturnal cramping is added to the history, medical management would include encouragement to walk to and beyond the point of pain, to engender collateralization, and elevation of the head of the bed to add hydrostatic pressure for better muscular perfusion. Trental (pentoxifylline) may also be prescribed to encourage better muscular perfusion and decrease the blood viscosity. If the process deteriorates in the tibial segment, grafting may be necessary if a patent runoff system remains available. If only the peroneal or one or both of the tibial vessels remains patent, an in situ saphenous vein bypass graft is the optimal procedure.

Atherosclerosis

A variant of arteriosclerosis is atherosclerosis, which is characterized by sclerosis of the wall associated with plaque formation known as atheroma. The focal plaque is composed of lipid deposits and blood cells that are fibrin bound to the arterial wall. Fibrosis also occurs in the subendothelial connective tissue of the intima. The homogeneous form has lipid deposits, particularly cholesterol and its esters, which are a continuum of the fatty streaks initially observed in adolescence. The heterogeneous plaque has lipids, proteins, carbohydrates, smooth muscle and macrophage-like cells, and blood cells and is usually denser, with predisposition to calcification.

Initially, cholesteryl esters accumulate within foam cells, found in the fatty streaks of juveniles, by enzymatic action on plasma-derived cholesterol. As the lesions become more fibrous and necrotic, large amounts of extracellular cholesteryl esters are found, and there is an increased amount of collagen synthesis. The endothelium receives its nutrients by diffusion from the blood within the lumen. Low-density lipoproteins pass through tight junctions between the endothelial cells by vesicular transport, whereas high-density lipoproteins do not pass this barrier. Focal injuries to the endothelium or enhanced epithelial cell turnover suppress prostacyclin production, an inhibitor of platelet aggregation, resulting in focal endothelial cell desquamation. The platelets then aggregate and release a growth factor that stimulates proliferation of smooth muscle cells. This proliferation also occurs in other endothelial cells when macrophages, which are derived from monocytes and accumulate large amounts of lipids, increase in numbers. Compounded by hyperlipidemia, the atherosclerotic lesion rapidly progresses.[16]

Either form obliterates the ostium to multiple small vaso vasorum, thereby weakening the arterial wall and predisposing it to aneurysmal formation. The lipid-rich plaque of atherosclerosis is usually found in the larger vessels, extending no further than the trifurcation of the popliteal arteries. Because of the projection of the plaque into the lumen, alteration of the laminar flow occurs. In addition, with the flow being slowest and having the least pressure at the periphery near the wall, the tendency for red cell and platelet accumulation is greatest.

Once the initial plaque is organized, the lesion may extend proximally and distally to form a mural thrombus. Platelets, on striking the proximal surface of the thrombus, release adenosine diphosphate (ADP), which binds with fibrinogen to enhance additional platelet adhesion. As the bloodstream passes rapidly through the stenotic segment, its forward velocity propels it to just past the far side of the thrombus, leaving a relative stagnant area of flow. This area is secondarily filled by eddy currents with the suspended and sludged platelets aggregating to the far side of the native plaque (Fig. 17-6). The spiraling of the laminar flow past the extended thrombus enhances a circumferential advancement of the plaque, leading to further occlusion. The sheer forces of blood streaming have also been thrombogenically implicated as a result of erosion of the intima, with plate-

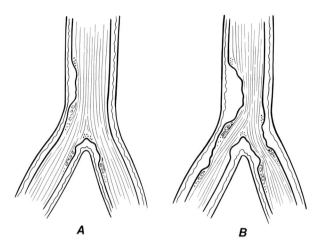

Fig. 17-6. Arterial thrombi formation at bifurcation levels. **(A)** Platelets strike and adhere to the proximal edge of thrombus with compression of laminar flow, and eddy current occurring at distal edge of thrombus. **(B)** Extension of thrombi with platelet aggregation, further compression of laminar flow that jettisons toward inner walls of bifurcating arteries. Outer walls exhibit refill by spiralling eddy currents, adding to stagnation and distal extension of thrombi as a result of platelet agglutination.

lets binding to the exposed collagen. Contributing factors to atherogenesis include cigarette smoking, hypertension, hyperlipidemia, obesity, genetic factors, age, and glucose intolerance.

Increasing plaque volume presents more complicating symptoms. At 50 percent stenosis claudication is identified, and 70 percent stenosis is characterized by rest pain. The decreasing perfusion volume and rate is insufficient to initially meet the muscular nutritional needs on demand, while further rationing of blood fails to meet the basal metabolic needs of other tissue. The overaccumulation of lactic acid and other metabolites as well as carboxyhemoglobin results in lowering the tissue pH, as detected by the sensory fibers, thereby initiating the pain complex.

With advancing stenosis, the blood volume proximal to the plaque is gradually diverted with increasing pressure to other bifurcating vessels or through nutrient muscular arteries. These natural conduits continue to dilate and serve as collateral vessels while shunting the blood to other, more distal patent arteries. If the bypass is short term and through naturally occurring anastomotic arteries, the pulsations may be preserved. However, if the diversion is through muscular nutrient arteries, the resistance to flow is considerable, resulting in dampening of pulsations and only passive flow. This cannot be identified by palpation or by pulse-detecting instrumentation such as oscillometry or segmental plethysmography (pulse volume recording).

Avoidance of risk factors is the best prophylaxis against the accelerated advancement of atherosclerosis. Discontinuance of smoking has been the most publicized risk-reducing measure recommended. Restrictions of low-density lipoproteins in the diet and increased consumption of bran cereals and fish oil have also been advocated to retard atherogenesis.

Treatment of claudicatory symptoms associated with moderate stenosis is directed to decreasing the blood viscosity and increasing the red cell flexibility. The only such hemorrheologic preparation currently available is pentoxifylline, which is taken three times daily following meals. This facilitates the flexion of red blood cells and propagation of pressure-reduced blood to the arterioles and increases perfusion. Since the microcirculation, which has the highest proportion of smooth muscles of all the vessels, remains dilated with reduced pressure and volume associated with atherosclerosis, thereby warranting lesser tonicity, usage of vasodilators is not indicated. These medications can only be expected to facilitate the dilation of collateral vessels.

Vessels with soft subtotal stenosis, identified ideally by real-time ultrasound imaging, may be dilated by the percutaneous transluminal angioplasty technique utilizing a balloon catheter to compress the plaque against the arterial wall, thereby reopening the channel. Totally or subtotally occluded arteries warrant bypass surgery using synthetic materials such as Dacron or Gore-tex or processed umbilical cord veins whose valves have been stripped and that have been treated so as to be immunologically inert. These are implanted from the prestenotic site to a patent poststenotic vessel exhibiting good runoff. It should be noted that the stenosed artery is left in place to allow any residual flow to occur, and that the grafts are always implanted side to side rather than end to end to minimize thrombogenicity.[17]

Another approach to bypass flow for stenotic lesions in the thigh or proximal leg segment is vein grafting. This procedure involves the surgical removal of the long saphenous vein while ligating the proximal and distal ends as well as any large feeder veins, reversing the vein to align the valves facing distally, and reimplantation to the artery. This procedure is physiologically unfavorable since the narrower end of the vein is implanted to the wide artery proximal to the stenosis while the wider end is anastamosed to the smaller patent artery distal to the stenosis. Finally, the in situ saphenous bypass procedure is the ideal option for multilevel stenotic lesions that present with patent arteries and good runoff at the ankle level. This procedure retains the anatomic position of the long saphenous vein along its entire course. The proximal end of the vein is ligated and severed; the vein is then anastomosed to the femoral artery. Distally the same freeing of the vein is accomplished, and the anastomosis is completed to an identified patent tibial or peroneal artery. The valves that face proximally are stripped in arterialization of the vein to allow distal flow. Unfortunately, the sectioned and exposed bases of valves are thrombogenic, with a propencity for future thromboses.[18]

If the medical status precludes extended surgical revascularization or adequate native vessel runoff is not appreciated by arteriography, lumbar sympathectomies have been performed, with ankle ischemic indices above 0.30 demonstrating a limb survival rate of 59 percent 2 years after surgery.

Thromboangiitis Obliterans (Buerger's Disease)

Thromboangiitis obliterans is an inflammatory condition of medium-sized arteries or veins leading to thrombotic occlusion and wound necrosis of the acral segments of the extremities. Medium-sized arteries in the distal third of the upper and lower extremities to the second bifurcation of the digital arteries, and vena communicantes, are subject to this form of stenosis. It is slightly more common in Jewish and Oriental males and is observed initially between the ages of 20 and 45. However, it affects many ethnic groups and no race or color is immune.

No immunologic or toxic basis has been identified clearly, although a history of cigarette smoking has been noted. The arteries and veins are involved segmentally and intermittently, with intervening areas of normal vessel morphology. The inflammatory process incites intimal proliferation leading to thrombosis, causing diversion of flow through developing collaterals. After years of crises, older segments undergo changes consistent with arteriosclerosis obliterans. This leads to distal ischemia associated with rest pain, coldness, and ulceration. Venous crises are associated with focal cutaneous inflammatory lesions about the sites of valves in the superficial veins.

Although life expectancy is not altered, partial amputations are common. Since the process involves the medium-sized vessels without residual native vessels exhibiting good runoff, bypass limb salvage procedures are impossible. The disease is rare in non-smokers. If patients continue to smoke, the disease tends to progress in spite of treatment. Patients who discontinue tobacco use tend to run a favorable course and exacerbations and new occlusions rarely occur. If associated vasospasticity is identified, cessation of smoking or usage of tobacco in any form is necessary. Relief of spastic tendencies may be effected by lumbar sympathectomy.

Arteriolosclerosis

The end circulation encompasses the arterioles and metarterioles. These vessels consist of all the tissue layers noted in larger arteries, with the muscular layer having the highest ratio. Therefore, they are collectively considered pressor vessels since the systolic head of pressure most dramatically decreases at this level. They are innervated by the autonomic nervous system and influenced significantly by metabolites and a humoral mechanism. The smooth muscles are circular, although they progress distally in a spiral distribution. The last smooth circular muscle fibers are considered precapillary sphincters, which dilate or constrict to allow or restrict flow through a capillary dependent upon the state of oxygen saturation of the local erythrocytes and the acidic pH of the serum with accumulated metabolites.

When proximal stenoses exist that decrease the systolic head of pressure to the arteriole level, the additional constriction mediated by the autonomic nervous system is superfluous. Such restriction of flow is compensated for by relaxation of the microvascular tonus by a process known as autosympathectomization. The arterioles and venules then remain dilated with a reduced rate of flow, even in the capillaries, resulting in relative stagnation that allows greater reduction of the oxyhemoglobin and darkening of blood. This microvascular bed in the subpapillary plexus, as observed clinically, results in dependent rubor. If the flow is further retarded and greater reduction occurs, cyanosis is noted. When vascular standstill is reached, the coloration progresses to black, consistent with full reduction and impending tissue necrosis. This color progression is also noted in blood-entrapped lesions such as ecchymoses and hematomas, as well as the blue toe syndrome due to cholesterol microembolization from more proximal atherosclerotic plaques.[19,20]

Arteriolosclerosis is most often associated with chronic hypertension and diabetes. The diabetic complication is further compounded by endothelial subintimal hyaline thickening of the basement membrane in the arterioles and capillaries. The reduction of vessel wall elasticity and luminal diameter begets retardation of flow that eventuates in rouleau formation of the erythrocytes. White blood cells, being of even greater diameter, also become entrapped and further worsen the ischemic process. Surrounding ischemic tissue is thought to release factors that activate these cells, thereby altering their mechanical and adhesive properties and further entrapping more white blood cells with progressive worsening of tissue ischemia. The shift in white cells under ischemic conditions is from lymphocytes to active granulocytes with pseudopodia and cytoplasmic irregularities. Such activation could arise from release of thromboxane or extended trapping under hypoxic conditions, leading to endothelial damage by production of oxygen free radicals and release of lysosomal enzymes.

Since this vascular deficit involves the most distal arteries, more proximal levels may be free of gross disease. The pressure head and pulsations may be normal to the pedal vessels in spite of digital ulcerations. Furthermore, the pedal pulsations may be abnormally high because of lateralization of the forward head of systolic pressure, which cannot be effectively distributed to the constellation of multiple microvascular beds.

Diabetes and hypertension are independent yet additive risk factors for atherosclerotic and arteriolosclerotic diseases. With hyperlipidemia and elevated levels of low-density lipoproteins (LDLs), the potential for lipid deposition is markedly increased. The α-adrenoceptor blockade preparation prazosin has been demonstrated to lower blood pressure without reducing cardiac output, to increase microvascular flow while lowering the peripheral resistance in arterioles and venules in cutaneous and musculocutaneous beds, and to decrease significantly the LDL levels with a downward trend in the ratio of LDLs to high-density lipoproteins. The hemorrheologic preparation pentoxifylline is also indicated to minimize the viscosity and tendency to rouleau formation. If this condition is compounded by more proximal stenotic plaques, those lesions should be surgically resolved to increase the pressure head to the end circulation.[21]

Acral cutaneous ulcerations also require prolonged care and all efforts to control contamination. When associated with infection, antibiosis, if effective at all, is administered for extended periods and at higher therapeutic doses since the amount reaching the lesion is minimized. Management of the pure form of arteriolosclerosis with only distal involvement is directed to avoidance of mechanical or thermal trauma since no additional circulatory reserve remains available for an inflammatory response leading to healing. Undue pressure from ill-fitting shoes or hose must be avoided since the superficial cutaneous vessels have only a marginal intravascular pressure head.

VENOUS DISORDERS OF THE LOWER EXTREMITIES

The venous system in the lower extremities consists of a deep system, a superficial system with interconnecting communicating veins, and perforating veins that originate from the superficial veins, penetrate the fascia, and anastomose with the deep veins. The deep veins consist of pairs, termed *vena communicantes*, that accompany the large arteries to the level of the popliteal and are designated by the same name as the accompanying artery. The more proximal deep veins have one vein per artery.

Each of these types of veins has unique conduit responsibilities with different potential pathophysiologic complications, including dilation, inflammation, and thrombosis. Clinically these may present as varices or thrombophlebitis, leading to potentially morbid complications of pulmonary embolization. Furthermore, even after resolution, deep phlebitis has the potential for scarring of valves, leading to chronic venous insufficiency and stasis ulcer formation.

Superficial Varicose Veins

The superficial veins originate as valveless venules in the cutaneous and subcutaneous tissues of the foot and leg. By a series of anastomoses the larger veins are clinically recognized along the medio- and lateroplantar borders of the feet. Dorsally the venous arch receives branches from the digits and forefoot and progresses laterally to form the short saphenous and medially to form the long saphenous vein. These vessels have valves and continue to receive anastomotic branches from other superficial leg veins as they progress proximally and interconnect with each other by communicating veins. They are supported by the fascia and skin, which is adequate under normal conditions.

The normal flow in the superficial system is from distal to proximal, with connecting perforating veins available to transmit excessive volumes to the deep venous system. Flow is augmented during muscular contraction, whereby the expansion of the muscle belly compresses the superficial veins against the resistance of skin. The valves are aligned and coapt in a plane parallel to the skin, thereby ensuring complete closure and cephalad direction of flow. Except in venous hypertension, the pressure head is usually under 70 mm Hg pressure. Since the superficial veins terminate at the popliteal or femoral veins, excessive pressure in the deep system precludes adequate emptying, leading to damage in the superficial vessels. This results in excessive pooling in the superficial veins and increased capacitance. Infrequent episodes of congestion do not lead to complications, whereas more frequent pooling episodes result in anatomic changes to accommodate the increased volumes. These changes typically are widening of the veins

in the transverse axis and elongation in the longitudinal axis. Dilation of the diameter of these veins results in clinically evident varices, and elongation results in a serpiginous distribution referred to as a map leg. Communicating veins also become engorged and dilated, and contribute to the clinical appearance. The increased hydrostatic pressure in these engorged veins is transmitted to the smaller, distal and superficial venules, which become secondarily dilated. These ectatic venules are called venectasia or telangiectasia, which connect to a central vessel that penetrates the dermis. On digital pressure they can be emptied and disappear.

Superficial varicosities develop as a result of inherent genetic weakness of the walls, or chronic pooling of blood. This may be attributed to occupations necessitating standing in one position for prolonged periods of time, thereby precluding adequate emptying, and working seated with flexture of the veins at the knee and hip levels, causing limited venous outflow. The terminal stage of pregnancy, with a gravid uterus pressing on the veins in the pelvic floor, leads to retarded outflow and pooling of blood, as does any soft tissue lesion, including neoplasm. Arteriovenous anastomoses with proximal instreaming of blood under high pressure also increase distal venous capacitance, leading to varicosities.

Treatment of the overt and fragile varices is total surgical removal of the superficial veins. Depending on location and flow characteristics, focal blowouts may be resected while leaving the balance of the vein in place. Management of nonsymptomatic or incipient stages of superficial varicosities is by pressure-gradient stockings to the knee level if the venous insufficiency is limited to the foot or leg, or graduated support pantyhose if the thigh segment is also involved.

Perforating Varicose Veins

Perforating veins are known to exist in the foot and are valveless up to the level of the ankle. Unidirectionality of flow from superficial to deep is preserved, however, by the repeated pumping action of alternate plantar and dorsiflexion of the feet and toes as well as compression of the superficial veins with weight bearing. The perforating veins in the leg conduct blood from the superficial saphenous system to the deep veins. They possess valves and are so named since they perforate the deep fascia. Three forms of openings exist for the passage of these veins: holes, funnels, and slits. As these veins pass through the deep fascia, they are accompanied by small cutaneous arteries, lymphatics, and cutaneous nerves. Although there exist many perforating veins, the three most clinically significant are located medially and connect the long saphenous to the deep system. These veins are called Cockett's veins and are spaced about 5 cm apart, with the most inferior one being just above the medial malleolus.

The perforating veins sometimes become secondarily dilated by a "blow-down" mechanism when chronic varicosities involve the superficial system. However, they dilate and become incompetent when excessive back pressure exists in the deep system, precluding adequate emptying and leading to focal edema. The reduced outflow increases the capacitance of the perforating veins, widening the lumen and precluding valvular apposition. The resultant distention of the perforating veins allows reversal of flow from the deep to the superficial veins. This focal increased volume in a sector of the superficial vein causes secondary dilation or "blow-out" at the site of the perforator, known as Dow's sign, and a clinical impression of a varicosity. The perforator defect may be differentiated from an undulating primary superficial varicosity by compression of the calf with its deep veins and auscultation for outward flow by the Doppler instrument. A primary undulating varicosity is diagnosed by percussion of another site while palpating the blow-out. If the two sites are a continuum of the same vein, containing the same column of blood, the percussive wave will be transmitted to the interrogated blow-out.

More distal varices can develop in the superficial veins secondary to increased volume and pressure from an incompetent perforator. The principle is akin to high volumes of blood under increased pressure from an A-V fistula or anastomosis emptying into a superficial vein, causing its dilation.[22]

With dilation of a perforating vein as it passes through the narrow opening in the fascia, the accompanying cutaneous artery is compressed. This leads to ischemia of the overlying skin and contributes to the stasis ulcerative process. Compression of the lymphatics results in focal edema while concomitant compression of the nerve yields the neuritic-type pain often described by patients. This is a result of expansive mechanical pressure on the superficial sensory fibers and transcient ischemia due to associated reduction of blood flow through the vasa nevorum. The vasa nevorum, as well as the vasa vasorum to the wall of the perforator vein, originate from the accompanying cutaneous artery.

Incompetent perforating veins with attendant clinical complications are ligated at their origin from the superficial veins to minimize strangulation of accompanying neurovascular structures at the fascial openings. These veins may also be ablated by sclerotherapy, which minimizes damage to associated nonvenous structures. In cases of a focal incompetent vein, local compression is sufficient, without the need for full-leg compressive bandagings or gradient compressive stockings.

Deep Varicose Veins

The deep veins originate as venules that receive blood from the digital and pedal capillaries of the osseous and muscular tissue as well as from the vasa nevorum and vasorum. These deep pedal veins also accept blood from the superficial vessels by way of the perforators. They are valveless at this level and usually are paired while accompanying the named arteries. The deep veins of the legs and thighs drain similar tissue and perforating veins, are paired to the level of the popliteal artery, and are bound by muscles and adjacent fascia or intermuscular septa. They possess valves that develop as hyperplastic ridges of endothelium that invaginate in the direction of flow, and extend into the lumen with some muscular fibers extending into the proximal third of the leaflets. The venous wall at this level is the thinnest that allows an embryonic outpocketing to form the deeper portion of a perforating vein. Valves are most commonly noted at points just distal to inflowing tributaries.

In the recumbant position, flow is noted to be spontaneous in the more proximal levels of the lower extremities and is rhythmic with respiration. As the abdominal pressure increases with inspiration, hesitation of flow is noted; as the abdominal pressure decreases with expiration, flow is reinstituted proximally to the pelvic veins. In the upright walking attitude, local muscular contractile activity overrides the diaphragmatic excursions and actively pumps and augments the flow of venous blood to more proximal levels. During the swing phase of gait the deep veins are engorged with blood, resulting in lesser propulsive pressure and greater transluminal diameter. During the weight-bearing phase the deep veins are compressed, resulting in decreased diameter and an increased propulsive pressure consistent with the systolic phase of the extremities' muscular pump.[23]

The deep veins of the thighs and legs can become varicosed as a result of chronic pressure from adjoining expansile soft tissue lesions such as cysts or compressive forces on the pelvic veins, such as in multiple pregnancies. These proximal veins rarely become varicosed de novo unless associated with a family history. The pedal and digital deep veins nearly never varicose except as a complication of more proximal insufficiency. All deep and perforating veins of the lower extremities may be subject to enlargement secondary to deep thrombophlebitis at any level (Table 17-1).

Treatment of these varicosities is directed at preventing extension and supporting the weakened vessels. Surgical removal is not indicated unless stasis causes frequent thromophlebitic crises with risks of loss of life from embolization or loss of limb as a result of extensive ulceration with concomitant infection and/or secondary limb-threatening compression of the arterial supply. Frequent daily uses of an intermittent limb compression pump to mobilize extravascular fluid accumulations as well as custom-fitted gradient support stockings provide satisfactory results.

Telangiectasia

Enlargement of the most superficial tegumentary venules is termed *telangiectasia, phlebectasia,* or *venectasia*. These vessels are about 1 mm in diameter, contain no valves, and have a wall composition of endothelium and elastic tissue. They drain venous blood from the subpapillary venous plexi, which in turn drain the vascular loops in the rete pegs of the dermis. These superficial venules unite into periodic central small veins that progress inward to anastomose with other larger superficial veins. The venous blood then is propagated to even larger superficial veins that may progress proximally or into perforating veins that direct the flow to the deep venous system.

In the natural state, the most superficial venules may become dilated and be seen clinically on the medial surface of the midfoot to the level of the medial malleolus as blue or red streaks. The coloration is due to stagnation of blood in these enlarged venules, with red signifying somewhat retarded flow and reduced hemoglobin, and blue indicating further sludging of flow and advanced reduction of hemoglobin. These findings may be evident by the age of 20. The earliest presentation of these engorged venules is relegated to the medial pedal area, which has the lowest concentration of intermediate-sized venules. Similar lesions with stellate distributions are evident on other surfaces of the

Table 17-1. Comparison of Various Thrombophlebitities

Location	Etiology	Complication	Risk	Treatment
Iliofemoral	Tumor compression	Phlegmasia cerulea dolens	Shock	Anticoagulation
	Iliac artery compression	Phlegmasia alba dolens	Gangrene	Thrombolysis
	Popliteal aneurysm	Deep varicosities	Death	Thrombectomy
Tibial soleal	Compartment syndrome	Postphlebitic syndrome	Pulmonary embolism	Anticoagulation
	Trauma	Stasis ulceration		Vena cava filter
	Infection	Superficial varicosities		Antibiotics
Perforator	Compartment syndrome	None	None	Rest, compresses
	Trauma			Anticoagulation
	Deep thrombosis			Ligation
Saphenous	Pregnancy	None	None	Rest, compresses
	Trauma, infection			Aspirin, steroids
	Familial history			Antibiotics

legs and thighs, more prominently in females, by the age of 30. These findings most probably are attributable to less support of these venules by estrogenated female skin. Males also may have such lesions but they are not brought to the clinician's attention and may be camouflaged by leg and thigh hair.

Telangiectasia also develop as a result of hypertension of the venules because of stagnation in larger veins.

The clinical confirmation of these lesions is by diascopy. A rigid transparent material, such as a glass slide or one's reading glasses, suffices as a diascope to identify these lesions. With compression of the involved skin, the blood is expressed from the engorged venules, and the venular streaks disappear. On removal of the diascope, refilling is noted immediately. The common draining veins are usually centrally located in spider-like distributions or at one end in linear-patterned ectatic vessels. Digital milking of these vessels, and sustained focal pressure with a blunt instrument over the central vein, temporarily empties these venules, with resultant disappearance of the lesion.

Other Venous Dysplasias

Hemangiomas

Congenital vascular malformations of the lower extremities are relatively rare. Superficial proliferative vascular lesions with increased mitotic activity are defined as hemangiomas. These lesions characteristically have enlarged subpapillary capillary and venous plexi, containing significant pockets of blood, are nonencapsulated, and are surrounded by connective tissue. They are termed *cavernous hemangiomas* and the coloration is a result of further deoxygenation of the sludged venous blood. The color is readily transmitted through the rather transparent epidermis. These lesions, although asymptomatic, are of cosmetic concern to parents or patients.

Amelioration of these lesions is by destruction of the superficial venous plexi. This may be accomplished by argon laser cautery more favorably than sclerotherapy. By either approach, the dilated superficial venules are collapsed and rendered nonpatent, with resultant near-normal skin coloration.

Angiodysplasias

Venous malformations that grow with the child and show normal endothelial mitotic activity are called venous angiodysplasias. They may involve the deep or superficial systems and could be considered analogous to arterial aneurysms. These dilated lesions are characterized by pain on dependency or walking, swelling, altered leg circumference in upright versus recumbent positions, subcutaneous or intracuticular venodilation, and spongy venous masses with local muscular atrophy. Dilations of the deep system are associated with atypical ultrashort perforating veins.[24]

Baseline examination procedures include Doppler insonation and partial oxygen tension determinations. Doppler flow studies demonstrate retarded passive flow unlike the rapid arterialized flow noted in A-V anastamoses or fistulas, from which these malformations must be differentiated since both present similar venous distention. The partial oxygen tension is lower than that of A-V anastomoses since there is no mixing of arterial blood with the venous system. Venous stress tests, such as Perthes' or Trendelenburg's, are unnecessary since the lesions become self-evident on standing erect or sitting with legs dependent.

Standing phlebograms with contrast media, conducted immediately following injection, 30 to 40 seconds later, and 3 minutes after the first radiograph, demonstrate these malformations. The degree of insufficiency is determined by the amount of dye remaining in the deep and/or superficial systems on the last radiogram. Treatment is by removal of the saccular or fusiform dysplastic lesions and ligation of the feeder perforating or communicating veins.

Superficial Thrombophlebitis

The superficial veins of the foot, the leg's saphenous system, and the superficial communicating veins are prone to injury leading to inflammation and thrombosis. Etiologic considerations include acute direct trauma, tightly fitting garters, stasis, extension of superficial or cutaneous ulcer infections, and injections of medications or abuse substances. The latter form of irritation is secondary to a rapid or high-dose infusion of a foreign substance into a slow-moving column of blood, causing focal endothelial injury. The puncture itself, if overly traumatic, also injures the endothelium and engenders thrombosis.

All forms of trauma, whether mechanical or chemical, as well as infection, incite an inflammatory reaction with aggregation of red blood cells. This may be clinically noted by rubor and calor of the skin overlying the involved vein. The resultant thrombus occludes the vessel, rendering it noncollapsible and, therefore, palpable as a denser cord along the distribution of the thrombosed vein. Pain is the usual presenting concern and is attributable to the venous back pressure as well as the focal intercellular edema.

Limb outflow disturbances are negligible because of the natural shunting of blood to the deeper veins via many perforators. Given the much smaller caliber as well as the lower propagative pressure of the superficial veins, embolization is an insignificant risk. Doppler insonation of the thrombosed site yields no signals demonstrative of spontaneity or augmentability of flow; if flow is heard, lymphangitis or cellulitis is the more likely diagnosis.

Treatment of superficial thrombophlebitis is directed to the pathogenesis of the condition. If the phlebitis is septic, antibiosis is required, whereas all other uncomplicated inflamed pedal and leg forms require aspirin for analgesia and mild anti-inflammatory effects. Nonsteroidal anti-inflammatory preparations may also be used for moderate to severe cases. Warm compresses and elevation to levels above the heart are additional measures taken, and individuals are dissuaded from ambulation. Superficial thrombophlebitis of the long saphenous vein at the thigh level is more serious because of the volume of blood that is transmitted from more distal segments and the greater caliber of the vessel predisposing to larger thrombi. The etiology of this condition requires greater interrogation, and heparin or anabolic steroids may be indicated since vessel wall plasminogen activator levels have been observed to be reduced with use of these drugs.

Perforator Thrombophlebitis

Thrombophlebitis solely of the perforator veins is observed infrequently. Fortuitous direct acute trauma to the epifascial end of the perforator vein incites the typical inflammatory response, eventuating in a thrombosis. Because of inflow stagnation, the thrombotic process extends to involve the local superficial vein and results in the puckered Dow's sign. Rubor and calor are limited to the junction site of the perforator and superficial veins, as is focal edema leading to shiny, stretched skin. Pain is no more pronounced than in superficial thrombophlebitis.

Perforator thrombophlebitis may occur secondary to deep vein thrombophlebitis by extension. Since deep thrombophlebitis occurs at valvular sites, and since valves are located just distal to anastomotic perforating tributaries, the inflow is readily obstructed, with stagnation resulting in thrombotic extension. The same end result occurs with gradually increasing pressure on the subfascial end of the perforating veins in compartment syndromes. The perforating veins of the leg are located medially and laterally to allow blood passage from superficial to deep veins. Therefore, injury to local muscle with resultant edema can compress the perforating veins passing the injured muscle. Extension of the inflammatory process as well as mechanical compression leads to perforator thrombosis.

Treatment of the primary form is supportive, with compression over the distended site and elevations. Reduction of platelet adhesiveness with aspirin therapy, as well as amelioration of the inflammation with nonsteroidal anti-inflammatory preparations, is recommended. In recalcitrant cases, minidose heparinization is advisable. Secondary forms of perforator thrombophlebitis are managed by direction of therapy to the primary condition.

Deep Thrombophlebitis

The endothelium of deep veins and other veins is nonthrombogenic and does not react with platelets. It has been proposed that the nonreactivity of intact endothelium is attributable to a negative electrostatic charge on the surface of cells as well as the secretion of prostacyclin and fibronectin. With venous wall damage and endothelial loss, the subendothelium is exposed and reacts both with platelets and the blood coagulation system. Vascular damage can occur in a number of ways, including mechanical trauma, thermal injury, immune complexes, enzymatic digestion, endotoxins, and viruses, as well as bacterial products.[25]

Stasis also predisposes to deep venous thrombosis by preventing clearance of activated coagulation factors by the liver and mixing of these factors with their inhibitors. Patients who are bedridden or immobilized by plaster casts or splints have stasis predisposing them to deep thrombosis. Since the soleal sinuses, and to a lesser degree the gastrocnemius sinuses, have negligible smooth muscles in the vessel wall and exhibit significant capacitance, restriction of these leg muscles engenders stasis, leading to thrombosis. Furthermore, with prolonged immobilization or lower extremity paralysis, atrophy of these large muscles decreases or ablates their contractile strength and capacity to function effectively as a venous pump. Stasis may also be associated with inadequate mobilization of blood, as in congestive heart failure, myocardial infarction, previous venous thrombosis, varicose veins, obesity, parturition, and postsurgical immobility.

Use of oral contraceptives has also been well recognized as an etiologic factor in deep thrombophlebitis. Estrogen-containing oral contraceptives produce venous dilation, result in reduced levels of plasminogen activator in the vascular endothelium, and increase a number of coagulation factors. An increased blood viscosity associated with high hematocrit readings, as in polycythemia, retards venous flow and contributes to the thrombotic tendency.

Primary thrombophlebitis is an inflammatory process initiated at the level of injury, which may be anywhere along the length of the deep vein. Thrombophlebitis secondary to increased viscosity, stasis, or a hypercoagulable state starts as a phlebothrombosis with platelet aggregates entwined with fibrin in the deep portions of valvular cusps that serves as an irritant leading to inflammation (Fig. 17-7). The luminal surfaces of valvular leaflets do not face the mainstream of flow, and blood contained in these valvular pockets is passively expelled with full muscular compression. These valves are typically located just distal to larger anastomosing muscular or perforating veins. If congestion of flow occurs from above, the extra volume and pressure is dissipated to these confluxing branches and burdens the valves. The deep venous wall at the valvular attachment sites distends and contributes to the stagnation. Endothelial cell slippage occurs, resulting in a nidus for inflammation leading to thrombophlebitis. The resultant thrombus composed of platelets and fibrin grows out of the valve pocket in the direction of flow. Later the thrombus attains sufficient volume to totally occlude the lumen, causing increased sludging of blood and extension of the thrombus distally and proximally. This extended thrombus is composed mainly of red cells enmeshed in fibrin (Fig. 17-8).

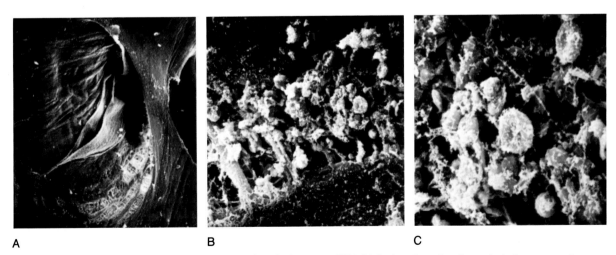

A   B   C

Fig. 17-7. Phlebothrombosis advancement in valvular cusp. **(A)** Initial microthrombus in pocket of venous valve. **(B)** Advanced thrombus with platelets and erythrocytes. **(C)** Fibrin-enmeshed cap of thrombus. (Courtesy of Gwendolyn J. Steward, Ph.D., Temple Medical Science Center, Philadelphia.)

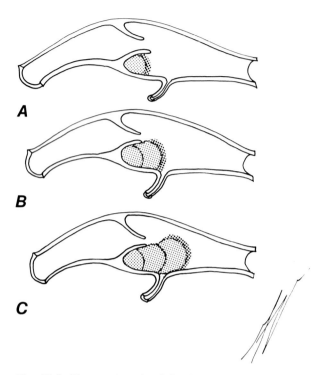

A

B

C

Fig. 17-8. Venous thrombosis leading to occlusion. **(A)** Initial thrombus in valvular pocket with fibrin-entrapped platelets and red blood cells. **(B)** Advancement of thrombus with continued stasis. **(C)** Thrombus extension blocking inflowing perforator vein.

The organized occluding thrombus incites perivascular inflammation with associated pain and tenderness. Distal swelling is secondary to limitation of outflow, and appearance of distended superficial veins is the result of redirection of blood through the perforators to the superficial veins. Should the thrombus obstruct the large femoral vein, which is the common outflow route for all the distal deep veins, a condition known as *phlegmasia cerulea dolens* results. This is characterized by pain, profound swelling, and cyanotic discoloration as a result of stagnation and reduction of hemoglobin in the entrapped red cells leading to tissue anoxia. With persistent back pressure reflected distally to the venules, metvenules, and even the capillaries, arterial spasm occurs, rendering the skin devoid of inflow. Clinically the skin appears pallored, and this stage is termed *phlegmasia alba dolens*.

The obvious complication of deep thrombophlebitis at the stage of organization is embolization. This occurs by active venous compression by local muscles or by passive compression, as in manipulation or rolling of the lower extremity. Increased pressure during hypertensive crises, reflected from the arterial side through anastomoses, may also break off the fragile tip of a non-fibrin-bound segment. The floating embolus is passed to the right side of the heart, then enters the pulmonary artery to be carried to either lung, and finally lodges in an arterial tributary too small to allow passage. The distal pulmonary tissue typically perfused by this tributary and its microvascular network undergoes ischemic changes, resulting in focal pulmonary infarction. Depending on the size of the embolus and the state of hypercoagulability, only local damage may occur, with some future lung scarring and overload of the right side of the heart leading to right-sided congestive failure. Total vascular standstill may also occur, resulting in death.[26]

The deep thrombus may spontaneously recanalize by lysis, or it may required medical intervention and long-term support of the injured veins. The most common lower extremity complication is the postphlebitic syndrome, which is characterized by brawny discoloration and lichenification of the skin. These result from the pressure-induced diapedesis of red cells into the extravascular compartments under the skin. The cells undergo a biodegradation process converting hemoglobin to hemosiderin while leaving an iron-pigmented discoloration. The concurrent inflammatory and cellulitic process leads to a cascading set of tissue reactions that eventuates in scarring and toughening of the integument.

Diagnosis of deep thrombophlebitis in the office setting is by history and clinical findings. Noninvasive studies include Doppler insonation of the veins during the nonorganizational stage, since compressive maneuvers are required that may dislodge a fragment. The traditional study for suspected leg deep thrombophlebitis is venous occlusive pneumatic or impedence plethysmography. Hospital-based procedures include fibrinogen scanning and ascending venography.

LYMPHATIC DISORDERS OF THE LOWER EXTREMITIES

The lymphatic system is composed of endothelium-lined channels containing valves as well as a series of nodes. The system arises from mesenchymal cells that differentiate into endothelium, thus forming the basis for the vessels. Enlarged segments of these channels, initially called sacs, are invaded by connective tissue that enmeshes the lymph cells and gives rise to the lymph nodes. Lymphatics are located throughout the body wherever other blood vessels are found, except in bone marrow; they are not located in cartilage, tendon, or nerve.[27]

At their origin, lymphatic capillaries may be open ended or closed. Either form has filaments on the abluminal surface of the endothelium that anchor these small vessels to adjacent tissue, thereby preventing their collapse during states of high external pressure, such as in advanced edema. The endothelial cells are connected to each other by abutment, overlap, or interdigitation. Periodically open junctions of about 30 nm or more are noted that serve as entry points for lymph-containing macromolecules. The endothelial cells also contain vesicles connected to the surface that presumably participate in the transport process.

The lymphatic capillary network empties into collecting channels that are originally thin walled. As these vessels anastomose, their luminal size increases, as does the thickness of the wall. Midsized lymphatics contain connective tissue and occasional muscle cells. Closer to the lymph nodes, the vessels are trilaminar, with the established media containing smooth muscle cells enabling the lymphatics to contract, while the adventitia contains collagen and elastin connective tissue. The adventitia is penetrated by vasa nevorum that innervate the smooth muscles, and vasa vasorum that nourish the thick wall. The lymphatic channels draining the lower extremities closely accompany the superficial and deep veins and bear similar names. The larger lymphatics posses tricuspid valves, with some widening of the vessels at these valvular sites.

Before entering the blood, lymph passes through several sets of nodes. The afferent channels divide before penetrating the node capsule and then enter the subcapsular sinus. Lymph flows through the cortical and medullary sinuses, which are lined with endothelium and which lie between aggregates of lymphocytes that form follicles and medullary cords. Within the sinuses are fibers and macrophages that screen the lymph, demonstrating ability for filtration and phagocytic action. After traversing the sinuses the lymph flows to the efferent vessels at the hilum of the node. Nodes are commonly located in the popliteal and inguinal regions, which drain lymphatic fluid from the deep and superficial channels, as well as at the iliac levels.

Larger lymphatic trunks located postnodally transmit lymph to the lymphatic duct, which ascends the torso posteriorly to pass through the diaphragmatic hiatus. The thoracic duct empties into the right jugular, subclavian, or innominate vein. There exist several lymphaticovenous anastomoses that allow earlier entry of lymph into the venous system when more proximal lymphatic channels are obstructed or ligated.[28]

Lymphedema

If retarded drainage of lymph occurs, extremity edema is observed. Decreased outflow may occur as a result of sectional aplasia or hypoplasia of lymphatic capillaries or obstruction leading to congestion, distention (lymphangiectasis), and lack of valvular coaptation. Any cause of edema increases the interstitial volume, which causes separation of connective tissue. The anchoring filaments attached to the adjacent connective tissue draw the lymphatic capillaries apart, thus increasing the lumen and allowing for greater intraluminal lymph volumes. If the lymph is not rapidly expelled, chronic distention of the lymphatic channels results in valvular insufficiency and lymph stasis. Overaccumulation of large protein molecules in the interstitium causes retention of more fluid, which eventuates in lymphedema. The skin and underlying structures are thickened, and fat is replaced by greatly dilated lymph spaces surrounded by fibrous tissue. The resulting structures are spongy because of the fibroblastic proliferation in the dermis, and digital pressure fails to rapidly express the albuminous fluid identified clinically as nonpitting edema.

Prophylaxis is the best treatment. Any lesions that compress and limit outflow through the major trunks and duct should be removed. Other causes of edema should be differentiated, supported by gradient hose or wraps, and reversed before secondary changes occur, leading to chronic lymphedema and its irreversible morphologic changes.

Congenital Lymphedema

Congenital lymphedema without any family history is noted at birth by diffuse swelling of the extremity. Initially the edema resolves with elevations, but with the advancing pathophysiologic and histologic changes described above, the circumference of the extremity increases. No cure or treatment is possible.

Milroy's disease is a congenital and familial form of lymphedema. It is manifested in other members of the family and is characterized by painless limb enlargement. It is limited to the legs and, initially, is pitting and reduceable with elevations. Later the cascading set of events leads to chronic lymphedema, resulting in permanent limb enlargement and dermal hyperplasia.

Lymphedema praecox presents most commonly in females during the growth spurt years when lymphatic development does not keep pace with expansion of other extremity tissue. This relative hypoplasia engenders lymph stasis, leading to chronic lymphedema. Initially swelling or heaviness of the foot, ankle, or leg is the presenting concern. The edema develops after prolonged periods of standing, in hot and humid weather, and during menstrual periods.

The edema is reversible with overnight rest and the limbs elevated to approximately 45 degrees, but as the chronicity is extended less edema is resolved, and many days of elevation may be required before the limb returns to normal appearance. Advancement of the edema may be delayed by appropriate support of the extremities with custom-fitted gradient stockings. Measurements of the extremities for support hose are conducted after several days and nights of elevation and immediately following limb decompression of residual edema with an intermittent compressive limb pump.

Secondary Lymphedema

Congestion of lymph nodes with external compression by tumors or internal obstruction by metastases results in slowly advancing lymphedema. Expansile lesions in the proximity of a channel or node restrict the low-pressured lymph flow normally propagated by lymphatic wall smooth muscle constriction or adjacent skeletal wall contraction. Metastatic cells are initially and painlessly trapped in the sinuses of the node, thereby causing local congestion. This results in tissue expansion just distal to the node, and eventually, with more acral lymphatic stasis, limb enlargement is noted throughout the balance of the extremity. The skin slowly becomes indurated.

Injury to lymphatic nodes or collecting channels in the proximity of the nodes, whether by surgical extirpation or trauma, results in sufficient loss of integrity to cause lymphedema. Injury to isolated peripheral channels or trunks is not as severe since the flow is usually rediverted to anastomotic vessels without any adverse sequelae.

Differentiation of primary from secondary lymphedema can usually be defined by a careful history. The integrity of the vessels or nodal dysfunction is defined by lymphangiography. Unilateral edema must also be differentiated from postphlebitic syndrome, A-V fistula or anastomosis, and chronic deep venous insufficiency; bilateral edema is differentiated from systemic conditions such as congestive heart or renal failure, hepatic cirrhosis, lipedema, and nutritional disturbances.

Treatment of secondary lymphedema is directed initially to the reversal of lymphatic flow restriction by surgical or medical means. Containment of the initial degrees of lymphedematous changes or prevention of the advancement of these morphologic changes is again addressed by custom-fitted gradient support hose for periods of ambulation. Home care for the non-weight-bearing periods or the nonambulatory patient is by elevation and intermittent compression pump. These measures mobilize the interstitial fluids, thus minimizing the integumentary changes and limb disfigurement.

Lymphangitis

Infections in the extremities result in a tissue response that is highlighted by vasodilation. This hyperperfusive state facilitates the arrival of leukocytes for phagocytitic activity. The dilation of arterioles is complimented by venular distention, and all the cardinal signs of inflammation are evident consistent with cellulitis. Focal edema, in response to the vasodilation and accumulation of infectious by-products, distends the local tissue. With retraction of the connective tissue, the anchoring filaments draw on the walls of the lymphatic capillaries, thereby widening the natural open wall junctions. This phenomenon, as well as increased lymphatic wall permeability, facilitates the entry of toxic by-products from the infected site into the lymphatic network. Such violation of the normally sterile lymph channels initiates an inflammatory response known as lymphangitis.

Once initiated, the inflammatory reaction continues up the channel in the normal direction of lymph flow. This process extends to levels rather remote from the infected site. The inflamed superficial lymphatic channel is visually identified by its ruborous appearance and is clinically termed *red streaking*. The pain at the infected site, due to local necrosis, pH alteration, and expansile pressure, is so intense that the inflamed lymphatic vessel remains relatively painless. If the infection continues, however, and the lymphangitis spreads to a node, pain ensues as a result of nodal congestion. This engorgement tenses the node, resulting in lymphadenopathy that is readily palpated as nodal firmness. Excessive compression of the node also yields pain. Lymphadenopathy may also less likely be caused by a filarial infection, which causes nodal scarring and renders the nodes nonfunctional for any filtration. This results in chronic and total lymphatic congestion with massive disfiguring hypertrophic changes in the extremity known as elephantiasis.

Treatment of superficial lymphangitis is with warm compresses to facilitate flow; however, all efforts are directed at resolution of the primary infection with appropriate antibiosis. Resolution of the lymphadenopathy should thwart the risk of chronic lymphedema and its disfiguring complications. If nodal or lymphatic trunk damage is irreversible, then an omental transposition to patent trunks has demonstrated anastomosing to occur. This allows drainage of the extremity through the new outflow pathway. If disfiguring hyperplasia has also occurred, all redundant skin and subcutaneous tissue is resected along with the nonfunctional superficial lymphatic collecting channels.

REFERENCES

1. Palmer T, Husum B: Blood pressure in the great toe with simulated occlusion of the dorsalis pedis artery. Anesth Analg 57:453, 1978
2. Needham T: The diagnosis and assessment of venous disorders in the office and laboratory. p. 103. In Hershey FB, Barnes RW, Sumner DS (eds): Noninvasive Diagnosis of Vascular Disease. Appleton Davies, Pasadena, 1984
3. Kemczynski RF: Clinical application of non-invasive testing in extremity arterial insufficiency. p. 343. In Kemczynski RF, Yao JS (eds): Practical Noninvasive Vascular Diagnosis. Year Book Medical, Chicago, 1982
4. Talbot SR: B-mode evaluation of peripheral arteries and veins. p. 351. In Zwiebel WJ (ed): Introduction to Vascular Ultrasonography. Grune & Stratton, New York, 1986
5. Beach KW, Phillips DJ: Doppler instrumentation for evaluation of arterial and venous disease. p. 11. In Jaffe CC (ed): Vascular and Doppler Ultrasound. Churchill Livingstone, New York, 1984
6. Phillips DJ, Baker DW, Strandess DE: Combined echo-doppler (Duplex) imaging. p. 272. In Bernstein EF (ed): Noninvasive Diagnostic Techniques in Vascular Disease. CV Mosby, St Louis, 1982
7. Pearce WH, Rutherford RB, Whitehill TA et al: Nuclear magnetic resonance imaging: its diagnostic value in patients with congenital vascular malformation of the limbs. J Vasc Surg 8:64, 1988
8. Nicolaides AN, Hobbs JT: Diagnosis of venous thrombosis by the I^{125} fibrinogen test. p. 213. In Bergan JJ, Yao JS (eds): Venous Problems. Year Book Medical, Chicago, 1978
9. Ryo UY: Radionuclide studies in arterial disease. p. 19. In Pinsky SM, Moss GS, Srinkantaswamy S et al (eds): Imaging of the Peripheral Vascular System. Grune & Stratton, New York, 1984

10. Lippert H, Pabst R: Arterial Variations in Man. J. F. Bergmans Verlag, Munich, 1985

11. Xu D, Wang G, Liu M et al: Anatomical analysis of the cause of skin necrosis of the great toe nail flap. Br Plast Surg 40:283, 1987

12. Green D, McFeeley ND, Kidawa A et al: Digital perfusion with tibial nerve block. J Am Podiatr Med Assoc 78:495, 1988

13. Richardson D: Effects of gravity on regional and capillary blood flows in the human toe. Microvasc Res 35:334, 1988

14. Wendt T, Van du Does R, Schrader R et al: Acute hemodynamic effects of the vasodilating and β-blocking agent Carvedilol in comparison to propranolol. J Cardiovasc Pharmacol 10:5147, 1987

15. Dormandy J: Clinical use of calcium antagonists in peripheral circulatory disease. Ann NY Acad Sci 522:611, 1988

16. St Claire RW: Pathogenesis of the atherosclerotic lesion: current concepts of cellular and biochemical events. p. 1. In Tulenko TN, Cox RH (eds): Recent Advances in Arterial Diseases. Alan R Liss, New York, 1986

17. Veterans Administration Study Group 141: Comparative evaluation of prosthetic, reversed, and insitu vein bypass grafts in distal popliteal and tibial-peroneal vascularization. Arch Surg 123:434, 1988

18. Andros G, Harris RW, Salles-Cunha SX et al: Bypass grafts to the ankle and foot. J Vasc Surg 7:785, 1988

19. Fine MJ, Kapoor W, Falanga V: Cholesterol crystal embolization: a review of 221 cases in the English literature. Angiology 10:769, 1987

20. Kumpe DA, Zwerdlinger S, Griffon DJ: Blue digit syndrome: treatment with percutaneous transluminal angioplasty. Radiology 166:37, 1988

21. Prout TE: Diabetes mellitus and hypertension: clinical perspectives. Md Med J 37:349, 1988

22. Pflug JJ: Chronic venous incompetence caused by stasis or intermittent hypertension via perforating veins. p. 113. In May R, Partsch H, Staubesand J (eds): Perforating Veins. Urban & Schwarzenberg, Baltimore, 1981

23. Hiesh J, Genton E, Hull R (eds): Venous Thromboembolism. Grune & Stratton, New York, 1981

24. Gorenstein A, Katz S, Schiller M: Congenital angiodysplasia of the superficial venous system of the lower extremities in children. Ann Surg 207:213, 1988

25. DiMinno G, Cerbone A: The antithrombotic potential of the vessel wall. Evidence from studies on patients prone to venous thrombosis. Hematology 73:75, 1988

26. Powers LR: Distal deep vein thrombosis. J Gen Intern Med 3:288, 1988

27. Montgomery RJ, Sutker BD, Bronke JT et al: Interstitial fluid flow in cortical bone. Microvasc Res 35:295, 1988

28. Abramson DI, Dobrin PB (eds): Blood Vessels and Lymphatics in Organ Systems. Academic Press, New York, 1984

Dermatologic and Soft Tissue Disorders

18

Daniel J. McCarthy, D.P.M., Ph.D.

Other chapters in this text describe a number of systemic diseases with lower extremity skin manifestations. Many such conditions have distinctive morphologic characteristics. Pemphigus, for example, is a term covering a wide range of more or less chronic bullous skin lesions that occur histologically in suprabasilar, subcorneal, and subepidermal locations. Because of its many variations, pemphigus may require immunofluorescent techniques for precise differential diagnosis.

Erythema multiforme with its variants may appear similar to pemphigus, but is an acute self-limiting disease.[1] Its etiologic agents are known to vary widely. Physical agents, drugs, fungal agents, bacterial and viral infection, neoplasia, and collagen vascular disorders must be considered as possible causes of vesiculobullous disorders in general.

Lupus erythematosus was first described by Biett in 1828. Osler in 1895 discussed the entity as a multisystem disease, and Keeperer in 1941 introduced the collagen disease concept. Since internal organs can be involved, systemic lupus erythematosus (SLE) has a potentially fatal outcome.[1] Its occurrence on the lower extremity is usually of the more benign discoid type, with raised, scaly, erythematous lesions. The so-called "butterfly rash" is more typical in the facial area. Podiatrists may be confronted with a nondeforming, effuse arthritis as one of the symptoms of SLE. These localized and systemic forms of the disease may require identification of antinuclear bodies or depressed serum complement values to confirm this often difficult diagnosis.

Scleroderma is yet another potentially fatal multisystem collagen disease that occurs in both localized and generalized forms (Fig. 18-1). Plaquelike morphea eruptions usually consist of a few well-defined, indurated, smooth ivory-covered plaques which are unrelated to deeper skin structures. Violaceous borders characterize newer, active lesions. A guttate morphea is less frequently associated with localized scleroderma. Small, circumscribed, chalk-white lesions with purplish borders are associated with scleroderma, and these lesion types tend to coalesce.

An encyclopedic discussion of systemic diseases that may have presentations in the lower extremities is beyond the scope of this chapter. Systemic involvement has been mentioned here as a reminder that certain lesions are symptomatic of generalized disease and not a localized entity. The subjects of lower extremity pruritus in general, ulcerations, malignancy, special integumentary concerns relating to diabetes mellitus and aging, skin trauma, and neurodermatitis, among others, have received attention in other chapters of this book. This chapter addresses the many other pedal dermatologic problems of a localized nature.

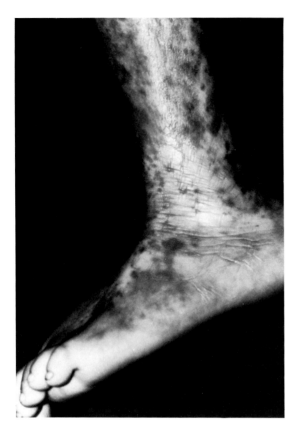

Fig. 18-1. Linear scleroderma. (Case courtesy of Dr. Port). (From McCarthy and Montgomery,[3] with permission.)

ANATOMY

The skin develops from both ectodermal and mesodermal components. In the case of the melanocyte, a specialized cell that imparts color to the skin and its appendages, embryologic derivation is by way of the neural crest ectoderm. The outermost layer of the skin is cellular and is called the epidermis; it is ectodermal in origin. The dermis, which is made up of matrix and fibers, underlies the epidermis and is mesodermal in origin. The two tissues interact as embryologic inductors, with mitosis of the epidermis being initiated by the "epidermal influencing factor," which is thought to be an elaboration of fibroblasts. Inhibition of epidermal cell mitosis is brought about from within the epidermis itself via the "epidermal chalone." The epidermis itself is separated from the dermis by a microscopic structure called the basal lamina, which is trilamellar and made up of both dermal and epidermal components.

The Epidermis

The epidermis is composed of four layers, which are in general committed to the process of keratinization: The strata basale, spinosum, granulosum, and corneum. The stratum lucidum described in earlier textbooks is now considered to be an artifact.

The stratum basale, the deepest layer, rests directly upon the basement membrane and the dermis proper. It consists of a single layer of high cuboidal cells with a dominant nucleus and nucleolus. The cytoplasm of these cells contains relatively few subcellular organelles or inclusions (Fig. 18-2).

The stratum spinosum is variably thick in the foot. It may be only two or three cells thick in the intertriginous spaces, but is commonly 20 or 30 cells thick in such dense regions as the heel and ball of the foot. The spinosal layer is progressively flattened as the free surface of the foot is approached. The longest dimension of both the cell and its now attenuating nucleus orients in parallel with the

The human integument is among the most physiologically complex of body structures. The skin together with its adnexa is the largest organ of the body.[2] It is not surprising, then, that many medical specialists in addition to dermatologists have great concern for the condition of the skin and examine it with great care and attention. Indeed, the skin may be considered to be a mirror of the patient's general state of health.

The skin of the human foot is subject to special stresses in terms of utilization, susceptibility to trauma, changes in nutritional status, and exposure to an often hostile environment.[3] Improper shoes and hosiery and poor hygiene either initiate or exacerbate many dermatologic foot conditions. Inherited and congenital factors can also predispose to podiatric dermatologic disorders.

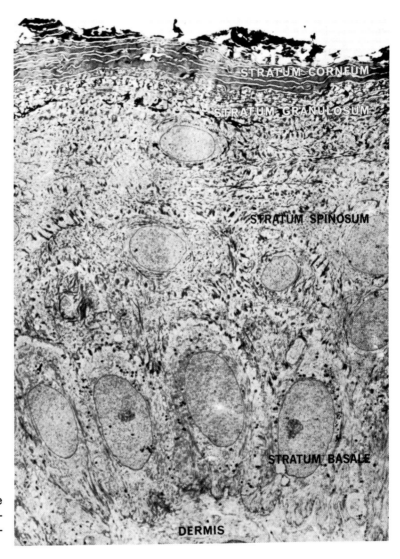

Fig. 18-2. Microscopic structure of the human skin. (From Zelickson A: Ultrastructure of Normal and Abnormal Skin, with permission.)

outer surface of the skin. The stratum spinosum is so called because electron-dense hemidesmosomes come together at tight junctions between keratinocytes. These clumps give the appearance of spines under light microscopy, but it is incorrect to say that intercellular bridges exist. Tonofilaments make their appearance in the stratum spinosum; these subcellular structures have important roles in keratinization.[2]

The stratum granulosum is so called because of microscopic clumps of keratohyaline, which give the cell a dense basophilic granular appearance.

These bodies become intimately associated with tonofilaments as part of the process of keratinization. Granulosum cells are quite flat, and their nuclei frequently bulge beyond the attenuated boundaries of the cell's cytoplasm. The number of cell layers that comprise the stratum granulosum may vary from one or two to four or five depending upon the location. The thickness of this layer is directly proportional to the degree of keratinization at the location involved.[3]

The stratum corneum is the outermost layer of epidermal cells. Its thickness also varies greatly according to its location. At the heel, for example, this layer is very thick, whereas on the dorsum of the foot it is quite thin. Nuclei and subcellular organelles are not normally seen in the stratum corneum. The intercellular spaces are periodic acid-Schiff (PAS) positive and wide, and the cells are stacked in basket-weave formation in this stratum. The cytoplasm of the stratum corneum is proteinaceous and sulfur rich. Its fibrous component is relatively sulfur poor.

Rete ridges are epidermal extensions of the epidermis, which extend finger-like into the dermis below.[2]

Special terminology is used to describe diseases of the skin. For example, hyperkeratosis is an abnormal thickening of the stratum corneum. Parakeratosis is the occurrence of nuclear remnant extending upward through the stratum corneum. Acanthosis is an abnormal thickening of the cellular layer of the epidermis, whereas acantholysis is the separation of cell layers within the stratum spinosum. Hypergranulosis and agranulosis refer to thickening or loss, respectively, of layers of the stratum granulosum.[3]

The Dermis

The dermis is that portion of the skin that underlies the epidermis and overlies the fibrofatty layer known as subcutaneous tissue. The dermis consists of a matrix, which is a PAS-positive mucopolysaccharide formed as one of the elaborations of the fibroblast. The fibroblast is also responsible for the biosynthesis of the fibrillar constituents of the dermis. These include reticular, elastic, and collagenic fibers, of which the last-named is the most widespread.[4]

The dermis is said to be composed of two portions. The pars papillaris is that part of the dermis which interdigitates and surrounds the rete pegs of the epidermis. It tends to have less density than deeper portions of the dermis. The pars reticularis is the deeper part of the dermis, which overlies the subcutaneous tissues and connects with the pars papillaris. It is said to be more fibrillar and has a more dense matrix than does the papillary dermis.[2]

The dermis contains a number of cell types. The fibroblast is native to this mesodermal tissue. This cell appears spindle shaped at the light microscopic level, but transmission electron microscopy reveals it as stellate. Its many subcellular organelles, including rough endoplasmic reticulum, Golgi apparatus, free ribosomes, and pinocytotic vesicles indicate that this cell is biosynthetically active. The pleomorphic nucleus also attests to this fact. Fibroblasts synthesize and excrete the dermal matrix and fibers, contribute to repair of the skin, and influence the epidermis in its replicative activities.[3] Other cells can also be identified within the dermis that migrate in response to physiologic and pathologic changes. These have significance in the diagnosis of disease. Basophils, eosinophils, neutrophils, and lymphocytes may be seen in greater and lesser numbers in the dermis. Histiocytes, giant cells, and certain tumor cells are among the numerous cells that can be identified microscopically in biopsies of skin tissue.[2]

Many exhaustive dermatologic and histologic textbooks provide a more complete discussion of cutaneous anatomy. Attention is drawn to the adnexa of skin as well. The structure and function of the hair, nails, sebaceous, and sudiferous glands are complex and need to be understood when these structures are involved in dermatologic conditions of the foot and leg.

CIRCUMSCRIBED SKIN HYPERPLASIAS

Helomata and Tylomata

Heloma and tyloma (corns and calluses) are aggregations of hyperkeratotic skin on the human foot. The acute and chronic pain produced by their presence was one of the principal causes of the emergence and success of podiatric medicine over a century ago.

Heloma

Heloma durum (hard corn) is a circumscribed area of hyperkeratotic tissue that occurs over bony prominences of the proximal and distal interphalangeal joints of the toes.[5] The region of hypertrophic stratum corneum is usually conical in shape, with the apex pointed downward so as to produce pain as the delicate sensory nerve endings are impinged upon.[6] Occasionally, heloma durum occurs deeper about the periphery, with a relatively atrophic center. The formation of an adventitious bursa in association with heloma durum is not uncommon, and small perineural fibromas are also an occasional finding.

In addition to hyperkeratosis and parakeratosis, microscopic examination of heloma durum biopsies usually demonstrates hypergranulosis, and acanthosis is a constant finding.[7] Elongation and hypertrophy of the epidermal rete pegs are also typical of this lesion.[8] Inflammatory infiltrates are usually lymphocytic in nature.

Heloma durum forms over pressure points of bony prominences, which are often hypertrophic and/or irregular, and arthritis and fixed deformity may occur at these locations as well (Fig. 18-3). Definitive treatment involves resection of appro-

priate portions of the offending bony involvement; most often, arthroplasty for resection of all or part of a phalangeal head is indicated.[3] Conservative care involves palliative reduction of the offending hyperkeratotic tissues. Adjunctive padding and dressings offer additional relief. Permanent shields of Latex or similar material made to a plaster of paris cast are especially useful in cases where surgery is inadvisable.[3]

Heloma molle (soft corn) is so named because of its macerated nature, resulting from moisture accumulations between the toes, where these lesions typically occur. The interdigital space between the fourth and fifth toes is the most common site of occurrence, as the fibular aspect of the base of the proximal phalanx of the fourth digit impinges upon the tibial aspect of the head of the proximal phalanx of the fifth toe.

Heloma miliare (seed corn) is a small, hyperkeratotic plug of tissue not related to bone. It may be due to focal irritation from footwear, but may also be associated with xerosis or similar dry skin conditions.[3]

Heloma vasculare is similar in many respects to heloma durum except that small blood vessels are pinched off into the heloma proper. They may bleed profusely when cut.[3]

Heloma neurovasculare resembles heloma durum and heloma vasculare except that nerve endings accompany the pinched-off blood vessels. The central portions of such lesions may be somewhat spongy, and they tend to be exquisitely tender.[3]

Porokeratosis Plantaris Discreta

Porokeratosis plantaris discreta is a plantar foot lesion that, like heloma, consists of a sharply circumscribed skin growth. The lesions are often exquisitely tender but are not associated with bony prominences. Earlier theories identified obstructed glandular ducts as producing these peculiar lesions. However, controversy has endured over many years regarding this point.

Tyloma

Tyloma or callus resembles heloma histologically in most respects. The stratum granulosum can be seen to be interrupted at some points.[9] Tyloma can

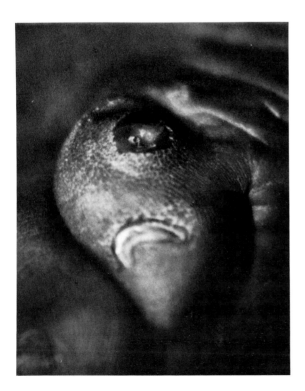

Fig. 18-3. Heloma durum at the proximal interphalangeal joint.

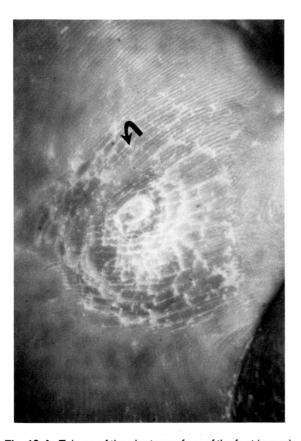

Fig. 18-4. Tyloma of the plantar surface of the foot (arrow).

occur anywhere on the foot where intermittent pressure is a problem, but it is most common over all or portions of the skin of the plantar aspects of the metatarsophalangeal joints (Fig. 18-4). Wherever special pressures may occur over a particular metatarsal head, a cornlike structure known as an intractable plantar keratosis (**IPK**) may develop. These lesions develop in response to increased weight-bearing demands to a particular area. These nucleated lesions are usually conical, with the apex pointed toward the bony prominence with which they are related. These lesions are associated most often with hypertrophy or hyperdeclination of the metatarsals or with interruption of the regular and normal geometric configuration of the metatarsal parabola.

Painful IPK may respond to surgical intervention.[3] Dorsiflexory wedge osteotomies, metatarsal head resections, and plantar condylectomies of the involved metatarsals are employed along with other procedures to correct the underlying structural faults involved in the formation of plantar callosities.

Tylomata of the forefoot are complex lesions. They are often the result of biomechanical faults involving the rearfoot or midfoot as well as the forefoot. Therefore, orthopedic correction using balanced inlays or functional orthoses may be required. Palliative reduction of calluses and padding and shielding of lesions are also beneficial.

In recent times, the use of shock-absorbing implants or injections of collagenic materials has been suggested. The interposition of such materials is intended to replace the fat pad and absorb shock at the points of overtraumatization of the plantar aspects of the involved metatarsophalangeal joints.

Clearly, the biomechanical implications of tyloma and even heloma are complex and beyond the scope of this dermatologically oriented discussion.

Verrucae

Verruca plantaris and verruca vulgaris are warty epidermal growths affecting the plantar surface of the foot as well as other pedal skin surfaces. These neoplasms are infectious acanthomas caused by an epidermotrophic DNA virus. The human papovavirus is immediately recognizable by transmission electron microscopy as having 72 individual capsomeres arranged in a skewed fashion in icosahedral form.[10] Although the papilloma virus appears to be morphologically constant, over 30 different serotypes exist. These different viruses tend to show different tissue specificities.

Verruca plantaris is a common podiatric presentation. They occur with great frequency among teenagers, often in epidemic proportions. The virus apparently penetrates the skin in association with some form of trauma and becomes an obligate parasite within individual keratinocytes.[3] Single lesions appear on the plantar surface of the foot as well-delineated, circumscribed lesions, which are painful upon lateral pressure. Such lesions are usually well covered with a layer of whitish-yellow hyperkeratotic and parakeratotic stratum corneum. When this layer is pared or débrided, the more spongy verruca proper is identified with its characteristic pinpoint bleeding.[3] Verruca vulgaris is not always associated with hyperkeratosis. It can occur almost anywhere on the foot—periungually, on the dorsum or interdigital areas of the toes, or elsewhere (Fig. 18-5). In such cases, judgment must be exercised in order to make the correct diagnosis. Many lesions such as pyogenic granuloma, arsenical keratosis, and amelanotic melanoma among others must be excluded. For these and other reasons, questionable lesions should be biopsied.

Biopsy at the light microscopic level demonstrates hyperkeratosis, parakeratosis, and inclusion bodies, which can be seen streaming outward through the stratum corneum. The stratum granulosum can be thickened peripherally, but is usually reduced and even interrupted in central parts of the lesions. The stratum spinosum frequently gives evidence of dyskeratotic changes, and focal vesiculation is common within these cells.[11]

The dermoepidermal interface is markedly altered in verrucae. Rete ridges are markedly elongated and centripetally oriented as if to converge upon a central point. The dermis demonstrates many small-caliber blood vessels, which ramify through the verrucae proper. Scanning electron microscopy of the dermoepidermal interface reveals that the verrucae are dome shaped in their three-dimensional structure. There is usually a central point at which an arteriole enters the lesion, and tiny venules exit the growth at various points about the periphery.[12]

Mosaic verrucae are a particularly difficult problem. Numerous satellite verrucae are seen disseminated about the original wart. These tend to coalesce into an extensive lesion of irregular depth and outline. Montgomery advises periodic applications of bichloroacetic acid to the more active points within mosaic verrucae and the use of 40 percent salicylic acid plaster to cover the entire extent of the lesion.[3] Normal contiguous skin should be shielded from the acid's action. The lesion is débrided and re-treated at regular intervals of 5 to 7 days. Care should be exercised that tissues do not become devitalized during the course of treatment.

There can be no doubt that suppression of the immune system to any degree adversely affects the outcome of pedal verrucae. The emergence of verrucae is a common finding in AIDS patients, who are severely immunologically compromised. Such lesions completely defy treatment. Lesser degrees of resistance to therapy are noted in some podiatric patients, and particularly among the older population.

Psychotherapy in various forms has been useful in treating verrucae. Posthypnotic suggestions and painting of lesions with otherwise innocuous substances are methods that have proved beneficial.

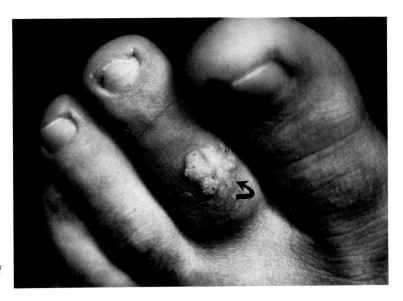

Fig. 18-5. Verrucae on the dorsal aspect of the second toe (arrow).

The application of intense cold by means of carbon dioxide ice or liquid nitrogen is a frequent treatment choice.[3] Electrodesiccation and currettage are established therapeutic modalities, as is negative galvanism.[13] The use of the carbon dioxide laser has become popular in more recent times. Ultrasound, irradiation, steroids, vitamins, and proteolytic enzymes have been useful in some cases.

A time-honored treatment for solitary verruca plantaris involves the palliative débridement of the tissues and application of one or two keratolytic acids. Aqueous solutions of monochloroacetic acid and 60 percent salicylic acid in ointment form are most commonly selected. The lesion is demarcated with protective shieldings of ⅛-inch adhesive felt and covered with an adhesive bandage. Débridement and re-treatment on a periodic basis are continued until the lesion is resolved.[3]

Surgical excision of well-demarcated lesions is an excellent treatment plan.[3] The region of involvement is aseptically prepared, and local anesthesia is obtained by local infiltration. The circumference of the lesion is sharply incised using a scalpel or tissue nippers to the level of the dermoepidermal interface. The lesion is then shelled out in toto using a correspondingly sized curette. Any small residual amounts of verrucous tissue are lightly cauterized by laser, fulguration, or chemocautery.[3]

Nevi

Nevi, commonly referred to as moles, are benign pigmented lesions of the skin. They normally appear after birth as proliferative aggregates of melanocytes or nevocytes which are morphologically normal.[1] Such lesions are characterized as either epidermal, junctional, compound, or intradermal. Halo and blue nevi are special variants of this general classification. A number of other, rarer types also exist. These include apocrine, connective tissue, eccrine, giant hairy, pigmented hair, pigmented giant, sebaceous, spider, strawberry, and vascular nevi.

Nevi appear variably as flat or slightly elevated, verrucoid, polypoid, dome shaped, and papillomatous lesions.[3] Sessile and halo characteristics may further modify their appearance. Nevi may be im-

possible to differentiate from lentigo in its various forms on the basis of clinical appearance alone.[1] Nevi need also to be differentiated from dermatofibroma, melanocytoma, histiocytoma, and minute forms of Kaposi's sarcoma.

Epithelial nevi are rare integumentary lesions. Jadassohn's sebaceous nevi are rare midline growths and are not likely to be a podiatric problem. They characteristically demonstrate yellowish unctuous nodules with granular, pitted surfaces.[1] Such lesions have the potential for malignant transformation into basal cell carcinomas. Patients with these lesions present at birth are associated with mental retardation, seizures, and other disorders.

Intradermal or dermal nevi concentrate all their melanocytic nevus cells within the dermis.[14] These cells are characterized as type A when they are seen uppermost in the dermis. They demonstrate abundant cytoplasm and much pigment. Cells of type C have neuron-like features, little pigment, and a clearer cytoplasm. They are observed deep within the dermis. Type B cells are intermediate in appearance. Dermal nevi occur in orderly nests and strands, and the epidermis is normal.[1]

Junctional nevi demonstrate nests above the basement membrane.[15] Melanocytes can be seen clustered within the epidermis proper.

Compound nevi demonstrate melanocytes in nests within the epidermis, which frequently is seen to bulge into the dermis. Orderly arrangements of nevus cells may occur as nests or strands within the dermis as well.[1]

Halo nevi are pigmented nevi that develop a peripheral ring of hypopigmentation. An intense inflammatory infiltrate is usually associated with halo nevi. Melanocytes are apparently replaced by Langerhans cells in halo nevi. The appearance of the halo around the nevus usually heralds the eventual disappearance of the nevus.[1]

Blue nevi are pigmented skin lesions with a royal blue to blue-gray coloration. These nevi are elevated nodules of regular outline (Fig. 18-6). Biopsy demonstrates elongated fibroblast-like, pigment-containing cells. They may extend to the papillary dermis from fibrous portions of the reticular dermis where they predominate.[3]

There are typically hundreds of various types of nevi on the human body. Obviously, excisional

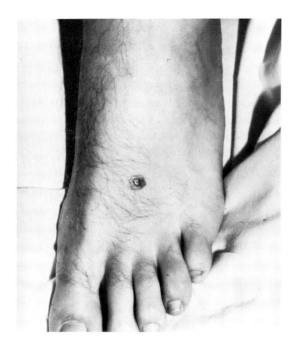

Fig. 18-6. Blue nevus. (Case courtesy of Dr. Laine.) (From McCarthy and Montgomery,[3] with permission.)

biopsy for all of these lesions is not warranted or practical. However, any pigmented lesion about which there is any question as a result of changes in morphology, coloration, tendency to bleed, or other changes should be subjected to excisional biopsy.[16] Shave biopsy and tissue-destructive approaches such as fulguration are contraindicated, since definitive microscopic examination is impossible.

HYPERHIDROSIS AND BROMOHYPERHIDROSIS

Profuse sweating of the feet is termed hyperhidrosis. The condition is not particularly associated with heat, although feet so affected often experience a burning sensation. Anxiety and stressful situations are frequently etiologic. Vasomotor instability and tachycardia can be found in many patients.

Hyperhidrosis is not a result of morphologic alterations in the sweat glands. There is little doubt that man-made materials used in the manufacture of shoes and hosiery contribute to the severity of the condition.

Bromohyperhidrosis occurs when the by-products of interactions between perspiration and bacteria cause the foot to be malodorous.[17] The foot often assumes a "galded" appearance, and the sock linings of shoes often rot away. Bromohyperhidrosis causes much social embarrassment, and for this reason patients seek professional help.

Obviously, advice concerning strict personal hygiene and proper care of footwear should be provided. Insoles containing charcoal granules are said to absorb perspiration and arrest the attendant odor. Commercially available foot powders may be of some assistance in milder cases.

Vasomotor conditions are associated with hyperhidrosis and may be treated with systemic or topical anticholinergic drugs.[18] However, side effects such as dryness of the mouth may be objectionable when the drugs are used systemically. Five percent diphemanil methylsulfate in a cream base (Prantal Cream) is a topical anticholinergic that might prove useful. Tranquilizing drugs may be of use in the management of anxiety when this state of mind produces vasomotor responses leading to hyperhidrosis.

Electrophoresis of aqueous aluminum or sodium chloride has been useful in more severe cases of hyperhidrosis. Fifteen to twenty-five percent zirconyl chloride or aluminum chloride in absolute alcohol can be used for topical application along with aqueous-alcoholic solutions with formalin, glutaraldehyde, and tannic acid.

VESICULOBULLOUS LESIONS

Eczema

Inflammatory responses of the skin to many endogenous and exogenous stimuli is given the general name of eczematous dermatitis.[1] Spongiosis is the histopathologic hallmark of eczematous dermatitis.[2] Eczematous dermatitis should be differentiated from the broader category of dermatitis.

Exogenous agents that induce eczematous dermatitis include dermatophytes (see section on "Dermatophytosis and Atopic Diseases"), infectious drainage, radiation- or light-induced causes, and chemical agents alone or in combination with photoallergic stimuli. Endogenous agents include drug eruption, products of fungal metabolism, and autosensitization by epidermal or exogenous products absorbed from sites of eczematous dermatitis.[1]

Areas of edema and erythema with minute vesicles of nonumbilicated clusters characterize acute eczematous dermatitis. Encrustations result from serum exudates of lesions. Chronic cases are characterized by lichenification.

Histopathologic findings in eczematous dermatitis are equivocal. Certainly, spongiosis or intercellular edema of the epidermis is a constant finding. Such regions coalesce to form vesicles of varying size. These lesions are suprabasilar. Chronic eczema presents a lymphocytic infiltrate of the dermis along with a nonspecific epidermal hyperplasia.

Acute phases of eczema are best treated initially with astringent antiseptic wet dressings. Corticosteroids, tar derivatives, and hydroxyquinoline are useful as the acute phase subsides. The itch-scratch cycle must be interrupted, and cold packs may be of assistance in this regard. Antihistamines may be useful systemically, but oral or parenteral corticosteroids are contraindicated.

Nummular eczematous dermatitis occurs most frequently on the lower extremities, although it is not restricted to this location. It is characterized by typical coin-shaped lesions composed of minute vesicles and papules, which tend to coalesce. Discrete patches may exhibit a central clearing. Acute lesions are characterized by exudation and encrustation; chronic lesions exhibit scaling and lichenification.

The etiology of nummular eczema is uncertain, but dryness and bacteria are most commonly implicated. Treatment emphasis is placed on the use of emollients and corticosteroids for their moisturizing and anti-inflammatory effects.[19] Pruritus in extensive involvements may require bed rest and sedation.

Contact Dermatitis

Podiatric practitioners frequently encounter cases of allergic eczematous contact dermatitis. Cutaneous eruptions are the results of sensitization by contact with specific allergens. Acute clinical presentations are characterized by varying degrees of erythema and papulovesicular lesions.[1] Lichenification and epidermal thickening are associated with more chronic stages of the disease. Areas of hypopigmentation or hyperpigmentation may also occur.[2]

In the early stages, contact dermatitis is directly associated with the site of exposure to the allergen (Fig. 18-7). The occurrence and severity of contact dermatitis affecting the lower extremities relate to the nature of the skin involved. The variable thickness of the skin, inclination to perspiration, friction, and/or pressure can influence the degree to which the skin manifests the dermatitis. For example, the thin skin of the dorsum of the foot is more prone to react to the dyes in hosiery than other, thicker skinned areas of the foot.

The distribution of the initial eruption on the foot often corresponds to the placement of the offending materials within the shoe.[3] Balance inlays with an allergen such as tannic acid may present an outline that mirrors the dermatitis on the plantar surface of the foot, with the medial longitudinal arch most affected. If contact dermatitis is treated ineffectively or left untreated, it may extend well beyond the region of initial involvement.[20]

Exanthematic and vesicular eruptions of the feet may be a form of systemic reactivity to contact allergens. Such a dermatitis can be wrongfully identified as a dyshidrotic eruption. These symptoms may occur following ingestion of small amounts of allergen. Anaphylactic manifestations associated with IgE-mediated systemic reaction seldom if ever occur.[1] Reference is made to the human leukocyte antigen system (HLA) in the discussion of atopy to follow. This material should be reviewed as it pertains to allergic sensitivity reactions in general.[21]

The diagnosis of contact dermatitis is made by careful history and physical examination. Patch testing is invaluable as a diagnostic tool. At this writing, kits prepared by Hollister-Stier Laboratories and Trolab of Denmark are restricted because

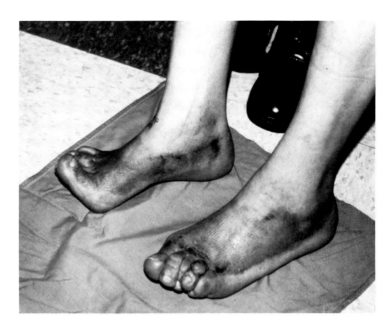

Fig. 18-7. Contact dermatitis as it may occur on the foot. (Case courtesy of Dr. L. Levy.) (From McCarthy and Montgomery,[3] with permission.)

of Food and Drug Administration concern over possible carcinogenesis.

In practice, one may take a suspected allergen for direct application to normal skin, usually the back or the arms, where the material is placed under a semiocclusive dressing. Materials from shoes or hosiery have been used in this manner. Patches are left in situ for 24 to 48 hours and interpreted 30 minutes after removing the dressing. Erythema is noted as a grade 1 response, and marked edema and/or vesicle formation constitutes the grade 4 response; grades 2 and 3 are intermediate.[3]

Skin biopsies may be of assistance in diagnosis as well. Perivascular round cell and histiocytic infiltrates may be present in the dermis. Vesiculation and the formation of fluid-filled spaces within the epidermis follow intercellular edema. Fibrin deposition within the reticular dermis, luminal narrowing in the microvasculature, and intradermal eosinophilia occur in later phases of contact dermatitis.

The obvious treatment for contact dermatitis is the expeditious removal of the offending allergenic material.[22] Symptomatic treatment in the form of conventional antipruritic and anti-inflammatory medications is usually indicated for contact dermatitis. Oral administration of antihistamines can be useful, and systemic corticosteroids may be considered in severe cases. Sedatives may also be indicated on a short-term basis in contact dermatitis.

Seborrheic Dermatitis

Dermatitis associated with oily or waxy conditions of the skin is called seborrheic dermatitis. Cholesterol and triglycerides are increased at the skin surface level, but actual serum fat levels usually remain normal. Histologically, seborrheic dermatitis may demonstrate accentuation of epidermal rete ridges, acanthosis, hyperkeratosis, and psoriasiform changes. Spongiosis and parakeratosis are usual epidermal findings.[1]

Seborrheic dermatitis is rare in the foot. Pityriasis rubra pilaris gives the appearance of seborrheic dermatitis, but is differentiated from it by the presence of papules and thickening of the skin of the sole of the foot.

Topical corticosteroids or tar preparations are useful for seborrheic dermatitis as anti-inflammatory and antipruritic agents. Keratolytic agents are employed to control scaling of the skin. Most cases of seborrheic dermatitis are self-limiting and will clear with time.

Drug-Induced Dermatitis

Adverse reactions to drugs are becoming an increasingly important medical problem with podiatric implications. In many instances, the skin is the responding organ to the sensitization process. In addition to the rash and itching, nausea, vomiting, diarrhea, drowsiness, drug fever, arrhythmias, and hyperkalemia may occur.[1] Women experience more drug reactions involving the skin than do men. Exanthematous or morbilliform rashes or hives along with pruritus are most commonly observed. Changes in epidermal pigmentation have also been associated with drug sensitivities.[23] Other lesions observed include acneform eruptions, alopecia, epidermal necrolysis, erythema multiforme, erythema nodosum, fixed drug eruptions, lichenoid skin changes, lupus erythematosus symptoms, photosensitive reactions, pigmentary skin changes, porphyria, and urticarial, vasculitic, and vesiculobullous lesions.

Antimetabolites such as 5-fluorouracil and methotrexate and most other metabolite-modifying drugs as well as most antibiotics demonstrate skin-reactive sensitization capabilities.[24,25] Alkylating agents, nitrosurea, vinca alkaloids, and a variety of common chemotherapeutic agents can produce drug sensitivity reactions.[1]

The pathogenesis of drug-induced eczema includes immunologic reactions, which are IgE-dependent or cell-mediated or cytotoxic responses. Some reactions are immune complex dependent. Alternatively, drug reactions that have a nonimmunologic basis involve activation of effector pathways. Drug interactions, overdosage, and cumulative toxicity must be considered along with the possibilities of side effects and environmental factors such as those involving photosensitivity.[1] Adverse reactions to drugs do not always occur immediately when the skin is the "shock organ." Such reactions may take up to a week to appear.

Treatment plans for adverse cutaneous reactions to drugs mandate immediate removal of the involved medication. Indeed, all drugs not absolutely essential to the patient's well-being need to be eliminated initially. Local and systemic medications employed for adverse drug reactions are essentially the same as for other eczematous conditions. Systemic corticosteroids are frequently employed, but their efficacy has not been well established.[1]

SCALING SKIN CONDITIONS

Lichen Planus

Violaceous, angular scaling, flat-topped, glistening papules are the characteristic lesions of lichen

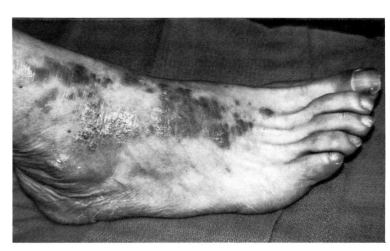

Fig. 18-8. Lichen planus as it may occur on the foot. (Case courtesy of Dr. Sander.) (From McCarthy and Montgomery,[3] with permission.)

planus. This condition involves the feet as well as the genitalia, the mucous membranes, and the flexor surfaces of the body (Fig. 18-8). Males and females are equally affected.[1] The etiology of the condition is unknown, but viral, immunologic, neurologic, and emotional factors have been cited.

The transparent, scaly lesion of lichen planus may demonstrate Wickham's striae, which are delicate networks of white lines or punctata. Localization of lichen planus on the soles of the feet is unusual, and lesions there may be of a more atypical appearance.[26] Scratching may induce the formation of new lesions. Occasionally hypopigmentation may occur, but hyperpigmentation is more characteristic of healed lesions.

Ungual involvement of lichen planus is heralded by flaking of tissues below the cuticle. Longitudinal splitting as well as ridges and grooves can be seen affecting the nail plate. Brownish discoloration, friability, and eventually onycholysis of the involved nails are later changes.

Biopsy of papules in lichen planus reveals thickening of the stratum granulosum along with degeneration and possible separation of the dermoepidermal junction. Subepidermal bullae may also be formed. Hyperkeratosis occurs in the presence of epidermal atrophy. The dermal infiltrate may be heavy and is composed of lymphocytes and histiocytes. Such infiltrates are sharply marginated and organize in close association with the epidermis.[2] The differential diagnosis includes psoriasis, localized neurodermatitis, cutaneous amyloidosis, and certain unusual presentations of Kaposi's sarcoma.

Treatment for lichen planus may be frustrating for both patient and physician. Spontaneous remission usually occurs within 8 to 12 months, however.[1] Regression of hypertrophic lichen planus lesions can be accelerated with corticosteroid preparations under occlusion. Intralesional injections of steroids have been of value, and triamcinolone has been employed where the nail matrix has become involved. Broad-spectrum antibiotics, heavy metals including arsenicals, antimalarials, vaccines, and vitamins have been employed in the treatment of lichen planus, but their efficacy has not been well established. The use of physical medicine in the form of x-ray and ultraviolet light has been prescribed on occasion.

Systemic administration of oral corticosteroids for limited periods (2 to 6 weeks) can be of use in acute or widespread disease. Griseofulvin was used and found beneficial in a British study.[1] Oral use of 8-methoxypsoralen in conjunction with ultraviolet light is still another approach to therapy. Symptomatic dermatologic care is employed adjunctively with these systemic approaches in the treatment of lichen planus.[1]

Psoriasis

Psoriasis is probably a genetic disorder controlled in part by environmental factors.[27] It is characterized by discrete erythematous papules and plaques. Characteristic silvery scales are typical in this most chronic of skin diseases. The nails may be involved in the erythematous scaling condition, in association with varying degrees of skin inflammation. Psoriatic arthritis is an unpleasant manifestation of the disease. Arthropathies often affect the distal interphalangeal joints.[1] The palms and soles of the feet are often involved with pustule formation, the exudates of which are sterile.

Skin biopsies in psoriasis reveal focal lymphocytic infiltrates in the papillary dermis. Dermal papillae proliferate upward into the epidermal region as the condition progresses.[2] A sevenfold increase of the dermoepidermal plane is accomplished by such extensions. This is reflected by increases in the equal number of cells making up the stratum basale of the epidermis. Along with this greatly increased area, individual cell mitosis is greatly increased within the epidermis in psoriasis.[28] Epidermal cell turnover time shortens from 5 days to only 2 days. In psoriasis, germinativum cell reproduction occurs every 37.5 hours, as compared to every 152 hours in normal skin.

Further biopsy findings include acanthosis and elongation of the rete ridges. The bases of all rete ridges are at an essentially constant level relative to that noted in the normal adjacent epidermis. There is therefore a relative reduction in the thickness of the involved psoriatic epidermis. Mitotic activity is augmented, and this phenomenon may even include fibroblasts and endothelial cells of the upper dermis. Accelerated cell transit time within the epidermis involved in psoriasis is responsible for the hyperkeratosis and parakeratosis observed. The stratum granulosum may be reduced or even focally absent within psoriatic lesions.

Polymorphonuclear leukocytes may invade the epidermis proper in psoriasis, whereas the round cell infiltrates remain typically confined to the dermis. Spongiosis, spongiform pustules, and subcorneal microabscesses (of Monro) are common to psoriatic skin.[2] Macroabscesses form from these microabscesses so as to literally lift off large sheets of cornified epidermis.[1]

The differential diagnosis in psoriasis should include such psoriasiform diseases as exfoliative dermatitis of various types, seborrheic dermatitis, and drug reactions of the skin.

Psoriasis exhibits the Koebner reaction, wherein psoriatic lesions arise at the sites of trauma. Such trauma may include excoriations, occupational exposures, exposure to sunlight, and (of podiatric interest) the application of adhesive tape.[1]

The course and prognosis of psoriasis are unpredictable except for its chronicity. Treatment is geared to the exacerbations that characterize the disease. PUVA, or the combined use of long-wave ultraviolet light and orally administered 8-methoxypsoralen in the controlled hospital setting, has proven beneficial.[29,30] The careful use of ultraviolet light alone has also proven helpful. The Goeckerman regimen combines ultraviolet light with daily applications of tar preparations used early in the treatment.

1,8,9-Trihydroxyanthracene (dithranol, trade name Anthralin) in 0.1 to 0.4 percent concentrations in zinc oxide paste may resolve plaques when applied twice daily. This and other intensive topical treatments are sometimes available at special day care centers.

Chemotherapeutic drugs have been employed in the treatment of psoriasis. Methotrexate is a systemic antimetabolite, and hydroxyurea inhibits DNA production.[1] They therefore reduce mitotic activity within the epidermis. However, these medications may produce serious side effects such as liver and renal failure or blood cell abnormalities. Their administration should be restricted to those especially qualified in their use.

DERMATOPHYTOSIS AND ATOPIC DISEASES

Infection of the skin and its adnexa by keratinophilic fungi is termed dermatophytosis. Tinea pedis is caused by *Trichophyton* and *Microsporum* species that involve the skin and nails, as well as *Epidermophyton* species that involve the skin.[3] The symptomatology and appearance of the clinical dermatophytoses are variable (Fig. 18-9). Treatment of such conditions is often difficult and frustrating because of recurrent or secondary infection as well as the devitalization of the skin of the foot that results from the chronic nature of the condition.

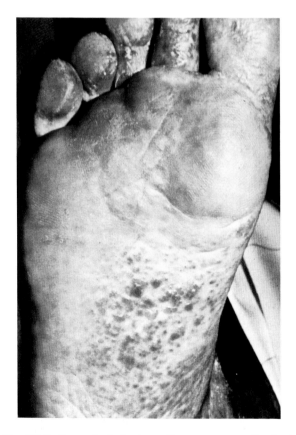

Fig. 18-9. Dermatophytosis as it may occur on the foot. (Case courtesy of Dr. Abramson.) (From McCarthy and Montgomery,[3] with permission.)

Dermatophytes are ubiquitous in the environment, and reinfection is common. This situation relates to poor hygiene and the tenacious presence of the organisms within shoes and hosiery. The warmth and moisture of skin encased within incubator-like footwear promote initial and recurrent dermatophytosis.

Trichophyton mentagrophytes is a common offender in infections of the interdigital area and is most frequently associated with athlete's foot. On hairless (glabrous) skin surfaces, it tends to involve large areas, forming flaky, ichthyosiform, ringworm-like lesions. In culture it is cottony and white or yellow with a flat surface. There is also a granular-appearing variety.[31]

Trichophyton rubrum is a variable, highly adaptable organism and is frequently implicated in mixed infections. It is most commonly found on the human foot but spreads easily to other regions. The clinical presentation is that of uninflamed diffuse or circinate scaling.[1] Such infections tend to be highly pruritic. Culture characteristics include a fluffy white surface type of growth with a red, nondiffusible pigment on the reverse side.[31] Some *T. rubrum* infections extend into the dermis so as to produce granulomatous lesions.[1]

Microsporum audouinii is most commonly seen in hairy regions such as the scalp and is relatively rare on the feet. The primary lesion is a red, round spot, which enlarges to become more pale and scaly. Cultures of *M. audouinii* present a cream-to-brown silky surface. Growth is slow and the color sometimes reddish-brown on the reverse surface.

Microsporum gypseum is most commonly associated with the scalp and is characteristically suppurative.[1] Such infections run an acute course. In culture, *M. gypseum* grows rapidly to produce a tan, powdery surface.

Epidermophyton floccosum involves other body locations as well as the foot. Its clinical appearance varies depending on the location infected. It is one of the most common offenders in athlete's foot. Lesions may appear fawn-colored or brown and scaly. It may mimic erythrasma, but it does not glow in Wood's light.

Culture characteristics vary for *E. floccosum*. Surfaces may be velvety, powdery, or fluffy and may be flat or folded. Surface coloration ranges from tan to olive-green, with reverse surfaces appearing tan to yellowish.

Candida albicans is not a true fungus but is classified as a yeast.[31] It favors moist surfaces such as the mouth and the vagina, although it may well involve the feet and toenails. It frequently involves the interdigital spaces.[1] Lesions may be pustular or ulcerative, and keratotic plaques sometimes occur.

In culture, *Candida* species produce opaque, cream-colored, raised colonies. Pseudo- and true hyphae as well as chlamydospores can be identified.[32]

Human Leukocyte Antigen System in Dermatophytosis and Other Skin Diseases

Measurable genetic traits are now known to affect the susceptibility to disease in general. Daussett discovered a system called the human leukocyte antigen (HLA) system in 1950. However, the importance of this system did not become fully realized until he received the Nobel prize in 1980.[33] Since the 1950s a number of diseases have been found to be related to the HLA genetic factors. These conditions include ankylosing spondylitis, which is known to be associated with HLA-B27 as well as other rheumatic, chronic inflammatory, and aberrant immunologic diseases.[34]

The human major histocompatibility complex (MHC) system is synonymous with the HLA system. The predominant host immune response to a donor's MHC antigen when exposed to foreign cells is graft rejection, as in cases of bone marrow, kidney, or heart transplantation. Therefore, the HLA system plays a major role in effecting transplant reactions as well as in predicting patients at risk for chronic rheumatic, inflammatory, and immunologic diseases.

Human chromosome 6 contains the genes of the HLA system. There are four identified gene loci, designated as HLA-A, -B, -C, and -D. Each HLA gene locus with multiple alleles controls a large number of gene products. There are five loci for HLA on chromosome 6. To date the following series of allelic genes have been identified: 20 HLA-A genes, 42 HLA-B genes, 8 HLA-C genes, 12 HLA-D genes, and 10 HLA-DR genes (DR stands for D-related antigens).[35] Antigens identified as HLA-DR types differ from the other antigens because they are found not only on B cells but also on monocytes, macrophages, and some bone marrow cells. They are not, however, detectable on most T cells. The other HLA antigens are present on the surface of B lymphocytes and are commonly known as B-cell antigens.

Mendelian laws direct the inheritance patterns of the HLA system. Each parent has two haplotypes, and one from each parent is transferred to the child. An HLA haplotype is the specific series of HLA alleles on the chromosome. HLA typing identifies an individual's phenotype. An HLA phenotype is the array of HLA antigens on the cell membrane. When the two haplotypes in a child are known, the child's genotype can be determined.

Relationship of Disease to the HLA System

Two possible mechanisms for the association of HLA and disease have been proposed. In the first hypothesis, HLA as a gene marker links with the immune response gene, which is associated with disease. In the second hypothesis, HLA antigenicity is similar to a virus or other microorganism such as a bacterium or fungus. The disease results because of decreased immunoreactivity toward the invading microorganism when the invader antigen resembles a person's own HLA or other self antigen.[36]

The immune response genes and susceptibility to disease can be explained by the relationship between HLA-DR and the immune response genes. The first report of human disease related to HLA typing was its association with Hodgkin's disease in 1967. Since that time HLA has been related to over 50 skin diseases as well as numerous arthritic and immunologic disorders.[34] This discussion emphasizes the relationship between HLA antigens and atopic diseases. This relationship developed among atopic diseases, genetic predisposition, the immune response system, and serum IgE levels which predispose certain patients to chronic dermatomycosis.

Specific IgE immune responses are associated with certain HLA haplotypes.[37] Human IgE antibody response is also related to the IgE serum level, which itself is controlled by a gene independent of the major histocompatibility locus. Therefore, the genetic control of the reaginic antibody formation is found to involve many separate genes. It is now believed that the synthesis of the immunoglobulin change by one locus acts in concert with a single gene controlling the overall production of the IgE molecules.[38] These two genetic control mechanisms are involved in specific reaginic production.

T and B Lymphocytes in Chronic Dermatophytosis of Genetically Predisposed IgE Atopic Diseases

A delicate balance exists between helper and suppressor subsets of T lymphocytes within normal human immunoregulatory networks. It is well documented that T and B cell function is normally modulated by a complex interaction between helper and suppressor T cells.[39] Overactive suppressor cells have been demonstrated in patients with hypogammaglobulinemia and other acute infectious diseases. Deficiencies in suppressor T cell function have been associated with autoimmune and collagen diseases. Consequently, the regulation of excessive IgE production may be due to an absence or deficiency of suppressor cells. These suppressor cells are T lymphocytes.

Abnormalities of IgE synthesis are associated with patients with atopic disease. T lymphocytes are depressed; therefore, depression of cell-mediated immunity is found as a clinical manifestation of atopy. These patients demonstrate decreased delayed hypersensitivity reactions to a panel of antigens, specifically trichophytin (an extract of *Trichophyton* cultures). Studies of atopics have shown a lack of delayed hypersensitivity reactivity, but an increased immediate hypersensitivity reaction to trichophytin. Studies of patients with chronic tinea pedis infections revealed 66 percent immediate and 33 percent delayed responses to trichophytin. Delayed reactivity to trichophytin in these patients was similar when tested with airborne and dermatophytic antigens other than *T. rubrum*. We can assume that delayed reactivity to trichophytin is related to the resistance to dermatophytic infections, and persons with immediate reactivity to trichophytin are more susceptible.

Individuals who demonstrate chronic tinea pedis or chronic onychomycosis showed a lack of delayed hypersensitivity. However, they frequently had occurrences of immediate hypersensitivity to trichophytin challenge.[40] Persons with longstanding tinea infections showed a higher immediate reactivity and diminished delayed reactivity.

Impaired T cell function must be considered a primary cause of the immunologic disturbances in certain kinds of atopy that are followed by a decreased resistance to dermatophyte infection.[41] This is usually followed by a clinical dermatophyte infection with a chronic course, especially in patients infected with *T. rubrum.*

The activation of B cells so as to produce IgE antibodies against any challenge is yet another mechanism to consider. Such encounters occur during an infection and may precipitate allergic disease. Allergic "breakthrough" may result from a temporary disturbance of the normal regulatory T-suppressor cell-dependent damping mechanisms on IgE sythesis controlled at the genetic level.[41]

Initial infections that occur may be due to a polyclonal B cell activator that results in hyperproduction of IgE and development of allergy in individuals who are genetically predisposed to atopic disease. Consequently, allergic sensitization may occur in individuals with genetically determined T cell deficiency upon allergenic stimulation during certain periods when T cell suppressor activity is unusually low, or the production of IgE by B cells may be increased because of mitogenic stimulation.

Chronic Dermatophytosis as Related to Genetic Atopy

Individuals suffering from hyperglobulin E syndrome usually have recurrent microbial infections, chronic dermatitis, or hyperimmunoglobulin E-associated disease. Patients with this syndrome show associated defects of T cell functions, neutrophil chemotaxis, or neutrophil phagocytosis. Serum inhibitors against lymphocytes or neutrophils inhibiting their function have also been found in patients with this syndrome. Patients present with chronic pedal dermatophytosis and onychomycosis; severe abscesses of the scalp, forehead, groin, and extremities caused by *Staphylococcus aureus;* as well as purulent rhinitis and severe dental caries.[42]

Relationships have recently been noted between atopy and chronic extensive infections from dermatophytes. Severe atopic dermatitis has been more or less constantly associated with generalized *T. rubrum* infection.[40] Jones in 1973 studied dermatophytosis in prison inmates and found that 40 percent harbored chronic extensive dermatophyte infections and were found to be atopic as well.[3] Their atopic manifestations were almost exclusively hay fever or asthma. Chronic dermatophytosis was three times more frequent in those inmates with atopic disease. Approximately 50 percent of patients in one group with chronic *T. rubrum* infection had a history of atopy. Other workers have reported the same frequency.

Specific predisposing factors associated with chronic extensive dermatophytosis include atopy, hay fever, asthma, diabetes mellitus, lymphoma, thymoma, Cushing's syndrome, primary immunodeficiency disease, and use of immunosuppressant medication.[33] The immunosuppression from systemic medications and topical steroids may be observed to heighten susceptibility to fungal infections, including dermatophytosis. These medications suppress the immune response.[42]

Impairment in the function of T-suppressor cells as well as B cells and macrophages leading to an imbalance between suppressor and helper T cells may be responsible for the hyperproduction of IgE.[39] Since the T cells are involved in delayed reactivity, and since delayed reactivity to trichophytin was reduced in patients with atopic disease, one might suspect that a relationship, which may be identified as the atopic-chronic-dermatophytosis syndrome, exists. This is evident in patients with a genetic predisposition for hyperproduction of IgE, as in atopic disease, which is controlled by HLA antigens, which in turn are genetically controlled from chromosome 6.

Patients with atopic-chronic-dermatophytosis are most commonly males with infections that begin during the second decade of life. Infections in patients presenting with clinical dermatophytosis are most commonly caused by *T. rubrum.* The chronic lesion is characterized by pruritus, erythema, scaling, and hyperkeratosis. The initial inflammation is usually intense but diminishes with time. The patient develops a moccasin-type, erythrodermic, hyperkeratotic foot lesion. Palmar and plantar skin surfaces develop painful fissures as well as tinea cruris and onychomycosis. The general description may be that of an exfoliative erythroderma.[43]

Patients with chronic-atopic-dermatophytosis have an increased serum IgE immediate hypersensitivity reaction to trichophytin, but the delayed reaction may be weak or absent.[44] Trichophytin-specific IgE may be identified by the RAST test. The immune responsiveness of the patient shows enhanced synthesis of IgE to trichophytin but failure to express cell-mediated immunity to trichophytin both in vivo and in vitro. There is a positive correlation between cellular immunity to dermatophytes and an intact host defense.

Additionally, there is an associated susceptibility to infection when the cellular immunity to trichophytin is compromised. As the fungal dermatophyte proliferates rapidly through the tissues, the host has little capacity to incite intense inflammation. However, an immunized host expresses cell-mediated immunity to dermatophyte antigen at the site of infection, and the skin becomes intensely inflamed. Development of intense inflammation results in the disappearance of the dermatophyte and subsequent resolution of the infection.[36] This suggests that host defense against dermatophytes requires intact cell-mediated immunity and an intense cutaneous inflammatory response of the delayed type.

Inflammatory changes are intense and may impede fungal invasion by damaging the epidermis and permitting inhibitory plasma factors to access the pathogen. In atopic patients with chronic dermatophyte infection, one finds that the infection is intensely inflamed for only a short period of time. This aborted inflammatory response suggests an altered host immunity, which is reflected in a diminished degree of inflammation.[45] During this period, there is usually a dramatic emergence of immediate hypersensitivity to trichophytin along with a disappearance of delayed hypersensitivity to the same allergen.

Delayed hypersensitivity to trichophytin decreases during the host-parasite interaction. This results in the infected lesions becoming less inflammatory. IgE measured at this point shows an increase in synthesis to the dermatophyte antigen and is found to be central to the defect in host resistance. It is believed that this mechanism predisposes the patient to the atopic-chronic-dermatophytosis syndrome. The basic mechanism includes the role of IgE in immune modulation of T-effector cells.

The mast cell and its complement of pharmacoactive mediators is deeply involved with IgE in the modulation of T-effector cell function in chronic dermatophytosis. During the infective stage of *T. rubrum*, water-soluble trichophytin diffuses into the dermis from the fungus. Trichophytin in the dermis binds specifically to sensitized T cells or specific antibody.[46] Therefore mast cell-fixed antitrichophytin IgE becomes a trigger that activates mast cell secretion of pharmacologic mediators. Histamine released locally would then act on antigen-activated T-effector cells. This in turn prohibits further activation and release of lymphokines or other mediators of inflammation. Histamine would therefore inhibit T-effector cell function and suppress delayed hypersensitivity-mediated inflammatory response.

An important mechanism for in situ immune modulation is the IgE mast cell mediator system. The IgE mast cell mediator modulation mechanism explains the basis of atopic susceptibility to dermatophyte infection as well as the decrease in inflammation concomitant with appearance of trichophytin-specific IgE and the antigen-specific nature of the cell-mediated immune defect.

It is interesting to note that the nonpathogenic molds also contain cross-reacting antigens. Many individuals with asthma and hay fever synthesize IgE early in life in response to inhalation of airborne molds and fungi. Many of these individuals examined for cell-mediated immunity to trichophytin or other antigens of airborne molds do not express cell-mediated responses. They are found to exhibit strong immediate hypersensitivity to airborne molds as well as to trichophytin antigens, but no delayed response. Therefore, although never infected with dermatophytes, these individuals exhibit the immune profile of the atopic-chronic-dermatophytosis syndrome patient.[36]

Sera collected from over 200 podiatrists demonstrated measurable immunologic response following inhalation of nail dust allergens; 30 percent produced high IgE values. Thus, although never infected with dermatophytes, these podiatrists exhibit the immune profile of the atopic-chronic-dermatophytosis syndrome patient. Should the skin of such individuals become infected with a dermatophyte, it logically follows that the cell-mediated immune mechanism would be diminished to trichophytin. Therefore, in the presence of cross-reactive IgE and by the modulation mechanism inhibiting T-effector cells, the delayed reaction would be diminished or inhibited.[47] Such responses result in highly susceptible at-risk patients with regard to fungal infection.[36]

Dermatophytosis causing chronic tinea pedis may be due to a combination of genetic and immunologic factors that limit the body's ability to fight the fungus causing athlete's foot. This discussion has described and identified certain genetic factors in terms of the preponderance of HLA types, which are genetic markers related to tissue rejection as well as genetic components causing persistent infection. This may explain why therapeutic plans are often ineffective when treating certain chronic dermatophytic infections.[42]

A more comprehensive understanding of the genetic predisposition of patients with altered immune mechanisms is needed. The type of genetically predisposed patient just described will present with a persistent resistant chronic dermatophytosis. This situation is difficult to understand and even more difficult to treat. Genetic immune defects of the HLA system appear to be the basic cause of perplexing difficulties associated with treating atopic skin diseases in podiatric medicine.

The reader is referred to Carl Abramson's review of this subject in *Podiatric Dermatology* for additional information. (Portions of this discourse on atrophy have been taken from this source[3] with permission.)

Therapeutic Approaches to Dermatophytosis

Systemic oral use of griseofulvin in dosages of 0.5 to 1.0 gram daily may be effective in dermatophytosis and onychomycosis. Side effects including gastrointestinal distress and neurologic symptoms should make one cautious and monitor the patient's progress with care.[48]

Ketoconazole in dosages of 0.2 to 1.2 grams daily may be effective against candidiasis and dermatophytosis. This oral medication also has significant potential for side effects over long periods of use.[49]

Topical therapies include nystatin, which when applied three times daily can be especially useful for candidiasis.[50] Tolnaftate as a 1 percent cream is useful topically in treating dermatophytosis. Miconazole in a 2 percent cream applied topically may be useful in treating dermatophytosis as well.

Over-the-counter remedies for tinea pedis are many and varied and are beyond the scope of this discussion. Brief mention should be made, however, of the several older formulary medications in use for superficial fungus infections of the foot. Compound ointment of resorcinol, Whitfield's ointment, 5 percent potassium permanganate foot soaks, and tincture of potassium iodate are examples of old remedies that prove useful on occasion.

Physical medicine can be of help in treating tinea pedis. Ultraviolet irradiation is fungicidal, and iontophoresis with aqueous solutions of copper sulfate can be excellent in treating resistant dermatophytosis.[3] Self-medication or previous overtreatment of fungus infections of the feet often brings patients to the podiatric office. Such cases should be treated with deference. Astringent mild wet dressings such as Burow's solution are useful in reducing inflammation. It is important in such cases to restore tissue vitality before embarking upon the indicated definitive treatment plan.[3]

PODIATRIC PARASITOLOGY

Scabies

Scabies is a common infestation of the human skin by *Sarcoptes scabiei* (mites). Spread of this mite is by interpersonal contact.[57] It frequently occurs in nursing homes and domiciliary institutions.

The scabies mite penetrates the skin and leaves subtle, noninflammatory burrows en route to egg-

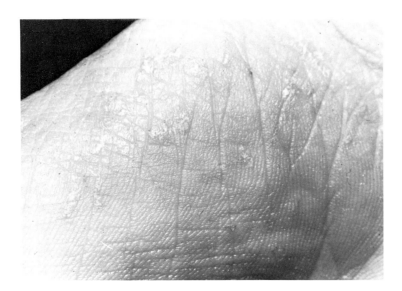

Fig. 18-10. Scabies at the burrowing stage in the human foot. (Case courtesy of Drs. Black and Fenske.) (From McCarthy and Montgomery,[3] with permission.)

laying sites (Fig. 18-10). The eggs hatch within a few days, leaving the skin infested with larvae. Interdigital spaces are commonly affected by scabies. Hyperkeratotic areas become loaded with larvae in Norwegian scabies. This acute form occurs most often in immune-compromised hosts.[3]

Differential diagnosis of scabies includes the eczemas and papular urticarias as well as superficial pyococcal infections. Diagnosis is made microscopically from skin scrapings taken from the involved sites.

Treatment of scabies requires sequestration of patients, enforcement of strict hygienic care, and frequent changes of clean clothing and bed linens. Hot, soapy baths along with daily applications of the antiscabetic material Kwell (lindane) on a 24-hour basis will kill the offending larvae. Postscabetic phenomena are to be treated symptomatically. Topical corticosteroids and intralesional injections are beneficial when nodular lesions occur.

Larva migrans is another skin condition characterized by nematode larvae that burrow under the human skin. In the United States, dogs and cats are the usual carriers of these intestinal hookworms. They are picked up through the feet of unshod individuals who walk through warm, damp sand or dirt where larvae are in the process of hatching.[3]

The entry points of the larvae in the skin are usually marked by reddish papules. Single or linear

eruptions mark the burrowing routes of the larvae. Pruritus and resultant excoriations lead to an initial nonspecific eczema, which can become secondarily infected. The larvae are microscopic and difficult to demonstrate. History and clinical findings are the usual means for diagnosis by the trained clinician.

Larva migrans is treated topically and systemically by thiabendazole (Mintezol). Care should be exercised in vigorously monitoring for side effects. Symptomatic treatment for the nonspecific eczema is indicated, and definitive treatment for bacterial infection with appropriate antibiotics should be instituted.

Hymenoptera, including ants, bees, and wasps, produce poisons that excite severe local and systemic reactions including episodes of life-threatening anaphylaxis. Fire ants are particularly noxious. Discrete pustules surrounded by erythematous rings are diagnostic. Oral antihistamines, cool compresses, and antipruritic lotions may be sufficient to deal with local symptoms. Sting kits are available for use when the precise etiology of the sting is known. Isoproterenol or other sympathomimetic drugs can be employed, and anaphylaxis should be treated with heroic medical measures using adrenalin and corticosteroids preferably in the hospital setting.

The class Arachnida includes the eight-legged

spiders. Reactions to spider bites are often delayed. Systemic reactions may take several days to appear. Muscle cramps and abdominal pains, nausea, vomiting, generalized weakness, dizziness, and sweating may occur.

The bite of brown recluse spiders may produce ulcerative or blistered lesions. The black widow spider's bite leaves two reddish puncta at the site.[3]

Spider bites are treated symptomatically. Neurotoxins are relieved by specific antisera. Muscle spasms respond to calcium gluconate injections and hot baths. Corticosteroids, antibiotics, and antihistamines are useful when indicated topically or systemically.

Fleas are blood-sucking parasites with the potential for transmitting parasitic, rickettsial, and bacterial disease. Flea bites appear as wheals or papules with hemorrhagic puncta. These lesions are irregularly clustered and highly pruritic. Eventually, bullae and small ulcerations occur.[3] A history of exposure to flea-infested environments is essential for diagnosis, since the presenting lesions are essentially nonspecific.

Burrowing fleas must be removed surgically. A sterile needle or other suitable probing instrument is useful. Cotton balls or gauze soaked with ether are lethal to the parasite. Antiseptic, antibacterial, and anti-inflammatory measures should be instituted as indicated. Obviously, vigorous treatment to rid the environment of fleas is required.

The order Acarina includes the tick, which is a large blood-sucking parasite. Ticks have leathery brown exteriors and prey upon many animals in wooded or grassy environs. Ticks attach themselves painlessly in order to suck blood from the host. Erythematous halos and/or small, pruritic nodules mark the site of attachment. Some ticks inject neurotoxins into the host, causing a reversible paralysis.[52] The leg is often involved in such sequelae.

The diagnosis of tick bite is confirmed by the actual presence of the tick or the single nodule seen at the site of the original attachment.

In treating tick infestation, it is important to remove the tick intact. Direct application of chloroform or the application of a hot nail or match will cause the tick to release its hold. Punch biopsy tools are useful in removing any part of the tick that might have been left in situ. Commercial repellents are available to spray on individuals and animals likely to be exposed to ticks, as they are found in wooded and grassy locations.

PYODERMA

Inflammatory and purulent reactions of the skin to the presence of pathogenic microorganisms are referred to as pyoderma (Fig. 18-11). Pyoderma may primarily involve cutaneous structures, or they may be secondary to systemic infections or infectious involvement of some other organ.

Normally, the skin represents a formidable obstacle to a hostile external environment, in part because of its keratinizing structure and its low pH of 5.5.[1] Sebaceous secretions contain material that is naturally antimicrobial as well as circulating immunoglobulins, which are additional factors that resist skin infection.

The integrity of the skin may, however, be compromised as a result of microangiopathy such as that observed in diabetes mellitus or peripheral vascular disease. Nutritional states such as protein depletion, avitaminosis, and starvation, commonly found in cases of alcoholism and substance abuse, can leave the skin more susceptible to skin infection.[3] Injudicious use of certain medications such as corticosteroids and antibiotics can also be deleterious.[53] Even the mental health of patients can be partly implicated with pyoderma along with poor skin hygiene.

The normal cutaneous flora consists of a number of organisms such as the aerobic diphtheroids, *Corynebacterium tenuis*, and *Corynebacterium minutissimum*. *Staphylococcus epidermidis* and to a lesser extent *Staphylococcus aureus* are also normal within limits on the skin. Gram-negative bacilli such as *E. coli*, *Proteus*, *Enterobacter*, and *Pseudomonas* species are native skin colonizers. Other transient organisms that cause no disease can also be found on the skin from time to time.

It appears that, among other factors, the number of organisms present affects the prognosis in pyoderma. An inoculum of 2 or 3 million organisms/

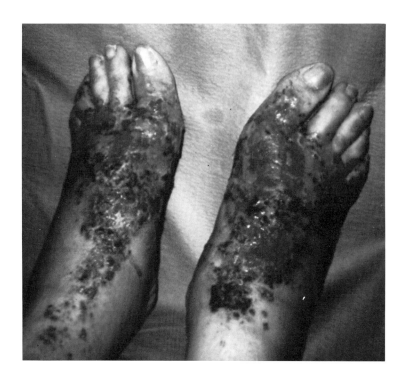

Fig. 18-11. Pyoderma at one stage as it affects the lower extremities. (Case courtesy of Dr. Brenner.) (From McCarthy and Montgomery,[3] with permission.)

ml[3] or greater is more likely to lead to pyoderma. Foreign bodies and trauma to the skin also favor the progression of skin disease.[54]

Most podiatric presentations of pyoderma are local manifestations. Primary pruritic dermatosis may lead to secondary pyodermas. The fingernails provide a means for self-inoculation when lesions are scratched. Unhappily, iatrogenic and nosocomial factors are etiologic in some pyodermas.

Erythrasma is a localized pyoderma of the interdigital space. The characteristic coral-red fluorescence under Wood's light is diagnostic of this condition, which responds well to the systemic use of erythromycin.[54]

Carbuncles and folliculitis are deep and superficial erythematous, indurated, and pustular lesions involving hair follicles. Boils and furuncles are deep abscesses, which frequently require surgical incision and drainage.

Paronychias are discussed elsewhere in connection with toenail involvements. This microbial infection of the posterior and lateral nail fold is caused by a variety of pathogens. The nail plate itself may act as a foreign body, thereby exacerbating the skin infection.

Ecthyma represents a deep expression of impetigo. Purulent ulcerations are covered by extensive encrustations. Streptococcal and staphylococcal species are commonly implicated.[55]

Impetigo may affect the lower extremities. Impetigo contagiosum is a highly contagious pyoderma associated with hyperhidrosis, heat, and poor personal hygiene. Vesiculopustular formations are superficially disposed just beneath the stratum corneum. Staphylococcal infestations are most often involved in bullous lesions.

Streptococcal impetigo presents as a spreading erythema in the lower extremities. Minute vesicles form pustules, which become encrusted. Removal of these crusts reveals red, weeping borders.[55] Cellulitis, lymphangiitis, and lymphadenopathy occur when pyodermas are left untreated or inadequate therapeutic plans are employed.[3]

Accurate diagnosis of the organism causing the pyoderma requires properly executed culture and sensitivity testing. Inappropriate antibiotic treatment can exacerbate pyodermas as well as other infectious conditions. The proper antibiotic, once known, may be used both topically and systemically.[56]

Proper, gentle cleansing of the pyoderma, using commercially available antibacterial agents such as dilute povidine-iodine solution, chlorhexidine gluconate (Hibiclens), and hexachlorophene (pHisohex) on a daily basis, is essential. Topical antibiotics, although useful initially, should be restricted to short-term use so as not to permit yeast overgrowth or sensitization.[3]

Astringent wet dressings, aqueous gentian violet in 2 percent solutions, or aqueous 5 percent silver nitrate solutions are beneficial in most cases. Aluminum subacetate soaks or wet dressings (Burow's solution) used four times daily for 10 minutes are astringent, antiseptic, and antipruritic. Changes in local pH, salinity, and dehydrating factors make Burow's solution especially useful in adjunctive treatment of pyodermas. Gentle débridement of encrustations by the podiatrist may accelerate the response of pyodermas affecting the foot. Once the pyoderma has resolved, the patient should be encouraged in aggressive self-care to ensure that the condition does not return.[57]

CONDITIONS OF THE TOENAILS (ONYCHOPATHY)

The human toenail is one of the special adnexal structures of the foot (Fig. 18-12). Its distal position on the toe, together with its being encased within the toe box of the shoe, exposes it to fre- quent microtrauma. As the population ages, certain trophic changes may also develop, and a number of diseases can affect the condition of the toenails. These and other factors are etiologic to a wide range of podiatric complaints classified as the onychopathies.

Onychocryptosis

Ingrown nails are most commonly associated with the hallucal nail borders but may occur on the lesser digits as well. Such complaints may occur at any time of life. Indeed, on several occasions, I have observed them in infants, where they were caused by tight-fitting "cute" booties. Predisposition to onychocryptosis may be a familial trait as the nails develop with an incurvated appearance.[3] The adjacent ungualabia (nail fold) frequently becomes hypertrophic as contiguous soft tissue structures become repeatedly inflamed. Trauma, improper footgear, and fragmentation of the nail as it is cut periodically also contribute to the incidence of the condition.

As the nail plate penetrates the ungualabia, inflammation and infection are initiated, and eventually purulent exudates may form. Chronic cases may present with exuberant granulation tissue at the site of nail impaction.

Onychocryptosis is the most common nail complaint seen in podiatric medicine.[3] Palliative treatment involves simple excision of the offending portion of the nail margin. It is important not to leave minute spicules behind during simple excision. Ju-

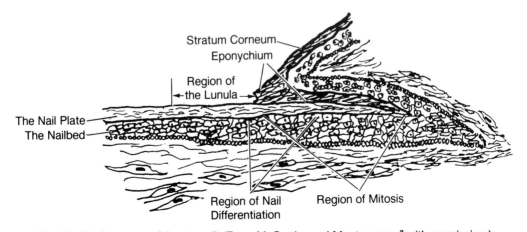

Fig. 18-12. Structure of the toenail. (From McCarthy and Montgomery,[3] with permission.)

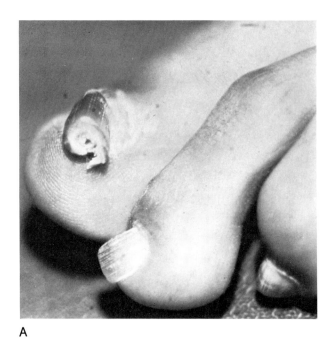

A

Fig. 18-13. **(A)** Onychocryptosis involving the great toenail. **(B)** Surgical excision.

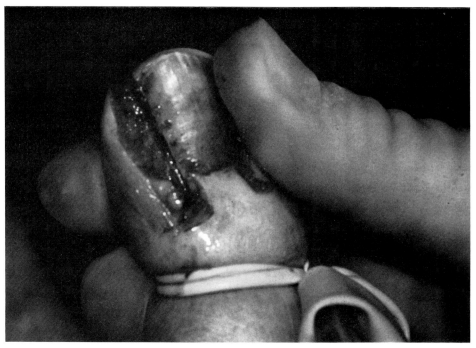

B

dicious use of the nail curette is of benefit in this regard. Granulation tissues may be excised whenever present, and silver nitrate cauterization can be useful. Antiseptic wet dressings or soaks such as aluminum subacetate or dilute aqueous povidine-iodine solution are useful topically. Local antimicrobial therapy is usually indicated as part of the home care regimen. Systemic antibiotics should be used sparingly. Their use should be supported by culture and sensitivity testing to identify the involved pathogen, and then only when infection is seen extending beyond the limits of the original complaint to involve the foot or the lower leg.

Chronic recurrent conditions are best treated surgically.[3] The matrix or growth center of the nail at the point or points of deformity should be excised or otherwise destroyed (Fig. 18-13B). Phenolization of the involved matrix portions has become a popular procedure in recent years. However, such treatment usually results in long-term drainage, and severe chemical burning can result if overused, especially among fair-skinned individuals.

The Winograd procedure or the Frost modification thereof involves excision of the offending portion of the nail, nail bed, nail matrix, and ungualabia. This type of permanent correction is a usually reliable surgical procedure, and healing is generally rapid in healthy surgical candidates.

Onychia

Onychia involves inflammation, which is usually associated with suppuration of the nail matrix.[3] Paronychia represents an advanced degree of onychia in which deeper structures become involved. Onycholysis frequently results from such involvements.

Onychia is usually associated with minimal or acute trauma to the part, but may be factitial in origin. Rarely, small skin parasites have been observed as the cause. The prognosis is good in healthy individuals, but nail deformity may be a sequela. When peripheral vascular disease or diabetes mellitus is involved, there may be a fulmination of the disease process, which can eventually threaten life and limb.[3]

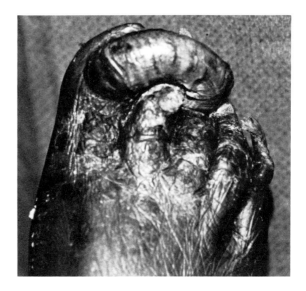

Fig. 18-14. Onychogryphosis of the human toenail.

Most onychias and paronychias respond to simple drainage of the suppurative material by removal of all or part of the involved nail plate. Wet dressings or soaks with aqueous solutions of aluminum subacetate or dilute povidine-iodine solutions are indicated. Occasionally systemic or local antibiotics may be indicated under conditions discussed earlier.

Onychogryphosis (Club Nail, Onychauxis, Ram's Horn Nail)

Trauma to the nail matrix and occasionally infection of the part result in hypertrophic changes to all dimensions of the toenail (Fig. 18-14). Such hypertrophic modifications may cause the nail to "hook" as it grows distally. For this reason, the deformity has been likened to convoluted rams' horns.[3] The mass of the hypertrophic nail produces localized pain, and it is not uncommon for the nail to encroach upon adjacent toes. Such self-induced trauma may produce lacerations and infections of contiguous structures.

Thorough palliative reduction of onychogryphotic nails by the skilled use of nail nippers and the podiatric burr often maintains the patient in comfort with an acceptable appearance for as long as 6 to 9 months following professional care, because these grossly hypertrophic nails tend to grow relatively slowly. Surgical intervention may benefit healthy patients who are distressed at the appearance and discomfort of onychogryphosis.[3] Avulsion of the offending nail plate and meticulous dissection of the total nail matrix under local anesthesia is usually elected. Single flap partial amputation of the distal hallux involving three-fourths or more of the ungual phalanx (Symes' type of procedure) is occasionally indicated when multiple associated complaints of the ungual phalanx are involved.

Onychomycosis

Pathogenic dermatophytes frequently involve the nails of both hands and feet. *Trichophyton* species, particularly *T. rubrum* and *T. mentagrophytes* are usually the offending organisms. *Candida albicans*, a yeast, may also be involved.[58]

Trauma, often of a comparatively minor nature,

to the distal part of the nail or its lateral margins allows for the introduction of the ubiquitous pathogens. Early infections are heralded by variously colored spots or striations.[3] Such involvements may be white, yellow, brown, or sometimes black, depending on the infecting organism. As the organism becomes established, the nail becomes totally involved (Fig. 18-15). It usually thickens and becomes dry and pithy in consistency. Adjacent toenails may become involved over time, causing much distress among cosmetically conscious individuals. Psoriasis can involve the toenails and may easily be mistaken for onychomycosis.[59]

When *Candida albicans* is involved, the nail plate region tends to demonstrate watery exudation.[58] *Candida* species produce whitish plaques on the involved nail plates.

Palliative treatment of onychomycosis is usually disappointing, perhaps because of poor patient compliance. The involved parts of the mycotic nail plates and contiguous infected soft tissues are débrided and/or burred when palliative approaches are elected. Topical fungicides are applied to the

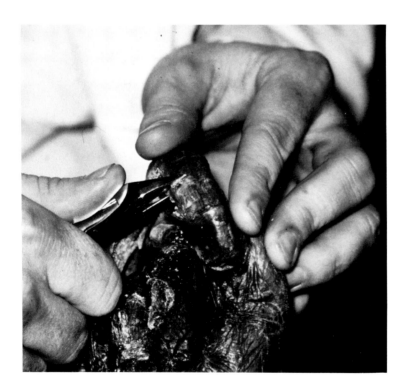

Fig. 18-15. Onychomycosis as it involves the hallucal toenail.

denuded nail and/or nail bed. Such fungicides are many and varied and are available with and without prescription. Undecylenic acid, tolnaftate, and clotrimazole are among the most commonly selected creams, solutions, and tinctures.

Oral administration of the systemic drugs griseofulvin and ketoconazole has proved successful in some treatments of onychomycosis. Since such treatments are of considerable duration when the nails are involved, it is important to monitor patients carefully throughout the course of treatment for potentially serious side effects (e.g., blood dyscrasias).

Surgical avulsion of the involved nail plate is frequently necessary. Such interventions expose the affected nail bed more advantageously to topical therapies. Secondary infection and postoperative pain are problems associated with nail avulsion. Urea creams and ointments have been effective in producing a chemical onycholysis when surgery is to be avoided. The action of urea compounds, however, requires that the involved nail plate be essentially totally undermined by the action of the fungus.

These four conditions—onychocryptosis, onychia and paronychia, onychogryphosis, and onychomycosis—constitute the principal podiatric complaints involving the toenails. Other disorders, dystrophies, and neoplastic disorders exist and will be defined and briefly discussed.

Onychyphemia

Hemorrhage may occur under the nail plate as a result of direct trauma. It is occasionally associated with diseases that affect bleeding time, such as hemophilia and avitaminosis C. Initially, subungual hemorrhages appear bright red and exquisitely tender because of the hydraulic pressures involved.[3]

Treatment should be instituted quickly to relieve the pressure and pain. This can be achieved by drilling one or several small holes with a dental burr. Appropriate analgesia should be instituted, using cold packs and medication if necessary after proper antiseptic precautions have been taken.

As the blood clot organizes, the color progresses from red to brown to black. Untreated cases may proceed to develop periostitis and formation of subungual exostosis. Isolated digital radiographs are necessary when fracture of the ungual phalanx is suspected.

Onychophosis

Onychophosis is synonymous with callus of the nail groove. Such conditions are invariably due to low-grade chronic trauma associated with improper, pinching footwear. Access to the callus within the nail groove usually requires excision of that portion of the nail that originally initiated the inflammation. Softening of the callous tissue may be achieved by a variety of softening solutions: Krausz recommends a 1 percent compound solution of cresol.[3] Podiatric débridement of the involved area is accomplished with instruments of the operator's choice. Curettage alone is seldom effective in removing the callus. It is wise to retreat the condition after several weeks, since the problem tends to recur rapidly.

Subungual Heloma

Subungual heloma may be associated with onychophosis. Inadequate examination of the nail groove may permit the patient to leave the office with the chief complaint left unattended. Once the offending portion of the nail and callus has been removed, the subungual heloma can be seen as a sharply circumscribed white to yellow mass, seldom exceeding ⅛ inch in diameter. Sharp dissection, using scalpel, chisel blade, and/or tissue nipper, is usually successful in removing subungual heloma.

Mild concentrations of salicylic acid ointments are useful in achieving chemical débridement of calloused nail groove with or without subungual heloma. Such lesions tend to reform as a result of inflammation and the attendant increase in epidermal cell production. Therefore, adequate follow-up care and prevention of inflammation and infection are essential.[3]

DYSTROPHIC CONDITIONS OF THE TOENAILS

Beau's Lines

Pathologic disturbances that affect the nail matrix may produce transverse furrows, called Beau's lines after the eighteenth-century French physician Joseph Beau. The condition proceeds distally from the posterior nail fold and is usually accompanied by discoloration of the looser distal portion. The condition is a sequela of acute systemic inflammatory disease as well as trauma and onychia.[3] It does not ordinarily require treatment.

Hapalonychia

Hapalonychia is that state in which the nail plate becomes rubbery and pliable. Chemical exposure, hyperhidrosis, and endocrine disorders have been implicated in this condition.[3]

Leukonychia

Nail plates exhibiting white spots (punctata) and/or streaks (striata) are said to exhibit leukonychia. The etiology is unknown.

Melanonychia

Pigmented longitudinal bands affecting the nails are called melanonychia striata.[60] The condition is thought to be congenital and involves the production of melanin extending from a small nevus situated within the nail matrix.

Onychatrophia

Reduction in the size, thickness, or texture of nails constitutes onychatrophia. Atrophic development of the nail is most common in the fifth toe and is usually congenital.[3]

Onychoschizia

The separation of the toenail into an outermost flaky layer and more normal strata proximally constitutes onychoschizia. The etiology is uncertain.

Onycholysis

The total separation of the nail plate beginning distally and proceeding proximally is termed onycholysis. It is to be differentiated from onychomadesis.[3] Onycholysis involves low-grade inflammation and occurs over a period of time. Onychomycosis, psoriatic nail involvement, and minimal traumatic episodes are the usual etiologies.

Onychomadesis

Onychomadesis involves separation of the nail plate beginning proximally. The condition is usually associated with acute trauma, onychia, or severe dermatitis. The process of complete separation occurs rapidly in onychomadesis and is much more inflammatory in nature than is onycholysis.[3]

Onychorrhexis

In onychorrhexis, longitudinal ridges and depressions occurring within the nail bed are reflected in the structure of the undersurface of the nail and in turn are seen on the upper nail surface. Nutritional disorders, aging, and dehydration of the nail substance have been associated with onychorrhexis.

NEOPLASTIC DISEASES ASSOCIATED WITH THE TOENAILS

Chondroma

Chondroma is a cartilaginous tumor infrequently observed in association with the ungual phalanx. The presence of chondroma produces deformity and erosion of the nail bed and contiguous tissues. Chondroma responds well to surgical correction. Growths associated with abnormal occurrences of cartilage are identified as enchondromata. Masses that arise from normal regions of cartilage development are identified as achondromata.

Glomus Tumors

Glomus tumors are relatively rare neoplasms of the dermis. They may occur within the nail bed and may be exquisitely tender. Such lesions are usually bluish since they involve a complex of minute muscular and vascular structures, which exert pressure upon plexuses of nerve endings (such as temperature sensory neurons) occurring on the distal parts of the toes.[3]

Granuloma Pyogenicum

Cherry-like nodules composed mainly of newly formed capillaries may occur in association with the nail folds or the nail beds. Such lesions may involute over all or part of the nail plate and are called "proud flesh," granulomatous tissues, or granuloma pyogenicum. Trauma and low-grade infection seem to be etiologic. These lesions bleed easily and may be excised and chemically cauterized with silver nitrate sticks.

Melanoma

Melanomas are malignant tumors which metastasize by way of lymphatic channels. When lower extremity lesions are involved, lymph nodes of the popliteal space are often spared, but the inguinal nodes most often reveal the presence of metastatic tumor cells. Melanoma may occur de novo in situ in association with the toenail or by malignant transformation of preexisting nevi. The prognosis is grave in tumors involving transforming melanocytes, and radical surgical excision or amputation is most often elected when digits are implicated.

The appearance of melanomas associated with toenails is highly variable. It may appear as the classic threatening black tumor mass, or it may be mistaken for subungual hematoma or an atypical mole.[59] Early acral lentiginous melanoma appears much like melanonychia striata as a darkly pigmented, striated lesion of the nail. The most insidious of malignant neoplasia are the amelanotic melanomas, which appear to have no dark coloration. They are frequently mistaken for squamous cell carcinomas of the nail bed or for benign nevus-like lesions of the nail or its contiguous soft tissue structures.

Periungual Fibroma

Fibrous tumors whose main constituent is collagenic connective tissue may involve the tissues contiguous to the toenails. Such tumors are benign, but surgical excision is indicated where pain or disfigurement is involved.[3] Periungual fibromas have been identified in association with both posterior and lateral portions of the ungualabia.

Subungual Exostosis

Trauma to the medial, lateral, and dorsal aspects of the ungual phalanges (usually that of the great toe) may produce a reactive periostitis. Such irritations may result in firm tumorous elevations of the cartilage or bone that grow progressively so as to elevate the nail plate itself. Subungual exostosis often assumes the radiographic appearance of a mushroom-like tumor. This type of lesion responds well to aggressive surgical resection of the mass.[3]

Periungual Verrucae

Verruca vulgaris has been discussed elsewhere in this chapter. These virally initiated growths may occur in a periungual or subungual location on the fingers or the toes. These lesions respond well to conventional therapies for verrucae. The atraumatic and avascular approach offered by laser therapy provides for a particularly attractive means of surgical intervention for these types of neoplasia, since they tend to be resistant to many treatment plans.

Table 18-1. Systemic Antibiotics Useful in Podiatric Dermatology

Group	Oral Form	Parenteral Form
Aminoglycosides		Gentamycin
Cephalosporins	Cephalexin	Cephalothin
	Cephradine	Cefazolin
Clindamycin	Clindamycin	Clindamycin
Chloramphenicol	Chloramphenicol	Chloramphenicol
Erythromycin	Erythromycin	Erythromycin
Penicillins	Penicillin VK	Penicillin G
		Procaine penicillin G
	Amoxicillin	Ampicillin
		Carbenicillin
	Dicloxacillin	Oxacillin

(From McCarthy and Montgomery,[3] with permission.)

DERMATOLOGIC THERAPEUTICS

The modes of dermatologic treatment for any given therapeutic plan demand consideration of the form the prescribed medication should take. Topical medicaments may be wet dressings, tinctures, paints, lotions, emulsions, creams, gels, ointments, powders, or fixed dressings such as the Unna paste boot. Systemic medications may take oral, rectal, and sublingual routes. Parenteral treatments include intramuscular, subcutaneous, and intradermal injections in dermatology. More rapid effects of systemic medications are achieved by intravenous or intra-arterial routes, but drug sensitivity reactions may be immediate and severe whenever they occur following injections.[3]

Systemic dermatologic medications include a wide range of antibiotics useful in pyodermas and other infectious processes involving the skin or its adnexa (Table 18-1). Care should be exercised in selecting antibiotics through culture and sensitivity testing. Gram stains of exudates are useful in making an immediate choice of initial medication.[3]

Systemic antifungal agents are available to deal with certain dermatophytes. Griseofulvin and ketoconazole have proven useful in selected cases. However, their side effects should be known, especially when long-term treatment as for onychomycosis is contemplated. Anti-inflammatory medications, long used for musculoskeletal conditions, also have a place in podiatric dermatology (Table 18-2). Analgesic, anti-inflammatory, and antipyretic actions make them efficacious in selected cases. Antihistamines are frequently employed for their antipruritic and analgesic effects. They are not particularly useful for exfoliative dermatitis in erythema multiforme.[3] Such diseases as atopic and contact- and drug-initiated dermatosis benefit from the use of antihistamines (Table 18-3).

Corticosteroids when used systemically for podiatric dermatologic conditions for their pronounced anti-inflammatory effects should be limited to short-term usage (Table 18-4). Their adverse effects in patients with psychoses, peptic ulcers, diabetes mellitus, and pregnancies are well known.[61]

Oral enzymes have been used for fibrinolytic and proteolytic effects by some podiatric physicians. Governmental agencies presently advise against their use in the systemic form, claiming that they are "less than effective."

Table 18-2. Systemic Nonsteroidal Anti-inflammatory Agents Useful in Podiatric Dermatology

Generic Name	Trade Name	Manufacturer
Fenoprofen calcium	Nalfon	Dista Products Co.
Ibuprofen	Motrin	Upjohn Company
Indomethacin	Indocin	Merck Sharp & Dohme
Naproxen	Naprosyn	Syntex Laboratories
Phenylbutazone	Butazolidin	Geigy Pharmaceuticals
Piroxicam	Feldene	Pfizer Laboratories
Sulindac	Clinoril	Merck Sharp & Dohme
Tolmetin sodium	Tolectin	McNeil Pharmaceuticals

(From McCarthy and Montgomery,[3] with permission.)

Table 18-3. Systemic Antipruritic-Antihistamine Agents Useful in Podiatric Dermatology

Drug Class	Generic Name	Trade Name	Manufacturer
Ethanolamines	Carbinoxamine maleate	Clistin	McNeil
	Dimenhydrinate	Dramamine	Searle
	Diphenhydramine HCl	Benadryl	Parke, Davis
Ethylenediamines	Tripelennamine citrate	PBZ Citrate	Geigy
	Tripelennamine HCl	PBZ HCl	Geigy
Alkylamines	Brompheniramine maleate	Dimetane	Robins
	Chlorpheniramine maleate	Chlor-Trimeton	Schering
	Dexchlorpheniramine maleate	Polaramine	Schering
Phenothiazines	Methdilazine	Tacaryl	Westwood
	Promethazine HCl	Phenergan	Wyeth
	Trimeprazine tartrate	Temaril	Smith Kline & French
Piperidines	Azatadine maleate	Optimine	Schering
	Cyproheptadine HCl	Periactin	Merck Sharp & Dohme
Miscellaneous	Cimetidine	Tagamet	Smith Kline & French
	Hydroxyzine HCl	Atarax	Roerig
	Hydroxyzine pamoate	Vistaril	Pfizer

(From McCarthy and Montgomery,[3] with permission.)

TOPICAL PREPARATIONS

Corticosteroids are used locally by intralesional injection or by topical application as lotions, creams, ointments, sprays, and impregnated occlusive dressings.[62] It is important to remember that corticosteroids mask the symptoms of infection and have a capacity for causing atrophy of the skin when used over long periods of time. Betamethasone, hydrocortisone, triamcinolone, prednisolone, and dexamethasone are among the many preparations available both as prescriptions and as over-the-counter remedies.

Antifungal agents frequently are employed in podiatric practice against *Epidermophyton, Microsporum,* and *Trichophyton* species. Haloprogin, tolnaftate, clotrimazole, and miconazole are ingredients in commonly prescribed creams and lotions. Mycostatin is useful for many candidal infections.[3] Many over-the-counter preparations are available, and some patients provoke complications of their dermatophytosis by self-medication. Undecylenic acid preparations are commercially available without prescription, and one should not forget such old reliable formulary preparations as Whitfield's

Table 18-4. Systemic Corticosteroids Useful in Podiatric Dermatology

Activity	Generic Name	Dosage
Short-acting		
Oral	Methylprednisolone	2, 4, 8, 16, 24, and 32 mg
	Prednisolone	5 mg
	Prednisone	1, 2.5, 5, 10, 20, and 50 mg
Injectable	Dexamethasone sodium phosphate	4 mg/ml
Intermediate-acting		
Oral	Triamcinolone	1, 2, 4, 8, and 16 mg
Injectable	Triamcinolone diacetonide	25 and 40 mg/ml
	Dexamethasone acetate	8 mg/ml
	Betamethasone sodium phosphate	6 mg/ml
Long-acting		
Oral	Dexamethasone	0.75, 4, 5, 20, and 25 mg
	Betamethasone	0.6 mg
Injectable	Triamcinolone hexacetonide	5 and 40 mg/ml
	Triamcinolone acetonide	10 and 40 mg/ml

(From McCarthy and Montgomery,[3] with permission.)

ointment and potassium permanganate soaks for use in selected cases.

Many topical antibiotic preparations for local skin infections are available. *Streptococcus pyogenes* and *Staphylococcus aureus* are common offenders in skin infections and respond to the use of topical antibiotics as a rule.[63] Triple-antibiotic preparations combining bacitracin, gramicidin, neomycin, and/or polymyxin B are available without prescription. Topical erythromycin, gentamicin, tetracyclines, and penicillins are commonly used, but the possibilities for sensitization should not be overlooked.

Pruritus is an aggravating dermatologic symptom that must be controlled to prevent complications arising from the itch-scratch cycle. Preparations of camphor, menthol, and phenol are useful older remedies, as are the calamine lotions with and without local anesthetic additives.[64] Local anesthetic creams and lotions alone as well as antihistamine products may also be used to good advantage. Tar preparations and, of course, corticosteroids, already mentioned, are commonly used to control itching symptoms.[63]

Topical antiseptics are useful in both treatment and prophylaxis against skin pathogens. Aluminum subacetate (Burow's solution) is astringent as well as antiseptic. Hexachlorophene, chlorhexidine, povidine-iodine, iodophores in general, aqueous alcoholic solutions of various types, and benzalkonium are among many other useful products available as local antiseptics.[3]

A number of preparations are used to exfoliate skin or to destroy localized benign neoplasia such as verrucae. Anthracin is used against psoriatic plaques. Cantharidin, 5-fluorouracil, and podophyllin have been used for different reasons as active against papillomas.[3] Keratolytic agents include resorcinol, retinoic acid, salicylic acid, sodium pyruvate, and mono-di-tri-chloroacetic acids are all variably destructive to integumentary structures. Silver nitrate varies in its action in proportion to its concentration. It is stimulatory and antiseptic in lower aqueous concentrations, but is destructive to skin at full strength.

Enzymes can be useful in topical applications for chemical débridement of diseased integumentary tissues. DNAse, fibrinolysin, and streptokinase-streptodornase are currently available.[64]

It has been a maxim of podiatric dermatologic treatment that if lesions are wet, they are to be dried, and if they are dry, they need to be moistened. Hyperhidrotic conditions usually respond to aluminum salts or compounds. Magnesium sulfate (Epsom salts), Burow's solution, solutions prepared with formalin or other aldehydes, glutaraldehyde, and methenamine salts are useful as astringents and antiperspirants.[65]

Skin moisturizing agents include 10 and 20 percent lotions and creams of urea. Corticosteroids may be added to these preparations to enhance their local effects. Euracin is a heavy preparation of vaseline petroleum jelly and has been found useful in treating anhydrous podiatric complaints.

REFERENCES

1. Fitzpatrick TB, Eisen AZ, Wolff K, et al: Dermatology in General Medicine. Vols. I and II. McGraw-Hill, New York, 1987
2. Pinkus H, Mehregan A: A Guide to Dermatohistopathology. 2nd Ed. Appleton-Century-Crofts, New York, 1969
3. McCarthy DJ, Montgomery R: Podiatric Dermatology. Williams & Wilkins, Baltimore, 1986
4. Arey LB: Human Histology. 4th Ed. WB Saunders, Philadelphia, 1974
5. Freed JD: Histologic post-mortem examination of bone hyperplasia accompanying digital hyperplasia. J Am Podiatry Assoc 59:467, 1969
6. Bonavilla CJ: Histopathology of heloma durum: some significant features and their application. J Am Podiatry Assoc 58:423, 1968
7. McCarthy DJ, Habowsky JEJ: Alterations in epidermal and dermal histo-differentiation in normal and hyperkeratinizing skin interpreted through histochemistry and anthropometric analysis. J Am Podiatry Assoc 1:2, 1975
8. McCarthy DJ, Habowsky JEJ: Alterations in skin morphology in heloma durum utilizing maceration technique for examination of epidermal-dermal interface. J Am Podiatry Assoc 62(8):303, 1972
9. Lemont H: Comments on the histologic differentiation of genetically and mechanically induced keratosis. J Am Podiatry Assoc 66(4):259, 1976

10. McCarthy DJ, Rusin J: The implications of ultrastructural modifications induced by cryocautery in pedal verrucae. J Am Podiatry Assoc 62:312, 1977

11. McCarthy DJ: A morphogenic and histochemical analysis of pressure prone verrucae of the human foot. J Am Podiatry Assoc 67:377, 1977

12. McCarthy DJ: Alterations in the morphology of dermo-epidermal interface of pedal verrucae as revealed by scanning electron microscopy. J Am Podiatry Assoc 66:505, 1976

13. Gibbs RC: Conservative management of plantar warts by gentle chemocautery. J Dermatol Surg Oncol 4:915, 1978

14. Zitelli JA: Histologic patterns of congenital nevi and implications for treatment. J Am Acad Dermatol 11:402, 1984

15. Becker SW: Critical evaluation of the so-called "junction nevus." J Invest Dermatol 22:217, 1954

16. Swerdlow AJ: Benign naevi associated with high risk of melanomas. Lancet 2:168, 1984

17. Shehadeh N, Kligman AM: The bacteria responsible for axillary odor. J Invest Dermatol 41:3, 1963

18. MacMillan FSK: Antiperspirant action of topically applied anticholinergics. J Invest Dermatol 43:363, 1964

19. Cone TE: Diagnosis and treatment: some diseases and syndromes and conditions associated with an unusual odor. Pediatrics 4:393, 1968

20. Fisher AA: Contact Dermatitis. 2nd Ed. Lea & Febiger, Philadelphia, 1973

21. Polack L: Immunologic Aspects of Contact Sensitivity (Monographs in Allergy. Vol. 15). S Karger, Basel, 1980

22. Adams RM: Occupational Skin Disease. Grune & Stratton, New York, 1983

23. Lebantine A, Almeyda J: Drug induced changes in pigmentation. Br J Dermatol 89:205, 1973

24. Porter J, Jack H: Amoxicillin and ampicillin equally likely. Lancet 1:1037, 1980

25. Parker CW: Drug allergy. N Engl J Med 292:511, 1975

26. Felner MJ: Lichen planus. Int J Dermatol 19:71, 1980

27. Abeles DC, Dobson RL, Graham JB: Heredity and psoriasis: study of a large family. Arch Dermatol 88:90, 1963

28. Cram DL: Psoriasis: Current advances in etiology and treatment. J Am Acad Dermatol 4:1, 1981

29. Warin AP: Photochemotherapy in the treatment of psoriasis and mycosis fungoides. Clin Exp Dermatol 6:651, 1981

30. Baker H: PUVA therapy for psoriasis. J R Soc Med 77:537, 1984

31. Joklik WK, Willett HP, Amos DB: Zinsser's Microbiology. 18th Ed. Appleton-Century-Crofts, Norwalk, CT, 1984

32. Finegold SM, Baron EJ: Diagnostic Microbiology. CV Mosby, St Louis, 1986

33. McCarthy DJ, Abramson C: Genetic aspects of chronic tinea pedis and related conditions. Curr Podiatry 12:11, 1982

34. Schaller JG, Hansen JA: HLA relationships to disease. Hosp Pract 5:41, 1982

35. Tait BD, Finlay RI, Simons MJ: Serum HLA typing: Tissue Antigens 17:129, 1981

36. Abramson C: A new look at dermatophytosis and atopy. In McCarthy DJ, Montgomery R (eds): Podiatric Dermatology. Williams & Wilkins, Baltimore, 1986

37. Bazin H, Platteau B, Pauwels R: Genetic control of the IgE reaginic immune response. Int Arch Allergy Appl Immunol 66:19, 1982

38. Matsumoto T, Gotoh Y, Narukami H, Honda M: Hyperimmunoglobulin syndrome with serum inhibitor against immune functions. Ann Allergy 46:86, 1981

39. Katona JM, Tata RT, Scanlon S, Bellanti JA: Hyper IgE syndrome with serum inhibitor against immune functions. Ann Allergy 39:295, 1980

40. Rajka G, Barlinn C: On the significance of tricophytin reactivity in atopic dermatitis. Acta Dermatol 59:45, 1979

41. Katz DH: The allergic phenotype: Manifestations of "allergic breakthrough" of IgE antibody production. Immunol Rev 41:77, 1978

42. Baer RL: Atopic Dermatitis. JB Lippincott, Philadelphia, 1955

43. Hernandez AD: An approach to the diagnosis and therapy of dermatophytosis. Int J Dermatol 19:540, 1980

44. Hunziker N, Grun R: Lack of delayed reaction in presence of cell mediated immunity in tricophyton hypersensitivity. Arch Dermatol 116:1266, 1980

45. Jones HE: The atopic-chronic-dermatophytosis syndrome. Acta Dermatol 91:81, 1980

46. Perelmutter L, Potvin L: Studies on T-lymphocytes of atopics and non-atopics. J Allergy Clin Immunol 65:223, 1980

47. Ozawa A, Ohkido M, Kimiyoshi T: Some recent advances in HLA and skin disease. J Am Acad Dermatol 4:205, 1981

48. Blank HD: Widespread *Trichophyton rubrum* granulomas treated with griseofulvin. Arch Dermatol 81:779, 1960

49. Borelli D: Treatment of pityriasis versicolor with ketoconazole. Res Infect Dis 2:592, 1980

50. Hernandez AD: An approach to the diagnosis and

therapy of dermatophytosis. Int J Dermatol 19:540, 1980

51. Orkin M: Scabies and Pediculosis. JB Lippincott, Philadelphia, 1977
52. Burgdorfer W, Keirans JE: Ticks and Lyme disease in the United States. Ann Intern Med 99:121, 1983
53. Biro L, Gibbs RC, Leider M: Staphylococcal infections. A study of incidence on a dermatological ward. Arch Dermatol 82:205, 1960
54. Sarkany I, Tapin D, Blank H: Erythrasma— common bacterial infection of the skin. JAMA 177:130, 1961
55. Moschella SL, Hurley HJ: Dermatology. 2nd Ed. WB Saunders, Philadelphia, 1985
56. Kallicks C: Diagnosis of Infected Lesions Associated with Abscesses and Ulcerations. Eli Lilly Series 2, Indianapolis, 1978
57. Rinaldi R, Sabca ML: A double controlled study: Betadine solution treatment of "athlete's foot": Arch Podiatr Med Foot Surg. 3(1):1, 1976

58. Zaias N: The Nail in Health and Disease. Medical and Scientific Books, New York, 1980
59. Calvert HT: Psoriasis and the nails. Br J Dermatol 75:12, 1963
60. Daniel CR, Osmont LJ: Nail pigmentation abnormalities: their importance and proper examination. Cutis 30:348, 1982
61. Storrs FJ: Use and abuse of systemic corticosteroid therapy. J Am Acad Dermatol 1:95, 1979
62. Arndt KA: Manual of Dermatologic Therapeutics. 3rd Ed. Little, Brown, Boston, 1983
63. Wilkowsker CJ, Hermans PE: General Principles of antimicrobial therapy. Mayo Clin Proc 58:6, 1983
64. Roenigk HH: Office Dermatology. Williams & Wilkins, Baltimore, 1981
65. Gordon HH: Hyperhydrosis treatment with glutaraldehyde. Cutis 9:375, 1972

Operative Care of Nail Disorders 19

John E. Laco, D.P.M.

Operative care of nail disorders is performed on a daily basis in the active podiatric practice. Many original procedures are presented to delineate philosophies and explain the popularity of certain procedures over other procedures.

ANATOMY

In order to understand the principles and reasoning behind nail surgery, it is necessary to understand the anatomy of the nail and surrounding structures. Common terminology involving the anatomy of the nail used during surgery can be confusing and can vary from clinician to clinician (Fig. 19-1).

Many of the techniques developed for nail surgery differ as a direct result of the controversy that seems to exist as to the exact location of the nail matrix, or as to which areas of the nail have the potential to become nail-producing cells. Some authors believe that a thin, cornified epidermoid layer secreted by the nail bed after nail matrix destruction may be mistaken for nail plate,[1,2] and this idea contributes to the controversy. Dixon dis-

cussed the possibility of nail production from areas other than the matrix and suggested that this may be the cause of recurrence after matrix excision.[3] There seems to be general agreement as to the posterior location of the matrix.[2,4,5-9] However, disagreement does exist as to the location of the matrix in the sagittal plane. Burns et al.[4] depicted the matrix as involving part of the eponychium (Fig. 19-1), whereas Keyes[10] and Heifetz[1] disagree. Another interesting point regarding the production of nail is mentioned in Bouché's discussion of the anatomy of the nail where the author refers to histochemical studies that divide the nail plate into three different areas from three germinal sites.[7] It is hoped that the controversy will be somewhat resolved here as different nail destructive procedures are discussed along with their respective results.

SUBUNGUAL HEMATOMA

One of the most simple procedures involving the nail is evacuation of a subungual hematoma. Evacuation will relieve the pressure that is applied to the nail bed and therefore reduce pain. One reported

499

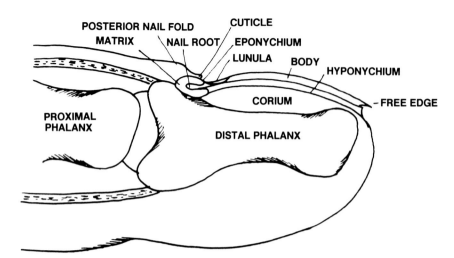

POSTERIOR NAIL FOLD
CUTICLE
MATRIX
NAIL ROOT
EPONYCHIUM
LUNULA
BODY
HYPONYCHIUM
PROXIMAL
PHALANX
CORIUM
FREE EDGE
DISTAL PHALANX

Fig. 19-1. Common terminology depicted in anatomical cross-section. (From Burns et al.,[4] with permission.) (Illustration by Marlene Burns.)

method is puncturing the nail with a red-hot paperclip, after applying antiseptic solution.[11] Probably a much easier way to puncture the nail over a subungual hematoma is to rotate a large-bore needle over the nail while applying light pressure. This evacuation will also eliminate any deforming force the hematoma may be applying to the nail itself.

ONYCHOLYSIS SECONDARY TO TRAUMA

Another common problem occurring during warm weather is separation of the nail plate from the nail bed as a result of trauma. The recommended treatment for this is complete nail avulsion. This will alleviate pain secondary to friction from the shoegear, and, it is hoped, allow a new nail to regrow without deforming forces that may be associated with the traumatized nail.

After the area has been suitably prepped and anesthetized, a spatula or periosteal elevator is used to separate any attachments the dorsal aspect of the nail may have with the proximal nail fold (Fig. 19-2A). The spatula is then used to separate the nail plate from the nail bed.[12] A hemostat may then be used to avulse the nail (Fig. 19-2B).

A popular variation of this technique involves avulsing the nail plate in a proximal-to-distal fash-

ion.[13] Many clinicians use a curved hemostat that is inserted beneath the eponychium and moved in a semicircular fashion so that the jaws of the hemostat are between the nail plate and nail bed. The hemostat is then opened to avulse the nail (Fig. 19-3).

ONYCHOCRYPTOSIS

Probably the most common type of nail surgery performed is the correction of ingrown nails.[14] The etiology of ingrown nails has been discussed and disputed throughout literature. Fowler has even challenged the term *ingrowing* and would prefer the term *embedded*.[2] Many authorities believe improper trimming of toenails can lead to ingrown nails.[1,3,15,16] The general consensus seems to be that toenails should be cut straight across and not curved or kept too short. Shoes — specifically, those that are too tight, small, or narrow for the foot — are listed as a causative factor for ingrown nails.[1,3,17,18] Soft tissue that is either in excess or growing in excess also has been blamed as the etiologic factor for ingrown toenails.[1,15,19-22] DuVries specifically suggested that there is soft tissue hypertrophy as a result of persistent trauma.[21] Polokoff believes the valgus component of hallux valgus allows the great toe to push against the second toe

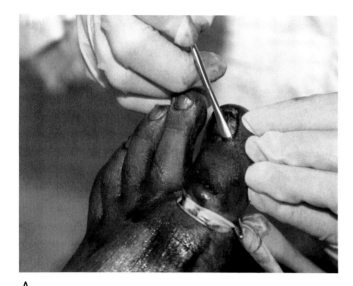

A

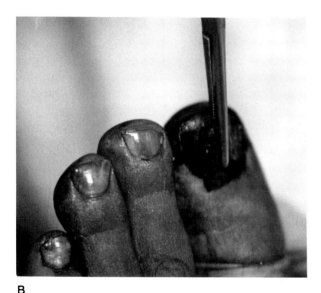

B

Fig. 19-2. (A) and **(B)**. Nail avulsion.

and is therefore the etiology for cryptosis of the lateral aspect of the hallux.[23] The same author also cited hypermobility of the first metatarsal segment as a cause of onychocryptosis. The reasoning behind this theory is that hypermobility of the first metatarsal allows the foot to roll medially. This medial rolling action allows the ground to exert a medial plantar force on the hallux during toe-off that in turn forces the great toe against the second toe. Trauma or microtrauma may also be an indirect factor in cryptosis. VanEnoo and Cane cited a case

of trauma leading to formation of a subungual exostosis that caused an increased curvature of the nail with resultant cryptosis.[24] Perlman also agrees that the pathogenesis of an ingrown nail is subungual exostosis.[25] In one case, Eibel suggested the possibility that a glomus tumor may have resulted in cryptosis.[26]

Some authors have divided ingrown nails into types. Frost[27] differentiated three types of lateral nail cryptosis: an incurvated nail, hypertrophic ungualabia, or an "ingrown nail." The ingrown nail

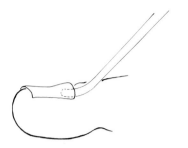

Fig. 19-3. Nail avulsion using curved hemostat.

designates a normal nail plate with a "fish hook" at the lateral border. Of course, combinations thereof may exist. Brown discussed three types of conformations of toenails: one with a gently rounded curvature, one with acute angles at the lateral margins, and one with excess curvature at the lateral ends.[28] Heifetz staged the ingrown toenail by clinical signs and symptoms.[1] The first stage of an ingrown toenail is one that reveals an inflammatory redness and swelling. The second stage reveals inflammatory secretions. The third stage of an ingrown toenail reveals granulation tissue. This leads into a discussion of a condition for which a large number of patients seek treatment every day.

PARONYCHIA

A common sequela of onychocryptosis is paronychia of the border. Regardless of the etiology, the nail may puncture the soft tissue and allow bacterial invasion. This ultimately leads to soft tissue infection. Resolution, as well as prompt termination of the propagation of the infection, is the primary concern of the clinician. Removal of the offending nail spicule is of primary importance. There are variations as to the appropriate procedure to be performed in specific time frames.

Many clinicians perform a partial or complete nail avulsion. The theory behind this procedure is that the "ulcer" of the nail is expected to heal by the time the new nail regrows. Further ingrowth, according to these clinicians, is not expected or can be prevented.[10] The argument against this proce-

dure performed solely by itself is not the failure of resolution of the paronychia, but the high recurrence rate of the ingrown nail. Palmer and Jones reported a 70 percent recurrence rate for ingrown nails after total nail avulsion and an 83 percent recurrence rate for an avulsion of a strip of nail.[29] They believe there are three reasons for this high recurrence rate. First, the lateral nail fold becomes large and fibrosed and the new nail grows into it. Second, the "pulp" tends to move dorsally. The third reason is that the nail is often thickened and less pliable. Dixon reported that two-thirds of the ingrown nails avulsed will recur.[3] Murray and Bedi reported the recurrence rate of symptomatic ingrowing toenails to be 64 percent following avulsion.[30] Regardless of the high recurrence rate for ingrown toenails, Murray and Bedi justify simple nail avulsion as a primary surgical procedure in cases of paronychia because it results in rapid relief of symptoms and eradication of infection.

A controversy arises as to when a permanent procedure for onychocryptosis involving a paronychia should be performed. Although a difference of opinion may exist, the general consensus is to eliminate the infection before performing a permanent nail procedure.[2,18,30,31] Postoperative sepsis has been reported as a complication when performing surgery on infected toes.[2,31] It is this author's opinion that before a permanent procedure is done for a cryptotic nail border, the infection must be resolved.

The following is a general guideline for treatment of paronychia and may have several variations pending the clinical scenario. A total nail avulsion should be used in the most extreme and chronic cases of paronychia. A total nail avulsion is also indicated where paronychia is coexistent with a severely dystrophic nail. These types of situations would dictate the use of appropriate antibiosis and antiseptic soaks. It should also be mentioned that in certain instances of chronic paronychia of long duration, a radiographic study of the toe may be indicated to rule out any bony involvement. When performing a total nail avulsion, the patient should be forewarned of the possibility of further nail deformity, as well as recurrence of the cryptosis.

If only one nail border is involved and eponychial inflammation and drainage are present, a strip of nail should be excised that should include the proximal aspect of the nail. This would again require appropriate antibiosis and antiseptic soaks. If the inflammation of the nail border is contained around the offending nail spicule, a partial oblique excision of the nail may be performed. Antiseptic soaks should help resolve the paronychia quickly. In this situation, the nail matrix is left intact and a permanent type of procedure may be scheduled in a shorter period of time after resolution of the infection. A large amount of variation in treatment of these conditions exists, and treatment depends on the patient's medical history, the physical examination, and the findings of the clinician.

PERMANENT TREATMENT OF ONYCHOCRYPTOSIS

There are many different approaches and techniques to treat and cure onychocryptosis. These variations are probably due, in part, to the controversy over the exact location of the nail matrix. Frost described three types of sharp procedures for an ingrown nail: nail lip reduction, excision of a piece of nail with subadjacent matrix, and a combination of these two.[18] Another sharp procedure is complete radical onychectomy with or without bone.[3] Much variation exists with regard to the destruction of the matrix, in which several modalities are employed. Devices and packing are also advocated by some clinicians. In some instances, permanent total nail ablation is advocated. Each of these variations is addressed in the following pages.

Conservative Care — Packing

Many authors have reported the use of cotton packing by clinicians as conservative treatment for onychocryptosis.[1,3,31,32] Heifetz stated that, if performed properly, it is the simplest and most effective means of conservative treatment.[1] McGlamry reported debriding the mildly cryptotic nail margins and smoothing the new nail edge.[32] The cleared nail groove is packed with antibiotic ointment and sterile cotton. The dressing is held in place with collodion or cohesive gauze. The packings are repeated until the free end of the nail can be cut even with the end of the nail groove. Obviously débridement and packing will have limited success with severely incurvated and cryptotic nails, but it should be taken into consideration when treating patients with peripheral vascular insufficency or diabetics with impaired circulation.

Devices

A number of devices have been created to treat onychocryptosis. In 1939, Linch devised a toenail splint to restore the normal curvature of the nail.[33] An instrument was also developed to facilitate its application (Fig. 19-4A–F). In 1949, Newman[22] devised a nail plate that is inserted surgically to ensure the formation of a normal nail sulcus (Fig. 19-5A–F). Farnsworth,[34] in 1964, described the application of a wire brace to flatten the nail and thereby relieve the onychocryptosis for a prolonged period of time (Fig. 19-6).

Currently, devices still receive a considerable amount of attention. Ilfeld and August reported elevating and separating the edge of the cryptotic nail from the soft tissue with a Teflon plastic strip approximately three-fourths of an inch wide and reinforced on one side.[35] The strip is glued to the toenail and provides a channel for the nail to grow. In 1979, an article in the *British Medical Journal* appeared discussing the gutter treatment for ingrown toenails.[36] The gutter treatment is designed to relieve pain and allow healing of the lateral nail groove. The gutter allows the soft tissue to reepithelialize and reform the nail groove in 8 to 12 weeks. According to the authors, some of the proud flesh and all the granulation tissue is excised from the nail groove with a V-shaped incision. The gutter is then applied down the lateral nail edge with an introducer. Sutures may be applied through the distal nail fold, the nail, or both to stabilize the gutter. The sutures are removed in 10 days and the gutter in 8 to 12 weeks (Fig. 19-7).

An interesting concept reported by Dixon[3] is the use of the Ilfeld technique[35] or application of commercially available nails after a resolution of paronychia following an oblique partial nail avulsion. The idea is to maintain a proper relationship of the

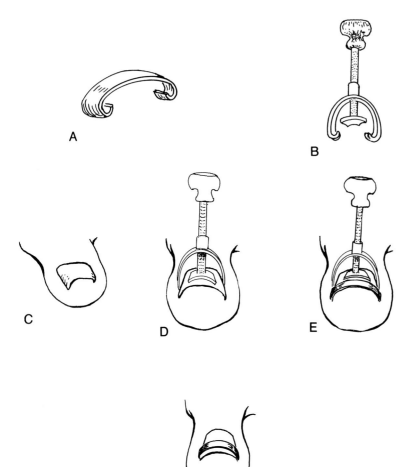

Fig. 19-4. (A–F) Toenail splint and device for application. (From Linch,[33] with permission.)

lateral aspect of the nail with the nail groove. Devices seem to have limited use currently because most patients are able to tolerate surgical procedures for permanent correction. The test of time and further studies will dictate their possible usefulness in the future.

Soft Tissue Reconstruction

Many authors have written or at least mentioned plastic nail lip procedures for the treatment of onychocryptosis.[1,3,10,17,20,27,37–40] In 1893, Howard[37] described "removing an elliptical wedge-shaped section" in the soft tissue of the toe, "to draw the soft tissue parts away from the nail when closed." According to Bartlett, the widest point of

the wedge should be at the level of the ingrown nail.[17] DuVries pointed out that room for the nail groove and the nail edge is created because the upper flap is pulled downward.[20] DuVries also pointed out that the incision may be extended to the opposite side of the toe for treatment of hypertrophy of the entire toe.

Frost stated that a plastic reduction of the hypertrophied lip may be performed in combination with his nail procedure.[27] Soft tissue resection may be gaining popularity in the medical field because there have been several articles recently written about this procedure.[3,38–40] There are limited data on the actual success and results of the procedure. Murray and Robb reported a cure rate of 60 percent using soft tissue resection on recurrent ingrown nails following avulsion.[40]

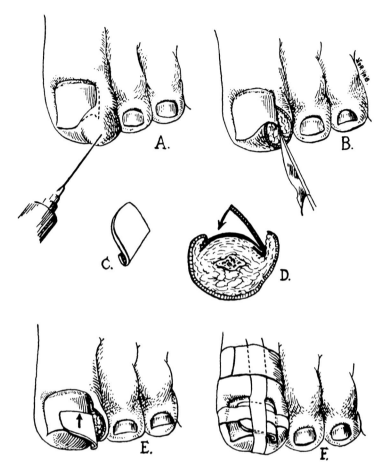

Fig. 19-5. Insertion of stainless steel nail plate. "**(A)** Novocain injected under pressure. **(B)** Incision of swollen, overgrown soft tissue along line of nail sulcus exposing ingrown portion of nail. **(C)** Nail plate made of light weight stainless steel. **(D)** Cross-sectional view of **E.** **(E)** Nail plate being put in place. **(F)** Operation completed with plate and tape properly placed. Note the relative size of plate and nail. The 60 degree angled corner of this plate projects beyond the soft tissue of the sulcus." (From Newman,[22] with permission.)

Soft Tissue Resection

Soft tissue resection as a treatment for onychocryptosis has many advocates. The variations as to the amount of tissue excised cover a wide gamut. Radical excision of the nail fold alone has been reported by different authors.[19,41,42] In 1984, Antrum[41] used this technique when conservative treatment failed, and for chronic and recurrent cases (Fig. 19-8). This procedure was performed even if infection was present. Any nail spicules or spikes are removed and the area heals by granulation. Ney[42] created two pedicle flaps before excising soft tissue (Fig. 19-9).

Review of the literature reveals that the most popular type of sharp tissue procedures for onychocryptosis are wedge resections. Zechel[43] advocated resection of the granulations and excising a wedge-shaped piece of hypertrophic tissue to create a space to allow the nails to grow forward (Fig. 19-10). The channel is packed with iodoform to prevent further production of granulation tissue. The opposite end of the resection spectrum is preferred by Herold and Daniel,[15] who perform a radical wedge resection. The wedge consists of any

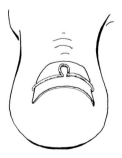

Fig. 19-6. Line diagram depicting wire brace by Farnsworth.[34]

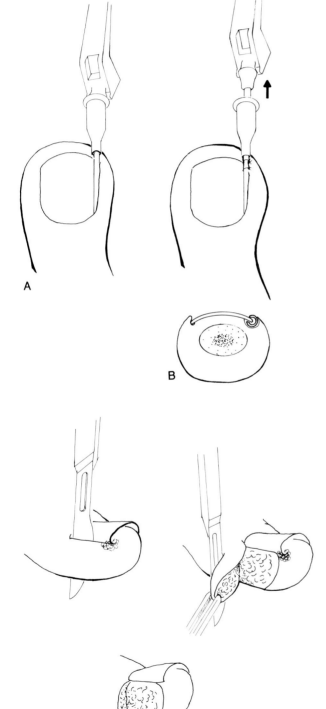

A

B

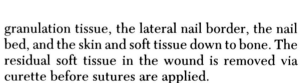

Fig. 19-7. The gutter treatment. (From Wallace et al.,[36] with permission.)

granulation tissue, the lateral nail border, the nail bed, and the skin and soft tissue down to bone. The residual soft tissue in the wound is removed via curette before sutures are applied.

Many authors in the past and recently have described wedge resection.[1,3,10,20,44,45] Usually the nail edge, matrix, and adjacent soft tissue parts are excised in a wedge. Keyes stated that the wedge is performed on the principle that ingrowth is caused by excessive width or convexity of the nail and hypertrophy of the nail wall.[10] Silverman reported symptomatic recurrence rates varying from 20 to 29 percent with wedge resections.[46] The most popular wedge resections used in the field of podiatry are the Winograd and Frost techniques.

Winograd Technique.   Review of the literature has revealed some discrepancies involving wedge resection and the original Winograd technique. As has been traditionally taught, Yale in his textbook *Podiatric Medicine* described the Winograd technique as a wedge-shaped resection that would in-

Fig. 19-8. Line diagram depicting radical excision of nail fold by Antrum.[41]

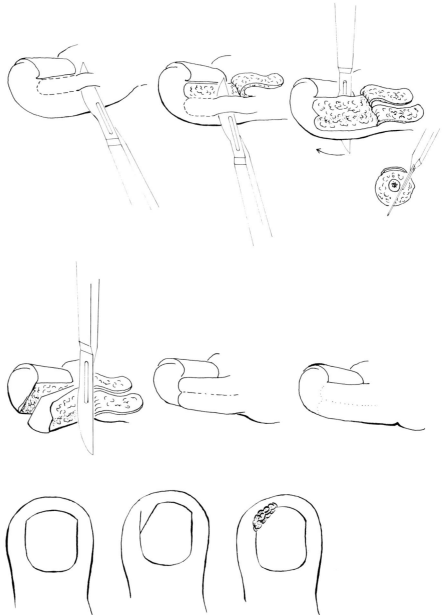

Fig. 19-9. Pedicle flaps used for soft tissue excision by Ney. (Redrawn from Ney.[42])

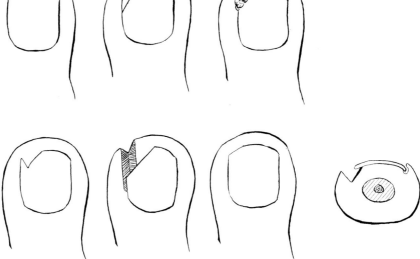

Fig. 19-10. Zechel's technique for wedge resection. (Redrawn from Zechel.[43]).

clude the matrix, offending nail, and nail lip.[47] Mercado in his textbook on *Forefoot Surgery* also depicted the Winograd technique as a wedge resection that includes the nail, plate, lip, bed, and matrix.[48] As pointed out by Burns et al., the traditional description of the Winograd technique in podiatry is indicated where there is an ingrown nail along with a hypertrophied and overlapping ungualabia.[4] The original procedure outlined by Winograd in 1929 and 1936 involves a small incision of the eponychium in line with the incision to be made in the nail.[49,50] The lateral soft tissue around the nail is retracted and preserved, and the matrix and nail bed are curretted. It was Winograd's[49] belief that the tissue surrounding the toenail was "in a state of chronic inflammation and will return to normal or nearly normal size after removal of the offending nail. . . ."

Keyes stated that the Winograd technique is based on the principle of permanently removing all of the ingrown portion of the nail, assuming the cryptosis was caused by excessive width or convexity of the nail and not by overgrowth of the nail wall.[10] In 1937, Heifetz advocated the method of Winograd with a few modifications in all cases of third-stage and most second-stage lesions.[1] (He defined the third stage as being a period of granulations and the second stage as being a period of drainage.) In 1945, Heifetz redescribed the procedure.[51] Excision of the matrix was performed using a scalpel instead of a curette, and the use of phenol after removal of the nail matrix was not mentioned, although it was originally described. Other modifications include correspondence in the *Medical Journal of Australia* that reports suturing the incision in the proximal nail fold.[52] In conclusion, it can be said that a wedge resection is not the true definition of the Winograd technique.

There have been varying reports on the results of the Winograd technique. Clarke and Dillinger reported 29 naval cases where the Winograd technique was used.[53] There were nine recurrences, two with symptoms. In 1936, Winograd reported a 15-percent recurrence rate after 18 months.[50] Although results are limited, in 1979 Murray advocated the original technique of Winograd as the procedure of choice for ingrown nails when the patient refuses to have a total proximal nail bed ablation performed and when there is only one nail border involved.[16]

Frost Technique. Many clinicians advocate and still use the Frost technique, which was originally described in 1950.[18] According to Frost, his technique is indicated for incurvated nails.[27] Interestingly enough, Frost did not recommend his procedure for all cases of onychocryptosis—for example, it was not recommended for hypertrophic ungualabia not associated with an incurvated nail. Mercado stated that the Frost technique is indicated for cryptosis when a nail is incurvated and there is little or no proud flesh.[48] Burns et al., however, stated that the Frost technique is primarily indicated where an ingrown nail coexists with a hypertrophied and overlapping ungualabia.[4]

The description of the Frost technique from the articles written in 1950 and 1957 is as follows.[18,27] The entire nail is split at the point where the incurvated nail begins its arc. A vertical incision is then made down to but not into the phalanx and extending beyond either edge of the nail. The inverted "L" is created by making an incision 90 degrees to the proximal end of the first incision. This incision should be through the dermis but not into adipose tissue. A flap is then underscored and created, taking care not to include any white, fibrous, glistening soft tissue, because this may indicate the nail root. A third incision is made parallel to the first, starting under the flap and extending distally. This incision becomes semielliptical as it courses to join the first incision at the distal aspect of the toe. The section of the nail, nail bed, and root is excised. Care is taken not to damage the periosteum. The area is inspected for white, glistening fibers, which are excised before the flap is replaced. No suturing is recommended according to Frost (Fig. 19-11A & B).

A noteworthy modification of the Frost procedure is the labiomatrixectomy procedure by Whitney.[8] Whitney removes a longitudinal wedge of "superfluous labile tissue," with a trial coaptation of the remodeled labium before the Frost incision is made and the nail plate, bed, and matrix are resected. Whitney recommends this procedure for adolescent patients with onychocryptosis who also have reactive hypertrophy of the paralabium.

Steinberg Trephine

In 1954, Steinberg designed a specific tool and technique to perform surgery on ingrowing nails.[31]

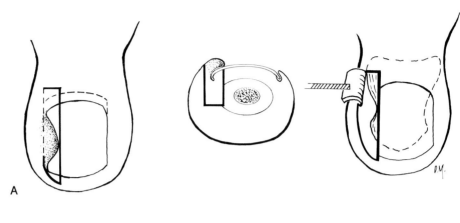

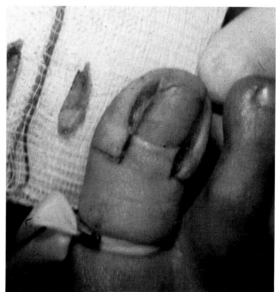

Fig. 19-11. (A) Frost nail procedure. As noted by Frost, skin flap does not include nail root. (From Frost,[27] with permission.) **(B)** Bilateral Frost procedure. (Courtesy of Drs. Ruff, Ruskusky, and Ward, Peoria, IL.)

The Steinberg trephine has an annular cutting head with a hollowed portion that holds a plug of excised tissue after transection by the head. After superficial débridement of loose infected tissue, a nick is made in the nail ⅛ inch from the border and an incision in the posteriolateral border of the eponychium is effected. After undermining the incision, the trephine is applied, engaging the nick. The trephine is manipulated with a boring action and is kept parallel and close to the phalanx. The plug of tissue should consist of nail, nail bed, infected granulations, and fibrous tissue. The cutting edge of the trephine is advanced under the previous incision until the leading edge is in front of the posterior extreme of the matrix. The instru-

ment is slightly retracted and raised perpendicular to the phalanx and the projecting cutting edge is pressed downward, severing the attachment of the plug. Steinberg then applies a Michel clip to the incision. Steinberg claims the advantages are immediate ambulation, minimum discomfort, and minimum operating time (Fig. 19-12).

Onychocryptosis Via Air Motor

Application of a high-speed burr to the matrix area for partial eradication of the nails is practiced by many clinicians. Perrone reported using a high-speed, low-torque air motor with a Busch burr to "erase" the nail matrix, and claims to use distinct

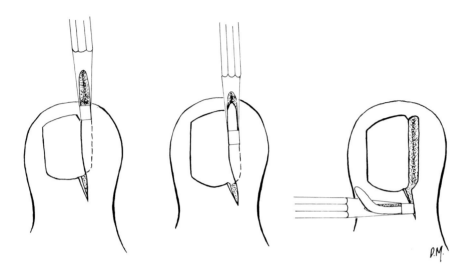

Fig. 19-12. The Steinberg trephine procedure. (From Steinberg,[31] with permission.)

sounds to determine when "erasure" of the nail matrix is complete.[54] Perrone reported that if a "bone noise" is not heard, recurrence is likely to take place. The burr is applied to the eponychial envelope only. Advantages of this technique are claimed to be decreased postoperative pain, immediate ambulation, and rapid healing time. Of 161 cases of partial matrix erasure, Perrone reported only one recurrence. Perrone also reported a healing time of 1 to 7 days with partial matrix erasure. This technique can also be used for complete eradication of nails.

Electrosurgery

Electrosurgery has been used to treat ingrown nails for many years. In 1938, Vernon described removing infected granulation tissue at the edge of the toenail with an electrocutting needle.[55] Recently an article in the *New Zealand Medical Journal* described treating acute paronychia with hyfriecator cautery.[56] A notable procedure used to treat cryptosis by some clinicians in the United States involves negative galvanic current (electrogalvanism). Polokoff described this procedure in 1935.[23] After removing the desired nail border and applying a dispersive electrode, Gardner used an unsharpened negative electrode in the shape of a saber that is applied to the matrix and nail bed.[57] The distal end of the electrode is below the eponychium while the body of the electrode lies on the nail bed. Care is taken not to touch the dermis above the matrix to avoid blistering. A notable advantage to the procedure is decreased postoperative pain. In a postoperative study, Gardner reported 10 recurrences in 176 nail borders.[57] Disadvantages of electrogalvanism include possible blistering of the integument and possible shedding of the nail plate. Variations in the milliamperage may occur. As the procedure is performed, the resistance to the current may drop, allowing more milliamperage than advisable. Variations in the texture of the skin may also require appropriate adjustments in the procedure. Another disadvantage may be that the patient may feel paresthesias in the limb. Care must also be taken to decrease the amperage before removing the electrode, because the patient may experience an uncomfortable shock if this is not done.

Gardner reported that events that occur at the negative electrode are release of hydrogen from the matrix cells and formation of "protein dissolving caustic sodium hydroxide." Other physical effects at the site are cataphoresis and electrophoresis, which are probably less important, according to Gardner.[57] Bouché reiterated the method of destruction of the nail matrix as a process of production of sodium hydroxide and low to moderate heat, which act by denaturing protein and dehydrating tissue.[7] Bouché also used a 5 percent acetic acid lavage to produce mechanical and chemical neutralization of the sodium hydroxide.

Cryosurgery

In September of 1984, Silverman reported using a liquid nitrogen cryoprobe to destroy the germinal matrix.[46] After suitable anesthesia and application of a tourniquet, the nail border was removed. A full-depth 0.5-cm incision was effected in the corner of the nail bed to allow insertion of the cryoprobe. The freezing process was continued until an area of frozen skin was apparent that was approximately 1.5 cm in diameter. This took approximately 90 seconds. The area was allowed to thaw, and application of warm sterile water was sometimes necessary. The freezing process was repeated in order to destroy granulation tissue. Two symptomatic recurrences and two cases of asymptomatic onychogryphosis occurred in 26 patients. The author suggested that the onychogryphosis was caused by a sublethal injury to the germinal matrix. It will be interesting to note further developments in the procedure.

Phenol and Alcohol Partial Nail Matrixectomy

To date, the most widely accepted and used procedure for the treatment of onychocryptosis is the phenol and alcohol partial matrixectomy. Advantages of the procedure include decreased postoperative discomfort,[58-60] simplicity,[61] low recurrence rate,[61] and cosmesis.[59] The decreased postoperative pain may be due to the neurolytic action of phenol.[60] Gallocher reported a success rate of 98.5 percent.[62] Robb and Murray reported a 5 percent recurrence rate with partial cauterization.[59] Suppan and Ritchlin reported a 98.7 percent success rate using phenol cauterization.[63] As can be easily noted from the preceding discussions, no other procedure can currently boast such success.

Some clinicians state that the procedure may be performed in the presence of local infection.[64] An-

other belief maintained by certain clinicians is that sepsis distal to the interphalangeal joint is not a contraindication since phenol is an antiseptic.[59] Other clinicians have stated that the procedure is indicated where there is no significant or gross hypertrophy of the ungualabia.[4,63]

However, this author feels that hypertrophy of the ungualabia is not a contraindication because a wider nail border may be resected to compensate for any recurrences that may develop due to possible soft tissue etiology (e.g., impingement of the soft tissue on the new nail border). Also, paronychia should be resolved before a permanent procedure is performed because many prominent clinicians have reported complications as a direct result of performing a permanent procedure on infected nail borders. It should be noted that it may be difficult to distinguish chronic irritation resulting in inflammation from local infection. Cauterizing the tissue with phenol may allow infection to propagate in the devitalized tissue and prolong healing time.

The phenol and alcohol partial matrixectomy procedure has been described on several occasions.[32,59,63,65,66] After suitable prepping and anesthesia, a Penrose drain is applied around the digit for hemostasis. It should be stated that a Penrose drain may not always be appropriate and should be used at the discretion of the clinician pending clinical findings of circulation and history of the patient. Excessive hemorrhaging will dilute and neutralize the phenol. The nail is split with an onychotome in the form of a #61 or #62 blade along the longitudinal striations of the nail. The split is usually initiated with a nail nipper. The width of the nail to be removed may depend on chronicity of the ingrown nail, amount of incurvation, and amount of nail lip hypertrophy. In certain instances, cosmesis may be a factor also. The nail is split completely under the eponychium. Splitting of the nail may also be accomplished with an English nail anvil up to the eponychium (Fig. 19-13). An onychotome is then required to split the nail beneath the eponychium. Although the instrument leaves a new nail border that is perfectly straight, it should be noted that an English nail anvil may cause onycholysis of the new nail border because the lower jaw of the instrument has a wedge and therefore a lysing action.

The nail portion to be removed is undermined

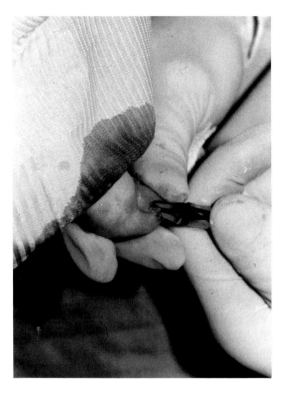

Fig. 19-13. English nail anvil application. (Courtesy of Dr. Silver, St. Louis Park, MN.)

and freed with a spatula or periosteal elevator. A hemostat is then applied to the nail underneath the eponychium and the nail border is removed by rolling the hemostat inward toward the center of the nail (Fig. 19-14). Fibrous tissues are resected with a curette and tissue nippers. Eighty-eight percent phenol is applied with cotton applicators, cotton pellets, or wisps of cotton twisted on toothpicks. There are many variations as to the amount of time of the application of the phenol. This is probably because each vehicle described will deliver different amounts of phenol to the area, and therefore necessary adjustments in time must be made. Usually hand-made toothpicks with cotton are applied three times for 30 seconds each time. Many experienced clinicians use appearance to determine amount of phenol application. The area is then flushed with alcohol, the tourniquet is removed, and an appropriate sterile dressing is ap-

plied. If the nail border is freed without excessive trauma, an eponychial envelope will be formed and application of the phenol to the matrix will be assisted. Care is taken not to apply phenol to nail folds because an unnecessary burn will occur to the exposed epidermis of the nail fold. Alcohol is used as a mechanical flush and it should be noted that phenol is solvent in alcohol.

Postoperative Care

Postoperative dressings vary from clinician to clinician by personal preference. A straw-colored exudate is expected to drain from the operative site,[58,59] and may be experienced for several weeks. In 1965, Cooper reported on Chymar (chymotrypsin) ointment, which is a product that contains proteolytic enzymes with neomycin and steroid in a water-soluble ointment base.[67] Cooper found that Chymar ointment used postoperatively decreased the healing time of partial phenol and alcohol matrixectomies to almost half that of topical antibiotics used postoperatively alone. Acker recommended using a combination of aqueous Zephiran (benzalkonium chloride) 1:750 solution, Metiderm aerosol, and Elase ointment (fibrinolysin plus desoxyribonuclease) immediately after surgery.[68] The dressing is changed every 3 to 4 days, and Elase is applied after painting with Zephiran Chloride solution. Fulp and McGlamry concluded that Travase (sutilains) could speed the healing process and reduce the postoperative drainage period if applied correctly.[64] Specifically, the dressing must be kept moist, agents that will deactivate the enzyme must be avoided, and the dressings changed every 6 to 8 hours to maintain a therapeutic level of enzymatic activity.

A study in the early 1980s involving Debrisan concluded that it is as effective in the postoperative care of phenol and alcohol nail procedures as other forms of postoperative care.[65] Debrisan consists of spherical hydrophilic beads comprised of cross-linked dextran. Other topicals that are routinely used by clinicians for partial phenol and alcohol procedures include otic Cortisporin (polymixin B-neomycin-hydrocortisone), Silvadene (silver sulfadiazine), Neosporin (polymixin B-bacitracin-neomycin) powder and cream, Furacin (ni-

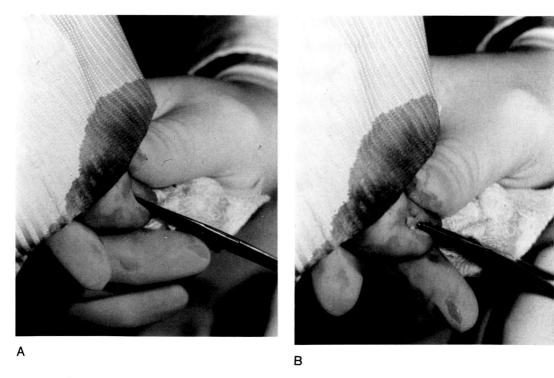

A

B

Fig. 19-14. Removing nail border with hemostat. (Courtesy of Dr. Silver, St. Louis Park, MN.)

trofurazone), and Betadine (povidone-iodine). An important point discussed by Greenwald and Robbins is that postoperative creams may be more beneficial than ointments.[69] Creams do not inhibit drainage and petroleum-based waterproof ointments do. Some clinicians may apply wicks or drains to the operative site to enhance the normal course of postoperative drainage. Rinaldi et al. specifically pointed out reduction in bacterial proliferation after matrixectomy using topical Betadine microbicides.[70]

Clinicians also vary on postoperative care. They may prefer to leave the dressing intact and apply dressing changes themselves or, after varying periods of time, have the patient change the dressing with appropriate topicals. Foot soaks are very popular after phenol and alcohol procedures. Again, personal preference will dictate what soaks are used, when they are initiated, how often they are performed, and if specified dressings with topicals are applied after the soaks. Various soaking agents include normal saline, Domeboro soaks, Epsom

salts, tea soaks, Betadine and water, vinegar and water, Pedi-Boro soaks, and warm soapy water soaks. An ionic solution will assist the draining process caused by the burn and therefore, it is hoped, decrease healing time. This author's personal preference dictates the use of Betadine soaks for the microbicidal activity that may be offered with this particular solution.

Disadvantages of the partial phenol and alcohol nail procedure are prolonged healing time[65] and extent of drainage.[9,65] Another disadvantage is acute reaction to phenol,[9] which may result in a phenol burn. Careless application of phenol, according to Yale, may result in Beau's lines.[66] Careless application of the phenol to surrounding integument may also result in undesirable and unnecessary destruction of soft tissue. As pointed out by Greenwald and Robbins, no chemical reaction occurs between isopropyl alcohol and phenol under the conditions of a matrixectomy and therefore neutralization refers to a physical or mechanical dilution.[69] This is yet another variable in the destructive process that may affect the results of the procedure.

Cameron described an interesting modification of the partial phenol and alcohol procedure referred to as *angular phenolization.*[71] According to Cameron, this procedure is indicated in severe or resistant cases and involves excision of the nail fold to a point level with the side of the nail before the actual partial phenol and alcohol matrixectomy is performed.

To summarize the phenol and alcohol partial matrixectomy, advantages include ease of performance, high success rate, and decreased postoperative pain, and disadvantages are prolonged healing time and drainage. Currently it is the most widely accepted and used procedure for onychocryptosis in podiatry today.

Sodium Hydroxide

A chemical matrixectomy procedure that is gaining popularity uses sodium hydroxide instead of phenol and alcohol. Travers and Ammon reported the advantages of sodium hydroxide over phenol to be predictability, high success rate, less drainage, faster healing time, and low recurrence ratios.[6] They reported 15 recurrences in 1,000 procedures. After proper anesthesia, the offending nail border is removed. The loose tissue is debrided and petroleum jelly is applied to the skin edges for protection. The 10 percent sodium hydroxide solution is applied with a cotton pellet to the nail bed for anywhere from 3 seconds to 3 minutes. According to Travers and Ammon, the application is continued, "until the capillaries of the nail bed visually coagulate." Neutralization occurs by application of 5 percent acetic acid. No tourniquet is used. The authors recommend lidocaine with epinephrine 1 : 200,000 or 1 : 300,000, which allows visualization of the capillaries as they coagulate. Destruction occurs via liquification necrosis.

Greenwald and Robbins pointed out that in this particular procedure, a true chemical neutralization occurs.[69] Brown applied a 10-percent sodium hydroxide solution with a thinned-out cotton-tipped applicator two times for a total of 20 to 25 seconds after hemostasis was obtained by pressure.[28] Brown used a 3-percent solution of acetic acid for neutralization.

Laser Treatment

The CO_2 laser produces infrared light that is invisible and is selectively absorbed by water in tissue.[72] The light is converted into heat energy, which vaporizes tissue.[72] A helium-neon aiming beam is used to direct the beam since the CO_2 laser light is invisible.[72] Advantages of the laser include precision control of depth and extent of surgical site, as well as sterilization and cauterization.[73] Borovoy et al. reported vaporizing the matrix with a 10- to 15-watt continuous wave and an average spot size of 2 mm after retraction of the eponychium. They reported no recurrence or infection in 93 partial nail avulsions, but do warn that care must be taken when vaporizing the matrix because traumatizing the periosteum can lead to periostitis.

Problems arising with laser destruction of the matrix include the need for precise destruction of the matrix without destruction of the periosteum, or "burning of bone." Visualization may be best accomplished with skin hooks retracting the eponychium. Other clinicians have suggested destruction of the eponychium overlying the matrix to solve this problem. Visualization of the matrix can be aided with the use of a microscope, control of hemostasis, and proper removal of the plume produced by the laser destruction.

Total Nail Ablation

Total nail ablation may be required for several reasons, ranging from recurrent ingrown toenails to dystrophic fungal nails to onychogryphosis. A deformed nail may be caused by damage to the nail bed or matrix.[9] Fowler classified onychogryphosis into two main types: thickening of the nail and thickening of the "sterile matrix," which is nail bed distal to the lunula.[2] Fowler reported that the characteristic onychogryphosis caused by fungal infections demonstrated thickening of both the nail and "sterile matrix" in combination.

There are many techniques for total nail ablation. Farber and South reported using urea ointment formulations for nonsurgical avulsion of nail dystrophies.[74] It should be stressed that, with any nail surgery, the patient should be treated conservatively if vascular insufficiency, increased susceptibility to infections, or other contraindications are elicited in the history or examination. Many of the procedures described for nail matrix destruction with onychocryptosis may be applied to total matrix ablation. These include onychotripsy,[54] the CO_2 surgical laser,[73] the phenol and alcohol chemical matrixectomy, and the NAOH chemical matrixectomy. Each of these have their obvious advantages and disadvantages. With the CO_2 laser, care must be taken not to "burn bone." Special instrumentation is required for onychotripsy. The phenol and alcohol procedure has prolonged draining and healing times. An attempt to resolve this dilemma has gone as far as applying split-thickness porcine xenografts to nail beds after phenol matrix destruction.[75]

Once again the problem of paronychia and performing total nail ablation arises. It is recommended that surgery not be performed until the active infection has been resolved. This may require partial or total nail avulsion with soaks and concomitant antibiotic therapy. Another problem that arises is prepping the toe for surgery. Some clinicians suggest a double scrub of the foot be performed, once before and once after total nail avulsion, to decontaminate subungual tissues.[76] This author also recommends the double scrub, especially if sharp matrixectomy procedures are executed. This may not be such an important prerequisite if phenol, sodium hydroxide, or the CO_2 laser is used because these procedures are grossly destructive anyway.

Kaplan Procedure

In 1960, Kaplan published an article about a procedure for total nail avulsion that was designed to eradicate club nail and produce satisfactory results without regard to etiology.[77] The following is a brief summation of the procedure as described by Kaplan. After proper surgical preparation, the great toe is anesthetized and the nail is avulsed. The foot is prepped and a tourniquet is applied. Two 1.5-cm incisions are effected in the medial and lateral aspects of the posterior eponychium and extend proximally. The area is retracted after sharp dissection at the nail level depth to expose the matrix. Another incision is effected connecting the nail folds distally. The nail bed is removed from the

phalanx using sharp dissection just distal to the tendon that includes the matrix. The phalanx is exposed and exostoses are removed. The eponychial flap is replaced and sutured. Of 359 cases reported by Kaplan, no failures were reported.

Mercado et al. described the Kaplan procedure in detail with additional modifications.[78] They used two incisions made just outside the nail grooves that are effected prior to underscoring the nail bed flap. After resection of the flap, two wedge sections are taken from both sides of the base of the phalanx to ensure complete removal of the matrix. These clinicians also resect the eponychium from the eponychial flap and reduce the size of the wound by placing two 3-0 plain catgut sutures across the two lateral margins of the wound. They reported a healing time that is equivalent to the healing time of an arthroplasty. They also stressed the complete denuding of the dorsum of the phalanx.

Zadik Procedure

Another procedure that has had so many modifications and variations that the original technique may be hard to identify is the Zadik procedure. Zadik described the procedure for treatment of onychogryphosis and cryptosis of the hallux.[5] A true Zadik procedure involves creating a skin flap, avulsing the nail, and resecting the nail bed proximal to the border of the lunula. The flap is advanced and sutured to the nail bed without tension. According to Zadik, the lateral nail folds are excised and corresponding coaptation with sutures is performed if the lateral nail furrows are deep. As with certain other total nail ablation procedures, nail bed resection is directed proximally and the nail bed distal to the lunula is undisturbed (Fig. 19-15).

Palmer and Jones reported a 28 percent recurrence rate when the Zadik operation was used for ingrown nails.[29] Robb reported a symptomatic recurrence rate of 29 percent when using Zadik's operation on children with nail dystrophy of the hallux.[79] Murray and Bedi reported a 16 percent symptomatic recurrence rate for ingrown toenails using the Zadik procedure,[30] and in 1979 Murray wrote another paper advocating the Zadik procedure.[16]

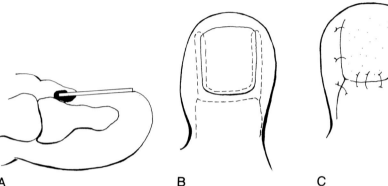

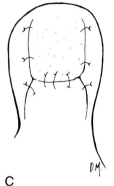

A   B   C

Fig. 19-15. Zadik procedure. (From Zadik,[5] with permission.)

Fowler Procedure

Fowler described a procedure for onychogryphosis and "bilateral embedded nails" where three flaps are created to expose the germinal matrix.[2] After proper anesthesia and application of a tourniquet, two one-half-inch incisions are effected at the junction of the nail fold and nail walls. Three flaps are dissected consisting of skin only, with the epithelium on the deep surfaces of the nail fold and walls left intact. The nail is removed. After retraction, a block of tissue is excised consisting of germinal matrix and the overlying deep layer of nail fold and nail walls. The flaps are sutured to cover the raw area or the majority of raw area (Fig. 19-16). Fowler reported three recurrences of a nail growth in 50 operations for onychogryphosis.

Whitney Acisional Matrixectomy

An "acisional" total matrixectomy procedure was reported by Whitney in 1968 for a hallux matrix resection.[76] The indications for use are hyperostosis in the matrix area, hyperostosis of the tuft of the distal phalanx, and chronic soft tissue changes that affect the nail bed and paralabial tissue. After anesthesia and application of a tourniquet, the nail is avulsed and the toe is rescrubbed. "Frost incisions" are effected on the bilateral borders, and the side flaps are undercut at the loose areolar tissue and retracted. The eponychium is trimmed before a transverse incision is effected at the level of the lunula. The central eponychial flap is freed and retracted and incisions are effected outside of the

posterior and lateral limits of the glistening matrix. The matrix is resected via sharp dissection. After total resection of the matrix, the skin flaps are sutured. The nail bed and the eponychial flap may be sutured, but gapping is acceptable if undue tension is present and nail bed undermining will not facilitate apposition (Fig. 19-17).

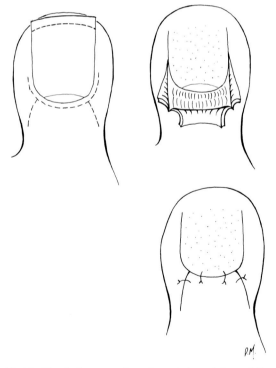

Fig. 19-16. Fowler's procedure for total excision of the germinal matrix. (From Fowler,[2] with permission.)

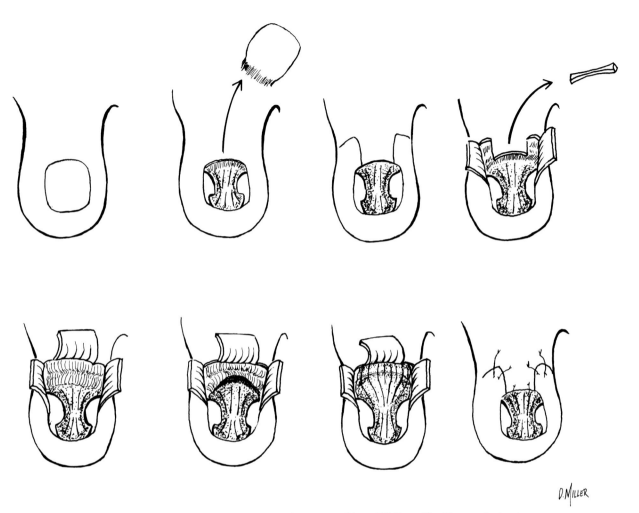

Fig. 19-17. Whitney acisional matrixectomy. (From Whitney,[76] with permission.)

Suppan Nail Technique No. 2

A very popular sharp nail procedure for complete removal of the nail matrix has been taught by Suppan since 1958. The advantages of the procedure as reported by Weisfeld are healing by first intention, complete visualization of the matrix to facilitate its excision, and no skin incisions.[9] The procedure as described by Weisfeld, referred to as the "Suppan Nail Technique No. 2," is as follows. After proper prepping, anesthesia, and hemostasis, the nail is avulsed. The remaining areas of hyponychium are debrided to prevent postsurgical recurrence. A #15 blade is placed parallel to the cor-

ium at the medial margin of the posterior nail fold and the blade is kept just deep to the nail fold. The blade is drawn laterally over the entire matrix (Fig. 19-18) and angled plantarly against the bone at the medial and lateral aspects of the incision. A transverse incision is made down to bone at the nail matrix and corium junction with the blade angled somewhat posteriorly. The matrix is resected in toto. The posterior nail fold may be sutured to the bed. It should be noted that the "envelope" of the nail matrix has to be excised. To fully understand the procedure, it is important to review the author's conception of the anatomy of the nail and sagittal location of the nail matrix (Fig. 19-19).

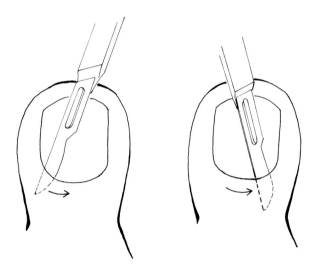

Fig. 19-18. Suppan nail technique no. 2.[9]

Terminal Syme Procedure

Clinicians have developed radical techniques for treatment of recalcitrant pathologies. In one case, a metatarsal phalangeal amputation is reported for a "distorted" toe with a hypertrophied nail that was painful and inflamed to the point of being disabling.[80] A less radical step, but comparatively radical with regard to other procedures, is the terminal Syme procedure. Murray stated that one indication for the terminal Syme procedure is recurrent cryptotic nail regrowth after a second attempt at proximal nail bed ablation.[16] Other indications include onychocryptosis, subungual osteoma, onychauxis, glomus tumors, circulatory dystrophies, mallet toe deformities, and macrodactyly.[81]

The procedure as described by Lapidus[82] involves a U-shaped incision surrounding the toenail and another incision that connects the two sides of the "U." The edge of the skin around the nail, the nail, and the matrix are totally resected. About one-half of the distal phalanx is resected, which leaves a long plantar flap that is turned up over the terminal phalanx and is sutured to the short dorsal flap. Lapidus advocated this procedure for onychogryphosis, subungual osteoma, and any nail pathology where total removal of nail is the procedure desired.

Thompson and Terwilliger stated that the advantage of the terminal Syme procedure in the treatment of recurring cryptosis is the completeness and permanency of the cure and the speed with which the cure is accomplished.[83] They also stress that "the ENTIRE nail bed, with an adequate margin, should be included in the excision." A controversy

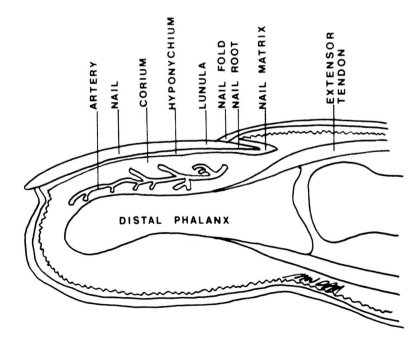

Fig. 19-19. Anatomy of the nail with a depiction of the, "envelope" or wrap-around characteristic of the "nail matrix."[9]

seems to exist over the toes for which this procedure is indicated. Based on the cosmetic results, some clinicians believe the procedure should be reserved for the lesser toes. Variations also exist as to the exact locations of the incisions and the amount of bone to be resected (Fig. 19-20). Usually one-third to one-half of the distal phalanx is excised, but the entire phalanx may be removed pending clinical findings.[81]

Procedure for Subungual Osteoma

Lapidus pointed out the possible recurrence of subungual osteoma and advocated resection of the distal part of the phalanx to prevent recurrence.[82] Because the terminal Syme procedure may not be cosmetically acceptable to patients, a less radical and disfiguring approach may be advised. After proper prepping, anesthesia, and hemostasis, the nail is avulsed. After rescrubbing the foot, the nail bed is incised along the longitudinal axis of the toe with the center of the incision being directly over or almost directly over the subungual osteoma. A fish-mouth incision is made anteriorly to facilitate sharp dissection of the nail bed from the distal phalanx in order to expose the osteoma. The osteoma is excised. To prevent recurrence it is suggested that a saucering be performed on the distal phalanx. Care should be taken so that the area proximal to the lunula and the lunular border is left undis-

turbed. The nail bed is replaced and sutured. This will allow minimal disruption of the nail bed and, it is hoped, allow the toenail to regrow without any disfigurement. No studies on results are currently available for this procedure.

Dilemmas in Total Nail Ablation

As stated in the beginning of the chapter, opinions vary as to the exact location of the nail matrix. This explains the large number of procedures devised to accomplish the same goal. Fowler pointed out that, when excising the matrix, the incisions must be kept clear of the lunula to avoid recurrences.[2] After reviewing the procedures and their respective results, it becomes apparent that the nail matrix is located proximal to and includes the lunular border. This must be true or procedures such as the Suppan Nail Technique for total nail ablation would not be successful. Further review of all of the procedures for nail matrix destruction may also lend credibility to the idea of a nail matrix "envelope."

Techniques also vary with respect to the resection of the periosteum. Some clinicians recommend complete eradication of the periosteum, whereas others believe the periosteum should be left intact because careful technique with good exposure will allow complete excision of the matrix. In actuality, the controversy involves risks versus benefits: the risk of tampering with the periosteum and all its functions versus the benefit of ensuring complete resection of the matrix. The resolution of this controversy is probably best answered by the ideas, beliefs, and personal experience of individual clinicians.

Another dilemma to be dealt with when performing total nail ablation is cosmesis. One clinician has reported synthesis of a prosthetic nail plate fabricated with dental acrylic polymer and monomer.[84] Prosthetic nails to date have not gained much popularity. Another problem regarding cosmesis and total nail ablation as described by Fowler[2] is "residual thickening of the sterile matrix. . . . " It should be noted that keratosis may form after certain total nail ablation procedures, such as phenol and alcohol matrixectomy, and the keratosis can easily and painlessly be debrided. Currently, cosmesis is a factor the individual patient must deal with.

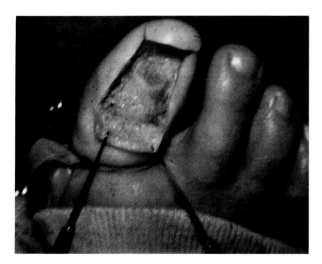

Fig. 19-20. The terminal Syme procedure. (Courtesy of Drs. Ruff, Ruskusky, and Ward, Peoria, IL.)

SUMMARY

Many different techniques and modes are used to treat nail pathology. Heavy emphasis has been placed on partial and total nail ablation because these procedures are commonly employed. Several operative procedures have been reviewed according to their original presentations to give the reader a clear perspective of original philosophies and salient points.

REFERENCES

1. Heifetz CJ: Ingrown toenail: a clinical study. Am J Surg, 38:298, 1937
2. Fowler AW: Excision of the germinal matrix: a unified treatment for embedded toenail and onychocryptosis. Br J Surg, 45:382, 1958
3. Dixon GL: Treatment of ingrown toenail. Foot Ankle, 3:254, 1983
4. Burns SA, Ketai RS, Ketai NH: Onychocryptosis. J Am Podiatry Assoc, 67:780, 1977
5. Zadik FR: Obliteration of the nail bed of the great toe without shortening of the terminal phalanx. J Bone Joint Surg [Br], 32:66, 1950
6. Travers GR, Ammon RG: The sodium hydroxide chemical matricectomy procedure. J Am Podiatry Assoc, 70:476, 1980
7. Bouche RT: Matricectomy utilizing negative galvanic current. Clin Podiatr Med Surg, 3:449, 1986
8. Whitney AK: An illustrated labiomatricectomy procedure. J Am Podiatry Assoc, 57:169, 1967
9. Weisfeld M: Illustrated technique for the complete removal of nail matrix and hyponychium without skin incisions (Suppan Nail Technique No. 2). J Am Podiatry Assoc, 65:481, 1975
10. Keyes EL: The surgical treatment of ingrown toenails. JAMA, 102:1458, 1934
11. Wee GC, Shieber W: Painless evacuation of subungual hematoma. Surg Gynecol Obstet, 133:531, 1970
12. Albom MJ: Surgical gems: avulsion of a nail plate. J Dermatol Surg Oncol, 3:34, 1977
13. Scher RK: Surgical avulsion of nail plates by a proximal to distal technique. J Dermatol Surg Oncol, 7:296, 1981
14. Miller TJ: A pilot of nail surgery. J Am Podiatry Assoc, 58:304, 1968
15. Herold HZ, Daniel D: Radical wedge resection in the treatment of ingrowing toenail. Int Surg, 49:558, 1968
16. Murray WR: Onychocryptosis. Principles of non-operative and operative care. Clin Orthop, 142:96, 1979
17. Bartlett RW: Conservative operation for the cure of so called ingrown toenail. JAMA, 108:1257, 1937
18. Frost LA: Root resection for incurvated nail. J Am Podiatry Assoc, 40:19, 1950
19. Vandenbos KQ, Bowers WF: Ingrowing toenail: results of weight bearing on soft tissue. US Armed Forces Med J, 10:1168, 1959
20. DuVries HL: Ingrown nail. Chiropody Rec, 27:155, 1944
21. DuVries HL: Hypertrophy of unguilabia. Chiropody Rec, 16:13, 1933
22. Newman RW: A simplified treatment of ingrown toenail. Surg Gynecol Obstet, 89:638, 1949
23. Polokoff M: Ingrown toenail and hypertrophied nail lip surgery by electrolysis. J Am Podiatry Assoc, 51:805, 1961
24. VanEnoo RE, Cane EM: Minimal incision surgery. Clin Podiatr Med Surg, 3:321, 1986
25. Perlman P: Don't Take Two Aspirin. Johnson Publishing Company, Boulder, CO, 1982
26. Eibel P: Unguis incarnatus complicated by glomus tumor. Can Med Assoc J, 93:811, 1965
27. Frost L: A definite surgical treatment for some lateral nail problems. J Nat Assoc Chiropodists, 47:493, 1957
28. Brown FC: Chemocautery for ingrown toenails. J Dermatol Surg Oncol, 7:331, 1981
29. Palmer BV, Jones A: Ingrowing toenails: the results of treatment. Br J Surg, 66:575, 1979
30. Murray WR, Bedi BS: The surgical management of ingrowing toenail. Br J Surg, 62:409, 1975
31. Steinberg MD: A simplified technique for the surgery of ingrowing nails. Surgery, 36:1132, 1954
32. McGlamry ED: Management of painful toes from distorted toenails. J Dermatol Surg Oncol, 5:554, 1979
33. Linch AO: Treatment of ingrowing toenail. South Surg, 8:173, 1939
34. Farnsworth FC: A treatment for convoluted nails. J Am Podiatry Assoc, 62:110, 1972
35. Ilfeld FW, August W: Treatment of ingrown toenail with plastic insert. Orthop Clin North Am, 5:95, 1974

36. Wallace WA, Milne DD, Andrew T: Gutter treatment for ingrowing toenails. Br Med J, 2:168, 1979
37. Howard WR: Ingrown toenail: its surgical treatment. NY Med J, 57:579, 1893
38. Kufdakis AD: Ingrown toenail surgery: a new procedure. Int Surg, 66:339, 1981
39. Crooke P: The ingrowing toenail. Aust Fam Physician, 10:808, 1981.
40. Murray WR, Robb JE: Soft tissue resection for ingrowing toenails. J Dermatol Surg Oncol, 7:157, 1981
41. Antrum RM: Radical excision of the nailfold for ingrowing toenail. J Bone Joint Surg, 66:63, 1984
42. Ney GC: An operation for ingrowing toenail. JAMA, 80:374, 1923
43. Zechel G: The fallacy of the ingrown toenail. Surg Gynecol Obstet, 131:117, 1970
44. Mogensen P: Ingrowing toenail. Acta Orthop Scand, 42:94, 1971
45. Palmer BV, Stevenson DL: Modified operation for ingrowing toenails (letter to the editor). Br Med J, 2:367, 1976
46. Silverman SH: Cryosurgery for ingrowing toenail. J R Coll Surg Edinburgh, 29:289, 1984
47. Yale JF: Podiatric Medicine. 3rd Ed. Williams & Wilkins, Baltimore, MD, 1987
48. Mercado OA: An Atlas of Foot Surgery. Vol. 1: Forefoot Surgery. Carolando Press, Oak Park, IL, 1979
49. Winograd AM: A modification in the technique of operation for ingrown toenail. JAMA, 91:229, 1929
50. Winograd AM: Results in operation for ingrown toenail. Il M J, 70:197, 1936
51. Heifetz CJ: Operative management of ingrown toenail. J Missouri Med Assoc, 42:213, 1945
52. Chambers DG: Ingrown toenails (letter to the editor). Med J Aust, 1:608, 1968
53. Clarke BG, Dillinger KA: Surgical treatment of ingrown toenail. Surgery, 21:919, 1946
54. Perrone MA: Nail matricectomy by onychotripsy with airmotor. J Am Podiatry Assoc, 60:92, 1970
55. Vernon S: Ingrown toenail: operation by electrosurgery. Am J Surg, 42:396, 1938
56. Dinesh D: Ingrowing toenail (letter to the editor). NZ Med J, 89:494, 1979
57. Gardner P: Negative galvanic current in the surgical correction of onychocryptotic nails. J Am Podiatry Assoc, 48:555, 1958
58. Ross WR: Treatment of the ingrown toenail. Surg Clin North Am, 49:1499, 1969
59. Robb JE, Murray WR: Phenol cauterisation in the management of ingrowing toenails. Scott Med J, 27:236, 1982
60. Shepherdson A: Nail matrix phenolization: a preferred alternative to surgical excision. Practitioner, 219:725, 1977
61. Wee GC, Tucker GL: Phenolic cauterization of the matrix in the surgical cure of ingrown toenails. Mo Med, 66:802, 1969
62. Gallocher J: The phenol alcohol method of nail matrix sterilisation. NZ Med J, 86:140, 1977
63. Suppan RJ, Ritchlin JD: A non-disabilitating surgical procedure for ingrown toenail. J Am Podiatry Assoc, 52:900, 1962
63. Fulp M, McGlamry ED: New enzyme aids phenol technique in nail surgery. J Am Podiatry Assoc, 62:395, 1972
65. Drago JJ, Jacobs AM, Oloff L: A comparative study of postoperative care with phenol nail procedures. J Foot Surg, 22:332, 1983
66. Yale JF: Phenol-alcohol technique for correction of infected ingrown toenail. J Am Podiatry Assoc, 64:46, 1974
67. Cooper C: Phenol-alcohol nail procedure: postoperative care. J Am Podiatry Assoc, 55:661, 1965
68. Acker I: Preventing the postoperative sequelae to phenolization of nail bed and matrix. J Am Podiatry Assoc, 58:351, 1968
69. Greenwald L, Robbins HM: The chemical matricectomy. J Am Podiatry Assoc, 71:388, 1981
70. Rinaldi R, Sabia M, Gross J: The treatment and prevention of infection in phenol alcohol matricectomies. J Am Podiatry Assoc, 72:435, 1982
71. Cameron PF: Ingrowing toenails: an evaluation of two treatments. Br J Med, 283:821, 1981
72. Apfelberg DB, Rothermel E, Widtfeldt A et al: Progress report on use of carbon dioxide laser for nail disorders. Curr Podiatry, 32:29, 1983
73. Borovoy M, Fuller TA, Holtz P, Kaczander BI: Laser surgery in podiatric medicine present and future. J Foot Surg, 22:353, 1983
74. Farber EM, South DA: Urea ointment in the nonsurgical avulsion of nail dystrophies. Cutis, 22:689, 1978
75. Elleby DH, Weil LS, Sorto LA, Smith SD: The use of porcine xenografts on nail beds following total nail avulsion and phenol chemomatrixectomy. J Foot Surg, 16:85, 1977
76. Whitney AK: Total matricectomy procedure. J Am Podiatry Assoc, 58:157, 1968
77. Kaplan EG: Elimination of onychauxis by surgery. J Am Podiatry Assoc, 50:111, 1960
78. Mercado OA, Dalianis G, Chulengarian J et al: Kaplan nail revisited. Curr Podiatry, 21:21, 1972
79. Robb JE: The results of surgery for nail dystrophy of

the hallux in children. Surg Infancy Child, 39:131, 1984

80. Field LM: An ultimate solution for a painful toe. J Dermatol Surg Oncol, 5:402, 1979
81. Gastwirth BW, Anton VM, Martin RA: The terminal Syme procedure. J Foot Surg, 20:95, 1981
82. Lapidus PW: Complete and permanent removal of toenail in onychogryphosis and subungual osteoma. Am J Surg, 19:92, 1933
83. Thompson TC, Terwilliger C: The terminal Syme operation for ingrown toenail. Surg Clin North Am, 31:575, 1951
84. Rosen S: Prosthetic nail plate. J Am Podiatry Assoc, 60:283, 1970

The Diabetic and Insensitive Foot 20

Richard M. Stess, D.P.M.
Vincent J. Hetherington, D.P.M., M.S.

DIABETES MELLITUS

Diabetes mellitus is a disease whose morbidity can be so insidious that only regular monitoring by both the general physician and the podiatrist can alert the patient to potential disaster. The podiatrists as well as other health care professionals who regularly treat patients with diabetes must integrate their individual skills with those of others if an impact upon morbidity is to be accomplished. It is necessary to develop a liaison with those physicians and allied health care providers with an interest in comprehensive health care. Only by such association can the incidence of foot ulcerations and amputation, which are increasing with alarming rapidity, be reduced.

Diabetes is not a rare, vague, exotic affliction that takes its toll on a few unfortunates. Rather, as the number of diabetics swells to over 13 million, representing approximately 4 percent of the population in the United States and steadily rising, there is concurrent steady inflation in expenditures of both personnel and health care dollars. If those patients with more mild degrees of glucose intolerance who have not yet been diagnosed were included in the statistics, the total would likely double or triple. The often-used figures of the number of hospitalizations required for patients with diabetic foot disease would suggest a serious wide variety of pathologic conditions that interplay, resulting in significant limb and life morbidity. The diabetic foot must be treated aggressively with every tool available both diagnostically and clinically. Great advancement in both areas is now being made, and it is imperative that the well-trained podiatrist either maintain expertise in the state of the art in the treatment of the diabetic foot or be prepared to refer that patient to those who do.

Despite the expenditures in both clinical and laboratory research, there remains in the late 1980s wide variances and controversy in the treatment of the diabetic foot. This discussion seems to originate from a significant lack of well-documented and evaluated methodologies. What one finds in practice at many of the major medical centers in the United States professing to be Diabetic Centers are often-used empirical remedies that have not been scientifically scrutinized and evaluated. One finds, for example, strong diverse opinions stated in two major diabetes textbooks regarding the use of warm foot soaks. One author favors soaks while another likens the use to heresy if practiced. Nei-

523

ther opinion has been put to a scientific test and evaluated in controlled studies. Unfortunate as it may be, many of the most common practices have never been evaluated and therefore their efficacy is suspect. It is necessary at this time to reevaluate diabetic foot disease, evaluate and study the natural history of the disease process, and develop effective diagnostic and treatment criteria whose results can be quantified. Only by such a methodical approach can we make a significant contribution to medical literature and have a positive impact on morbidity.

Examination

The method of examination of the diabetic patient must be comprehensive, organized, and well documented. Only by setting strict methodology will the practitioner be able to more thoroughly evaluate the patient; also, he or she will be able to determine the progression of the disease. This examination will serve as a reference for both past episodes and future sequelae. The practitioner must have every tool available in order to understand the totality of the foot pathology.

The initial history should make reference specifically to the following diseases: hypertension, retinopathy, renal failure, myocardial infarction, angina, cirrhosis, radiculopathy, intermittent claudication, and impotency. Additionally, any history of lower extremity vascular surgery, foot ulceration, or foot surgery should be carefully reviewed and documented. Once the review of systems and past medical history is obtained, a more detailed diabetic history becomes necessary in order to obtain an appreciation for the current status of the disease. This portion of the history should include the following:

Type of diabetes (see Table 20-1)
Year diabetes mellitus was diagnosed
Number of years since the diagnosis
Types of medication and dosages
History of hemorrhagic callous, foot ulcerations, amputations
Type of footwear, insoles, or orthotic devices the patient has worn
Smoking history
Alcohol consumption

Table 20-1. Classification of Diabetes

Insulin-dependent diabetes (type 1)
Non-insulin-dependent diabetes (type 2)
Secondary diabetes
Gestational diabetes

The history should include the patient's subjective data as to the sensation in his or her feet, specifically if the patient feels good sensation, burning, tingling, or any shooting pain. It is surprising how infrequently this information is recorded, and how it proves so useful as a reference years later.

The lower extremity examination for known diabetic patients is in some ways more complete than that for the nondiabetic patient. The development of this examination has been based on an appreciation of a cross-sectional research study conducted at the Veterans Administration (V.A.) Medical Center in San Francisco.[1] The study revealed that 34 percent of the patients examined were considered to be insensate (the inability to sense the 5.07 Semmes-Weinstein Aesthesiometer probe for at least three of six plantar locations). It was also of note that 15 percent of the 100 patients surveyed had either a history of foot ulceration or amputation (digital, ray, below knee, above knee). All of these patients were insensate, strongly suggesting the influence of neuropathy in diabetic foot disease.

Diabetic Lower Extremity Physical Examination

Patients should have their height and weight recorded at least every 3 months. The percentage of ideal body weight should be calculated. These findings should be utilized as references and referred to annually at a minimum.

Routine dermatologic examination, including a careful notation of any and all hyperkeratotic lesions, should be performed. Care should be taken to locate and measure all such lesions. If a patient presents with a foot ulceration at the initial visit the examiner should carefully outline the lesion on clear acetate, as well as recording the width and length of the lesion. In order to fully appreciate the state of an ulcer the wound should be classified according to the Wagner scale[2] (Table 20-2).

Table 20-2. Classification of Diabetic Foot Ulceration by the Wagner Method[2]

Grade	Description
0	Skin of the foot is intact, bony deformity may be present.
1	Superficial ulcer.
2	Deep ulcer extending to bone, ligament, tendon, joint capsule, or fascia.
3	Ulcer with deep abscess, osteitis, or osteomyelitis.
4	Gangrene of the toes or forefoot.
5	Gangrene of the whole foot.

Equally important, specific reference should be made to the following: date the ulcer was first noted to be open, area, depth, ulcer floor and edge, surrounding skin, and discharge.

This reference provides a systematic inspection rather than allowing the examiner to attempt to recall the appearance of the ulcer in subsequent visits. Additionally, specific reference should be made to the presence of anhydrosis, tinea, onychomycosis, and varicosities. The integrity of the skin and nails must be thoroughly examined for any break in continuity because this can lead to infection, particularly in ischemic and neuropathic feet. All hyperkeratotic lesions should be carefully examined for underlying hemorrhage, which is often the precursor to ulceration. The pedal nails should be inspected for any ingrowing portions, and careful note should be taken of hypertrophic or onychomycotic nails because it is not uncommon for subungual infections to develop in insensate feet secondary to excessive shoe pressure. Finally, any signs of recent injury to the skin from direct shoe irritation or acute trauma require careful, thorough inspection.

Role of Vascular Changes

Vascular changes in the development of foot ulceration in the diabetic foot can be the result of three mechanisms: autonomic neuropathy, microvascular insufficiency, and occlusive peripheral vascular disease. The role of autonomic neuropathy in the development of diabetic foot complications has received more interest recently in both the clinical and research communities. The local manifestations of autonomic neuropathy in the diabetic foot can be manifest as medial vascular calcification,[3-6] and neuropathic edema. It has

been associated with an increased incidence of ulceration[7] and the development of a painful neuropathy.[8]

Long-term sympathetic denervation has been shown to cause structural damage to the peripheral arteries. The effects of long-term sympathectomy include smooth muscle atrophy in the involved vessels, leading to ultimate structural changes in the arterial tree.[3] This increase in blood flow has been implicated as an important factor in the development of Charcot's joint and pedal ulceration.[9] The mean venous PO_2 in the feet of subjects with neuropathy and ulceration was significantly higher in controls or diabetics without ulceration or evidence of peripheral neuropathy. Several authors have compared this abnormal blood flow with arteriovenous shunting.[10,11] Ward et al. postulated that, as a result of faster flow due to arteriovenous shunting, flow in the small distal vessels is inadequate.[12] This situation, complicated by abnormalities of platelet function and fibrinolysis, may become critical in the slower blood in the smaller vessels.

Watkins and Edmonds further suggested that increased flow results in rarefaction of bone, making it more prone to damage even after mild trauma.[3] Such rarefaction of bone, coupled with loss of sensation and proprioception, permits abnormal stresses that normally would be prevented by pain. It is by this mechanism that the autonomic neuropathy contributes to the formation of Charcot's joint.

Abnormally high blood flow, vasodilatation, and arteriovenous shunting that results from sympathetic denervation lead to abnormal venous pooling. The neuropathic edema that develops interferes with the normal mechanism of skin function and predisposes the patient to the development of pedal ulcerations. There is also experimental as well as clinical evidence suggesting a direct relationship between sympathetic denervation and the incidence of neuropathic ulceration.

Autonomic neuropathy may also result in complications in the insensitive foot through the development of anhidrosis and dyshidrosis, which could also lead to the development of skin fissures and pedal ulcerations.

At present there exist a variety of opinions as to the contribution of microvascular and macrovascular disease to the development of diabetic foot complications. There is little doubt, however, that both microvascular and macrovascular disease are a significant cause of morbidity or mortality in patients with diabetes.

Conrad concluded in a study of diabetic and non-diabetic individuals that in diabetes there appears to be an increase of arteriosclerosis in the calf musculature.[13] Arteriosclerosis in the diabetic appears to occur more distally and progresses in a distal-to-proximal fashion. This distal-to-proximal margin and progression results in the development of a less effective collateral circulation. However, Conrad thought that there was insufficient evidence to favor the existence of small vessel disease and that changes in the capillary permeability could not be backed up by conclusive evidence. She believed that the decrease in blood flow to the digits could be accounted for by increased resistance in the more proximal calf arteries.

Colwell[14] and others[15-25] attribute microvascular disease, probably best termed *microvascular insufficiency,* in the diabetic to a combination of factors. These factors include all the changes listed in Table 20-3. A combination of these changes may contribute to diabetic microvascular insufficiency; however, the exact nature and effect on the diabetic lower limb is still very controversial.[26] At present no clinical or other method to evaluate the presence and severity of microvascular insufficiency is available.

Screening Tests in the Vascular Evaluation

Vascular laboratory evaluation is imperative in the diabetic patient. From the vascular evaluation one can decide how much circulation exists in the extremity, and if the circulation is adequate to allow treatment of the problem or vascular reconstruction surgery is indicated.

Table 20-3. Factors That May Contribute to Diabetic Vascular Insufficiency

Hyperplasia of the basement membrane
Functional changes in the endothelium
Endothelial injury
Increased platelet adhesion and aggregation
Increased plasma viscosity
Increased fibrinogen levels
Tendency for red blood cell aggregation
Altered fibrinolysis

Some simple screening tests for initial evaluation include obtaining an ischemic index or ankle-arm or ankle-brachial index and the pulse reappearance time. A normal value for the ankle-arm index is considered to be 0.9 or greater. However, vessel wall rigidity and vascular calcification associated with diabetes result in abnormally high values when determining the ankle-arm ratio; therefore, additional testing is required prior to any invasive therapy.[27]

In certain cases some form of stress testing, such as the postreactive hyperemia test, may be useful. Digital plethysmographic studies have also been found helpful in determining the ability of a diabetic patient to heal a foot lesion or wound. If one were considering surgical correction of a deformity, Doppler evaluation, including an ankle-toe index,[28,29] could be performed. Laser Dopplers[30] and transcutaneous oxygen tension measurements are also useful in the evaluation of the diabetic dysvascular limb and may be more reliable than Doppler pressure and wave form evaluations.

Another useful screening test is the pulse reappearance time.[31] In this simple test a pneumatic tourniquet is placed on the calf or thigh. A recording of the preocclusion photocell wave form is obtained. The pneumatic tourniquet is then inflated to 100 mm Hg above the systolic pressure. The pressure is maintained for approximately 3 to 4 minutes and the tourniquet is released. Time required for reappearance of the pulse wave is monitored. The reappearance of the toe pulse is instantaneous or in less than 1 second in normal subjects. In diabetic patients significant delays can occur ranging from 10 to 120 seconds. Generally the reappearance time is closely related to the severity of the disease.

Both electronic and liquid crystal thermographic equipment has been utilized to demonstrate several changes that occur in patients with foot ulceration and particularly in patients with neurotrophic changes. The patients who demonstrate loss of protective sensation should undergo thorough vascular analysis with those instruments capable of quantifying both major arterial disease and microvascular changes.

Doppler imaging, magnetic resonance imaging, and spectroscopy can potentially provide much information regarding the viability of the limb; however, they should be considered experimental at this time. Noninvasive vascular testing is discussed in greater detail in Chapter 17 of this text.

Other Factors in Vascular Function

The role that edema plays in gangrenous lesions of the foot has been studied by Lithner and Tornbolm.[32] In 48 percent of their cases a "close temporal relationship" between development of edema and development of gangrene was observed. Edema of different etiology was observed in 46 percent of the patients with gangrene, cardiac decompensation with edema being of particular importance. Multiple gangrenous lesions were more common in patients with cardiac insufficiency, and occasional occurrence of only one lesion was especially common in patients with signs of arterial insufficiency. Edema of the feet and legs in diabetic patients should be treated; the edema, if possible, should be prevented.

Certain peripheral and autonomic neuropathies contribute to the viability of the limb and should be evaluated and considered during examination. Neurologic examinations should include evaluation of vibratory sensation, joint position, sharp/dull and warm/cold discrimination, muscle reflexes, and muscle strength. Brand describes the use of the Semmes-Weinstein Asthesiometer to quantify cutaneous protective sensation.[33] It is believed that during repetitive stress the normal sensate individual is aware of subsequent repeated trauma to the skin and underlying tissues. As a result of this they can alter their gait and stride as a protective means. The patient who has loss of this protective sensation threshold and continues to traumatize local regions of the foot is in danger of callus formation, foot ulceration, and possibly eventual amputation because of the inability to sense pain. It was shown by Holewski et al. that patients who are unable to sense the 5.07 monofilament nylon Semmes-Weinstein Asthesiometer probe at three of six plantar sites were at significant risk of developing a plantar foot ulcer or experiencing some form of infection or amputation.[34] It has therefore become customary to routinely evaluate all diabetic patients with these probes. Certain other methods known for evaluation and quantifi-

cation of peripheral neuropathy are not nearly as well suited for routine, inexpensive clinical use.

Two methods for monitoring autonomic neuropathy are measuring the R-R interval on a standard electrocardiogram during the Valsalva maneuver[35] and heart rate monitoring during deep breathing and upon standing up. Heart rate variation on deep breathing was more sensitive in the diagnosis of autonomic neuropathy,[36] and thus has been utilized to substantiate its presence. Although not performed on a routine basis, the technique has shown significant results among those patients who have experienced major foot complications. Also, the loss of the Achilles tendon reflex has been shown to be quite common in the diabetic population at highest risk of foot ulceration and amputation.

Diabetics may present with multiple neuropathies, including those most commonly affecting the lower extremity, classic polyneuropathy and mononeuropathy. Polyneuropathy is the most characteristic of the diabetic neuropathies. At least 5 percent of adult diabetics show this disorder. The patient complains of sensory disturbances manifested with parathesias such as burning of the feet and tenderness of the calf. It may begin distally and spread proximally. Initially the disturbance is primarily sensory and in the classic stocking distribution. These patients will show varying degrees of diminished touch, pain, vibratory, and joint position sense, with depressed reflexes. Mononeuropathy is believed to be the result of vascular occlusion of an arterial supply to a peripheral nerve. Peroneal palsy is the most common disorder to occur, but the femoral nerve may also be involved. Clinically the patient may present with a motor sensory and reflex impairment in the distribution of a specific peripheral nerve.

Biomechanical Examination

The clinical evaluation of the diabetic patient must include a biomechanical examination that takes into account the influence of specific foot characteristics and structure. It has been shown by sonographic examination that diabetic patients who suffer from neuropathy have atrophic plantar fat pads.[37] Significant numbers of hammer toe deformities with accompanying limitation of dorsi-flexion existed in the San Francisco V.A. cross-sectional study.[1] Brand conducted an experiment that suggested that tissue will most likely break down at those areas of high pressure that experience repetitive stress.[33] It becomes important, therefore, to appreciate radiographically, clinically, sonographically,[37,38] or by other means the anatomic regions of the foot and their inherent biomechanics if an effective treatment plan is to be formulated.

Weight-bearing studies have been performed by various authors on the neurotrophic foot. Stokes and co-workers[39,40] found that in diabetics peak loads were shifted laterally on the foot and increasing abnormalities in loading occurred with a corresponding evidence of peripheral neuropathy. They considered their most striking finding to be the reduction of load of the toes that was significantly present in the diabetic even without evidence of ulceration. Position of maximum load was found in each case to correspond to the position of the ulcer in patients who did develop neuropathic ulcers. Callosities did occur at sites of heavy loading. Stokes et al. theorized that lateral shifting and weight-bearing could be due to weakness of the muscles or loss of coordination as a result of a loss of physiologic impulses from the tendon receptors and denervation of the intrinsic muscles. Barrett and Mooney found that lesions of the plantar aspect of the forefoot showed high pressure in areas of ulcer formation,[41] supporting Stokes et al.'s findings. This was also confirmed by Sabato et al. in ulcers in patients with leprosy.[42] Ctercteko et al. differed from that of the Stokes group in that they found a medial shift in loading in the metatarsal region.[43] They also found significantly greater forces acting on the first ray area in diabetics both with and without ulceration. One difference noted between ulcerated and nonulcerated diabetics was that in the group of ulcerated diabetics the heel was less heavily loaded. Ctercteko et al.'s study did, however, agree with the Stokes et al. study in that all ulcers in the metatarsal region occurred at the sites of maximum force and that the peak force was also significantly greater in the ulcerated feet. No significant differences between contact time and no correlation to the severity of the neuropathy was obtained in their study. This anterior displacement of body weight was also not noted by Burman

and Perls[44] in 1958. Ellenberg in 1968 attributed the hammering and contracture of the digits in the diabetic with neuropathy to imbalances and weakness of the intrinsic muscles of the foot.[45] Pati and Hehera found, in 57 cases of metatarsal head ulceration in leprosy, that clawing of the digits was associated with 50 of the cases and amputation of the toe in the remaining seven.[46]

The EMED system (Novel Electronics Inc, Minneapolis MN), the Pedobarograph (Biokinetics, Bethesda, MD), and the Electrodynogram (Langer, Deer Park, New York) have been developed for evaluation of plantar foot pressure analysis (Fig. 20-1). Each system displays certain characteristics that the practitioner must evaluate as to their usefulness in clinical practice. Certainly the data obtained from each system must be evaluated as to accuracy and reproducibility. There is little doubt that the measurement of plantar foot pressures is an essential technology in the treatment of the diabetic patient. Its usefulness will be demonstrated in screening regions of the foot for increases in time or pressure and in the evaluation of the effectiveness of therapeutic modalities (i.e., surgery, foot orthotic devices, and shoe modifications). The study of foot biomechanics and the influences of foot structure will gain wider acceptance and be more appreciated with the use of these new tools. However, to date there have been only limited numbers of studies performed at very few centers. Based upon the evaluation of data by Betts et al.,[47] Rogers et al.,[48] Ctercteko et al.,[43] there is little doubt that evaluation of plantar foot pressures can be accomplished only by instrumentation that allows the practitioner to quantify the forces to the foot. It is hoped that, as the technology develops and improves, the cost of the instrumentation will be reduced, allowing for wide distribution and greater acceptance by the medical community. With the acceptance of the data obtained from this technology it is anticipated that care to the diabetic patient will be positively influenced.

Prevention and Treatment of Diabetic Foot Disease

The care of the diabetic patient with foot disease is often episodic, and if we are to be successful in impacting the morbidity, major changes must be

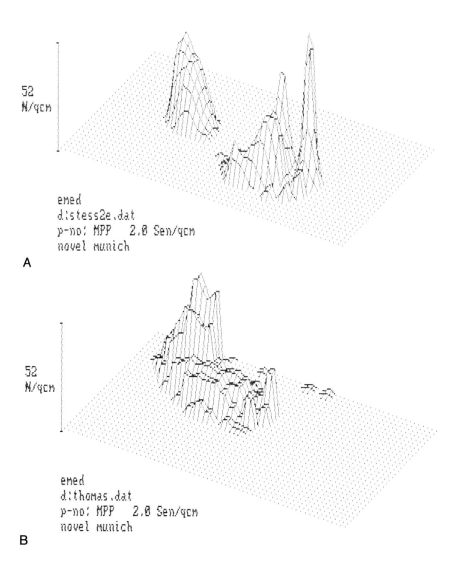

52
N/qcm

emed
d:stess2e.dat
p-no: MPP   2.0 Sen/qcm
novel munich

A

52
N/qcm

emed
d:thomas.dat
p-no: MPP   2.0 Sen/qcm
novel munich

B

Fig. 20-1. Examples of peak pressures of a normal foot **(A)** and a Charcot's joint foot **(B)** demonstrating marked abnormality of weight distribution in ambulation.

made in screening, outpatient care, inpatient care, prophylactic footwear, and education of both physician and patient. It is important that those patients who are at high risk be identified as early as possible in order for the first stages of education to be undertaken. All too often the practitioner learns that the diabetic patient has not been seen on a regular basis and has not been educated as to the "do's" and "don'ts" of diabetic foot care. Both written pamphlets on foot care and verbal reinforcements should be provided to the patient regularly. The patient should also be shown how to examine his or her own feet, and certainly should be taught the warning signs of impending danger. The

diabetic educational program must be regularly repeated and reviewed. The diabetics who have been screened for neuropathy and found to be insensate will require more intensive education about the potential sequelae and methods of prevention.

All physicians should regularly examine their patients' feet, but a recent study[48a] indicated that a surprisingly small number of physicians actually do so. With the increasing aged population podiatrists and physicians should prepare themselves for effective methods for screening diabetic patients. Certainly the easiest method for determining relative status of the feet of the diabetic patient is to establish the presence of protective sensation threshold. The Von Frey method using the 5.07-mm monofilament nylon probe to map plantar sensation will allow rapid general assessment of the existence of neuropathy. General screening with reference to the autonomic, circulatory, and biomechanical systems should be performed on all diabetics who demonstrate any loss of protective sensation.

General guidelines as to hygiene and maintaining the integrity of skin should be practiced by patients. No studies have demonstrated the benefits or ill effects of foot soaks. Until such studies are conducted it would seem reasonable that no excessive soaking of the foot should be performed and that regular use of water-based moisturizing emollients should be encouraged. Those diabetic patients with normal cutaneous sensation and intact pedal pulses can be instructed on proper nail care. Patients with nail pathology who demonstrate compromised sensory and circulatory systems should seek professional care on a regular basis. Diabetic patients should *never* use commercially available keratolytic preparations and should never attempt to remove hyperkeratotic tissue themselves. All too often the precursor to gangrene and amputation is the nonhealing diabetic ulcer. The ulcer when presented should be treated vigorously and yet with great caution. All wounds should undergo culture and sensitivity testing of the deepest structures. Most diabetic wounds are polymicrobial, with both aerobic and anerobic bacteria.[49-52] If possible a satisfactory specimen from the subcutaneous tissue should be obtained. Osteomyelitis of the foot in diabetic patients is a common finding that holds significant mortality. Radiography, routine hematology, bone scans, and blood cultures should be obtained if one suspects osseous involvement. Before any decision regarding treatment is made, care must be taken to review the vascular, radiographic, and neurologic findings. Based upon all the presented factors, ulcers should then be graded according to a scale such as Wagner's.[2] All shoes likewise should be evaluated as to their contribution to excessive pressure. At this point a decision can be made regarding whether to manage the patient as an outpatient or as a hospital inpatient. All patients with acute ulcerations in the presence of infection should be hospitalized immediately. Any delay in admitting the patient could result in disaster. Consultations with vascular and orthopedic specialists should be made as soon as possible if appropriate. Once the acute phase of an ulcer has been controlled, the wound and all surrounding callous tissue should be thoroughly debrided. The peripheral margins of the ulcers should be traced onto clear acetate in order to monitor healing on a weekly basis. This débridement should be performed weekly or more frequently if necessary, and appropriate accommodation in shoes or healing sandals should be made.

Diabetic insensate patients with unresponsive plantar ulcerations should be considered candidates for a total contact cast as described by Brand.[33,53,54] The foot is well protected and rested in a plaster cast. If applied properly, the cast transfers retrograde forces and pressures to forces that are distributed uniformly to the foot and leg, while the piston affect of standard plaster casts is eliminated. The hazard of this cast, which has only minimal padding, is the potential abrasive effects of the plaster against bony prominences. These areas must be thoroughly padded with orthopedic felt. All toes should be protected using foam and lambs wool between the digits. Great care should be taken in applying the plaster of Paris to avoid wrinkling or tenting. Because the casts have proven to be quite successful, certain modifications have been made in order to improve ambulation and decrease the number of complications directly attributed to the cast. One modification has been to apply to the foot and lower one-third of the leg a polyurethane resin–impregnated fabric in sock design (Scotch Sock manufactured by 3M). This sock is applied to the foot after the first plaster shell layer has dried. It also allows for easier removal of the cast. The second major change in the cast that significantly contributes to better ambulation is the application of polyurethane resin–impregnated foam to the plantar aspect of the cast as a replacement for the wooden platform soleplate and rubber heel method. This synthetic impregnated foam serves as both a soleplate and a walker while only adding a few ounces to the total weight of the cast. These two modifications have resulted in casts that are 20 to 30 percent lighter, stronger, and more easily applied while providing the patient greater ease in ambulation.

Reconstructive foot surgery may be indicated for

those patients who are predisposed to ulcer formation because of excessive pressures exerted by underlying bony deformities. Prolonged union time may occur in diabetes after fracture; this is especially true with displaced fractures and those fractures treated by closed reduction. This prolonged fracture healing can be explained at the cellular level by the effects of insulin and diabetes on bone and mineral metabolism. The effect is present for both primary bone healing and healing with bone callus formation.

When in the judgment of the surgeon reconstructive foot surgery is necessary, then all steps should be made to stabilize the patient medically prior to the procedure. It again becomes a team effort between the internist and the podiatrist to ascertain a satisfactory result. The patient should be made well aware of all risks and hazards of the procedures being contemplated. The podiatric surgeon should also contemplate the functional role of the foot following surgery in order to assure satisfactory long-term results. In certain patients an amputation may become necessary. Often the surgeon is called upon to perform amputation in the face of ischemia. The podiatric surgeon is frequently called upon to perform amputation in the face of recurrent ulceration, osteomyelitis, and infection. Again at this point in the treatment plan, the multidisciplinary team assuming the care for the diabetic patient should prepare the patient medically and emotionally for the procedure.

The team of diabetic health care providers working together should at a minimum include a physician, podiatric physician, nurse, nutritionist, pedorthist, prosthetist, psychologist, and physical therapist; a variety of other allied health care providers may also be involved. This team is charged with the responsibility of education, prevention, primary health care, emotional support, and rehabilitation. Such a working unit of professionals may be difficult to achieve; however, those who have experience in treating diabetics understand the complexities of conditions that will be faced in treating the "diabetic foot." The diabetic foot has been shown to undergo structural changes that result in abnormal stresses being placed on the forefoot. Likewise the foot that has been afflicted with an ulcer with or without boney changes will produce abnormal forces in a dynamic state. The dia-

betic foot must be supported with reduction of high-pressure zones. The biomechanics of the diabetic foot must be addressed with the purpose of reducing regions of high pressure. A 1983 study by Boulton et al. found that 51 percent of neuropathic feet had abnormally high pressures underneath the metatarsal heads compared with 17 percent of the feet of diabetic controls.[55] The entire weight-bearing surface of the foot should be utilized to more evenly distribute the weight.

The patient who has a diabetic ulcer may require any of several custom shoes and orthotic devices depending on the stage of healing of the ulcer (Table 20-4). The podiatric physician should anticipate and plan for obtaining both shoes and orthotic devices as early as possible. Various shoe modifications such as metatarsal bars and rocker soles can be quite useful and should be considered if indicated. It must be made very clear that each case is managed individually and there is no one perfect shoe for all feet. There have been no definitive studies performed to date that have shown the relative therapeutic effectiveness of one shoe versus another. The practitioner must keep abreast of all the new innovations in footwear and materials. New designs and materials, such as the San Francisco V.A. custom shoe, make custom shoes more cosmetically appealing to the patient and certainly more affordable (Fig. 20-2).

The rate of recurrent foot ulcerations among neuropathic diabetic patients is quite high. There

Table 20-4. Orthotic Devices and Shoes Available for Diabetic Patients with Healing Ulcers

Healing Phases	Orthotic Devices and Shoe Types
Initial	1. Custom molded insole or microcellular insole (e.g., Pelite, PPT, Spenco) 2. Healing sandal
Early	1. Accommodative insole in extra-depth shoe. (Pelite, PPT, Spenco, microcellular rubber) 2. Custom-molded sandal
Long-standing	1. Custom-molded shoe 2. Custom-molded sandals, nonthong type 3. Orthopedic shoe with custom-molded insole and rocker sole 4. Semiflexible orthotic devices 5. Regular shoes with over-the-counter insoles 6. Extra-depth shoes with custom accommodative insoles

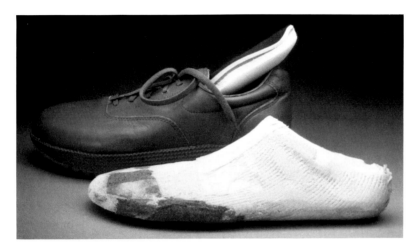

Fig. 20-2. The San Francisco V.A. shoe, a new design in custom-molded footwear. A resin-impregnated fabric (Scotch Sock®) is adapted and utilized as a custom last. The polyurethane midsole is injected and assumes the contour of the foot shape. An insole of Pelite and Spenco is utilized to cushion and protect the plantar surface of the foot. This type of custom shoe is accepted very well by patients because of the improved cosmetic appearance as well as the moderate cost.

are rough estimates that between 30,000 and 50,000 amputations are performed annually and approximately half of these are in diabetic patients. The economic impact of caring for diabetic patients in the United States is enormous and can only be expected to grow as the aged population increases. It behooves the specialists of the foot to make every effort to reduce the number of amputations not only for economic reasons but also to lower the numbers of diabetics who suffer from high levels of recurrent foot ulcers and mortality. Effective multidisciplinary diagnostic and treatment centers appears to be a method to accomplish this goal. Amputation is advisable in cases of advanced peripheral vascular disease, life-threatening infection, and unstable osseous deformity.

The perioperative risk of the diabetic patient are several (Table 20-5). In the case of elective foot surgery on a diabetic patient a glycosolated hemo-

globin determination should be performed preoperatively. If the result is extremely high it is advisable to postpone the surgery to allow for correction of the hyperglycemia and reduce the risk of postoperative complications, including infection (Fig. 20-3). A rapid decrease in insulin requirement occurs postoperatively (e.g., after drainage of an abscess). However, an increased need for insulin postoperatively may also be indicative of infection. Urine glucose monitoring is not a reliable method for following postoperative patients.

Protein-calorie malnutrition affects both the morbidity and mortality of patients undergoing surgery.[56-58] Dickhaut et al. used a simple method to estimate the severity of the nutrition deficit by the measurement of serum albumin.[58] In 23 diabetic patients undergoing a Symes amputation only 43 percent (or 10) of the patients healed. Seven of the 10 had a serum albumin level of 3.5 g/dl or greater. In contrast, to the 11 patients in whom only 2 amputations healed, with a serum albumin of less than 3.5 g/dl. In addition, the impaired humoral and cell-mediated immunity that accompanies malnutrition decreases a patient's ability to fight infection.

Immune deficiency in the diabetic has been reported by various authors.[59-65] The polymorphonuclear leukocyte appears to be the cell in which the malfunction occurs. The etiology on a cellular basis is unclear. In experimental models hyperglycemia alone leads to decreased phagocytosis, de-

Table 20-5. Perioperative Risks of Diabetic Patients

1. Autonomic neuropathy
   - Difficulty in maintaining stable blood pressure
   - Postural hypotension
   - Painless myocardial infarction
2. Increased sensitivity to drugs
3. Coronary artery disease (three to four times as frequent in age-matched population)
4. Nephropathy
   - Difficulty metabolizing and excreting drugs
   - Fluid and electrolyte imbalance
5. Nutritional imbalance

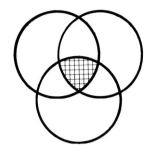

Bacteria
−Virulence
−Innoculum

Host Defense Mechanisms
−Cell Mediated Immunity
  Dysfunction
−PMN Dysfunction
−Hyperglycemia
−Protein − Calorie
  Malnutrition

Enviornment
−Skin
−Ulceration
−Neuropathy
−Vascular Disease

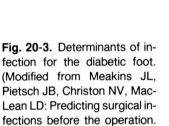

Fig. 20-3. Determinants of infection for the diabetic foot. (Modified from Meakins JL, Pietsch JB, Christon NV, MacLean LD: Predicting surgical infections before the operation. World J Surg, 4:439, 1980, with permission.)

creased intracellular killing of bacteria, and decreased diapedesis. Depression of cell-mediated immunity (T cell function) has also been reported; this defect in leukocyte function may also be in part responsible for defects in wound healing occurring in the diabetic in the absence of infection.[66]

THE INSENSITIVE FOOT

As noted by Hetherington,[67] "the insensitive foot is best defined as an extremity without a warning mechanism for intricate external and internal environmental changes." The external environmental changes include the home or work place, occupation, floor surfaces, and shoegear. The internal environment encompasses altered musculoskeletal function, deformity, vascular disease, neurologic disease, and skin dysfunction. The primary deficit is neurologic dysfunction.

A list of those disorders resulting in insensitivity is presented in Table 20-6. The signs and symptoms associated with the insensitive foot are listed in Table 20-7. Many forms of evaluation and therapy are common to both the patient with diabetic foot complications and the patient with insensitive feet. In patients with peripheral insensitivity a thorough history and physical examination as previously outlined should be performed.

The Pathogenesis of Soft Tissue Lesions

The pathogenesis of soft tissue lesions in the insensitive foot is closely related to the biomechanical properties of the skin.[68,69] The skin serves various functions as a result of its complex constituents. Among these functions are adaptability and the absorption and dissipation of energy.

In order to function properly the skin must have adequate sensibility and vascularity. The skin can be regarded as a series of networks that consist of collagen and elastic fibers and vascular and neural elements.[68] The collagen fiber network functions so that, if stretched in any direction, most of the fibers will orient themselves along the lines of stretch. At low loads few fibers may be involved. As the load increases the recruitment of additional fibers is needed to resist further tissue extension. The elastic fibers act as an energy storage device, or spring, to return the collagen to its relaxed position.

The interstitial fluid serves to lubricate this mechanical mechanism and serves as a buffer against sudden changes. It is also important in dissipation of heat. Interstitial fluid is forced out of the tissue during deformation and returns during a recovery period. This function has been compared to that of a shock absorber. Increases in the amount of interstitial fluid increase the resistance of skin to adaptation.

The mechanisms or pathogenesis of the develop-

Table 20-6. Outline of Diseases and Processes Resulting in an Insensitive Foot

1. Neuropathy associated with systemic diseases
    Diabetes mellitus
    Uremia
    Amyloidosis
2. Neuropathy associated with nutritional disturbances
    Alcoholism
    Pernicious anemia
3. Neuropathy associated with infectious diseases
    Leprosy
    Syphilis
    Poliomyelitis
4. Neuropathy on a vascular basis
    Cerebral vascular accident
    Spinal cord infarction
    Diabetic mononeuropathy
    Arteritis
    Peripheral vascular disease
5. Hereditary motor and sensory neuropathy (HMSN)
    Roussy-Lévy disease
    Charcot-Marie-Tooth disease
6. Hereditary sensory and autonomic neuropathy (HSAN)
    Hereditary sensory neuropathy
    Congenital sensory neuropathy
    Dysautonomia (Riley-Day syndrome)
7. Cerebellar degeneration
    Friedreich's ataxia
8. Motor neuron disease
    Amyotrophic lateral sclerosis
9. Diseases of the spinal cord
    Spina bifida
    Syringomyelia
10. Trauma
    Spinal cord injury
    Peripheral nerve injury
    Spinal root trauma
11. Compressive neuropathy
    Spinal cord tumor
    Peripheral nerve compression
12. Toxic neuropathy
    Lead poisoning
13. Other
    Cerebral palsy

(From Hetherington,[67] with permission.)

Table 20-7. Signs and Symptoms Associated with the Insensitive Foot

Paresthesias
Hypesthesia
Anesthesia
Nocturnal cramping
Diminished or absent deep tendon reflexes
Diminished or absent vibratory sensation
Diminished or absent temperature or pain sensation
Anhidrosis
Callus formation
Ulceration
Intrinsic muscle atrophy
Digital deformity
Cavus foot deformity or pes valgus deformity
Increased skin temperature
Edema
Change in function (foot-drop)

(From Hetherington,[67] with permission.)

ment of plantar ulcers have been discussed by Brand[33] and Hall and Brand[70] and include:

1. Continuous pressure
2. Concentrated high pressure
3. Repetitive mechanical stress
4. Excessive heat or cold.

In addition, ischemia, thermal injury, sinus tract formation, and skin fissuring are also mechanisms for the initiation of pedal ulceration.

The ulcerations that arise from continuous pres-sure are of a local ischemic nature, such as the de-cubitus ulcer of a heel. Another area of occurrence of this type of lesion is over a bony prominence such as the first metatarsal-phalangeal joint in a patient with poor shoe fit. The constant pressure exerted by the shoe over the bony prominences causes a compression of the capillary blood flow leading to ischemia followed by necrosis.

Skin defects that are a result of continuous pres-sure are caused by lack of blood supply. Kosiak pointed out that intense pressures of short duration are as detrimental as low pressures applied for ex-tended periods.[71] Regardless of the type of mecha-nism, necrosis results from ischemia. As a result of ischemia irreversible tissue damage occurs.

Concentrated high pressure as a result of a pene-tration injury causes an initial break in the skin that can act as a focus.

Repetitive mechanical stress sets off a sequence of events that result in the development of ulcer-ations (see Fig. 20-4). Repetitive mechanical stress or cyclical biomechanical trauma that exceeds the mechanical limits of the skin and subcutaneous tis-sue results in inflammation, which, if rest is not provided, will become severe. Following the in-flammation, autolysis of the soft tissues will occur. The formation of a seroma or hematoma ensues within the deeper layers of the subcutaneous tissue and the dermis. Dissection of the subcutaneous tis-sues occurs with pressures from walking, and the continued pressure and injury will eventually lead

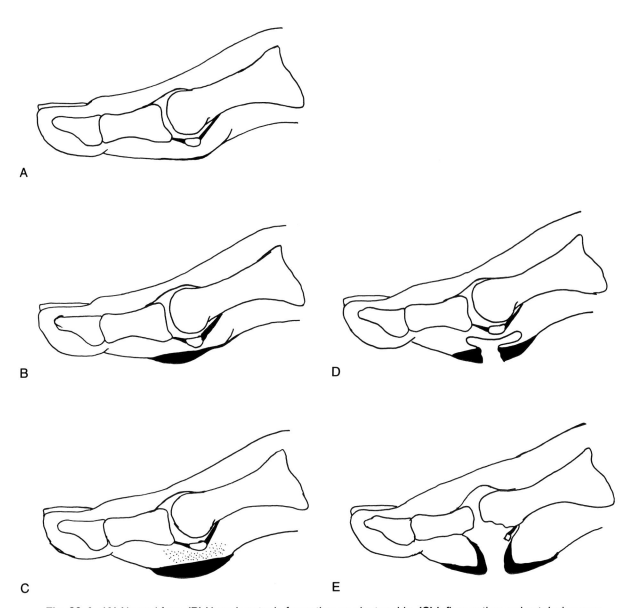

Fig. 20-4. (A) Normal foot. **(B)** Hyperkeratosis formation on plantar skin. **(C)** Inflammation and autolysis occur with subsequent dissection of the soft tissue by seroma or hematoma. **(D)** Ulceration (fundamental). **(E)** Ulceration, infection, and exposure of capsule, tendon, and bone (complicated). (Modified from Delbridge L, Ctercteko G, Fowler C et al: The aetiology of diabetic neuropathic ulceration of the foot. Br J Surg, 72:1, 1985, with permission.)

to breakdown of the skin and rupture of the lesion through the plantar surface of the foot. Continued aggravation leads to enlargement and deepening of the lesion, and subsequent infection readily occurs. These ulcers are predominantly located on the plantar surface of the foot and are frequently referred to as *mal perforans* ulcers (Fig. 20-5). This type of ulceration, although it occurs predominantly on weight-bearing surfaces can occur on dorsal digital surfaces in association with hammer toe deformity.

Manley and Darby,[72] in their research on mechanical stress and the development of foot ulcerations in rats, included the following:

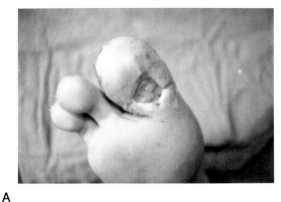 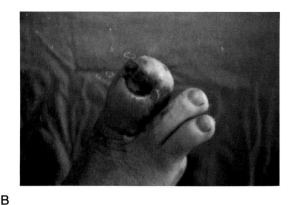

A   B

Fig. 20-5. Typical diabetic mal perforans ulcers in a diabetic foot that has undergone multiple digital and ray amputations. Note the extreme hyperkeratosis surrounding the ulcer. This tissue must be debrided aggressively and regularly if healing is to be achieved via conservative therapy.

1. Repetitive mechanical stress of a magnitude and repetition rate within physiologic limits can stimulate the formation of foot ulcers, if the foot is subjected to a significant number of stress repetitions.
2. With the increase in the daily number of repetitions a shorter time period is required for ulcer formation.
3. Denervation predisposes to the formation of plantar ulcers.

The presence of edema interferes with the delivery of nutrients to the area because there is an increased distance from the capillary to the cell and a decrease in the rate of diffusion proportional to this distance. The removal of metabolites and cell debris would also be impaired in the presence of edema. These findings are also supported by the work of Beech and Thompson[73] and that of Bergtholdt.[74,75]

Thermal injury may also cause tissue destruction and necrosis in the insensate foot. These burns are often painless incidents with noticeable swelling, blistering, or tissue loss as the presenting complaint. Patients who sustain a burn of the foot and are unaware of this injury can, often as a result of unintentional neglect, convert a partial-thickness tissue loss to a full-thickness tissue loss by continued ambulation on the foot and the development of infection.

Osseous and Radiographic Changes

Osseous changes associated with the diabetic or insensitive foot can be of two types: atrophic and hypertrophic arthropathy. This type of neuropathic destruction of joints, or Charcot's joints, has been well described in the diabetic by Forgács.[76,77] The signs and symptoms associated with neuroarthropathy are listed in Table 20-8.

Atrophic or *reabsorptive arthropathy* exhibits radiographically osteoporosis, atrophy, destruction, and disappearance of bone substance. Dislocation of the joints has also been noted to occur. The joints are usually free of osteophytes, eburnation, and the fragmentation that is seen with the hypertrophic arthropathy.

Table 20-8. Signs and Symptoms of Neuropathic Osteoarthropathy

Swelling
Warmth
Erythema
Good vascularity
Neurologic deficit
Joint hypermobility
Crepitation
Tarsal subluxation (rocker bottom)
Digital subluxation
Hyperkeratosis
Infection and ulceration

(From Hetherington,[67] with permission.)

Pogonowska and co-workers discussed the reabsorptive type of arthropathy that is initially described as affecting the forefoot in diabetic patients.[78] The process affects the metatarsals and phalanges. Pogonowska et al. summarized the radiographic changes to include:

1. Osteoporosis
2. Juxta-articular cortical bone defects
3. Osteolysis
4. Apparent destruction of the entire bone (bone loss)
5. Reconstruction occurring
6. Slight periosteal reaction (new bone formation)
7. Sclerosis of the shaft of the bone.

To this list Newman added pathologic fracture and spontaneous dislocations.[79] Reinhardt, in studying radiographic residual evidence of healed diabetic arthropathies, found Freiberg-like lesions, shortening of the proximal phalanx of the great toe, and joint ankylosis to be common in the foot. Many of these so-called changes that were related to diabetic osteopathy occur in other types of neuropathic osteopathy, including alcoholic neuropathy[81,82] and the distal absorption seen in bones of the foot in leprosy.[83,84]

Kraft et al., in discussing the diabetic foot, stated that in the reabsorptive type of arthropathy the bone becomes sclerotic, simulating osteomyelitis.[85] Schwartz and co-workers postulated that the reabsorptive type of arthropathy is due to autosympathectomy in addition to impaired sensation.[86] Osteomyelitis often resembles changes in the neurotrophic foot. In many patients with vascular insufficiency, the bone may appear normal on x-ray evaluation even when osteomyelitis is present. The presence of only a mottled lytic lesion can be the most frequent and sometimes the only positive finding. The soft tissues should be examined for the presence of air or gas, arterial calcification, and soft tissue swelling.

Radiographically the bones may appear to exhibit penciling or a "sucked candy" deformity. The pathologic process is usually gradual reabsorption of the metatarsals and phalanges of the foot commencing at the distal end, progressing gradually toward the base, and terminating with a distal

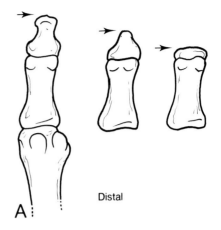

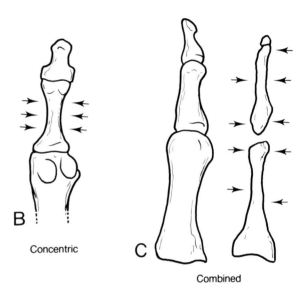

Fig. 20-6. Methods of absorption of the small bones. (Modified from Enna CD: The foot in leprosy. p. 299. In McDowell F, Enna CD (eds): Surgical Rehabilitation in Leprosy. Williams & Wilkins, Baltimore, 1974, with permission.)

pointed deformity. The epiphyseal ends are lost and the remaining points may tend to become sclerotic. The joints may take the appearance of the mortar-and-pestle deformity. Absorption of the small long bones in the foot manifests in one of three ways: distal absorption, concentric absorption, or a combination of these two (Fig. 20-6).

In contrast *hypertrophic arthropathy* may present with a pes planus–type deformity. This type

of bone destruction usually involves the tarsometatarsal, midtarsal, subtalar, and ankle joints. Horibe
et al. studied these changes in the patient with
Hansen's disease.[87] Those involving the ankle, subtalar, and tarsometatarsal joint are usually associated with some type of trauma such as a sprain or
fracture. Direct trauma was not as evident in those
patients with midtarsal joint involvement. Horibe
et al. further noted that ankle involvement was
likely to follow peroneal nerve motor loss with
foot-drop and postulated that leprotic patients
without protective sensations and with loss of
motor function are likely to suffer inversion injuries resulting in neuroarthropathy. They also reported that most patients with midtarsal joint involvement presented with paralysis of the tibialis
posterior. This they believed concentrated stresses
on the talonavicular joint during gait, resulting in
navicular collapse. The incidence of trauma as a
major factor in participation neuroarthropathy in
the ankle and tarsometatarsal joint was also established by Sinha et al.[97] in the diabetic; however,
involvement of the metatarsophalangeal joints in
most instances was not associated with trauma.[88]
They reported the tarsal and tarsometatarsal joints
(60 percent) to be most commonly involved, followed by the metatarsophalangeal joints (31 percent) and ankle (9 percent). Of 101 patients 24 had
bilateral disease.

Painless fractures and fracture dislocations of the
lower extremity involving the calcanus, midtarsal
joint, tarsometatarsal joint, leg, and knee are frequently reported in patients with insensitivity.[89–93]

Epiphyseal separation may occur in children.[94]
The injuries if unrecognized may lead to severe
disability in susceptible individuals.[95]

The radiographic presentation of neuroarthropathy has been discussed in numerous
sources.[79,87,96–102] Frykberg pointed out that in
every case the primary factor is loss of joint sensation.[103] The joint is subjected to extreme ranges of
motion, which results in capsule and ligament
stretching and joint laxity and instability. Further
weight-bearing on this unprotected extremity
leads to subluxations, dislocations, and osteochondral fragmentation. Continual trauma develops a
vicious cycle. Normal inflammatory mechanisms
produce joint swelling and hyperemia, which leads
to further instability and reabsorption. When these

Charcot's joints are left untreated, continued destruction occurs creating more fragmentation, dislocation, and deformity. (Fig. 20-7). Forjacs[76,77]
classified the changes in three stages:

Stage 1: The initiation of symptoms occur, there
is subluxation of the joints, osteoporosis
occurs, and cortical defects become obvious.
Stage 2: The deformity progresses with osteolysis, fracture, and periosteal elevation or new
superiosteal bone formation.
Stage 3: First healing stage, where reconstruction occurs with the subsiding of swelling; re-
organization of cortical defects and ankylosis
of the joints may occur.

The etiology of the development of Charcot's
joints is multifactorial (Fig. 20-8). It occurs in
the presence of a denervated foot and appears to
have a higher incidence in those patients with
pronounced autonomic neuropathy. Repetitive
trauma to this foot type leads to continued destruction and gross foot deformity.[103]

The diagnosis of osteomyelitis of previously diseased bone is difficult (Table 20-9). Radiologic distinction between osteomyelitis and bone changes
due to neuropathy is difficult. Radioisotopic evaluation of the neurotrophic foot can be somewhat
unreliable.[104–108] Difficulty occurs with the interpretation of the technetium scan as a result of previous bone disease secondary to neurotrophic destruction. Focal uptake may reflect not
osteomyelitis, but the actual repair process initiated against the neuropathic process. An infection
from a contiguous source with an underlying bone
disease process can give the radioisotopic appearance of acute osteomyelitis when in fact one is
dealing with soft tissue ulceration with infection
and neurotrophic bone deformity. In patients
without neurologic disease a matched defect on
both the technetium and gallium scans could be
indicative of acute osteomyelitis. Great care must
be taken when interpreting technetium scans of the
neurotrophic foot. Glynn also noted a marked accumulation of gallium in neuroarthropathy.[109]
Thus, although radioisotopic studies can be helpful
in evaluating the neurotrophic foot, care must be
given to their interpretation, and occasionally bone
biopsy is required to make a definitive diagnosis of

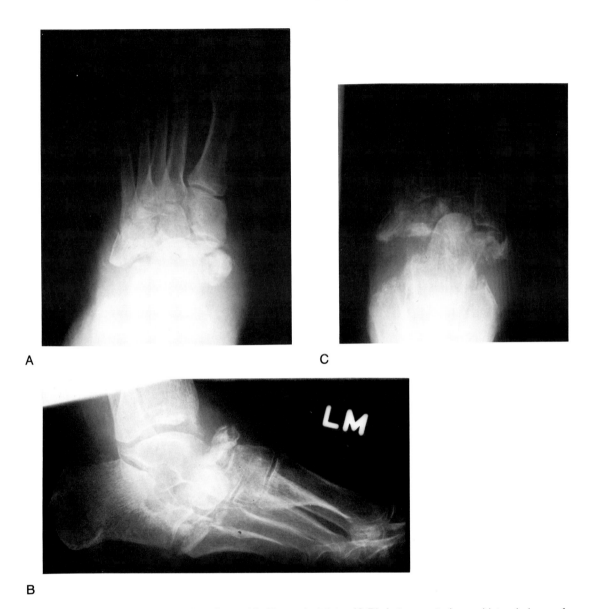

Fig. 20-7. Radiographic findings in a foot with Charcot's joints. **(A,B)** Anteroposterior and lateral views of a Charcot's joint demonstrating marked destruction of midfoot. **(C)** The same patient approximately 10 weeks later demonstrating continuance of destructive process. *(Figure continues.)*

osteomyelitis.[110] Future methods of radioisotopic detection of infection may prove valuable, such as the white blood cell scan.[111]

Burgtholdt recommended temperature assessment as a program to demonstrate changes in temperature pattern in the foot.[75] Increased activity or ill-fitting footwear can be detected by increased temperature; this method, what Bergtholdt termed a *pain substitute*, can detect areas sensitive to ulceration. Thermography is also useful in the early diagnosis of Charcot's joints because of the increased heat in the area of the involved joints.

Thermography in the management of the insensitive foot can prove invaluable in detecting areas of inflammation prior to the time at which ulceration will occur. Liquid crystal thermography is a

D

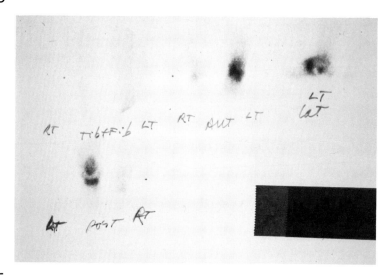

E

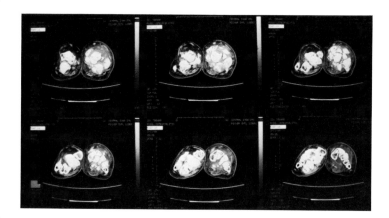

F

Fig. 20-7 *(Continued).* **(D,E)** Technetium bone scan of the same patient in flow study (D) and static scan (E). No osteomyelitis is present. This scan is reflecting only the Charcot process. **(F)** Computed tomography scan of the same patient dramatically demonstrates the destructive process.

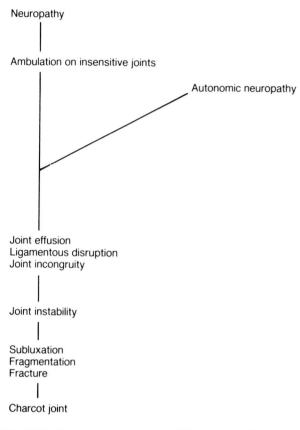

Neuropathy

Ambulation on insensitive joints

Autonomic neuropathy

Joint effusion
Ligamentous disruption
Joint incongruity

Joint instability

Subluxation
Fragmentation
Fracture

Charcot joint

Fig. 20-8. Sequence of events and factors contributing to the formation of a Charcot's joint. (From Hetherington,[67] with permission.)

Table 20-9. Comparative Radiographic Appearances in Osteomyelitis Seen in or Mimicked by Neuropathic Bone Disease

Osteomyelitis	*Neuropathic*
Bone destruction present	Bone destruction and fragmentation
Increased soft tissue density	Increased soft tissue density
Changes in bone density with early sclerosis and osteoporosis in later progression	Sclerosis may be present and osteoporosis may present as diabetic osteolysis
Progressive reabsorption of bone occurs	Progressive reabsorption usually is not present
Sequestra formation occurs	Sequestra formation may be mimicked by fragmentation
Subperiosteal new bone formation occurs	Subperiosteal new bone formation occurs

(From Hetherington,[67] with permission.)

convenient method for in-office evaluation (VJ Hetherington, unpublished data; see also refs. 112 and 113). Xeroradiography may also be helpful in the evaluation of the soft tissue in this foot type. Arterial calcifications, in duration of small-sized arteries, and intra-articular bone fragments and periosteal reactions in osteoarthropathy are easily identified by xeroradiolography.[114] Sinography may also be of benefit in evaluation of this foot type.[115]

A Logical Approach to Management

The insensitive foot may be classified into three types in terms of management (Fig. 20-9). The first is the foot with no ulcerations with or without bony deformity and no evidence of active bone destruction. The second type is the foot in which active bone destruction is occurring. The third type is that of the ulcerated foot with or without a bony deformity. These ulcerations can further be classified as fundamental or complicated.

In 1982 Enna classified the first type, the insensitive foot with no ulceration with or without bony deformity and no active bone destruction, into four categories as they related to the need for orthotic care[116]:

Category 1 presents with only one deficit, loss of plantar sensation. A soft insole of microcellular rubber, such as Spenco, is provided as a mean of prophylaxis.

Category 2 presents with two defects, loss of plantar sensation with deficiency of the subcutaneous soft tissue. This may be associated with scarring of the plantar skin. In this foot type, a molded material such as Plastazote, with or without a layer of microcellular rubber, would be advantageous to the patient. The use of such material would require a shoe with extra depth to accommodate the thickness of the insole.

Category 3 presents with three deficits: the two previously noted and gross deformity. This foot type may require surgical intervention, which may include both resection of prominent osseous structures and, in some cases, judicious arthrodesis of involved joints.

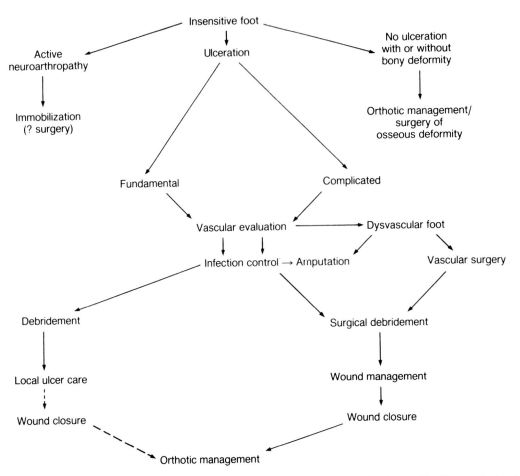

Fig. 20-9. Logical approach to managing the insensitive foot. (From Hetherington,[67] with permission.)

Molded shoes with the appropriate insole materials would be required to manage this type of deformity.

Category 4 presents with a short, deformed, and rigid foot. A molded shoe is fabricated to the dimensions of the foot. In this type of deformity the sole of the shoe requires adjustment to add a rocker mechanism to assist gait and reduce the forces interacting with the insensitive foot.

The use of insoles and shoes as outlined here is also applicable to the follow-up care of patients after the development of superficial or deep ulcerations that have been adequately and thoroughly treated.[117-120]

The second type of insensitive foot is one in which patients present with active neuroarthropathy.[121] Initial treatment after the diagnosis is made depends upon the development of early or late signs. Localized warmth is the cardinal sign in these changes. Rest is required until clinical and radiologic evidence of healing is seen. Lennox advised bed rest followed by non-weight-bearing on crutches followed by partial weight-bearing and then the use of gait-assistive devices over a period of some weeks until union is achieved.[122] He pointed out, however, in that practice such ideal treatment may not be feasible. At a minimum the use of plaster immobilization is recommended until radiographic evidence of union is achieved. Care must be taken to mold the foot in a good functional position, avoiding deviation. Lennox pointed out that the initial period of immobilization may be as long as 3 to 4 months and that shortcuts often increase the risk of failure.

Return to activity should be gradual, and the patient should be followed frequently after the removal of the cast for the development of heat and swelling. If incomplete healing occurs the need for further immobilization is indicated. Arthrodesis of major foot joints may be indicated in select cases. The aims of surgery are: (1) to simplify and stabilize the remaining skeleton, (2) to restore the foot to a plantargrade position without deviation, (3) to restore a functional foot for ambulation, and (4) to prevent further deformity. The use of bone grafts and internal or external fixation may also be indicated.

The third type of insensitive foot, that with ulceration, can be divided into fundamental and complicated (Table 20-10). In the fundamental type simple ulcers and soft tissue infection may be present. A complicated ulcer is one that extends past the

subcutaneous tissue into the deeper layers of the foot. It is associated with deep plantar space infection and or infection of underlying structures such as bone and muscle.

In these patients, appropriate neurologic and vascular laboratory evaluation should be performed. In those patients with a dysvascular foot, proper referral for vascular reconstruction or the decision for amputation should be given priority in the initial management. Control of the active infection should be treated by the use of specific and appropriate parental antibiotics. In the fundamental uncomplicated ulcer, the goal of local care is to remove necrotic tissue, reduce the existing bacterial level, and promote healing. Management of this type of ulcer involves:

1. Treatment of soft tissue and skin infection if one has established itself. This is primarily accomplished with the use of intravenous antibiotics. A positive culture does not necessarily mean an infection of an invasive or systemic nature. Colonization of the ulcer must be a consideration. Look for evidence of systemic infection and deep local infection, such as abscess formation. The course of the infection should be followed with regular white blood cell counts and differentials. Systemic antibiotics are not indicated for bacterial colonization.
2. Local care of the ulcer with topical agents.[123] Included in these are topical enzymes, Silvadene, and other topical antibiotics; biologic dressings such as porcine and amnion; and nonbiologic dressings. Mechanical débridement can be obtained by the use of wet-to-dry dressings. Whirlpool therapy followed by a vigorous rinse has been found to reduce the bacterial count.[124]

It is recommended that care be taken to ensure that proper anaerobic cultures are taken. There has been a poor correlation of results of testing between specimens obtained from swabs of the ulcer and those obtained with needle aspirates or curettage.[50] Also, surgical débridement is often required for drainage and definitive treatment of infection because intravenous antibiotics do not always eradicate the organism in deep tissues.

Table 20-10. A Comparison of Fundamental Versus Complicated Ulcerations

	Fundamental	Complicated
Tissue involvement	Superficial: skin/subcutaneous tissue	Deep: extends to muscle, tendon bone
Ulcer activity	Stable	Progressive
Infection	Local soft tissue Infection only Cellulitis, skin only	Systemic infection Osteomyelitis Plantar space infection abscess
Blood supply	Adequate	Inadequate or signs of ischemia
Bone	No active osseous bone disease	Active noninfected bone disease
Healing capacity	Potential for self-closure	Delayed healing
Wound care	Local	Requires coverage Requires débridement
Clinical types	Continuous pressure Repetitive trauma Concentrated high pressure Ischemic	Continuous pressure Repetitive trauma Concentrated high pressure burns 1, 2, 3 Ischemic Traumatic vascular Sinus complicated

Appropriate dressing technique is indicated in the management of these ulcers. The dressing should provide the following functions: protection, compression, immobilization, and access for the application of medication as so desired. The dressings should be so constructed that three layers are maintained: the initial contact layer that conforms to the defect, an absorptive layer that will pull the secretions of the wound from the overlying surface of the first layer, and a fixation layer to maintain the context of the first two layers.

The key to care of these ulcers is good mechanical débridement. Wet to dry dressings using normal sterile saline have been found to be most beneficial, in conjunction with minimal sharp débridement at bedside. Other types of dressings useful for débridement are dry-to-dry and wet dressings and Dakin's solution.[123]

One of the keys in allowing these patients to return to normal function is total-contact weight-bearing. This is especially true in patients with neuroarthropathy. Total-contact weight-bearing allows the weight of the foot to be better and more evenly distributed and does not allow areas of focal pressure to build up, which may lead to ulceration. Casting for the treatment of these types of ulcers has been advocated by various authors; however, a risk of potential infection may be concealed by a plaster cast. It is an easy appliance to fabricate in the office and is a most helpful adjunct to the management of these patients.

Management of the complicated ulceration requires precise and accurate surgical treatment.[125-128] Débridement and resection in the necrotic tissue, including tendon and bone, is required. This is accomplished usually with a radical débridement with a ray resection or amputation of an infected digit. Radical débridement is exactly what the term means, radical excision of all necrotic tissue and infected tissue. This includes bone, tendon, and muscle. All necrotic tissue must be removed in order to allow healing. A large area may have to be resected and the wound deepened. The guidelines that have been established for radical débridement include:

1. never sacrifice blood supply
2. allow adequate incisions for drainage
3. avoid weight bearing areas if at all possible.

After radical débridement, depending on the amount of exposure that is required, treatment usually consists of local wound management until a healthy granulating basis is obtained. Débridement may be required on more than just one occasion. Exposed bone will cover spontaneously with granulation tissue followed by epithelium or will sequestrate and then cover providing there is adequate circulation at the wound site.[129]

After débridement wound closure may be obtained by various methods.[130-142] Certain cases may be closed with the use of in-and-out drains, and some may be treated as open contaminated wounds. Other methods of wound closure include the use of skin grafts and flaps. A split-thickness skin graft to the sole of the foot may be used, but this is generally not preferred in areas of weight-bearing. Plantar rotational flaps, transferring muscle that is then covered with a split-thickness skin graft, may also be used.

Various foot deformities may be found in patients with neurologic disease and insensitivity.[143] These include clubfoot, flatfoot, foot-drop, hammer toe, and any of the talus deformities (talipes calcaneus, cavus, valgus, and varus). Correction of these static and dynamic deformities must be given consideration in order to prevent recurrent and difficult-to-manage problems.

REFERENCES

1. Holewski JJ, Moss KM, Stess RM et al: Prevalence of foot pathology and lower extremity complications in a diabetic outpatient clinic. J Rehab Rehabil, in press, 1989
2. Wagner WF: The diabetic foot. Orthopedics, 10(1):163, 1987
3. Watkins PJ, Edmonds ME: Sympathetic nerve failure in diabetes. Diabetologia, 25:73, 1983
4. Bevan RD, Tsuru H: Long-term denervation of vascular smooth muscle causes not only functional but structural change. Blood Vessels, 16:109, 1979
5. Goebel FD, Fuessl HS: Monckeberg's sclerosis after sympathetic denervation in diabetic and non-diabetic subjects. Diabetologia, 24:347, 1983

6. Edmonds ME, Morrison N, Laws JW, Watkins PJ: Medial arterial calcification and diabetic neuropathy. Br Med J, 284:928, 1982

7. Deanfield JE, Daggett PR, Harrison MJG: The role of autonomic neuropathy in diabetic foot ulceration. J Neurol Sci, 47:203, 1980

8. Archer AG, Roberts VC, Watkins PJ: Blood flow patterns in painful diabetic neuropathy. Diabetologia, 27:563, 1984

9. Boulton AJM, Scarpello JWB, Ward JD: Venous oxygenation in the diabetic neurotrophic foot: evidence of arteriovenous shunting? Diabetologia, 22:6, 1982

10. Borowski M: An experimental study on the role of arteriovenous anastomoses in the pathogenesis of trophic ulcer. Arch Immunol Ther Exp, 21:363, 1973

11. Edmonds ME: The neuropathic foot in diabetes, Part 1: Blood flow. Diabetic Med, 3:111, 1986

12. Ward JD, Simms JM, Knight G et al: Venous distention in the diabetic neuropathic foot (physical sign of arteriovenous shunting). J R Soc Med, 76:1011, 1983

13. Conrad MC: Contributions of large and small vessel disease to severe ischemia of the lower extremities in diabetics and nondiabetics. Vasc Diagn Ther, 2:17, 1981

14. Colwell JA: Studies on the pathogenesis of diabetic vascular disease. J SC Med Assoc, 77:267, 1981

15. McMillan DE: Deterioration of the microcirculation in diabetes. Diabetes, 24:944, 1975

16. Arenson DJ, Sherwood CF, Wilson RC: Neuropathy, angiopathy, and sepsis in the diabetic foot (Part two: Angiopathy). J Am Podiatry Assoc, 71:661, 1981

17. Janka HU, Standl E, Schramm W, Mehnrt H: Platelet enzyme activities in diabetes mellitus in relation to endothelial damage. Diabetes, 32:47, 1983

18. Sinziner H, Silberbauer K, Kaliman J, Klein K: Vascular prostacyclin synthesis, platelet sensitivity, plasma factors and platelet function, arteriopathy with and without diabetes mellitus. p. 93. In Noseda G, Lewis B, Paolett R (eds): Diet and Drugs in Atherosclerosis. Raven Press, New York, 1980

19. Bern MM: Platelet functions in diabetes mellitus. Diabetes, 27:342, 1978

20. Williamson JR, Kilo C: Small vessel disease: diabetic microangiopathy. Angiology, 31:448, 1980

21. Williamson JR, Vogler NJ, Kilo C: Microvascular disease in diabetes. Med Clin North Am, 55:847, 1981

22. Williamson JR, Kilo C: Capillary basement membranes. Diabetes, 32:96, 1983

23. Friedericki HHR, Tucker WR, Schwartz TB: Observations on small blood vessels of skin in the normal and in diabetic patients. Diabetes, 15:233, 1966

24. Banson BB, Lacy PE: Diabetic microangiopathy in human toes. Am J Pathol, 45:41, 1964

25. Feingold KR, Siperstein MD: Diabetic Vascular Disease. p. 309. Year Book Medical Publishers, Chicago, 1986

26. LoGerfo FW, Coffman JD: Vascular and microvascular disease of the foot in diabetes. N Engl J Med, 311:1615, 1984

27. Emanuel MA, Buchanan BJ, Abraira C: Elevated leg systolic pressures and arterial calcification in diabetic occlusive vascular disease. Diabetes Care, 4:289, 1981

28. Hauser CJ: Tissue salvage by mapping of skin surface transcutaneous oxygen tension indeces. Arch Surg, 122:1128, 1987

29. Bongard O, Kranenbuhl B: Predicting amputation in severe ischemia: the value of transcutaneous PO_2 measurement. J Bone Joint Surg [Br], 70:465, 1988

30. Karanfilian RG, Lynch TG, Zirul VT et al: The value of laser Doppler velocimetry and transcutaneous oxygen tension determination in predicting healing of ischemic forefoot ulcerations and amputations in diabetic and nondiabetic patients. J Vasc Surg, 4:511, 1986

31. Fronek A, Bernstein EF: The pulse reappearance time: an index of overall blood flow impairment in the ischemic extremity. Surgery, 31:376, 1977

32. Lithner F, Tornblom N: Gangrene localized to the feet in diabetic patients. Acta Med Scand, 215:75, 1984

33. Brand PW: Management of the insensitive limb. Phys Ther, 59:8, 1979

34. Holewski JJ, Stess RM, Graf PM, Grunfeld C: Aesthesiometry: quantification of cutaneous pressure sensation in diabetic peripheral neuropathy. J Rehab Res Dev, 25:1, 1988

35. Ewing DJ, Clarke BF: Diagnosis and management of diabetic autonomic neuropathy. Br Med J, 285:916, 1982

36. Mackay JD, Page MMcB, Cambridge J, Watkins PJ: Diabetic autonomic neuropathy: the diagnostic value of heart rate monitoring. Diabetologia, 18:471, 1980

37. Gooding GAW, Stess RA, Graf PM et al: Sonography of the sole of the foot: evidence of loss of foot pad thickness in diabetes and its relationship to ulceration of the foot. Invest Radiol, 21:45, 1986

38. Gooding GA, Stess RM, Graf PM, Grunfeld C: Heel

pad thickness, determination by high resolution ultrasonography. J Ultrasound Med, 4:173, 1985

39. Stokes IAF, Faris IB, Hutton WC: The neuropathic ulcer and loads on the foot in diabetic patients. Acta Orthop Scand, 46:839, 1975

40. Stokes IAF, Hutton WC: The effect of the diabetic ulcer on the load bearing function of the foot. p. 245. In Kenedi RM, Cowden JM (eds): Bedsore Biomechanics. University Park Press, Baltimore, 1976

41. Barrett JP, Mooney V: Neuropathy and diabetic pressure lesions. Orthop Clin North Am, 4:43, 1973

42. Sabato S, Yosipovitch Z, Simkin A, Sheskin J: Plantar trophic ulcers in patients with leprosy. Int Orthop, 6:203, 1982

43. Ctercteko GC, Dhanendran M, Hutton WC, Lequesne LP: Vertical forces acting on the feet of diabetic patients with neuropathic ulceration. Br J Surg, 68:608, 1981

44. Burman M, Perls W: The weight stream in Charcot disease of joints. Bull Hosp Joint Dis, 19:31, 1958

45. Ellenberg M: Diabetic neuropathic ulcer. J Mt Sinai Hosp, 35:585, 1968

46. Pati L, Hehera F: Metatarsal head pressure (MHP) sores in leprosy patients. Lepr India, 53:588, 1981

47. Betts RP, Franks CI, Duckworth T, Burke J: Statis and dynamic foot-pressure measurements in clinical orthopaedics. Med Biol Eng Comput, 18:674, 1980

48. Rodgers MM, Cavanagh PR, Sanders LJ: Plantar pressure distribution of diabetic feet. p. 343. In Johnson B (ed): Biomechanics X. Human Kinetics Publishers, Champaign, IL, 1987

48a. Dailey T, Yu H, and Rayfield E: Patterns of foot examination in a diabetic clinic. Am J Med, 78(3)371–374, 1985

49. Louie TJ, Bartlett JG, Tally FD, Gorbach SL: Aerobic and anaerobic bacteria in diabetic foot ulcers. Ann Intern Med, 85:461, 1976

50. Sharp CS, Bessman AN, Wagner FW et al: Microbiology of superficial and deep tissues in infected diabetic gangrene. Surg Gynecol Obstet, 149:217, 1979

51. Sapico FL, Canawati HN, Witte JL et al: Quantitative aerobic and anaerobic bacteriology of infected diabetic feet. J Clin Microbiol, 12:413, 1980

52. Walsh CH, Campbell CK: The multiple flora of diabetic foot. Ir J Med Sci, 149:366, 1980

53. Coleman WC, Brand PW, Birke J: The total contact cast. J Am Podiatry Assoc, 74:548, 1984

54. Walker SC, Helm PA, Pullium G: Total contact casting and chronic diabetic neuropathic foot ulceration: healing rates by wound location. Arch Phys Med Rehabil, 68:217, 1987

55. Boulton AJM, Hardisty CA, Betts RP et al: Dynamic foot pressure and other studies as diagnostic and management aids in diabetic neuropathy. Diabetes Care, 6:26, 1983

56. Kay SP, Moreland JR, Schmitter E: Nutritional status and wound healing in lower extremity amputations. Clin Orthop Rel Res, 217:253, 1987

57. Dreblow DM, Anderson CF, Moxness K: Nutritional assessment of orthopedic patients. Mayo Clin Proc, 56:51, 1981

58. Dickhaut SC, DeLee JC, Page CP: Nutritional status: importance in predicting wound-healing after amputation. J Bone Joint Surg [Am], 66:71, 1984

59. Eliashiv A, et al: Depression of cell-mediated immunity in diabetes. Arch Surg, 113:1180, 1978

60. Robertson HD, Polk HC: The mechanism of infection in patients with diabetes mellitus: a review of leukocyte function. Surgery, 75:123, 1974

61. Repine JE, Clauson CC, Goetz FC: Bacteriocidal function of neutrophils from patients with acute bacterial infection and from diabetics. J Infect Dis, 142:869, 1980

62. Nolan CM, Beaty HN, Bagdage JD: Further characterization of the impaired bactericidal function of granulocytes in patients with poorly controlled diabetes. Diabetes, 27:889, 1978

63. Bagdade JD, Stewart M, Walters E: Impaired granulocyte adherence. A reversible defect in host defence in patients with poorly controlled diabetes. Diabetes, 27:677, 1978

64. Bagdade JD, Root RK, Bulger RJ: Impaired leukocyte function in patients with poorly controlled diabetes. Diabetes, 23:9, 1974

65. Rayfield EF, Ault MJ, Keuson GT et al: Infection and diabetes: the case for glucose control. Am J Med, 72:439, 1982

66. Goodson WH, Hunt TK: Wound healing and the diabetic patient. Surg Gynecol Obstet, 149:600, 1979

67. Hetherington VJ: The insensitive foot. In McGlamry ED (ed): Fundamentals of Foot Surgery. William & Wilkins, Baltimore, 1987

68. Gibson T, Kenedi RM: Biomechanical properties of skin. Surg Clin North Am, 47:279, 1967

69. Daly CH: Biomechanical properties of dermis. J Invest Dermatol, 79:17, 1982

70. Hall OC, Brand PW: The etiology of the neuropathic plantar ulcer. J Am Podiatry Assoc, 69:173, 1979

71. Kosiak M: Etiology and pathology of ischemic ulcers. Arch Phys Med Rehabil, 40:62, 1979
72. Manley MT, Darby T: Repetitive mechanical stress and denervation in plantar ulcer pathogenesis in rats. Arch Phys Med Rehabil, 61:171, 1980
73. Beach RB, Thompson DE: Selected soft tissue research. Phys Ther, 59:30, 1979
74. Bergtholdt HT: Temperature assessment of the insensitive foot. Phys Ther, 59:18, 1979
75. Bergtholdt HT: Measurement in tissue response in rat footpad from repetitive mechanical stress. In Brand PW, Mooney V (eds): The Effects of Pressure on Human Tissues. Report III. Rehabilitation Services Administration, Washington, DC, 1977
76. Forgacs S: Clinical picture of diabetic osteoarthropathy. Acta Diabetol Lat, 13:111, 1976
77. Forgacs S: Bones and Joints in Diabetes Mellitus. Martinus Nijhoff Publishers, The Hague, Netherlands, 1982
78. Pogonowska MJ, Collins LC, Dobson HL: Diabetic osteopathy. Radiology, 89:265, 1967
79. Newman JH: Non-infective disease of the diabetic foot. J Bone Joint Surg, 63B:593, 1981
80. Reinhardt K: The radiological residua of healed diabetic arthropathies. Skel Radiol 7:167, 1981
81. Miller RM, Hunt JA: The radiological features of alcoholic ulceroosteolytic neuropathy in blacks. S Afr Med J, 54:159, 1978
82. Thornhill HL, Richter RW, Shelton ML, Johnson CA: Neuropathic arthropathy (Charcot forefeet) in alcoholics. Orthop Clin North Am, 4:7, 1973
83. Riordan DC: The hand in leprosy: a seven year clinical study. Diabetes, 42A:683, 1960
84. Enna CD, Jacobson RR, Rausch RO: Bone changes in leprosy: a correlation of clinical and radiographic features. Radiology, 10:295, 1971
85. Kraft E, Spyropoulos E, Finby N: Neurogenic disorders of the foot in diabetes mellitus. Am J Roentgenol Rad Ther Nucl Med, 124:17, 1975
86. Schwarz GS, Berenyi MR, Siegal MW: Atrophic arthropathy and diabetic neuritis. Am J Roentgenol Rad Ther Nucl Med, 106:523, 1969
87. Horibe S, Tada K, Nagano J: Neuroarthropathy of the foot in leprosy. J Bone Joint Surg [Br], 70:481, 1988
88. Ainna et al.
89. Coventry MB, Rothacker GW: Bilateral calcaneal fracture in a diabetic patient. J Bone Joint Surg [Am], 61:462, 1979
90. El-Khoury GY, Kathol MH: Neuropathic fractures in patients with diabetes mellitus. Radiology, 134:313, 1980
91. Giescke SB, Dalinka MK, Kyle GC: Lisfranc's frac-
92. ture dislocation: a manifestation of peripheral neuropathy. Am J Roentgenol, 131:139, 1978
92. Williams B: Orthopedic features in the presentation of syringomyelia. J Bone Joint Surg [Br], 61:314, 1979
93. Fath MA, Hassanein MR, James JIP: Congenital absence of pain. J Bone Joint Surg [Br], 65:186, 1983
94. Schneider R, Goldman AB, Bohne WHO: Neuropathic injuries to the lower extremities in children. Pediatr Radiol, 128:713, 1978
95. Kristiansen B: Ankle and foot fracture in diabetics provoking neuropathic joint changes. Acta Orthop Scand, 51:975, 1980
96. Bruckner FE, Howell A: Neuropathic joints. Semin Arthritis Rheum, 2:47, 1972
97. Sinha S, Munichoodappa S, Kozak GP: Neuroarthropathy in diabetes mellitus. Medicine, 51:191, 1972
98. Wolf DS, Raczka EK, Shevlin AM: Charcot's joint in a juvenile-onset diabetic. J Am Podiatry Assoc, 67:200, 1977
99. Sella AJ: Diabetic neurosteoarthropathy of the tarsus. Conn Med, 43:70, 1979
100. McNamara G, Shor RI: Diabetic neuropathic osteoarthropathy. J Am Podiatry Assoc, 73:485, 1983
101. Weissman SD, Weiss A: Diabetic neurotrophic osteoarthropathy (Charcot joint). J Am Podiatry Assoc, 70:196, 1980
102. Harris JR, Brand PW: Patterns of disintegration of the tarsus in the anaesthetic foot. J Bone Joint Surg [Br], 48:4, 1966
103. Frykberg RG: The diabetic Charcot foot. Arch Podiatr Med Foot Surg, 5:15, 1978
104. Hetherington VJ: Technetium and combined gallium and technetium scan in the neurotrophic foot. J Am Podiatry Assoc, 72:458, 1982
105. Park HM, Wheat LJ, Siddiqui AR et al: Scintigraphic evaluation of diabetic osteomyelitis: concise communication. J Nucl Med, 23:569, 1982
106. Maurer AH, Chen DCP, Camago EE et al: Utility of three phase skeletal scintigraphy in suspected osteomyelitis. J Nucl Med, 22:941, 1981
107. Thrall JH, Geslien GE, Corcoron RJ, Johnson MC: Abnormal radionuclide deposition patterns: adjacent to focal skeletal lesions. Radiology, 15:659, 1975
108. Clark WD, Fann TR, McCrea J, Venson JN: Uses of bone scanning in podiatric medicine. J Am Podiatry Assoc, 68:621, 1978
109. Glynn TP: Marked gallium accumulation in neurogenic arthropathy. J Nucl Med, 22:1016, 1981
110. Sugarman B, Hawes S, Musher DM et al: Osteo-

myelitis beneath pressure sores. Arch Intern Med, 143:683, 1983

111. Propst-Proctor SL, Dillingham MF, McDougall IR: The white blood cell scan in orthopedics. Clin Orthop, 168:157, 1982

112. Sandrow RE, Torg JS, Lapayowker MD, Resnick EJ: The use of thermography in the early diagnosis of neuropathic arthropathy in the feet of diabetics. Clin Orthop, 88:31, 1972

113. Matlin SR: Liquid crystal thermography. Arch Podiatr Med Foot Surg, 1:235, 1974

114. Popmynaloua H, Yaneja R, Koev D et al: Xeroradiology of the diabetic foot. Rev Roman Med Endocr, 19:249, 1981

115. Goldman F, Manzi J, Carver A et al: Sinography in the diagnosis of foot infections. J Am Podiatry Assoc 71:497, 1981

116. Enna CD: Rehabilitation of leprous deformity. Annu Rev Med, 33:41, 1982

117. Block P: The diabetic foot ulcer: a complex problem with a simple treatment approach. Milit Med, 146:644, 1981

118. Seder JI: Management of foot problems in diabetics. J Dermatol Surg Oncol, 4:708, 1978

119. Singleton EE, Cotton RS, Shelman HS: Another approach to the long term management of the diabetic neurotrophic foot ulcer. J Am Podiatry Assoc, 68:242, 1978

120. Brenner MA: An ambulatory approach to the neuropathic ulceration. J Am Podiatry Assoc, 64:862, 1974

121. Goldman F: Identification, treatment, and prognosis of Charcot joint in Diabetes mellitus. J Am Podiatry Assoc, 72:485, 1982

122. Lennox WM: Surgical treatment of chronic deformities of the anesthetic foot. p. 350. In McDowell F, Enna CD (eds): Surgical Rehabilitation in Leprosy and in Other Peripheral Nerve Disorders. Williams & Wilkins, Baltimore, 1974

123. Noe JM, Kalish S: Dressing materials and their selection. p. 37. In Rudolph R, Noe JM (eds): Chronic Problem Wounds. Little, Brown and Co, Boston, 1983

124. Bohnannon RW: Whirlpool versus whirlpool and rinse for removal of bacteria from venous stasis ulcer. Phys Ther, 62:304, 1982

125. Robson MC, Edstrom LE: Conservative management of the ulcerated diabetic foot. Plast Reconstr Surg, 59:551, 1977

126. Kritter AE: A technique for salvage of the infected diabetic gangrenous foot. Orthop Clin North Am, 4:21, 1973

127. Rice JS: Diabetic infection, ulceration and gangrene. J Am Podiatry Assoc, 64:774, 1974

128. LaPorta GA, Richter KP, Marzzacco JC: Local radical amputation in the foot for arterial insufficiency. J Am Podiatry Assoc, 67:192, 1977

129. Brown PW: The fate of exposed bone. Am J Surg, 137:464, 1979

130. Singer A: Surgical treatment of mal perforans. Arch Surg, 111:964, 1976

131. Wexler MR, Barlev A, Peled IJ: Plantar split-thickness skin grafts for coverage of superficial pressure ulcers of the foot. J Dermatol Surg Oncol, 9:162, 1983

132. Kipp LJ: Hynes reverse dermal skin graft. J Foot Surg, 15:26, 1976

133. Shapiro GD, Brownstein M, Coulter KR, Woodcox LH: Non-diabetic neurotrophic ulcer of the heel. J Foot Surg, 21:285, 1982

134. Morain WD: Island toe flaps in neurotrophic ulcers of the foot and ankle. Ann Plast Surg, 13:1, 1984

135. Hartwell SW: Local flaps of the foot and leg. p. 497. In Grabb WC, Myers MD (eds): Skin Flaps. Little, Brown and Co, Boston, 1975

136. Curtin JW: Functional surgery for intractable conditions of the sole of the foot. Plast Reconstr Surg, 59:806, 1977

137. Colem LB, Buncke HJ: Neurovascular island flaps from the plantar vessels and nerves for foot reconstruction. Ann Plast Surg, 12:327, 1984

138. Snyder GB, Edgerton MT: The principle of the island neurovascular flap in the management of ulcerated anesthetic weightbearing areas of the lower extremity. Plast Reconstr Surg, 36:518, 1965

139. Ger R: Newer concepts in the surgical management of lesions of the foot in patients with diabetes. Surg Gynecol Obstet, 158:213, 1984

140. Nelson EW, Scurran B, Turek D et al: Reconstruction of plantar heel defects. J Am Podiatry Assoc, 73:235, 1983

141. Scheflan M, Nahai F: Reconstruction. p. 585. In Mathes JJ, Nahai F (eds): Clinical Applications for Muscle and Musculocutaneous Flaps. CV Mosby Co, St Louis, 1982

142. Mathes SJ, Nanai F: A systemic approach to flap selection. p. 3. In Mathes SJ, Nahai F (eds): Clinical Applications for Muscle and Musculocutaneous Flaps. CV Mosby Co, St Louis, 1982

143. Lang-Stevenson AI, Sharrard WJW, Betts RP, Duckworth T: Neuropathic ulcers of the foot. J Bone Joint Surg [Br], 67:438, 1985

Disorders Associated With Aging $\qquad$ 21

Arthur E. Helfand, D.P.M.

Aging and its social as well as medical relationships have become a significant area of concern in the American health care system. The American population is growing older. Modern medical science has extended life spans while focusing on retaining quality of life. With that segment of the population 65 years and older growing more rapidly than any other, the need for podiatric care for the elderly and the need to recognize the relationship between foot health and mobility has been brought into sharper focus. Foot care and the ability to remain active are directly related to the quality of life of our aging society.

In 1900, only 1 in 10 Americans was age 55 or over, and 1 in 25 was age 65 or over. By 1984, 1 in 5 was at least 55 years old, and 1 in 9 was at least 65 years of age. Our older population has grown twice as fast as the rest of the population over the last two decades. The number of persons 65 and over is expected to rise from 27.4 million in 1984 to 58.8 million by the year 2025. The number of "old old" Americans, those 85 and over, is expected to be seven times as large by the middle of the next century as it is today. By the year 2000, half of our elderly population will be more than 75 years of age. Elderly women will continue to outnumber elderly men, and by the year 2010 there are expected to be 22 retired persons for every 100 working individuals; this will change the scope of the labor force.

About half of the elderly live in eight states, five of which — California, New York, Florida, Pennsylvania, Illinois, and Ohio — house colleges of podiatric medicine. Projections of future needs in education, research, and clinical service present a significant opportunity to the podiatric profession and its educational system.

Elderly persons have less cash income than those under 65 years of age. They are more likely to be poor. With the potential for catastrophic illness, the economic picture becomes even more serious, particularly given that the majority of health care dollars are expended in the final year of life. The old old (those over 85 years of age) have even less money than the young old, yet funding for services after age 85 might even be more critical. With a significant reliance on Social Security for income and benefits, the share contributions from the American work force continues to fall, creating a crisis in the system.

Retirement has become an expected part of life. In 1900, the average American male spent 3 percent of his lifetime in retirement. By 1980, he was spending 20 percent. Although 65 has been considered as the primary age of retirement, today almost two-thirds of the working population retire before the age of 65. In 1985, three-quarters of workers 65 and over were in either (1) managerial and professional; (2) technical, sales, and administrative support; or (3) service occupations. Most elderly persons prefer to maintain some part-time work after retirement. For those elderly who become unemployed, the financial loss is even greater.

Most elderly persons view their health in a positive manner. Even with multiple chronic illnesses, they tend to want to keep going. One in five are known to have at least a mild degree of disability; perhaps the term *functional disability* better describes such limitations of activity. Over half of the old old have no disability, but the likelihood of disability increases with age. Cognitive impairment is more common in the elderly. Three out of four elderly die from heart disease, cancer, or stroke. Thus, health care needs to be directed toward comfort rather than cure. Informal support systems by family members continue to be a major need to keep the elderly in noninstitutional settings. The elderly account for 30 percent of all hospital discharges and one-third of the country's health expenditures, even though they constitute only 11 percent of the population. The average out-of-pocket expense for health care for the elderly in 1984 was $1,059 annually, and total per capita spending for health care for the elderly in 1984 was $4,202, demonstrating the need for concern and for planning. In fiscal year 1986, 28 percent of the federal budget, or $273.1 billion dollars, went to programs benefiting the elderly.

Most elderly men today are married and live in a family setting. Most elderly women are widows. The educational gap that used to exist between the elderly and the nonelderly is closing and will continue to close. With increasing age, Americans tend to rent rather than own their homes, and most of the elderly live in older homes. They also tend more to live in inadequate housing, lacking privacy and basic telephone service. The elderly are also more likely to vote and are a potential political force.

The cost of health care for the elderly is almost equal to federal expenditures on retirement. Although 65 years of age today is not considered old, from a statistical point of view, it represents the line between old and young—the start of Medicare benefits, the start of Social Security benefits, and the time when the golden years are to begin.

As health care providers, we must become involved in the planning for the health and social needs of our future elderly, so that we can remain responsible contributors to the quality of life.

PRIMARY PODIATRIC CARE

Through the active years, the human foot undergoes a significant degree of use, trauma, misuse, and neglect. The stress of society, the normal aging process, multiple systemic diseases, focal impairments, and environmental factors help create foot problems in the elderly. It has been estimated that painful feet are a leading cause of discomfort in the elderly. The ability to move about and remain an active and viable member of society is easily lost as a result of impairments, conditions, and deformities involving the feet. Keeping the elderly walking is a major goal for the podiatric practitioner as a member of the health care team.

To the elderly, inability to remain mobile translates into social segregation, a loss of efficiency, declining health, and resultant emotional and personality changes. Out of health, out of time, out of usefulness, and out of enjoyment characterize those changes related to foot impairment and disability. What may well be left is life without quality. Foot problems, especially in the elderly, produce immobility, which in turn limits self-respect and increases the potential for social poverty.

As practitioners, we cannot always cure or make things right again. However, we can help the elderly establish new goals for their lives and activities that maximize their capacity to cope with life and their living environments. We can help the elderly achieve and maintain the dignity of age, for this is all that may be left to them in life.

Many factors contribute to the development of foot problems in the elderly. Some are the amount of walking the individual does; the duration of hospitalization or institutionalization; previous types of foot care; environmental factors; emotional adjustments; current medications and therapeutic programs; associated systemic and localized disease processes; and past foot conditions and pedal manifestations of disease.

The average aging patient is usually taking more than one drug at any given time, and sensitivities and reactions to drugs differ from those of younger people. Local infections are more common because of related conditions and the anatomic location of the foot itself. Atrophy, degeneration, avascularity, and neuropathic changes are more common.

There may be a lower threshold of physical and emotional stress, and there is often more confusion about health care needs. The patient usually has more than one chronic disease or condition, is gradually deteriorating, and has a more difficult time adjusting to social and environmental changes. There is a tendency to defer early examination and care as well as to minimize health education as a means of prevention. Exacerbations of preexisting conditions are more common in the elderly. Injuries to the lower extremities are more common, as is the potential for limb loss.

The problems of delivering and financing podiatric services for the elderly are similar to those in other medical specialties. However, comprehensive programs must include primary podiatric care as a primary service and allow early and direct patient entry for diagnosis and management. Outreach, education, and the social elements of care for the elderly must include the above components and offer primary physical care to deal with complaints. Appropriate support must also include administrative policies, reimbursement, staff education, records (utilization, review, and quality assurance), laboratory services, radiology, pharmaceutical services, health education, and social services.

The key to developing a podiatric program for the elderly lies in the ability of community practitioners to recognize problems, look for abnormal findings, listen to the complaints of the patient, and set a series of goals for the patient, to include but not be limited to the following:

1. Improve healing
2. Reduce pain
3. Maintain and increase ranges of motion
4. Maintain and improve muscle effort
5. Encourage walking
6. Prevent complications
7. Keep the elderly ambulatory
8. Provide comfort

The problems associated with aging and the management of the elderly population will increase in the years to come. Planning comprehensively and being involved in the system should permit the elderly to retain their dignity and to remain active, needed, wanted, and respected members of society.

ELEMENTS OF THE PODOGERIATRIC EVALUATION

In the examination of elderly patients who present with foot complaints, symptoms, or findings, it is essential to establish an appropriate and comprehensive data base. Name, sex, age, date of birth, address, phone number, sex, marital status, referring and/or primary care practitioner, and the individual responsible in an emergency all should be identified and recorded. The patient's Social Security number as well as any other insurance carrier information should also be obtained for the record.

The patient's height and weight should be recorded, with notation made of any recent or sudden changes. The chief complaint should provide the initial focus for the evaluation and immediate treatment needs. The reason why the patient is seeking care is important, as discomfort may be the reason for the visit but may not be the most critical entity clinically. If comfort is not provided at the initial visit, the elderly patient may not seek management for other, more serious problems.

The present illness and condition should be explored for duration, location, severity, prior treatment, and general symptoms. There needs to be a systems review focusing on the cardiovascular, metabolic, peripheral vascular, neurologic, dermatologic, and musculoskeletal systems. A past medical history should be recorded to include previous infections, operations, fractures, injuries, asthma, allergies, and drug sensitivities, particularly those related to lower extremity involvement. A past podiatric history should also be recorded and include any care for foot conditions and related ailments, as well as methods of commercial and/or self-care.

An occupational history should include military exposure, geographic locations visited, present occupation, the percentage of weightbearing, and plane of support surfaces, such as flooring. The social history should include the use of tea, coffee, alcohol, and tobacco; sleeping habits; sedatives and hypnotics; narcotics and other drugs; chemical or substance abuse; hobbies and interests; and the patient's reaction to the current illness, condition, or state of health.

The subjective symptoms should be identified as clearly as possible, with assistance from family or others when necessary. Hyperkeratotic lesions should be clearly identified as to type and location. Their relation to foot deformities and abnormalities should be noted. Dermatologic abnormalities should also be noted and may include clinical infections, tinea, xerosis, ulceration, atrophy, and other dermatologic changes.

Onychial changes should be noted, including those associated with age such as onychauxis, onychogryposis, onychomycosis, involution, onychopathies, and other related nail dystrophies, deformities, changes, and diseases.

Peripheral vascular findings should include pedal and related pulses, color, temperature changes, trophic manifestations, edema, varicosities, night cramps, claudication, fatigue, burning, pain, and other indicators of a compromised vascular supply. Vascular function tests may be indicated. These should also be related to cardiovascular and hypertensive disease.

The neurologic evaluation should include gait, reflexes (patellar, Achilles, superficial plantar), ankle clonus, and vibratory sense as well as any other impressions. Vertigo, ambulatory dysfunction, use of gait-assistive devices, and functional disability should be noted. Motor function, muscle strength, proprioception, pain, and tactile sensation are all essential. Local muscle wasting, atrophy, and reduced muscle power can be clues to the patient's ability to deal with the activities of daily living.

A drug history should be taken and includes the use of antihypertensives, antidiabetics, cortisone, sedatives, topicals, antibiotics, cardiovascular drugs, and antihistamines as well as other related drugs. The information recorded should be as specific as possible.

The foot orthopedic, biomechanical, and pathomechanical evaluation should include foot type, gait, postural deformities, palpation for pain and swelling, ranges of motion, angulations, and muscle power. Radiographic findings should be noted as indicated. Clinical deformities such as hallux valgus, hallux rigidus, digiti flexus, pes planus, valgus or varus deformities, bursitis, and other clinical syndromes should be noted, particularly when they affect weightbearing and ambulation.

The type of stockings and footwear used should be noted, particularly in relation to deformities that may be present. Current or previous use of orthotics should be noted.

The summary of findings, impressions, special notations, and projected immediate treatment and long-range management suggestions should be noted and explained to the patient and the patient's family, as appropriate.

Pain is a significant finding and may be masked as discomfort. One can be reasonably sure that the elderly patient will have pain upon seeking care, unless there has been a specific referral as, for example, a diabetic being referred for periodic primary care. Because the foot is many times the focal point of psychosocial problems, complaints such as tension, anxiety, known phobias, inability to concentrate, fears, and worries may well relate to the onset and course of foot problems in the elderly. As an example, most diabetics in their later years know someone who has lost a limb or part of a foot as a complication of diabetes. Thus, denial of what might appear to be minor symptoms or care needs can precipitate greater problems for the elderly patient. Frank discussion of treatment needs and goals is an essential element of the podiatric evaluation. What is important is to identify attainable goals and treatment aims. The periodic management of geriatric foot problems is an element of care that can provide both comfort and prevention, as well as a total therapeutic approach for the elderly patient, similar to the management of any other chronic disease or condition.

RISK FACTORS

The elderly patient's ambulatory status is often compromised or limited by physical deterioration, the patient's environment, and social poverty. Being old and developing chronic diseases create additional stress for the pedal extremities. A general lack of health education, inability to provide self-examination and self-care, limited care programs, and perhaps society's belief that foot problems and care are not an important health issue increase the level of functional disability and ambulatory dysfunction as a part of the aging process. Certain diseases are known to have a high risk of precipitating foot conditions and augmenting complications, which can be catastrophic. Diabetes mellitus is an example. The primary known risk factors include but are not limited to those listed in Table 21-1.

A key element in developing diagnostic and total care programs is to relate the foot problems to the degree of risk, associate the changes with the ambulatory dysfunction and functional disability, and relate future activities to the functional needs of

Table 21-1. Primary Risk Factors for Podiatric Problems in the Elderly

Diabetes mellitus
Arteriosclerosis
Ischemia
Chronic induration
Cellulitis
Lymphedema secondary to disease (e.g. Milroy's disease, malignancy)
Buerger's disease
Chronic superficial phlebitis
Deep venous thrombosis
Venous stasis
Peripheral neuropathies
Malnutrition
Alcohol, chemical, and substance abuse
Malabsorption
Pernicious anemia
Carcinoma
Toxic states
Multiple sclerosis
Uremia
Chronic renal disease
Chronic obstructive pulmonary disease
Cardiac disease and congestive heart failure
Hypertension
Edema
Trauma
Leprosy
Neurosyphilis
Hereditary diseases
Mental illness
Mental retardation
Thyroid disease
Milroy's disease
Hemophilia
Anticoagulant therapy
Stroke
Degenerative joint disease
Gout
Rheumatoid arthritis
Scleroderma
Arteritis
Intractable pain

the patient and efforts to maintain the patient's dignity.

ONYCHIAL CHANGES ASSOCIATED WITH AGING

Disorders of the toenails are common in the elderly. They may result from severe trauma or repeated microtrauma or appear as a result of the aging process itself, diseases of the toenails, or the residuals of systemic, cutaneous, or functional diseases. Onychial changes are directly related to infection, dietary deficiencies, drug reactions, vascular insufficiency, metabolic diseases such as diabetes mellitus, and degenerations. Toenails undergo changes much more often than do fingernails, due to trauma, the environment, and the forces associated with ambulation.

Management of disorders of the aging toenail must include care of those tissues that support the nail structure as well as the nail plate itself. A key factor in the elderly is to minimize discomfort and pain and not expose the patient to risk due to associated vascular, metabolic, or nutritional changes. Atrophy, hypertrophy, and dystrophy are changes generally associated with most nail conditions in the elderly.

Onychia is an inflammation of the soft tissue adjacent to the nail plate. It may involve the medial and lateral nail grooves and/or the posterior nail wall or eponychium. Its presence in the elderly may be the residual of repeated microtrauma or the initial sign of a purulent process. Complications arising from systemic diseases, such as diabetes mellitus, may exhibit such changes as an early sign of impending necrosis. Initial management should include the use of tepid saline compresses and povidone-iodine (Betadine) compresses, and the minimizing of trauma to the area. If the etiology is pressure from the toenail, appropriate débridement should be performed.

Paronychia in the elderly patient combines an inflammatory response with infection. It is a serious problem as the potential for bone involvement increases with age and the presence of such diseases as diabetes mellitus and ischemia. Radiographs, incision and drainage, culture and sensitivity, saline or Betadine compresses, and systemic antibiotics are appropriate considerations. Minimizing trauma to the area is also an essential element of management. The use of a surgical shoe, such as the Darby shoe, is a valid consideration. The patient should be closely monitored, and hospitalization is suggested if cellulitis is apparent.

Onychauxis results in a hypertrophic thickening of the toenails. Its etiology may be repeated microtrauma, a history of significant trauma, prior inflammation, nutritional changes, or risk diseases, which provide a focus for disturbances in nail growth. The toenail becomes laminated and thick, and there is usually an exaggeration of the longitudinal striations in the nail plate (onychorrhexis). Some degree of onycholysis is usually noted, and the nail becomes opaque rather than translucent. Subungual keratosis is also common. Management consists of mechanical débridement every 60 days. Mild keratolytics, such as 20 percent urea (Carmol-20), can be employed to reduce the residual soft tissue keratosis in tissues surrounding the nail plate. Onychomycosis is a common etiologic and complicating factor. Where the condition becomes painful to the point of limiting ambulation and producing some degree of functional disability, surgical removal of the nail plate should be considered. Where there is a significant degree of subungual pain present, particularly on palpation or from the toe box of a shoe, radiographs should be taken to identify any evidence of subungual spur, exostosis, or deformity of the tufted end of the distal phalanx. Management in these situations is usually surgical. Tube foam or lamb's wool can also be used as protective dressings to help reduce pressure to the area.

Onychogryposis or ram's horn nail is the end result of neglected or untreated onychauxis. The nails become grossly deformed, hypertrophic, and laminated. The length and deformity may be so extensive that the toenail encircles the end of the toe and even forms a toe cap to the plantar surface of the foot. Débridement and partial or total avulsion should be considered as initial management, with the determination based on the degree of onycholysis and hypertrophy. The condition of the toenails may reflect general neglect of the patient's health. Autoavulsion is also a factor with trauma. Subungual keratosis and idiopathic subungual hemorrhage are related complicating factors. Onychomycosis is a common complication and etiologic factor.

Many systemic diseases produce changes in the nail plate. One of the most common of the dystrophies is diabetic onychopathy. There is pronounced onychorrhexis. Idiopathic subungual hemorrhages are common and many times are the initial complicating sign pointing to hemorrhage in other organs, such as the eye and the renal system. Some degree of onychauxis and onychophosis is noted. Onycholysis and, with subungual hemorrhage, onychomadesis are usually present. Subungual keratosis and xerotic changes are also associated with diabetic onychopathy. Management consists of débridement and the use of emollients to produce a mild keratolytic effect. In the presence of subungual hemorrhage, monitoring should be maintained and related to other complicating factors.

Patients with hypothyroidism usually demonstrate a slower rate of nail growth. Onycholysis is more common, and a spoon-shaped appearance can also be demonstrated. Atrophy is common in the vascularly impaired patient. Pterygium is more common with vasospasm and is associated with Raynaud's disease and scleroderma. Diffusion of the lunulae is demonstrable in chronic organic vascular disease in the elderly.

Patients with rheumatoid arthritis will present with dry and brittle toenails. Onychorrhexis is more common and subungual keratosis may become pronounced. Onycholysis is also present in the elderly and provides a focus for the development of onychomycosis.

Onychomycosis or tinea ungulum is a fungal infection of the nail plate and its subungual structures. It is more common in the toenails. Onychomycosis is caused by repeated microtrauma and by environmental factors related to footwear, which create a dark, warm, moist area that serves as a medium for infection. It is more common in the elderly and becomes chronic. Clinically the infection may appear as a superficial white mycosis that is easily débrided and treated with a topical fungicide such as Halotex solution, Funginail, or other similar preparations. Usually, however, this superficial form is not treated and goes on to invade the nail plate, creating the tissue destruction and deformity commonly seen in elderly patients. The mycosis destroys the nail plate, and as it invades the matrix area, disturbances of nail growth are noted as hypertrophy. The affected areas also serve as a focus of chronic infection for residual tinea pedis.

Left untreated and unmanaged, the residual deformity can produce pain, limited ambulation, inflammation, and other complicating factors. As the nail plate begins to disintegrate, dystrophic changes are noted as hypertrophy, deformity, discoloration, distortion, onycholysis, and a granular appearance of the nail plate itself. Subungual keratosis and débris are common. Although the etiologic agent is usually tricophyton, monilial involvement can be present and is more commonly associated with diabetes mellitus. A characteristic musty odor is also present and increases with the opaque yellowish-brown color. Scaling and xerosis are common in the nail folds. Left unmanaged, hypertrophic onychomycosis and onychogryposis develop.

Management is a more appropriate term than treatment in these cases. For the most part, by the time this condition is diagnosed in the elderly, a cure is not possible. Care should be considered equal in importance to that of any other chronic infective process in another part of the body. Local and periodic débridement, the use of mild keratolytics, and the use of topical fungicides in solution are appropriate. In uncomplicated cases a 60-day utilization factor is appropriate. Systemic antifungal agents seem to have less effect on the geriatric toenail, probably because of vascular insufficiency and other systemic nutritional changes. Avulsion and total removal of the nail and matrix may also be considered when complications are a factor and pain persists as a result of deformity and hypertrophy. Continuing assessment and management are key elements of care.

Ingrown toenails in the elderly patient are usually associated with one of two primary problems. The first is inappropriate care, usually self-care. The second is involution or incurvation of the toenails, which creates pressure on the lateral nail folds leading to onychophosis and penetration of the nail folds.

The classic ingrown toenail presents with swelling, redness, and infection. Purulent material can be isolated with drainage. A fragment of the nail plate penetrates the lateral nail wall. Left untreated, periungual ulcerative granulation tissue develops, complicating the management of this condition. With involuted or incurvated toe nails, the residual deformity is C shaped when viewed distally. Pressure from the nail, hypertrophic changes, onychophosis, or external causes such as shoes or stockings give rise to a feeling of fullness in the toe and pain. If the patient attempts self-care, the residual fragment then creates the classic ingrown toenail within a short time.

When there is an abscess, the area needs to be drained and managed with compresses, such as Domeboro, (aluminum acetate solution), saline, or Betadine, and the use of appropriate systemic antibiotics as indicated. Periungual granulation tissue can be excised or cauterized by electrosurgery or with chemical caustics such as 75 percent silver nitrate. The offending segment of nail must be removed from the soft tissue. Follow-up measures must be completed to prevent retraction of tissue as the nail grows forward. The use of mild keratolytics such as Carmol-20, Lac-Hydrin, or Keralyt Gel will aid in the reduction of onychophosis and provide some flexibility to hypertrophic nail tissue.

When the clinical picture is one of marked swelling, deformity, and granulation tissue, or the involuted deformity is extensive, partial or total excision of the nail and matrix is indicated. Either surgical excision or a combined approach utilizing CP Phenol or similar caustics to destroy the matrix area is used. The pyogenic granulation tissue, which is ulcerative in character, also needs to be removed and the area subsequently treated with silver nitrate. Caution must be taken where there is vascular insufficiency, diabetes mellitus, or other risk factor diseases, as this singular condition, improperly managed by either the patient or the practitioner, can result in necrosis, gangrene, and the loss of a limb.

Periungual or subungual abscess can be the residual of trauma, disease, or nail dystrophy. Regardless of the cause, incision and drainage, Betadine compresses, and systemic antibiotics should be employed as indicated.

Subungual hemorrhage in the elderly is the result of two primary etiologic factors. The first is direct trauma. Recent subungual hemorrhages will appear reddish, and onycholysis may be noted. If the hemorrhage is the residual of older trauma, the color will appear much darker. Management to some degree depends on the symptoms. Radiographs should be taken to rule out fracture. If the patient is in significant pain and the hemorrhage is recent, a small hole can be drilled in the dorsal surface of the nail to permit drainage. Older hemorrhage that has coagulated does not need to be drained and should grow distally as the nail grows. Onychomadesis and onycholysis may be present, and autoavulsion of the toe nail is a possibility, depending on the extent of the subungual hemorrhage.

The second primary etiologic factor is associated with diseases such as diabetes mellitus or associated with patients on anticoagulant therapy, which produce hemorrhage into the tissues. In these cases, drainage is contraindicated and the patient only needs to be observed as the nail grows forward. Onychomadesis and onycholysis as well as autoavulsion are feasible in these cases. If the nail becomes loosened, the free segments should be removed to prevent additional trauma.

Subungual heloma, when identified in the elderly patient, is usually related to the presence of a subungual spur or exostosis located on the superior surface of the distal phalanx of the toe. A hypertrophy of the tufted end of the distal phalanx may give rise to similar symptoms. Radiographs should be taken to isolate bone pathology. Associated pathologies such as subungual hemorrhage, subungual melanoma, glomus tumor, or subungual ulceration should be ruled out. Management consists of partial removal of the dorsal nail segment, débridement of the keratotic tissue, and measures to remove pressure from the area.

In the presence of subungual exostosis or spur, surgery may be used to remove excess bone, as continuing pressure on the subungual area will continue to produce localized hyperkeratosis, discomfort, and pain.

Some of the other dystrophic changes that are common in the elderly patient include onychoschizia, which is a splitting of the nail plate. The etiology is usually one of a variety of dermatologic entities including onychomycosis, nutritional disturbances, and psoriasis, and the condition is aided by the ingestion of gelatin on a daily basis.

Beau's lines (transverse changes on the nail) may appear when nail growth is interrupted for a short period of time, usually by some systemic trauma. The most common causes are acute myocardial infarction, cerebral vascular accidents, and severe emotional shock. No specific treatment is required other than monitoring of the patient.

Onychorrhexis is an exaggeration of the longitudinal striations in the nail plate and is related to systemic diseases, the most common being diabetes mellitus. Onycholysis is the freeing of the nail from the distal segment; onychomadesis is the freeing of the nail from the proximal segment or eponychium. These conditions are related to other nail conditions such as onychomycosis and reflect part of their symptom complex.

Hapalonychia is a softening of the nail plate, usually related to mycotic infection or nutritional disturbances. Extreme hyperhidrosis can also be a factor in the development of this condition.

Patients with psoriasis will usually present with onychial changes that resemble mycotic infections. Punctate depressions in the nail plate are usually present. It is not unusual for the elderly psoriatic also to have mycotic involvement, making the nail changes and subsequent management more difficult.

Pterygium is also a common hyperkeratotic clinical finding noted in the elderly. It represents a hyperplastic keratin dysfunction involving the eponychium. Débridement and the use of mild keratolytic emollients, such as Carmol-20 or Lac-Hydrin, will help control this condition, which can be painful for the elderly patient.

The clinical finding of necrosis of the distal segments of the toes and nails, associated with diabetes mellitus and vascular insufficiency, represents the potential for limb loss and its medical and social sequelae.

HYPERKERATOTIC LESIONS IN THE ELDERLY

The major functions of the human foot can be generally classed as static and dynamic. The foot is an organ of weightbearing, propulsion, and locomotion, and it carries an extensive workload throughout life. The foot is relatively rigid and is forced by society, the environment, one's occupation, and the activities of daily living to undergo significant stress over a lifetime. The residual effect coupled with the normal process of aging, degeneration, and disease as a final stress, can be decompensating and produce both functional disability and ambulatory dysfunction.

Civilization has forced the foot to function on hard, flat surfaces, which for the most part do not absorb shock. In addition, the repeated tissue trauma associated with occupational stress and the environmental factors associated with walking do not provide for a compensatory element of weight diffusion or dispersion over the entire foot or an equal percentage of compensation for both feet. There are limits placed on total foot function, particularly on the intrinsic function of the foot. The best example is that of atrophy of the interossei and the resulting digital contractures. The foot, for the most part, is maintained in a single attitude, and when disease and aging become a factor, discomfort, pain, and a limitation of activity can be severe enough to change one's life-style and possibly leave the patient a ward of society.

Stress and repeated tissue trauma result in osteitis, periostitis, synovitis, capsulitis, fasciitis, myositis, arthritis, and fibrositis. Pain changes ambulation. Trauma, disease, and aging produce atrophy and deformity. The body responds by what is initially a protective mechanism, namely, the development of hyperkeratotic lesions as space replacements and shock absorbers. Subsequently these become pathomechanical, with the keratotic areas acting as foreign bodies. As morphologic variations become more apparent in the elderly, the residuals of the biomechanical and pathomechanical changes become more symptomatic. The physiologic changes related to gait magnify these problems.

The ability to adapt to stress is lessened in the elderly. This maladaptation is accelerated by the presence of risk diseases that produce pedal symptoms, signs, and complications. As the neuromuscular and vascular systems demonstrate changes, symptoms become more severe. The systemic stressors most commonly affecting the elderly are the aging process itself, diabetes mellitus, arteriosclerosis, and arthritis.

The mechanical stressors are generally some form of macrotrauma, which is trauma significant enough to cause a fracture or soft tissue tear, and microtrauma, which results in a gradual onset of discomfort, pain, ambulatory dysfunction, and residual functional disability. Occupation, overweight, posture, gait changes, the activities of daily living, and foot-to-shoe last incompatibilities are all nonsystemic stressors.

Force, compressive stress, tensile stress, shearing stress, friction, elasticity, and fluid pressure are the primary factors related to the development of hyperkeratotic lesions in the elderly. Certain broad principles should be considered in managing hyperkeratotic lesions in the elderly patient. It is obvious that the foot can not be divorced or segmented off from the rest of the body, nor can the foot itself be segmented. As in the old spiritual, the foot bone is truly connected to the head bone. The foot is an end organ of stance and locomotion, and any residual of systemic disease or any mechanical, positional, or rotational change that produces stress may produce a hyperkeratotic lesion in the elderly. In a sense, these hyperplastic and hyperkeratotic changes comprise parts of a syndrome that is progressive in nature.

Treatment should be directed toward eliminating the cause or compensating for the biomechanical, pathomechanical, dermatologic, or systemic changes that affect the feet of the elderly. There is a need to identify the etiologic factors as early as possible and to prevent complications where existing lesions are identified. The principles of primary, secondary, and tertiary prevention all apply. Management must include appropriate lubrication and hydration to maximize skin tone. Stress areas, which create the potential for dermal irritation, must be controlled. The principles of weight diffusion and weight dispersion should be followed to maximize weight and pressure redistribution so as to provide a uniform ambulatory pressure. It should be remembered that there are variations among individuals and, from time to time, within an individual in the capacity to adjust to change. The primary goals in the elderly in dealing with biomechanical and pathomechanical problems are to restore maximum function, relieve pain, and maintain the maximum level of independent function.

Many of the most common foot complaints of the elderly patient are focused on the presence of hyperkeratotic lesions (corns and calluses). The types of lesion generally seen include heloma durum (hard corn), heloma molle (soft corn), heloma miliare (seed corn), heloma neurofibrosum (neurofibrous corn), heloma vasculare (vascular corn), and tyloma (callus). In the absence of overlying cutaneous disease, the lesions are usually symptomatic and secondary to some existing deformity or biomechanical or pathomechanical abnormality combined with excessive pressure to a circumscribed area. The pressure may be a bony abnormality, foot-to-shoe last incompatibility, a deformity such as digiti flexus (hammer toe), hallux valgus or bunion, or changes in the method of weightbearing and weight transmission, as in the case of pronation, rotational deformities, hypermobility, plantar flexion deformities, calcaneal varus, equinus, and forefoot varus deformities.

In foot-to-shoe last incompatibility, the shape of the foot and its direction or flare do not follow the design or last (model) of the shoe. For example, most older people tend to walk with their feet pointed outward, adding to stability and presenting a wider base of support, as in the pediatric patient. Most shoes, however, are directed or flared inward. The result is like putting a right foot into a left shoe. Problems develop not because of disease but because of an incompatibility between the foot and the shoe.

Tyloma (callus) is a broad-based hyperkeratotic lesion, similar to heloma, caused by hyperplasia of the keratin layer and generally associated with a more diffuse pressure. Like all hyperkeratotic lesions, callus is a normal body reaction to external or internal stresses placed on the skin or on the patient. The stress may be compressive (such as shoe compression or last incompatibility), tensile (such as digital deformities and compensatory pronation, with or without fixation, which pulls one part from another), or shearing (caused by parts sliding on each other, creating friction). Linked to these problems are the elasticity and fluidity of soft tissue, which can act as a normal protective mechanism for body parts in general and the foot in particular.

Degenerative loss of the plantar fat pad, digital contractures, spur and hyperostotic formation, arthritic changes, and functional adaptations are significant in the development of hyperkeratotic le-

sions. Usually, the initial skin lesion is a tyloma. Where the etiologic factor is permitted to remain and intervention and modification are not instituted to prevent, modify, or manage the problem, the pressure becomes greater, a central nucleus develops, and a heloma is generated.

Heloma molle is an excellent example of such a progression. The usual etiology is some change in normal toe alignment, which permits the head of one of the phalanges to be compressed against the base of or adjacent to a phalangeal or metatarsophalangeal articulation. There is usually an associated condylar enlargement of one or both of the areas in juxtaposition. Continued pressure and compression from associated footwear can create the lesion, which may become inflamed, infected, and ulcerated. Necrosis in the diabetic or vascularly impaired patient many times surfaces from this scenario.

Management may involve periodic débridement, the use of emollients and mild keratolytics, and the use of silicone molds or other orthotic devices to reduce pressure and help modify the alignments and weight-bearing forces. Surgical excision of bony enlargements and joint reconstruction also deserve fair consideration. In most cases, management, including débridement, when instituted early on, is the best approach to dealing with these chronic conditions.

In many cases these lesions have existed for many years, and neither patient nor practitioner should expect an instant cure. These conditions may require periodic treatment to maintain patient comfort.

Primary care in the elderly most often involves providing comfort and relieving pain; these are clearly primary goals in managing the elderly patient, as total cure and restoration to a predisease state may not be feasible.

The approach to the management of hyperkeratotic lesions involves identifying the type of lesion, establishing the etiologic factors, and developing a proper long-range plan of therapy. Management often will include periodic débridement of the keratotic lesions. Given the chronicity of the condition, management is no different from the approach to treating hypertension, diabetes mellitus, or exacerbations of degenerative joint disease. Radiographs taken in weight-bearing positions are of value when compared to radiographs in non-weight-bearing positions. Because the foot is an organ of stance, weightbearing, and propulsion, assessment in functional positions is required as part of the diagnostic workup. Initial management usually consists of débridement, an emollient such as Carmol-20 or Lac-Hydrin to both hydrate and lubricate the skin and provide a mild keratolytic effect, and the use of protective padding to remove pressure. The involvement of the patient in a home care program is essential. The same is true for institutionalized patients.

Patients should be warned not to utilize any commercial corn cure products, which use strong concentrations of acid to produce their keratolytic effect. Inappropriate use generally produces a second-degree chemical burn, loss of tissue, and the potential for infection. For the patient with diabetes mellitus or arterial insufficiency, this minor trauma can precipitate limb loss. Unfortunately, warning labels are usually printed so small that the average elderly patient is unable to read them.

Various materials such as felt, foam rubber, sponge rubber, plastics, and leather, and newer materials such as Plastazote, Spenco, Sorbathane, and similar products that provide both weight diffusion and weight dispersion, can be employed to help reduce pressure. Paddings of different types are employed for plantar orthotics, to help restore a neutral function of the foot. Crest padding and silicone molds may be useful in the presence of digital deformities and contractures. Latex shields can also be employed for these deformities. If the patient is physically able to tolerate it, surgical revision should also be considered when the deformity is marked, when pain is persistent, and when surgery can prevent future extension of the impairment and complications. The patient's ability to adapt postsurgically to changes in ambulation is a factor in the decision.

Choice of footwear is also a consideration in the initial management of keratotic lesions, regardless of the etiology. When there is a clear shoe-related incompatibility, changes should be recommended. Use of the Extra Depth Inlay shoe, Thermold or Ambulator-type shoes, bunion last shoes, the classic orthopedic last, or a standard shoe that has been relasted, deserves consideration. The newer athletic shoes offer an excellent alternative for many elderly patients as a general walking shoe. The object is to select a shoe that will eliminate pressure and generally fit the contour of the foot as it exists, with its deformities.

COMMON SKIN PROBLEMS IN THE AGING FOOT

The most common clinical signs observed in the skin of the geriatric foot include dryness, scaling, and atrophy. The etiologic factors are varied and multiple and include the normal aging process, systemic disease, and environmental factors. The skin demonstrates diminished sebaceous activity, diminished hydration of the epidermis, metabolic and nutritional alterations, and dysfunction in keratin formation. There is an associated loss of hair and of skin elasticity, and the toenails become striated and brittle. There are multiple degenerative changes related to aging and disease, and pigmentary changes are common. The presence of any form of vascular occlusive disease may result in color changes ranging from pallor to cyanosis. Increased deposition of hemosiderin can frequently be demonstrated. If the stress of ambulation is added, keratin dysfunction becomes magnified as a reaction to pressure and as a space replacement.

Pruritus is common in the elderly patient. It may be related to disturbed keratin formation, dryness, scaliness, decreased sebaceous activity, environmental changes, and defatting of the skin as a result of hot baths. It must be differentiated from chronic tinea and various forms of neurogenic and emotional dermatoses. Treatment should be directed toward moderation in bathing habits and the use of emollients, which lubricate and hydrate the skin. If pruritus is related to tinea, an appropriate antifungal agent should be instituted. Antihistamines in adjusted doses can also be employed to break the scratch reflex. Appropriate care should be taken with patients with prostatic disease and with those patients taking multiple medications, to avoid adverse drug interactions. Topical steroids are also of value in selected patients.

The complaint of dry skin is more often heard in the winter and in colder climates. Emollients for hydration and lubrication provide relief. Oil and water baths are also beneficial. However, the patient should be cautioned that these products in bath water may make for a slippery tub, and precautions should be taken to minimize potential falls.

Fissured heels can create a serious problem for the elderly patient, particularly when there is an associated degree of vascular insufficiency. Devitalized skin presents an excellent avenue for bacterial invasion and infection. Superficial tinea should be considered a possibility when there is diffuse keratosis along the marginal areas of the heels. Atrophy of the skin and repeated microtrauma will also precipitate stress marks in the heel, which are the early signs of calcaneal fissuring. Management should be directed toward closing the fissures and preventing their recurrence. Emollients and the use of heel cups to reduce pressure should be employed. Poly-foam and plastic cups are available, and the choice of treatment depends on the degree of soft tissue present and patient tolerance. Topical antifungals such as Vioform-HC ointment (iodochlorhydroxyquin), Lotrisone, or Loprox (ciclopirox) are indicated with mycotic infections. Antibiotics and reduced weightbearing should be considered in the presence of infection. The possibility of contact dermatitis should also be considered in longstanding cases and appropriately managed. In patients with a diminished vascular supply, physical modalities such as whirlpool, low-voltage therapy, and exercise can be used for mechanical débridement and to improve the local vascular status. Topical enzymes are of value to help provide chemical débridement of the fissured areas. Local stimulants such as compound tincture of benzoin or gentian violet help to improve epithelialization. Protection also includes the use of heel protectors during bed rest and the use of Plastazote sandals or shoes to reduce pressure and stress to the calcaneal areas during weightbearing and ambulation. Local débridement when indicated should be performed judiciously, as the calcaneal area is poorly supplied vascularly, and the risk of necrosis should be minimized.

Hyperhidrosis, or excessive sweating, is not as common in the elderly as in younger patients. When present, it may be associated with tinea, inappropriate footwear, the use of stockings that do not absorb perspiration, fabrics in shoes and as orthotic coverings, and emotional factors. Local management involves daily foot hygiene and the use of an absorbent foot powder. Peroxide and alcohol swabbing and the use of 10 percent formalin solutions are also of value in resistant cases. Dry-Sol (20 percent aluminum chloride) is another product that can be used topically to manage excessive perspiration.

Bromohyperhidrosis is a form of excessive sweating characterized by a fetid odor due to the bacterial decomposition of sweat. The therapeutic approach is similar to that for hyperhidrosis. Deodorants and, at times, topical neomycin may be needed during the initial period of care. Shoes should also be changed daily and permitted to air dry in sunlight when possible.

Contact dermatitis from shoe dyes or various forms of foot covering material should be considered when the patient presents with a circumscribed area of inflammation, pruritus, and urticarial lesions. A history of allergy may also be a predisposing factor. Treatment should be directed toward eliminating the etiologic agent and providing management for the dermatologic lesions present. The use of a shoe test kit can be of assistance in identification of the agent. Mild compresses of Burow's solution, saline, or even cool milk can help reduce the inflammation. Antihistamines can be employed to help control pruritus, but the dosage should be titrated to meet the needs of the elderly patient. Topical steroids or other related medications can be employed. The key element must be the elimination of the causative agent.

Superficial infections or pyodermas should be considered serious in the elderly and treated early in their development. Given the various degenerative changes associated with aging, any break in the skin can result in a bacterial infection. Treatment consists of tepid saline or Betadine compresses and appropriate topical and systemic antibiotics to manage the infection. Bed rest and hospitalization may be required early on for the patient with systemic risk diseases, such as diabetes mellitus and peripheral arteriosclerosis, to prevent significant tissue damage.

Tinea pedis may present in any one of its clinical

varieties — acute vesicular, subacute vesicular, chronic hyperkeratotic, and interdigital. Smears and cultures may be employed for identification, but the clinical presentation alone should prompt treatment. In the acute stages, astringent compresses and topical antifungals should be employed. Solutions and creams tend to be of greater value for the nonkeratotic types, and ointments more effective with keratotic tinea. When secondary bacterial infection is present and some degree of cellulitis is noted, appropriate systemic antibiotics should be instituted. Delay in management may result in serious infection in the elderly patient at risk. Systemic antifungals tend to be more effective in the younger patient and in lesions other than the lower extremity. In addition, because the elderly are usually taking more than one drug at any given time, drug interactions are more common. Decreased vascular supply also inhibits the systemic response. Castellani's paint or gentian violet is effective in interdigital areas, but their color tends to mask the clinical signs. Clotrimazole, tolnaftate, undecylenic acid, iodochlorhydroxyquin, and haloprogin are examples of topical antifungals. When the tinea is monilial in origin, antimonilial topicals should be utilized. The topical use of antifungal foot powders is an appropriate preventive approach, particularly in the presence of hyperhidrosis. This protocol for prevention is particularly useful in institutions for the elderly.

The vast majority of ulcerative lesions in the foot of the elderly patient are the result of pressure or biomechanical or pathomechanical dysfunction and are usually associated with a concomitant systemic disease, such as diabetes mellitus or peripheral arterial insufficiency. Associated angiopathy, dermatopathy, and neuropathy are major contributing factors, as is atrophy of the plantar structures. Deformities related to joint change and degenerative joint disease are precipitating factors. In all cases, the presence of a systemic disease mandates control of that problem. Laboratory and radiographic studies should be followed by bone scans if indicated. Initial management should consider bed rest, management of the related disease process, and early hospitalization to avoid amputation. Judicious débridement may be surgical or chemical, if indicated. Drainage should be established as indicated. Topical enzymes are of value when prop-

erly controlled. Antibiotics should be prescribed when infection is present and may be suggested as a prophylactic measure. Physical measures such as whirlpool or low-voltage therapy should be prescribed to assist in healing. Every attempt should be made to remove weightbearing from the ulcerative site. This includes the use of a Plastazote sandal or shoe, a Thermold shoe, an Extra Depth Inlay shoe with an appropriate orthotic, or a molded shoe in the secondary stages of management. The use of a surgical shoe such as the Darby shoe in the acute stages of management is appropriate when dressing changes are performed on a daily or periodic basis. Reduction of weightbearing, establishment of drainage as indicated, and débridement of the overlying keratotic tissue as indicated are essential.

Attempts to improve the vascular supply are indicated and may include physical modalities and procedures as well as medications that produce a vasodilatory effect. Ulcers in the diabetic patient are usually painless and are accompanied by diffuse hyperkeratotic formation. The arteriosclerotic ulcer, however, is generally very painful and will usually exhibit early local necrosis and gangrene. Ultimate success depends on proper diagnosis and management together with the full cooperation of all health providers, the patient, and his or her family.

Localized pressure ulcerations may also be present and are related to keratotic formation. There is usually a pressure area, subcallosal hemorrhage, and pain prior to the development of the ulceration. Local débridement and drainage, the removal of pressure, and the use of topical compresses such as tepid saline or Betadine usually provide rapid healing. The key is to prevent such lesions from developing in the future.

Verrucae are not common in the elderly. Plantar verruca needs to be differentiated from neurofibrous keratosis, intractable plantar keratosis, heloma, and porokeratosis. Plantar verrucae that are clustered and multiple are referred to as mosaic warts because of their clinical appearance. These warts usually present as an encapsulated lesion with pinlike bleeding points. This lesion is more recalcitrant in the elderly patient.

Single lesions can be managed by a variety of methods, including surgical excision, currettage, electrodesiccation, fulguration, negative galvanism, and a variety of caustics for chemical cautery. These preparations include Duofilm, Veranol, salicylic acid, and silver nitrate, among others. Destruction with acids is by liquefaction and minimizes residual scars.

Mosaic verrucae are best managed by the daily application of 10 percent formalin followed by a mild keratolytic such as Keralyt Gel. This tends to dehydrate the lesions and provide a mild keratolytic effect.

Xerosis tends to be protracted in the elderly and may be related to pruritus. The use of emollients such as Carmol-20 and Lac-Hydrin along with hydration provides adequate control of this problem if the patient fully complies.

Other skin conditions that may occur in the aging foot, such as psoriasis, neurodermatitis, erythema nodosum, pigmented and purpuric dermatoses, stasis dermatitis, herpes, and atopic dermatitis, are discussed in Chapter 18. The primary concern in management of any condition in the elderly is to recognize the potential for complications, the relationship to multiple systemic diseases, and the need to titrate medication dosages.

PRIMARY BIOMECHANICAL AND PATHOMECHANICAL FOOT PROBLEMS

Digiti flexus or hammer toe may involve any or all of the lesser toes. The deformity can result from a variety of factors, including atrophy or contracture of the interossei, rotational deformities, the residuals of degenerative joint disease or rheumatoid arthritis, hyperostosis, and condylar prominence, associated with arthritic change. Pain is usually the result of inflammatory changes and may be associated with bursitis, capsulitis, and tendinitis. Heloma formation is common dorsally and distally and is related to foot or gait changes, rotational deformities, tissue atrophy, and shoe-to-last incompatibility. Ulceration and possible sinus formation can be anticipated with continuous pressure to localized areas.

Management should be directed toward care of the keratotic and ulcerative lesions, changes in footwear, the use of protective orthotics, crest molds, silicone molds, and consideration of surgical procedures to revise and modify the deformity.

Hallux valgus is a complex of changes, symptoms, and deformities that are generally referred to as a "bunion deformity." The condition usually involves a varus deviation of the first metatarsal, valgus deviation of the hallux, lateral displacement of the plantar sesamoids under the first metatarsal head, tendon contractures, adventitious bursa formation, rotation of the great toe, and some bony enlargement. In many cases, the rotational deformity coupled with the residuals of degenerative joint disease displaces the stress of weightbearing and propulsion from the plantar surface to the medial aspect of the hallux, increasing the forces of deformity. The pain that develops is usually of an inflammatory nature, associated with repeated microtrauma to the soft tissues and joint swelling. When symptoms are not a factor, the patient's concern focuses on the cosmetic appearance of the foot.

Management in the elderly patient should be directed toward relief of pain and restoration of maximum function. Given that the elderly women usually maintain a sense of style, their cosmetic concerns still need to be discussed so that an understanding can be reached on what is best for the patient's total well-being. Because of the longstanding character of this condition in the elderly and its possible hereditary and degenerative etiology, conservative therapy should be considered initially. A bunion last shoe can be prescribed to help compensate for and accommodate the deformity. Orthotics and shields can be constructed to modify pressure to the joint. Local steroids and physical measures such as ultrasound, whirlpool, and exercise can be employed to manage the acute and subacute inflammatory process. Proper concern should also be directed to compensating the associated rearfoot changes biomechanically and to helping provide a more normal gait pattern. It should be noted that the longer the patient has the problem, the better are the chances that the patient has made some adjustment in ambulation to compensate for the deformity. The various surgical procedures that have been identified to revise and modify the "bunion joint" comprise a text in themselves. Justification for surgery should be based on the symptoms present and the functional needs and general medical condition of the patient. The key consideration is the ability of the patient to manage and withstand the changes following surgery. The selection of a specific procedure is a matter of individual professional judgment, and every procedure will involve some modification and customizing. Concern should also be directed to the patient's ability to adjust to the changes that will occur in gait following surgical revision of a major propulsive joint, and to postoperative management of related foot problems.

Hallux limitus appears clinically and radiographically as a monoarticular degenerative arthritis of the first metatarsophalangeal joint. When no motion is demonstrable in the hallux joint, the condition is termed hallux rigidus. It is many times associated with hallux valgus. Clinically there is marked limitation of extension of the great toe due to dorsal and/or lateral lipping and spur formation at the periarticular segments of the joint. Movement creates a chronically inflamed joint, resulting in pain on movement especially during the propulsive phase of gait.

Treatment, following appropriate radiographic examination, includes the use of analgesics; nonsteroidal anti-inflammatory drugs; physical modalities such as ultrasound, whirlpool, and transcutaneous electrical nerve stimulation (TENS) for pain; local steroid injections; and orthotics and shoe modifications to limit dorsiflexion or extension and trauma to the first metatarsophalangeal joint. A steel plate can also be prescribed for placement in the shoe, between the outsole and the insole, from the sulcus anterior to the head of the proximal phalanx to the sulcus posterior to the head of the first metatarsal head, which will limit motion as identified. An orthotic with the same configuration can also be used in place of the shoe modification. Surgical revision should be considered when conservative measures fail, in keeping with the functional needs of the patient.

At times, repeated microtrauma to the plantar surface of the first metatarsal head may result in clinical inflammation of the sesamoids in the flexor hallucis brevis tendon. It can be more symptomatic in the elderly because of atrophy of the plantar structures as well as degenerative joint changes. Where pain is acute and sudden in onset, the possibility of fracture must be considered, and bilateral radiographs should also be taken to verify bipartite sesamoids.

Sesamoiditis can generally be managed with local steroid injections and physical modalities such as ultrasound during the acute phase, and the use of analgesics and mild heat together with padding and/or orthotics to suspend pressure and weightbearing in the area of involvement. The "dancer's pad," a ¼- to 3/16-inch felt pad applied to the foot, usually provides immediate relief. Thermold and Extra Depth shoes are excellent choices for footwear modification to provide for weight diffusion and dispersion.

Digiti quinti varus or tailor's bunion involves a varus deviation of the fifth toe and a valgus deviation of the fifth metatarsal, along with an enlargement of the fifth metatarsophalangeal joint. Its pathomechanics are similar to those involved in hallux valgus. The principles of management are also similar. However, the pain is not usually as acute because of the different requirements of the fifth toe in gait and function. Local steroid injections, analgesics, mild heat, and ultrasound as well as shoe modifications are initial suggestions for care. Surgery may be considered in cases of inability to relieve pain, protracted ambulatory dysfunction, and functional disability.

Diffuse pain in the ball of the foot is another common foot complaint among the elderly. The term *metatarsalgia* has been used to describe the problem of pain in the metatarsal head area. An attempt should be made to identify the causes. Some possible factors are a short first metatarsal segment or ray, hypermobility of the first segment, loss of the anterior metatarsal fat pad, traumatic anterior metatarsal bursitis, tendinitis, tenosynovitis, capsulitis, fasciitis, and the residuals of rheumatoid and degenerative arthritis. Gout should also be considered in cases where pain is severe enough to keep the patient awake at night. Forefoot and rearfoot compensatory factors are also taken into consideration.

Management should be directed toward the cause; comparative radiographs in weight- and non-weight-bearing positions are of marked value. Physical modalities including ultrasound, whirlpool, heat, and low-voltage therapy are indicated during the acute phase. Analgesics, non-steroidal anti-inflammatory drugs, local steroid injections, and orthotic compensation for the biomechanical or pathomechanical changes will help reduce trauma and prevent exacerbations of pain. Where there are changes in metatarsal length configuration, producing a maldistribution of weight transmission during function, functional orthoses or molds that either diffuse or redistribute weight may be used to compensate.

Interdigital neuritis and neuroma (Morton's neuroma) may produce a burning pain that is exaggerated by compression factors such as footwear. The patient generally complains of electric shock-like pain radiating from the metatarsal head area to the distal portion of the toe. Neuritis generally responds to management that includes the use of local anesthetics, local steroids, and physical modalities. Orthotics can also be employed to change the intermetatarsal head relationships, and a change in shoe last and size is useful to remove the compression factor. The neuroma usually does not respond to conservative management and requires surgical excision.

Heel pain in the elderly may result from many causes, one of which is an exaggeration and hyperostosis of the posterosuperior surface of the calcaneus, known as Haglund's disease. Shoe pressure from the heel counter precipitates a retrocalcaneal bursitis or a retro-Achilles bursitis (also known as a "pump bump"). Continuing pressure from the counter of the shoe is a precipitating factor in the development of the bursa.

Plantar calcaneal spurs can be demonstrated on radiography and usually involve the medial plantar tuberosity. Pain is usually related to subcalcaneal bursitis and a chronic plantar myofasciitis. This results from repeated and continuous microtrauma and a continual pulling on the posterior attachment of the plantar fascia.

Management of posterior calcaneal conditions includes the use of heel lifts, physical modalities such as ultrasound, orthotics, steroid injections locally, and consideration of surgical excision of the hyperostosis. Removal of all pressure from the posterior portion of the heel, however, generally resolves the symptoms. Once the patient is comfortable, an appropriate shoe modification can be constructed to compensate for the deformity and pain.

Management of plantar heel pain in the elderly patient includes the use of physical modalities, such as ultrasound, whirlpool, radiant heat, and low-voltage therapy, to reduce inflammation. Local steroid injections via a medial approach are indicated during the acute phase, when the patient can pinpoint the pain. Analgesics, nonsteroidal anti-inflammatory drugs, and muscle relaxants can be used to reduce pain and spasm. Heel pads, heel cups (plastic or poly-foam), shoe modifications, and orthotics that reduce the tension on the plantar fascia and the percentage of weightbearing on the medial tuberosity of the calcaneus are also indicated. The primary biomechanical aim is to provide some elevation in a superior, lateral, and posterior direction. The choice of method and material is secondary to this principle. Materials such as Spenco, Sorbathane, and Plastazote, all reduce shock to the plantar structures and help compensate for tissue atrophy. In most cases, heel pain can be managed by nonsurgical means. When pain becomes intractable, surgery may be appropriate.

Trauma may produce fractures of the foot. Management consists of appropriate radiographic review followed by immobilization. Postfracture care is most important in the elderly, for any degree of immobilization and prolonged disuse usually results in some degree of patient decompensation, functional disability, and ambulatory dysfunction. In many cases, fractures involving the foot that are neither compound nor significantly displaced can be immobilized by materials other than plaster casts, for example, surgical shoes, the Darby shoe, flexible casting such as strapping and padding with shoe modification, digital splinting, and silicone molds, or a rigid protective material such as Celastic. At times, this provides a better end result for the elderly patient, as ambulation can be maintained with walking aids such as crutches, canes, and walkers. Isometric exercises in the cast will help reduce disuse atrophy and minimize the recovery period. A key element in the management of fractures involving the foot is the elderly patient's future functional needs and ability to adapt to treatment while maintaining dignity and the ability to function for oneself.

A variety of conditions that present in the elderly

are residuals of earlier disorders and occupational activities. Some of these conditions include pes planus, pes valgo planus, imbalance, subtalar or calcaneal varus, forefoot varus, equinus, and plantarflexed first ray. When not of a congenital or inherited etiology, these biomechanical and pathomechanical changes cause pain and discomfort which are modified by the functional needs of the patient. Where deformity exists, compensation is usually the best approach, and time needs to be provided for a slow adjustment to change. Where pain is persistent, arthritic and soft tissue inflammation should be considered.

In most cases, physical modalities and exercises are of marked value. Shoe selection should meet the functional needs of the elderly patient and change to meet their desired use. Orthotics should be functional and provide accommodation and compensation for the conditions noted. Care must also be taken to provide for the loss of soft tissue, which is common in the elderly patient. Shoe modifications often can be the simplest and most cost effective measure. Adequate footwear that gives proper support and protection is increased in value when accompanied by the use of molds, inlays, and shielding material, which provides for weight diffusion, weight dispersion, and other modifications that redistribute weight.

When recommending a shoe for the elderly patient, it must be determined whether the patient is one who lives at home and is involved in a near-normal life-style, or one who is confined to either the home or an institution and whose activity is significantly limited. The prime concerns should be personal comfort, protection, support, last compatibility, and provision of a shoe that will be functional and permit modifications for existing deformities and impairments as well as permit the use of an orthotic, if indicated.

It should be noted that the "orthopedic shoe" is not corrective but rather compensatory, particularly in the elderly patient. Care must be exercised in the use of these shoes so that they do not take the place of other forms of treatment. Where deformity is protracted and extensive, as that resulting from advanced arthritic changes, and surgical revision is not possible to maintain the patient in some functional form, the molded shoe, the Thermold shoe, the Ambulator, the Extra Depth shoe, or an-

other similar shoe may provide a viable alternative. The shoe should be considered as an article of clothing and should meet the functional needs of the patient. Slip-on styles are more acceptable to many elderly patients who are not able to bend and tie their laces. Long shoe horns should also be available for the elderly as dressing aids. Full covering of the foot, particularly the heel and long plantar areas, is advisable during ambulation to provide stability and help minimize falls, which can occur when footwear is inappropriate for a specific activity. It is of prime concern that shoes and stockings meet the requirements of the patient. It is also important to remember that shoes by themselves do not cause foot impairment unless there is a major sizing or last incompatibility (an example would be a broken shank). It is the aging process, disease, years of use and abuse, and changing functional requirements that create most foot complaints and problems.

When deformities such as hallux valgus exist, special shoes or modifications should be suggested to compensate for the deformed and altered foot contours. The "bunion last" is the best example of such a shoe. It provides a modified shape and additional material, usually a soft leather, over the hallux joint, to permit the deformity to be housed without excessive pressure. In the elderly, a most important factor in shoe fit is foot-to-shoe last compatibility.

Most women wear high heels and pumps in their youth. Depending on the height of the heel and the length of time the shoes are worn, a short heel cord is the result in the elderly patient. High heels also change the weight-bearing surface of the foot and reduce the total area of contact with the plane of support. This reduction in contact causes greater stress on the plantar structures, particularly in the forefoot. Many older women may still need some heel height, but this should be limited to a broad medium heel ($\frac{8}{8}''$ to $1\frac{2}{8}''$), which offers greater stability to the foot. Medial and lateral heel flares can also be added to increase stability if indicated.

Mention should be also made of the "molded shoe." A made-to-order shoe generally will resemble a standard shoe with special sizes or modifications built in. A molded shoe usually conforms to the shape of the foot, and the insole or inner surface conforms to the total weight-bearing area of the foot. Its basic advantages are that it reduces shock, is shaped to fit the deformed foot, and provides a greater distribution of stress to help compensate for painful conditions. Evaluation and prescription should be judicious, and commercialism should be avoided to protect the safety of the patient. The Thermold shoe, the Ambulator, the Extra Depth shoe, and the Plastazote shoe are stock shoes that offer most of these advantages at a low cost. Broad toe lasts with high toe boxes and a wedge-type sole are the basic characteristics of all of these types of footwear.

Caution should be exercised in the use of plaster casting for shoes in the elderly. As plaster sets, heat is generated. Thus, patients with open lesions and vascular impairment might do better in modified stock lasts rather than with plaster casting, which adds risk to what should be a nonrisk procedure.

FOOT CONDITIONS AS RESIDUALS OF SYSTEMIC DISEASE

Although in many diseases foot symptoms present as the initial complaint, the usual presentation in the elderly is one of overt abnormality and a multiplicity of symptoms, signs, and clinical findings relating to multiple chronic diseases and conditions. Complaints are often motivated by ambulatory dysfunction and functional disability related to foot problems. The patient usually does not seek care initially unless there is significant pain; often an individual who has seen the patient has a keen index of suspicion and provides a referral. The patient is often faced with complications arising from multiple sources at the same time; this makes primary podiatric care for the elderly anything but routine, no matter how common the condition. Foot problems related to systemic manifestations and complications should not be taken lightly and should be managed to maintain the functional activity and total health of the patient.

Foot infection, with or without necrosis or gangrene, is by far the most serious complication in the elderly patient. It may be related to systemic dis-

ease or result from neglect or improper self-care of a local foot problem. Residual deformities of earlier conditions together with the aging process itself, provide an excellent medium for the development of foot infections in the elderly. Foot infections are the most common precipitant of amputation, which may reduce the patient's will to live, resulting eventually in the loss of a life. The National Diabetes Advisory Board has estimated that 50 to 75 percent of all amputations in the diabetic can be prevented with proper foot care. The same projection can easily be made for the elderly patient. To some degree, the loss of a limb in an elderly patient is even more critical from a social standpoint. Most elderly persons are unable to cope with such a traumatic loss and are unable to adapt to the use of a prosthesis, let alone a significant degree of self-care.

Most of the causes of foot infection can be classed within a few categories:

Trauma, such as a cut or abrasion, or as a result of crushing, blistering, or pinching, which causes a break in the skin

Neglect, such as poor hygiene, use of ill-fitting footwear, foot-to-shoe last incompatibilities, and a lack of self-care due to functional disability and/or poor vision

Changes due to the aging of the skin, such as fissuring, dryness, hyperkeratosis, and atrophy

Metabolic changes associated with systemic diseases, such as diabetes mellitus, peripheral vascular insufficiency, advanced arteriosclerosis, chronic renal failure, and decompensation

Primary and secondary skin diseases

Surgical procedures, particularly when vascular impairment develops as a complicating factor.

Osteoarthritis or degenerative joint disease can usually be identified in the elderly patient in its primary form or secondary to trauma, inflammation, or metabolic changes. The associated relationship among chronic trauma, strain, and obesity is well reflected in the weight-bearing joints of the foot. Osteoporosis and postmenopausal syndromes can also be demonstrated in the same individual.

The primary findings in the foot include pain, stiffness, swelling, limitation of movement, and deformity. These usually produce some degree of functional disability and ambulatory dysfunction. Clinically, diagnostic associations may include plantar fasciitis, calcaneal erosions and spur formation, periostitis, osteoporosis, stress fractures, tendinitis, and tenosynovitis. When osteochondritis and avascular necrosis have been present in youth, the result is an arthritic joint in the later years.

Existing deformities such as pes planus, pes cavus, and digital deformities such as hallux valgus, hallux limitus, and digiti flexus create increased pain, limitation of motion, and a reduction in the ambulatory tolerance of the patient. The primary factor to consider is that osteoarthritis in the foot is usually secondary to repeated microtrauma and may be precipitated by inadequate and inappropriate foot care at earlier ages.

Clinically, gouty arthritis may produce symptoms in any joint of the foot and should always be suspected where intense pain is present without trauma or is precipitated by minimal trauma. The primary manifestations in the elderly are related to chronic tophaceous gout and include chronic painful and stiff joints, soft tissue tophi, a loss of bone substance, deformity, and functional impairment.

Rheumatoid arthritis in the elderly patient usually presents as the end stage of the disease, with exacerbations of pain, joint swelling, stiffness, muscle wasting, and marked deformity.

Residual deformities of the forefoot include but are not limited to the following:

Hallux rigidus
Arthritis of the first metatarsophalangeal joint
Hallux valgus
Cystic erosion
Sesamoid erosion
Metatarsophalangeal dislocations, deformities, and hyperkeratosis
Digiti flexus
Fused interphalangeal joints
Phalangeal reabsorption
Extensor tenosynovitis
Rheumatoid nodules
Bowstring extensor tendons with valgus displacement
Ganglions.

Residual deformities of the rearfoot include but are not limited to the following:

Talonavicular arthritis
Rigid pronated foot
Ankle arthritis
Subtalar arthritis
Tarsal arthritis
Subachilles bursitis
Subcutaneous nodules
Plantar fasciitis
Spurs
Achilles tendon shortening.

Osteoporosis can be demonstrated radiographically by a significant loss of bone mass, increased bone lucency, and loss of the normal trabecular pattern. The bones have a washed-out appearance, and the cortex may resemble an eggshell. The prime concern is related to stress fractures, pain and discomfort, deformity, and complications related to any projected surgical procedure involving the foot.

Diabetes mellitus is well known to be complicated by multiple pedal manifestations. Very often, foot symptoms in an individual who is not known to be diabetic will lead to the detection of the disease itself. With the increased prevalence of diabetes, particularly among the elderly, the disease can always be suspected when there are multiple foot complaints and symptoms that resemble the usual complications of the disease. The pedal manifestations are related to multiple systems and often include such symptoms and signs as paresthesias, sensory impairment, motor weakness, reflex loss, neurotrophic arthropathy, muscle and soft tissue atrophy, diminished or absent pedal pulses, and the clinical findings of peripheral arterial insufficiency, angiopathy, dermatopathy, neuropathy, and diabetic onychopathy. Other clinical findings include tinea pedis, chronic inflammation and infection, ulceration, and terminal necrosis or gangrene. Diabetic onychopathy is almost universal and is related to microangiopathy. Idiopathic subungual hemorrhages are common in the diabetic and may manifest before other hemorrhagic abnormalities appear in the ocular and renal systems.

Neurotrophic and diabetic ulcers in the elderly patient are usually resistant to treatment and require a multifaceted approach. They can often be prevented by appropriate management of pedal lesions and a realistic approach to preventive care and health education. For example, ulceration can be precipitated by continuous pressure causing focal vascular impairment, penetration of tissue with trauma, and continued friction with thrusting and shearing of the plantar structures. Rest, control of any infection present, appropriate débridement (chemical and surgical), and measures to remove or redistribute weightbearing are indicated. Use of a surgical shoe, Plastazote shoe, Darby shoe, or orthotics may be appropriate management. Again the principles of weight diffusion and weight dispersion are to be considered. Prevention of future ulcerations is essential. Many patients can be maintained by conservative means for long periods of time even with an ulcerated lesion. Amputation is usually considered when there is systemic toxicity, uncontrolled infection, or marked vascular degeneration leading to advanced necrosis and gangrene. End artery occlusion is usually the precipitating factor in the loss of a limb.

Peripheral vascular insufficiency is present at some point in the majority of elderly patients, to varying degrees. Overt indications of decreased arterial supply in the feet are muscle fatigue, cramps, claudication, pain, coldness, pallor, paresthesias, burning, atrophy of soft tissues, trophic dermal changes such as dryness and loss of hair, onychopathy, absent pedal and related pulses, and decreased readings in vascular function studies. Calcification can be demonstrated during the course of a diagnostic radiographic study ordered for other purposes. Arch pain is often mistaken for some pathomechanical problem and blamed on so called "arch problems," when the real problem is one of local ischemia. The final result of severe arterial occlusion is gangrene, which is many times self-demarcating. Environmental factors and personal habits that place the patient at risk should be eliminated.

Edema, related either to cardiorenal disease or to dependency, may be the first indication of impending arterial complications. The loss of the anatomic landmarks is a significant finding, especially when accompanied by other clinical manifestations.

The patient leaving bed following a long period of hospitalization or immobilization should have adequate supportive measures for the feet and legs. Edema due to a combination of inactivity, dependency, immobilization, pain, and venous insufficiency may give rise to substantial complications. Venous insufficiency, with or without varicosities, usually leads to chronic stasis and ulceration with its associated dermatologic manifestations. Topical infections of the foot and lower leg in the elderly patient should be considered a serious complication, given early treatment and management.

Paresis of the lower extremity, often the end result of a cerebral vascular accident, may result in foot-drop, trophic changes, and changes in the weight-bearing areas on the foot, which the individual may not have difficulty compensating for. Changes in ambulatory status include spasticity, which produces abnormal relationships with the plane of support, especially where residual deformity is present. Associated peripheral neuropathies produce changes in the normal position sense and lead to trauma to the foot and lower leg due to a lack of coordination. Inability to functionally adapt to gait and related system changes creates situations that can turn minor foot lesions into ulcerations. In the poststroke patient, special care needs to be provided to the foot, and shoe selection deserves serious consideration.

FOOT HEALTH EDUCATION FOR THE ELDERLY

Attention must be paid to health education for the elderly, which is the first form of preventive medicine. Health education must include more than the basic rules for foot care. It must deal with the mechanics of delivery, the quality of service, standards of care, professional qualifications, continuing education, and reimbursement for services. Education must be a multidisciplinary effort and emphasize the total patient, the family, and the community. Excellent media promoting such concepts include *Feet First* and *Long-Term Care Facility Administration,* published by the U.S. Public Health Service; *Functions and Educational Qualifi-*

cations for Podiatrists in Public Health, published by the American Public Health Association; and *Pedal Health Training Guide for Long Term Care Personnel,* published by the American Podiatric Medical Association.

SUMMARY

Podogeriatric management has as its prime concern the total patient and the appropriate utilization of all health-related personnel in a team approach to patient care. The key element is making comprehensive care and services readily accessible to the elderly.

It is essential to listen when an elderly person complains about his or her feet and to respond quickly. The prevention of foot problems in the elderly is the responsibility of the patient, his or her family, the community and society, and all of the related health professionals that have added years to life.

Throughout life, there must be purpose and activity and a feeling of usefulness, appreciation, and comfort. Foot health is necessary to help achieve the basic goals of dignity and self-respect during the golden years of life.

SELECTED READINGS

Baran R, Dawber RPR: Diseases of the Nails and Their Management. Blackwell Scientific Publications, Oxford, England, 1984

Beaven DW, Brooks SE: Color Atlas of the Nail in Clinical Diagnosis. Year Book Medical Publishers, Chicago, 1984

Calkins E, Davis PJ, Ford AB (eds): The Practice of Geriatrics. WB Saunders, Philadelphia, 1986

Davidson JK: Clinical Diabetes Mellitus. Thieme New York, 1986

Esidorfer C (ed): Annual Review of Gerontology and Geriatrics. Vol. 4, Springer, New York, 1984

Helfand AE (ed): Clinical Podogeriatrics. Williams & Wilkins, Baltimore, 1981

Helfand AE, and Bruno J (eds): Rehabilitation of the Foot. Clinics in Podiatry. Vol. 1. No. 2. WB Saunders, Philadelphia, 1984

Helfand AE (ed): Public Health and Podiatric Medicine. Williams & Wilkins, Baltimore, 1987

Jahss MH (ed): Diseases of the Foot. WB Saunders, Philadelphia, 1982

Kozak GP, Hoar CS Jr, Rowbotham JL, et al: Management of the Diabetic Foot. WB Saunders, Philadelphia, 1984

Levin ME, O'Neal LW (eds): The Diabetic Foot. 3rd Ed. CV Mosby, St Louis, 1983

Libow LB, Sherman FT (eds): The Core of Geriatric Medicine. CV Mosby, St Louis, 1981

McCarthy DJ (ed): Podiatric Dermatology. Williams & Wilkins, Baltimore, 1986

Neale D (ed): Common Foot Disorders, Diagnosis and Management. Churchill Livingstone, Edinburgh, 1981

Reichel W (ed): Clinical Aspects of Aging. 2nd Ed. Williams & Wilkins, Baltimore, 1983

Samitz MH: Cutaneous Disorders of the Lower Extremities. 2nd Ed. JB Lippincott, Philadelphia, 1981

Samman PD, Fenton DA: The Nails in Disease. 4th Ed. William Heinemann Medical Books, London, 1986

Steinberg FU: Care of the Geriatric Patient. 6th Ed. CV Mosby, St Louis, 1983

U.S. Department of Health and Human Services: Feet First (publication no. 0-388-126). Government Printing Office, Washington, DC, 1970

White House Conference on Aging. Final Report of the 1981 White House Conference on Aging. Vol. 3. Government Printing Office, Washington, DC, 1981

Williams TF (ed): Rehabilitation in the Aging. Raven Press, New York, 1984

Wilson LB, Simson SP, Baxter CR (eds): Handbook of Geriatric Emergency Care. University Park Press, Baltimore, 1984

Witkowski JA (ed): Diseases of the Lower Extremities. Clinics in Dermatology. Vol. 1. No. 1. JB Lippincott, Philadelphia, 1983

Yale I (ed): Podiatric Medicine. 2nd Ed. Williams & Wilkins, Baltimore, 1980

Yale I, Yale JF: The Arthritic Foot and Related Connective Tissue Disorders. Williams & Wilkins, Baltimore, 1984

The Pediatric Patient

22

General Pediatric Podiatry

Vincent J. Hetherington, D.P.M., M.S.
Janis Lehtinen, D.P.M.
Franz Grill, M.D.

EMBRYOLOGY AND DEVELOPMENT

Human limbs develop in the fourth week of gestation with the appearance of the primitive limb buds. The limb bud is an ectodermal sac filled with mesoderm. The ectoderm gives rise to the skin and its adnexia and the mesoderm to the muscular and bone system. Subsequent to development of the limb the distal tip of the ectodermal nodule thickens. This thickened layer of ectoderm becomes known as the apical ectodermal ridge.[1] It appears first for the upper limbs and subsequently for the lower limbs. As the limb buds develop the upper extremities are usually just slightly ahead of the lower extremities.

When growth of the extremity begins vigorous cell duplication occurs with perceptible vascularization. The ectoderm is dependent upon the underlying mesoderm to supply nourishment by way of the mesoderm's numerous blood capillaries and intracellular substance. The limb bud elongates by the proliferation of mesenchyme contained within the ectoderm. New mesoderm arises in situ by mitotic activity, with the greatest such activity occurring in the zone of progress behind the apical ectodermal ridge.[2] The apical ectodermal ridge is important in directing limb development, and any insult to the ridge or its functions will result in some type of limb malformation. In the deeper tissues of the mesoderm, zones of thickening occur at varying distances from the ectoderm, representing the outline of the early skeleton of the extremities.

Development of the vascular system begins with the formation of a marginal vein. The rudimentary arteries develop in the direction of the nutritional requirements of the growing extremities.[1] These are oriented not in the direction of the longitudinal axis of the growing limbs, but on a diagonal. In the middle of the second month the nerves as well as the blood vessels are developing. Blood vessels and nerves extend into the limb buds from the central axis of the embryo. The ingrowth of the blood vessels precedes the ingrowth of nerves. The lumbosacral plexus is formed and nerves grow into the posterior limb during the first half of the fifth week of gestation. Skeletal differentiation usually begins in the region of the hip and extends distally and proximally. This differentiation immediately precedes ingrowth of the nerves of the limb. Skeletal structures therefore serve in part to guide the nerves in their distribution.

Muscle differentiation immediately follows the entrance of a motor nerve into a given region.[3] The bulk of the musculature differentiates in situ from mesenchymal condensations on the flexor and extensor aspects of the limb cartilages. The myotomes probably make a contribution to the more proximal musculature, but there is no evidence that they migrate beyond these regions.[2] Development of the intrinsic musculature of the foot is usually from mesenchyme.

According to Bohm, at 4.5 weeks the lower extremities differentiate into foot, leg, and thigh regions.[4] At 5 weeks there is distinct differentiation into a knee bend and an area known as the foot plate. By the sixth week there is a foot plate, a leg component, and perceivable toe rays. At this point the thigh is a direct extension of the torso with a slight bend for the knee, and the foot is a direct extension of the leg with no noticeable bend at the ankle area.

At the fifth to sixth week the thigh and knee are rotated outward. The foot is separated from the leg by a slight constriction, but it is still essentially in a straight line with the leg. The dorsal surface of the foot faces laterally and the plantar surface faces medially. No digits are truly identified (Fig. 22-1). The condensations for the tibia and fibula are present with the talus lying between them. The navicular is distal to the talus, but lies obliquely and somewhat medially to it. The calcaneal area is a direct extension of the fibula and is not rotated beneath the talus. The second through fifth metatarsals are severely adducted. The first metatarsal is at a 50 degree angle to the long axis of the foot.[4] Between the seventh and ninth weeks a very important rotation occurs: the lower extremities rotate 90 degrees inward.[5,6] This allows for the knee and the dorsum of the foot to face dorally and me-

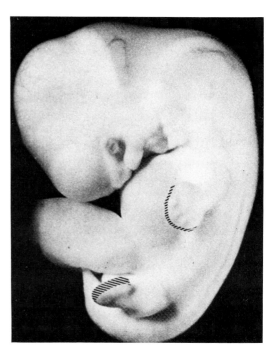

Fig. 22-1. Human embryo approximately 36 days old demonstrating position of limb development. (From Swinyard and Pinner,[1] with permission.)

dially as opposed to facing laterally. After this rotation occurs the toes, fingers, and elbow and knee joints develop (Fig. 22-2). However, considerable torsion within the tarsal and other foot bones must occur during later gestation, to bring the foot to its position at birth and subsequently through childhood to the adult. Figure 22-3 outlines the changes which will continue to occur after birth until adulthood. From the second month on the toes become well developed. The webbing between them is reabsorbed and prominence of the heel begins to develop.

At 3.5 months a dorsiflexion begins to occur at the ankle joint region. The digits are fully differentiated, the heel is distinct, and joints are beginning to form. The growth flexion of the knee and growth torsion of the foot gradually increase. The importance of an intact blood supply in the development of the lower limb has been stressed by several authors.[7,8]

Some of the details of chondrification and ossification are presented by O'Rahilly and colleagues[9] (Table 22-1). They noted that the tarsus can be distinguished as condensed mesenchyme at ap-

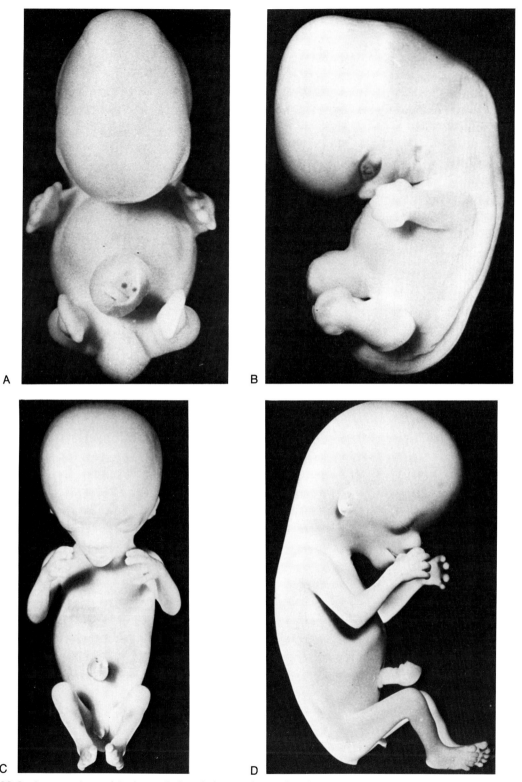

Fig. 22-2. A comparison of the lower limbs of a human fetus after the rotation development has occurred. **(A** and **B)** Fetal age approximately 36 days. **(C** and **D)** Fetal age approximately 90 days. (From Blechschmidt E: The early stages of human limb development. p. 19. In Swinyard CA (ed): Limb Development and Deformity: Problems of Evaluation and Rehabilitation. Charles C Thomas, Springfield, IL, 1969.)

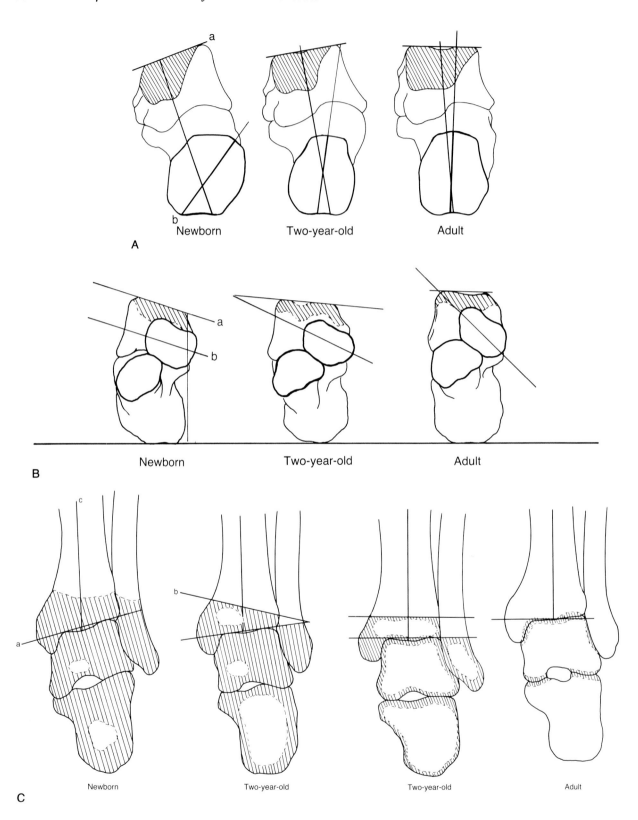

A

Newborn   Two-year-old   Adult

B

Newborn   Two-year-old   Adult

C

Newborn   Two-year-old   Two-year-old   Adult

Lateral   Medial

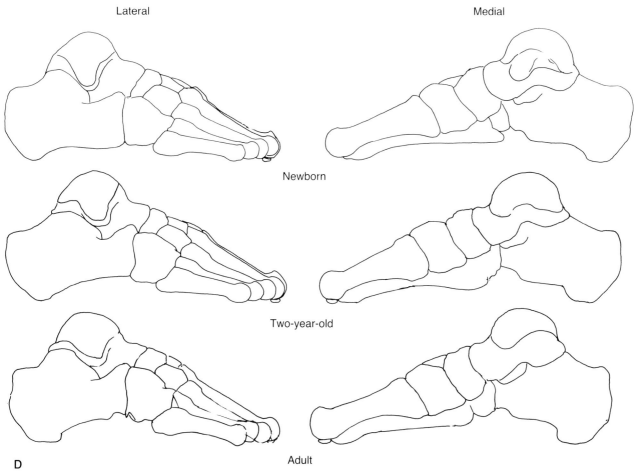

Newborn

Two-year-old

D   Adult

Fig. 22-3. (A) Frontal plane rotation of the calcaneus. *A*, long axis of the posterior surface of the heel; *B*, inclination of the talar dome. **(B)** Talar neck rotation. *A*, inclination of the talar dome; *B*, long axis of the talar head. **(C)** Frontal plane development of the ankle. *A*, plane of talar dome; *B*, plane of distal tibial epiphysis; *C*, long axis of the leg. **(D)** Development of the foot (arch) from medial and lateral views. *(Figure continues.)*

proximately the fifth postovulatory week. Within a few days the individual tarsals begin to chondrify in a definite sequence. Chondrification of the metatarsals begins at the same time. This is followed by chondrification in proximal-distal sequence of the three rows of phalanges.

Many of the accessory bones evident in the adult have been observed in cartilaginous form in the embryo and fetus. O'Rahilly et al. also reported examples of bipartism of the medial cuneiform, tarsal coalition, and symphalangia.[9] The initiation of the development of synovial joints by the formation of interzones occurs at approximately the end of the embryonic period, at week 7 or 8. Where the limb cartilages articulates the perichondrium

blends to form the interzone. External to the interzone, capsular and synovial thickening differentiate from the adjacent mesenchymal materials. The interzone or cavitation is reabsorbed and a synovial cavity is formed.[2] Cavitation, or formation of the joints, commences in most joints of the foot during the second week of the fetal period (Table 22-1).

Ossification commences in the foot in the embryonic period proper and continues into postnatal life. The first elements usually to show signs of ossification in the foot are the distal phalanges. Ossification of the big toe begins as early as 7 weeks, in the embryo. During the fetal period bone collars are discernible in each of the metatarsals and pha-

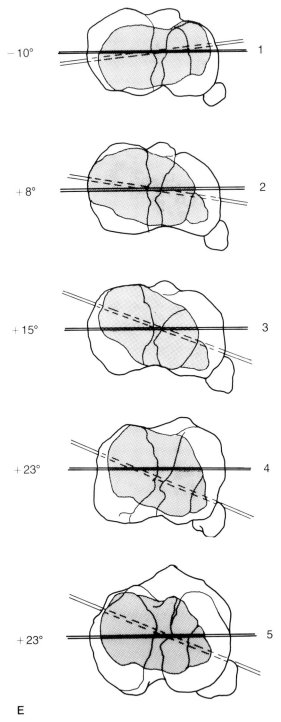

Fig. 22-3. *(Continued)* Tibial torsion. *1,* birth; *2,* 6 months; *3,* 3 years; *4,* 10 years; *5,* adult. (**A–E** Redrawn from Praktische Anatomie, Bein Und Statik, Erster Band. In Teil V, Lang J, Wachsmuth W (eds). Springer-Verlag, Berlin, 1972)

Table 22-1. Early Development of the Lower Limb

Feature	Stage	Mm.	Postovulatory Weeks	Authors
Lower limb bud	13	3.0–6.0	4	Streeter (1945)
Foot plate	15	6.0–11.0	4½	Streeter (1948)
Ectodermal ridge	15–18	6.0–18.0	4½–5	O'Rahilly, Gardner and Gray (1956)
Mesenchymal hip bone	16	9	5	Bardeen (1905)
Mesenchymal femur, tibia, fibula	17	8.6–14.5	5	O'Rahilly, Gray and Gardner (1957)
Mesenchymal foot	17–18	8.6–18.0	5	O'Rahilly, Gray and Gardner (1957)
Chondrifying femur, tibia, fibula	17–18	8.6–18.0	5	O'Rahilly, Gray and Gardner (1957)
Chondrifying hip bone	18	12	5	Bardeen (1905)
Chondrifying foot	18–23+	11.7–32.2	5–7	O'Rahilly, Gray and Gardner (1957)
Mesenchymal patella	20	18.5–25.0	6	O'Rahilly, Gray and Gardner (1957)
Chondrifying patella	21	19.0–26.4	6	O'Rahilly, Gray and Gardner (1957)
Ossifying femur, tibia	22–23	23.0–32.2	6½–7	O'Rahilly, Gray and Gardner (1957)
Cavitation in hip	?	28	7	Gardner and Gray (1950)
Cavitation in knee	?	30	7	Gray and Gardner (1950)
Cavitation in ankle	?	30	7	Gardner, Gray and O'Rahilly (1959)
Ossifying fibula	?	29–35	7	Noback and Robertson (1951)
Cavitation in foot	?	30–?	7–?	Gardner, Gray and O'Rahilly (1959)

(From O'Rahilly et al.,[9] with permission.)

langes. Ossification in the tarsus, unlike the carpus, begins before birth. The first tarsal bone to exhibit calcification is the calcaneus, followed by the talus. Postnatal ossification occurs with the cuneiform and navicular appearing in infancy. The medial cuneiform and navicular may each develop from two centers.[9] Epiphyseal centers appear in the metatarsals and the phalanges during infancy and early childhood. Secondary centers of ossification appear during childhood in the tubercalcanei, the lateral tuberosity of the posterior process of the talus, and the tuberosity of the fifth metatarsal (Table 22-2).

LIMB MALFORMATIONS

Limb malformations may result from both genetic and environmental factors. Such malforma-

Table 22-2. Times of Appearance of Postnatal Ossific Centers in the Foot (Median Ages in Years)

Bone	Appearance		Complete Radiographic Fusion	
	Female	Male	Female	Male
Tibia, distal end	⅓	⅓	15	16
Fibula, distal end	¾	1	15	16
Tuber calcanei	5	7–8	14	15
Top of tuber	11	13	14	?
Talus, lateral tubercle of posterior process	8	10	10	12
Lateral cuneiform	⅓	⅓		
Medial cuneiform	1	2		
Intermediate cuneiform	2	2		
Navicular	2	3		
Metatarsal epiphyses	2–4	2–4	15	16
Tuberosity of 5th metatarsal	10	12	13	14
Phalangeal epiphyses	1–4	1–4	14	15
Sesamoids	9	12		

(From O'Rahilly et al.,[9] with permission.)
(Data from: Flecker H: Am J Anat 87:163, 1950; Hubay CA: Am J Roentgenol 61:493, 1949; Mainland D: Anatomy as a Basic for Medical and Dental Practice. Hamilton, London, 1945.)

tions may be congenital (i.e., evident at birth) or may occur postnatally. Crossan and Wynne-Davies[10] developed a classification of congenital developmental disorders:

1. Chromosomal abnormalities (e.g., Down's syndrome).
2. Single-gene disorders (e.g., osteogenesis imperfecta).
3. Disorders of multifactoral inheritance, which include both genetic and environmental components (e.g., congenital dislocation of the hip and club foot).
4. Malformation syndromes, which include neurofibromatosis. Crossan and Wynne-Davies defined these malformation syndromes to include disorders with structural bone defects of multisystem involvement. They may have a pattern of inheritance, but the frequency of sporadic cases indicates nongenetic origin in many instances.
5. Nongenetic disorders due to teratogens (e.g., thalidomide and rubella virus).

Crossan and Wynne-Davies found in their study an association of genetic and environmental components for talipes equinovarus and talipes calcaneovalgus. They suggested that the genetic factors somehow caused defective formation of connective tissue. This defective connective tissue resulted in abnormal mobility of the feet at some stage of intrauterine development. The intrauterine environmental factors in these conditions may well be related to malplacement, application of abnormal pressure, or abnormal positioning in the uterus. Crossan and Wynne-Davies suggested that the deforming environmental forces, which were transient, positioned the abnormally mobile feet in equinovarus at a vulnerable time in their development. When the deformity becomes set subsequent muscle development is inhibited and is inadequate to overcome the deformity. It was also suggested that if the deforming force was exerted later in fetal life it could account for less severe calcaneovalgus deformity or postural talipes equinovarus, both of which are easily correctable and tend not to recur. Other authors support the theory of a multifactoral form of inheritance for congenital dislocation of the hip and clubfoot.[11,12]

Studies by Wynne-Davies[13] on talipes equino-varus, talipes calcaneovalgus, and metatarsus varus found that the incidence of these deformities is 1 : 1,000. If one child in a family had the deformity the chances of a second child having it were 1 : 35 for talipes equinovarus and 1 : 20 for talipes calcaneovalgus and metatarsus varus. Wynne-Davies[14] cited Leonard's findings that tarsal coalitions appear to be inherited in a dominant manner. Leonard's analysis revealed about 40 percent of first-degree relatives to be affected. It was interesting to note, however, that the onset of spastic flatfoot in association with tarsal coalition is unexplained and apparently only occurs in a small proportion of those with such a defect, perhaps one-fourth of the total cases. Johnston[15] also presented a seven-generation pedigree of a family showing hallux valgus. The anomaly appeared to be transmitted as an autosomal dominant with incomplete penetrance of the gene.

Postnatal limb malformations are a result of biomechanical forces. Such deformations[16] are abnormalities in form, shape, or position of the body caused by biomechanical molding. The molding forces may be intrinsic or extrinsic. The infant, because of its rapid growth and the liability of its tissues, is more susceptible to molding by constraining pressure.

Biomechanical molding may also occur in utero, resulting in fetal constraint, which normally develops as the fetus fills out the uterine cavity in late gestation. Several factors may result in fetal constraint (Fig. 22-4). Intrinsic forces contributing to deformation include both diseases of the central and peripheral nervous systems and congenital muscle diseases that cause general hypotonia, which does not cause deformation but increases fetal susceptibility to extrinsic forces. As Dunne and Clarren[16] pointed out, other conditions, such as meningomyelocele, that cause congenital muscle imbalance directly predispose the infant to deformity without the need for contributing extrinsic pressure. It is not unusual for the constrained infant to present with a pattern of deformation. Foot deformities associated with this type of restraints are common and include calcaneovalgus, metatarsus adductus, some forms of clubfoot, and overriding digits.

Fetal position has also been implicated as a cause of right- and left-sided foot disorders. McDon-

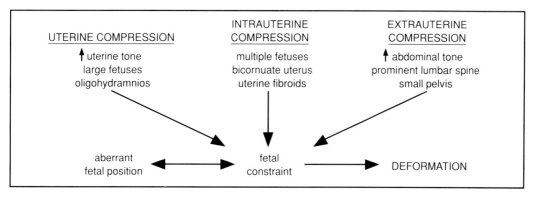

Fig. 22-4. Deformation results from fetal constraint produced by multiple factors. (From Dunne and Clarren.[16])

ough[17] has shown that positional deformities that predominate on the right leg and foot differ from those of the left, and that these deformities show direct relationships to fetal positioning. McDonough hypothesized that the fetal environment in left-sided carry presents a strong posterior uterine wall and osseous superstructure influencing the medial functional range for the maturing fetal leg. The right limb is accordingly encouraged into a predominantly lateral range of motion with a potential for right foot abutment on an anterior uterine wall. With increasing confinement and attempts at lateral rotation of the right leg the foot is placed into a position of calcaneovalgus. This coincided with the finding that calcaneovalgus was predominantly a right-sided phenomenon and was associated with lateral torsion. The statistics of this series also show that right-sided calcaneovalgus dominated over left-sided with 19.6 to 3.9 percent incidence, respectively. Conversely, unilateral metatarsus adductus is most frequently left-sided, associated with medial tibial torsion. Metatarsus adductus was found to predominate on the left side, 17.6 percent of cases versus 5.8 percent occurrence on the right side. A windswept deformity with right lateral torsion and left medial torsion was also predominant.

The description of congenital limb malformations has often used various terminology and classifications, with some degree of confusion resulting. The classification presented here was developed by Swanson[18] (Table 22-3). As the author stated, this classification employs simple, easily remembered descriptive terminology. According to this system the defects can be categorized as follows:

1. Failure of formation of parts (arrest of development)
2. Failure of differentiation (separation) of parts
3. Duplication
4. Overgrowth
5. Undergrowth
6. Congenital constriction band syndrome
7. Generalized skeletal abnormalities

Table 22-3. Classification of Foot Malformations According to Swanson et al.

Failure of formation of parts
  Longitudinal arrest
    Tibial ray deficiency
    Central ray deficiency
    Fibular ray deficiency
Failure of differentiation of parts
  Syndactyly
  Clinodactyly
  Arthrogryposis multiplex congenita
Duplication
  Polydactyly
    Preaxial
    Axial
    Postaxial
    Mixed
Overgrowth
  Macrodactyly
Undergrowth
  Brachymetatarsia
  Brachydactyly
    Brachydactyly
    Brachymesophalangia
Constriction band syndrome
General skeletal disorders

(From Masada et al.,[19] with permission.)

Failure of formation of parts can be either transverse or longitudinal. Longitudinal defects may be tibial, central, or fibular. In category two, failure of differentiation of parts, synostosis and syndactyly would be included. Although this category was described predominantly for the hand, it has been accepted as a classification for congenital malformation of the hand and foot.[18,19]

Generalized skeletal abnormalities include bone dysplasias, dystrophys, and dysostosis. A dysplasia is an intrinsic bone disturbance wherein the effects are mostly on bones of endochondral ossification. There is early closure of the epiphyseal plates and limb growth is stunted. Intramembranous bones develop normally; however, although these infants have normally shaped heads, there are some characteristic facial abnormalities. Examples of dysplasia are achondrodysplasia and autosomally inherited dwarfism. Dystrophies are generalized metabolic diseases, such as ricketts, and may be primary or secondary. Dystosis is a generized mesodermal or ectodermal disturbance.

HISTORY AND PHYSICAL EXAMINATION

History

The podiatric history should include a perinatal history and a history of the progression of the child through the developmental landmarks. These landmarks include the times at which the child began crawling and walking (Table 22-4). A history of any "growing pains" should also be elicited. An in-depth family history should be obtained as indicated. In view of a family history of lower limb

Table 22-4. Selected Developmental Milestones

Gross Motor Skills	Fine Motor Skills
1 Month	
Has incomplete head control	Follows to midline
Has tonic neck reflex	Fixes both eyes on light
4 Months	
Turns from back to side	Brings object to mouth
Rolls over	Follows 180 degrees visually
6 Months	
Sits without support	Transfers object
Has reciprocal leg pattern	Picks up spoon
9 Months	
Crawls freely	Shakes bell
Pulls self to stand	Develops pincer grip
12 Months	
Walks with assistance	Can release object voluntarily
Climbs	Follows simple commands
15 Months	
Lets self down from standing to sitting	
Attains standing position unaided	
18 Months	
Throws and catches ball	
Creeps backward down stairs	
21 Months	
Squats	Turns knob
Walks up and down stairs	Begins hand preference
24 Months	
Alternates feet walking upstairs	Turns pages singly
Runs	Likes to take things apart

(From Drennan JC: Evaluation of neuromuscular disorders. p. 2. In: Orthopedic Management of Neuromuscular Disorders. JB Lippincott, Philadelphia, 1983, with permission.)

deformity it is often helpful to question and examine other siblings or members of the family. A history as to shoe wear should be obtained. The shoes should examined for any abnormal wear patterns.

Assessment of Gait

The development of gait is preceded by both reflex and learned responses in the child. Initially this may begin as observation of the response to reflexes of normal development. This is often followed by attempts at weight shifting and the development of the parachute or protective extension reactions. These enable the child to use extension of his or her arms for weightbearing and support in sitting and crawling without falling over.[22] Independent sitting often develops at 6 to 8 months of age. This is followed by crawling, which is followed by upright locomotion holding onto furniture, often referred to as "cruising." A child may begin walking as early as 10 months, but the average time is 12 to 13 months of age.

The feet of the beginning walker are usually markedly pronated. There is a wide-based gait for support, and a tendency to lift the feet up and down in a form of placement rather than a true walk.[23] At 2.5 to 3 years a normal heel-strike gait may develop, followed by the development of a somewhat normal propulsive phase of gait at about 4 years. As trunk stabilization improves the base of gait narrows and the length of step becomes longer. At approximately 2 years of age several differences between the standing and walking child and the infant can be determined immediately. These include the reduction in the amount of bowing of the legs, the external malleolar position, and the fact that the joints of the hip and knee can be fully extended.

In stance the child usually shows marked pronation. Calcaneal stance position can have anywhere from 4 to 10 degrees of eversion.[23] In gait, children less than 2 years of age usually have a greater knee flexion and more ankle dorsiflexion during the stance phase. Reciprocal arm swing and heel strike are present in most children by the age of 18 months.

Sutherland and colleagues[24] reported that important factors in the development of a mature gait

pattern are increase in length of limbs and greater limb stability, manifested by an increased duration of a single-limb stance. A mature gait pattern as determined by these criteria is well established by age 3. However, although this may occur grossly, Menkveld and coworkers[25] have shown that a flat foot position in single-leg support with decreased rotation about the longitudinal axis of the foot is the final sign of immaturity as a child assumes an adult walking pattern. Their data show that subtle development of a gait pattern occurs after age 7 and continues into adolescence.

Abnormal gait patterns are briefly outlined in Table 22-5.

Gait analysis in the young child can be difficult. This may be due to a variety of reasons, such as the strange environment, new people, an effort to "walk normally," shyness, or embarrassment. Also, when a child walks holding a parent's hand the gait is altered significantly. Therefore it is recommended that gait evaluation be performed initially by watching the child walk into the treatment room or down the office or clinic corridor. Children should then be observed walking with their shoes both on and off. Base and angle of gait should be observed, as well as general body symmetry and

Table 22-5. Abnormalities of Gait

In-toe gait
    Internal femoral torsion
    Internal femoral position
    Internal tibial torsion
    Metatarsus adductus
    Cavus foot
Out-toe gait
    External femoral torsion
    External femoral position
    Flatfoot
Toe-walking (equinus)
    Habit
    Osseous equinus
    Gastrocnemius or gastrocnemius-soleus equinus
    Short limb (unilateral)
Pathologic gait patterns
    Steppage
    Waddling
    Hysterical
    Spastic
    Ataxic
    Familial
    Delayed walking
    Antalgic

motion. Additionally, it is often useful to have the child walk fast and run and walk on both the toes and the heels. These latter tests may be useful in evaluating muscle strength and detecting disorders of the neuromuscular system.

Physical Examination of the Neonate

Examination of the neonatal infant should proceed in a systematic and gradual fashion. Initial examination should include neurologic evaluation, especially of the startle, Moro, and grasping reflexes. Overall observation of the child for asymmetry of activity is also performed. The child is then observed for any gross deformities. These may range from obvious congenital amputations to minor deformities such as syndactyly. If more than two to three minor congenital deformities are detected than further evaluation for a major congenital defect should be considered.[20]

The limbs of the child should be evaluated from segment to segment.[21] The position of the thigh should be examined relative to that of the body. The position and alignment of the leg and femur at the knee joint should also be evaluated. Relationship of the foot to the ankle and the ankle to the leg should also be evaluated. The positioning of the rearfoot should be inspected and any abnormalities recorded. Range of motions should be described. One must keep in mind that the range of motion for the neonate is different from that of the developing child and the adolescent. Range of motion of the knee should not be limited or restricted. If this occurs it would lead to consideration of a congenital dislocation of the knee; however, this would be associated with a gross deformity.

Examination for congenital dislocation of the hip should also be performed. This includes clinical examination as well as radiographic and ultrasonic evaluation when indicated. Clinical tests for the evaluation of congenitally dislocated hip include the limited abduction test. There are normally 50 to 90 degrees of abduction of the hip; less than 50 degrees is a positive limited abduction test. This test is usually performed with the child lying on his or her back and abducting both limbs. In the Galeazzi or Allis test the two knees are placed together with the knees bent and the heels on the examining surface. If one knee is lower than the other, there is a significant likelihood of a congenitally dislocated hip.

In another test for congenitally dislocated hip, the child supine with the knee flexed to 90° the examiner grasps the femur and abducts the thigh while pushing the greater trochanter toward the midline. If the hip relocates the examiner will feel a pop or click (Ortolani's sign). As this motion is reversed another pop or click will be felt as the hip dislocates. Therefore the hip dislocation is reduced by abduction and the "click" occurs as the femoral head slides into the socket over the posterior rim of the acetabulum. So the Ortolani's sign is a relocation sign of a dislocated hip. Many texts describe this click as audible; however, more often than not it is a palpated click. Barlow's test is performed by adducting and rotating the femur until a click or pop is felt. The Barlow test is carried out to detect an unstable hip in the newborn, so Barlow's test is a dislocation test.

Two additional tests for congenital dislocation of the hip include the telescoping sign, in which the femur is pushed back and forth gently and a telescoping effect occurs on the deficient hip. Telescoping of greater than 1.5 inches is usually significant. Posterior examination of the child revealing an asymmetry of the gluteal folds also may be indicative of congenitally dislocated hip. Usually the side with the higher gluteal fold is the side of the congenital dislocation.

Physical Examination of the Young Child

Physical examination of the lower limbs of the child also proceeds in a gradual and orderly fashion. After observation for a gross asymmetry one should look for disorders that are visible in stance, such as shoulder drops, pelvic tilt, and curvature of the spine as seen with lordosis or kyphosis. Examination of the hips may be performed with the child sitting on the examination table with the legs dangling over the free end. With the limb forming the pointer in an imaginary protractor the degree of internal and external rotation is estimated with the hip flexed and extended (Fig. 22-5). The end range of motion is assessed for sponginess or abrupt hardness. An estimate of the degree of femoral torsion that is present may be obtained using Ryder's test.[26]

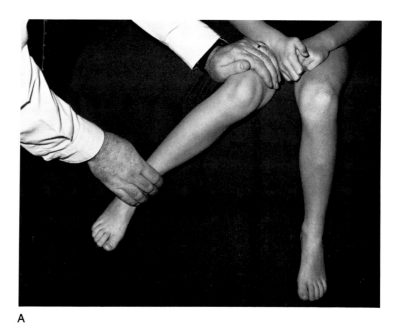

A

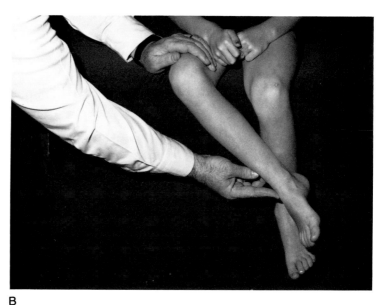

B

Fig. 22-5. (A) Testing internal hip rotation.
(B) Testing external hip rotation.

This estimate is performed on the examining table with the hip in an extended position. The greater trochanter is palpated laterally and the point at which it is felt most laterally may be read off protractor-style, as previously described for hip rotation, to yield the degree of torsion. As suggested by McCrea, these tests should be performed in conjunction with each other to verify the clinical findings, and the data of both should be supportive.

Any discrepancy found between the measurement of hip rotation and Ryders test requires reevaluation.

Examination of the knee should be performed to determine abnormal position and mobility at the knee joint. The patient may then be examined in the standing position for genu recurvatum and knee position, such as genu varum and genu valgum. The measurement for genu varum and val-

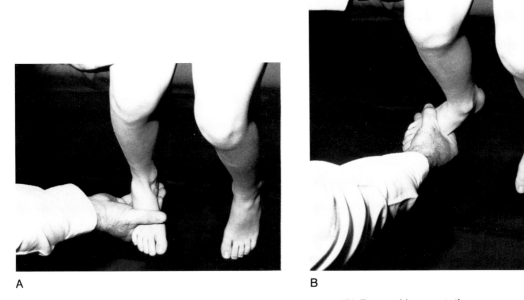

Fig. 22-6. (A) Internal knee rotation. **(B)** External knee rotation.

gum is usually performed with the child in the supine position. In a child with genu varum the medial malleoli usually touch first, whereas in a child with genu valgum the knees are the structures that touch first. The appearance of genu varum and valgum is part of the normal physiologic development of the child; however, pathologic conditions need to be carefully evaluated.

Genicular position or rotation should also be evaluated (Fig. 22-6). There is a varying degree of transverse plane motion that will be present in the child's knees. This is more noticeable at birth and reduces with normal development. In the adult there is usually less than 5 degrees of transverse plane rotation. This motion has been described as being equal in internal and external rotation at the knee. The test of transverse plane motion is usually performed with the hip flexed and then extended, as recommended by McCrea.[26] When the foot is held in a neutral position the knee is in the frontal plane. The foot is then rotated medially and laterally and the degree of rotation in each position is read off an imaginary protractor with the foot as the pointer. Tibial torsion is considered to be normal with greater internal rotation than external rota-

tion; this is defined as an internal genicular position, which is the cause of an adducted gait. If the range of motion increases with the hip flexed versus extended, then muscular tightness may account for this asymmetry of motion. If the rotation is uneffected by a motion of the hip then ligamentous involvement of the knee joint may be suspected.

The next segment to be evaluated is the tibia. Tibial torsion is reflected directly as malleolar torsion or position. It is measured with the child in the supine position, with the knee extended in the frontal plane (Fig. 22-7). The foot is held in its neutral position with the ankle at 90 degrees. Care should be taken to prevent inadvertent malpositioning of the foot, which may lead to an inaccurate reading. Both malleoli are bisected and these serve as the point of measurement. Measurements may be taken with a goniometer or estimated.

Ankle joint dorsiflexion and plantar flexion should also be measured (Fig. 22-8). Dorsiflexion should be measured specifically with the knee both flexed and extended in order to separate the various components of a subtissue rearfoot equinus. When performing this test it is ideal to keep the

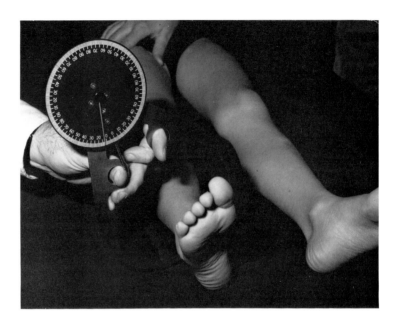

Fig. 22-7. Clinical measurement of tibial torsion.

subtalar joint in its neutral position. Subtalar joint evaluation for the total range of motion, including quality and direction, should also be evaluated. Subtalar joint position may best be evaluated in the stance examination, and is reflected in the calcaneal stance position, which is measured both in relaxed and in neutral position (Fig. 22-9). An additional test called the lateral malleolar index, described by Whitney (personal communication), is a measurement of the relationship of the lateral aspect of the calcaneus to the lateral malleolus. These two structures will be aligned on the same plane in a normal foot.

Evaluation of the relationship of the forefoot to the rearfoot in terms of varus or valgus deviation of the forefoot should also be performed. This becomes increasingly more significant when dealing with the older child and adolescent.

Asymmetrical forms of foot problems such as flatfoot may be the result of unequal limb length. Estimates of limb length may be obtained by measurement of the limb from the anterior superior iliac spine to the medial malleolus and from the umbilicus to the medial malleolus. This will help differentiate true from apparently discrepancy, the latter of which may be caused such problems as pelvic tilt and spinal disorders. Accurate measurement of limb length can only be done radiographically.

SPECIAL PROBLEMS IN THE PEDIATRIC PATIENT

Limp and Foot Pain

Limp may be a common complaint in the pediatric patient.[28] The causes can range from relatively minor problems, such as a simple ingrown toenail, to major and potentially catastrophic problems, such as hidden neoplasms. Fields[29] classified limp according to specific location, nonspecific location, and age (Table 22-6).

Foot pain in the child can result from a wide variety of pathologies: extrinsic problems, structural and inflammatory conditions, trauma, or neoplastic changes. Gross[30] has suggested a list of more common causes of foot pain in children (Table 22-7). Some of these are discussed in more detail below.

Growing Pains

Leg aches or pain in the legs and often in the foot have been attributed to so-called growing pains. The child may be affected as early as age 5, but

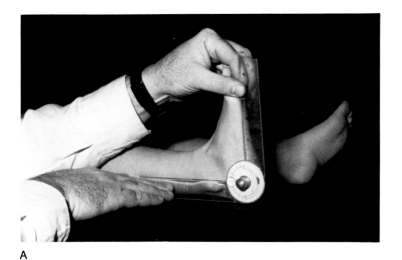

A

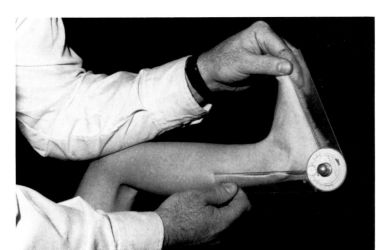

B

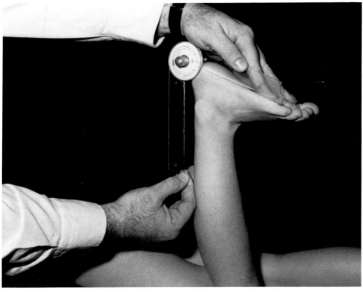

C

Fig. 22-8. Measurement of ankle joint dorsiflexion. **(A)** Knee extended. **(B)** Supine position, knee flexed or alternately. **(C)** Prone position, knee flexed.

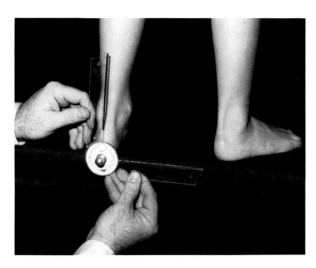

Fig. 22-9. Measurement of relaxed calcaneal stance position.

growing pains are most pronounced between ages 8 and 12. As Peterson[31] pointed out, "some children have vague nebulous discomfort in the limbs for which no cause can be found." Underlying causes for this discomfort can be many and varied. A diagnosis of growing pains is usually arrived at by exclusion of other pathologies, as listed in Table 22-7.

Growing pains have been defined as consisting of intermittent annoying pain or ache usually located in the muscles of the legs and thighs. These pains may be accentuated by increased activity. The pain is usually not associated with local tenderness, erythema, or swelling. There is usually a lack of objective findings. However, pain of unknown origin in the pediatric patient cannot be ignored and written off as growing pains.[32] In order for a child's pain to be classified as growing pains the results of the physical examination, laboratory studies, and radiographic evaluation must be normal.

Baxter and Dulberg[33] attributed growing pains to a benign clinical entity of unknown etiology. They did find, however, that these growing pains responded to conservative therapy with muscle stretching. In the study group there was a more rapid resolution of symptoms of the growing pain in the 18-month period when compared to a controlled group. The stretching exercises involved stretching of the quadriceps, calf, and hamstrings.

Table 22-6. Limp Relating to Specific Location

Location	Cause
Brain	Cerebral tumor
	Attention seeking device
Back	Trauma
	Iliac adenitis
	Acute appendicitis
	Neoplasms
	Herniated nucleus pulposus
	Osteitis
	Scheuermann's disease of the spine
	Spondilolisthesis
	Scoliosis
Hip	Transient synovitis
	Congenital dislocation of the hip
	Slipped femoral capital epiphysis
	Legg-Calvé-Perthes disease
	Coxa vara
	Fracture
	Trochanteric bursitis
	Soft tissue infection
	Referred from back
Knee	Scurvy
	Hemophilia
	Anaphylactoid purpura
	Sickle cell anemia
	Acute leukemia
	Erythema nodosum
	Thrombophlebitis
	Synovitis
	Osgood-Schlatter disease
	Osteochondritis dissecans
	Chondromalacia
	Congenital discoid meniscus
	Referred from hip
	Fracture
	Ruputured tendo achillis or plantaris
	Muscle group paralysis
Ankle	Fracture/sprain
Foot	Sever's disease
	Tarsal coalition
	Calcaneal spurs
	Köhler's disease
	Plantar lesions
	Freiberg's disease
	Soft tissue infection
	Poliomyelitis
	Fracture/sprain
	Foreign body

(From Fields,[29] with permission.)

Inflammatory Causes of Foot Pain

Pediatric Osteomyelitis

Osteomyelitis may occur as a result of several mechanisms: (1) blood-borne, or hematogenous, infection, (2) direct extension via soft tissue infection or ulceration, and (3) open fracture. In chil-

Table 22-7. Common Causes of Foot Pain in Children

Extrinsic
  Ill-fitting shoes
  Ingrown toenail
  Foreign body
Structural
  Hypermobile flat foot with tight heel cord
  Peroneal spastic flat foot (tarsal coalition)
  Accessory navicular (prehallus)
  Pes cavus
  Osteochondroses (?)
  "Relaxed" flat foot (?)
Inflammatory
  Osteomyelitis
  Juvenile rheumatoid arthritis (JRA)
  Rheumatic fever
Trauma
  Stress fracture
  Fractures
  Sprains (adolescents)
  Achilles tendonitis
Tumors
  Osteoid osteoma
  Ewing's sarcoma
  Synovial sarcoma

(From Gross,[30] with permission.)

dren the predominant forms of osteomyelitis are bacterial and hematogenous.

The primary organism that causes osteomyelitis is *Staphylococcus;* however, in children under 2 years of age it is *Streptococcus.* In the evaluation of children with hematogenous osteomyelitis it is important to look for the primary source of infection. These sources of infection may be a sore throat, ingrown toenail, infection in the oral cavity or a tooth, or urinary tract or soft tissue infection (Fig.

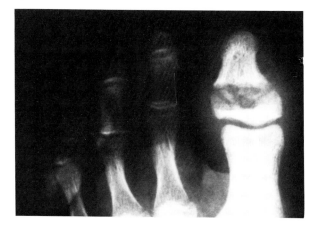

Fig. 22-10. Osteomyelitis of the great toe secondary to an improperly treated ingrown toe nail.

22-10). It is often useful to identify the site and perform a culture when identified.

The clinical picture will vary depending on the patient's age, underlying disease, resistance, localization, extent of disease, and virulence of the organism. There is a rapid onset and the child will become acutely sick. Motion will be present at the adjacent joint depending upon the degree of muscle guarding. The lesion will be palpable and painful. In the initial stage of hematogenous osteomyelitis the joint is not septic.

Evaluation of a child with suspected osteomyelitis or septic arthritis should include a thorough history and physical exam. Laboratory evaluation should include a white blood cell count with differential, erythrocyte sedimentation rate, and blood cultures. Aspiration may be performed for Gram stain and culture. Aerobic and anaerobic cultures should be made. In the older child a bone scan is indicated. However, in the early stages of osteomyelitis a bone scan may be reported as normal or demonstrate photopenia as a result of local bone ischemia. In the presence of a normal technetium bone scan a second scan with gallium-67 citrate–or indium-111–tagged white blood cells may be required to make the definitive diagnosis. Once a patient has been started on antibiotics after the appropriate wound cultures and needle aspirates, when indicated, have been drawn, if no response to antibiotics has occurred in 38 to 48 hours bone biopsy by an open method should be performed.[35,36]

The presence of a photopenic or cold lesion with ischemic osteomyelitis is an ominous sign. If the radiopharmaceutical cannot enter the site of the infection it is unlikely that the antibiotic will be able to do so either. The ischemia results from the pressure generated within the bone because of the expansion of the pus. In these cases, or when a soft tissue abscess is identified, surgical drainage should be performed to minimize bone damage and deformity.[36]

Puncture wounds of the foot should also be handled with great care because subsequent development of osteomyelitis has been reported. Fisher and associates[37] have shown a significant incidence of *Pseudomonas aeruginosa* osteomyelitis in children following puncture wounds. A relationship was noted between the growth of *Pseudomonas* in the spongy inner layers of the soles of sneakers and the development of this infection.

Growth disturbances have also been reported secondary to the development of osteomyelitis. A report of two cases of osteomyelitis of the calcaneus following routine heel puncture resulted in growth disturbance of the heel.[38]

Juvenile Rheumatoid Arthritis

Juvenile rheumatoid arthritis must be considered in the differential diagnosis of foot pain. Initial presentations may be somewhat insidious. Juvenile arthritis in the foot may mimic several diseases, such as osteomyelitis.[39] It may be associated with a variety of systemic diseases. Juvenile rheumatoid arthritis is a term used to describe the condition of chronic synovitis in children.[40]

Dhanendran et al.[41] found that gross changes in the force distribution under the foot were detected in patients with juvenile rheumatoid arthritis. It was found that these individuals walked predominantly on their heels, midfoot, and lateral metatarsal heads. Reduction in great toe loading was the most significant and consistent change. The patients in this study all had juvenile rheumatoid arthritis with widespread involvement of the feet, but none of them had observable deformities of the lower limbs.

Osteochondrosis

Osteochondrosis was best defined by Brower as a condition in which a primary or secondary ossification center in the growing child undergoes aseptic necrosis with gradual reabsorption of dead bone and replacement by reparative osseous tissue.[42] This disease process may involve several sites in the lower extremity. These include the hip (Legg-Calvé-Perthes disease), the tibial tubercle (Osgood-Schlatter disease), the calcaneus (Sever's disease; Fig. 22-11A), the second metatarsal head (Freiberg's disease), the medial tibial epiphysis (Blount's disease), and the tarsal navicular (Köhler's disease; see Fig. 22-11B).

The osteochondroses may be articular, nonarticular, or physeal[43] (Table 22-8). The articular osteochondroses may cause alterations in the shape and form of a joint. They also may result in a later degenerative arthritis. Irregularities may occur as a result of either primary or initial involvement of articular and epiphyseal growth cartilage (Freiberg's disease) or secondary or initial necrosis of all or part of a bony nucleus of an epiphysis (e.g., Köhler's disease). Nonarticular osteochondroses may occur at tendon attachments, ligament attachments, or impact sites (e.g., Sever's disease). Physeal osteochondroses affect the longitudinal growth plates of the tibia (e.g., Blount's disease).

The etiology of the osteochondroses is not well known, but they may be related to trauma and interruption of the vascular supply to the involved bones. Interference with the epiphyseal vessels may result in varying degrees of necrosis of deeper layers of cartilage cells. This interferes with bone formation within the epiphyseal nucleus and interferes with both chondrogenesis and osteogenesis. The nonspecific pathologic changes observed in the osteochondroses are characterized by disorderly endochondral ossification and reparative osteogenesis. In general all stages in replacement of the necrotic bone have been observed, including revascularization, granulation, osteoclasis, ingrowth of osteoid, and remodeling.

Freiberg's disease is usually characterized by pain upon weightbearing and may be associated with any effusion of the joint in the acute stages. In the early stages, tenderness over the head of the metatarsal or over the metatarsophalangeal joint may be the only physical sign. A technetium scan will reveal a hot spot over the affected metatarsal head.[44] As the problem progresses, deformity occurs with expansion and flattening of the head of the metatarsal and at times the base of the proximal phalanx. This is followed by further deformity and arthritis. Initial treatment may involve non-weight-bearing ambulation in the early stages; surgical intervention may also be indicated.

Helal and Gibb[44] cited McMasters, who determined that a chondral or osteochondral impingement lesion may be produced by the base of the proximal phalanx under conditions of forced dorsiflexion. McMaster's initially performed this research in order to understand the incidence of hallux rigidus. However, he suggested that this might also account for the development of the lesion in Freiberg's disease. McMasters noted that there was

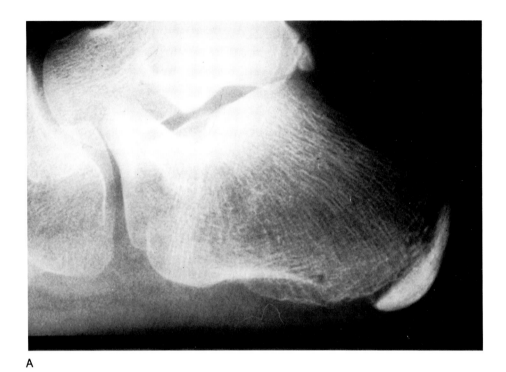

A

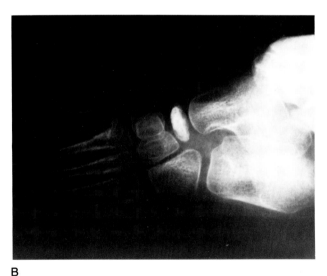

B

Fig. 22-11. (A) Radiographic presentation of Sever's disease. (B) Radiographic presentation of Köhler's disease.

a striking similarity in the lesions found in both conditions, but noted that the separated osteochondral fragment was much larger in Freiberg's disease than in hallux rigidus.

Osteochondrosis of the tarsal navicular was described by Köhler.[45] The most common symptoms of *Köhler's disease* are pain and limp. Tenderness in the area of the tarsal navicular is the most consistent finding; it may be accompanied by swelling and heat. Specific decreases in the ankle or subtalar joint are noted. In a study by Williams and Cowell[46] the age of onset of symptoms ranged from 2 to 9

Table 22-8. Classification of the Osteochondroses

I. Articular Osteochondroses
   A. *Primary* involvement of articular and epiphyseal cartilage and subjacent endochondral ossification (*e.g.*, humeral condylosis. Freiberg's disease)
   B. *Secondary* involvement of articular and epiphyseal cartilage as a consequence of avascular necrosis of subjacent bone (*e.g.*, LCPS, Köhler's, osteochondritis dissecans)
II. Nonarticular Osteochondroses
   A. At tendon attachments (*e.g.*, Osgood-Schlatter disease)
   B. At ligament attachments (*e.g.*, vertebral ring, epicondyles)
   C. At impact sites (*e.g.*, Sever's disease)
III. Physeal Osteochondroses
   A. Long bones (*e.g.*, tibia vara)
   B. Vertebrae (Scheuermann's disease)

(From Siffert,[43] with permission.)

Table 22-9. Differential Diagnosis of Childhood and Adolescent Heel Pain

A. Overuse/overgrowth/traumatic
   1. Calcaneal apophysitis
   2. Contusion/strain
   3. Stress fracture of calcaneus
   4. Fracture of calcaneus
B. Developmental
   1. Tarsal coalition
C. Inflammatory
   1. Tendinitis (Achilles, patellar, flexor hallux longus)
   2. Plantar fasciitis
   3. Retrocalcaneal bursitis
   4. Periostitis
   5. Os trigonum inflammation
D. Infectious
   1. Soft tissue infection
   2. Abscess
   3. Calcaneal osteomyelitis
E. Rheumatologic
   1. Juvenile rheumatoid arthritis
   2. Reiter syndrome
   3. Miscellaneous
F. Tumorous
   1. Benign
      a. Osteoid osteoma
      b. Osteochondroma
      c. Chondroblastoma
      d. Bone cyst (solitary or aneurysmal)
   2. Malignant (very rare)
      a. Leukemia
      b. Metastatic
G. Neurologic
   1. Tarsal tunnel syndrome

(From Micheli and Ireland,[47] with permission.)

years. The average age at presentation was 5 years and 10 months: 6 years and 2 months in the male and 4 years and 6 months in the female. This was thought by these authors to be consistent with the early appearance of the navicular in the female. The radiographic findings commonly seen with Köhler's disease are an increased density and flattening of the navicular. Also, a trabecular pattern may occur and fragmentation has been reported. Treatment by immobilization in a short-leg weight-bearing cast appeared to result in earlier improvement. However, in Williams and Cowell's series all patients eventually had spontaneous reconstitution of the navicular and excellent functional recovery.

Perhaps the most common of the osteochondroses is that in the calcaneal epiphysis *(Sever's disease).*[47] Pain is the chief complaint. Tenderness to palpation of the posterior and inferior aspect of the heel is usually found, and medial lateral compression of the heel may cause discomfort. Usually no erythema, skin changes, swelling, or other local abnormalities are noted. A gastrocnemius-soleus equinus can be found in most patients. Therapy includes initial restriction of activity depending upon the severity of symptoms. Anti-inflammatory agents are not indicated. An exercise regimen including flexibility exercises for the gastrocnemius and soleus muscles is indicated. A base-of-heel cup, a heel pad, and at times a heel lift may be indicated.

Orthotics may be used to control any of the biomechanical foot faults. The differential diagnosis of heel pain in children and adolescents is presented in Table 22-9.

PEDIATRIC LOWER EXTREMITY DEFORMITIES

It is important to note that the descriptions presented in this section of this chapter are brief and of an overview nature. Many of the specific deformities are covered in more detail in other chapters in this text.

Torsional and Angular Deformity

The etiology of torsional deformities may be either hereditary or secondary to intrauterine position. Deformity due to intrauterine position usually has a better prognosis than the genetic, or hereditary, type. The hereditary type will usually occur in other members of the family.[48] In discussing torsional deformity of the femur the following four terms are commonly used:

1. Medial femoral torsion
2. Medial femoral position
3. Lateral femoral torsion
4. Lateral femoral position

"Torsion" is used in reference to an osseous problem and "position" relates to a soft tissue problem involving the hip joint. Lateral femoral torsion is an unusual finding; medial femoral torsion is more common. Either condition may result in rotational problems in a child.

Rotational Problems

Lateral femoral rotational problems are usually positional in nature. External rotation contracture usually appears early in life, followed by internal femoral torsion occurring after the age of 12 to 18 months. The knee joint examination usually reveals transverse plane hypermobility in the infant and young child. A limitation of motion at the knee joint can occur that involves the contracture of the posterior fibers of the knee capsule and relates to genicular position. This may also involve the soft tissue and muscle of the knee joint, which will cause an internal rotation of the tibia.

The most useful method for screening a child with rotational problems was probably first described by Staheli.[48-50] Four areas are evaluated: hip rotation, foot-to-thigh angle, foot progression angle, and the foot. *Hip rotation* is measured with the patient in a prone position with the knees flexed and the pelvis held level. Medial rotation refers to the angle between the vertical and the axis of the tibia with maximal internal rotation of the hip. (The legs are allowed to fall into full internal

rotation by gravity alone.) Lateral rotation is measured from the same position allowing the patient's legs to cross. Tibial rotation is assessed using the *foot-to-thigh angle.* The angular difference between the axis of the thigh and the foot is observed with the patient prone and the knees flexed to 90 degrees. It is important that the view of the foot and thigh be from directly above. The *foot progression angle* is the angle that is formed by the long axis of the foot relative to the line of progression of the child's gait. The *foot* is examined for the presence of foot deformity, such as metatarsus adductus. A rotational profile can be developed from this evaluation and compared to establish norms. The normal values were established through the study of approximately 1,000 patients, with normal considered to be within 2 standard deviations from the mean.[48]

In addition to rotational deformities, the knee malalignment syndrome can occur in a patient who has medial femoral torsion and lateral tibial torsion. In this individual the foot progression angle may be normal but the patellae are medially rotated during gait. Positional effects during sleeping and sitting make a significant contribution to the deformity. These habits often have to be changed in order to achieve effective therapy (Fig. 22-12).

Angular Problems

Difficulty can arise in distinguishing rotational from angular problems. At birth a varus position of the knee is present that reduces to become initially straight, then develops into a valgus attitude. This valgus position gradually reduces to about 5 to 8 degrees in the adult. This varus-to-valgus attitude can result in the presence of a physiologic flatfoot that may or may not require treatment.

The appearance of bowing is a physiologic process in the young child. It can be difficult for the parents to understand as they picture the child with a future appearance of bow legs.[51] Often no more than an evaluation and reasssurance are required as therapy. The appearance of bowing is secondary to the external rotation at the hip joints, the normal physiologic bowing of the femur, and the internal rotation of the tibia. Passive correction of the rota-

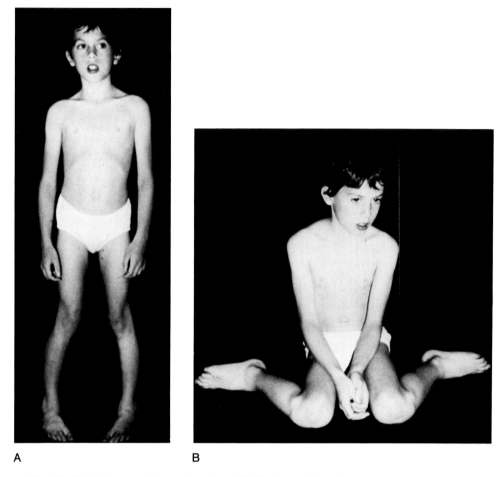

Fig. 22-12. (A) Internal femoral torsion. **(B)** Sitting position that maintains the deformity.

tional positioning by placing the foot and tibia in external rotation from the long axis of the knee and internally rotating the femur will eliminate this bowed appearance in the child with physiologic bowing.

Knock knees may also be predominantly a physiologic variant.[52] However, pathologic forms do exist, such as Blount's disease, which may be infantile or juvenile; ricketts, which may be primary or secondary; and knock knees associated with short stature, which may be associated with some form of dysplasia. In children with pathologic deformity a thrust at the knee joint is often evident in gait. This thrust demonstrates instability of the knee joint (Fig. 22-13).

Treatment

In the treatment of rotational and angular deformities several things should be kept in mind:

1. The need for treatment
2. The proposed benefit from the treatment
3. The effectiveness of the treatment

Nonoperative methods of therapy include shoe wedges, gait plates, twister cables, Denis-Browne bars, Ganley splints, Filauer splints, and casting.

Although these devices do not provide treatment they can be an adjuvant to treatment in the correction of sitting, sleeping, and postural habits that maintain these deformities. Moreland[53] demon-

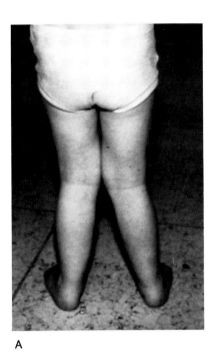

A

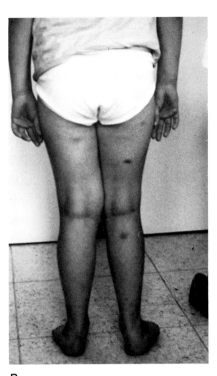

B

Fig. 22-13. Two examples of genuvalgum in children of different ages. The marked pronatory effect on the subtalar joint is evident.

strated that it would be unlikely that significant rotational changes could be produced with longitudinal growth in humans by external means. He also demonstrated, using load cells, that in children wearing Denis-Browne splints torsional load occurred only while the child was awake, and was present equally in both directions.[54]

Surgical therapy usually requires some form of angular or derotational osteotomy. The value of conservative therapy is limited. It has predominantly proved to be ineffective.

Flatfoot

Flatfoot may be classified into two main categories, physiologic and pathologic, as outlined in Table 22-10.[55] The distinction between the categories is largely related to the development of symptoms. Symptoms secondary to the development of flatfoot can be quite varied. In the young child they can range from muscle cramps, particularly in the calf or anterior portion of the leg, to discomfort in

the arch in the heel area. Occasionally more structural problems such as knee, hip, and low back pain may develop. In the examination of the flexible foot one should look for the presence of ligamentous laxity.

Therapy

The majority of flatfeet respond to conservative management using a variety of techniques. Ther-

Table 22-10. Classification of Flatfoot

Physiologic
  Developmental
  Familial
  Racial
Pathologic
  Congenital
    Calcaneovalgus
    Vertical talus
    Tarsal coalition
    Short Achilles tendon
    Skewfoot
  Traumatic
  Neurologic

apy depends upon several factors, including the type of flatfoot, the age of the patient, and the severity of the deformity.[26,56]

The primary goal in treatment with an orthotic is to maintain joint congruity and alignment. A simple method for evaluating positioning of the foot is the lateral malleolar index as described by Whitney.[27] The lateral malleolar index measures the distance from the lateral malleolus to the lateral aspect of the calcaneus. Normally these are in line with one another in the foot with normal joint alignment and congruity.

Treatment is usually not required in those children who presents with asymptomatic flatfoot. However, treatment should be considered in those children who have severe flatfoot deformity. This includes a marked valgus of the calcaneus a medial longitudinal arch in which the foot is in flat contact with the ground, and marked transverse abnormality of the forefoot on the rearfoot.

Physiologic Flatfoot

Physiologic flatfoot has sometimes been referred to as developmental flatfoot because it is secondary to rotational and angular deformities that are part of normal development. A family history of a tendency toward the development of flatfoot may occur. In these families the adults sometimes have hypermobile flatfoot but are predominantly asymptomatic. There can also be a racial predominance to the development of flatfoot.

Pathologic Flatfoot

Congenital Flatfoot *(Congenital Flexible Flatfoot).* *Calcaneovalgus* Calcaneovalgus is usually present at birth and has been reported to occur in 1 in 1,000 births. This deformity is characterized by excessive dorsiflexion and eversion of the foot on the leg (Fig. 22-14). The foot may be sitting in a markedly valgus position or may assume in the older child a somewhat more neutral position. When dorsiflexing and everting the foot, the dorsal and lateral aspect of the foot can be made to touch the anterior surface of the leg. There is limited plantar flexion of the ankle joint. Controversy exists as to whether this foot should be treated. Left untreated, it has been hypothesized that this will develop into a hypermobile flatfoot.

Congenital hypermobile flatfoot presents with a valgus position of the heel to a varying degree, prominence of the head of the talus medially with abduction of the forefoot, and lowering of the medial longitudinal arch. The degree to which the foot compensates depends upon the orientation of the axis of the subtalar and midtarsal joints. This concept of planal dominance and the biomechanics of flatfoot has been discussed elsewhere in this text. Biomechanical examination is necessary to outline

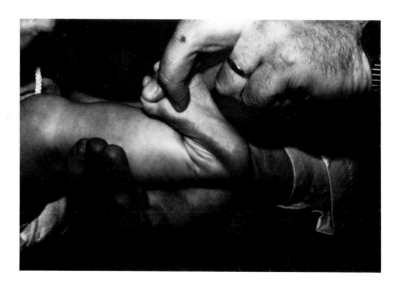

Fig. 22-14. Calcaneovalgus congenital.

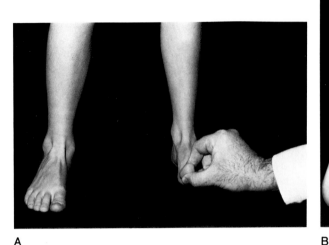

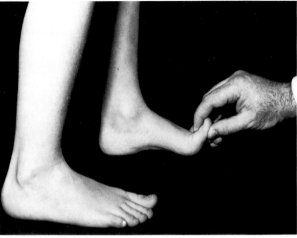

A

B

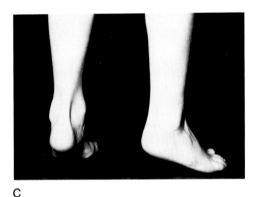

C

Fig. 22-15. (A) Great toe extension test (front view); **(B)** (side view.) **(C)** Resupination test.

the various etiologic factors in the development of the hypermobile flatfoot. These factors are presented in Chapter 37.

Methods of distinguishing hypermobile flatfoot from rigid flatfoot are the great toe extension test and the resupination test (Fig. 22-15). The great toe extension test is performed by dorsiflexing the great toe while the patient is standing. Rose et al.[57] demonstrated that passive extension of the great toe in the normal foot results in (1) elevation of the medial longitudinal arch and (2) lateral rotation of the tibia. A normal test requires both to be present; an intermediate result is when no tibial rotation is demonstrated, and a negative result occurs when no elevation of the arch or tibial rotation is seen. Formation of a medial longitudinal arch is a positive result showing flexibility of the foot. The *resupination test* is performed with the individual

standing on his or her toes. Development of a medial arch configuration is a positive result showing that the foot is flexible. Radiographically a flexible flatfoot shows an increased talocalcaneal angle in both the dorsoplantar and lateral views and a plantar-flexed attitude to the talus.

Fortunately most cases of calcaneovalgus respond to conservative therapy. This includes manipulation of the foot by the parents at every diaper change; the parent is instructed to plantar flex and invert the foot gently. In moderate cases strapping and taping may be of some use, and in severe cases casting in a neutral position and eventually a plantar flexed position may be useful. It is important to remember when using taping, strapping, or manipulation that the proper plantar flexion of the foot must occur, and not just motion at the midfoot.

Vertical Talus. Vertical talus is a congenital de-

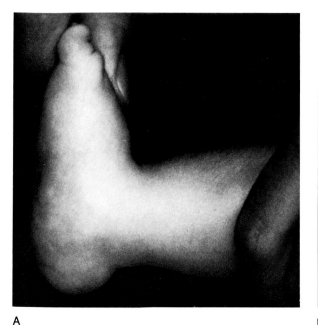

A

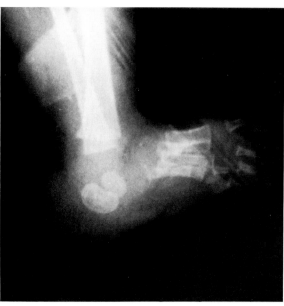

B

Fig. 22-16. Clinical **(A)** and radiographic **(B)** appearance of vertical talus.

formity in which there is dislocation of the talonavicular joint. The talus appears vertical and the navicular articulates with the dorsal aspect of the talus (Fig. 22-16). Two types of vertical talus have been described: type I, with an intact calcaneocuboid joint, and type II, with disruption of the calcaneocuboid joint associated with complete dislocation of the forefoot on the rearfoot.[58]

Vertical talus has been associated with several congenital and neurologic diseases. It may also occur in an idiopathic form that is believed to be secondary to in utero position. Marked anatomic malalignment of the structures of the leg is also part of the deformity.[58–60]

Vertical talus must be differentiated from oblique talus because the course of oblique talus can be approached conservatively.[61] In management of vertical talus, the primary key is to reduce the dislocation at the talonavicular joint and to maintain this joint in its reduced position. Conservative treatment may be tried initially and should be attempted preoperatively to allow stretching of the soft tissues.

In surgical management posterior release is usually required due to severe equinus. Usually there is a reversal of the calcaneal inclination angle radio-graphically. In type I vertical talus, below the age of 1 year usually a soft tissue release will be helpful. Past 1 year, in order to maintain the position of the talonavicular and subtalar joint a subtalar bone block may be required. Type II is often recalcitrant and some type of fusion may be required at an older age to provide lasting correction.

Tarsal Coalition. Tarsal coalition is the result of a congenital tarsal anomaly that is possibly genetic in origin (Fig. 22-17). Anatomic locations of tarsal coalitions are listed in Table 22-11 along with their reported incidences.[62,63]

The different types and histologic structures of coalitions as developed by Buckholz are presented in Table 22-12.

The initial symptom associated with tarsal coalition or limitation of motion due to arthrodesis is pain. Development of symptoms is often related to the onset of the coalition or the restriction of motion, and the development of secondary symptoms is associated with functional adaption.[64,65]

Treatment of tarsal coalition initially includes immobilization, which may be accomplished by nonweightbearing initially followed by a partial to full weight-bearing cast. Treatment may also involve the use of local injection therapy into the

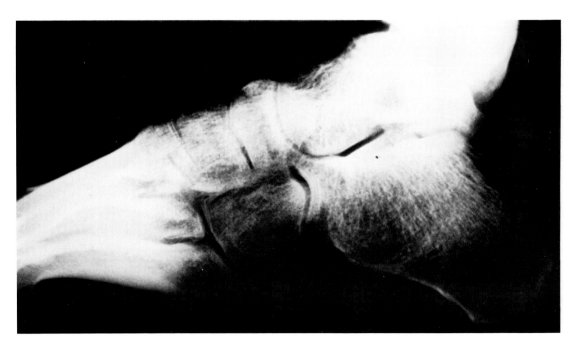

Fig. 22-17. Calcaneonavicular coalition.

area of the sinus tarsi. Tibial and peroneal blocks also help relieve discomfort and may reduce spasms. Use of anti-inflammatory agents may also prove helpful. Surgical intervention is required for those patients who do not respond to conservative therapy.[66,67] Surgical intervention may include resection of the bar or joint arthrodesis depending on the anatomic location of the bar and extent of secondary arthritic changes.

Peroneal spastic flatfoot may be associated with tarsal coalition,[62] and is a result of a spasm of the peroneal muscles, acting as a guarding or splinting mechanism, that forcibly pronates the foot. Peroneal spastic flatfoot may be due to a variety of conditions, including trauma, arthritis, infection, and tarsal coalition (Table 22-13). Initial evaluation of the tarsal coalition includes radiographic evaluation. Certain specialized radiographic methods are

Table 22-11. Relative Incidences of Tarsal Coalition

Calcaneonavicular (common)	43.6
Talocalcaneal	48.1
Anterior facet (rare)	
Middle facet (common)	
Posterior facet (rare)	
Talonavicular (rare)	1.3
Calcaneocuboid (rare)	1.3
Other	5.7
Naviculocuboid (rare)	
Massive tarsal coalitions	

(Anatomic locations modified from Mosier and Asher,[62] with incidence data from Stormont and Peterson.[63])

Table 22-12. Types and Histologic Structures of Tarsal Coalition

Coalitions
A. Types
  1. Synarthrosis—fusion occurring within an anatomical joint
  2. Synostosis—tissue extensions joining one bone to another from outside the anatomical joints
  3. Synarthrostosis—coexisting synarthrosis and synostosis
B. Histological structure
  1. Fibrous
  2. Cartilaginous
  3. Osseous
Arthroereisis
A. Accessory ossicles—inconstant sesamoids that may block motion
B. Accessory processes—apparently remnants of incomplete morphological bone formation; the process is continuous with the parent tarsal bone
C. Conglomerants—accessory ossicles that are fused to an anatomical parent bone

(From Buckholz JM: Peroneal spastic flatfoot. p. 338. In McGlamry ED (ed): Fundamental of Foot Surgery. Williams & Wilkins, Baltimore, 1987, with permission.)

Table 22-13. Differential Diagnosis of Peroneal Spastic Flatfoot

1. Coalitions
   a. Calcaneonavicular (common)
   b. Talocalcaneal
      (1) anterior facet (rare)
      (2) middle facet (common)
      (3) posterior facet (rare)
   c. Talonavicular (rare)
   d. Calcaneocuboid (rare)
   e. Naviculocuboid (rare)
   f. Massive tarsal coalitions
2. Arthritis of the tarsus
   a. Rheumatoid
   b. Gout with subtalar urate deposits
   c. Osteoarthritis
   d. Post-traumatic
   e. Tuberculous in which an early stage may be limited to part of a joint
3. Inflammation of the tarsus
4. Infection of the tarsus, which may lead to bone ankylosis
5. Large bone-mass malformation of the sustentaculum leading to a block in motion; this may be difficult to diagnose radiographically
6. Acromegaly
7. Fibrosarcoma
8. Osteochondral fracture of the undersurface of the talar head
9. Osteitis deformans
10. Osteochondritis dissecans
11. Osteochondrodystrophy (Morquio's disease)
12. Iatrogenic, usually causing only secondary radiographic signs[a]
    a. Overzealous cast correction of club foot
    b. Grice procedure
    c. Gallie subtalar arthrodesis
    d. Postoperative subtalar arthrodesis
13. Occupational strain leading to spasm
14. Rigid flat foot, which is the same as peroneal spastic flat foot but without the spasm
15. Relaxed or flexible flat foot. This deformity exists in childhood: the mid-tarsal joint is hypermobile, and pain may develop in adolescence or later, caused by excessive ligament strain and traumatic arthritis

(From Mosier and Asher,[62] with permission.)

[a] It is important to remember that these secondary radiographic signs are not specific for tarsal coalition. They are associated with limited subtalar motion, and any condition that decreases subtalar motion may result in similar radiographic signs.

required to accomplish this. These include the Harris Beath, or ski jump, view to demonstrate the posterior subtalar joint facets, and Isherwood[68] views, which are a series of multiple oblique exposures at varying degrees into the subtalar joint. Tomography and more recently computed tomography scanning and magnetic resonance imaging have proved to be of great value.[69]

Short Achilles Tendon. Flatfoot may also be secondary to a short Achilles tendon or the equinus foot, often referred to as the equinovalgus foot deformity.[70,71] This is often associated with either gastrocnemius or gastrocnemius-soleus equinus. As a result of tightness of this muscle compensatory pronation of the foot is required. This often results in dislocation or subluxation of the subtalar and midtarsal joints. Treatment may require lengthening of the Achilles tendon or gastrocnemius recession.

Skewfoot. Another deformity that may be classified in the congenital pathologic type of flatfoot is the skewfoot, sometimes referred to as the "S"-shaped foot, serpentine foot, and "Z" foot deformity. Skewfoot is defined as a complex foot deformity with adduction of the forefoot from the tarsal-metatarsal articulations (metatarsus adductus); the midfoot is in an abducted position relative to the rearfoot and the rearfoot is in a pronated or valgus attitude.[72] Peterson[73] pointed out that skewfoot must be distinguished from that foot with only metatarsus adductus.

The etiology of skewfoot is somewhat unclear. It has been suggested that it may result from an inadequate or improperly applied plaster cast for the treatment of metatarsus adductus. A second hypothesis is that in a patient with untreated metatarsus adductus or varus walk, a twisting effect occurs pushing the hindfoot laterally into calcaneovalgus. A congenital basis for the deformity is also suggested. In this author's experience a 3-month-old infant was examined who had clinical metatarsus adductus and calcaneovalgus. This author has also seen a case in which there was a familial history in the development of skewfoot (Fig. 22-18).

Peterson[73] stated that surgical therapy for skewfoot must address both the forefoot and rearfoot deformities. It has been pointed out that the early supple deformity may become rigid with time. Stabilization of the rearfoot as well as reduction of the metatarsus adductus is recommended. Peterson was careful to point out that "the natural history of untreated cases is unknown, and the wisdom on any treatment for the deformity might be questioned. Long term followup of untreated patients would be beneficial." Berg[72] reported on the identification, classification, and conservative management of metatarsus adductus in skewfoot. He reported that adduction of the forefoot associated with a lat-

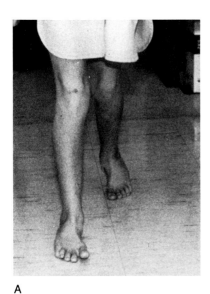

A

Fig. 22-18. (A) Skewfoot deformity in a 9-year-old child. **(B)** Radiographic appearance of skewfoot anteroposterior *(left)* and lateral *(right)* views.

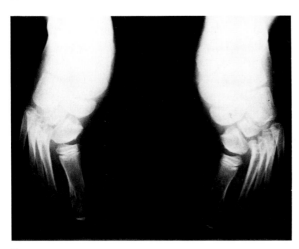

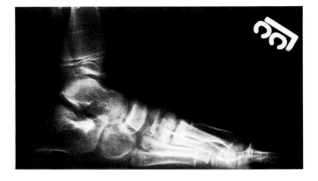

B

eral translation of the middle part of the foot or valgus deformity of the hindfoot or both requires a statically significant increase period in the time for treatment in a cast in order to obtain correction of the forefoot. It was also noted that in the treatment of these patients, whether it be for simple metatarsus adductus or the complex skewfoot deformity, a higher incidence of flatfoot was found at follow-up when a Denis-Browne bar was used as part of the treatment regimen.[72]

Traumatic and Neurologic Flatfoot. Other forms of pathologic flatfoot may be traumatic, such as rupture of the tibialis posterior tendon (although this is uncommon in children, it has been reported), or

associated with neuromuscular diseases such as cerebral palsy (Fig. 22-19).

Cavus Foot

There are multiple etiologies for cavus foot as well as several morphologic varieties. A thorough patient evaluation is required in the assessment of cavus foot prior to any consideration for therapy.

Cavus foot may be idiopathic or may be associated with a variety of congenital and/or neurologic diseases.[74,75] The development of cavus foot is not usually seen before the age of 3 years but may occur (Fig. 22-20). It may begin as a flexible deformity and over time, through functional adaption,

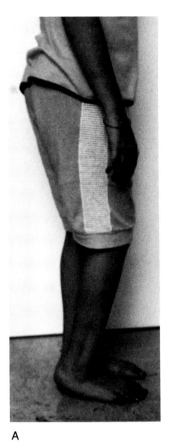

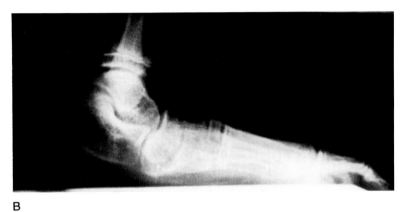

A   B

Fig. 22-19. Spastic flatfoot secondary to cerebral palsy. **(A)** Clinical presentation. **(B)** Note marked equinus of rearfoot on radiography.

turn into a rigid deformity. Traditionally, cavus foot has been associated with Charcot-Marie-Tooth disease and Friedreich's ataxia. However, Exner[76] pointed out, on the basis of personal observation, that he has found that in infancy patients with either of these diseases may have an extreme pes valgoplanus, implying that the cavus foot develops secondarily to the dynamic imbalance with function over time. An etiology involving dynamic imbalance was also supported by Sabir and Lyttle.[77]

The treatment of cavus foot must be directed at managing both the static and dynamic (muscular imbalance) components of the deformity. Early treatment of cavus foot begins with the accurate diagnosis of any underlying disease process. Initial treatment in younger patients may involve passive stretching, manipulation with casting, and the use of orthotics and bracing. Surgical intervention is based upon the deformity and the symptoms. The individual who is functional with a cavus foot, has no plantar lesions, and is experiencing no discomfort does not appear to be a candidate for surgery. The patient with deformity associated with pain and or instability, contractures of the toes that are fixed and unable to function normally in gait require surgical intervention. It is important to remember that, with neuromuscular disease, in addition to correcting the structural deformity, the dynamic imbalances may need to be corrected with the use of appropriately planned muscle and tendon transfers. Surgical management in the younger patient initially may begin with a plantar release, including the plantar fascia and the first layer of the intrinsic muscles.[78] Osseous procedures are recommended for the correction of osseous deformity and to allow stabilization of an unstable foot, especially prior to tendon transfer.[79-82]

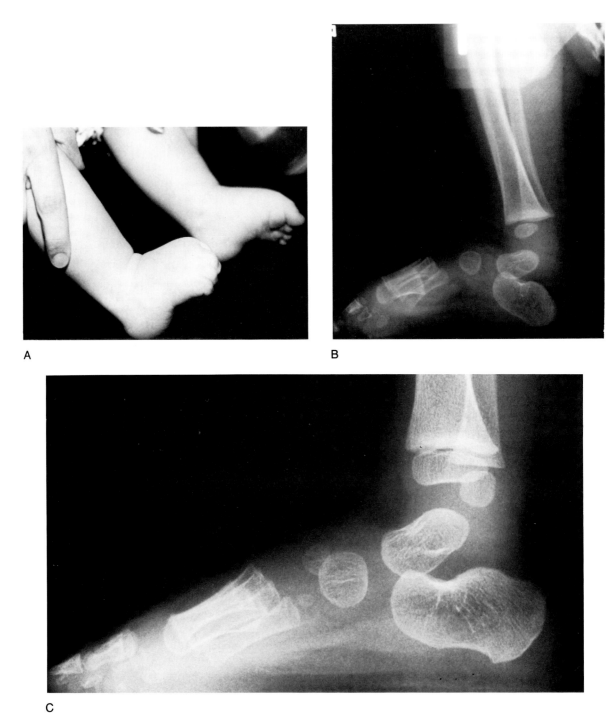

A

B

C

Fig. 22-20. (A) Congenital idiopathic cavus foot in infant. The clinical picture and x-rays are not of the same patient. **(B)** Initial radiographic evaluation. **(C)** Approximately 1 year posttherapy by gentle casting and manipulation.

Metatarsus Adductus

Metatarsus adductus is a common congenital problem seen in the pediatric patient. It is a transverse plane deformity of the metatarsals occurring at the level of the tarsometatarsal joints. The child may present with a "C"-shaped appearance to the foot with a marked lateral prominence at the base of the fifth metatarsal. Upon examination the medial side of the foot is concave and the lateral border is convex. The forefoot cannot be abducted into a neutral position; it may also be in a position of marked varus, hence the term *metatarsus varus*. Metatarsus adductus may be either flexible or rigid; however, the degree of flexibility or rigidity does not appear to correlate with the outcomes of conservative therapy. A functional metatarsus adductus may also be caused by hyperactivity of the abductor hallucis and the short flexor muscles. Metatarsus adductus may also be associated with congenital hip dysplasia and may not occur as the sole orthopedic presentation.

Metatarsus adductus is commonly treated as one of those deformities that the child will "outgrow." Although there is controversy in the literature regarding metatarsus adductus, as Kling and Hensinger[52] pointed out there does not appear to be a method to determine prospectively which feet will resolve spontaneously and which will not; "Non treatment cannot be prescribed for an obvious foot deformity in a child that has a 14% chance of being a persistent deformity later in life and which can be corrected only by a surgical procedure."

The treatment of metatarsus adductus begins with the early recognition of the deformity. As with clubfoot therapy, treatment may begin in infancy. For mild deformities passive stretching by the parents may help promote spontaneous correction. In the foot that demonstrates marked or severe deformity, serial plaster casting in conjunction with stretching prior to the application of a cast is the method of choice. Casting is continued until the metatarsals can be abducted past the midline bisection of the foot and there is reduction of the initial clinical appearance to a more normal foot configuration (Fig. 22-21). In the normal infant stroking of the lateral aspect of the foot will often cause the child to abduct the metatarsals of the forefoot; when the child is able to abduct the meta-

tarsals past the midline after such stroking sufficient correction has been obtained. Maintaining the correction after casting by the use of several commercially available devices or the use of outflair, lace-up, high-top orthopedic oxfords is recommended. Careful fit and the use of padding within these shoes or devices help to maintain the corrected position.[83]

Children may be cast from birth up to the age of 18 months. Greatest success is obtained within the age group from birth to 8 months. The older the child the longer the casting treatment time required to obtain correction of the deformity. In those children who have residual deformity or were untreated and are experiencing symptoms surgical intervention is warranted.

Surgical intervention in the younger child may consist of tarsal, metatarsal, and intertarsal joint release.[84,85] This method may be successful until the squaring off of the metatarsal bases occurs, which may be as late as age 4 or 5. Past this age correction of the deformity can only be obtained by the use of multiple metatarsal osteotomies.[86] An alternative procedure described by Johnson[87] involves chondrotomies of the metatarsals. This procedure was also recommended in place of the soft tissue mobilization of the tarsal, metatarsal, and intermetatarsal articulations.

Juvenile Hallux Valgus

Juvenile hallux valgus is defined as a hallux abductovalgus deformity that occurs in a patient below the age of 20 years (Fig. 22-22). Hallux valgus in the adult may begin in childhood but does not become symptomatic in childhood or adolescence. Juvenile hallux valgus may be the presenting complaint of a child with metatarsus adductus. The intermetatarsal angle in these patients may be small, but they present with a symptomatic bunion and deviation of the great toe. In this deformity, there is an increase in adduction of all the metatarsals as opposed to only the first metatarsal as in a metatarsus primus adductus.

Etiology

In the child, metatarsus primus varus or metatarsus primus adductus has been associated with

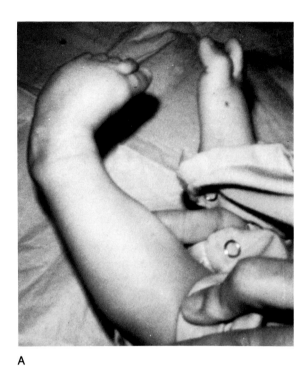

A

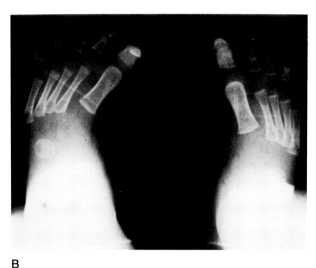

B

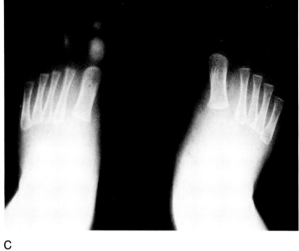

C

Fig. 22-21. **(A)** Severe metatarsus adductus. **(B** and **C)** Radiographic appearance of metatarsus adductus before **(B)** and after **(C)** manipulation and casting.

juvenile hallux valgus. Bohm[4] described the early stages of embryologic development of the first metatarsal. The proximal end of the first metatarsal is at the medial border of the first cuneiform and forms an angle of 50 degrees with the long axis of the embryonic foot, with the remaining metatarsals being in marked adduction. This adduction is seen in the fetus up to the fourth month, gradually re-

ducing until birth. Shoe-deforming factors are considered to be secondary deforming forces in the development of metatarsus primus varus. Hawkins et al.[88] believed that there was a tendency to underestimate the significance of congenital metatarsus primus varus in the development of adolescent hallux valgus deformity. Simmonds and Menelaus[89] also associated metatarsus primus

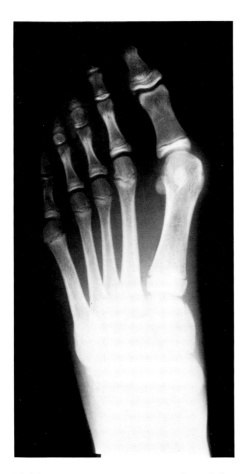

Fig. 22-22. Juvenile hallux abductovalgus deformity.

transferred to the lateral axis of the great toe. Because there was no extensor sheath to fix the tendon to the metatarsal, contraction would increase the deformity. Once the process has started, the lateral displacement of the first digit must increase. They stressed that the deformity was caused primary by displacement of the great toe with widening of the intermetatarsal angle secondarily.

Another theory presented the abductor hallucis as a factor in the development of metatarsus primus varus. Schubert[94] and Tangen[95] suggested that muscle imbalance produced faulty weightbearing and contributed to the formation of metatarsus primus varus and hallux valgus. These authors believed that metatarsus primus adductus resulted from rotation of the great toe changing the line of force of the abductor hallucis tendon. The plantar dislocation of this tendon therefore acts as a plantar flexor of the first metatarsophalangeal joint and places an adductory and valgus rotation onto the great toe.

Another contributing factor to the development of juvenile hallux valgus is ligamentous laxity, such as that in Ehlers-Danlos syndrome.[96] Goldner and Gaines[97] noted a congenital hallux valgus with a short first ray skin contraction and severe deviation of the toe. They stated that the skin contractures and severe deviation of the toe should be treated early. Soft tissue releases and skin grafting may be necessary. Osteotomy with bone graft to elongate the ray may also be required.

Hallux valgus may also result from a disturbance in the metatarsal parabola. A short first metatarsal is prone to the development of hallux valgus; however, both long and short first metatarsal relative lengths have been implicated in the development of hallux valgus. Intermetatarsal angles tend to be higher in those individuals with shorter metatarsals as opposed to those with unusually long first metatarsals.

The biomechanics of the child's foot greatly contribute to hallux valgus formation. The pathomechanical problem most often associated with juvenile hallux valgus is a hypermobile and lax flexible flatfoot deformity with abnormal pronation. This is most noticeable in the child or patient with hallux valgus with a marked rearfoot equinus deformity, who compensates via pronation and demonstrates early heel off and marked unlocking of the midtar-

varus with juvenile hallux valgus. They noted, as did Bonnie and Macnab[90] that metatarsus primus varus is the important aspect needing correction in adolescence to avoid recurrence of the deformity and is a factor in the breakdown in the forefoot.

Truslow,[91] in describing the zig-zag foot and the diamond-shaped foot, cited metatarsus primus varus as the primary anatomic variant and adduction of the hallux as secondary. Lapidus[92] classified hallux valgus into three groups with the most predominant group showing a congenital predisposition to metatarsus primus varus.

Hardy and Clapman[93] presented another theory suggested by Emslie. Their paper suggested that some factor caused a lateral displacement of the distal phalanx of the great toe. They proposed that the pull of the extensor hallucis longus tendon was sal joint. A propulsive gait in children usually develops after age 4 or 5.

The pathomechanical development of hallux abductovalgus was described by Root and co-workers.[98] Stage one is characterized by sagittal and frontal plane subluxation of the first metatarsophalangeal joint. This is accompanied by hypermobility of the first ray, instability of the hallux in propulsion, and toe off in the propulsive phase occurring off the medial plantar aspect of the hallux, and lateral subluxation of the great toe. This is followed in stage two by the hallux abductus deformity; at this stage functional adaptation may occur. Subluxation in the juvenile foot leads to the formation of abnormal bone structure. Juvenile bone rapidly adapts to abnormal changes and positions by changing shapes, following Wolfe's law. Stage three initiates the formation of metatarsus primus varus or metatarsus primus adductus and displacement of the sesamoids. Stage four results in endstage hallux valgus with dislocation of the metatarsophalangeal joint.

Patient Evaluation

The evaluation of hallux valgus in the juvenile begins with a thorough clinical and radiographic examination of the patient.

Clinical Examination. A thorough biomechanical evaluation of the adolescent or young adult presenting with juvenile hallux valgus is mandatory. The etiology of the flexible flatfoot must be known before treatment can be instituted. Muscular evaluation, especially muscle testing, may elucidate the etiology of juvenile bunion deformity. A dynamic imbalance of the muscles of the foot can lead to the development of a flexible flatfoot as seen with anterior tibial weakness or paralysis, and disorders involving the posterior tibial tendon. A flatfoot may also be neurologic in origin, such as that associated with cerebral palsy or spasticity of the gastrocnemius muscle or gastrocnemius-solus complex.

The first metatarsophalangeal joint in juvenile hallux valgus must be evaluated for limitation of motion, including not only direction and quality of motion, but whether the joint is tract bound. The integrity of the soft tissue of the foot should be examined as part of the differential diagnosis. Patients presenting with suspected ligamentous laxity should be evaluated to determine if it is contributing to the deformity. Too often, only the first metatarsophalangeal joint is given consideration and the remainder of the foot is not treated as a functional unit.

Radiographic Examination. Radiographic evaluation should be conducted using standard angle and basic gait, dorsoplantar, lateral, and axial sesamoidal views. The following points should be evaluated in the dorsoplantar view. The *metatarsus adductus angle* is evaluated to determine the amount of metatarsus adductus and the possibility of a metatarsus adductus deformity; the metatarsus adductus angle is 14 to 16 degrees in a normal adult foot. In an evaluation of a juvenile an increase greater than 25 degrees is significant enough to contemplate surgical intervention. Surgical intervention may also be necessary when the foot is symptomatic with a mild increase of metatarsus adductus angle in a child beyond the age at which casting is practical for the treatment of the metatarsus adductus.

The *talocalcaneal angle* is an indication of the degree of pronation present in the rearfoot. A talocalcaneal angle of 25 degrees is considered abnormal. Abduction of the cuboid in a dorsoplantar view is indicative of midtarsal joint pronation.

Goldner and Gaines[97] recommended that the *angle formed between the articular surfaces of the first cuneiform and first metatarsal* be measured. If the angle measured is 0 to 25 degrees, realignment and correction of the first metatarsal may be done by osteotomy of the first metatarsal base. If the angle is 25 degrees or greater, a triangular resection of the cuneiform would be required.

Interangle Relationships The relationship of intermetatarsal, hallux abductus, and interphalangeal angles was studied by Hardy and Chapman.[99] They examined normal children from ages 4 to 15; the male-female ratio was approximately 1:1. Their findings revealed the following. The mean hallux abductus angle was 12.0 ± 5.1 degrees. There was no significant difference between the distribution for each sex. When broken down into age groups a progressive increase in lateral displacement of the great toe was observed with increasing age. The mean first metatarsal angle was 7.4 ± 2.1 degrees; the mean male value was 7.33 ± 2.04 degrees and that for females 7.55 ± 2.06 degrees. This difference was found to be statistically significant. No significant increase in the intermetatarsal angle with advancing age in males occured; however, a significant increase with age was seen in the females in this study. The mean interphalangeal angle was 2.7 ± 0.5 degrees; there was no significant difference between the sexes. This displacement decreased with increasing age.

In comparing the children with normal adult controls, a slow increase in displacement of the hallux with age was revealed in the children. This occurred before the age of 14. The intermetatarsal angle increases after the age of 15, and the decrease in interphalangeal angle takes place before the age of 15. Expected ranges for hallux abductus and intermetatarsal angles measured in children and in adults considered by Hardy and Chapman to be normal are listed in Table 22-14A. The mean values are given in Table 22-14B.

Comparison of the mean ranges for the interphalangeal and hallux abductus angles shows no significant difference between children of ages 14 and 15 and adults. A significant difference was seen when comparing the hallux abductus angle of 4 and 5 year-old children with that of adults. The intermetatarsal angle mean value showed a significant difference when compared to adults for both the 4- to 5- and 14- to 15-year-old age groups. A progressive increase in the hallux abductus angle from 4- to

5-year-olds to adults was observed; however, this increase was not seen from 14- to 15-year-olds to adults.

Hardy and Chapman[99] also found the first metatarsal in cases of hallux valgus to have a greater relative metatarsal protrusion than that of the controls. Of the patients studied in 1951, 45 percent indicated an onset of 20 years or less and 30 percent indicated an onset of less than 15 years for their deformity. The authors noted that for a high degree of valgus of the digit and a low intermetatarsal angle, the first metatarsal tends to have greater relative protrusion than the second; in cases of low degree of valgus and high intermetatarsal angle the second metatarsal has a greater relative protrusion. Lundberg and Sulja[100] agreed with Hardy Chapman's results regarding the relative protrusion of the first metatarsal and hallux valgus. However, metatarsus primus varus can lead to an apparent shortening of the first metatarsal.

Treatment

Piggott,[101] in his studies of adolescent hallux valgus, classified first metatarsophalangeal joints into three groups that most surgeons are familiar with: congruous, deviated, or subluxed. In his study he could produce little or no evidence that metatarsus primus varus was the underlying causes of hallux valgus. It was concluded that the structural prognosis of hallux valgus in the adolescent was as follows. Congruity of the joint surfaces can be regarded as normal and indicates that progressive deformity will not occur. Deviation may or may not progress to subluxation, and subluxation indicates that deterioration is likely. Piggott also noted that subluxation of the first metatarsophalangeal joint was seen before closure of the metatarsal and phalangeal epiphysis.

Goldner and Gaines[97] believed that treatment should be initiated while the joint is congruous. They further divided juvenile hallux valgus into congenital cases, with deformity observed in the newborn, and adolescent cases, in which the deformity becomes more evident because of periods of rapid growth between the ages of 8 and 15. Deformity occurs at the extreme of the adolescent group

Table 22-14. Interangle Relationships in Children and Adults

	Child (4–15 Years)	Adult[a] (20+ Years)
A. Expected Ranges		
Hallux abductus angle	2–22°	4–28°
Intermetatarsal angle	3–12°	3–15°
B. Mean Values		
Intermetatarsal angle	7.4± 2.1°	8.5°
Hallux abductus angle	12.0± 5.1°	15.7°
Interphalangeal angle	2.7± 0.5°	—

(Data from Hardy and Chapman.[99])
[a]Considered by Hardy and Chapman to be normal.

from ages 16 to 20 as a result of a final growth spurt, increased weight, and the influence of external forces. Goldner and Gaines also noted that the first cuneiform – metatarsal angle may be horizontal but the epiphysis widens laterally.

In an adult the correct treatment of hallux valgus deformity must be chosen after careful examination both clinically and radiographically. The growing foot of a juvenile adds another dimension to foot surgery; if the proper procedure has not been chosen, the condition may recur after surgery. Thus, a slightly elevated intermetatarsal angle at the time of examination in a child may need greater reduction because of its tendency to increase with age.

Several surgical reviews have been written regarding common procedures performed for juvenile hallux valgus.[102–108] Some procedures have become more popular than others in the management of juvenile hallux valgus. Unfortunately, at times the one-key-fits-all-doors theory is still applied. The correct procedure(s) in any case must be chosen on the basis of clinical and radiographic findings. The procedures can be classified into four categories: proximal osteotomies, distal osteotomies, phalangeal osteotomies, and soft tissue procedures.

Proximal osteotomies are of two basic types, osteotomy of the first metatarsal base or osteotomy of the first metatarsal – cuneiform joint. Osteotomy of the first metatarsal base may be one of three kinds: opening or closing wedges or crescentic osteotomies. These osteotomies are used to correct hallux valgus deformities with an increased intermetatarsal angle. Closing wedge and crescentic osteotomies have a tendency to shorten the metatarsal, and an opening osteotomy is used to gain length for a short metatarsal and requires bone grafting. The metatarsal parabola must be considered in addition to the intermetatarsal angle; in the child, the osteotomy should be performed distal to the epiphyseal plate. Osteotomies of the first metatarsal-cuneiform joint are used in patients with increased metatarsus-cuneiform joint angles. This type of osteotomy was described by Lapidus[92] and Goldner and Gaines.[97] This will reduce the intermetatarsal angle and again cause changes in the metatarsal parabola.

Distal metatarsal osteotomies perform four basic functions. They decrease the intermetatarsal angle, they can realign structural joint abnormalities such as abnormal proximal articular set angles, and they can shorten or maintain the length of a metatarsal. Distal osteotomies are of the Mitchell, Wilson, Austin, or Reverdin (and its various modification) types. The Reverdin-type osteotomy is used in correction of abnormally high proximal articular set angles. This may also be accomplished by biplane osteotomies of the Wilson, Mitchell, or Austin types. Reduction of the intermetatarsal angle can be accomplished by lateral displacement osteotomies. The degree of reduction is smaller than that with the proximal osteotomies, and therefore the lateral displacement osteotomy is used with intermetatarsal angles ranging from 12 to 16 degrees. Distal osteotomies may cause a significant decrease in metatarsal length and therefore should not be used with excessively short metatarsals.

Phalangeal osteotomies are used to correct and increase interphalangeal angles or distal articular set angles. *Soft tissue balancing procedures* such as the McBride procedure may be used in conjunction with metatarsal osteotomies, but are not often used alone in the adolescent.

These procedures are often done in conjunction with correction of other foot deformities such as equinus or flatfoot. It should be explained thoroughly to the patient and parents that even with the above precautions all procedures do not stop recurrence; postoperative biomechanical control is mandatory to aid in maintaining the correction. An important fact to bear in mind, if adequate correction is to be achieved and maintained, is that the child's foot continues to grow. Surgery in the younger child should be reserved for those cases that are symptomatic.

Care must be taken in the performance of procedures to correct juvenile hallux valgus because complications may result. These complications, as with the adult, may include limitation of motion postoperatively, metatarsalgia secondary to shortening, or iatrogenic metatarsus primus elevatus. The latter has been reported to be a significant problem following Mitchell-type procedures. The Austin procedure has been found to be a useful distal osteotomy in this type of patient.[108]

Digital Problems

BRACHYMETATARSALIA/ CONGENITAL SHORT METATARSAL

Brachymetatarsalia is a congenital shortening of one or more metatarsals. This deformity is not uncommon, with shortening of the first metatarsal (metatarsis primus atavicus) being the most frequently encountered and shortening of the fourth metatarsal occurring second most frequently according to Tachdjian.[128] Metatarsus varus and talipes equinovarus may be associated with a shortened first metatarsal, although either occurring as a primary deformity is rare.[128] Shortened metatarsals are also seen in patients with pseudohypoparathyroidism and pseudopseudohypoparathyroidism.[129]

SYNDACTYLISM

Syndactylism may occur as a developmental defect as a result of an arrest of fetal development between the sixth and eighth weeks. Etiologies may include a nutritional deficiency, ring constriction syndrome, indiscriminate use of radiation, and perhaps thalidomide.[130] It may be classified as complete when the web extends to the end of the digits involved and incomplete when it does not. When there is only soft tissue in the web it is classified as simple; when the web contains abnormal bone it is termed complicated.[131] Syndactylism is seen more commonly in males; the overall incidence is 1 : 1,000 to 1 : 3,000.[132]

CONGENITAL CURLY TOE (VARUS TOE)

Congenital curly toe is a common defect in which one or more toes are bent plantarward, medially deviated, and rotated laterally at the distal interphalangeal joint.[133] Therefore, the terminal portion of the affected toe curls under the adjacent toe. This is usually bilateral, symmetric, and associated with a high familial incidence.[128]

CONGENITAL DIGITUS MINIMUS VARUS

Congenital digitus minimus varus, a common familial deformity referring to an overriding fifth toe, is caused by subluxation of the fifth metatarsophalangeal joint dorsomedially with hyperextension and adduction of the fifth toe across the base of the fourth toe.[128] Therefore the extensor tendon is shortened, the dorsal skin surface between the fourth and fifth toes is taut, and the capsule of the metatarsophalangeal joint is contracted dorsomedially.[133] This is often bilateral.

MICRODACTYLISM

Microdactylism (small or underdeveloped toes) may be due to an embryologic arrest and is frequently seen in association with other conditions, such as Apert's disease or Streeter's dysplasia.[134] Usually this does not cause any major deformity or disability and treatment is not necessary.[133]

MACRODACTYLISM

Macrodactylism refers to hypertrophy or gigantism of one or more toes.[128] It may be caused by neurofibromatosis or by congenital hyperplasia of lymphatic or adipose tissue.[133]

POLYDACTYLISM

Polydactylism is the term for supernumerary digits on the foot. It can be preaxial (meaning medial to the great toe), postaxial (lateral to the fifth toe), or central. Polydactylism can be transmitted as an autosomal-dominant trait or through mutant genes and is more common in blacks and females. Other common associated defects include tibial hypoplasia, Ellis–van Creveld chrondroectodermal dysplasia, and Jenne's infantile thoracic dystrophy. These conditions should be excluded by a thorough history, physical, and workup.[128]

CONGENITAL HALLUX VARUS

Congenital hallux varus is the deformity that includes medial deformity of the great toe at the metatarsophalangeal joint. There are three types described in the literature. The first is primary type, which is not associated with any other congenital anomaly. A tight fibrous band extends from the medial side of the great toe to the base of the first metatarsal that pulls the great toe medially. The second type is associated with congenital deformities of the forefoot, including hallux varus with metatarsus varus, hallux varus with an isolated brachymetatarsalia of the first metatarsal, and hallux varus with supernumerary bones or toes.[128,135,136] The third type includes hallux varus with skeletal developmental abnormalities such as seen in diastrophic dwarfism.

EPIPHYSEAL PLATE INJURY

In considering physeal injuries, classification is of paramount importance in communicating to the physician the extent of the injury. This aids in the determination of the appropriate method of treatment and improves the potential outcome of the injury. Classification of physeal injuries has been described by Poland,[109,110] Weber,[111] Aitken,[112] and Salter and Harris.[113] In this section the Salter-Harris classification of physeal injuries is reviewed since it is the most widely used (Fig. 22-23).

Salter-Harris Classification

Type I

In this injury the epiphysis is completely separated from the metaphysis without radiologic evidence of a metaphyseal fragment attached to the displaced epiphysis. It is produced by a shearing or avulsion force and is commonly seen in infants.[114,115] It may occur in pathologic fractures associated with rickets, scurvy, or osteomyelitis.[116] Reduction is usually not necessary and growth is not usually disturbed.

Type II

In this injury the fracture plane travels transversely through the cartilage plate for a variable distance before exiting through the metaphysis on the side opposite the initiation of the fracture. It is produced by a shearing or avulsion force and is the most common physeal fracture. It is found frequently in children over the age of 10.[117-121] When seen on x-ray, the metaphyseal fragment is referred to as the Thurston Holland sign.[122] In a Type II injury, reduction is easily achieved and growth is usually not arrested.

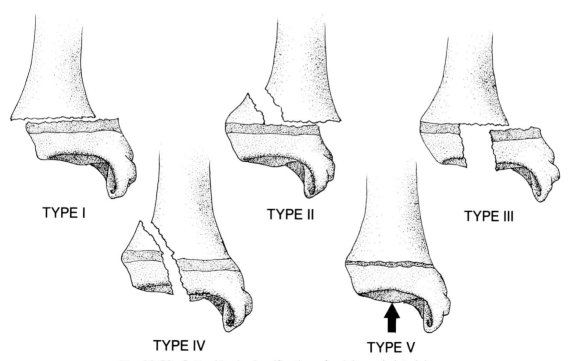

Fig. 22-23. Salter-Harris classification of epiphyseal plate injury.

Type III

In this rare injury, an intra-articular fracture of the epiphysis occurs in which the fracture plane travels through the epiphysis to the physis, where it then runs parallel with the growth plate to the periphery. It is produced by an intra-articular shearing force. Without anatomic reduction, there is a higher incidence of growth arrest.[113,123]

Type IV

In this injury, the fracture plane begins at the articular surface of the epiphysis, travels through the physis, and exits through the metaphysis. It is very important to achieve perfect anatomic reduction, preferably with open reduction and wire fixation; otherwise bony bridging across the physis may occur, leading to an early partial growth arrest.[113,123]

Type V

In this rare injury, a severe compression force is transmitted through the epiphysis to a segment of the physis, crushing the physeal cells. It is usually not suspected until later when a growth arrest develops.[124] Prognosis is poor with this type of injury.[113] Two nontraumatic causes for this injury are metaphyseal osteomyelitis (infection)[125] and epiphyseal aseptic necrosis (circulatory embarrassment).[126]

Rang's Type VI Epiphyseal Injury

In this injury, a peripheral bruise or injury to the perichondral ring or associated periosteum at the edge of the physis may cause an osseous wedge to develop between the epiphysis and metaphysis, leading to a partial growth arrest or angular deformity.[127]

Congenital Talipes Equinovarus

Franz Grill, M.D.

The term *talipes equinovarus* is derived from Latin: *talipes* is a combination of the words *talus* and *pes; equinus* means "horselike" (the heel in plantar flexion), and *varus* means inverted and adducted. In a not only descriptive but specific definition based on pathologic findings, the clubfoot is a medial and plantar displacement (subluxation or dislocation) of the talocalcaneonavicular joint (Fig. 22-24).

ETIOLOGY

Since the first written description by Hippocrates around 400 B.C. the congenital clubfoot has proved to be a challenge for any orthopedic surgeon as well as a subject with controversial and unresolved aspects. It is a complex deformity involving all of the bones of the foot. The incidence is 1 : 1,000 live births. The sex ratio is approximately 2 males to 1 female. It is more often unilateral than bilateral.

The genetics of congenital idiopathic talipes equinovarus is not yet well defined. Bailey reported a multifactorial inheritance pattern.[137] The incidence of clubfoot deformity among first-degree relatives is 20 to 30 times higher than the normal incidence. The incidence of the deformity changes depending on racial background and in the Polynesian population is 6.81 : 1,000 births.

The etiology of congenital talipes equinovarus remains unclear and controversial, although many theories have been advanced. Primary muscular imbalance, primary rotational deformity of the talus, a localized form of arthrogryposis, and a neuromuscular disease are being discussed as possible causes for the deformity. Histologic studies of muscles in congenital clubfoot have been disappointing and conflicting. In 1981 Handelsmann and Badalmente studied, with the electron microscope, 90 muscle biopsy specimens that were obtained from 13 patients who had clubfoot.[138] They reported the presence of ultrastructural abnormalities, which they interpreted as being of neurogenic origin, in all of the muscle samples that were examined. They concluded that an underlying neurogenic disorder could be important in the pathogenesis of congenital clubfoot.

Ponseti and his coauthors reported studies demonstrating an abnormality of the fascia and sheath of the posterior tibial muscle.[139] In contrast, Bill and Versfeld[140] studied specimens electromyographically that were obtained from muscle in 25 patients who had idiopathic clubfoot. They con-

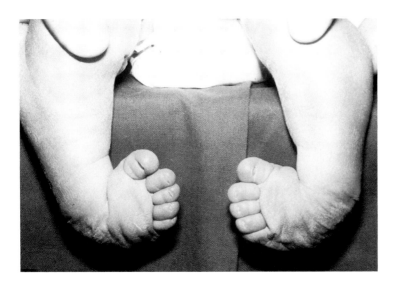

Fig. 22-24. Congenital talipes equino-varus. (first category, stiff-stiff) feet.

cluded that, with conventional electromyographic techniques, they were unable to demonstrate the presence of abnormalities suggesting neuropathic or myopathic changes in patients who had congenital idiopathic clubfoot. The same conclusion was published by Irani and Sherman, who dissected 11 extremities with equinovarus in stillborns and found no primary abnormalities of nerves, vessels, muscles, or tendon insertions.[141] In every specimen the neck of the talus was found to be short and distorted and the anterior portion of the talus was found to rotate in a medial and plantar direction. The deviation of the anterior end of the talus was believed to be the primary fault.

PATHOLOGIC ANATOMY

The pathologic changes observed in talipes equinovarus may be either primary (congenital) or secondary (adaptive). Bony deformities, articular malalignments, and soft tissue changes were investigated by dissections of more than 40 talipes equinovarus cases in fetuses in different stages of fetal development by several authors.[142–147] These dissections have shown that the principal structural deformity in clubfoot is medial and plantar deviation of the neck of the talus. On the inferior surface

of the talus the anterior and middle facets are distorted and fused into a single misshapen articular surface that is tilted medially and downward. The calcaneus is much less deformed than the talus. However, determining the relative positional relationship between the bones of the hindfoot is more difficult than simply describing the morphology of the individual bones. Dissection techniques destroy the various restraining ligaments, thus destroying the exact rotational alignment of the bones. To understand the deformity, a functional analysis of clubfoot deformity compared to a normal foot can be helpful.

Functionally speaking a foot can be divided into three entities: (1) the lower leg with tibia and fibula, forming the ankle mortise; (2) the talus; and (3) the entire subtalar region. The lower leg is the origin of muscles, nearly all of which have their insertions on the foot (i.e., on the subtalar plate). The talus is located between the lower leg and the subtalar foot region and its development is influenced by a balanced or unbalanced action of the muscles running from lower leg to foot. Whereas in the normal foot the relationship of pronators and supinators is well balanced (Fig. 22-25), in the case of clubfoot deformity — irrespective of the cause — the fetal foot is in the equinovarus position and a muscular imbalance in favor of supinators is seen with the posterior tibialis muscle in the leading role. The function of the tibialis posterior is a three-dimensional one (Fig. 22-26), and one has to

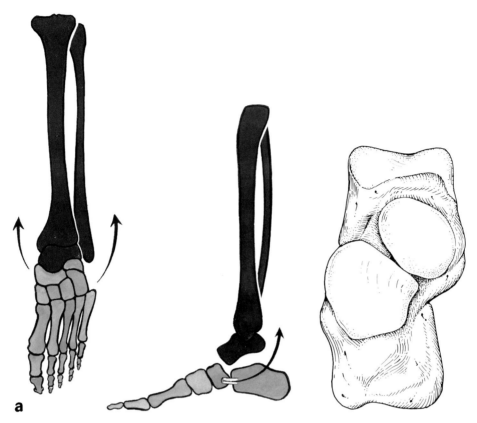

Fig. 22-25. (A) Normal foot. The relationship of the pronators and supinators is well balanced. **(B)** In a normal foot in neutral position the articular surface of the calcaneus for the cuboid is well to the lateral side of the long axis of the leg.

keep in mind that this muscle does not have its insertion on the navicular bone only, but also plantarly from the base of all metatarsals to the calcaneus. The medioplantar insertion of the tibialis posterior results in an equinus position with plantar flexion and ventralization of the talus (nutcracker effect) in the ankle joint, in the sagittal plane. Consequently, the anterior one-quarter to one-third of its superior anterior surface is uncovered. That means that the wider anterior part of the dome of the talus is outside the ankle mortise, and the narrower posterior part therefore has more latitude in the ankle joint (Fig. 22-27A). In the frontal plane the activity of the tibialis posterior results in a supinating position of the whole subtalar foot (Fig. 22-27B), and in the horizontal plane in a subtalar horizontal internal rotation (Fig. 22-27C). The center of this rotation is the interosseous talocalcanea ligament. The internal rotation of the entire subtalar region results in an approximation of the calcaneus to the fibula (Fig. 22-27D). This subtalar rotation consequently has to be considered a principal component of the clubfoot deformity and explains the frequently observed internal rotation, which is never a result of internal torsion of the lower leg. Confirmation of this rotation is possible clinically as well as by computed tomography (Fig. 22-28).

The internally rotated position of the clubfoot has always been the subject of controversy. The internal torsion of the tibia, the internal rotation of the talus in the bimalleolar joint, the external rotation of the tibia, and the abnormal position of the tibiofibular syndesmosis resulting in retroposition

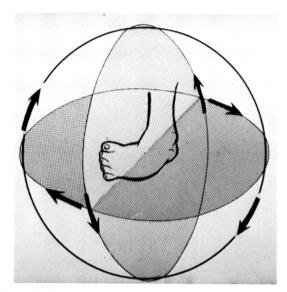

Fig. 22-26. Three-dimensional function of the tibialis posterior.

of the fibula have been postulated as possible causes for the internal rotation deformity in clubfoot. The internal rotation of the calcaneus beneath the talus was emphasized and reported first by Bösch[148] in 1953, and was also stressed by McKay in 1982.[149] This was also reported by Simons and Sarrafian in a 7-month stillborn fetus that had a congenital clubfoot.[14X]

With the rapid growth of the tarsal bones in the fetus, the pull of the contracted calcaneonavicular and tibionavicular ligaments and the posterior tibial tendon will progressively displace the navicular medially and plantarward toward the medial malleolus. An accessory articulation may even develop. The talus on its medial side is narrowed by the navicular and medial malleolus and the fibrocartilage between. Its growth expansion is now limited on the medial side, and there is more growth expansion on the lateral convex side, which leads to an external rotation of the body of the talus.

By an analysis with three-dimensional computer modeling Herzberg and his colleagues[150] found that the clubfoot talus showed 14 degrees of external rotation of its body and 45 degrees of internal rotation of its neck, compared to 5 degrees of internal rotation of the talar body and 25 degrees internal rotation of the talar neck in a normal foot. The calcaneus in a clubfoot is internally rotated 20 to 30 degrees; in a normal foot the calcaneus is externally

rotated 5 degrees. This rotation in relation to the bimalleolar axis can be shown clearly by means of computed tomography (Fig. 22-28A). The cuboid bone has to follow the position of the navicular, talus, and calcaneus, thus developing a deformity that is located not only medially but also laterally (Fig. 22-28B). The cuneiforms as well as the metatarsals contribute to the deformity as a result of the primary deformity. The foot is composed of two columns. The lateral column consists of the os calcis, cuboid, and fourth and fifth metatarsals. The medial column consists of the talus, navicular, three cuneiforms, and the first, second, and third metatarsals. Since the medial and lateral columns are joined, a displacement on the medial side cannot take place without displacement on the lateral side (Fig. 22-28B).

Around the skeletal deformity can be found soft tissue contractures according to the shape and position of the bones. The soft tissues on the medial and posterior aspects of the foot and ankle are shortened. The Achilles tendon inserts more medially and anteriorly on the calcaneus, owing to the lateral shift of the posterior part of the heel. On the plantar aspect of the foot the plantar aponeurosis as well as the abductor hallucis, the short toe flexors, and the abductor digiti quinti are shortened. (A cavus deformity in a clubfoot, however, is usually not seen before walking.) The most important soft tissue contractures are the plantar calcaneonavicular ligament, the tibionavicular ligament, the superior medial and plantar parts of the talonavicular capsule, the posterior tibial tendon with its wide insertions, the master knot of Henry that envelopes the flexor hallucis longus and flexor digitorum longus tendons as they cross each other, the posterior talocalcaneal ligament, the posterior capsule of the tibiotalar joint, the Achilles tendon, and the interosseous ligament. Of special interest is the posterior calcaneofibular ligament. This ligament is very strong. Whereas in a normal foot it takes an oblique direction, in a clubfoot it is extremely shortened and runs in a vertical direction. According to Hosking and Scott,[147] the release of this ligament frees the mobility of the subtalar joint and increases dorsiflexion of the ankle joint by 45 percent. The pathologic changes vary according to the severity of the bony and articular deformity and the degree of soft tissue contracture.

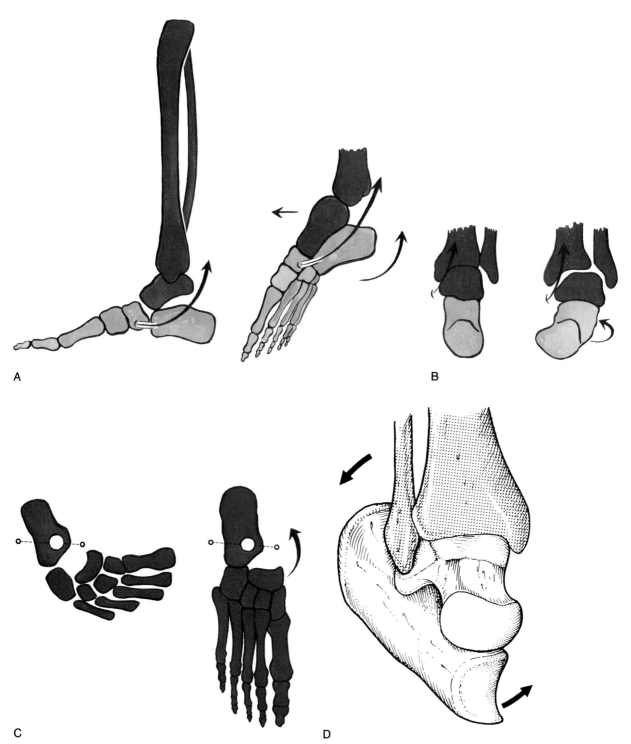

Fig. 22-27. **(A)** Clubfoot, sagittal plane: the medioplantar insertion of the tibialis posterior results in an equinus position with plantar flexion and ventralization of the talus (nutcracker effect). In this position the posterior part of the superior articular surface of the talus, which is narrower than the frontal part, articulates with the ankle mortise. **(B)** Clubfoot, frontal plane: the activity of the tibialis posterior results in a supinating position of the whole subtalar foot. **(C)** Clubfoot, horizontal plane: the activity of the tibialis posterior results in a subtalar horizontal internal rotation. The center of this rotation is in the area of the interosseous talocalcanear ligament. **(D)** The medial rotation of the calcaneus in the horizontal plane displaces its posterior tuberosity laterally toward the fibular malleolus and brings the anterior end of the calcaneus beneath the head of the talus instead lateral of it.

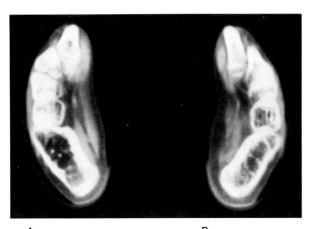

A   B

Fig. 22-28. Computed tomography of a clubfoot. **(A)** The medial displacement of the calcaneus in the horizontal plane with lateral positioning of its posterior tuberosity toward the fibular malleolus is demonstrated. **(B)** A displacement on the medial side (talonavicular joint) cannot take place without displacement on the lateral side. The tomograph shows clearly the dislocation of the cuboid in relation to the calcaneus.

CLASSIFICATION

It is important to differentiate talipes equinovarus from postural clubfoot. In the latter type of foot the deformity is mild and can be readily corrected to neutral position by passive manipulation. Free passive dorsal flexion is possible. In the congenital form it is of importance that talipes equinovarus may be associated with multiple congenital malformations, or be a part of a generalized developmental syndrome (constriction band syndrome, diastrophic dwarfism, arthrogryposis, Freeman-Sheldon syndrome, Larsen's syndrome). The idiopathic clubfoot also must be distinguished from acquired types of clubfoot, which in the newborn is relatively easy. Causes of acquired talipes equinovarus are either neuromuscular (meningitis, polio, spinal deformities, cerebral palsy, diastematomyelia) or posttraumatic (spinal or sciatic nerve damage, lower leg trauma, Volkmann's contracture, distal tibial epiphysial damage).

In the idiopathic clubfoot an ideal type of classification has yet to be found. There are several degrees of severity that cannot be calculated and quantified objectively.

All classifications of congenital talipes equinovarus are determined by the degree of manual reducibility as well as the morphology of the deformity itself. At birth the best classification remains the clinical one. The examination must be very methodical. The deformity in itself is not the most important factor; rather, its reducibility is most important. One must take time to examine the child, locate the position of the external malleolus, test the mobility of all joints, and note any visible skin creases, the presence (if any) of plantar cavus retraction, and the degree of equinovarus intensity and of stiffness. Some severely deformed feet have a significant potential for reducibility and therefore will easily be corrected. Others, more mildly deformed, are stiff and will be more difficult to treat. Dimeglio and colleagues[151] have outlined four categories of feet.

Category 1: The Stiff-Stiff Foot

The foot is generally short and stiff. It is still called "teratogenic." Reducibility of the horizontal and sagittal planes does not exceed 20 percent. The equinus deformity is severe; varus of the calcaneus exceeds 45 degrees. There often exists a severe posterior bend, an inner bend, and plantar retraction. This group accounts for approximately 15 to 18 percent of clubfoot cases. These feet are often considered to represent a somewhat limited form of arthrogryposis (distal arthrogryposis syndrome). This type of clubfoot is often bilateral. A unilateral stiff-stiff foot is always very suspect and warrants an investigation into medullary damage and in particular dysraphism. It is in this category that the poorest results, as well as recurrence, are found.

Category 2: The Stiff-Soft Foot

The percentage of reducibility is less than 50. The foot is resistant but partially reducible as regards the horizontal and sagittal planes. This category is by far the one most frequently encountered, representing nearly 60 percent of all cases.

Category 3: The Soft-Stiff Foot

This category of clubfoot represents 20 to 25 percent of all cases. The reducibility is considerable, exceeding 50 percent on the horizontal and sagittal planes. The varus angle is less than 20 degrees. Generally the foot is long. In this category, when treatment has been well done, successful results exceed 90 percent.

Category 4: The Soft-Soft Foot

This foot may also be called postural or resolvent, and does not require surgery. Orthopedic treatment using casts or physiotherapy, when well carried out, is sufficient.

RADIOGRAPHIC FINDINGS

The purpose of roentgenography is to define precisely the anatomic relationship of the talocalcaneonavicular, tibiotalar, midtarsal, and tarsometatarsal joints. X-ray examination at birth is not a practice used by all, but it can be a valuable diagnostic tool. X-rays can help in noting small malformations of the metatarsals, hypoplasia of the talus and os calcis, or even a discrete abnormality, subtle as it may be, of the fibula or the tibia.

It is only toward the sixth month of life that an x-ray examination can give meaningful information. The best x-rays are those in which the foot is in a dynamic position, to test its reducibility. Anteroposterior and lateral x-ray studies are usually sufficient. It is imperative that the patient's feet be placed in identical positions and that a standard technique be utilized. The placing of the feet in the maximally corrected position according to the technique described by Simons[146] is recommended. The child is placed in a sitting position with his or her knees and hips flexed at right angles, and the feet pressed on the cassette with their medial borders parallel and touching each other. The forefoot is manually pushed into maximal abduction and the ankle into maximal dorsiflexion, or as far as the equinus deformity will allow. An anteroposterior roentgenogram is made with the x-ray tube angled 30 degrees from the perpendicular to the cassette. Lateral radiographs are made with the foot in maximum dorsiflexion. In the anteroposterior projection the anteroposterior talocalcaneal angle (normally 20 to 40 degrees), the talocalcaneal divergence (0 to +1), the calcaneal–second metatarsal angle (15 to 20 degrees), and the navicular position before and after ossification are measured. On the lateral radiograph the lateral talocalcaneal angle (35 to 50 degrees), the calcaneal–first metatarsal angle (140 to 180 degrees), the tibiotalar angle (dorsiflexion 70 to 100 degrees; plantarflexion 120 to 180 degrees), the tibiocalcaneal angle (dorsiflexion 25 to 60 degrees), and the navicular position are measured according to the level of the talus (Fig. 22-29).

It must be accepted that it is always a very difficult task to achieve an excellent x-ray of a clubfoot, and that roentgenographs obtained can only partially reflect reality.

TREATMENT

The objectives of the treatment of talipes equinovarus are: (1) to achieve concentric reduction of the dislocation of the talocalcaneonavicular joint; (2) to restore normal articular alignment of the tarsus and the ankle; (3) to establish muscle balance and maintain the reduction; and (4) to provide a mobile foot with normal function and weightbearing. There is no doubt that treatment of the clubfoot deformity has to be started immediately after birth, within the first days of life. With only very

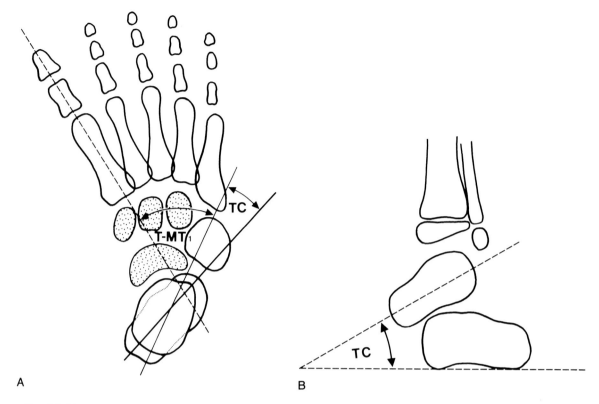

Fig. 22-29. Measurements of angles in the roentgenogram of a clubfoot. **(A)** Anteroposterior view. *TC,* talocalcaneal angle (normal 20 to 40 degrees); *T-MT$_1$,* talo–first metatarsal angle (normal 0 to 15 degrees). **(B)** Lateral view. *TC,* talocalcaneal angle (normal 35 to 50 degrees).

few exceptions primary treatment should always be conservative.

Conservative Treatment

Conservative treatment can be performed by casting or by physiotherapy combined with taping and splinting. Since the time of Hippocrates the classical concept of clubfoot treatment has consisted of exerting pressure on three points of the foot: the forefoot from medially, the hindfoot from medially, and the head of the talus from laterally. Bösch revealed the contradictions of the classical redressment treatment as early as 1950.[152] Bösch's method was new insofar as he exerted pressure on the calcaneus from laterally, and thus intuitively

corrected the most important deformity, the subtalar horizontal internal rotation.[153–159] It is the objective of conservative treatment to normalize the development of the muscles by way of stretching the soft tissue contractures, to establish a dynamic balance of the muscles and to relocate the navicular anterior to the talus (Fig. 22-30).

As far as the application of pressure is concerned, the correctional forces are the opposite of the forces of the deformity. In a one-step maneuver, pressure is applied with one index finger on the craniolateral aspect of the calcaneus, from externally to medially, to move the calcaneus away from the fibula and out of equinus and varus. This manipulation is supported by the exertion of pressure with the other index finger or thumb on the lateral arch at the level of the calcaneocuboid joint. Thus

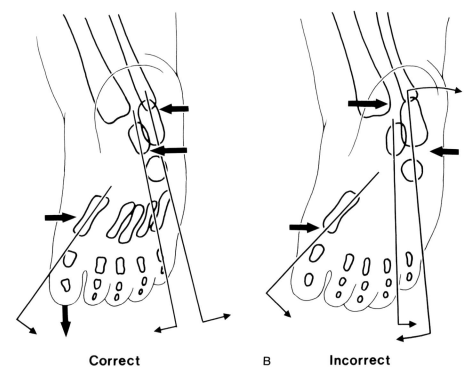

A   **Correct**   B   **Incorrect**

Fig. 22-30. Conservative treatment of clubfoot by exertion of pressure (drawing according to original by Bösch.[152]) **(A)** Bösch's method: exertion of pressure on the posterior tuberosity of the calcaneus from laterally (craniolaterally) "away from the fibula" and plantar-lateral at the processus anterior of calcaneus, thus correcting varus, equinus, and medial rotation. **(B)** Classical method is counteractive to correction; the calcaneus is pressed even more into its pathologic position below the talus.

the anterior part of the calcaneus is elevated and the varus corrected (Fig. 22-31). With this manipulation it is possible to get a correction of the varus, the subtalar rotation, and perhaps in some cases also the equinus. Emphasis is placed on the fact that a common mistake has to be avoided—obtaining correction by pressure from laterally against the cuboid and from medially against the calcaneus and forefoot. This is counteractive to correction because the anterior end of the calcaneus is pressed even more into its pathologic position below the talus; the posterior end of the calcaneus (i.e., the posterior surface of the calcaneus) is pressed farther out into its incorrect position in the direction of the fibula and the false rotation of the foot is reinforced. It is also important to know that a rocker-bottom deformity can be the consequence of increased pressure on the forefoot against the equinus position. In the correction of the equinus

position, patience must be exercised. Nevertheless, the correction should be a one-step maneuver; that means that there is no use correcting first adduction and then supination in full equinus and keeping this equinus position strictly throughout the first weeks of treatment.

By correcting the deformities mainly from the hindfoot (the forefoot is only manipulated by stretching and gentle abduction) there is no danger of producing a rocker-bottom deformity. Above-knee plaster casts should be used routinely and the cast has to be changed as frequently as possible. This is usually two times a week within the first 3 weeks of life and then once a week. The foot should be corrected within 6 to 8 weeks. To determine correction it is necessary to use x-ray monitoring.

After a successful correction femur-tibia splints are applied, and the parents have to perform regular physical exercises. Treatment is carried out pas-

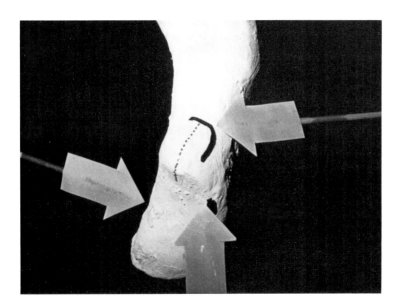

Fig. 22-31. Exertion of pressure: where and how to do it.

sively and actively by manipulation of the joints and stimulation of the muscles responsible for pronation. If the foot is not corrected by conservative methods in 6 to 10 weeks or if there is relapse of the deformity, surgical correction is indicated. If feet with positional deformity (grade IV) are eliminated, about 85 percent of all clubfeet require surgical correction, so the chance of correction of a clubfoot by manipulation is fairly poor. Nevertheless, the treatment with manipulation and plaster is important because it facilitates handling of the soft tissues and provides a better starting point should surgery become necessary. It must be stated, however, that casting may lead to problems by using excessive pressure and omitting joint manipulations when changing plasters. Joints that do not get moved become stiff.

A new concept of conservative treatment that was introduced by Bensahel in France[160-162] seems to give better results than casting, by combining continuous manipulations and taping. This is a meticulous treatment to be done on a daily basis, necessitating expert hands. After several months of treatment, if the evaluation shows a satisfactory correction the foot is held in the corrected position in a special above-knee splint that should be worn for 18 hours daily, until walking age. The use of a Denis-Browne splint should not be recommended, because of the possible recurrence of equinus de-

formity. Passive stretching and manipulation have to be performed on a regular basis. Corrective tarsopronator (Antivarus) shoes are used when the child starts walking. To make sure that the deformity has been corrected sufficiently, the following criteria for correction should always be kept in mind: normal shape of the foot, no rocker-bottom deformity, no medial or dorsal skin crease, free dorsiflexion in the ankle joint of 20 degrees, normal alignment of the foot and leg, and normal roentgenograms. However, if there is no evidence of continued improvement or response to conservative treatment at an age of 3 to 6 months, surgery should be performed.

Operative Treatment

Many operative procedures have been described in the literature and nearly all have merit. Nevertheless, the surgical approach for the clubfoot correction today is still controversial. This is because we do not know the etiology, even experts on this topic do not agree on pathomorphology, there are different methods and quality of preoperative management, and—last but not least—no two clubfeet are alike. Consequently, each foot must be evaluated carefully and dealt with in the appropriate manner. It is surely a mistake for the surgeon to adapt all feet to a particular operation. To a certain degree clubfoot surgery has to be an "à la carte" treatment.

There are some facts that should be kept in mind before surgery is decided on and performed. Walking and weightbearing on an uncorrected clubfoot increases the deformity. With any operation the joints that are released become more rigid than before. Undercorrection leads to relapse, and overcorrection to severe foot problems during adolescence without the possibility of repair. The first operation should be the last. There is no surgical method that results in a normal foot in shape *and* function. In general, excellent results are exceptional. Nevertheless, any clubfoot should be afforded an adequate, strictly followed treatment.

Operative correction immediately after birth should be the exception. This is supported by the fact that in a newborn anesthesiologic and surgical problems spell a higher risk of poor outcome because of the very small anatomy. Therefore, only few authors advocate surgical correction immediately after birth. The first operation is indicated when conservative treatment fails to show further success. In most cases this is between the ages of 2 and 6 months (average age 3 months). Turco[163] advocated not performing the first surgical correction before walking. He suggested waiting to see the fully developed deformity, which one is then able to correct in one surgical intervention, thus avoiding reoperations. A further argument to postpone the procedure to an age of 12 to 24 months is to minimize the risk of operating on unrecognized neuromuscular or other nonidiopathic clubfeet and on patients with a plantar-flexed talus.

Where surgical treatment is concerned, several "cultural" influences as well as strategies are superimposed. An English strategy, based on Attenborough's principles,[164] was taken up by Lloyd-Roberts and co-workers.[165] This strategy is dominated by an early posterior release around the third month of life, with elongation of the Achilles tendon, tibialis posterior and flexor, with postero-internal release, posterolateral release, and liberation of the peroneal "sheath." This surgery is often sufficient, but further surgery may become necessary during the growing years for internal release and plantar release.

The strategy defended by Turco[163,166,167] is mainly inspired by Codivilla's work. The first phase, posterior release, includes cutting of the calcaneoperoneal (i.e., posterior calcaneofibular) or tibioperoneal (i.e., posterior inferior tibiofibular) ligaments, and is completed by a second internal phase that consists of subtalar release.

The strategy defended by Simons and McKay involves extensive surgery, straight away, often facilitated by a Cincinnati incision, that elongates practically all the tendons, opening up the foot quite extensively. While McKay[149] preserves the interosseous talocalcaneal ligament, Simons[143] prefers to cut this ligament and pays meticulous attention to repositioning of the bones in order to avoid overcorrection by pin fixation of the talocalcaneal, calcaneocuboid, and talonavicular joints, and uses X-rays taken during the operation (Fig. 22-32).

The "à la carte" strategy is defended by the French school, where posterior and internal release operations are almost always performed but where further interventions, be they plantar, mediotarsal, or calcaneocuboid, are carried out only as necessary. In the experience of the author and in the German school dominated by Imhäuser, in the majority of cases lengthening of the Achilles tendon combined with posterior capsulotomy with particularly exact preparation, and cutting of the peroneal tendon sheath and the posterior calcaneofibular ligament, has proved to be a sufficient method to treat clubfeet at an age of 3 to 6 months, provided that a perfect alignment of the forefoot with reduction of the talonavicular joint could be achieved by conservative methods. Overlengthening, especially of the Achilles tendon, should be strictly avoided because of the danger of producing a disabled foot that is not fit for toe-walking and sport activities. The Achilles tendon should always be sutured under tension in slight equinus (5 to 10 degrees). In patients who have bilateral clubfoot posterior release can be performed simultaneously. A circumferencial release according to McKay or Simons should always be done too, 2 to 3 weeks later.

Tendon Transfers

Tendon transfers are never indicated in the initial treatment of a clubfoot, but they may be of

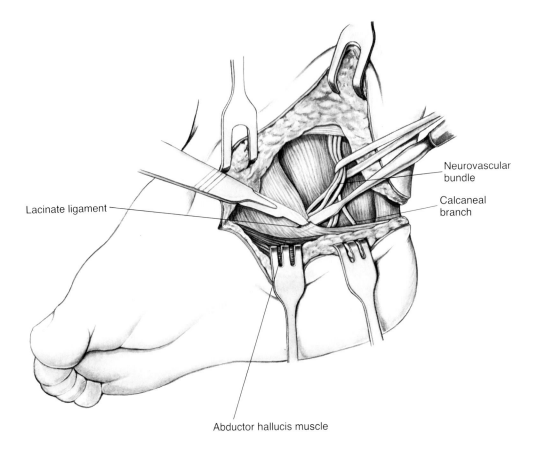

Lacinate ligament

Neurovascular bundle

Calcaneal branch

Abductor hallucis muscle

A

Fig. 22-32. (A) After incision of the subcutaneus tissue the superficial medial dissection is performed. The abductor hallucis is dissected from its underlying tissue and the lacinate ligament is incised from the level of the malleolus distally to the area where it passes into the midfoot. Then the neurovascular bundle is prepared and mobilized medially and retromalleolarly. A vessel loop can be inserted around the bundle for retraction. By blunt dissection the deep insertions of the abductor hallucis are also freed and the tendon sheath of the flexor digitorum communis is prepared. The tendon then is dissected out of its sheaths as far as proximal, distally to the master knot of Henry (crossing with the flexor hallucis longus).

In a similar manner the tibialis posterior tendon sheath is opened. Care has to be taken not to cut the retromalleolar part of the tendon sheath and to perform a Z-lengthening of tibialis posterior tendon distal to the preserved part of the sheath. The flexor digitorum communis is not lengthened. *(Figure continues.)*

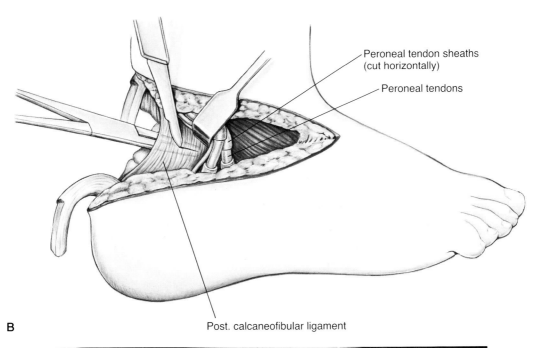

Peroneal tendon sheaths
(cut horizontally)

Peroneal tendons

B

Post. calcaneofibular ligament

Retracted
peroneal
tendons

Post. fibulo-
calcanear lig.

C

Fig. 22-32. *(Continued)* **(B** and **C)** Lateral release. Before the deep structures (e.g., the talonavicular and the subtalar joints) on the medial side are released the lateral and posterior dissection is performed. The sural nerve is dissected and retracted posteriorly. The retinaculum peroneum is cut, the peroneal tendon sheets are incised, and the tendons are retracted. The posterior calcaneofibular ligament is released. The bifurcated ligament is cut, and a complete capsulotomy of the calcaneocuboid joint is performed from dorsally and from the plantar aspect, with care being taken to spare the lateral calcaneocuboid ligament.

Before the capsulotomy of the lateral side of the talocalcaneal joint and the opening of the talonavicular joint from laterally is performed, the posterior release has to be done. (It is also possible to perform the posterior release before the lateral release, but to get the tibiotalar joint reduced, the posterior fibular calcaneal ligament must be cut first.) *(Figure continues.)*

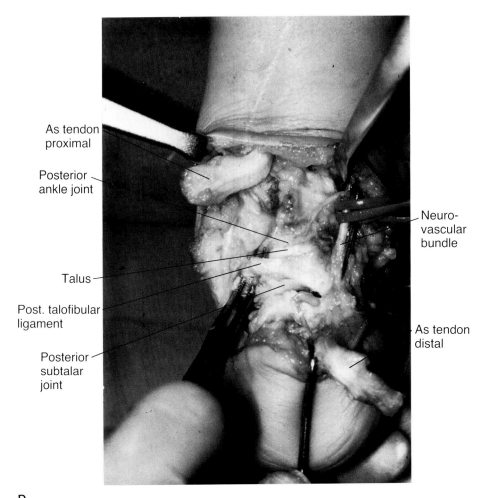

As tendon proximal

Posterior ankle joint

Neuro-vascular bundle

Talus

Post. talofibular ligament

As tendon distal

Posterior subtalar joint

D

Fig. 22-32. *(Continued)* **(D)** Posterior release. The Achilles tendon is incised either in the coronal or in the sagittal plane. The dissection should be extended as far proximal as possible. Depending on the severity of the deformity a lengthening of 2 to 5 cm should be performed. The flexor hallucis longus muscle is identified and its tendon sheath is cut as distal as possible. The flexor hallucis and the peroneal muscles are retracted and the posterior capsulotomy of the ankle joint is performed. The level of the capsulotomy is most easily found by using the tip of an instrument to feel the joint. The best access is on the fibular corner. The capsule is cut by using scissors.

The next structure to be released is the posterior capsule of the subtalar joint.

By traction on the calcaneus with a hook and dorsal extension of the forefoot the talus will be reduced in the ankle mortise. If this is not properly performed, the posterior talofibular ligament, which if possible always should be preserved, has to be cut to allow further opening of the ankle joint. *(Figure continues.)*

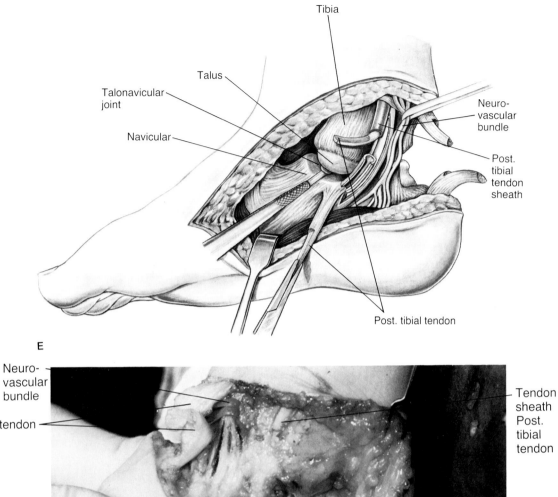

Tibia

Talus

Talonavicular
joint

Navicular

Neuro-
vascular
bundle

Post.
tibial
tendon
sheath

Post. tibial tendon

E

Neuro-
vascular
bundle

As tendon

Tendon
sheath
Post.
tibial
tendon

Talus

Navicular

Post.
tibial
tendon

Flexor digit comm.

F

Fig. 22-32. *(Continued)* **(E** and **F)** Deep medial dissection. With the help of the distal portion of the lengthened tibialis posterior tendon it is relatively simple to expose the talonavicular joint, which is most frequently parallel with the longitudinal axis of the foot. All ligamentous connections between the navicular and talus are now severed. Care must be taken not to dissect proximally onto the talar neck where the blood supply enters the talus.

The talonavicular capsule incision on the medial side must be connected with the incision on the lateral side of the foot.

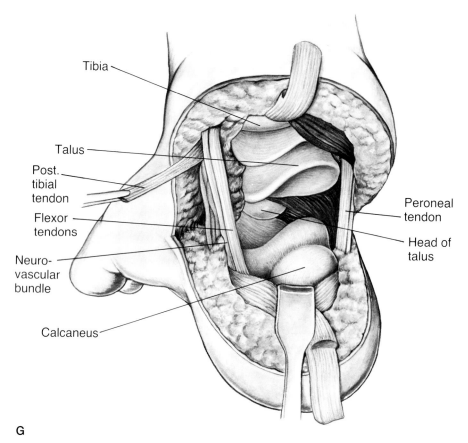

G

Fig. 22-32. *(Continued)* **(G)**   If after the complete talocalcaneonavicular release it is not possible to achieve a normal alignment of the foot it will be necessary to perform a release of the talocalcaneal interosseal ligaments, which should be cut step by step with sharp scissors. Then it is possible to correct all the components of the deformity. The correct position of the foot is kept by fixing the talus and calcaneus and the navicular and talus with two threaded pins.

To get the forefoot aligned additional surgery, such as lengthening of the flexor hallucis longus tendon, the Steindler procedure, and osteotomy of the second and third metatarsal may have to be performed.

The skin closure in corrected and neutral position of the foot sometimes is very difficult or impossible. Therefore it is advantageous to suture the foot in an equinus position and to make the first plaster cast, which should always be an above-knee cast, in an appropriate equinus position. By changing the casts on the third and sixth postoperative days it is then easily possible to correct the equinus without the risk of skin necrosis. *(Figure continues).*

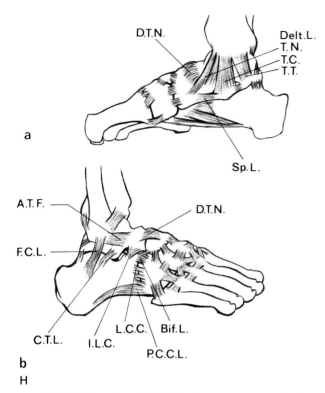

Fig. 22-32. *(Continued)* **(H)** For better conceptualization of what to cut the anatomy of the ligaments of the foot from medial and lateral is illustrated.

(a) Clubfoot from medial aspect: *Sp.L.*, spring ligament; *D.T.N.*, dorsal talonavicular ligament; *Delt.L.* deltoid ligament; *T.N.*, tibionavicular fibers; *T.C.*, tibiocalcaneal fibers; *T.T.*, posterior talotibial fibers.

(b) Clubfoot from lateral aspect: *A.T.F.*, anterior talofibular ligament; *I.L.C.*, interosseous ligament; *C.T.L.*, lateral talocalcaneal ligament; *Bif.L.*, bifurcated ligament; *D.T.N.*, dorsal talonavicular ligament; *L.C.C.*, lateral calcaneocuboid ligament; *F.C.L.*, fibulocalcaneal ligament; *P.C.C.L.*, plantar calcaneocuboid ligament.

benefit under special circumstances. The muscles available for transfer are the anteriotibial (whole or half), posteriotibial, flexor digitorum longus, and extensor hallucis longus.

The lateral transfer of the anterior tibial tendon was recommended by Garceau,[168] if there is weakness or absence of the peroneus longus and brevis muscles. The author recommends the lateral transfer of only half of the anterior tibial muscle to the cuboid or the base of the fifth metatarsal. Transplantation of the tendon of the posterior tibial mus-

cle from its insertion on the medial aspect of the foot, through the interosseous membrane anterior to the middle of the dorsum of the foot, has been advocated by Gartland[169] to correct the supination of the forepart of the foot that may occur during gait. However, it is doubtful that the transferred tendon can function as a dorsiflexor during walking. Anterior transfer of the posterior tibial tendon has an extremely limited place in the treatment of idiopathic talipes equinovarus. Its sole indication is unquestionably muscle imbalance in which the evertors and dorsiflexors of the ankle and foot are weak, and the strong invertors and plantar flexors pull the foot into equinovarus position.

Release Involving the Forepart of the Foot

In 1988 Heyman et al.[84] described release of the tarsometatarsal and intermetatarsal joints for correction of residual adduction of the forepart of the foot in metatarsus adductus as well as for congenital clubfoot. This procedure is performed infrequently because the deformity may recur, or residual stiffness of the forepart of the foot may develop.

Procedures on Bone

In children over 6 years of age, in cases of relapse, soft tissue operations very often are ineffective and must be combined with bony procedures. The most common method is the *Dillwyn-Evans–type collateral operation* that was described by Evans in 1961.[170] A superomedial incision is made, and the navicular is mobilized on the talus by dividing the capsule of the talonavicular joint superiorly, proximally, and inferiorly. The tibialis posterior tendon is divided. Through a separate inferomedial incision the plantar fascia is divided and stripped forward. The calcaneocuboid joint is then exposed through a lateral incision and the joint surfaces are excised as a laterally based wedge. It is important not to excise too much bone because this will produce overcorrection into valgus. The lateral column of the foot is shortened by this method, and it is also possible to correct any supination deformity. The calcaneocuboid arthrodesis is secured with a single staple.

The *osteotomy of the calcaneus* was devised by Dwyer to correct the varus deformity of the hindpart of the foot.[171] It consists of an opening wedge osteotomy of the calcaneus. A wedge of bone is inserted medially to fully correct the varus deformity. Slight overcorrection should be attempted.

Berman and Gartland advised *osteotomy of the base of the metatarsals* for structural deformity of the forepart of the foot.[172] An opening wedge osteotomy of the first cuneiform combined with a radical plantar release to correct residual adduction of the forepart of the foot has been described by Hofmann.[173]

Triple arthrodesis should be regarded as a last-resort wedge procedure and should be reserved for older patients who have painfully stiff feet. This operation should not be done before an age of 12 years.

The aim of these surgical procedures is to establish a plantigrade foot and to compensate for the discrepancy in length between the medial and lateral parts of the foot by shortening the lateral side. In feet with a fixed and inadequate reduction of the calcaneus relative to the talus, a satisfactory alignment can be achieved only by overcorrection at the midtarsal joint. The effect of all these operations or of correction in adolescence by triple arthrodesis with wedge excision is to produce a much shortened foot.

An alternative method is the correction of severely relapsed or neglected clubfeet by an external fixator. With the Ilizarow ring fixator it is possible to correct even severe talipes by gradual distraction. The duration of the period of the correction depends on the deformity and varies from 4 to 10 weeks (Fig. 22-33).

Postoperative Treatment

The postoperative care is as important as the surgery. Loss of surgical correction during postoperative care is often the cause of an unsuccessful outcome. The common factor in these cases is the failure to maintain the normal orientation of the tarsal bones while remodeling stable articular sur-

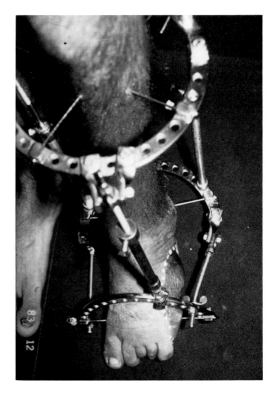

Fig. 22-33. Neglected clubfoot after correction with Ilisarov device in situ.

faces. The following are some of the faults that result in surgical failure: inadequate internal fixation, internal fixation lost early in postoperative care, discontinuation of plaster immobilization too soon after surgery, loss of correction in plaster after removal of internal fixation, and below-knee cast immobilization after removal of internal fixation. Loss of correction in plaster after removal of internal fixation is more likely to occur in infancy. After removal of the cast, specially fitted orthopedic shoes should be worn for at least 1 year. Also, night splints should be used for at least 1 year, until a balance between pronators and supinators is established. Physical exercises to achieve mobility, and to avoid stiffness, are a must.

The goal in treating clubfoot deformities should be to achieve a flexible, painless plantar grade foot that can utilize regular shoegear.

REFERENCES

1. Swinyard CA, Pinner B: Some morphological considerations of normal and abnormal human limb development. In Swinyard CA (ed): Limb Development and Deformity: Problems of Evaluation and Rehabilitation. Charles C Thomas, Springfield, IL, 1969
2. Fitzgerald M: The limbs. p. 75. In: Human Embryology: A Regional Approach. Harper & Row, New York, 1978
3. Baradeen CR, Lewis WH: Development of the limbs, body wall and back in man. Am J Anat, 1:229, 1901
4. Bohm M: The embryologic origin of club-foot. J Bone Joint Surg, 11:229, 1929
5. Tuchmann-Duplessis H, Haegel P: Skeleton and muscles. p. 2. In Tuchmann-Duplessis H, Haegel P (eds): Illustrated Human Embryology—Organogenesis. Springer-Verlag, New York, 1974
6. Bleschschmidt E: Human embryology. p. 160. In Blechschmidt E (ed): The Stages of Human Development Before Birth. WB Saunders, Philadelphia, 1961
7. Hootnick DR, Packard DS, Levinsohn EM, Casy R: Soft tissue anomalies in a patient with congenital tibial aplasia and talo-calcaneal synchrondrosis. Teratology, 36:153, 1987
8. Atlas S: Intra-osseous vascularization of talus and calcaneus in human embryos and fetuses. Anat Clin, 2:13, 1980
9. O'Rahilly R, Gardner E, Gray DJ: The skeletal development of the foot. Clin Orthop Related Res, 16:7, 1960
10. Crossan JF, Wynne-Davies R: Research for genetic and environmental factors in orthopedic diseases. Genet Environ Factors, 210:97, 1986
11. Wang J, Palmer RM, Chung DS: The role of major gene in clubfoot. Am J Hum Genet, 42:772, 1988
12. Yang H, Chung CS, Nemechek RW: A genetic analysis of clubfoot in Hawaii. Genet Epidemiol, 4:299, 1987
13. Wynne-Davies R: Family studies and the cause of congenital club foot talipes equinovarus, talipes calcanco-valgus and metatarsus varus. J Bone Joint Surg [Br], 46:445, 1964
14. Wynne-Davies R: Heritable disorders in orthopedics. Orthop Clin North Am, 9(1):3, 1978
15. Johnston O: Further studies of the inheritance of hand and foot anomalies. Clin Orthop Related Res, 8:146, 1956
16. Dunne KB, Clarren SK: The origin of prenatal and postnatal deformities. Pediatr Clin North Am, 33(6):1277, 1986
17. McDonough MW: Fetal position as a cause of right and left-sided foot and leg disorders. J Am Podiatry Assoc 71(2):65, 1981
18. Swanson AB: A classification for congenital limb malformations. J Hand Surg, 1:8, 1976
19. Masada K, Tsuyuguchi Y, Kawabata H, et al: Terminal limb malformations: analysis of 532 cases. J Pediatr Orthop, 6:340, 1986
20. Leppig KA, Werler MM, Cann CI, et al: predictive value of minor anomalies, I association with major malformations. J Pediatr, 110:531, 1987
21. Ganley J: Lower extremity examination of the infant. J Am Podiatry Assoc, 71(2):92, 1981
22. Jordan RP: The neuromotor development of bipedal locomotion in the normal infant. J Am Podiatry Assoc, 71(2):84, 1981
23. Tax HR: Locomotion and the child patient. J Am Podiatry Assoc, 67(2):96, 1977
24. Sutherland D, Olshen R, Cooper L, Woo S L-Y: The development of mature gait. J Bone Joint Surg 62:336, 1980
25. Menkveld SR, Knipstein EA, Quinn JR: Analysis of gait patterns in normal school-aged children. J Pediatr Orthop, 8:263, 1988
26. McCrea JD: Pediatric Orthopedics of the Lower Extremity: An Instructional Handbook. Futura Publishing Co, Mount Kisco, NY, 1985
27. Whitney A: personal communication.
28. Hensinger RN: Limp. Pediatr Clin North Am, 33(6), 1355, 1986
29. Fields L: The limping child. J Am Podiatry Assoc, 71(2):60, 1981
30. Gross RN: Foot pain in children. Pediatr Clin North Am, 33(6):1395, 1986
31. Peterson H: Growing pains. Pediatr Clin North Am, 33(6):1365, 1986
32. Ehrlich M, Zaleske D: Pediatric orthopedic pain of unknown origin. J Pediatr Orthop 6(4):460, 1986
33. Baxter MP, Dulberg C: "Growing pains" in childhood—a proposal for treatment. J Pediatr Orthop 8:402, 1988
34. Vaughan PA, Newman NM, Rosman MA: Acute hematogenous osteomyelitis in children. J Pediatr Orthop, 7:652, 1987
35. Karlin JM: Osteomyelitis in children. Clin Podiatr Med Surg, 4(1):37, 1987
36. Conway JJ: Radionuclide bone scintigraphy in pe-

diatric orthopedics. Pediatr Clin North Am, 33(6):1313, 1986

37. Fisher MC, Goldsmith JF, Gilligan PH: Sneakers as a source of *Pseudomonas aeruginosa* in children with osteomyelitis following puncture wounds. J Pediatr, 106:607, 1985

38. Borris L, Helleland H: Growth disturbance of the hind part of the foot following osteomyelitis of the calcaneus in the newborn. J Bone Joint Surg [Am], 68:302, 1986

39. Schaller JG: Arthritis in children. Pediatr Clin North Am, 33:1565, 1986

40. (Arthritis Foundation Handbook)

41. Dhanendran M, Hutton WC, Klenerman L, Witemeyer S, Ansell BM: Foot function in juvenile chronic arthritis. Rheumatol Rehabil, 19:20, 1980

42. Brower AC: The osteochondroses. Orthop Clin North Am, 14(1):99, 1983

43. Siffert R: Classification of the osteochondroses. Clin Orthop Related Res, 158:10, 1981

44. Helal B, Gibb P: Freiberg's disease: a suggested pattern of management. Foot Ankle, 8(2):94, 1987

45. Köhler A: A frequent disease of individual bones in children, apparently previously unknown. MMW (Muench. Med. Wochenschr.) 55:1923, 1908

46. Williams G, Cowell H: Kohler's disease of the tarsal navicular. Clin Orthop Related Res, 158:53, 1981

47. Micheli L, Ireland ML: Prevention and management of calcaneal apophysitis in children: an overuse syndrome. J Pediatr Orthop 7:34, 1987

48. Staheli LT: Torsional deformity. Pediatr Clin North Am, 33(6):1373, 1986

49. Staheli LT, Corbett M, Wyss C, King H: Lower extremity rotational problems in children. J Bone Joint Surg, 67(1):39, 1985

50. Engel GM, Staheli LT: The natural history of torsion and other factors influencing gait in childhood. Clin Orthop Related Res, 99:12, 1974

51. Wilkins KE: Bowlegs. Pediatr Clin North Am, 33(6):1429, 1986

52. Kling TF, Hensinger RN: Angular and torsional deformities of the lower limbs in children. Clin Orthop Related Res 176:136, 1983

53. Moreland MS: Morphological effects of torsion applied to growing bone, an in vivo study in rabbits. J Bone Joint Surg [Br], 62:230, 1980

54. Moreland MS, et al: Denis Browne splint: torsion or no torsion (abstract). J Pediatr Orthop, 8:105, 1988

55. Staheli LT: Evaluation of planovalgus foot deformities with special reference to the national history. J Am Podiatr Med Assoc, 77:2, 1987

56. Spencer AM, Person VA: Casting and orthotics for children. Clin Podiatry 1(3):621, 1984

57. Rose GK, Welton EA, Marshall T: The diagnosis of flat foot in the child. J Bone Joint Surg [Br], 67:71, 1985

58. Coleman S, Stelling F, Jarrett J: Pathomechanics and treatment of congenital vertical talus. Clin Orthop Related Res, 70:62, 1970

59. Lamy L, Weissman L: Congenital convex pes valgus. J Bone Joint Surg 21:79, 1939

60. Specht E: Congenital paralytic vertical talus. J Bone Joint Surg [Am], 57:842, 1975

61. Lembach L, Leibowitz L: Oblique talus. J Am Pediatr Med Assoc, 76(4):214, 1986

62. Mosier K, Asher M: Tarsal coalitions and peroneal spastic flat foot. J Bone Joint Surg [Am], 66:976, 1984

63. Stormont DM, Peterson HA: The relative incidence of tarsal coalition. Clin Orthop Related Res 181:28, 1983

64. Lahey MD, Zindrick MR, Harris EJ: A comparative study of the clinical presentation of tarsal coalitions. Clin Podiatr Med Surg, 5(2):341, 1988

65. Conway J, Cowell H: Tarsal coalition: clinical significance and roentgenographic demonstration. Radiology 92:799, 1969

66. Scanton P: Treatment of symptomatic talocalcaneal coalition. J Bone Joint Surg [Am], 69:533, 1987

67. Danielsson LG: Talo-calcaneal coalition treated with resection. J Pediatr Orthop 7:513, 1987

68. Isherwood I: A radiological approach to the subtalar joint. J Bone Joint Surg [Br], 43:566, 1961

69. Beckley DE, Anderson PW, Pedegana LR: The radiology of the subtalar joint with special reference to talo-calcaneal coalition. Clin Radiol, 26:333, 1975

70. Hall J, Salter RB, Bhalla SK: Congenital short tendo calcaneus. J Bone Joint Surg [Br], 49:695, 1967

71. Harris RI, Beath T: Hypermobile flat-foot with short tendo achilles. J Bone Joint Surg [Am], 30:116, 1948

72. Berg E: A reappraisal of metatarsus adductus and skewfoot. J Bone Joint Surg [Am], 68:1185, 1986

73. Peterson H: Skewfoot. J Pediatr Orthop 6:24, 1986

74. Mayer PJ: Pes cavus: a diagnostic and therapeutic challenge. Orthop Rev, 7(8):105, 1978

75. Brewerton DA, Sandifer PH, Sweetnam DR: "Idiopathic" pes cavus. Br Med J, 2:659, 1963

76. Exner GU: Knick-plattfuss bei morbus friedreich und morbus Charcot-Marie-Tooth-Hoffman. Z Orthop, 125:298, 1987

77. Sabir M, Lyttle D: Pathogenesis of pes cavus in Charcot-Marie-Tooth disease. Clin Orthop Related Res 175:173, 1983

78. Sherman FC, Westin GW: Plantar release in the correction of deformities of the foot in childhood. J Bone Joint Surg [Am], 63:1382, 1981

79. Levitt RL, Canale ST, Cooke AJ, Gartland JJ: The role of foot surgery in progressive neuromuscular disorders in children. J Bone Joint Surg [Am], 55:1396, 1973

80. Bradley GW, Coleman SS: Treatment of the calcaneocavus foot deformity. J Bone Joint Surg [Am], 63:1159, 1981

81. Gudas CJ: Mechanism and reconstruction of pes cavus. J Foot Surg, 16:1, 1977

82. Altennuber J, Grill F: Treatment of pes cavus with the V-osteotomy according to Japas. Estratto da Chirurgia Del Piede, 8:341, 1984

83. Tax H, Albright T: Metatarsus adducto varus—a simplified approach to treatment. J Am Podiatry Assoc, 68:331, 1978

84. Heyman C, Herndon C, Strong J: Mobilization of the tarsometatarsal and intermetatarsal joints for the correction of resistant adduction of the fore part of the foot in congenital club-foot or congenital metatarsus varus. J Bone Joint Surg [Am], 40:299, 1958

85. Stark JG, Johnson JE, Winter R: The Heyman-Herndon tarsometatarsal capsulotomy for metatarsus adductus: results in 48 feet. J Pediatr Orthop, 7:305, 1987

86. Berman A, Gartland J: Metatarsal osteotomy for the correction of adduction of the fore part of the foot in children. J Bone Joint Surg [Am], 53:408, 1971

87. Johnson JB: A preliminary report on chondrotomies—a new surgical approach to metatarsus adductus in children. J Am Podiatry Assoc, 68:808, 1978

88. Hawkins FB, Mitchell CL, Hedrick DW: Correction of hallux valgus metatarsal osteotomy. J Bone Joint Surg 27:387, 1945

89. Simmonds FA, Menelaus MB: Hallux valgus in adolescents. J Bone Joint Surg [Br], 42:761, 1960

90. Bonney G, Macnab I: Hallus valgus and hallux rigidus. J Bone and Joint Surg [Br], 34:366, 1952

91. Truslow W: Metatarsus primus varus or hallux valgus. J Bone Joint Surg 7:98, 1925

92. Lapidus PW: Operative correction of the metatarsus varus primus in hallux valgus. Surg Gynecol Obstet, 58:183, 1934

93. Hardy RN, Clapman JCR: Hallux valgus—

predisposing anatomical causes. Lancet, 1:1180, 1952

94. Schubert DA: The role of the abductor hallucis in metatarsus primus varus associated with hallux valgus. J Am Podiatry Assoc, 53:752, 1963

95. Tangen O: Hallux valgus. Acta Chir Scand, 137:151, 1971

96. Contamposis JD: Generalized ligamentous laxity. p. 81. In Smith SD, DiGiovanni JE (eds): Decision Making in Foot Surgery. Yearbook, Chicago, 1976

97. Goldner JL, Gaines RW: Adult and juvenile hallux valgus: analysis and treatment. Orthop Clin North Am, 7(4):863, 1976

98. Root ML, Orien WP, and Weed JH: Normal and Abnormal Function of the Foot. Clinical Biomechanics, Vol II. Clinical Biomechanics Corp. Los Angeles, CA, 1977

99. Hardy RH, Clapman JCR: Observations on hallux valgus. J Bone Joint Surg [Br], 33:376, 1951

100. Lundberg BJ, Sulja T: Skeletal parameters in the hallux valgus foot. Acta Orthop Scand, 43:576, 1972

101. Piggott H: The natural history of hallux valgus in adolescence and early adult life. J Bone Joint Surg [Br], 42:749, 1960

102. Helal B, Gupta SK, Gojaseni P: Surgery for adolescent hallux valgus. Acta Orthop Scand 42:271, 1974

103. Mitchell L, Fleming JL, Allen R, Glenney C, Sanford GA: Osteotomy–bunionectomy of hallus valgus. J Bone Joint Surg [Am], 40:41, 1958

104. Auerbach AM: Review of distal metatarsal osteotomies for hallux valgus in the young. Clin Orthop Related Res, 70:148, 1970

105. Dooley BJ, Berryman DB: Wilson's osteotomy of the first metatarsal for hallux valgus in the adolescent and the young adult. Aust NZ J Surg, 43:255, 1973

106. Haddas RJ: Hallux valgus and metatarsus primus varus treated by bunionectomy and proximal metatarsal osteotomy. South Med J, 68:684, 1975

107. Wilson JN: Oblique displacement osteotomy for hallux valgus. J Bone Joint Surg [Br], 45:552, 1963

108. Grill F, Hetherington V, Steinbock G, Altenhuber J: Experiences with the chevron (V–) osteotomy on adolescent hallux valgus. Arch Orthop Trauma Surg, 106:47, 1986

109. Poland J: Traumatic Separation of the Epiphyses. Smith, Elder and Co., London, 1898

110. Poland J: Traumatic separation of the epiphyses in general. Clin Orthop, 41:7, 1965

111. Weber BG (ed): Treatment of Fractures in Chil-

dren and Adolescents. Springer-Verlag, New York, 1980

112. Aitkin AP: Fractures of the epiphyses. Clin Orthop, 41:19, 1965

113. Salter RB, Harris WR: Injuries involving the epiphyseal plate. J Bone Joint Surg [Am], 45:587, 1963

114. Chand K: Epiphyseal separation of distal humeral epiphysis in an infant. J Trauma, 14:521, 1974

115. Rogers LF, Rockwood CA, Jr.: Separation of the entire distal humeral epiphysis. Radiology, 106:393, 1973

116. Silverman FN: Follow-up notes on articles previously published in the journal. Recovery from epiphyseal invagination: sequel to an unusual complication of scurvy. J Bone Joint Surg [Am], 52:384, 1970

117. Cooperman DR, Spiegel PG, Laros GS: Tibial fractures involving the ankle in children. J Bone Joint Surg [Am], 60:1040, 1978

118. Lynn MD: The triplane distal tibial epiphyseal fracture. Clin Orthop, 86:187, 1972

119. Marmor L: An unusual fracture of the tibial epiphysis. Clin Orthop, 73:132, 1970

120. Shelton WR, Canale T: Fractures of the tibia through the proximal tibial epiphyseal cartilage. J Bone Joint Surg [Am], 61:167, 1979

121. Torg JS, Ruggiero RA: Comminuted epiphyseal fracture of the distal tibia. Clin Orthop, 110:215, 1975

122. Holland CT: A radiographical note on injuries to the distal epiphyses of the radius and ulna. Proc R Soc Med, 22:695, 1929

123. Kling T, Bright RW, Hensinger RN: Medial malleolar fractures in children: a case for open reduction. In: Proceedings of 49th Annual Meeting, AAOS, New Orleans, 1982 (abstr)

124. Peterson H, Burkhart S: Compression injury of the epiphyseal growth plate: fact or fiction? J Pediatr Orthop, 1:377, 1981

125. Trueta J: Studies of the Development and Decay of the Human Frame. WB Saunders, Philadelphia, 1968

126. Selke AC: Destruction of phalangeal epiphysis by frostbite. Radiology, 93:859, 1969

127. Rang M: The Growth Plate and Its Disorders. Williams & Wilkins, Baltimore, 1969

128. Tachdjian MO: The Child's Foot. WB Saunders, Philadelphia, 1985

129. Tachdjian MO: Pediatric Orthopedics, Vols. 1 and 2. WB Saunders, Philadelphia, 1972

130. Hancock PA, Flory RJ: Syndactyly — a review of the literature. J Am Podiatry Assoc, 61:1, 1974

131. Rogala EJ, Wynne-Davis R, Littlejohn A, Gormley R: Congenital limb anomalies: frequency and aetiological factors. J Med Genet, 11:221, 1974

132. Bunnel S (cited by) Barksy AJ: Congenital Anomalies of the Hand and Their Surgical Treatment. Charles C Thomas, Springfield, IL, 1959

133. Tax HR: Podopediatrics. Williams & Wilkins, Baltimore, 1980

134. Kohler HG: Congenital transverse defects of limbs and digits. Arch Dis Child, 37:263, 1962

135. Thomson SA: Hallux varus and metatarsus varus. Clin Orthop, 16:109, 1960

136. Farmer AW: Congenital hallux varus. Am J Surg, 95:274, 1958

137. Bailey T: Inheritance pattern of Talipes Equinovarus. J Bone Joint Surg (Am) 40, 1966

138. Handelsman JE, Badalmente MA: Neuromuscular studies in clubfoot. J Pediatr Orthop, 1:25, 1981

139. Ponseti I, et al: Congenital club foot: the results of treatment. J Bone Joint Surg [Am], 45:261, 1963

140. Bill PLA, Versfeld GA: Congenital clubfoot: an electromyographic study. J Pediatr Orthop, 2:139, 1982

141. Irani RN, Sherman MS: Pathological anatomy of club foot. J Bone Joint Surg [Am], 45:45, 1963

142. Settle GW: The anatomy of congenital talipes equinovarus: sixteen dissected specimens. J Bone Joint Surg [Am], 45:1341, 1963

143. Simons GW: The complete subtalar release in clubfeet. Orthop Clin North Am, 18(1):667, 1987

144. Simons GW: Complete subtalar release in club feet Part I — a preliminary report. J Bone Joint Surg [Am], 67:1044, 1985

145. Simons GW: Complete subtalar release in club feet Part II — comparison with less extensive procedures. J Bone Joint Surg [Am], 67:1056, 1985

146. Simons GW: The diagnosis and treatment of deformity combinations in clubfeet. Clin Orthop, 150:229, 1980

147. Hoskin SW, Scott W: A study of the anatomy and biomechanics of the ankle region in normal and club feet (talipes equino varus) of infants. J Anat, 134:227, 1982

148. Bösch J: Operative oder konservative Klumpfußbehandlung. Zf Orth und Grenzgeb 83:8, 1952

149. McKay DW: New concept of and approach to clubfoot treatment: Section I — principles and morbid anatomy. J Pediatr Orthop, 2:347, 1982

150. Herzenberg J, Caroll NC, Christofersen MR, Eng Hin Lee, White ST, Munroe R: Clubfoot analysis with three dimensional computer modeling. J Pediatr Orthop 8:257, 1988

151. Dimeglio A, Bensahel H, Catterall A: Clubfoot —

the search for a consensus. E.P.O.S.-Meeting, Amsterdam 1988

152. Bösch J: Biologische Grundlagen Konservativer Klumpfußbehandlung. Zf Orth und Grenzgeb 85:429, 1954
153. Bösch J: Klumpfussbehandlung nach Kite. Verh. Deutschen Orth. Gesellschaft, Stuttgart, 1955
154. Bösch J: Biologische Grundlagen konservativer Klumpfussbehandlung. Z Orthop Grenzgeb, 85:429, 1954
155. Bösch J: Zur Technik der Klumpfussbehandlung. Z Orthop Grenzgeb, 94:159, 1900
156. Bösch J: Die konservative Klumpfussbehandlung des Säuglings und Kleinkindes. Med Orthop Technik, 6:150, 1974
157. Bösch J: Zur Abhängigkeit der Valgusstellung der Ferse von der Stellung des oberen Sprunggelenkes. Arch Orthop Unfall-Chir, 50(Suppl):330, 1959
158. Bösch J: Die Calcaneuosteotomie beim Ballenhohlfuss. Arch Orthop Unfall-Chir, 73:149, 1972
159. Bösch J: Wodurch wird der Klumpfuss rebellisch. Arch Orthop Unfall-Chir, 50:11, 1959
160. Bensahel H: La reeducation dans le traitement du pied bot varus equin. Encylcopedie medico-chirurgicale (Paris) 6428 B(10) -4-9-12
161. Bensahel H: A propos de six cents pieds bots. Chir Pediatr, 21:335, 1980
162. Bensahel H: The functional anatomy of clubfoot. J Pediatr Orthop 3:191, 1983
163. Turco VJ: Resistant congenital club foot—one stage posteromedial release with internal fixation. J Bone Joint Surg [Am], 61:805, 1979
164. Attenborough CG: Severe congenital talipes equinovarus. J Bone Joint Surg [Br], 48:31, 1966
165. Lloyd-Roberts GC, Paterson H, Catterall A: Medial rotational osteotomy for severe residual deformity in club foot. J Bone Joint Surg [Br], 56:37, 1974
166. Turco VJ: Current management of clubfoot. p. 218. A.O.S. Instructional Course Lectures, Vol. 0.
167. Turco VJ: Surgical correction of the resistant club foot. J Bone Joint Surg [Am], 53:477, 1971
168. Garceau GJ: Transfer of the anterior tibial tendon for recurrent club foot. J Bone Joint Surg [Am], 49:207, 1967
169. Gartland JJ: Posterior tibial transplant in the surgical treatment of recurrent clubfoot. J Bone Joint Surg [Am], 46:1217, 1964
170. Evans D: Relapsed club foot. J Bone Joint Surg [Br], 43:722, 1961
171. Dwyer FC: The treatment of relapsed club foot by the insertion of a wedge into the calcaneus. J Bone Joint Surg [Br], 45:67, 1963
172. Berman A, Gartland JJ: Metatarsal osteotomy for the correction of adduction of the fore part of the foot in children. J Bone Joint Surg [Am], 53:498, 1971
173. Hofmann AA: Osteotomy of the first cuneiform as treatment of residual adduction of the fore part of the foot in club foot. J Bone Joint Surg [Am], 66:985, 1984

SUGGESTED READINGS

Addison A: The review of the Dillwyn Evans type collateral operation in severe clubfeet. J Bone Joint Surg [Br], 65:14, 1983

Adam A: Tibialis posterior transfer in relapsed club foot. J Bone Joint Surg [Br], 45:804, 1963

Atlas S: Some new aspects in the pathology of clubfoot. Clin Orthop Related Res, 0:224, 1900

Baumann JU: Zur Behandlung und Varus-Fehlstellung des Rückfusses

Beatson TR: A method of assessing correction in club feet. J Bone Joint Surg [Br], 48:40, 1966

Bechtold CO: An embryological study of associated muscle abnormalities. J Bone Joint Surg [Am], 32:827, 1950

Benacerraf BR: Antenatal sonographic diagnosis of congenital clubfoot: a possible indication for amniocentesis. J Clin Ultrasound 14:703, 1986

Benghachem M: L'Osteotomie du calcaneum chez l enfant. Technique, indications et resultats. Ann Chir, 36, 1982

Bost FC: Plantar dissection. J Bone Joint Surg [Am], 42:151, 1960

Brougham DI: Use of the Cincinnati incision in congenital talipes equinovarus. J Pediatr Orthop, 8, 1988

Browne RS: Anomalous insertion of the tibialis posterior tendon in congenital metatarsus varus. J Bone Joint Surg [Br], 61:74, 1979

Bunning PSC: A comparison of adult and foetal talocalcaneal articulations. J Bone Joint Surg [Br], 61:74, 1979

Burns AE: Revised tarsectomy for correction of relapsed clubfoot. J Foot Surg, 3:275, 1984

Capener N: Congenital clubfoot. (Proceeding and Reports of Councils and Associations.) J Bone Joint Surg [Br], 44:956, 1962

Cerulli G: Results of manipulative treatment of congenital clubfoot. Communication to the 61st Congress of the Italian Society of Orthopaedic Surgery and Traumatology, Milan, October 1976

Cobey JC: Standardizing methods of measurement of foot shape by including the effects of subtalar rotation. Foot Ankle, 2:30, 1981

Colburn RC: Flat talus in recurrent club foot. (Proceedings and Reports of Councils and associations.) J Bone Joint Surg

Commerell J: A new approach to the untreated or relapsed club foot in adults. (Proceedings and Reports of Councils and Associations.) J Bone Joint Surg

Cowell HR: Genetic aspects of club foot. J Bone Joint Surg [Am], 62:1381, 1980

Cowell HR: The management of club foot. J Bone Joint Surg [Am], 67:991, 1985

Crawford AH: The Cincinatti incision: a comprehensive approach for surgical procedures of the foot and ankle in childhood. J Bone Joint Surg [Am], 64:1355, 1982

Czeizel A: Confirmation of the multifactorial threshold model for congenital structural talipes equinovarus. J Med Genet, 18:999, 1981

Dekel S: Osteotomy of the calcaneus and concomitant plantar striping in children with talipes cavo-varus. J Bone Joint Surg [Br], 55:802, 1973

Denham RA: Congenital talipes equinovarus. (Proceedings and Reports of Universities Colleges, Councils, and Associations.) J Bone Joint Surg [Br], 49:583, 1967

Denham RA: Early operation for severe congenital talipes equinovarus. (Proceedings and Reports of Universities, Colleges, Councils, and Associations.) J Bone Joint Surg

DeRosa GP: Results of posteriomedial release for the resistant clubfoot. J Pediatr Orthop, 6:590, 1986

Dietz FR: Morphometric study of clubfoot tendon sheaths. J Pediatr Orthop, 3:11, 1983

Dietz FR: On the pathogenesis of clubfoot. Lancet, 1,1985

Doskocil M: Recommendations for modified surgical treatment of pes equinovarus based on embryological findings. Acta Chir Orthop Traum Cech, 49:4, 1982

Drummond DS: The management of the foot and ankle in arthrogryposis multiplex congenita. J Bone Joint Surg [Br], 60:96, 1978

Duncan WR: Surgical reconstruction of cominuted fractures of the calcaneus. Early operation for severe congenital talipes equinovarus. (Proceedings and Reports of Universities, Colleges, Councils and Associations.) J Bone Joint Surg [Am], 49:1475, 1967

Dunn HK: Flat-top talus. J Bone Joint Surg [Am], 56:57, 1974

Dwyer FC: Osteotomy of the calcaneum for pes cavus. J Bone Joint Surg [Br], 41:80, 1959

Flinchum D: Pathological anatomy in talipes equinovarus. J Bone Joint Surg [Am], 35:111, 1953

Franke J: Die operative Behandlung des angeborenen Klumpfusses. Beitr Orthop Traumatol, 32:600, 1985

Franke J: The use of an instrumental distractor in the treatment of severe relapsed or neglected club feet.

Fried A: Recurrent congenital club foot. J Bone Joint Surg [Am], 41:243, 1959

Ganley JV: Corrective casting in infants. Clin Podiatry, 1(3):501, 1984

Ghali NN: The results of pantalar reduction in the management of congenital talipes equinovarus. J Bone Joint Surg [Am], 65:1, 1983

Gray DH: A histochemical study of muscle in club foot. J Bone Joint Surg [Br], 63:417, 1981

Greider TD: Arteriography in club foot. J Bone Joint Surg [Am], 64:837, 1982

Green ADL: The results of early posterior release in resistant club feet. J Bone Joint Surg [Br], 67:588, 1985

Grice DS: An extra-articular arthrodesis of the subastragalar joint for correction of paralytic flat feet in children. J Bone Joint Surg [Am], 34:927, 1952

Grill F: Die konservative Klumpfussbehandlung nach Bösch. Paper presented at the Foot Surgery Congress, Vienna, 1983

Grill F: Clubfoot therapy according to Bösch: conservative and operative aspects. Arch Orthop Traum Surg, 1984

Grill F: The Ilizarov distractor for the correction of relapsed or neglected clubfoot. J Bone Joint Surg [Br}, 69:593, 1987

Grill F: Neue Aspekte der operativen Klumpfussbehandlung—Technik und Erfahrungen mit dem Cinnatizugang. (Arbeit zusammen mit GroBbötzl G.)

Haicl Z: Empirical hazard in pes equinovarus. Acta Chir Orthop Traum Cech, 38:205, 1971

Haicl Z: Our experience with pes equinus congenitus according to Turco. Acta Chir Orthop Traum Cech, 50:530, 1983

Handelsmann JE: The muscles in club foot—a histological, histochemical and electron microscopic study. J Bone Joint Surg [Br], 59:465, 1977

Harrold AJ: Treatment and prognosis in congenital club foot. J Bone Joint Surg [Br], 65:8, 1983

Hassler WL: Tarsometatarsal mobilization for resistant auction of the fore part of the foot. J Bone Joint Surg [Am], 52:61, 1970

Hehne HJ: Die Calcaneus-Osteotomie nach Dwyer bei der Varusfehlstellung des Rückfusses. Z Orthop, 117:202, 1979

Henkel H-L: Die Muskulatur beim angeborenen Klumpfuss.

Henkel H-L: Operation nach Evans

Herold HZ: Tibial torsion in untreated congenital club-foot. Acta Orthop Scand, 47:112, 1976

Hersh A: The role of surgery in the treatment of club feet. J Bone Joint Surg [Am], 49:1684, 1967

Hjelmstedt EA: Arthrography as a guide in the treatment of congenital clubfoot. Acta Orthop Scand, 51:321, 1980

Hjelmstedt EA: Talo-calcaneal osteotomy and soft-tissue procedures in the treatment of clubfeet. Acta Orthop Scand, 51:349, 1980

Hootnick DR: Congenital arterial malformations associated with clubfoot. Clin Orthop Related Res, 167:160, 1982

Hörenz L-V: Behandlung der angeborenen Fussdeformitäten im Rahmen der Frühtherapie. Beitr Orthop Traumatol 33:129, 1986

Hutchins, PM: Tibiofibular torsion in normal and treated clubfoot populations. J Pediatr Orthop, 6:452, 1986

Index Subject index of clubfoot

Imhäuser G: Was bedeutet ein verkleinerter Winkel zwischen Talus- und Kalkaneuslängsachse im Röntgenbild des angeborenen Klumpfusses. Arch Orthop Unfall-Chir, 88:163, 1977

Ippolito E: The treatment of relapsing clubfoot by tibialis anterior transfer underneath the extensor retinaculum. Paper presented at the 2nd Orthopaedic Clinic, University "La Sapienza", Rome, 1900

Jahss MH: Tarsometatarsal truncated-wedge arthrodesis for pes cavus and equinovarus deformity of the fore part in the foot. J Bone Joint Surg [Am], 62:713, 1980

Jahss MH: Bone procedures—dorsal osteotomy

Kaplan EB: Comparative anatomy of the talus in relation to idiopathic clubfoot. Clin Orthop, 85:32, 1972

Karlin JM: The Cincinnati incision. J Am Podiatr Med Assoc, 76:386, 1986

Kite JH: Some suggestions on the treatment of club foot by casts. J Bone Joint Surg [Am], 45:406, 1963

Kordos J: Our experience with conservative treatment of pes equinovarus. Acta Chir Orthop Traum Cech, 48:527, 1981

Kummer F: Technical note: a brace for the radiological evaluation of talipes equinovarus. Bull Hosp Joint Dis Orthop Instit, 47(2), 1987

Leder K: Sonographische Beurteilung der subtalaren Rotation beim congenitalen Klumpfuss

Lehman WB: The Surgical Anatomy of the Interosseous Ligament of the Subtalar Joint as It Relates to Clubfoot Surgery

Lehman WB: Hard Tissue Surgery

Letko E: Analysis of the heredity of pes equinovarus. Acta Chir Orthop Traum Cech, 51:410, 1984

Lichtblau S: A medial and lateral release operation for club foot. J Bone Joint Surg [Am], 55:1377, 1973

Loeffler F: Ursachen und Behandlung von schweren an-

geborenen Klumpfussen und von Klumpfussrezidiven. Arch Orthop Unfall-Chir, 52:200, 1960

Lusskin R: The technique of dynamic adhesive strapping for congenital clubfoot. Bull Hosp Joint Dis Orthop Instit, 47, 1987

Main BJ: An analysis of residual deformity in club feet submitted to early operation. J Bone Joint Surg [Br], 60:536, 1978

Mattner H-R: Unsere Erfahrungen mit unterschiedlichen Methoden der operativen Klumpfussbehandlung

McKay DW: New concept of and approach to clubfoot treatment: Section II—correction of the clubfoot. J Pediatr Orthop, 3:10, 1983

McKay DW: New concept of and approach to clubfoot treatment: Section II—evaluation and results. J Pediatr Orthop, 3:141, 1983

Meehan PL: Part II—anatomy and nonoperative management of the congenital clubfoot. A.A.O.S. Instructional Course Lectures, Vol 0.

Miller JH: The roentgenographic appearance of the "corrected clubfoot." Foot Ankle, 6:177, 1986

Miller MG: Posterio tibial tendon transfer: a review of the literature and analysis of 74 procedures. J Pediatr Orthop, 2:363, 1982

Mir GR: Residual forefoot adduction in treated congenital talipes equinovarus. J R Coll Surg Edinburgh 29:285, 1984

Mittal R: The surgical management of resistant club foot by rotation skin flap and extensive soft tissue release. Int Orthop (SICOT), 11:189, 1987

Nather A: Conservative and surgical treatment of clubfoot. J Pediatr Orthop, 7:42, 1987

Ono K: Anterior transfer of the toe flexors for equinovarus deformity of the foot. Int Orthop (SICOT), 4:225, 1980

Otis JC: Gait analysis in surgically treated clubfoot. J Pediatr Orthop, 6:162, 1986

Otremski I: Residual adduction of the forefoot. J Pediatr Orthop, 7:149, 1987

Palarcik J: Talipes equinovarus congenitus. Acta Chir Orthop Traum Cech, 46:123, 1979

Pandey S: "T"-osteotomy of the calcaneum. Int Orthop (SICOT), 4:219, 1980

Paulos L: Pes cavovarus. J Bone Joint Surg [Am], 62:942, 1980

Peleska L: Surgical treatment of talipes equino-varus deformity—a commentary. Acta Chir Orthop Traum Cech, 45:483, 1978

Porat S: The history of treatment of congenital clubfoot at the Royal Liverpool Childrens Hospital: improvement of results by early extensive posteromedial release. J Pediatr Orthop, 4:331, 1984

Porter RW: Congenital talipes equinovarus: I. Resolving

and resistant deformities. J Bone Joint Surg [Br], 69:822, 1987

Rogdveller B: Talipes equinovarus. Clin Podiatry 1:477, 1984

Rosen H: The measurement of tibiofibular torsion. J Bone Joint Surg [Am], 37:847, 1955

Rybka V: Treatment of congenital equinovarus (club-foot) deformity by stages. Acta Chir Orthop Traum Cech 43:511, 1976

Ryöppy S: Neonatal operative treatment of club foot. J Bone Joint Surg [Br], 65:320, 1983

Salzer M: Die operative Klumpfussbehandlung mit Transfixation des Rückfusses. Z Orthop, 106:368, 1900

Scheel PF: Fehlerquellen in der operativen Behandlung des Säuglingsklumpfusses.

Scholder P: Die wachstumsbedingte Knochenremodellierung beim angerborenen Klumpfuss.

Sedgwick WG: Congenital diastasis of the ankle joint. J Bone Joint Surg [Am], 64:450, 1982

Shapiro F: Gross and histological abnormalities of the talus in congenital club foot. J Bone Joint Surg [Am], 61:522, 1979

Sherman FC: Plantar release in the correction of deformities of the foot in childhood. J Bone Joint Surg [Am], 63:1382, 1981

Slavik J: Congenital talipes equinovarus as a problem. Cesk Pediatr XXI:807, 1966

Slavik J: Clubfoot and its relapse. Acta Chir Orthop Traum Cech, 34:74, 1967

Slivika M: Surgical treatment of pes equinovarus at the Department of Orthopaedics, Medical Faculty, Bratislava. Acta Chir Orthop Trauma Cech, 45:23, 1978

Smith RB: Dysplasia and the effects of soft tissue release in congenital talipes equinovarus. Clin Orthop, 174:304, 1983

Strach EH: Club-foot through the centuries. Prog Pediatr Surg, 20, 1900

Sudmann E: Features resisting primary treatment of congenital clubfoot. Acta Orthop Scand, 54:850, 1983

Suppan RJ: Correction of severe adult congenital talipes equinovarus. J Am Podiatry Assoc, 71:454, 1981

Swann M: The anatomy of uncorrected club feet. J Bone Joint Surg [Br], 51:263, 1969

Tayton K: Relapsing club feet. J Bone Joint Surg [Br], 61:474, 1979

Thomas W: Über die Translokationsoperation der Peronaeus-brevis-Sehne beim Klumpfuss. Z Orthop, 116:378, 1978

Toohey JS: Distal calcaneal osteotomy in resistant talipes equinovarus. Clin Orthop Related Res, 197:224, 1985

Tönnis D: Elektromyographische und histologische Untersuchungen zur Frage der Entstehung des angeborenen Klumpfusses

Vesely J: Surgical treatment of severe recidivating deformities in pes equinovarus (clubfoot). Acta Chir Orthop Traum Cech, 49:63, 1982

Victoria-Diaz A: Pathogenesis of idiopathic clubfoot. Clin Orthop Related Res, 185:14, 1984

Waisbrod H: Congenital club foot. J Bone Joint Surg [Br], 55:796, 1973

Wedge J: A method of treating clubfeet with malleable splints. J Pediatr Orthop, 3:108, 1983

Wynne-Davies R: Talipes equinovarus—a review of eight-four cases after completion of treatment. J Bone Joint Surg [Br], 46:464, 1964

Wynne-Davies R: Aetiology and interrelationship of some common skeletal deformities. J Med Genet, 19:321, 1982

Yadav SS: Observations on operative management of neglected club-foot. Int Orthop (SICOT), 5:189, 1981

Zimny ML: An electron microscopic study of the fascia from the medial and lateral sides of clubfoot. J Pediatr Orthop, 5:577, 1985

Composite Radiographic Findings for Pediatric Foot Deformity

Appendix

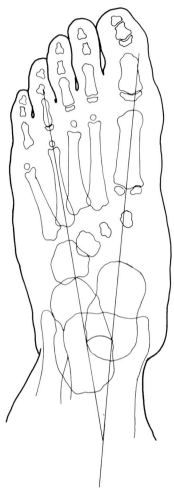

NORMAL CHILD'S FOOT

Transverse Plane. Talocalcaneal angle *(angle A)* 30 to 50 degrees in infants; 15 to 50 degrees in children. Midtalar line *(line a)* coincides with first metatarsal head and shaft. Midcalcaneal line *(line b)* coincides with fourth metatarsal head and shaft.

Sagittal Plane. Talocalcaneal angle *(angle A)* is an acute angle of 15 to 50 degrees. Midtalar line *(line a)* coincides with first metatarsal; no angle formed. Inferior calcaneus – fifth metatarsal angle *(angle B)* is obtuse (150 to 175 degrees), apex up.

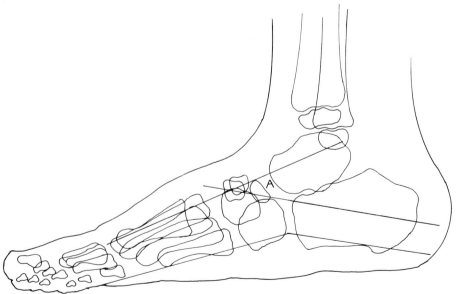

CLUBFOOT

(Left) Transverse plane. Talocalcaneal angle is reduced. Midtalar line is lateral to first metatarsal head and shaft. Midcalcaneal line is lateral to fourth metatarsal head and shaft. **(Right)** Sagittal plane. Talocalcaneal angle is reduced, or parallel lines. Midtalar line forms obtuse angle apex downward with first metatarsal line. Inferior calcaneus–fifth metatarsal angle is obtuse (>175 degrees), apex downward.

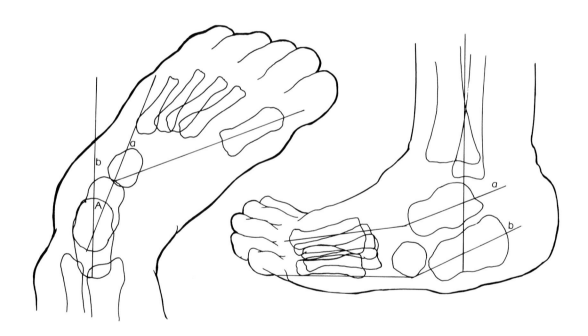

CAVUS FOOT

(Left) Sagittal plane.   Talocalcaneal angle is increased. Midtalar line passes dorsal to first metatarsal head; with first metatarsal line forms angle with apex upward. Inferior calcaneus – fifth metatarsal. Angle is increased, apex upward. **(Right)** Transverse plane.   Talocalcaneal angle, midtalar line, and midcalcaneal line are relatively normal unless adductus of forefoot is a major plane of compensation.

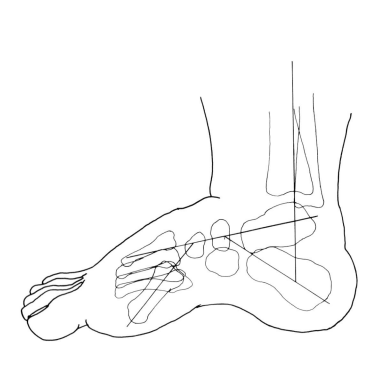

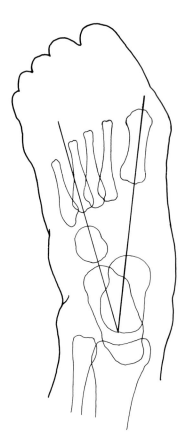

FLATFOOT

(Left) Sagittal plane.   Talocalcaneal angle is increased. Midtalar line falls plantar to first metatarsal head. Inferior calcaneus – fifth metatarsal angle is obtuse, apex upward; however, equinus may cause reversal of angle. Additionally demonstrated are lateral diagrams of oblique talus and vertical talus. **(Right)** Transverse plane.   Talocalcaneal angle is increased. Midtalar line is medial to first metatarsal. Midcalcaneal line varies.

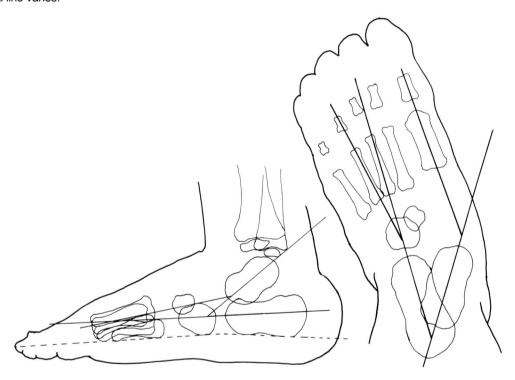

METATARSUS ADDUCTUS

(Left) Sagittal plane. Talocalcaneal angle is normal, midtalar line varies, and inferior calcaneus – fifth metatarsal angle varies dependent upon rearfoot positioning. **(Right)** Transverse plane. Talocalcaneal angle is normal to increased. Midtalar line forms angle with first metatarsal, moves laterally with respect to first metatarsal. Midcalcaneal line passes lateral to normal position.

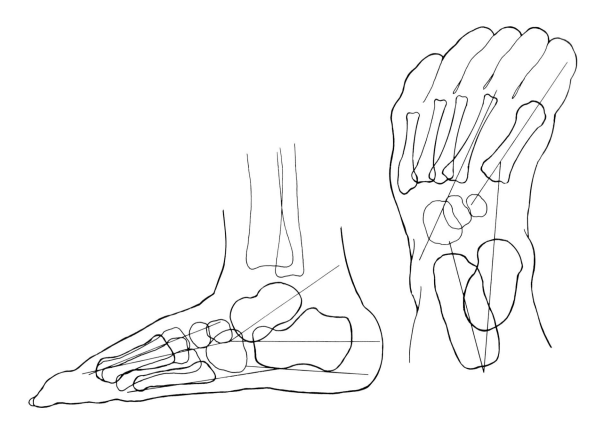

SKEWFOOT

Transverse Plane.   Talocalcaneal angle is increased. Midtalar line falls medial to first metatarsal. Midcalcaneal line passes lateral to normal position. (Sagittal plane.   Talocalcaneal angle, midtalar line, and inferior calcaneus – fifth metatarsal same as for metatarsus adductus.)

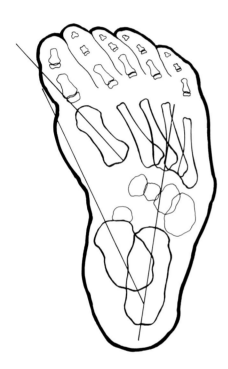

Podiatric Sports Medicine

23

Phillip Perlman, D.P.M.

In the 1970s, interest in aerobic fitness set off a running boom, and many sedentary Americans began running and competing in athletic events. Because athletic competition invariably leads to injuries, there was an increase in sports-related injuries. The podiatrist, because of his or her familiarity with lower extremity pathology, became the primary caregiver in many cases. The aim of sports medicine is to treat the pathology of the injury, but also to allow the individual to return to his or her previous level of fitness.

PLANTAR CALCANEAL PROBLEMS

History

Typically, a patient with heel spur/plantar fasciitis entity (Fig. 23-1) will describe increased amount of time or effort in a sport (the "too much, too soon, too fast" syndrome). Early morning dull, achy plantar heel pain is classic. Initially, these symptoms are of short duration and occur the morning following exercise. Patients either disre-gard these symptoms or attribute them to a "stone bruise." In intermediate stages of the disease, any walking after prolonged rest will consistently produce pain. If the patient continues to exercise in the late stages of the disease and allows the problem to go untreated, a seemingly monumental number of symptoms involving numerous tissues develop. This is caused by the athlete running through the pain.

In sports requiring consistent gait patterns—walking, running and aerobics—the patient can quickly move from early-stage symptoms to late-stage symptoms in a matter of weeks. Many athletes will provide a history and are aware of defensive gait patterns that develop as a result of increased pain. Typically, a more supinated gait pattern is acquired in an attempt to take pressure off the medial calcaneal area. This quickly developing defensive gait pattern is responsible for the early development of tarsal tunnel syndrome medially, and strains and tension placed on the peroneus longus and brevis laterally.

In cases of extreme defensive gait, the patient may develop a toe-walking attitude (apparently believing that what doesn't touch the ground can't possibly get hurt). This defensive gait affects the posterior tibial tendon/posterior muscle group, and exacerbates the primary disease.

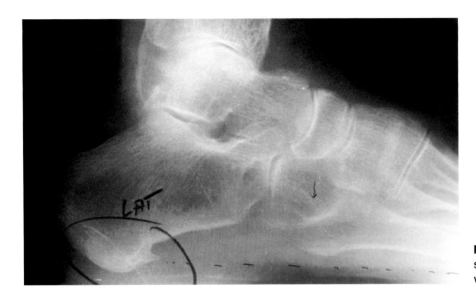

Fig. 23-1. Plantar calcaneal spur. (From Subotnick (1988), with permission.)

Evaluation

In terms of physical examination, the secondary symptoms involving the posterior tibial tendon and the lateral muscle group are discussed later in this chapter.

Although much of the plantar heel may hurt, point tenderness should be found at the medial plantar tuberosity of the calcaneus. Deep palpation at this site will typically elicit profound pain. In a number of cases, plantar calcaneal enlargement may be observed. If fluctuance and pain are noted on light palpation, one might suspect an adventitious bursa.

Dorsiflexing the hallux and evaluating the long flexor should also be done to evaluate for a partial rupture, pull, or herniation of the individual tendon and/or muscle group. Although there is often a suggestion of arch symptoms provided by the patient, seldom is there any physical pain noted on deep palpation of the deep plantar structures or when the hallux is placed in an extended position.

Beyond the physical examination, lateral x-rays should be taken to rule out fractures or tumors of the calcaneus. In cases of intractable, unremitting pain, a bone scan may be needed to rule out the possibility of stress fracture. Finding a well-developed spur on x-ray is of dubious value, because as much as 30 percent of the population may have a plantar heel spur without symptoms. Many of these patients will have no history of heel pain.

Athletes, no matter how fit, fall prey to the same diseases as the general public. Therefore, laboratory studies to identify systemic disease (e.g., gout, collagen diseases, and diabetes) may be necessary.

Pathogenesis

The commonly held opinion is that heel spur formation is the result of a long-term process involving a segment of the plantar fascia pulling off the periosteum, followed by bleeding and then by calcification, resulting in a spur. Authors have suggested that "in many cases, the spurring is a consequence and is not the cause of the inflammation."[1] Cryometic studies have shown that the attachment of the plantar aponeurosis is not always at the site of exostosis formation. Frozen section studies have associated the flexor hallucis brevis muscle with plantar calcaneal spur.

Therapy

The prevailing attitude regarding treatment disregards pathogenesis and revolves around reducing the rate of traction of the plantar soft tissue on the heel. Initially, the use of adhesive tape to reduce foot motion is an easy, cost-effective means of reducing pain. For most patients tape applied every 3 days is sufficient to significantly reduce symptoms. Family members can be taught to tape, thus avoiding unnecessary office visits. However, no matter what protective measures are used, skin breakdown is likely to occur.

For the patient with bursa or mild heel spur pain, reduction of symptoms can occur simply by the use of heel cups or quarter-inch felt aperture pads. An orthotic is the most appropriate treatment for the patient with defensive gait and resultant secondary symptoms.

Mechanically, the typical heel spur patient presents with a high degree of rearfoot varus (tibial varum and subtalar varus). A fully pronated subtalar joint is generally not sufficient to get the forefoot plantargrade. (Note that in cases of large amounts of rearfoot varus, resulting in a fully pronated subtalar joint, the posterior calcaneus will during gait still appear inverted.) As a result, midtarsal joint pronation becomes necessary. Soft tissue is then put on a stretch, which results in plantar calcaneal inflammation.

Conversely, patients with calcaneal eversion past the vertical as a result of forefoot varus, talipes equinus, or flexible forefoot valgus are less likely to have heel spur symptoms. In general, this situation seems to produce the myriad upper foot and leg pathologies.

Neutral shell orthotics made from Rohadur (Fig. 23-2) or other rigid materials work best in dealing with "straight ahead"–type repetitive sports such as walking, running, and jogging. After several weeks of wearing an uncorrected orthotic, the patient is seen on the track. In this situation, site

lines (strips of padding felt) are placed on the heel of the running shoe, and rearfoot and temporary forefoot posts are added to the orthotic using ⅛th-inch felt padding on temporary casts or shims. Permanent posting is undertaken based on office examinations and the patient's positive response to temporary shimming. Finally, in lateral motion sport situations (racquet sports, jumping sports, aerobics, etc.) that rigid devices are difficult to tolerate and more flexible orthotics and posts become necessary.

Beyond mechanical control of the foot, patients are encouraged to become involved in their own treatment. This especially is true in a patient with possible heel bursitis and/or inflammation of the posterior tibial nerve. In addition, patients are encouraged to stretch the posterior muscle group via the straight knee stretch and stretch the soleus and posterior tibial muscle group via the bent knee stretch. Stretching is extremely helpful in treating pain- and exercise-produced tightness. Additionally, the sprained ankle stretch is excellent for tightness and spasm of the lateral muscle group.

Heel spur care, like many other forms of treatment, seldom produces overnight cures. Rather than viewing treatment as success or failure, one considers treatment based on a continuum. Heel spur is a typical "directional"-type disease: As long as the patient is going in the direction of getting better and symptoms are reducing, more invasive care should be avoided.

No matter what the doctor's or patient's prejudices are, as much as 20 percent of patients undergoing a conservative regimen (tape/orthotics and physical therapy) will require further care. For that patient in whom treatment itself has reached a plateau and can seemingly go no further, or for the

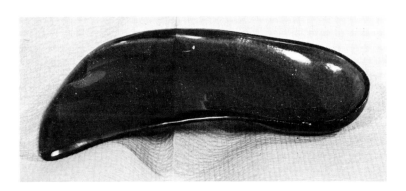

Fig. 23-2. Rohadur neutral shell orthotic with deep heel cup. (From Subotnick (1988), with permission.)

patient who is receiving no benefits from initial conservative care, the use of injectable steroids is mandatory. The initial injections afford the most relief and subsequent injections are much less effective.

The patient with heel spur as a result of high rearfoot varus foot would be well served simply by keeping up the heel contact area of the shoe with a shoe-caulking compound. Providing this care will reduce overstriding, which puts the foot in a less than desirable position, although there is no true "heel spur" shoe per se.

Training

A reduction in training of more than one level is unnecessary (see Table 23-2, below). Extended rest is of little treatment value and of possible detriment.

Finally, when all else fails, heel spur surgery and/or plantar fascial release is necessary for up to 10 percent of patients who have severe symptoms and choose to continue their athletic regimen. The biggest pitfall in heel spur surgery for athletes is convincing the patient that a substantial amount of time must be allowed for tissue to recover. Postoperatively walking with an inverted gait is common. If the patient continues to run in a defensive, supinated manner 6 to 12 months after surgery, he or she then becomes susceptible to all manner of stress fractures in the lateral column.

PROBLEMS INVOLVING THE POSTERIOR CALCANEUS

Calcaneal Apophysitis

Calcaneal apophysitis in children proves that excesses, to any degree, will produce penalties that will not go unnoticed by the body, even in a seemingly indestructible age group.

Evaluation/History

The child with a calcaneal apophysitis will present with a variety of symptoms involving numerous tissues. The initial pains are fairly straight-

forward in that there is dull tenderness associated with the posterior calcaneus. These early symptoms go unnoticed by the child or are attributed as "growing pain" by the parents.

As in untreated heel spur syndrome, a large portion of children with calcaneal apophysitis quickly develop histories suggesting secondary symptoms of both the posterior tibial nerve and the lateral muscle group.

Physical Examination

The pain involving the primary disease, calcaneal apophysitis, can be reproduced by deeply palpating the medial and lateral borders of the proximal one-third of the calcaneus. It is not uncommon in chronic apophysitis to be able to palpate tenderness along the posterior tibial nerve. The visible swelling seen in the adult is rarely noticed in children with palpable nerve pain. When examining the subtalar joint in the prone position, it is common to note a momentary catch as the foot is inverted; this is likely the juvenile version of the lateral muscle tightness seen in heel spur syndrome in adults.

Radiographic examination, although helpful in correlating biomechanical examination findings, is of no value in supporting the diagnosis of calcaneal apophysitis.

Pathogenesis

Much like heel spur syndrome in the adult, calcaneal apophysitis in children represent a traction epiphysis. Most frequently this disease is associated with jumping and situations in which the posterior muscle group is placed on a stretch (e.g., the position of a down lineman in the case of football).

Therapy

The child with calcaneal apophysitis generally responds to the high-dye basketweave taping system at the initial visit. A well-made orthotic device that compensates for biomechanical abnormalities will normally provide total relief of pain. Regular taping, icing, and stretching is seldom necessary in treatment of children. On rare occasions, children can be aggressive enough athletically to produce stress fractures. Failure to respond to mechanical care would suggest the need for a bone scan.

Posterior Calcaneal Pain in Adults

The two most common complaints involving the posterior calcaneus in the adult are a retrocalcaneal exostosis/bursitis and Achilles tendonitis (Fig. 23-3) with or without involvement of the retrocalcaneal bursa.

Evaluation

With the patient in the prone position, observe the posterior calcaneus. In the case of retrocalcaneal exostosis the palpable pain generally occurs laterally. On physical examination, a well-circumscribed area of erythema and posterior tenderness can be found. Conversely, in the case of Achilles tendonitis one can palpate crepitus upon dorsi/plantarflexion of the foot. By palpating the lateral aspects of the tendon one might be able to elicit pain, and nodules may be palpated along the ten-don sheath. It is not unusual to see a substantial amount of edema in the posterior aspect of the tendon and the calcaneus. Finally, the attachment of the Achilles tendon to the calcaneus should be palpated. It is not uncommon for this and the bursitis that lies posteriorly to produce pain on palpation.

Pathogenesis

In the case of both diseases shoes play a major factor in both the cause and eventual treatment of associated symptoms.

Therapy

Retrocalcaneal exostosis bursitis, known as "pump bump," is a classic biomechanical/shoe problem. Typically the patient with this entity has a high calcaneal inclination angle or elevated rear foot varus or both. The shoes usually involved in

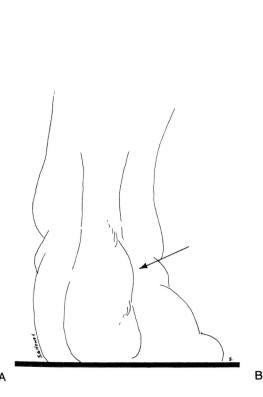

A

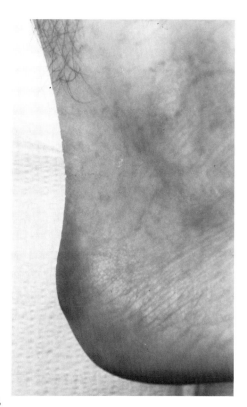

B

Fig. 23-3. (A) Retrocalcaneal exostosis and irritation of the Achilles tendon. Note lateral compression of the ankle and subtalar joints, resulting from excessive pronation. **(B)** Example of inflamed retrocalcaneal exostosis caused by irritation from running shoes. (From Subotnick (1988), with permission.)

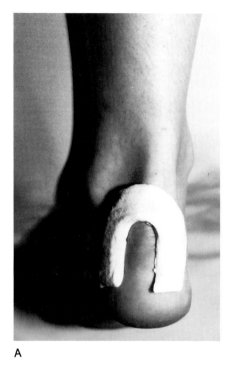

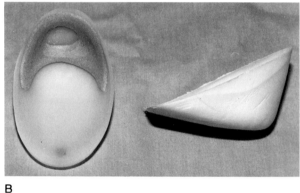

A   B

Fig. 23-4. Pads for painful retrocalcaneal exostosis or bursitis ("pump bump"). The pad may be applied to the foot **(A)** or placed directly into an orthotic device **(B)**. (From Subotnick (1988), with permission.)

the problem, women's pumps and men's loafers, fit from heel to toe; otherwise, they would slip off the heel. Thus, treatment involves:

1. Finding shoes that allow the posterior counter of the heel to hit the calcaneus in a better place.
2. Applying a tongue pad to the tongue or vamp of a shoe to keep the shoe from rubbing on the heel (Fig. 23-4).
3. Wearing shoes that fit from ball to heel, which are less likely to produce stress on the heel.

This is a rare syndrome in adults over 25. It is possible that these individuals may have eventually found more appropriate shoes. It is more likely that the foot goes through less range of motion as individuals age and therefore less stress is placed on the posterior calcaneus. This is also generally a rare athletic shoe–related problem.

In runners, Achilles tendonitis has by and large been successfully treated by the running shoe industry. In the early 1970s, running shoes had little

if any heel lift. Today, only a minimal number of companies produce a low-profile-heeled shoe.

Rather than purchase higher heeled shoes, the runner/walker/jogger may elect to simply use a quarter-inch to three-eighths-inch heel rise in both shoes. Multiple pieces of cardboard equaling $\frac{3}{8}$-inch can be used initially, and one-third of the total material can be removed on a weekly basis. Such a temporary measure may be ideal for the individual participating in sagittal plane sports because permanent elevation of the heel can change both the foot and shoe mechanics and produce a whole new set of problems. For the individual in lateral motion sports, a simple device such as heel lifts can be catastrophic because increasing the heel of a tennis shoe can predispose the athlete to lateral ankle sprains.

Attempting to match orthotic care and shoes to specific sport and specific injury is not possible. Orthotic devices and shoes represent variables in the individual's athletic program. The aim of mechanical care is to find the combination of shoes and

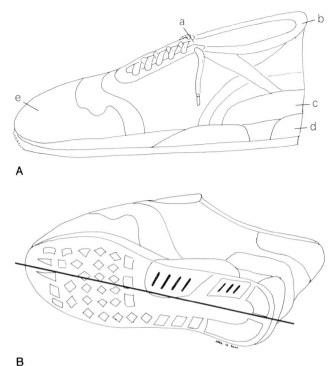

A

B

Fig. 23-5. Characteristics of a running shoe. **(A)** Side view: *a*, well-padded tongue; *b*, molded Achilles pad; *c*, firm heel counter; *d*, flared and beveled heel; *e*, high, rounded toe-box. **(B)** Bottom view showing straight last and studded sole. Running shoes are not suitable for cutting sports, because the high heel increases lateral instability. (From Subotnick (1988), with permission.)

orthotic devices that will aid the patient in returning to his or her previous level of fitness. Shoes/orthotic devices should act as a constant in athletic training formulas so that when (not if) an athlete develops new injuries, the patient will more likely look at training as the cause.

Based on this concept the following suggestions might be true for any shoe-related sport[2]:

1. Make sure any and all foot aids are brought to the shoe store at the time of purchasing shoes to ensure compatibility.
2. Do not wear running shoes (Fig. 23-5) for lateral motion sports; as heel height increases so does lateral instability.
3. Make sure wear spots (lateral posterior heel) are kept up with shoe caulking compound so overstriding is reduced. However, avoid resoling.

4. Purchase multiple pairs of the same shoes for consistency.
5. Purchase popular proven styles because new and overly expensive models may not be available next year.
6. Be prepared to switch new shoes often, because research indicates that at the 300- to 400-mile mark as much as 50 percent of shock absorbency is lost.

Beyond shoe advice, the patient must be willing to do a great deal of icing of the Achilles tendon after exercise. Preexercise icing, however, can be dangerous because the anesthetic qualities of ice can mask symptoms.

Although stretching is always advised, overstretching produced by training room incline boards is to be avoided because this places increased stress on both the tendon and the tendon attachments to the calcaneus. This form of overstretching in the patient with a genetic shortage of the gastrocnemius or soleus will exacerbate symptoms unnecessarily.

A short course of basketweave taping may serve as a helpful adjunct to patient self-care. More permanent mechanical care via an orthotic device is generally unnecessary in most cases. Orthotic devices are of least value in their relationship to sagittal plane motion and it is difficult to treat this problem biomechanically. Conservative treatment involving cortisone injections is contraindicated because injections may lead to evulsion of the tendon from its attachment.

Fracture of the Posterior Process

An unusual situation is the patient who presents with the history of Achilles tendonitis, but, upon evaluation, no positive findings are noted at the Achilles tendon or its attachment to the calcaneus except for generalized edema and posterior calcaneal pain. Forceful plantarflexion-eliciting pain coupled with bilateral radiographs (and possible bone scans) will suggest either a posterior process fracture or localized symptoms of reflex sympathetic dystrophy. Forceful flexion or muscle testing of the flexor hallucis longus and producing posterior superior calcaneal pain may also be a positive finding in the disease because of its anatomic relationship with the bone.

From a pathologic standpoint, there are several etiologic possibilities. The most common is an individual who plantarflexes the foot on a regular basis. The best examples would be the foot used as the take-off leg to the bar in the case of a high jumper, or situations in which the individual is jumping a great deal, or in ballet, where the foot is plantarflexed. With trauma, the possibility of a fracture of the posterior process of the talus resulting from a profound plantarflexion inversion sprain is a possibility. In the pronation syndrome, adduction plantarflexion of the talus on a continual basis could produce an irritation and possible disuse atrophy of the posterior process itself. Conservative care involving ice, light immobilization such as taping, or even below-knee cast-type immobilization may be used. The fracture has a poor history of healing, and removal of the fragment is probably in the patient's best interest.

TARSAL TUNNEL SYNDROME

In my schooling, I was constantly told by an elderly lecturer that, "when in doubt think of gout." Today in sports medicine a similar warning concerning the posterotibial nerve as a primary and secondary cause of symptoms is useful. A familiar story of a direct blow to the posterotibial nerve leading to classic pain, anesthesia, and paresthesia is not the nice, typically packaged history one elicits from an athlete. The symptoms of posterotibial neuritis more often present either as primary overuse injury without a history of trauma or as a problem secondary to a chronic disease state.

In the medial ankle, patients will often describe a burning, lancinating type of pain that is exacerbated by exercise and diminishes with rest. Often patients may be able to trace the course of the nerve with their fingers when describing the pain. In rare cases, the patient may also be able to correlate the burning and anesthesia of digits with medial malleolar symptoms. An inordinate number of patients with posterior nerve symptoms have a history of posterotibial shin splints/posterotibial myo-

sitis. Since both exist anatomically in the same compartment, such a relationship should not be unexpected.

Evaluation

Initial physical exam should entail direct palpation into the laciniate ligament area. Because of its anatomic location, palpation must be heavy enough to elicit pain. The course of the nerve should be digitally traced (Valleiux's points). In a similar manner, the calcaneal nerve branch should be deeply palpated. This examination is superior to the classic Tinel's sign, which is elicited by percussion with a neurologic hammer. After testing the posterior tibial nerve and its calcaneal branch, one should apply similar digital pressure on the lateral calcaneal periosteal area to allow the patient to better judge the examination. As a cautionary note, athletes who are highly involved in self-treatment should be cautioned against continual palpation of this area because this can exacerbate the problem.

Continuing the physical examination, one should place the foot at right angles to the leg with both legs in a similar position. Through observation one may note a slight bulge over the laciniate ligament area. Light palpation will confirm visual findings. In the case of positive findings, one should be able to rule out varicosities and ganglionic cysts from those involved with the posterotibial nerve. The dorsum of the hands may be used to compare temperature in the two lower extremities and to detect an elevated temperature in the affected area. Muscle testing with palpation of the posterior tibial and flexor hallux tendon should be carried out to evaluate for the presence of crepitus and/or loss of tendon integrity. Next, the fore-foot exam should be performed (see discussion under "Neuroma," below). Finally, either by physical examination or by additional history-taking it should be determined that there are no problems more proximal (e.g., sciatica) to the involved posterotibial nerve.

Beyond physical examination, one should be prepared to take an anteroposterior and a lateral radiograph of the ankle to rule out possible bone involvement. Hematologic studies should be performed to rule out systemic diseases such as the arthritides and diabetes mellitus. At some point it may be necessary to run nerve conduction and electromyographic studies. These tests are probably unnecessary on initial visits but become more critical later if conservative care fails and more invasive treatment becomes necessary.

Pathogenesis

From a medical standpoint and for the purposes of identification, tarsal tunnel syndrome/posterotibial neuritis represents a medical continuum. Posterotibial neuritis is more representative of a low-grade neuritis that might be classified as stage I disease. In this classification, during the initial stages the patient can identify intermittent burning pain that occurs after exercise. As the disease process continues, the patient can more easily identify both the pain and its location. In the final stages of the process night pain occurs, and the possibility of a bona fide medical pathology (tarsal tunnel syndrome) is a reality.

Essentially pain, swelling, and resultant inflammation occurring over a long period of time produces scar tissue. It is then that nerve conduction studies will identify the amount or indicate the degree to which the nerve is potentially irreversibly trapped by scar tissue.

Therapy

Initially, the athlete with posterotibial nerve involvement may present with a plethora of symptoms in many locations, making the problem appear unmanageable. Fortunately, this is not the case because most nerve symptoms reduce with successful treatment of the primary disease.

The application of ice affords almost immediate relief of many neuritis symptoms. By the use of cold packs, icing is easily managed by the patient. Several wraps of Ace bandage are applied to the area and the cold pack is placed in the medial malleolar area and is secured with the remaining Ace bandage. This produces an "ice envelope" dressing that (1) allows the ice to be held in place; (2) does not allow the ice to touch the skin directly, thereby reducing tissue damage; and (3) allows the patient to both move and ice at the same time, which may have a synergistic effect.

The difficulty with ice as a form of therapy, no matter what the disease, is that it does not feel good. Patients would much rather heat an area because that produces a feeling of well being. It is common to find that, after initial improvement has been made with ice, patients stop using it. Compliance is best achieved if the athlete is initially told that icing, if not done with regularity, will have to be replaced by anti-inflammatory drugs, which are even less desired by athletes in general.

Patient self-treatment in the form of flexibility training is also quite helpful in reducing muscle/tendon spasms associated with defensive gait. Besides traditional posterior and lateral muscle group stretches (Fig. 23-6A & B), putting the ankle through a series of figure-eights is helpful to maintain flexibility. A more productive and inviting form of flexibility is to have the patient "write" the alphabet with the foot.

Beyond self–physical therapy, a dramatic reduction of symptoms can be achieved by simply limiting foot/ankle motion by application of a basketweave taping system.

1. Tape disallows motion requiring less defensive gait and resultant muscle spasms.
2. Tape will control end ranges of motion and thus treat underlying mechanical problems.
3. Tape by its nature will produce local compression of the tarsal tunnel area, thus aiding icing.

As an adjunct or in place of orthotic therapy, tape can be applied twice weekly. For example, if applied Monday, the tape should be removed Thursday night and reapplied Friday; remove the tape Sunday night and reapply on Monday. This allows the skin at least 8 to 10 hours between tapings to recover.

Women, because of their increased range of motion and flexibility, may be more difficult to treat. Other forms of motion control than tape and orthotic devices are often necessary. Ace bandages and slip-on ankle braces with metal stays can be added as necessary to reduce range of motion and assist treatment well after symptoms have reduced.

Should conservative treatment fail, more invasive care may need to be provided. In this case a nerve conduction study should be performed to determine the baseline status of the nerve. Such documentation is necessary in the case of multiple steroid injections and/or surgery performed on the nerve itself. Unroofing the ligament and freeing the trapped nerve does not hold a high success rate

Before

Running

Approximately 9 Minutes

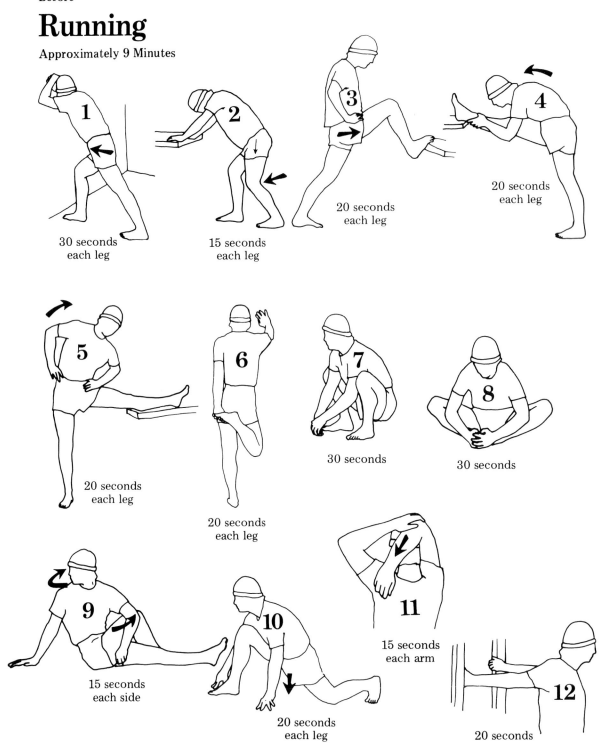

30 seconds
each leg

15 seconds
each leg

20 seconds
each leg

20 seconds
each leg

20 seconds
each leg

20 seconds
each leg

30 seconds

30 seconds

15 seconds
each side

20 seconds
each leg

15 seconds
each arm

20 seconds

Fig. 23-6A. Typical stretching exercises to be performed before running. (From Anderson RA: Stretching. Illustrated by Jean Anderson. Anderson World Publishing, Fullerton, CA. © 1975 Robert A. Anderson and Jean E. Anderson.)

656

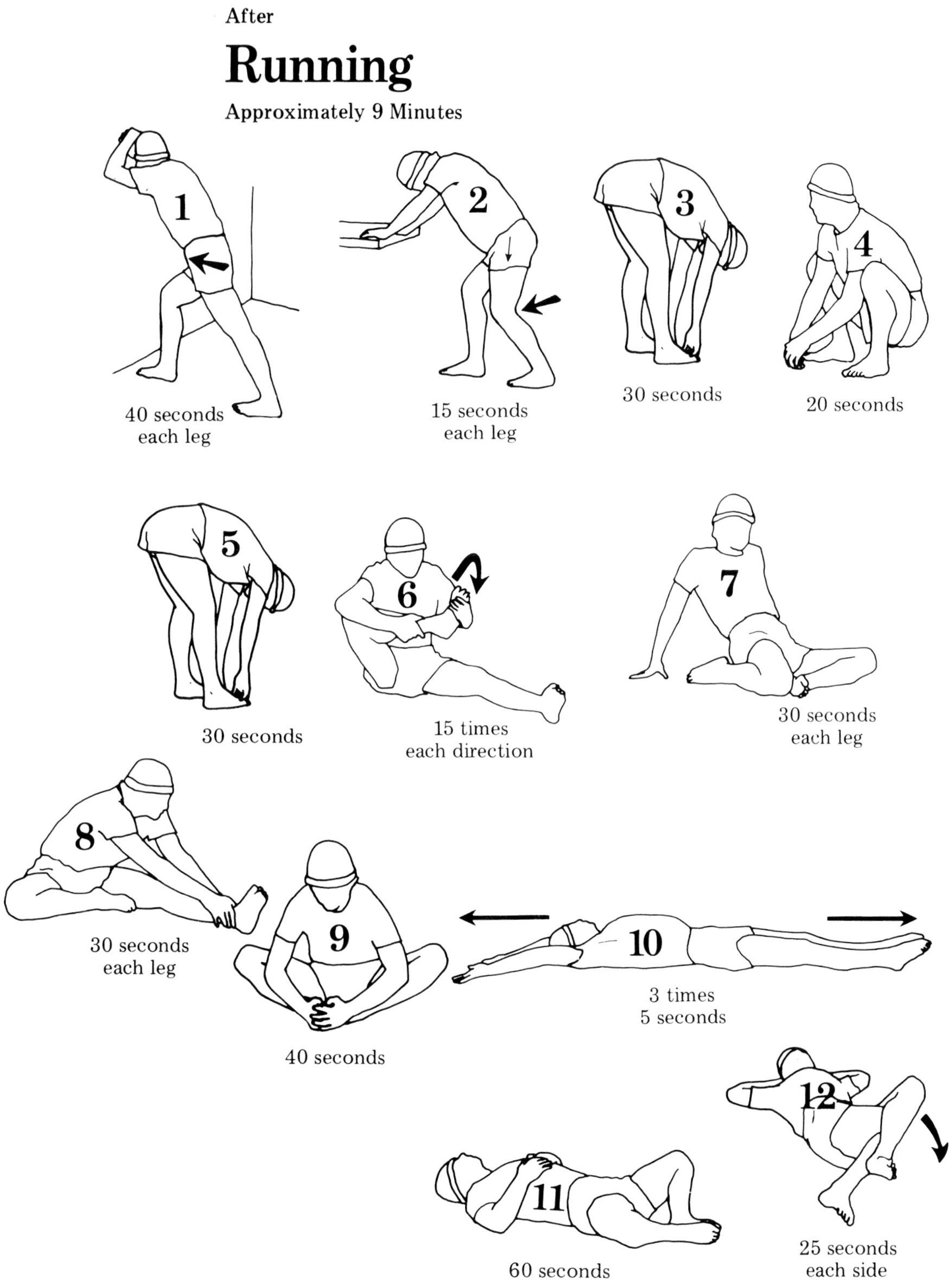

After

Running

Approximately 9 Minutes

Fig. 23-6B. Typical stretching exercises to be performed after running. (From Anderson RA: Stretching. Illustrated by Jean Anderson. Anderson World Publishing, Fullerton, CA. © 1975 Robert A. Anderson and Jean E. Anderson.)

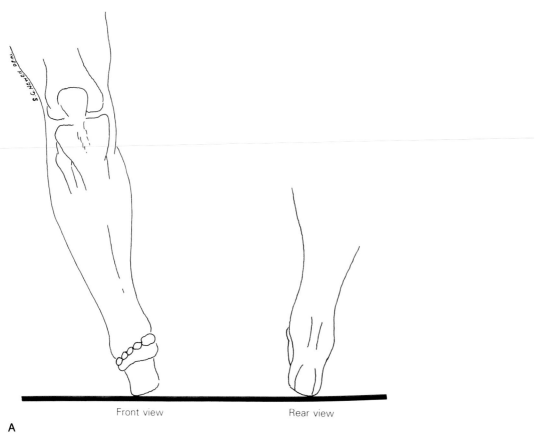

Front view   Rear view

A

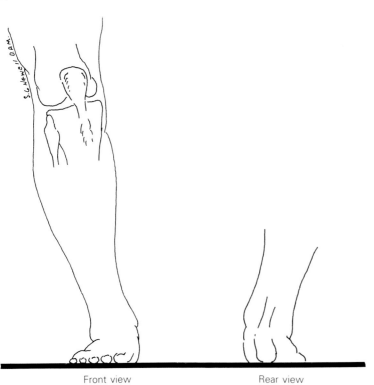

Front view   Rear view

B

Fig. 23-7. Effect of terrain on supination and pronation. **(A,B)** On a flat surface, supination occurs at heel contact and pronation at midstance. *(Figure continues.)*

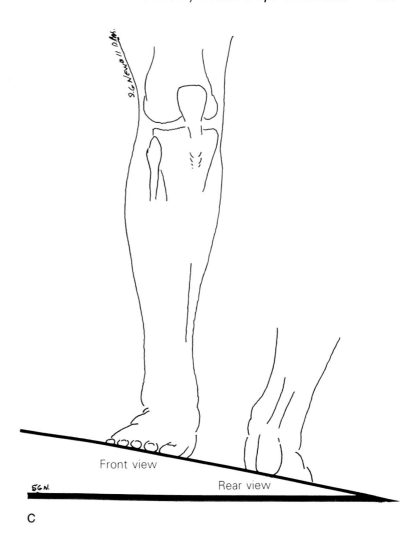

Front view

Rear view

Fig. 23-7 *(Continued).* **(C)** Running on a banked surface increases pronation. (From Subotnick (1988), with permission.)

C

in the athlete. First, postoperative bleeding and resultant scar may not leave the tissues in any better condition. Second, failure to reduce all motion short of a triple arthrodesis and ankle fusion still allows some motion and the possibility of additional scar tissue.

In summarizing care, it is necessary that the patient be involved in icing, flexibility, and exercises, and use modalities that reduce range of motion. Next, the patient may find it necessary to permanently modify the amount of training or change to an activity that is less irritating to the problem.

The following are specific training suggestions that are helpful in the treatment of runners:

1. Avoid running on grassy trails or sand. Even though the surface is softer the excessive motion produced by the varied terrain is impossible for most motion aids to control.
2. Running on sidewalks may be better than running on the softer yet highly canted roads. When running toward traffic, highly crowned roads cause the uphill right foot to overpronate and the downhill left foot to oversupinate (Fig. 23-7). It may be added that if a unilateral condition exists, running against traffic may be a treatment for the problem as long as one does not get hit by a car, which is the ultimate running injury.

3. Avoid jumping sports and situations where the foot is highly supinated.
4. Avoid the instability produced by high-heeled shoes.
5. Guard against over palpation of the nerve.

STRESS FRACTURES

Whether it be a fracture of a metatarsal, fibula, or any other lower extremity bone, general principles remain the same. By patient history, the most consistent finding in this disease entity is consistent unremitting pain. Unlike soft tissue pain, which may abate during some part of the exercise, stress fracture pain resolves only when the activity is halted. In the case of metatarsal stress fracture the patient will identify dull, sometimes throbbing forefoot pain that becomes progressively more intense with exercise. Although the patient may recall an event that may have caused the injury, generally there is no history of trauma.

Athletes often heroically continue to train after sustaining a multitude of nagging and painful injuries; however, this is not the case with metatarsal stress fractures. A large percentage of athletes read a number of self-treatment magazine articles and are quite cognizant of this phenomenon, and justifiably fear it, because it is the one entity that abruptly curtails athletic training. As a result, the patient will hide his or her fears and make the physician sort out the information. Essentially, the patient has sought treatment to confirm his or her own diagnosis. For this reason, and in the case of all sports medicine diseases, it is helpful after taking the patient's history to simply ask the patient for his or her opinion of the problem.

Evaluation

As in the case of Morton's neuroma, there may be enough signs of edema with a stress fracture to obliterate observation of the extensor tendons. Conversely, a lack of edema in no way rules out the diagnosis. Extensor tendon tightness might be encountered, but rarely is there any crepitus. Also, there is little pain on movement or palpation of the metatarsophalangeal joints. Intermetatarsal interspaces may be mildly positive for tenderness as a result of generalized edema. Palpation of each metatarsal shaft is critical. While palpating the individual metatarsals dorsally, the examiner's eyes should be fixed on the patient's facial expression. In this way the appropriate metatarsal can be identified with surprising accuracy on physical examination. An often used and ineffective student examination involves application of the tuning fork to the affected metatarsal. In the case of most forefoot swelling any application of force in any area may produce pain.

Radiographs should be taken at right angles, with comparison of the asymptomatic foot, to confirm the diagnosis. Any periosteal elevation of the metatarsal shaft should be suspect. As a matter of course, initial negative radiographs should be followed up 1 week later. Positive radiographic findings should be followed 2 to 3 weeks later to check for the expected appearance of bony callus. Rarely in the case of metatarsal stress fracture is a bone scan necessary. This is not the case with stress fractures of large extremity bones such as the tibia and fibula.

Pathogenesis

Although patients chose to believe in the single event theory (I ran a race too hard and fractured my bone), stress fractures are not single-event syndromes. Bone is an adaptive structure that changes based on forces acting upon it. As a classic overuse injury, stress fractures represent a failure of the bone to respond fast enough to changes of exercise patterns. In summary, in athletic situations where the steps are always the same (i.e., running and walking) and there is substantial biomechanic pathology, it is obvious that overexercise in addition to the nature of bone physiology make stress fracture an inevitable result.

In addition to the above pathogenesis, a special consideration should be given to female athletes based on endocrine/osteoporosis concerns. This is critical should there be any history of previous stress fractures.

Treatment

Regardless of the location of the stress fracture, the physician has two basic options as to therapy.

Ultimately these choices are based on trust and the doctor-patient relationship.

The first and safest option for the doctor is to stop all patient activity and immobilize the affected part. Salter, in his approach to this problem, disdains immobilization as a negative factor in the healing process.[3] Total immobilization via the below-knee cast disallows key forms of ongoing aerobic cross-training activity such as pool training. Such overtreatment can result in both psychological trauma and physiologic reduction of bone and muscle mass as well as loss of aerobic fitness.

The second option of allowing more movement places a premium on doctor-patient communication. Pain is the best indicator as to the effectiveness of treatment. In using the immobilization ladder (Table 23-1), the physician bases the amount of activity the patient may undergo on the patient's description of pain. A common example is a runner/triathalonist sustaining a metatarsal stress fracture. Seldom does this individual need any immobilization. This allows for participation in the other two (swimming/cycling) sports. Should the athlete continue to experience pain associated with normal walking, more restriction of movement is necessary. Note that in relationship to the immobilization ladder, two intense methods (Unna boot and a postoperative shoe) may be as effective as one heavier form of immobilization (below-knee cast). The doctor who chooses to allow the patient the luxury of maintaining a substantial level of fitness should meticulously chart such communications.

Once primary bone healing has taken place and the patient has been able to walk substantial distances without symptoms, preventive care should be undertaken. A well-constructed orthotic device based on both the patient's abnormal biomechanics and individual style of gait should be produced.

Table 23-1. Immobilization Ladder

Heavy forms of immobilization
   Above-knee casting
   Below-knee casting
   Crutches/total non-weight-bearing
      EXAMPLE: Bivalve posterior splint
Medium Immobilization
   Gelocast in the postoperative shoe
   Adhesive tape in the postoperative shoe
      EXAMPLE: Air splint
Light immobilization
   Adhesive tape/orthotic ankle braces with metal stays

In summary, because of the prevalence of metatarsal stress fractures, any pain severe enough to stop the athlete should be suspect. Second, the edema that is traditionally found in most fracture cases may not be present in this entity. Finally, when stress fractures are suspected negative radiographs almost always require the use of bone scans to convince patients to curtail or modify training patterns.

MORTON'S NEUROMA

Evaluation

An individual with Morton's neuroma will classically describe "burning pain in the ball of my foot; it makes me take my shoes off and I massage my foot and it feels better." The pain, which is generally dull and sometimes throbbing, generally affects only the middle three digits.

In many cases there is a long history of this pain pattern. Not unusual is the presence of plantar hyperkeratotic lesions with a history of professional and/or self-care. In the absence of lesions, patients generally attribute the pain to arthritis.

Nearly all patients in time see some relationship between their forefoot pain and shoes. Any shoe that can impart lateral stress against the metatarsal (ski boots) or shoes that put more stress on the forefoot (spike heels, cowboy boots) are suspect. Generally wearing no shoes or running-type shoes reduces the pain substantially.

Although the typical history of chronic pain exists on occasion, patients will present with a history of a single event that exacerbates an already existing chronic problem. Situations such as spading a garden, starting an aerobic dance class, or jumping rope are typical examples whereby increased stress on the forefoot exacerbates pain. Should no such history exist, patients exhibiting this pain pattern will generally initially attribute their pain to a misstep, resulting in the classical self-diagnosis of a "stone bruise."

On physical examination of the acutely painful condition, physical findings may be consistent with a "hot neuroma." In this situation, there may be enough forefoot edema to mask the extensor tendons. Pain may be severe enough to disallow nearly any weight-bearing in shoes.

In examination of the forefoot, one should palpate the plantar aspect of each metatarsal head. The range of motion should be determined and palpation of the metatarsal shafts should be performed. Deep pressure between the toe web and each intermetatarsal interspace (especially the second and third) will produce a "Chandelier's sign." Having the patient stand and producing dorsal pressure into the intermetatarsal interspace with an eraser may produce similar findings. Students, out of fear of hurting the patient, generally do not press hard or deep enough to elicit symptoms, thus missing the possible diagnosis. The easiest test to perform is to squeeze the forefoot laterally and have the patient determine which interspace hurts. Moving adjacent metatarsals in the sagittal plane and attempting to notice a click (Moulder's sign) is unrewarding. Also less than ideal is observing a radiographic separation of the metatarsal heads due to "the traditionally" enlarged nerve (Sullivan's sign). Radiographs certainly are of value in ruling out metatarsal stress fracture as well as joint disease and foreign bodies.

Pathogenesis

There are a number of theories that have been proposed as to the prevalence of third interspace neuromas. First, metatarsals 1 through 3 and 4 and 5 work as separate segments or columns, causing excessive stress on the third interspace nerve. Root proposed the idea that symptoms resulted from shearing forces at the propulsive phase of gait.[4] Other factors, such as an anatomic variant of the third interspace nerve or simple retrograde force produced as a result of hammer deformities, all have been implicated in the production of the problem. Regardless of which theory is accepted, the best pathologic explanation is the medical term *neurofibrolipoma* (Fig. 23-8), which indicates a normal nerve with fibrous and fatty tissue invested around it. Using the analogy of the growth of tree rings may be the easiest and most acceptable explanation for patients. In summary, the key to evaluation is to separate the nerve problem from typical

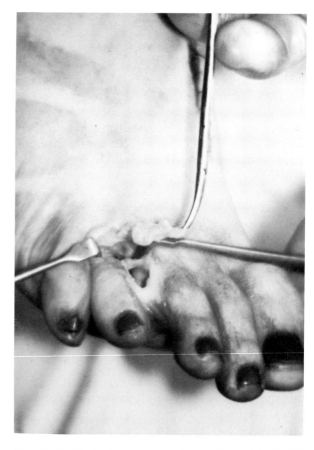

Fig. 23-8. Morton's neuroma. (From Subotnick (1988), with permission.)

problems of skin, bursa, bone, and joint, and possible contributory systemic disease.

Treatment

The easiest nonthreatening initial visit care should include instructions as to icing (15-minute time intervals, two to five times a day) and application of metatarsal pads to the skin. This author's personal preference is ⅛th-inch adhesive-backed felt padding. Students who insist on using quarter-inch padding with skived edges have found that self-applications of these pads can produce a substantial amount of grief (relief).

Continuance of this mechanical care may include simple padding of the bottom of the shoe with similar materials or the application of a metatarsal pad to the underside of the Spenco insole. Besides shock-absorbing qualities, Spenco, because of its ability to reduce shear, is not only helpful as a temporary orthotic device but reduces the slippage of the foot off a rigid orthotic.

Should symptoms stop short of a total cure, a more sophisticated orthotic device based on biomechanical examination can be produced. When conservative care produces less than total reduction of symptoms or the patient presents with a highly inflamed "hot neuroma," the treatment of choice is injectable cortisone. A number of clinicians suggest producing a cocktail by adding hyaluronidase to B-12, a local anesthetic/cortisone preparation. For many, the injection with its resultant temporary reduction of inflammation, allows ongoing conservative therapy (i.e. icing, padding, orthotic care) to ultimately be successful.

Certainly a dangerous and nonproductive treatment suggestion in the athlete is changing shoes. As long as the shoe fits properly, a change of shoes is most likely to produce new and unwanted changes in running gait. Since this is a street shoe problem, such shoe change suggestions should be avoided. The only exception is when patients buy inexpensive shoes that have no flexibility or shock absorption at the forefoot.

In suggesting street shoes, certainly shoes that tie as opposed to loafers will put less stress on the forefoot. Likewise, attempting to purposely misfit the shoe by fitting the individual a half-size longer and applying a tongue pad is occasionally helpful. It is rare that the individual will psychologically and aesthetically tolerate a traditional rocker bottom addition to a street shoe.

From the standpoint of training, it is rare that reduction of training schedule is helpful in treating this problem unless the condition is acute. In this case, cross training in terms of an exercise bike or swimming are helpful during the acute period.

SESAMOIDITIS

Although first metatarsophalangeal joint symptoms involving hallux valgus/hallux rigidus occur with great frequency in the general public, problems involving the sesamoids are commonly seen in the athlete. It is not unusual for the athlete to attribute sesamoid pain to preexisting hallux valgus deformities. The patient will cite a history of vague medial first metatarsophalangeal joint pain associated with no history of trauma. Activities that require jumping are more commonly associated with these symptoms. In many cases, the patient will have pain for a prolonged period of time, thinking that the problem is a "stone bruise" that will eventually resolve.

Evaluation

On physical examination, hallux valgus/hallux rigidus may exist. In putting the first metatarsophalangeal joint through a range of motion, the tibial and fibular sesamoid can be located and individually palpated for pain. Lateral pressure against each of the sesamoids should be attempted to ascertain the possibility of arthritis of the sesamoid/first metatarsophalangeal joint apparatus.

X-ray studies in the anteroposterior, lateral, lateral oblique, and axial views will help to define the morphology, position, and presence of possible osteoarthritis. Not infrequently, bone scans may be necessary to confirm a diagnosis of fracture/stress fracture. Laboratory studies are occasionally necessary to separate systemic disease, such as arthritides, from a local condition.

Pathogenesis

The first, most critical cause of sesamoiditis relates to jumping sports such as basketball, because these result in direct trauma to the bone. Next, more obscure but as important, are those mechanical problems whereby the first metatarsal is positioned to absorb more stress. Such is the case with plantar flexed first ray and forefoot valgus. Finally, more obscure are those sesamoid problems that result from a combination of hallux varus, hallux valgus, and their related biomechanical causes.

Treatment

Initial response to protective padding generally suggests a simple diagnosis of sesamoiditis, thus reducing the need for possible bone scans. Patients can easily be taught to ice and pad the affected part. In many cases, simple Spenco insoles with appropriate additional sesamoid-protective padding will provide enough relief to make sophisticated orthotics unnecessary.

LATERAL ANKLE PROBLEMS

In attempting to narrow discussion of lateral foot and ankle problems, it is first necessary to eliminate those acute problems associated with lateral ankle sprains, such as (1) dislocations/fractures of the bone, (2) avulsion of the lateral collateral ligaments, (3) disruption of muscle/tendon apparatus, and (4) lateral foot and ankle instability secondary to any or all of the above.

Resultant differential diagnosis involving chronic lateral ankle pain would most surely include (1) sinus tarsi pain; (2) traction injuries and symptoms related to the dorsal lateral cutaneous nerve; (3) peroneal tendonitis; and (4) for a lack of a better term, cuboid arthralgia.

First, a history of anesthesia and paresthesia should help diagnose problems associated with a *dorsal lateral cutaneous nerve* or any branch of the common peroneal nerve. Pathologic symptoms involving this nerve commonly result either from a single incidence involving a lateral ankle sprain that may rupture the nerve or artery, or from chronic rubbing of the nerve against a bony prominence. Standard neurologic examination certainly would include response to sharp, dull, and direct palpation of the nerve itself starting from the head of the fibula. As noted by Lerman et al., "The dorsal lateral cutaneous nerve may be easily observed and palpated if the foot is plantar flexed and inverted; it lies anteromedial to the fibular malleolus."[5] Nerve conduction studies and electromyographic testing should confirm the diagnosis.

The course of the disease is variable depending upon the degree of damage. During convalescence, the part should be protected by a variety of immobilization aids similar to those suggested in treatment for stress fractures.

Tendonitis involving the peroneus longus and brevis is rarely an isolated problem, and usually occurs as a result of a guarded gait caused by the initial injury. When it does occur, the patient generally is able to trace the course of the tendon and will volunteer a history of crepitus and possibly one of trauma. Examination of the frontal plane motion of the subtalar joint and palpation of the tendon should confirm crepitus and altered range of motion.

A red flag should go up when a patient suggests that the tendonitis in his or her foot or leg is so painful as to make exercise impossible. Stress fractures of the fibula are quite common. Treatment for this injury is the same as for any tendon injury, and its response to care is more likely to be based on the severity of primary disease.

Whereas nerve and tendon injuries are fairly easily identified by the patient and doctor, such is not the case in *sinus tarsi syndrome.* Patients will describe a history of vague, generalized pain located at the dorsal, lateral aspect of the sinus tarsi. Injecting the affected joint with a local anesthetic and radiopaque dye can confirm the diagnosis (1) by noting the disruption of the joint and (2) by noting the reduction of symptoms.[6] It is thought by some authors that the sinus tarsi canal and its fatty plug and neurovascular elements are responsible for the pain. The origin of the problem is often a single episode of trauma.

As intriguing and as esoteric as the previous problems are, as a group they represent a minority of the chronic lateral ankle problems seen in practice. Most frequently, the patient with lateral ankle pain will describe low-grade symptoms that appear during the normal day's activities. Patients will relate symptoms to changes of shoegear (especially high heels), morning inflexibility, recent ankle turns, and especially pain on stepping on the threshold of the carpet (the metal attachment of the junction of the carpet/linoleum). The symptoms of this *cuboid arthralgia* are located at the dorsal aspect of the fourth/fifth metatarsal cuboid articulation. This is the same area of symptoms associated with pain with sinus tarsi syndrome.

On physical examination, there is seldom any palpable pain or edema noted. If the problem has lasted for several weeks, it is possible to palpate some tenderness along the course of the peroneus longus and brevis tendons. The only confirmatory physical examination test is dorsal pain at the fourth/fifth metatarsal cuboid articulation produced by forced dorsiflexion of the calcaneal cuboid joint. Because of the prevalence of stress fractures on the lateral side of the foot associated with exercise, such examination should not be undertaken until x-rays have ruled out obvious bone pathology.

There are two separate etiologies for this problem. The first is an obvious defensive response of the peroneal tendons to the post-sprained-ankle syndrome. Highly inverted positions will incite the midtarsal locking mechanism, creating stability in the foot, but the soft tissue will suffer. The second and more subtle etiology is oversupination as result of varus positions of an orthotic, heel lifts, or extreme amounts of subtalar joint compensation action as a result of rigid forefoot valgus. In all of these cases, supination, microtrauma, and resultant spasm or tightness of the peroneal group produce the syndrome.

This particular entity is seen and treated by many practitioners in the manipulative sciences. While simple manipulation is adequate for the nonathlete, normal exercise trauma makes one-time manipulative treatments in the athlete difficult. Good results can be obtained by applying basketweave/low-dye taping systems, changed every 3 days (with or without ⅛-inch cuboid pad), to the cuboid area, and by gentle heating and stretching of the peroneal muscle. In general, this problem is easily self-treated by the patient, seldom indicating the use of long-term care such as orthotics, which may, in fact, cause or exacerbate this problem.

ATHLETIC TRAINING

For many students/doctors of medicine, the treatment of athletes holds great appeal. However, it is quite possible for the practitioner to be the great doctor/diagnostician of our time and still not be able to develop a sports medical practice. Without some basic knowledge of sports/fitness, it is impossible to answer the inevitable last question of the patient visit: "But doctor, what can I do now?"

The easiest way to view athletic training is as an ever-extending ladder. Getting motivated to start the first rung (exercise) is hardest but once on the ladder it becomes increasingly easier. Care must be taken to systematically move up the ladder slowly, one rung at a time, lest one fall off and become injured.

The first rung, and the key to any aerobic program, is the ability to walk 2 to 4 miles two to four times a week. If the individual is so cardiovascularly unfit that walking is physically stressful, the common disclaimer of consulting with the family doctor is in order.

For the individual entering into an exercise program, self-monitoring via target heart rate is mandatory. Using the formula of 220 minus the patient's age, multiplied by two-thirds, will result in expected beats/per minute, called the target heart rate.

In the conditioned but injured athlete, walking, besides being injury provoking, tends to not be aerobic. With this individual, alternative exercise such as pool training (running in the deep end of the pool by treading water using flotation devices) will stimulate an aerobic workout.

Once the athlete is able to negotiate running 3 miles on a regular 3- to 5-day/week basis, he or she has achieved rung two. This says the individual can run at an aerobic pace for 20 minutes every other day for three nonconsecutive times a week. If unable to run all 2.5 to 3 miles without pain, the patient should return to the first rung of the ladder and walk.

Rung three is achieved when the patient finds that an aerobic workout every other day is not enough. This rung is simply satisfied by running two consecutive days once a week. This now puts aerobic activity at 4 to 5 days a week. The temptation next to exercise without days off should be avoided by all but Olympic-bound athletes.

Rung four is the level at which 4 to 6 days of athletic activity is nice but the times spent is insufficient or unsatisfying. Why do people run more than 3 miles? Folklore says that the first 3 miles are

Table 23-2. The Athletic Training Ladder

Rung 1	Walk 2 to 4 miles two to four times a week
Rung 2	Run 3 miles every other day
Rung 3	Run 3 miles five to six times a week
Rung 4	Run 5 to 6 miles once a week
Rung 5	Run 5 to 6 miles five times a week
Rung 6	Run 1.5 times normal distance or do interval training

for the heart and the next 3 are for one's head. It is assumed this statement refers to the "runners high," a theoretical endorphin reaction that produces a feeling of well-being. Although there are books written about how one moves from 3 miles to 5 to 6 miles on a regular basis, the patient should avoid the nickel-dime method, that is, adding 1 mile to each run. Rather, it is easier to gauge the penalties of doing this new distance in the form of a single long run.

Achieving rung four, then, says the individual can run a long run once a week without problems. As a half-step the individual may find that a long run twice a week is acceptable. Then, over a period of time all of the 3-mile runs can be converted into 5 to 6 mile runs. This now means the individual can run 5 to 6 miles five to six times a week.

Rung five not only is beyond the scope of many individuals but this chapter as well. Simply stated, the individual at this level either runs longer (1.5 to 2 times the usual daily distance, or more) or does speed training on a track.

It is possible and mandatory that both the doctor and the patient negotiate an exercise program based on the patient's aerobic fitness and present injury status. This can be achieved using the athletic training ladder concept, as summarized in Table 23-2.

REFERENCES

1. McCarthy DJ, Gorecki GF: The anatomical basis of inferior calcaneal lesion. J Am Podiatry Assoc 69:536, 1979
2. Cook SD, Kester MA, Brunet ME, Haddad RJ: Biomechanics of running shoe performance. Clin Sports Med 4:619, 1985
3. Salter RB, Bhalla SK: Congenital short tendocalcaneus. J Bone Joint Surg [Br] 49:695, 1967
4. Root M, Orien W, Weed J: Normal and Abnormal Function of the Foot, Vol. II. Clinical Biomechanics Corp., Los Angeles, CA, 1977
5. Lerman B, Garnish L, Bellam H: Injury to the superficial peroneal nerve. J Foot Surg 23:334, 1984
6. Fried A, Dobbs B: Sinus tarsi synovectomy. J Am Podiatr Med Assoc 75:445, 1985

SUGGESTED READINGS

Hlavac H: The Foot Book. World Publications, Mountain View, CA, 1977.
Nicholas JA, Hershman EB: The Lower Extremity and Spine in Sports Medicine. Vol. 1 & 2. CV Mosby Co., St. Louis, 1986.
Subotnick SI: Sports Medicine of the Lower Extremity. Churchill Livingstone, New York, 1988.

The Handicapped and Disabled Podiatric Patient

24

Leonard A. Levy, D.P.M., M.P.H.

Appropriate emphasis must be given to the foot health needs of those society members designated as handicapped or disabled. Physical problems that are disabling often involve the foot and its associated structures. However, there are also physical and nonphysical conditions not directly involving the foot or the lower extremity that either prevent access to professional foot health care, greatly reduce such access, or require special methods to accomplish diagnosis and treatment.

Handicapped and disabled individuals are often unable to carry out the necessary activities to provide normal foot hygiene or cannot independently seek professional foot health services when needed. This may be due to limitations of hearing, sight, manual dexterity, or ambulation; diminished cognitive powers; or certain neuropsychiatric disorders. Such problems may also arise in individuals who are disabled with severe cardiac, respiratory, neurologic, renal, musculoskeletal, or hematologic conditions and those in the terminal stages of life.

Handicapped or disabled patients may be found in any age group, from early childhood to the elderly. With advances in medical technology and increased attention to the special problems of handicapped persons, many people who would have prematurely died because of a medical condition leading to or associated with their disability now survive and often live a full life span. In addi-

tion, since more people are living longer, they become possible victims of diseases and disorders that may lead to various degrees of disability. Another phenomenon to consider is that the use of automobiles, and of various types of machinery in the home and workplace, because of human error, operational abuse, or mechanical failure, has resulted in an increasing number of injuries that not infrequently include the creation of thousands of newly handicapped individuals yearly.

Some providers of foot health care may not routinely see severely handicapped patients. It is possible that, like the rest of the population, these physicians will share certain common responses that may include embarrassment for the patient and for the doctor, feelings of guilt that he or she is in good health, guilt that this fact makes the doctor happy and even a sense of fear of contagion. All this may result in a generalized adverse reaction by the doctor, even though he or she is fully aware of the fact that there is no danger of acquiring the disease or disorder through the doctor-patient association.

The feelings of unease may be compounded even more in patients with moderate to severe communication disorders. Such patients may be mentally retarded or have aphasia, cerebral palsy, cleft lip or palate, sensory defects, or injuries to the central nervous system resulting from stroke, tumor, or trauma. Communication with such patients can vary from adequate to marginal. However, like others, these patients may require periodic foot care. In some instances podiatric problems may not be recognized by the health care team, including the podiatrist responsible for foot care, because of the patient's inability to communicate adequately. Sometimes this can be at least partially compensated for by closer examination of the foot to identify visible or palpable conditions or giving patients who can partially communicate, even if poorly, the time it takes to describe their complaint. In other cases the physician may have to rely on someone who accompanies or who spends considerable time with the patient. This is particularly helpful when the patient talks in a manner that the physician may not understand but that is understandable to the person accompanying the patient. In such cases, the physician should not assume or act as if the patient cannot communicate by leaving him or her out of the conversation. This could severely hamper a potentially good patient-doctor relationship and be very deleterious to the treatment plan that is established. Parents, other family members, an attendant, or close friends need to be given support and encouragement since they could be valuable members of the team attending to the patient's needs. They may be better able to communicate with the patient and are often in a position to provide certain prescribed care.

In many handicapped individuals foot health hygiene is grossly inadequate as a result of lack of patient education combined with the physical or mental incapability to properly carry out appropriate foot care. It is essential to educate the patient and, if necessary, the person who helps care for the patient. Without such instruction the risk of the handicapped patient developing foot problems could be elevated considerably.

The patient's physical and mental status will help determine the extent and type of treatment that should be rendered. It should be emphasized that a treatment plan based on such an individualized assessment may range from the ideal to a holding pattern. Often consulting with the physician responsible for the overall health care of the patient can be most invaluable in establishing such a therapeutic regimen. Making promises or undertaking therapeutic procedures that are impractical or impossible, provoked by sympathies and the pressures from patients and their families, should be avoided. Because we are sometimes forced to treat patients who are handicapped in less than ideal environments (e.g., at home, while they are in a wheelchair, in an ill-equipped nursing home) physicians must accept that they are performing a valuable service to these patients even though the care rendered under such conditions is less than textbook perfect. Of course under such circumstances physicians should be particularly careful to explain their reasoning and the shortcomings of such care to the patient and the patient's family when the treatment plan is presented. In the overwhelming majority of these situations patients and their families are very aware of these problems and very appreciative of the efforts of the podiatric physician.

MULTIDISCIPLINARY APPROACH

The rapid development of cooperative approaches to health problems is the inevitable result of the scientific and technical advances in medical care in general. This is the hallmark that has led to the evolution of the so-called health care team. Multidisciplinary cooperation allows for the best use of knowledge and skills and frees families and patients from taking full responsibility for coordinating their own health care.

To care for handicapped and disabled individuals a multidisciplinary approach is essential, and its absence is a disservice to patients. To cooperate effectively professionals must be prepared to spend extra time in consultation with colleagues from other disciplines. They must also communicate with patients and their families to make sure there is an understanding of the problems, the treatment needed, its limitations as well as capabilities, and how the therapeutic regimen is carried out.

The podiatric physician must be psychologically prepared to become involved in the long-term care of the handicapped patient. Most typically, there are no quick remedies or rehabilitative surgical procedures that will eradicate the handicap. Health professionals must be prepared to establish and accept goals for both the patient and themselves that are less than ideal. Even this level of success, however, can be extremely gratifying to both handicapped patients and their families.

COMMON PODIATRIC PROBLEMS IN NEUROLOGIC DISORDERS

It is certainly well beyond the scope of this book and this chapter to describe all the numerous neurologic and neuromuscular disorders that can lead to an individual becoming handicapped and how such disabilities may impact on podiatric medical practice. A few common conditions have been selected that may help to emphasize what might create special problems in the podiatric medical management of patients who also may have a neurologic disorder.

Epilepsy

One of the most prevalent of neurologic disorders is epilepsy, a term usually employed to describe the outward manifestations of many different underlying disorders of the central nervous system. Depending on the source and location of the problem, the condition may manifest itself in major or minor focal seizures, which may be primarily sensory or primarily motor, and partial seizures, which are generally referred to as temporal lobe seizures, in which there may be visual or auditory phenomena frequently associated with motor automatisms. Finding the drug or combination of drugs that will produce the maximum control of the attacks with minimal or no side effects is frequently accomplished. Many such individuals can still have attacks in specific circumstances, particularly when they are under considerable stress. The apprehension or anxiety created in anticipation of a podiatric procedure or the actual performance of such a procedure itself could constitute a sufficient amount of stress in some patients to be a cause for concern.

Therefore, it is advisable that, when contemplat-ing foot surgery or some other potentially stressful procedure, the neurologist or other physician who is responsible for the control of the patient's epilepsy be contacted. Such a contact would be for the purpose of discussing the nature of the procedure and whether general anesthesia will be necessary, and to ascertain whether the patient's epilepsy has been under good control. Relying solely on the patient or family of the patient to provide honest and complete information regarding the occurrence of symptoms is not always adequate. Older teenagers, for example, may not be entirely truthful in revealing any difficulties they may have had. This often is because of their fear that such a revelation of even a minor seizure may result in their inability to acquire an automobile driver's license. The ability to measure the serum level of anticonvulsants has provided the physician with a far better way of ascertaining whether the patient can be expected to remain free or relatively free of symptoms.

For the most part, patients with epileptic seizures tolerate podiatric procedures quite well. It is rare to hear of a problem encountered during the course of foot surgery. However, when patients subject to seizures undergo surgery under general anesthesia, the surgeon must be aware that it is not unknown for such individuals to have a convulsion when coming out of anesthesia. Seizures almost never occur during the induction or duration of the anesthetic.

Seizures of the greatest concern during the care of patients being treated for foot disorders are those of the major motor variety, but focal motor seizures occasionally may also be a problem. Some doctors may not be adequately aware of the automatic behavior of persons suffering from temporal lobe epilepsy. Unless they have been alerted to the diagnosis, they may conclude that the patient has a psychiatric condition. Here again it is particularly useful to have specific information from the physician responsible for the medical care of the patient.

Cerebral Palsy

Cerebral palsy is a term that has been used to characterize nearly every central nervous system disorder in early life resulting in either spastic or athetoid movements or both. Most neurologists, however, use the term to refer to the consequences of disturbances occurring during the perinatal period, particularly trauma or asphyxia, and varying greatly from patient to patient. In some patients the spastic weakness involves only the lower extremities, whereas in others it involves both upper and lower extremities, with or without bulbar involvement. More severely handicapped individuals may also have difficulty in swallowing and speech. These patients can have generalized or focal convulsions and varying degrees of intellectual deficit. Because of communication problems it is frequently difficult to determine their relative level of intelligence, and therefore their ability to cope independently with the problems of normal daily living, much less their ability to understand why foot health care is important.

Treating many patients with cerebral palsy requires special consideration. For example, for those who are spastic and have problems with coordination as a result of cerebellar or extrapyramidal tract injury, it is difficult to maintain the positions that may be necessary to accomplish even simple procedures on the foot. Through the cooperation of the physician responsible for the patient's medical care, it may be possible to alleviate temporarily some of the motor difficulty in patients with spastic or atheototic cerebral palsy. This may be accomplished by using medications such as muscle relaxants or tranquilizers while attempting to perform the procedure.

Parkinsonism and Huntington's Disease

Muscular rigidity and tremor may be found either together or alone in older patients with Parkinson's disease. The etiology of this disorder is still not known, but it appears that the basic abnormality is one of failure of the midbrain to produce dopamine, an essential neurotransmitter. Dopamine, when properly balanced with acetylcholine produced elsewhere in the nervous system, enables the person to perform smooth voluntary motor activities. Some patients are treated with medications such as levodopa and carbidopa, which control symptoms by replacing the deficient dopamine. This type of medical therapy often results in a marked reduction in rigidity and in improved movement, but is not so effective with regard to the tremor. Procedures for the care of foot problems are sometimes more easily performed in these patients. The cooperation of the physician treating the parkinsonism is invaluable in developing a plan for the treatment of such patients with foot problems.

Chorea is another form of involuntary movement seen in adults with Huntington's disease. It involves almost continuous small movements of some part of the body, including the distal portions of the limbs. Medication such as haloperidol can sometimes achieve some reduction in the amount of movement, aiding the podiatrist in performing foot care procedures. These patients have an insidious onset of their disease which may permit normal activity for years but ultimately they develop cortical degeneration with intellectual deficits and dementia.

LOGISTICS OF PATIENT CARE

Patients with certain neurologic and musculoskeletal handicaps, as well as many frail, debilitated individuals, may not be able to get around without the use of a wheelchair. Those who use a wheelchair may be confined to that device or may be capable of being transferred with or without assistance to the treatment chair or table. Patients not confined to a wheelchair do not present major problems as to office design, space, and equipment. Those confined to wheelchairs may have problems gaining access to the office or treatment facility if there are no ramps, elevators, and barrier-free doors. Once inside, however, patients who can be transferred to the treatment chair or table usually are moved quite easily, with some assistance. Those patients not able to be easily moved from their wheelchair can usually be examined and treated, even if with difficulty, by raising the limbs onto a footstool to the degree possible. Setting the footstool on a small wooden box may permit easier access to the lower extremities for both examination and treatment.

When a patient can be transferred from a wheelchair to the treatment chair or table, extreme care must be taken to avoid injury to assistants and to the patient. A family member who is familiar with transfer techniques can be most helpful in carrying out this procedure. In some instances, patients themselves can be very helpful. For those who cannot, position the wheelchair, if possible, adjacent to the treatment table, making sure the wheels are locked. The person who does the greatest amount of lifting should stand behind the patient, placing their arms beneath those of the patient. An assistant or family member should stand facing the patient with their hands beneath the knees of the patient. The patient is then in the best position to be lifted to the table or chair.

If care is provided in an environment where a treatment chair or table is not available, such as in a house, a skilled nursing facility, or even some hospitals, a lounge-type chair is often quite suitable. Making a patient comfortable and arriving at a good position for care to be provided is not difficult with that type of chair design. Cerebral palsy and parkinsonism patients with severe contractures of their arms, legs, or bodies may require support no matter where they are receiving foot care; this can be achieved by using small pillows or folded blankets. Physical restraining straps are not recommended unless a patient would feel more comfortable supported in this fashion. When this is the case, such support can best be accomplished with Velcro fasteners attached to nylon straps. Both patient position and the comfort of the doctor must be sacrificed or greatly compromised when a patient who is wheelchair-bound must remain there for treatment, particularly when there are contractures of the lower extremities. Occasionally one may try to treat such patients with foot problems while they are positioned horizontally, but this sometimes is not practical because of respiratory problems that people with these conditions may have.

In patients with advanced Parkinson's disease, treatment may be compromised to some extent. However, simply providing maintenance care or placing the patient on a holding program can be of great service to the patient. Epileptic patients, unless the epilepsy is associated with cerebral palsy, are treated as normal, although medically compromised, patients. Many patients with severe mental retardation who are not amenable to treatment in the office should be referred to a hospital or similar environment for foot care.

SELECTED READINGS

Finkelstein HB, Abraham MA, Crismali NC, Scherer RB, Tabak, BA: Basic Concepts of Physical Therapy for the Lower Extremity. Dr. William Scholl College of Podiatric Medicine, Chicago, 1983

Koningsberg I: A Final Report of the Symposium on the Special Patient Evaluation Management Treatment, The University of Texas Health Science Center at Houston — Dental Branch, April 10–12, 1980

Krusen FH, Kottke G, Stillwell K, Lehmann, JF: Handbook of Physical Medicine and Rehabilitation. 3rd Ed. WB Saunders Co, Philadelphia, 1982

Rusk H: Rehabilitation Medicine. 4th Ed. CV Mosby Co, St. Louis, 1977

Behavioral Medicine and the Podiatric Physician

25

Leonard A. Levy, D.P.M., M.P.H.

Health professionals specializing in the foot need to be aware that they do not treat feet, but rather people who have foot problems. How patients are approached and treated is not only a function of the foot pathology or systemic conditions that affect the foot. In providing health care it is also necessary to include cultural, social, economic, and behavioral considerations in patient management and assessment. Insensitivity to these factors can result in patient noncompliance or the inability of doctors to convince them to accept a necessary treatment plan.

Recalcitrance, noncompliance, or neglect, while often not life or limb threatening, can be devastating to people with serious foot health problems. With growing populations of at-risk patients, such as the elderly and chronically ill, social and psychological barriers can seriously delay seeking care by people with infections, ulcerations, and other potentially limb-threatening foot conditions. Tomb pointed out that 60 percent of patients needing mental health care are being treated by physicians for physical illness. He also indicated that 50 percent of patients in a psychiatric clinic population have an undiagnosed medical conditions.[1]

Patients who seek care for foot problems may have a concurrent psychiatric disorder such as depression, confusion, memory loss, anxiety, personality changes, or psychosis. These may not have any direct relationship to the pathogenesis of their foot problem. However, failure to be aware of the presence of these behavioral disorders can adversely affect podiatric care because of lack of patient compliance or little understanding by the physician of the implications of these behavioral conditions for the management of the foot disorder. In some instances, the podiatrist learns from patients or their family of the presence of the psychiatric problem. In many situations the patients may not be aware of these behavioral disorders, so that the physician is not fully aware of the patient's mental health state or its potential implications for podiatric management.

Conversely, the podiatric physician may focus attention on the foot and completely overlook the patient as a whole. This could be because of little interest or lack of knowledge about the importance of both normal and abnormal behavior in patient assessment and management. It may also be that the physician may have an inadequate background

Table 25-1. **Behavioral Problems Associated with Medical Disorders That May Have Manifestations in the Lower Extremity**

Behavior Manifestation	Medical Condition	Lower Extremity Sign/Symptom/Treatment Response
Anxiety	Hyperthyroidism	Fine tremor, hyperactive Achilles reflex
	Hypothyroidism	Dry skin, hypoactive Achilles reflex
	Hyperparathyroidism	Bone pain
	Hypoparathyroidism	Tetany
	Hypoglycemia	Tremor
	Cushing's syndrome	Postcorticosteroid therapy
	Infection	Infection in foot
	Porphyria	Neuropathy
Depression	Hypothyroidism	Fine tremor, hypoactive Achilles reflex
	Pernicious anemia	Neuropathy
	Infection	
	Diabetes mellitus	Neuropathy, peripheral vascular occlusive disease
	Cushing's syndrome	Postcorticosteroid therapy, diabetic state
	Hyperparathyroidism	Bone pain
	Hypoparathyroidism	Tetany
Mixed psychotic-hysterical symptoms	Multiple sclerosis	Neuropathy, muscle weakness
	Systemic lupus erythematosis	Arthritis, red nodules, purpura, periungal erythema
	Hyperthyroidism	Fine tremor, hyperactive Achilles reflex
	Porphyria	Neuropathy

in behavioral medicine, to the point where those patients who require a mental health professional are not recognized or appropriately referred.

PHYSICAL CONDITIONS WITH ASSOCIATED PSYCHIATRIC SYMPTOMS

The foot care provider should be aware of the physical conditions that may have associated psychiatric psychological, or common behavioral symptoms. Problems associated with medical disorders that may have manifestations in the lower extremity are shown in Table 25-1.

BEHAVIORAL ASPECTS OF CONDITIONS ASSOCIATED WITH PODIATRIC PROBLEMS

The Addiction of Cigarette Smoking

In spite of more intensive antismoking campaigns championed by governmental agencies, voluntary health organizations, and others, the use of tobacco continues to be one of the major health hazards in the nation. While perhaps proportionally fewer people are cigarette smokers, the addictive quality of nicotine makes the smoking habit often one of the most difficult to overcome. While sometimes successful, behavior modification techniques often fail because of the great dependency people acquire for the substances in the cigarette.

As a result of this behavior people are far more likely to develop lung cancer and heart disease as well as peripheral vascular disorders. Peripheral vascular occlusive disease has received virtually no attention by the media and health agencies with regard to its strong association with cigarette smoking, despite the fact that the Surgeon General has concluded that smoking cigarettes is the single most important factor associated with it. In spite of overwhelming evidence supporting the conclusions of the Surgeon General, the general public still is unaware of them. The lack of public attention to this side effect of cigarette smoking makes it more difficult for the doctor who is trying to prevent occlusive vascular disease in patients who may be at risk of having it or to treat those who already are victims of the condition.

One of the most dramatic examples is the case of patients with thromboangiitis obliterans (Buerger's disease), a condition that usually becomes asymptomatic upon cessation of smoking. Progression of disease may cease and disease process usually reverses. Yet many who have the condition continue to smoke in spite of warnings that their feet and legs are in jeopardy as well as their upper extremities. The author has seen patients with all four limbs amputated who were holding a cigarette at the end of their prosthetic arms. Such patients refused to or could not modify their behavior to the point where they completely stopped smoking. In many instances the patient will cut down smoking or give it up for short periods of time, but not enough to reverse or arrest the progress of their vascular condition. In other cases patients will cheat or frankly lie to their doctors about whether they are still smoking. Smokers often need a great deal of encouragement by their doctors when efforts to stop smoking are being made.

In some instances the doctor needs to be blunt in advising patients, indicating to them that they can choose to have their cigarettes or their legs, but not both. Unfortunately some doctors do not emphasize the importance of ceasing cigarette smoking in peripheral vascular disease patients. Referring patients who need help in their attempts to stop smoking to support groups, hospitals, or other smoking cessation clinics, and in some cases to individual mental health professionals (e.g., psychiatrists, psychologists), can sometimes be successful.

In any event, behavioral modification programs that attempt to get smokers to stop their habit have become more popular in our society, but still are in need of new psychological and or medical approaches to dramatically increase their success rate.

Weight Disorders and Obesity

Those who see patients with foot problems know that many such conditions are aggravated and sometimes caused by the burden of excessive weight. Patients with heel spurs, for example, are often far more symptomatic when they are overweight. In addition, people with abnormal pronation, as seen in pes valgoplanus, who are obese have in many instances more discomfort. The burden of added weight on the foot in the obese patient can be an important if not major cause of stimulation to the bones to produce degenerative changes more rapidly as well as to make such osteoarthritic conditions more painful.

Patients who are successful in weight reduction, and especially those who are able to modify their behavior to remain at a lower, more acceptable weight, often find considerable relief from foot symptoms in these biomechanically associated conditions. Although there may be genetic and physiologic factors leading to excessive weight, usually poor eating habits are a most important reason. Emotional conflicts and other psychological problems often need to be addressed in order to assist patients to modify their diet and lose weight. Without addressing these issues through the assistance of a qualified mental health professional, little progress may be made or the patient may go through one or more crash diet regimens. These may have the risk of endangering their general health in the process; also, after reaching some predetermined weight goal, patients often revert to their former diet, gaining back all the weight that they had lost.

The Foot and Sexuality

The relative sexual attractiveness of the feet has also been associated with foot problems, including deformity. Since ancient times and persisting even to the early part of this century, female infants in China often had their feet bound. This resulted in feet that, although difficult to walk with, were considered to be sexually attractive. The deformity created by this practice was covered by a decorative shoe or boot that, as a result of the foot binding, was very small. Shoes today further establish the foot as a part of human sexuality, especially, but not only, in women. High heels, for example, help place the calf in what is considered to be a more shapely position that is attractive to the opposite sex. A combination of cultural and social practices, greatly influenced by designers and the mammoth shoe industry, have resulted in styles considered sexually attractive, but often compromising foot health and comfort to some degree. Women with foot problems and even deformities often resist wearing shoes that would be more comfortable for fear of not being sexually attractive, referring sometimes to their aversion to "old ladies'" shoes.

The practice of wearing open-toed shoes or sandals, which exposes part or almost all of the foot, influenced the use of polish on toenails and even decorative rings on toes. Exposing the foot through the use of such shoes and the practice of going to public beaches has made many people more sensitive to how their feet look. Discolorations of toenails or other dystrophies, while probably overlooked by most in the past, are more likely to be upsetting today. Fashion magazines feature articles not only on shoes, but also on how feet should look and feel.

Less attention has been paid to the foot as a part of human sexuality. This includes the pleasurable feeling in some people when their feet are rubbed or massaged. Like other forms of massage, this may help some people feel generally relaxed or make overworked feet feel better; it may also be a sensual or erotic experience. Manually stimulating the feet in this manner may also be a component of sexual foreplay. In addition, touching the leg and foot of a sexual partner further emphasizes the potentially erotic role of the foot during lovemaking.

Whether patients consent to have certain procedures performed on their feet by the doctor is a function of their concern about such issues as pain and disability, but may also be a function of how the procedure may affect relationships with their partners. Having a bandage on the foot for a long period of time may be considered to be offensive to the patient, perhaps even a sexual turnoff. A cast postoperatively or after foot and ankle trauma may be even more of a turnoff to some as well as an inconvenience to lovemaking to others. Conversely, because these symbols of disability may result in receiving more attention both from lovers and others, the patient may outwardly or unconsciously enjoy the added attention that may result. One of the most common questions and concerns that patients have about foot surgery, even if it is a relatively minor procedure, is when they will be able to wear shoes that they feel make them look most attractive.

Another concern that both men and women often voice is about being unable to engage in their normal physical fitness activity. Not only is this a concern about the health status of their heart and lungs or about the loss of the euphoria that serious runners sometimes experience during running, but it is also a concern that somewhat prolonged disability from a foot disorder or foot surgery may result in gaining weight and becoming less appealing to the opposite sex.

Somatic and Nonsomatic Foot Symptoms

Although it is true that not everything that results in foot pain is psychosomatic, it is also true that some foot problems can be psychological in origin. It also should be emphasized that people with minor or severe psychiatric disturbances can have a concomitant, essentially nonrelated somatic disorder. Obviously, in treating a somatic foot disorder in a patient who also happens to have a behavioral condition, the ability of such a patient to cope with the foot problem may be markedly affected. Pain, for example, may be more pronounced or the patient may use it to get attention more than would be expected of the normal individual.

Caution needs to be taken about labeling patients as being emotionally disturbed when the doctor is unable to find an obvious somatic cause for a foot problem. The author participated with a colleague, Dr. Marvin D. Steinberg, in a dramatic case that emphasizes this axiom. A 13-year-old girl had been brought to his office by her parents. Dr. Steinberg was informed that she had had severe foot pain for several months with no apparent somatic cause and had finally been to a psychiatrist, who diagnosed the problem as being emotional in nature. The child permitted no one to ever touch the bottom of her foot and was reassured by Dr. Steinberg that he would not palpate that area. Instead, a posterior tibial block was given and within several minutes the child remarked that she was no longer experiencing pain in her foot. She then permitted Dr. Steinberg to palpate the plantar aspect of her foot deeply and a focal hard area was felt. A small incision into the plantar tissues was made and with a hemostat a splinter of wood of considerable size was removed. There had been no evidence on the outer skin of any entry point, area of inflammation, swelling, or other tissue reaction. The child's so-called emotional problem had been cured.

Of course, there also are stories of patients with what appears to be little evidence of a foot condition, but who complains of severe pain. The presence of an emotional illness must not be overlooked in such instances. Such patients might best be referred to a psychiatrist, perhaps after discussing the problem with their general physician.

A number of patients with no organic disease may have conversion disorders or hysterical neuroses. For example, a patient may have paresthesias, numbness, or paralysis affecting the foot. This could be a somatic reaction to some emotional problem. The somatic presentations (e.g., paralysis) may help the patient avoid doing something distasteful, such as working in a job that is very stressful. Such patients can be difficult to differentiate from malingerers. In many instances, the malingering patient improves dramatically when a workers' compensation claim or third-party action is concluded and a cash settlement results.

Factitiously induced ulcers may occur as a result of psychogenic factors causing patients to experience itching. Pruritus associated with atopic eczema and urticaria may also be exacerbated because of psychosocial stress. Psoriasis is an example of another condition frequently seen in the feet that may be exacerbated during stress.

Patients with diabetes mellitus who have emotional problems and difficulties coping with their disease may neglect their diet, discontinue necessary medication, and fail to observe good foot hygiene as well as other appropriate foot health care. The risk of such patients developing generalized and podiatric complications runs high. Sometimes this is done consciously or unconsciously by patients so that they may be placed under the protection of a hospital to avoid facing their daily problems themselves.

Drug Abuse and the Podiatric Patient

Some patients with little or no foot problem will seek podiatric medical care and feign severe pain or encourage a surgical procedure in order to obtain narcotics or other addicting drugs. Often quite desperate, such addicted individuals can be quite skilled and persistent enough to convince a doctor to provide them with the prescription they want or perform the surgery so that the possibility of acquiring drugs is high for relatively long periods of time. These patients go to great lengths in convincing their various physicians to prescribe drugs for them. They often will do whatever they can to manipulate their doctor. It is important to recognize them without retribution. Such patients need to receive help from mental health professionals with experience in treating victims of substance abuse. Calling one of many local substance abuse associations found in most communities may be extremely helpful in acquiring advice as to how best to direct the patient to such services.

SOCIOECONOMIC IMPLICATIONS FOR FOOT HEALTH CARE

How people cope with their foot problem is often a function of their socioeconomic status. Some individuals will not seek help early because of their socioeconomic depression, which may include a lack of education about health care in general. Such people might not seek out any health care unless their problem becomes painful or is otherwise uncomfortable. Obviously, in the diabetic with insensitivity in the foot as a result of neuropathy this could be devastating, since an ulcer communicating with underlying areas of bone could be left untreated by the patient because of lack of discomfort.

In addition to the relative lack of awareness by the socioeconomically disadvantaged, there also may be a different series of priorities that they may have when compared to more affluent members of society. It is known, for example, that the incidence of foot problems is greater among the poor than the rest of the population.[2] Poorer individuals are often more concerned about food and shelter or other members of their family. They may place themselves last, in some instances, in matters of health care. Even when they do seek out health care they may be less likely to follow directions or to return for appointments. This may not be to spite the doctor or those who administer health facilities. Rather, it may be because of their preoccupation with other basic activities of daily living, perhaps simply day-to-day survival. This, combined with poor educational opportunity and less access to certain health care services, leads to a socioeco-

nomically disadvantaged class that seeks out care episodically.

REFERENCE

1. Tomb DA: Psychiatric presentations of medical disease. p. 107. In Psychiatry for the House Officer. Williams & Wilkins, Baltimore, 1981
2. Greenberg L: An assessment of foot health problems and related manpower utilization and requirements. J Am Podiatr Assoc 67:102, 1977

SELECTED READINGS

Bowden CL, Burstein AG: Psychosocial Basis of Medical Practice. Williams & Wilkins, Baltimore, 1974

Cadoret RJ, King LC: Psychiatry in Primary Care. CV Mosby Co, St Louis, 1974

Levy LA, Levine PA: A curriculum in the behavioral sciences relevant to the primary care role of podiatric medicine. J Podiatr Med Educ 11(2):4, 1980

Tomb DA: Psychiatry for the House Officer. Williams & Wilkins, Baltimore, 1981

Section IV

PATIENT MANAGEMENT

A. Clinical Procedures

Basic Operative Procedures: Technique and Instrumentation

26

J. Colin Dagnall, L.H.D., F.Ch.S.

HISTORICAL BACKGROUND

The practice of podiatric medicine developed from the work of European craftsmen, commencing in the 16th century, who (reacting to medical indifference) relieved troublesome excresences on the human foot.[1] The first chiropodist appeared in 1785, when David Low in London pirated a French text and had the word coined to describe his calling as a corn-cutter.

A classic text by Lewis Durlacher (1792–1864) published in London and Philadelphia in 1845 described his rational approach to corns and callosities.[2] In the preface to his book Durlacher confessed:

Although I have devoted nearly thirty years' practical experience to the investigation, and have tried various chemical and other remedial agents, yet I have never been able to discover any certain cure for corns. . . . the operations for their relief require as much skill and dexterity as are necessary for the performance of those of greater importance; and fatal consequences have frequently occurred from the want of proper treatment and attention.

I fear the public will be somewhat disappointed at the paucity of the remedies I employ, and still more at not finding a certain panacea for corns. . . . my experience has led me to prefer the use of nitrate of silver, cold water, spirit lotions, and soap plaster, as the most efficient remedies . . .

Ernest G.V. Runting (1861–1954) was the third generation of a British family of chiropodists. Following Durlacher, he made major contributions to the discipline,[3-5] and commenced his 1925 book, *Practical Chiropody:*

No matter what aptitude a chiropodist may show in dealing with general affections of the foot, or what operating skill he may have developed, there can be no doubt that one of his greatest assets is the capacity for being able, cleverly and painlessly, to enucleate a corn.[4]

Runting followed and added to the techniques of Durlacher, and his book can be read with profit today as outlining the approach to "corns, bunions, the diseases of nails, and the general management of the feet."

The scope of podiatric practice today might seem to have little in common with the "straight chiropody" of our predecessors, but skillful technique is as necessary in enucleating a corn, or removing the splinter in onychocryptosis, as it is in performing a triple arthrodesis.

CORNS AND CALLUS

The ability of the epidermis to respond to intermittent friction and pressure with an increase in the thickness of the keratotic outer layer is a useful function of the skin. Callus on the foot can be useful, and its overenthusiastic removal can be to the patient's detriment. It is unfortunate if the patient subsequently reports: "That toe was always trouble free until you removed the hard skin."

However, when the intermittent pressure is greater than the ability of the skin to cope with it by simple thickening, then the process begins (and it is a complicated one) that leads to the pathologic condition described as a corn. There seems little to be gained by adopting the term *heloma.*[6]

Often the process of inflammatory reaction leading to the formation of a corn can be one of its most painful stages. Once the nucleus of the corn is established, what Durlacher described as "a sac or sheath" develops below and around the corn. This can result from the organization of the epidermal or dermal tissues and can be a fully developed adventitious bursa.

Corns have been classified, somewhat arbitrarily, as:

1. Hard corn
2. Vascular corn
3. Neurovascular corn
4. Soft corn
5. Seed corn

The formation of a vascular corn involves the pushing up of enlarged capillaries into the callus mass. It is doubtful if there is involvement of nerve endings or fibers in the so-called neurovascular corn.

Seed corns, as Lake pointed out,[7] are less dependent on pressure (indeed, they can occur on non-weight-bearing skin) and affect largely patients with abnormally dry skin. To quote Lake:

Seed corns are unique in character, and are much less common. They are frequently multiple, and affect, principally, the heel and plantar arch in individuals having an abnormally dry skin. Their de-

velopment does not appear to be so intimately dependent upon pressure as does that of the other types. They resemble callosities, with, here and there, separate nuclei about the size of a millet seed. These nuclei often contain a crystalline material, which, upon analysis, proves to be cholestrin mixed with a small amount of debris, not, as is frequently taught, uric acid or urates.[7]

A corn may form over the scar of an operation or injury when it is subjected to pressure.

Another type and site was described by Lake:

A hybrid between a corn and callosity is often seen where the prominence of certain tendons presses the skin against the shoe. These occur most frequently in women, the commonest being those of the tendons of tibialis anticus and extensor longus hallucis, where they pass under the strap of the shoe, and that over the tendo Achillis, where it is rubbed by the heel of the shoe.[7]

When the tendon has a synovial sheath, care must be taken in enucleating the corn because the sheath may be penetrated. Sometimes the corn is in effect a keratotic plug filling a sinus opening into the sheath.

The removal of keratosis is the first step in attempting to returning the skin to normality. The early practitioners from the 17th century developed considerable skill in the use of cutting instruments to "remove" corns, and yet detailed discussion of the techniques has been neglected.[8]

In the treatment of corns emphasis must be placed on the need to influence the often multiple causes. Older practitioners concentrated on treating corns as entities, whereas today there is less interest in the lesions themselves. However, as Durlacher and Runting showed, technique in the use of scalpels can become highly skilled. The continuing local treatment when all that is possible has been done with a cutting edge is of equal if not greater importance.

Scalpel Technique

Until World War II, chiropodists used solid scalpels of high-quality steel, and there were many individual preferences as to the shape of the blade. Creating and maintaining an edge, by honing and stropping, required considerable skill. Once ac-

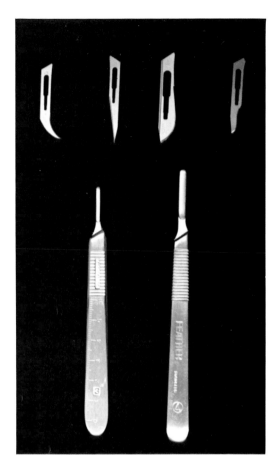

Fig. 26-1. Scalpel handles (*bottom*, no. 3 and no. 4) and various blades used in operative podiatric procedures (*top left to right*, nos. 12, 11, 20, and 15).

quired, that skill resulted in cutting edges superior to what is available today.[9] Now we are largely dependent on replaceable scalpel blades. The need for presterilized, one-use blades is also necessitated by the growing incidence of hepatitis B and AIDS. Stropping of new replaceable blades can enhance the edge, but then there is the problem of resterilization.

For removal of large areas of callus I use no. 20 blades on a no. 4 handle; for finer work on callus a no. 11 blade, which can also be used for enucleation, on a no. 3 handle; and for enucleation and on interdigital lesions, a no. 15 blade on a no. 3 handle (Fig. 26-1). It is important to use a handle compatible with the make of blade, and to discard it

when wear results in even slight movement of the blade.

Comparable to solid scalpels for particularly fine work, the "Beaver" range of scalpel blades and handles is useful (Fig. 26-2). Blade no. 67 and chisel no. 62 on handles nos. 3K and 3H may be used for complete dissection of a corn, and sectioning the edge of a nail plate. For those who favor a chisel-type blade for the débridement of callus, blades nos. 83, 85, and 88 on handle no. 4S give good results.

There are variations in the cutting edge of unused replaceable scalpel blades, and it is unwise to continue working with a new blade if its keeness is doubtful; and they should be discarded for a new blade if there is drag on the callus.

Operative Technique

There are two schools of thought about the removal of corns and callus: working on the lesions with no prior preparation, or softening the lesion first by using compresses of 5 percent potassium hydroxide solution, or 1 percent saponated solution of cresol. Pretreatment whirlpool baths also has some softening effect.

I prefer not to attempt any preoperative softening. However, the use of fluids to "highlight" the demarcation of nucleus and callus, and the junction with normal skin, is useful. Swabbing the operative area with water helps visualization of the extent and distribution of the variable keratotic thickness. Old-time chiropodists often had their own secret "corn stain" and would offer to sell the "magic formula." Most were only variations of 2 percent iodine in 70 percent alcohol. Application of such a solution prior to operating, and after initial callus débridement, is helpful to enucleation, particularly when total dissection is practiced.

Callus

For the removal of plaques of callus, skin tension should be secured by the fingers of the left hand. The scalpel handle is held just below the blade by the thumb and forefinger, and the shaft rests on the little finger. This allows for a side-to-side cutting movement, with minimal downward pressure. Flexibility at the wrist allows removal of graduated

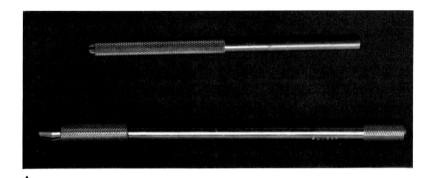

A

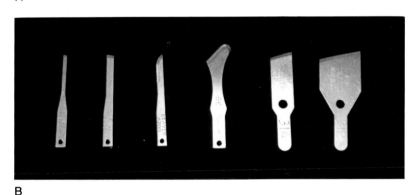

B

Fig. 26-2. *Top,* Beaver blade handles. *Bottom,* Beaver blades (left to right, nos. 6100, 6200, 6700, 86, 314, and 312).

slices of callus, commencing at the center of the lesion and working toward the edges. If the larger blades, nos. 22 or 24, are used initially, a no. 11 blade can be used for final débridement.

Heavy keratosis on the margins of the heel responds to the same technique. Dorsiflexion of the foot with traction applied by the thumb gives skin tension. Although the use of appropriate burrs in a drill handpiece is preferred by some, a simple board covered with sandpaper or long-lasting abrasive material can be useful for quick final smoothing of heel callus.

Corns

All techniques for the enucleation of corns are variations of the following methods: (1) entire dissection, (2) partial dissection; and (3) minute section. Of primary importance is the need to fix the lesion by the use of the left hand. In the case of dorsal digital lesions flexion of the toe can be useful. The thumb and index finger are used to apply tension in opposite directions to, in the words of Runting, "always ensure tensity of the area."

Complete Dissection. This requires considerable skill but it allowed 18th- and 19th-century chiropodists to acquire a considerable reputation. It is particularly appropriate to corns on the plantar surface and well-developed, sharply demarcated, corns on the toes.

The area is highlighted by the use of water or the iodine stain. After fixation of the lesion by thumb and finger tension an initial incision is made at the exact junction of the surrounding callus and the normal skin, using the no. 15 blade or the "Beaver" no. 6700. Mouse-tooth forceps are used to grasp the incised keratosis and enough tension is applied to lift the margin of the lesion. The scalpel is held like a pen between the thumb and index finger, the shaft resting on the second finger. Delicate cutting strokes are made, slowly extending deeper and around the lesion, maintaining traction on the forceps to expose the demarcation of the tissues. Sometimes it can be useful to revert to finger tension. With patience the nucleus and its surrounding callus can be removed in one piece.

Partial Dissection. This is the more usual method,

which requires considerably less skill. The superficial and surrounding callus is first removed using a no. 11 blade, concentrating at first on the edges of the callus (operating "downhill") and removing graduated sections until only the nucleus, or nuclei, remain. It is then usually easy to enucleate the corn using a no. 15 blade and forceps (or skin tension), as in entire dissection.

Minute Section. With this technique, after removal of all the callus small sections of the nucleus are lifted out by a cutting process. Forceps are not used and the skin is held in a state of tension until a complete clearance is achieved.

Removing Surrounding Callus. It used to be believed that there was merit in removing the nuclei and leaving all the surrounding callus as a protection to the denuded area. However, as Runting wrote, the theory:

> . . . is now exploded, it being recognized that the cavities and surrounding walls do not maintain the same contour for long after the operation. The edges which were intended for protection are compressed into an induration which, in itself, is a source of pressure and discomfort, so that the corns again rapidly develop.[4]

Special Problems. In the case of *vascular corns,* a compromise usually has to be made by removing all the keratotic points between the vascular papillae. Care must be taken to try to avoid cutting the vascular parts, unless a deliberate decision is made to do so with the aim of creating a more severe reaction when a coagulant chemical is then applied.

Interdigital corns often present other problems. Keratosis that has been saturated in sweat has a whitened appearance with a rubbery texture. Painting with compound tincture of benzoin in advance of operating allows the scalpel blade to bite into the abnormal tissue. A no. 15 blade, and good skin tension, allows small sections at a time to be removed. Pausing while other work is done allows the air to dry the exposed layers, and more tincture can be applied if necessary. Attempting to remove all of a soft corn is usually unnecessary because bleeding can so easily occur. The application of a silver nitrate solution, usually 25 percent, and ideally relieving pressure by slitting a shoe, or supplying a splint boot, is as important as the operative procedure. Of course, not all interdigital corns are soft; typical hard corns are common in the area.

Corns *below a nail plate* are easy to enucleate once the overlying nail has been removed. The putty-like appearance of subungual corns under a transparent nail plate is obvious. Subungual exostosis is a rare condition and it can be differentiated from a corn because digital pressure over the area gives a characteristic yielding in the case of a corn, and rigidity with an exostosis. Usually, a "V" can be cut into the free edge of the nail with nippers, taking care to avoid shortening the corners of the nail. The use of a no. 11 blade gripped in the four fingers, using the thumb as a stop and a forward paring action, allows the nail to be removed to expose the corn. Good exposure of the nucleus and surrounding callus should be achieved. The margins of the scooped-out nail should not press on the area where keratotic change has taken place.

The minute nuclei that develop *in the nail sulci* are best enucleated with a no. 11 blade. Firm traction on the nail fold with the thumb, while the index finger provides anchorage on the other side of the toe, exposes the lesion. A lateral graduated section of the nail may need to be removed to gain access to the corn. However, if this can be avoided it is wise to do so, because there can be subsequent trouble as the narrowed plate grows forward. Fine straight nippers can start the section, which can be continued proximally with the "Beaver" no. 6200 chisel.

Similarly, *pinpoint corns* can occur in the grooves of the lesser toenails. The fifth nail is particularly liable to such a corn, often concealed until the thickened apology for a nail plate is reduced—this lesion used to be known in Britain as Durlacher's corn. When lesser nails are thickened they can become embedded in a mass of callus, and thorough, often deep, removal is needed to relieve discomfort.

Multiple seed corns can present a daunting operative task. The no. 15 blade is appropriate for their enucleation. They are sometimes the exception to my practice of not attempting prior softening, because compresses of 5 percent potassium hydroxide solution applied for a few minutes can make "shelling" them out easier. One can also apply circles of 40 percent salicylic acid plaster, slightly larger than the lesions and secured by adhesive strips. The patient is asked to keep the foot dry for two days and then retain the dressing. A week or so later the softened nuclei can be more easily enucleated.[10]

Postoperative Treatment of Corns

Footwear

Good, and patient, scalpel technique is but the first part of the local, conservative, treatment of corns. It will give the patient immediate relief, and there is no doubt that interest in open surgery has led to its relative neglect. However, the corn is a symptom of the trauma resulting from unsuitable footwear, or abnormalities in the foot or its function, or both combined.

Maurice D. England (1909–1980), senior lecturer at the London Foot Hospital, used to teach: "There are no foot problems, only shoe problems."[11] I was taught nothing as valuable as that largely (but not always) true maxim. Consideration of function, structure, and malfunction by biomechanical assessment, and consideration of footwear, is vital if cure, or at least stabilization, as opposed to palliation, is desired.

Slitting shoes as an emergency measure gives excellent results.[12] I learnt from Durlacher that there is a time, in acute cases, to stop fighting the shoe; in the interests of the patient it is simpler to annihilate it. We can sometime do far more good when we use a scalpel (kept for that purpose) to incise the shoes than when we use it on the foot.

Cutting a hole or criss-cross is not necessary; a simple slit is all that is needed, of a length so that the shoe opens ½ inch beyond the affected area. A no. 11 blade will cut easily, even through a man's toecap stiffener. Infections and ulcerations of toes, interdigital lesions, bursitis, onychocryptosis, and plantar lesions associated with a retracted toe are conditions that often demand *complete* absence of pressure. Incising the shoe is often the logical treatment; it gets quick results, and also makes the patient take the foot and its trouble seriously.

Silver Nitrate

Almost 40 years of practice have taught me that

Durlacher was right when he praised silver nitrate for the treatment of corns. The changes in the tissues below the thickened stratum corneum are not dealt with by enucleation.[13] Once the corn has become established the degrees of pressure required to perpetuate it are trivial to those required to produce it in the first place. As Runting wrote:

> . . . the complete cure of a corn depends entirely upon the restoration to the normal of the underlying tissue. The lining sac must be obliterated and the depressed papillae restored to their more or less normal dimensions. This may be achieved by two or more different methods. If a corn were removed from the foot of a person who, for some other reason, was confined to bed for a lengthy period, the filling-up of the cavity would be brought about by Nature's own effort. However, if the patient were still using the foot, and perfect protection were assured by a sufficiently easy shoe and proper padding, the addition of a stimulant to the cavity would be, in most cases, all that would be needful to ensure restoration.[4]

The stimulant to the cavity *is* silver nitrate. John Higginbottom,[14] in 1865, wrote: "The nitrate of silver is not a caustic in any sense of the word. It subdues inflammation and induces resolution, and the healing process. It preserves rather than destroys the part to which it is applied, even where the skin would eventually slough."

For macerated, interdigital soft corns a 25 percent solution of silver nitrate is the medicament of choice. The solution is well worked into the tissues (slight bleeding is not a contraindication); it gives quick relief by contraction of the sweat-laden tissues. Here, as in all cases of applications of silver nitrate in strength, it must be remembered that the quickly forming eschar limits the action of the chemical. Removal of the coagulum, and a further application, ideally within a few days, is needed to ensure continuity of action, although even a single application is often effective.

Digital hard corns can be treated with a 25 percent solution or even with the moistened 95 percent hardened silver nitrate stick (although it is wise to moisten the skin rather than the stick). Complete obliteration of the fibrous lining below the nucleus can result from regular application and, of course, modification of pressure. As well as coagulating effete material, silver nitrate has a stimulating effect on the surrounding tissues by the hyperemia it produces. Dorsal vascular corns respond well to the application of the 95 percent stick if the case is seen at regular intervals, say weekly.

For plantar hard corns with dense underlying fibrous tissue it must be admitted that silver nitrate is not as effective as applications of 20 percent pyrogallol in a stiff ointment base. However, by frequent applications of 95 percent silver nitrate and careful operating, it is possible to obtain a good result, and by obviating the need to retain a dressing and keep the foot dry it can be more convenient for the patient than the use of pyrogallol ointment. Vascular plantar corns respond well to generous applications of the 95 percent stick, as does heavy plantar callus, particularly the type macerated with sweat. Indeed, in all cases of keratosis associated with excessive sweat gland activity the result of silver nitrate is exceptionally good, and the relief given is often spectacular.

Bursitis

When an adventitious bursa has developed below a corn (the dorsal aspect of the fourth toe is the classic site), with organization of a synovial membrane, further problems can arise. The nucleus often communicates with the bursal sac and, when removed, reveals a sinus. Obliteration of the sinus is needed before the corn can resolve. Removal of all pressure by slitting a shoe, or supply an open-toed support boot, is often a particular need for bursal corns.

It can be necessary to first reduce the acute bursitis by hypertonic saline soaks, or applications by the patient of Burow's solution. Then, repeated applications of 25 percent silver nitrate, on a thinned wooden applicator, are worked into the sinus (on occasion the hardened 95 percent stick can accelerate the process but this can cause a painful reaction). Whenever silver nitrate is used patients should be warned of a possible reaction and advised to use hypertonic saline soaks without removing any dressing. Once the sinus has been destroyed, suitable footwear, and perhaps a replaceable latex or silicone rubber protective device, can prevent a recurrence of the condition.

A more drastic approach to a bursal corn with sinus formation is to use 40 percent salicylic acid ointment in a stiff base to bring about coagulative necrosis of the abnormal and surrounding tissues. When the healing process is complete the tissues can return to normal and sometimes the bursa itself has been obliterated. However, it is not always wise to attempt to destroy or surgically dissect out the bursa. Providing the patient is likely to subsequently take care with footwear — the *right* shoe for the *right* occasion — the bursa can have a protective function.

TREATMENT OF VERRUCAE

It is important to differentiate between the varying types of lesions classified under the heading verrucae (warts). The painful space-occupying, encapsulated lesion (which can occur on non-weight-bearing sites) responds well to treatment. Mosaic lesions and verrucae vulgaris do not, and are often better left untreated to await spontaneous resolution.

For the inwardly developing lesion, the term *myrmecia* is useful to distinguish this group; I favor chemotherapy using a saturated solution of monochloroacetic acid.[15] The overlying keratosis should not be debrided but merely scarified, using a no. 15 blade, to assist absorption of the acid. As much acid is applied (using a wooden applicator stick or a glass capillary tube) as the lesion can be induced to absorb. About a week later the effects of coagulation-necrosis can be seen. An incision is made at the margin of the reaction, using a no. 15 blade, the edge is grasped with a hemostat, and, using the scalpel, the lesion, with its margin of normal skin, can be dissected out cleanly.

Curetting the lesion is an alternative treatment. An incision is made with a no. 15 blade at the exact junction of the lesion and normal skin, and an appropriate-sized curette is used to scoop out the encapsulated lesion. Silver nitrate or liquefied phenol can be applied to the cavity.

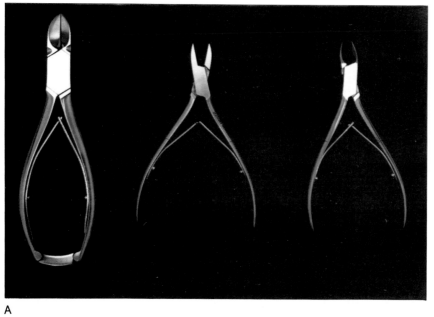

A

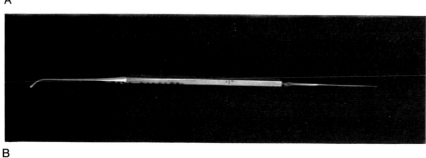

B

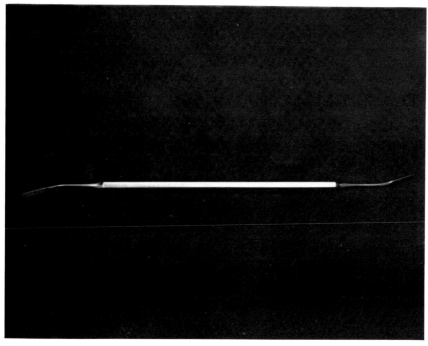

C

Fig. 26-3. (A) (left to right), Nail nipper, nail splitter, tissue nipper. **(B)** Probe and packer, double ended. **(C)** Double-ended nail or bone rasp, angular, file inside and outside. *(Figure continues.)*

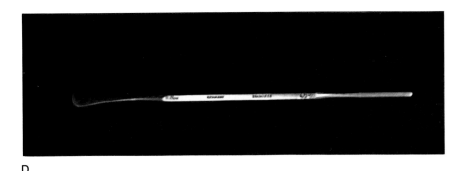

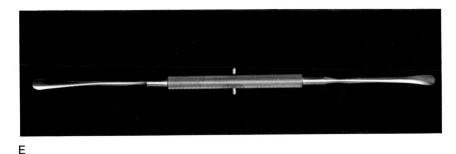

Fig. 26-3. *(continued)* **(D)** Spatula and packer. **(E)** Freer elevator.

TOENAIL CONDITIONS

Many troublesome nails are best dealt with by partial or total eradication, but there is still a need for conservative therapy. Nineteenth century practitioners had much skill in dealing with nails, and we can learn much from the writings of Durlacher,[2] Runting,[5] and Joseph et al.,[16] for example. Durlacher demonstrated his operation for "the nail growing into the flesh" at the London Hospital of Surgery in 1827, and the *Lancet*[17] described it as being "a most important improvement in this department of operative surgery."

Cutting of nails that are within the limits of normality is often badly done by both patients and some practitioners. The aim should be to preserve the lateral corners just clear of the sulci and not to disturb the invagination of the nail edge with the fibrous sheath of the sulci. The free edge can usefully have a concave shape to minimize pressure.

There are many nail nippers available but one with a concave edge is the type I find most useful. It is important that the edges should be sharp to avoid

dragging on the nail. If the initial cut is made just inward from a corner and the center scooped out without including the other corner, the corners can then be cut flush with the end of the toe. Fine straight-edge nippers, an excavator, a Black's file, a nail packer, a nail chisel, and a smoothing file are basic equipment (Fig. 26-3A–C).

Hypertrophied Nails

In onychauxis and onychogryphosis the bulk of the nail can be removed with the nippers. Probing with the excavator will determine the point at which the nail is attached to the bed, and a wisp of animal wool or a length of ribbon gauze can be slipped under the free edge and pulled back to mark the area of attachment.

The left thumb and index finger grasps the toe and the nail to prevent movement of the nail and lifting traction on it by the nippers. Clipping into the side of the nail at a transverse striation and then applying steady pressure on the handles of the nipper splits the nail transversely. Occasionally the nail will split only part way across, and then a similar cut can be made into the other lateral edge to complete the separation.

Subungual debris should be cleared away and the bulk of the remaining nail reduced to the minimal thickness possible, including the plate under the posterior fold, unless there is a good attachment of the eponychium, in which case it can be wise to leave it undisturbed. However, if the bulk of nail below the nail fold is judged to be a possible cause of discomfort to the patient then the eponychium can be carefully detached with the excavator and a nail plate elevator to gain access to reduce the concealed nail.

Reduction of nail bulk is usually achieved by the use of electrically driven rotary burrs. A low-torque motor is required, and many burrs (few designed specifically for podiatric use) are available. A forward stroking movement of the burr is employed and downward pressure on the burr should be avoided. The burr should be frequently dipped in a container of alcohol to cool it. Burrs should be frequently renewed, although diamond burrs are long lasting but slower in reduction. All burrs must be cleaned after each use and then sterilized.

The problem with reduction by burrs is the dust produced. Practitioners can become allergic to the inhaled dust, and there is the possibility of fungal organisms gaining ingress to the respiratory system, although most epidermophytes will only infect stratum corneum or nail plate.[18] Thus it is probably wise not to grind nails unless an efficient dust extraction system, monitored regularly for efficiency, is available. It has also been suggested that the heat generated during grinding can damage the nail bed and also render it more susceptible to fungal infection.

Well into the 20th century chiropodists reduced nails quickly and efficiently by paring them with a scalpel, and many developed instruments for the purpose. Having routinely used a drill for many years, I find I am now increasingly following their example. A new no. 11 blade is used, the handle gripped by the four fingers and forward paring movements are made. The thumb is held at the end of the toe to act as a stop for the blade. Some advise the precautionary use of a rubber thumb stall, but I have never found it necessary. The other hand flexes the toe and holds it firmly. With practice it is surprisingly easy to quickly reduce even bulky and very hard nails. Obviously the blade is discarded as frequently as required to make the process speedy and minimize drag on the nail plate. Lesser nails are particularly easy to reduce with scalpel paring, and with more control and quicker than when using a burr.

Nails that are involuted often have thickened shoulders and these can be reduced in a controlled way by scalpel paring. In fact, when it is possible to preserve the full area of the nail, with the corners clear of the sulci, paring is often better than drilling, which can so weaken the nail edge that a portion can subsequently break away.

Onychocryptosis

The conservative treatment of onychocryptosis is the removal of the embedded nail splinter; the management of the swelling (due to a foreign body reaction of the tissues to the embedded keratin); the control of the exuberant granulation tissue; the treatment of the rare infection; and the subsequent "training out" of the nail edge.[19] The technique for the removal of the splinter advocated by Durlacher[2] is the method of choice.

It is often necessary to reduce swelling by hypertonic saline soaks and/or Burow's solution compresses for a few days. If sectioning of the nail is to be attempted without first inducing local analgesia, careful technique is essential to make the procedure tolerable to the patient.

The lateral flap can be pulled away from the nail edge by downward traction by the thumb. The nail groove is gradually packed tightly with cotton wool and then hydrogen peroxide, 10 volumes, is applied to the pack with a pipette. The release of oxygen causes the pack to swell, thus pressing the soft tissue away from the nail; this procedure can be repeated several times with fresh packing until the nail edge is exposed. Maintaining maximum traction of the flap, the excavator is used to locate the point of entry of the splinter. Using a fine solid scalpel, and starting just proximally to the entry point, the nail is cut proximally to distally with the aim of producing a graduated edge. The minimal amount of nail possible should be removed to avoid problems with subsequent training out of the nail.

The alternative operative approach is to make a

nick with fine nippers in the free edge of the nail and then split back with a nail chisel. It is more difficult to maintain control by this method and to ensure a smooth, graduated edge. After the section has been removed the resulting edge is smoothed with a Black's file.

When there is considerable swelling of the toe, local analgesia is needed in order that the splinter can be located precisely and that the subsequent proximal-to-distal removal of the section can be accomplished. Without local analgesia it often seems easier to section the nail backward with a chisel, and less painful for the patient, but a graduated (easy to train out) edge rarely results.

If local analgesia is induced exuberant granulations can be excised before or after removal of the splinter and then sealed by the application of silver nitrate. Packing the nail to hold the flap away is necessary. Footwear pressure should be avoided, and the nail should be checked regularly over the subsequent months until the corner of the nail has grown clear of the sulcus.

Avulsion of the Nail Plate

Total avulsion of the nail plate is still often done by forcing one blade of a hemostat under the free edge, locking the instrument, and with a twisting motion of the wrist tearing the nail off. Soft tissue damage is considerable, bleeding can be profuse, and this method of ripping off a nail plate is recorded only to condemn it.

An understanding of the structure of a nail should suggest the method of removing the plate from its purely physical connection with the nail bed. The plate can be likened to the outer skin of an orange, the nail bed to the inner white skin, and the tissues below the bed to the flesh of the orange. The eponychium attaches the posterior nail to the dorsal area of the base of the nail plate, and the hyponychium lies under the plate just before it develops its free edge and it is continuous with the nail bed and covered with epidermis. In the sulci, if normal structure is present, the lateral edges of the plate are tightly invaginated in the fibrous sheath lining the sulci. Thus, the dead horny nail plate is very tightly held to the toe by a very clever locking of keratotic tissue. The nail plate itself cannot touch

the germinal layer of the epidermis, nor of course dermal tissue, or they would react to it as a foreign body. It is useful to compare the nail apparatus and the hair follicle, for the structure and function is basically identical; the living matrix of the follicle produces cells that die and are welded on to the base of the dead keratinous hair shaft, which is kept away from living tissue by the lining of the follicle. We all know how painful it is to pluck out a hair; the same applies to a nail plate.

The technique of removing a nail plate with minimal damage to the underlying tissues involves carefully breaking the invaginating sheath at all the borders of the nail. The eponychium is detached from the plate with a no. 15 scalpel blade and then both ends of a nail packer (Fig. 26-3) can be used to complete the separation and lift the posterior fold from the plate, thus opening up the nail matrix chamber. The same procedure is followed at the free edge of the plate to detach it from the epidermis and the hyponychium. Using a nail excavator the lateral edges are freed in the sulci; the back of the Black's file can be useful because it gives more bulk to press under the lateral edge. Then a Locke nail elevator or a McKay elevator is pressed under the free edge, lifting upward at the same time against the undersurface of the plate. With backward pressure and side-to-side movement of the elevator the seal of the plate to the bed is broken. Brute force should never be used; if there is resistance, particularly in the corners where the plate is continuous with the matrix, the excavator should again be used. Once separation is obviously complete, a hemostat can be clamped onto the free edge and a gentle pull forward breaks the connection with the matrix at the base of the nail.

Subungual Hematoma

If seen within a few days of the injury, a hematoma can be easily dealt with by drilling two holes in the nail plate to release the blood. An alternative approach is to use the no. 11 scalpel blade to pare away a small area over the hematoma until the fluid is released.

Should the injury be sufficient that it is obvious there has been a break in continuity of the plate with the matrix, with the result that eventually the plate will be shed, it is in the interest of the patient that the plate be removed as soon as its natural detachment makes that possible with minimal trauma to the surrounding tissues. Often within a week or so, particularly if the fluid has been drained, the toe becomes painless and the plate seems firmly attached, and it can be tempting to leave well enough alone so that months later the "old" plate will shed on its own. That is a mistake because it interferes with the formation of the "new" plate beneath. Early removal of the plate, advice to the patient about footwear, and follow-up checks every month or so can help to improve the chances of a trouble-free "grown out" nail.

REFERENCES

1. Dagnall JC: A history of chiropody-podiatry and foot care. Br J Chirop 48:137, 1983
2. Durlacher L: A Treatise on Corns, Bunions, the Diseases of Nails, and the General Management of the Feet. Simpkin, Marshall, London, 1845
3. Runting EGV: Battalion Chiropody Training and Practice. Scientific Press, London, 1918
4. Runting EGV: Practical Chiropody. Scientific Press, London, 1925
5. Runting EGV: The treatment of corns. Lancet 1:51, 1927
6. Dagnall JC: Corn or heloma. Br J Chirop 25:42, 1960
7. Lake NC: The Foot. Baillière, Tindall and Cox, London, 1952
8. Scullion PG: Scalpel technique in removing heloma and hyperkeratosis. J Foot Surg 23:344, 1984
9. Kemp CE: Chiropody Instruments, Their Use and Maintenance. Actinic Press, London, 1951
10. Addante JB, Marks JH: Saponated solution of cresol as a softening agent. Footprints 40:11/3, 1986
11. England MD: Footwear for Problem Feet. Disabled Living Foundation, London, 1973
12. Dagnall JC: Shoe incisions. Br J Chirop 31:89, 1966
13. Dagnall JC: Chiropodial uses of silver nitrate. Br J Chirop 38:154, 1973
14. Higginbottom J: A Practical Essay on the Use of the Nitrate of Silver, in the Treatment of Inflammation, Wounds, and Ulcers. John Churchill, London, 1865
15. Dagnall JC: Monochloroacetic acid and verrucae. Br J Chirop 41:105, 1976
16. Joseph A, Burnett EK, Gross RH: Practical Podiatry. First Institute of Podiatry, New York, 1918
17. Diseases of the nails. Lancet 12:702, 1826–27
18. Davies RR, Ganderton MA: Allergic hazards in chiropody. Chiropodist, 30:89, 1975
19. Butterworth RF: Conservative treatment of onychocryptosis. Br J Chirop 53:45, 1988

Orthodigita Techniques

27

Kendrick A. Whitney, D.P.M.
Alan K. Whitney, D.P.M.

To fully appreciate the importance of orthodigita, and the role of the orthodigital specialist in today's practice, we should first understand why the profession has avoided and retreated from this speciality for the past 50 years. Certainly surgery has overshadowed the more conservative orthodigital approach, and as the surgical barriers lowered and training became more readily available, an absolute need for conservative orthodigital measures was virtually eliminated. Although we applaud the surgical advances that have taken place and agree that surgical intervention may often be the best course of treatment, we strongly caution that it may as often not be the best solution to the problem. For this reason we present a systematic approach to the evaluation and treatment of orthodigital problems that we hope will provide the optimal therapeutic result.

Another reason orthodigita may have become merely an afterthought in today's practice is that pioneers and advocates in the field, such as Dr. Harry Budin, have been few and far between. Budin, truly the "father" of orthodigita, laid a sound foundation with his unsurpassed book on the *Principles and Practice of Orthodigita*, published in 1939.[1] His works have certainly inspired us to champion Budin's efforts toward the advancement and appreciation of this highly complex field of study, which needs the revitalization it so justly deserves.

Perhaps the most damaging of all to the orthodigital speciality have been those who understand orthodigita least, and yet silently or vocally tend to belittle those associated with orthodigita as doctors who could not make it as surgeons and had to settle for orthodigita.

It is our sincere hope that we may be able to dust off old cobwebs, dispel misconceptions, and restore the necessary role of orthodigita in today's practice by providing a logical approach to the assessment of digital problems that, in turn, provides the template for appropriate therapy. It is important to recognize that the role of orthodigita is becoming increasingly important as we begin to face more surgical constraints and liabilities. As a sound alternative for the patient who selects not to undertake surgical intervention, as well as for the "at-risk" patient, the orthodigital choice becomes preferable. We discuss the importance of the orthodigital examination in distinguishing the structural from the positional digital deformity and in revealing those influences that affect the outcome of the planned program of digital therapy.

ORTHODIGITAL EVALUATION

While it is a generally accepted approach to direct one's attention immediately to examination of the presented digital concern, the orthodigital specialist refrains from this temptation in order to gain an overall perception of the problem and its development. The various therapeutic options for orthodigital care and control first require a thorough history and orthopedic evaluation of the lower extremities. Careful inquiry should be directed toward a relevant history of foot and digital complaints, which may include the patient's occupational and avocational demands, shoegear style and habits, and injuries and operations. A generalized assessment of lower extremity structure and function should always precede a definitive orthodigital examination because postural imbalance and limb deformity have a decided influence on digital alignment and tensions.

The decision as to whether the operative or nonoperative approach is indicated should be predicated on clear principles and findings with regard to the specific nature of the digital problem. Often, the digital deformity develops in response to a basic foot defect or dysmorphism wherein the digits grip or claw in an effort to compensate the deficiency. This would clearly indicate a need for mechanical accommodation and rebalancing as opposed to the choice of a surgical intervention. On the other hand, some digital problems reflect a chronic, structural adaptation or actual gross deformation that most certainly call for surgical solution. Our primary concern, then, becomes an attempt to discern between the purely positional and the frankly structural digital deformity.

As part of our orthopedic evaluation, we have found a technique of *sway testing,* developed by one of the authors (**AKW**), to be useful in assessing the location and direction of foot imbalance that creates the reactive digital deformity. With the pa-

tient standing erect, the digits are observed as to any clawing or gripping activity that may reflect compensation for imbalance. We then redirect the patient's center of gravity from side to side and from front to back until the most relaxed and well-aligned digital attitude is observed. In this manner we can determine the direction or vector of postural imbalance and can estimate its probable source.

Another technique we commonly employ, in conjunction with the sway testing, is that of *functional block testing,* which involves the use of blocks and wedges of varying size and shape. Once we have identified the probable locus of imbalance producing the digital distortion, we restore a more ideal foot-to-body relationship by placing appropriate wedge and blocks beneath the suspected area of foot force deficiency (Fig. 27-1). When

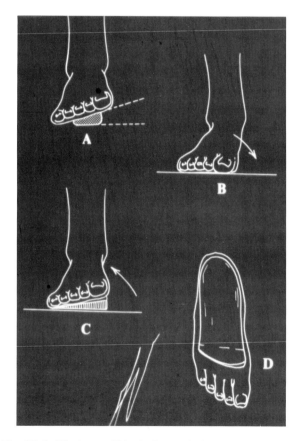

Fig. 27-1. Wedge and blocks beneath the suspected area of foot force deficiency.

proper balance has been restored, the involved digits tend to return to their normal relaxed alignment.

Depending on the degree of digital response to such functional tests, one gains a fairly accurate idea of the therapeutic case needs and the probable response to the same.

Following the functional evaluation and testing for foot and limb influences upon faulty digital alignment and tension, the toes are directly scrutinized as to their anatomic and physiologic status. Careful observation of the toes, noting the location and direction of deformities, is accompanied by a survey of skin lesions, tensions, and tendon contractions. Perhaps the most important aspect of the orthodigital evaluation, however, is a manual appraisal of reducibility of the existing digital deformity. The reactive resistance to realignment will largely determine the best treatment approach and its prognosis (Fig. 27-2). An estimation of the deforming resistance can be rather misleading if the situation is only judged when the foot is at rest. Under weight loading, during stance, the digits may become functionally tense, and such tension forces are greatly exaggerated in the presence of postural imbalance, as we have previously indicated. So any analysis of realignment ease and po-

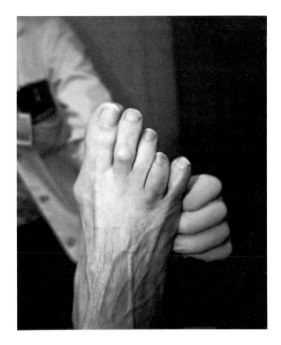

Fig. 27-3. "The digital lineup."

tential must be assessed under weight-bearing conditions.

The structural or anatomic status of the digits should be carefully studied in terms of aberrant digital length pattern as well as for comparative size, shape, and contour of the toes. We utilize what we refer to as "the digital lineup," whereby the examiner manually straightens the digits to reveal their actual anatomic length pattern, which has often been greatly obscured by the acquired deformation (Fig. 27-3). Exposure of such anatomic aberrations may suggest the need for surgical reconstruction as contrasted with digital realignment. It is astounding how frequently an unduly long digit can camouflage itself by contraction with underlapping so as to lie on a common "line of gripping" (Fig. 27-4).

The patient's footgear is surveyed for causative or aggravative factors, and must also be viewed as either favorable or detrimental with respect to the impending orthodigital treatment program. A careful survey of both the inner and outer surfaces may prove diagnostic from the standpoint of appropriate style, fit, flare, and heel height. For example, the inflare-lasted shoe applied to the rectus-type

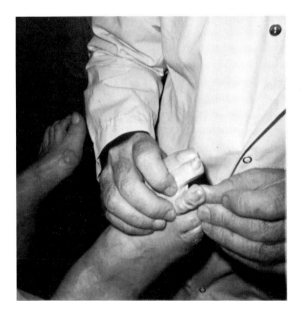

Fig. 27-2. Reactive resistance to realignment.

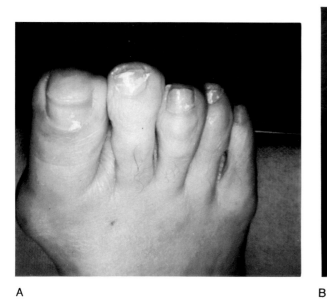
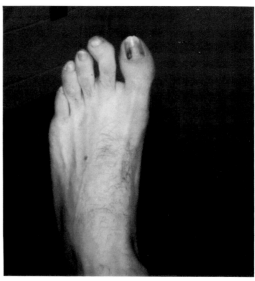

A   B

Fig. 27-4. "Line of gripping."

foot will, without doubt, cause havoc by way of adductory impingement upon the fifth toe and its metatarsal. A useful technique, devised by one of the authors (KAW) educates the patient with regard to improper shoe fit. The sole of the presented shoe is traced on a clear sheet of plastic, which is then superimposed over the patient's dorsoplantar standard radiograph to demonstrate how the patient's complaints may arise from shoe-foot conflict. An orthodigital evaluation would not be considered complete without obtaining standard, comparative dorsoplantar radiographs, but some care should be taken not to overexpose the distal forefoot region.

PRELIMINARY ORTHODIGITAL CARE AND TESTING

Nowhere is the need for preliminary neutralization of abnormal forces more essential than in the care and rehabilitation of the toes. If the human foot organ supports and balances the body, it is only with the rather precise assistance of digital gripping actions and reactions. In the presence of overall foot malalignment and improper loading, the toes do not and cannot maintain their anatomic or functional integrity. It is therefore clinically essential to control foot and lower limb mechanics before attempting to deal with the digits. To fail in this is to invite orthodigital disappointment or failure.

While there are many possible approaches to preliminary foot rebalance and control, we find the technique of *functional test padding*[2] to be most straightforward and effective. With this approach, a pad array, suggested from the orthopedic findings, is temporarily inserted into the presented or selected shoes (Fig. 27-5). A positive response to such test padding often indicates the need for more permanent orthotic devices, which can be fashioned and fitted later on in the treatment program.

Digital realignment involves a realistic assessment of deformative forces and their resistance to correction. Manual realignment of the toes during rest appraisal is usually misleading, because under static loading the same digital units become surprisingly intractable. We suggest, in all but the most simple of presented problems, that one

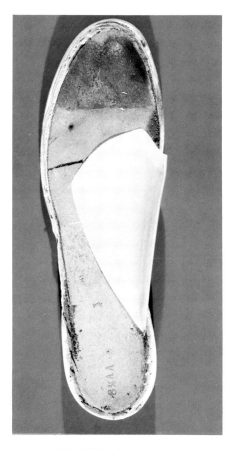

Fig. 27-5. A pad array.

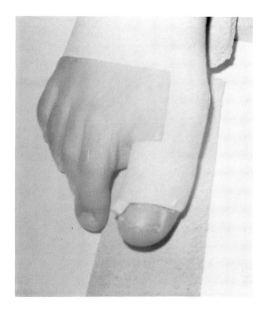

Fig. 27-6. Hallux retention taping.

should test digital reducibility under weight-bearing conditions. A most common pattern of malalignment is represented by the case of hallux abductus with an overlapping second toe. The hallux can often be test-realigned through the use of hallux retention taping (Fig. 27-6), but the dorsal displacement of the second toe may be a relatively greater challenge. We have found a so-called *digital band splint* (Fig. 27-7) to be quite useful for this purpose, but it is true that second metatarsophalangeal joint subluxation or frank dislocation is a very formidable opponent. In such cases, progressive digital traction visits, or even a preliminary soft tissue surgical release, must be performed to facilitate the digital realignment, which may then be retained through use of our digital band splint or the original Budin rubber toe splints or slings. As a preliminary to a urethane mold–type device, we find that a dry polyurethane foam version can offer

a unique combination of tensile and compressive forces without actual molding by latex solution (Fig. 27-8). Such urethane foam splints have proven a simple and effective mode of initial testing, both of the digital restitution and of the patient's attitude and response to wearing such a digital encumbrance.

The just-alluded-to matter of patient tolerance for digital devices and the individual capacity to daily don and remove them, plus the occasional idiosyncratic skin response to materials applied directly over the toes, are potent factors influencing the success of an orthodigital venture. Some patients reject encircling devices on the basis of a mild claustrophobic tendency, whether recognized or not, making it clinically judicious to apply such preliminary digital prototypes in advance of any serious or expensive treatment program.

At some early juncture an appropriate shoe must be sought and approved as a "treatment shoe" that will not obstruct the process of toe realignment and will provide the space for the devices required to do the task. In practice, however, the shoe requirements become apparent as progress is made and may not be initially essential. The vital concern, with regard to suitable footgear, is the patient's awareness and cooperation with respect to the need for proper digital housing.

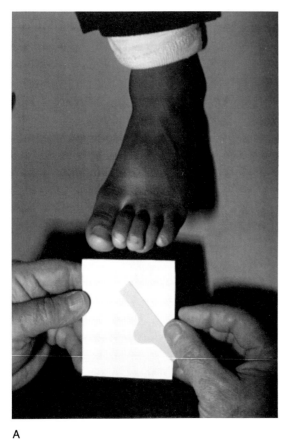

A

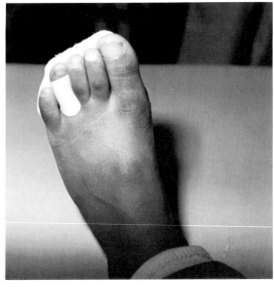

B

Fig. 27-7. Digital band splint.

DEFINITIVE ORTHODIGITAL DEVICES AND TECHNIQUE

Traction Therapy

One of the oldest of the physical modalities is that of traction therapy. Primitive peoples no doubt gained the benefits of body traction when they climbed up vines or suspended themselves from boughs. It has been said that yawning and stretching may represent a physiologic means of joint distraction. Whatever its early origin and development, traction force applied to the joints of the spine and extremities remains an accepted mode of physical therapy. An early type of device for traction to the first metatarsophalangeal joint involved suspension of the foot within a special frame in which the hallux was attached by means of a wire mesh finger trap. The weight of the foot and leg became the tractive force.

One of the first controlled applications of digital traction was practiced by Budin some 50 years ago. Budin devised a digital traction machine that, through a series of office traction visits, served to gradually reduce the extent of digital deformities and restore motion lost through injury, chronic articular stress, and arthritis. The authors have selectively utilized digital traction therapy as a component of their orthodigital programs, over a substantial period of time, with gratifying results. Although some hold that the benefits of digital

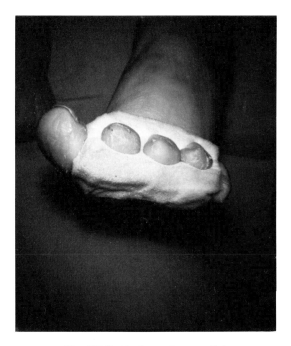

Fig. 27-8. Urethane foam splint.

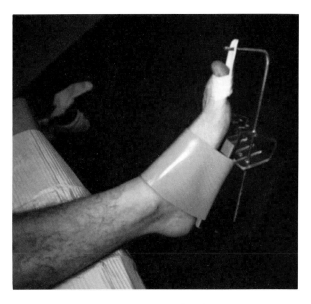

Fig. 27-9. Digital traction therapy.

traction therapy are temporary, it is our belief that when foot function and footwear are improved, the benefits of traction can be prolonged. One of the authors (AKW) devised a unique traction device with which multiple digits can be treated and such treatment rendered without the necessity of moving the patient from the treatment chair or table (Fig. 27-9).

Traction therapy is contraindicated at joints presenting with acute pain, inflammation, infection, or neoplasms, and it should be applied with caution at sites where the bone substance is fragile or pathologically suspect. We have not had experience with traction at recent bone implant sites, but would suggest the possibility of implant displacement if such force is applied too early or with too much intensity. In any case, radiographs should be obtained before traction therapy is rendered.

With apprehensive patients, some preliminary form of relaxation or tranquilization is recommended for the reason that unrelenting muscular tension prohibits the benefits and purposes of tension force application. We also believe that, at the initial visit, traction should be relatively mild and reassuring so as to gain patient confidence and relaxation.

A typical traction visit involves a comfortable, semireclined patient upon whose involved toes a traction grip is taped or the digit is inserted within a wire mesh finger trap if such are available (Fig. 27-10). We have not been able to locate a sufficiently large wire mesh trap to fit the average hallux. If the skin is oily or otherwise slippery, an alcohol prep wipe cleanses the digit before the grip is applied. The traction device is placed over the foot and, if the holding cuff is loose, the addition of Plastazote "choker pads" serves to tighten the security. Traction rods are then inserted and attached to the digital grips or wire mesh traps, and traction is commenced by pulling the traction rod from the holding plate until the desired initial force is attained. We advise a milder "starting force" for about 1 minute to allow the muscles to relax and the articular interface to separate. It would seem that the distractive force does not become effective until the intra-articular synovial tension is overcome, signaled by actual disengagement of component joint surfaces. When this occurs a more pronounced traction force may be applied, but we recommend a milder initial visit application of

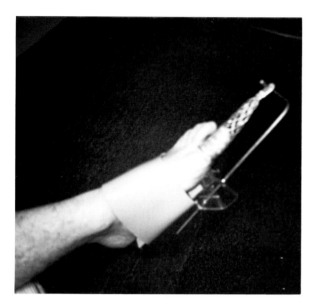

Fig. 27-10. Typical traction treatment.

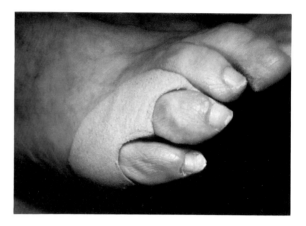

Fig. 27-11. Urethane mold device worn as retentive night splint.

force. There are differences of opinion as to the optimal traction treatment time and interval between traction visits, but it is our feeling that a visit duration of 10 to 15 minutes repeated once or twice a week is sufficient to gain results in the average case. How many such visits are needed will, of course, depend upon the individual problem and the rapidity of patient response. Following each traction application we like to apply brief light massage to the affected joint area. Posttraction instructions are given to forestall anxiety over normal reactions to tissue distention.

Urethane Mold Therapy

The urethane mold is an orthodigital innovation now some 25 years old that has been utilized for the correction and control of digital and metatarsal malalignments and their associated lesions. This technique, developed by one of the authors (AKW), has been shown of great value for the postoperative retention of attained realignment, and has also proven to benefit the digital and distal metatarsal amputee.

A suitably designed block of polyurethane foam

is impregnated with a special synthetic molding latex, applied over the involved digits, wrapped in plastic, and dynamically shaped by the patient during function. The completed device is easily adjusted and corrected during subsequent office visits. It is comfortable to wear and is relatively durable provided it is handled with reasonable care. Essentially, the urethane mold represents an effective and versatile medium of force applications when used with knowledge, imagination, and judgment; it is likewise limited by lack of these same qualities.

The *indications* for the urethane mold device can be grouped into four basic categories:

1. Correction and prevention of digital malalignments and their associated secondary skin lesions in children, adults, and even the elderly. These splints are extremely useful for the retention of postoperative gains, and they may additionally be worn as retentive night splints (Fig. 27-11).
2. Protection of painful lesions and sites of trauma in the average case and in the insensitive or otherwise at-risk patient with neurogenic, metabolic, or peripheral vascular disease (Figs. 27-12 and 27-13).
3. Functional stabilization of the arthritic, ataxic, myodystrophic, or similar form of postural instability and dynamic dysbasia (Fig. 27-14). For the care of digital and metatarsal fractures, this

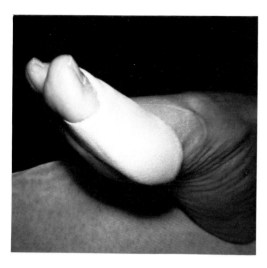

Fig. 27-12. Protection of painful lesions and sites of trauma in the average case.

type of molded splint has demonstrated a valuable role. Its application as a compression mold to minimize postoperative edema has been clearly documented by McGlamry et al.[3]

4. Prosthetic substitution for amputated or congenitally absent digits and metatarsals is a particularly well-suited indication for such mold application, which preserves alignment of the remaining digits while promoting improved functional stabilization of the amputee extremity (Fig. 27-15).

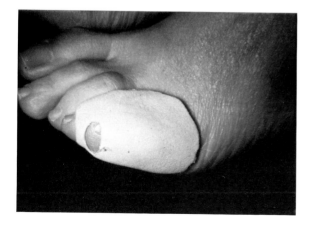

Fig. 27-13. Protection of painful lesions and sites of trauma in the insensitive or otherwise at-risk patient.

Although there are seldom any true *contraindications* to the urethane mold, there are certain cautions in its application. A small number of individuals show a sensitivity to the liquid latex used for molding. One should not be misled, however, by an occasional "minor setting reaction" that may be experienced during the molding process but that will often quickly subside. It is a clinical truism that a definite percentage of patients are mildly to moderately claustrophobic and tend to reject any constriction or encirclement by way of clothing or devices. An initial "dry foam" test application will generally reveal such a tendency before the definitive mold is undertaken. Many elderly, arthritic, or otherwise infirmed patients display justifiable difficulty in removing and replacing their digital molds. In many instances a simpler compromise in design is necessary. A companion or relative can sometimes be recruited as an aide. Then, too, daily removal of the digital device may not be an absolute requisite.

Designing of the polyurethane foam falls easily into the classification of crests, shields, slings, and combinations of these basic elements. Apertured crests are developed when a discreet realignment of digits is desired. Generally speaking, three adjoining apertures are needed for forceful digital realignment and control, although, within the confines of the shoe, fewer apertures may suffice (Fig. 27-16). The shoe itself is a dominant molding influence that must be calculated into the planning process. For the molding visit, the snuggest shoe, not the roomiest, is recommended because the device molded in the larger shoe will not usually be comfortable within the confines of the dressier shoe.

At the *molding visit* the patient is comfortably reclined or semireclined. The forepart of the foot is precleansed of any surface oils and detritus that might be undesirably impregnated in the molded device. The designed foam block is placed in a plastic bag into which a small amount of Vultex solution is poured. Manual mixing of the synthetic latex liquid throughout the open-celled polyurethane foam accomplishes a thorough coating of the foam matrix. Next, the wetted foam block is removed from its plastic bag and blotted of excess latex with a plastic-backed paper towel. Then using plastic gloves, the operator positions the latexed foam over the involved toes (Fig. 27-17). Final scissor

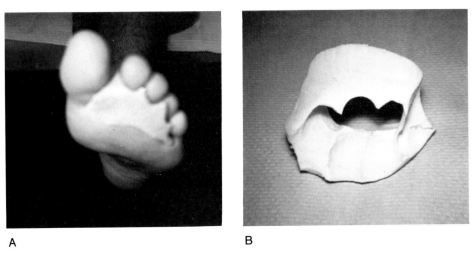

A   B

Fig. 27-14. A. Functional stabilization. **B.** Molded splint.

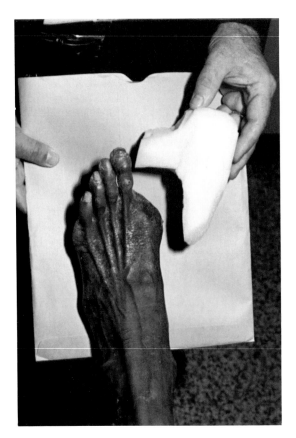

trimming of any excess foam bulk is undertaken, following which two plastic bags are wrapped over the forefoot and taped securely in place to prevent any contact of the Vultex with the patient's stockings. Before the patient's hose and shoe are reapplied, all possible trapped air is manually extruded from the bags to minimize bulk and promote the molding process. The patient is instructed to remove the wrapping and the newly molded device before retiring, but not before 4 or 5 hours after the office visit. The device is then reapplied and worn

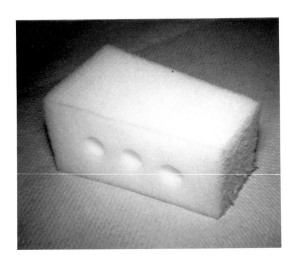

Fig. 27-15. Prosthetic substitution for amputated or congenital absence of digits and metatarsals.

Fig. 27-16. Design with three adjoining apertures for forceful digital realignment and control.

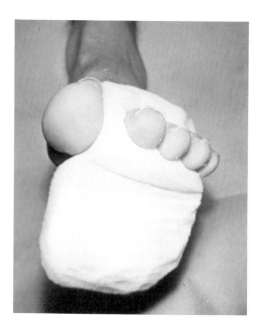

Fig. 27-17. Latex foam positioned over the involved toes.

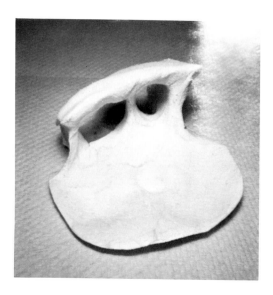

Fig. 27-18. Remolding visit.

daily until the next office visit, which should be scheduled within a week. Printed instructions are given to prevent any misunderstanding or problems associated with this relatively unique therapy.

At the second or *remolding visit*, the device is checked and evaluated as to its intended comfort and function. Irritations or problems are eliminated and the device is cosmetically refined (Fig. 27-18). Once, again, the device is placed in a plastic bag to which more of the Vultex solution is added and squeezed firmly into the molded device. The device is then removed from the bag, blotted of excess latex, reapplied to the foot and covered with a fresh plastic bag. When the remolded device has dried after several hours, the plastic cover is to be discarded. The patient is instructed to wear the device daily, or as otherwise indicated, and to return for a "silicone coating" visit in 2 weeks.

The *silicone coating visit* accomplishes two basic purposes; it checks on the comfort and function of the completed device and it protects the surface of the mold against contamination and deterioration by providing a thin, flexible silicone coating. At this visit the device is coated with a special silicone liquid preparation using a cotton-tipped applicator and allowed to air dry for several minutes. It is then

dispensed to the patient in a plastic bag and should not be worn until the next day, when the coating has completely dried (Fig. 27-19).

If the urethane mold device is utilized for corrective realignment of the digits, it is not usually silicone-coated until all corrections have been accomplished.

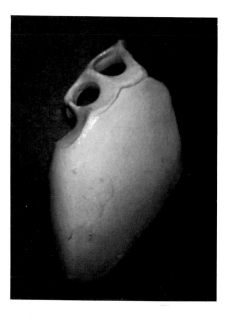

Fig. 27-19. Device coated with special silicone liquid preparation.

The Silicone Mold

The silicone rubber molding technique is of undoubted English origin and early development. Within the past 15 or 20 years, however, American podiatrists have adopted this valuable digital and metatarsal device. We have recently used a newer method that combines two silicone putty compounds (the base and catalyst) to produce a most dependable mold within several minutes. The development of this recent reliable molding kit and technique should be largely credited to Dr. C. Starrett of the Orthopedic Department at the Pennsylvania College of Podiatric Medicine in Philadelphia.

Basically, the silicone rubber molded device is an attractive, durable, flexible mold that is applied directly to the involved digits, covered with a plastic bag to avoid adhering to the stockings, and encouraged to finally "set" with the shoes on during weight-bearing function. Therefore, it can be regarded as a dynamic mold but the timing is somewhat delicate because if the mold completes its "setting process" before the patient replaces his or her shoes and begins ambulation, the mold will not be dynamically shaped.

At the application visit the patient should be comfortably semireclined and the toes appropri-

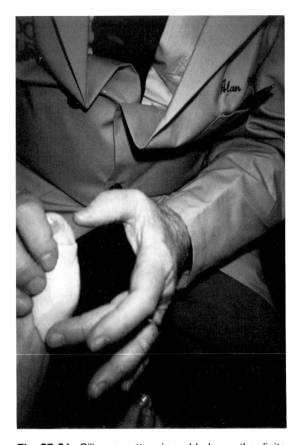

Fig. 27-21. Silicone putty mix molded over the digits.

ately cleansed. The proper amounts of the two silicone putty components are withdrawn from their containers and manually mixed until the colors are well blended (Fig. 27-20). The silicone putty mix is now molded over the digits as planned and man-

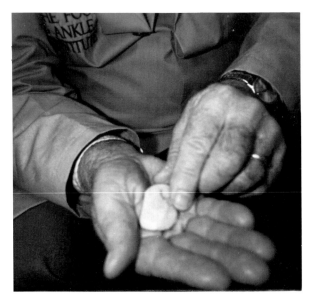

Fig. 27-20. Mixing of the silicone putty components.

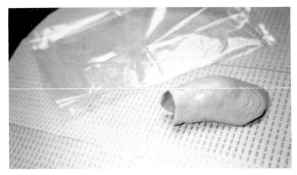

Fig. 27-22. Silicone putty mix formed into its intended shape.

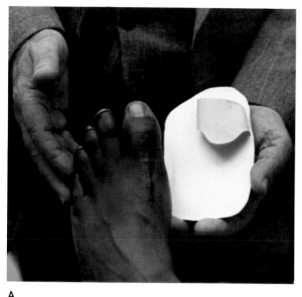 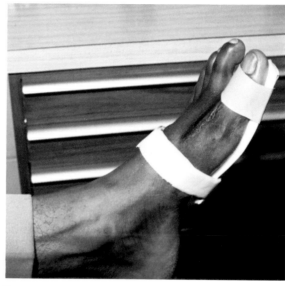

A　　　　　　　　　　　　　　　　　　B

Fig. 27-23. Retentive splinting to maintain digital realignment.

ually formed into its intended shape (Figs. 27-21 and 27-22). The forepart of the foot is wrapped in a plastic bag, the hosiery and shoes are replaced, and the patient is instructed to walk immediately to induce the dynamic final set of the device.

ORTHODIGITAL RETENTION AND MAINTENANCE

Once the digital realignment has been attained, it is imperative that the hard-won correction be preserved. Such retentive effort must be persistently maintained, day and night, for months and for years if necessary.

Some milder cases may require mere observation, and the digital restitution may be quite long lasting, whereas other cases will need retentive splinting for extended periods of time (Fig. 27-23). When a muscular imbalance exists, the retentive efforts should be considered permanent until or unless the muscular inequity is overcome. Most patients will not complain if they must wear a retentive device, because they feel a continuously com-

fortable toe is far better than the painful one they used to have.

Retentive devices are classed as those worn during the day and those worn at night. While the retentive daytime splint may be identical to the device employed for correction of the digital distortion, more likely it is a simplified version of the earlier corrective splint. For example, an apertured urethane mold for realignment of the intermediate toes may be replaced by a simpler ure-

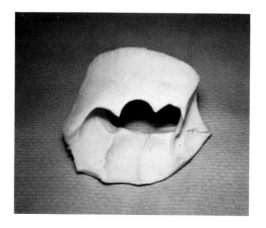

Fig. 27-24. Urethane mold "slit crest."

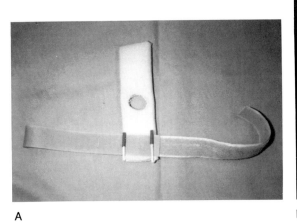

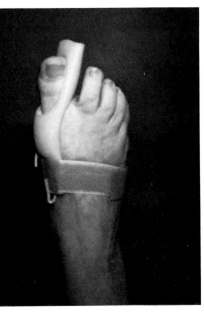

A   B

Fig. 27-25. Wire/foam night splint.

thane mold "slit crest" once the correction has been obtained (Fig. 27-24). A night splint may often consist of the same daytime device worn at night, or it may be a special device fashioned specifically for the resting patient. A most effective device is represented by the so-called wire/foam

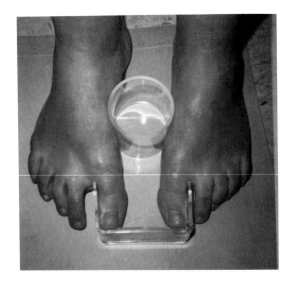

Fig. 27-26. "Hallexercist."

night splint (Fig. 27-25). Such forceful frame-type splints should be applied somewhat gently at first until the patient has become adapted to the change, to avoid an acute cramplike reaction that wakens the patient during the night. A light sock should be worn over the splint so as to circumvent an entanglement with the bedding or the spouse.

Exercises and exercise aids are often part of the well-organized orthodigital program. We have had success with two basic forms of home exercise: a digital gripping exercise and the single foot balancing exercise. In the digital gripping exercise, the patient is instructed to "make a fist" with the toes, through which effort the intrinsic foot muscles are actively contracted. Such toe gripping is to be maintained for a slow count of five, followed by a brief relaxation, and then repeated five times. We have found that if an average patient will persist with this exercise once a day, the digits regain much of the flexibility and strength they formerly possessed. The single foot balancing exercise involves having the patient balance on each foot for a minute or so each day to improve foot mobility and balancing capacity. The human foot's capacity for precision balancing of the body becomes most apparent when one performs this simple exercise.

There are also some home exercise aids and devices that should be mentioned as components of the overall treatment program. One such device is the "hallexercist," devised by us, which is but a version of many other similar and effective instruments of the past (Fig. 27-26).

or her successes are measured in millimeters over extended periods of treatment time.

CONCLUSION

In general, we would conclude with the admonition that the digital therapy discussed herein is for the well-trained foot specialist who is mechanically inclined and who is patient by nature, because his

REFERENCES

1. Budin HA: Principles and Practice of Orthodigita. Strathore Press, New York, 1941
2. Whitney AK: Biomechanical Footwear Balancing. Pennsylvania College of Podiatric Medicine, Philadelphia, 1979
3. McGlamry ED: Post Operative Use of Urethane Moulds. J Am Podiatry Assoc 58(4):169, 1968

Padding and Taping Therapy 28

Alan K. Whitney, D.P.M.
Kendrick A. Whitney, D.P.M.

PADDING AND SHIELDING

Padding and protective shielding has been a highly individualistic and empirically evolved system developed by each practitioner as he or she confronts the presented problems of podiatric practice. Certain basic and well-known pads have been passed along from generation to generation, originating from sources often too ancient to trace. The "general metatarsal pad" is one such example; it was designed to restore a distal metatarsal[1] arch, which has since been shown to be an anatomic/biomechanical nonentity. However, even though the condition it was designed for has been disproven, this particular pad will undoubtable survive, even thrive, in the foot health service community. Many specific pads have apparently evolved from a particular concept or theory of foot function, their developers having found a practical projection of their ideas that was clinically applicable and successful. Dudley Morton's first metatarsal platform is a good example of this type of pad development. Empirical satisfaction with a particular pad seems, in certain cases, to have generated a suitable theory to explain the clinical success with similar case problems.

Regardless of their exact purpose, nature, and origin, all podiatric padding applications represent relatively discrete, regional force elements that are calculated to protect or functionally influence the foot mechanisms within the existing confines and restriction of footwear.

The basic purposes of foot or shoe padding can be divided into the simpler protective shielding needs and the more complex mechanical applications affecting foot function. Herein, we classify pads into protective, functional, and substitutive categories, the latter of which may be aptly described as amputee "fillers" for the congenital or acquired partial loss of foot or toe substance. The more sophisticated removable pads, devices, and inserts, however, are considered to be foot orthoses and prostheses, which are beyond the scope and intent of this presentation.

The authors feel strongly that foot padding should be used as a bridge to the definitive surgical solution or orthopedic program rather than a substitute for the optimal treatment regimen. A thorough patient history and orthopedic examination should be performed to help avoid being hopelessly trapped in the chiropodical routine of periodic débridement and adjunctive padding. Once the nature of the problem is better understood

709

through careful assessment and evaluation, the practitioner will be able to select the appropriate pad elements. The principles and techniques used in selecting and designing the optimal pad should be based on the region of the foot to be treated and the particular need, whether it be one of a protective, functional, or substitutive nature.

Whether a proposed pad is applied directly upon the foot or toes, or cemented within the patient's shoe, is largely a matter of choice and practice style. As a general guideline, we advise padding the shoe when possible so as to circumvent the hygienic and irritative complications of skin occlusion that may become more distressing than the original condition. It is equally evident, however, that precise digital or metatarsal shielding is often only possible by means of direct pad application and retention on the involved skin site. Conversely, larger elements intended for foot support and rebalance have no business being wrapped on the foot and secured with bulky bandages when they could be more easily and efficiently inserted into the patient's footwear. Moreover, an off-the-foot padding approach facilitates the procurement of requested radiographs and the institution of prescribed physical therapeutic measures.

Principles of Pad Design and Application

The *padding material* selected to perform a job is important in the matter of force recruitment and redistribution, because it is apparent that a pad cannot apply more influence than the compressive resistance inherent in the chosen material. Soft foam rubber sheeting, for example, can produce the same pressure as that from firm sponge rubber but requires a far greater bulk to achieve a similar mechanical effect. Therefore, within the space limitations of the average shoe the firmer materials are more logically utilized.

The *pad foundation* (shoe counter and shank support) is a decisive factor that governs the effect of a pad placed in the middle section of the typical heeled shoe, because any flexible pad can exert no more force than it can gain from the surface upon which it rests. For this reason, a so-called wedgie-type shoe sole provides an ideally firm foundation

for supportive midfoot padding needs. A pad applied to give support to the medial aspect of the longitudinal arch often lacks the necessary backup resistance from the medial counter of the shoe. When such improved medial counter force is required, an extended, reinforced medial counter is prescribed.

The *pad design* (i.e., size, shape, thickness, contour) is of great significance in the consideration of the specific clinical effect and benefit of a particular pad. In general, the space constraints are of constant concern, but it should be remembered that the instituted force must be adequate for the intended purpose, and, if the presented shoe is unduly restricting, a roomier one should be prescribed. Pad size and shape should be commensurate with the protective, supportive, or other need for which it is intended. A metatarsal pressure problem will require a pad that is specifically tailored to the contour of the individual metatarsal length pattern (Fig. 28-1a). It can be generalized that a broader pad will better serve to redistribute focal noxious pressure than a smaller, ringlike design (Fig. 28-1b). Abrupt pad corners and "dog-ears" are to be avoided in favor of smoothly rounded shapes and forms, and for similar reasons all pad edges should be carefully beveled. The thickness of a pad or shield will vary with the prominence to be protected and with the corrective force indications (Fig. 28-1c). Once again, space limitations, shoe support, material firmness, and compressibility all play a role in the final effect.

Pad apertures are the dells that subtract focal pressure concentrations and permit a redistribution of such force over a broad area. These apertures and cutouts are designed to conform to the offending prominence or lesion with their surrounding edges appropriately beveled to eliminate excessive edge pressure and irritation.[2] If the aperture is too remote from the site to be protected, it fails to protect (Fig. 28-1d); when the aperture is too small, its intimacy causes continued irritation on the sensitive area immediately surrounding the part to be protected. Protective apertures designed in shoe padding are usually longitudinally ovoid or distally opened cutouts to allow for the fore-and-aft foot shifting within the footgear during dynamic function (Fig. 28-1e).

It is almost unnecessary to mention that with foot

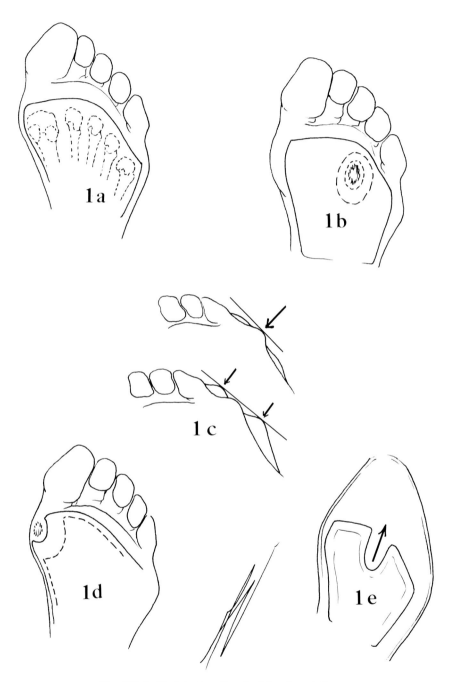

Fig. 28-1. Pad design. See text for description.

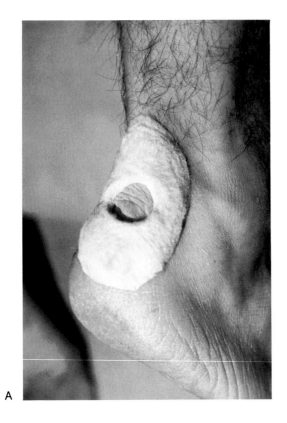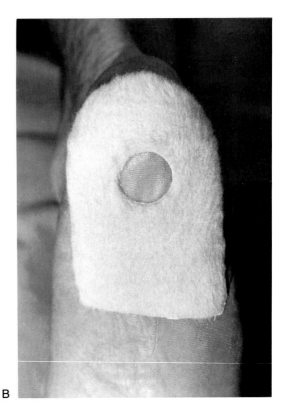

Fig. 28-2. (A) Posterior calcaneal shield. **(B)** Plantar calcaneal shield.

or toe padding proper skin cleansing and preparation is important, as are the adherents and the retentive bandaging techniques. A skin adherent will not only allow for a more secure contact between foot and pad but will also provide a thin protective film to help prevent maceration and to create a less favorable climate for fungal growth.

Types of Padding

Protective Shielding

Protective shielding may be regionally classified as rearfoot, midfoot, forefoot, and digital. Such shields are most commonly made of felt or foam rubber sheeting and are adhered directly upon the foot and digits.

1. Protective rearfoot shields
   a. Posterior calcaneal shield (Fig. 28-2A)

   b. Plantar calcaneal shield (Fig. 28-2B)
   c. Medial/lateral calcaneal shield
2. Protective midfoot shields
   a. Dorsal cuneometatarsal joint shield (Fig. 28-3A)
   b. Medial navicular tuberosity shield (Fig. 28-3B)
   c. Plantar cuneometatarsal joint shield
   d. Lateral fifth metatarsal base shield (Fig. 28-3C)
3. Protective forefoot shields
   a. Dorsal bunion shield (Fig. 28-4A)
   b. Medial bunion shield (Fig. 28-4B)
   c. Plantar sesamoid shield (Fig. 28-4C)
   d. Plantar lesser metatarsal shield (Fig. 28-4D)
   e. Lateral bunionette shield (Fig. 28-4E)
4. Protective digital shields
   a. Dorsal hallux shield (Fig. 28-5A)
   b. Plantar-medial hallux shield (Fig. 28-5B)
   c. Plantar hallux shield (Fig. 28-5C)
   d. Lesser digital shields (Fig. 28-5D–F)

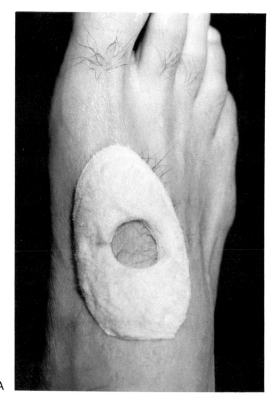

A

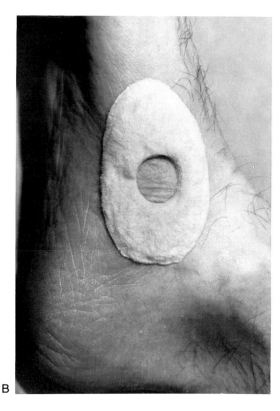

B

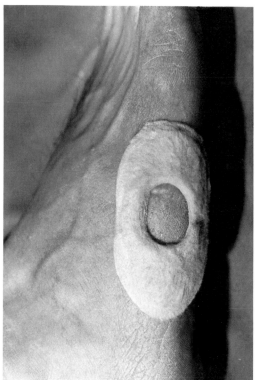

C

Fig. 28-3. (A) Dorsal cuneometatarsal joint shield. **(B)** Medial navicular tuberosity shield. **(C)** Lateral fifth metatarsal base shield.

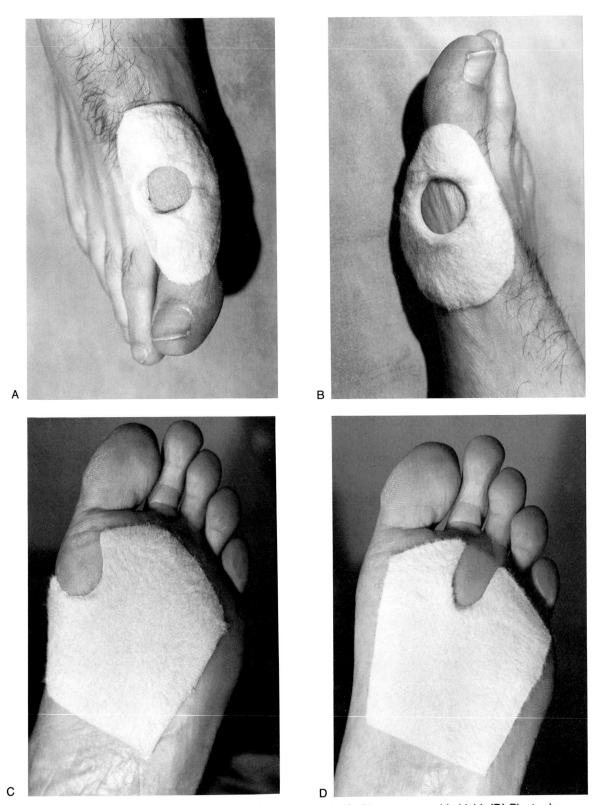

Fig. 28-4. (A) Dorsal bunion shield. **(B)** Medial bunion shield. **(C)** Plantar sesamoid shield. **(D)** Plantar lesser metatarsal shield. *(Figure continues.)*

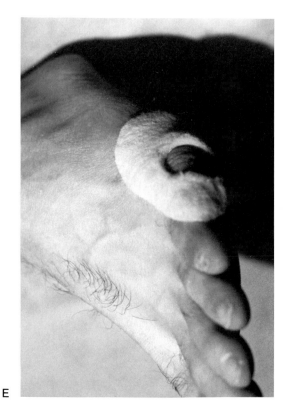

E

Fig. 28-4 *(Continued).* **(E)** Lateral bunionette shield.

Functional Padding

Functional padding includes the mechanical elements, regionally applied and preferably inserted in the shoe with rubber cement, the intent of which is to support, balance, realign, or otherwise influence the function of the foot and lower extremity. We offer a regional classification and terminology that divides the plantar aspect of the foot and shoe insole into nine sectors of prospective pad application (Fig. 28-6). For each of these regions, suggested pad types are illustrated along with a brief descriptor as to their clinical selection and intent.

The authors have utilized a system of "functional test padding" to attain initial symptom relief while testing individual tolerance and functional response to the pad application.[3] If such applied forces produce relief and promote improved function, a more permanent orthosis can be prescribed and recommended with confidence. For this system of test padding a somewhat firm, pressure-moldable material called SBR (styrene-butadiene resin)° has been used by us for several years with great satisfaction. Pads designed from this material will compress to about one-half their original thickness within a few days. During trial use, when an initially gratifying response diminishes as the pad compacts, it can be assumed that the initial pad thickness is indicated. However, when the initial response is adverse or uncertain but the situation improves with pad compression, it can reasonably be deduced that a milder correction is warranted.

1. Functional rearfoot pads
   a. Medial heel wedge pad (Fig. 28-7A)
   b. Central heel elevation pad (Fig. 28-7B)
   c. Lateral heel wedge pad (Fig. 28-7C)
2. Functional midfoot pads
   a. Medial longitudinal pad
      —Talonavicular (scaphoid) pad (Fig. 28-8A)
   b. Central cavus (saddle) pad (Fig. 28-8B)
   c. Lateral longitudinal pad
      —Cuboid pad (Fig. 28-8C)
3. Functional forefoot pads
   a. Medial forefoot pads
      —Varus pad (Fig. 28-9A)
      —Varus/extension pad (Fig. 28-9B)
      —Varus/flange pad (Fig. 28-9C)
      —Varus/extension/flange pad
   b. Central forefoot pads
      —Met balance pad (Fig. 28-10A)
      —Met balance/extension pad (Fig. 28-10B)
      —Met balance/flange pad (Fig. 28-10C)
      —Met balance/extension/flange pad
   c. Lateral forefoot pads
      —Valgus pad (Fig. 28-11A)
      —Valgus/extension pad (Fig. 28-11B)
      —Valgus/flange pad (Fig. 28-11C)
      —Valgus/extension/flange pad

Corrective Pediatric Padding. This is a preferred approach of many practitioners to the care of foot malalignments in younger children during the period of structural and functional foot immaturity. Such an approach is exceedingly useful because of

---

° SBR (styrene-butadiene resin) R8402 S-SBR vacuum-formable material. Available from Rubatex Corp., Bedford, VA.

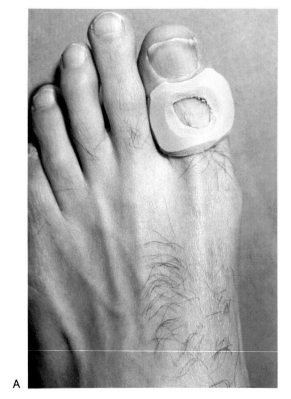

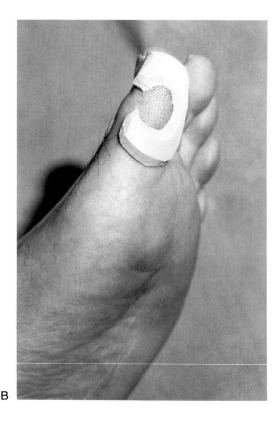

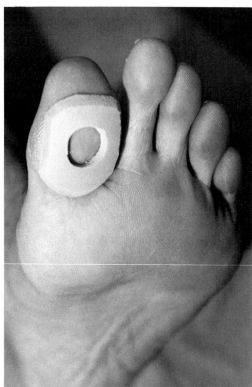

A

B

C

Fig. 28-5. (A) Dorsal hallux shield. **(B)** Plantar-medial hallux shield. **(C)** Plantar hallux shield. *(Figure continues.)*

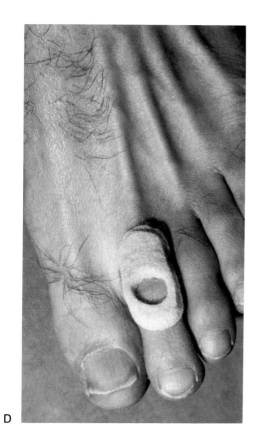

D

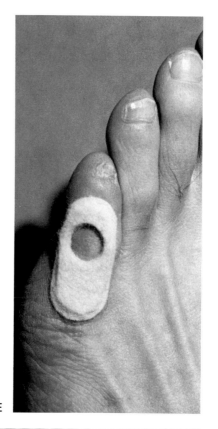

E

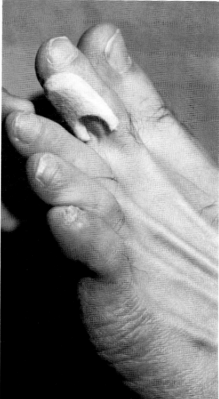

Fig. 28-5. *(continued).* **(D-F)** Lesser digital shields.   F

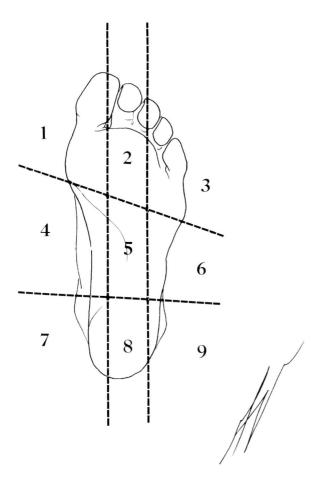

Fig. 28-6. Nine sectors of prospective pad application.

partial forefoot amputee. A cone-shaped pad can be heated and formed over the stump of the trans-metatarsal amputee; such a pad can then simply be inserted within the toe box of the patient's shoe or could be worn directly on the foot beneath the hosiery.

Historical Padding Perspective

It may be of interest to review a few of the many pads introduced over the years by foot practitioners who matched their theories with their pads or, conversely, their pads with their theories.

The Meyer *metatarsal pad* was essentially pear shaped and devised to restore a "depressed anterior metatarsal arch." Closely associated with Meyer's contribution was the Schaeffer *longitudinal pad,* which presumably led to the development of the medially flanged longitudinal arch support. The first metatarsal *extension platform* of Dudley J. Morton compensated for inadequate weightbearing by the first segment (Fig. 28-12A). L. Schreiber and H. Weinerman, in the 1950s, advocated a *medial or lateral balance pad* for forefoot varus or valgus, respectively. Somewhat earlier, there was the *pocket pad* advocated by E.C. Meldman to help stabilize the lateral forefoot and, more specifically, the basal joint of the fourth metatarsal. The C. Leydecker *heel leveling pad* and *lateral forefoot* pad were apparently employed to improve female foot function in the steeply elevated dress pump style of footgear.

The *cuboid pad* may have multiple origins in various concepts of lateral longitudinal arch stability, the pivotal role of the fourth and fifth cubometatarsal joints, and the occurrence of calcaneocuboid joint subluxation. Thus, one can cite the concepts and contributions of William Koppe, J.M. Hiss, and Dr. Locke (the Canadian bonesetter) as proponents of some version of a cuboid pad. F. Carlton had his "muscular" medial tarsal pad,[4] which was placed against the medial aspect of the talocalcaneal articulation. More recently, we have witnessed the advent of the *cobra pad,* which appears to be an evolution of the prior Schwartz meniscus and Helfet heel seat versions of calcaneal pronation control (Fig. 28-12B). Also worthy of note were the *segment rebalance pads* of M. Polokoff and C. Turchin (Fig. 28-12C) and the so-called *pontoon pads* of R.

its simplicity, adjustability, and economic advantage to young parents, but caution is always due when and if such padding forces are insufficient to accomplish the mechanical aims and needs of the case.

Substitutive Filler Padding

Substitutive filler padding is often of esthetic and functional benefit to the partial foot or toe amputee who, predictably, has stuffed old paper or foam wadding into his or her shoes to serve as a functional buttress and to help prevent the upturning of the vacant toe box. The insertion filler-type pads and moldable inserts are greatly appreciated. Softer to medium-density Plastazote is a most useful moldable padding material that can be roughly shaped and then heat-conformed to the digital or

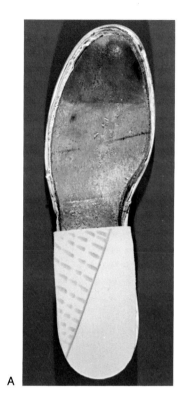

A

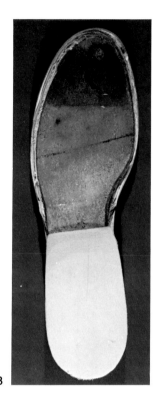

B

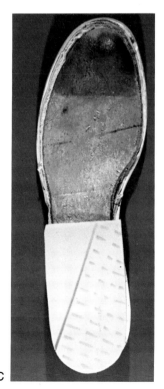

C

Fig. 28-7. (A) Medial heel wedge pad. **(B)** Central heel elevation pad. **(C)** Lateral heel wedge pad.

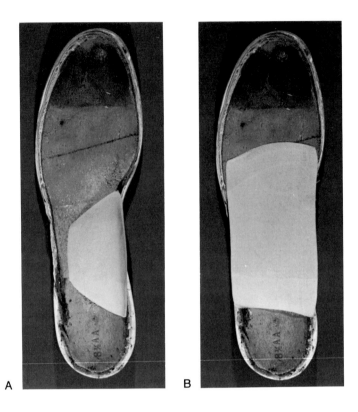

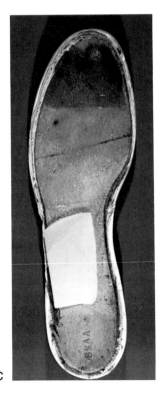

Fig. 28-8. (A) Talonavicular (scaphoid) pad. **(B)** Central cavus (saddle) pad. **(C)** Cuboid pad.

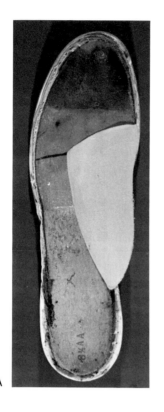
A

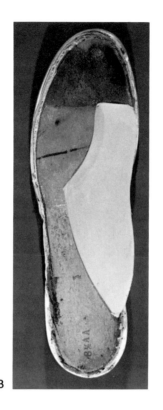
B

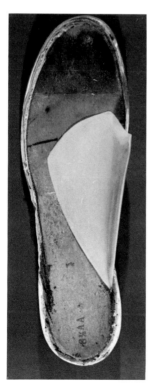
C

Fig. 28-9. (A) Varus pad. **(B)** Varus/extension pad. **(C)** Varus/flange pad.

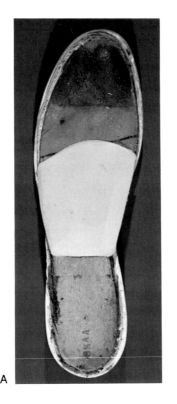

A

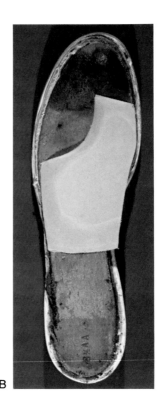

B

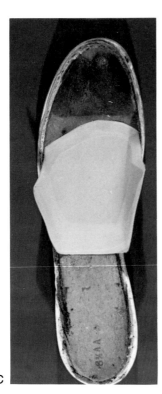

C

Fig. 28-10. **(A)** Met balance pad. **(B)** Met balance/extension pad. **(C)** Met balance/flange pad.

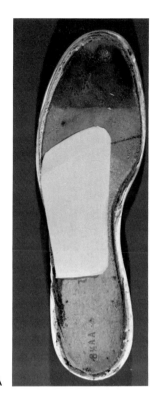

A

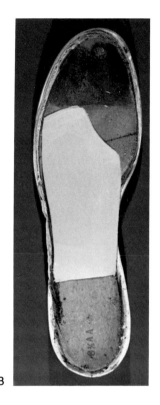

B

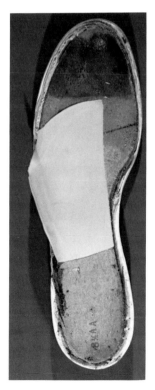

C

Fig. 28-11. (A) Valgus pad. **(B)** Valgus/extension pad. **(C)** Valgus/flange pad.

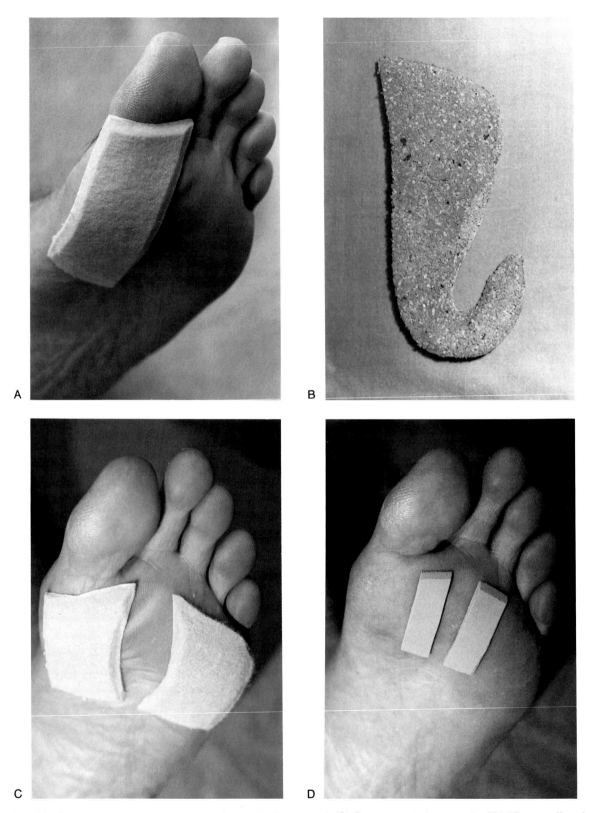

Fig. 28-12. (A) Metatarsal extension platform. **(B)** Cobra pad. **(C)** Segment rebalance pads. **(D)** ''Pontoon'' pads.

724

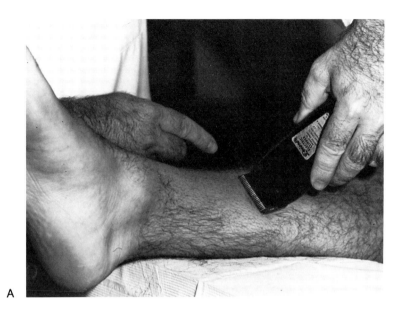

A

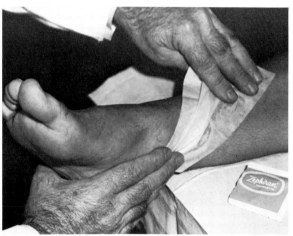

B

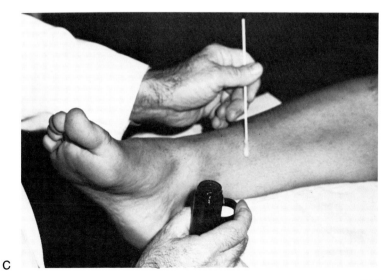

C

Fig. 28-13. Preparation of the skin surface to be taped. **(A)** Shaving hair from taping areas. **(B)** Cleansing skin. **(C)** Applying skin adherent.

Sansone (Fig. 28-12D). A relatively controversial theory of neuropodology was proposed by E. Davis, who used small *button pads* to nullify reflexive functional influences.

These examples are but a sample of existing and extinct pad designs and elements of the distant and more recent past. Numerous other individuals, not mentioned here, deserve much credit for their padding innovations through which significant relief to footsore patients and podiatric progress have been attained.

ADHESIVE TAPING

Adhesive taping for control of abnormal joint tension and position has long been practiced in podiatry. Simple foot and ankle injuries are greatly benefited by "relative immobilization" while preserving the obvious advantages of ambulation. In light of modern orthopedic theory and practice, the test control of "neutral joint position" is a sensible preliminary to a more definitive disposition. In the empirical past, many practitioners attempted and achieved foot realignment through persistent application of adhesive tension.

Indications and Contraindications

Adhesive taping therapy can be utilized for symptomatic/supportive bracing, relative immobilization, corrective realignment, and accommodative neutralization. *Symptomatic/supportive* bracing is used for the relief of pain associated with an abnormal amount, duration, or disposition of weight-bearing stress. Subluxatory joint manifestations and muscle fatigue can be contained through tension taping.[5] *Relative immobilization* of uncomplicated foot and ankle sprains, by adhesive strapping, has proven its value in the field of sports medicine and for the care of industrial injuries. *Corrective realignment* of subtalar, midtarsal, and hallux malposition is attainable to varying degree through persistent application of tensive taping. *Accommodative neutralization* or rebalancing of

the intractable foot deformity is initially accomplished through a combination of tensive stabilization and plantar posting that permits estimation of probable clinical response to the repositioning.

Contraindications to adhesive taping include idiosyncratic responses to adhesive tape and its components, which at times is aggravated by hyperhidrosis. If tape must be employed in such cases, it should be applied over roller gauze bandaging. Superficial wounds and various ischemic, congestive, or other preulcerative states are not favored by adhesive dressings, which may even induce mechanical and microbial wound disruption. Also, podedema from the effect of constricting tape edges and encircling straps can pose a distinct problem. An awareness of the potential problem permits avoidance of such a complication.

Preliminary Considerations and Procedures

Regardless of the specific strapping to be employed, one is well advised to consider some general principles and questions concerning the nature and stage of deformity and the physical and psychological capacity of the patient for correction. In other words, one estimates the individual potential for change with a realistic acceptance of the intractable.[6]

To what extent is manual realignment possible? What is the nature and source of the encountered resistance?

Would a preliminary "soft tissue release" facilitate the desired alignment or is a bone procedure required?

Is manipulative therapy or tractive mobilization indicated and is the intent pain relief or increased range of motion?

Would muscle stimulation, stretching, or strengthening exercise be beneficially prescribed in this case?

What is the relative potential for tissue change (plasticity) in this patient?

What corrective forces can be recruited from the supporting surface? Do the current or prospective shoes provide adequate shank and counter strength?

Which corrective or accommodative plantar paddings should be instituted along with adhesive therapy? Would neutralizing heel wedges, rebalancing forefoot posts, appositional cavus padding, or segmental metatarsal platforms be suitable in this particular case?

What exterior shoe modifications can be prescribed as mechanical adjuncts to lower extremity function?

With acute injuries, is a fracture or dislocation present? Has a complete tendinous or ligamentous separation occurred? How much reactive myospasm and edema can be anticipated? Is Gelocast bandaging appropriate or would firm plaster immobilization be a better therapeutic selection?

If chronic, is arthritis, paralysis, or myodystrophy a concomitant feature?

Prestrapping Procedure

Skin preparation for adhesive taping therapy includes the following three steps[7]:

1. Shave hair from prospective taping areas (Fig. 28-13A).
2. Cleanse skin with skin prep packets (Fig. 28-13B).
3. Apply skin adherent using cotton-tipped applicators (Fig. 28-13C).

Basic Strapping Patterns

Subtalar Joint Control

This strapping pattern is most useful for the relative immobilization of common medial or lateral sprains involving the ankle and subtalar joints. For initial symptomatic and supportive relief of chronic subluxatory rearfoot changes, edema, and associated muscular fatigue, the taping serves as a temporary "rest dressing." More recently, this form of stirrup splinting has been utilized for the test control or neutral subtalar position.

Strapping Procedure.

1. Determine optimal subtalar joint position in accordance with presented symptoms, evident in-stability, or the neutral joint position estimation.
2. Prepare the skin surface to be taped.
3. Technique
   a. Apply three 2-inch vertical stirrup straps (Fig. 28-14).
   b. Apply one 2-inch short plantar strap (Fig. 28-15).
   c. Apply three 2-inch anterior leg straps (Fig. 28-15).
   d. Apply the notched 2-inch dorsal strap (Fig. 28-16).
4. Powder the finished dressing (Fig. 28-17), and dispense adhesive taping instructions (verbal and printed) to the patient (see later in chapter).

Midtarsal Joint Control

Indications for the control of midtarsal joint position and tension include the typical plantar sprains and strains generally associated with increased and prolonged weight-bearing stress, especially in faulty footgear. Primary instability or a compensatory hypermobility at the midtarsal joint complex can be temporarily contained by adhesive taping. In the milder, tractable cases of foot malalignment, such persistently applied adhesive tension dressings are of value.

Strapping Procedure.

1. Determine desired midtarsal apposition by manual palpation of joint congruency (Fig. 28-18), and by manipulative estimation of reposition potential (Fig. 28-19). Tractographic "sighting" is further helpful for appraisal of renmant forefoot posting needs (Fig. 28-20).
2. Prepare the skin surface to be taped.
3. Technique
   a. Apply two 1-inch horizontal harness straps (Fig. 28-21).
   b. Apply three 2-inch short plantar straps (Fig. 28-22).
   c. Apply the distal 2-inch plantar cover straps (Fig. 28-23).
   d. Apply two more 1-inch horizontal harness straps (Fig. 28-24).
   e. Apply the 2-inch dorsum strap (Fig. 28-25).
4. Powder the finished dressing (Fig. 28-26) and dispense the adhesive taping instructions to the patient.

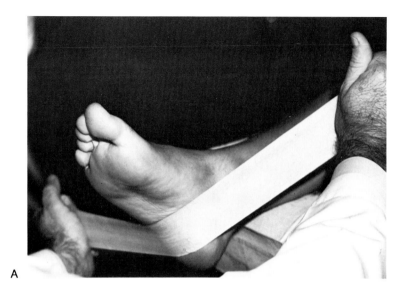

A

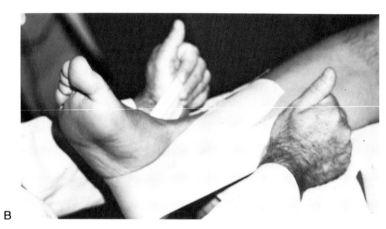

B

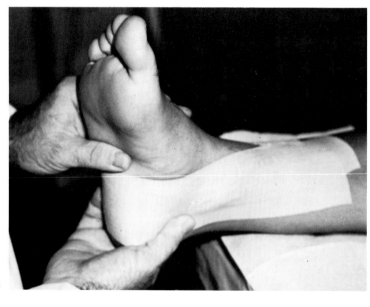

C

Fig. 28-14. Application of three 2-inch vertical stirrup straps. **(A)** Initial strap. **(B)** Additional straps. **(C)** Completed appearance.

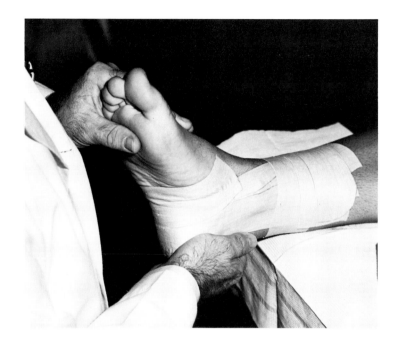

Fig. 28-15. Application of one 2-inch short plantar strap and three 2-inch anterior leg straps (completed appearance).

Hallux Control

Hallux alignment is often the vital ingredient in the preservation or restitution of forefoot function. In both midstance and propulsion, the hallux consecutively "buttresses" and "windlasses" the medial longitudinal foot structure. Hallux abductovalgus represents a medial metatarsophalangeal "blow-out" with secondary lateral jamming of the articulation. Trial adhesive tape realignment relieves both local and remote symptoms while serving as a functional test of the new position.

Strapping Procedure.

1. Manually determine the improved hallux position with realistic awareness of shoe style limitation and requirements. As the great toe is drawn medialward, the relative resistance to intermetatarsal angulation is noted as an index of obstruction to hallux correction. In such instances, preliminary "adductor release" can be considered in the milder cases, whereas an osseous reconstruction may be needed in more advanced conditions.
2. Prepare the skin surface to be taped.

3. Technique:
   a. Apply the cushioned 1-inch hallux anchor strap (Fig. 28-27).
   b. Apply the 2-inch metatarsal anchor band (Fig. 28-28).
   c. Apply the medial 1-inch hallux tension strap (Fig. 28-29).
   d. Apply the plantar-medial 1-inch hallux tension strap (Fig. 28-30).
   e. Apply the dorsomedial 1-inch hallux tension strap (Fig. 28-31).
   f. Apply the top 1-inch hallux anchor strap (Fig. 28-32).
   g. Apply the top 2-inch metatarsal anchor strap (Fig. 28-33).
4. Powder the dressing (Fig. 28-34) and dispense adhesive taping instructions to the patient.

Strapping Variations and Adjunctive Padding

Rearfoot control variations

1. Gibney strapping (Fig. 28-35A)
2. High-dye strapping (Fig. 28-35B)

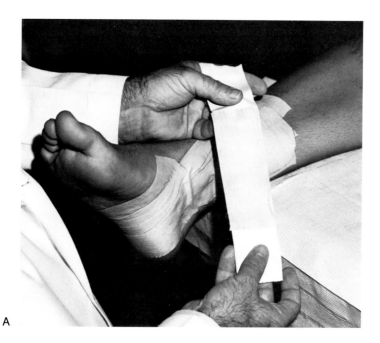

A

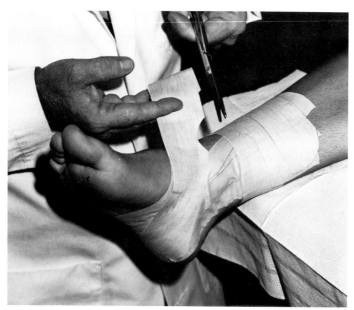

B

Fig. 28-16. Application of notched 2-inch dorsal strap. **(A)** Dorsal strap. **(B)** Notching of strap.

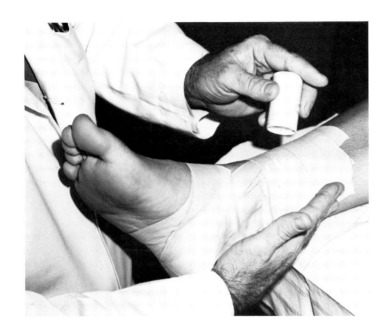

Fig. 28-17. Application of powder to the finished dressing.

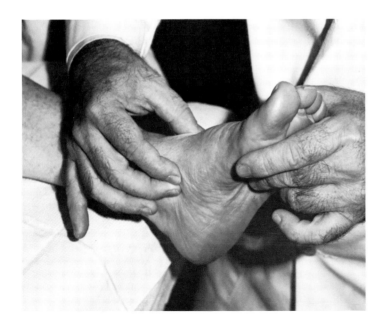

Fig. 28-18. Determination of midtarsal apposition of manual palpation of joint congruency.

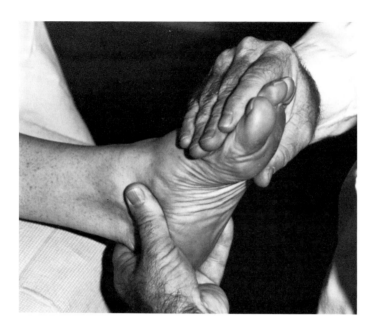

Fig. 28-19. Determination of midtarsal apposition by manipulative estimation of reposition potential.

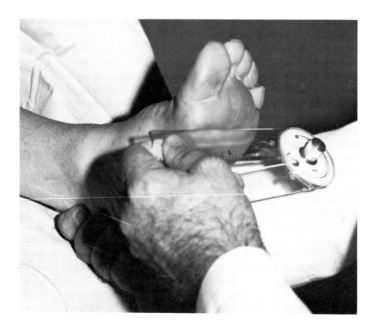

Fig. 28-20. Appraisal of remnant forefoot posting needs by tractographic ''sighting.''

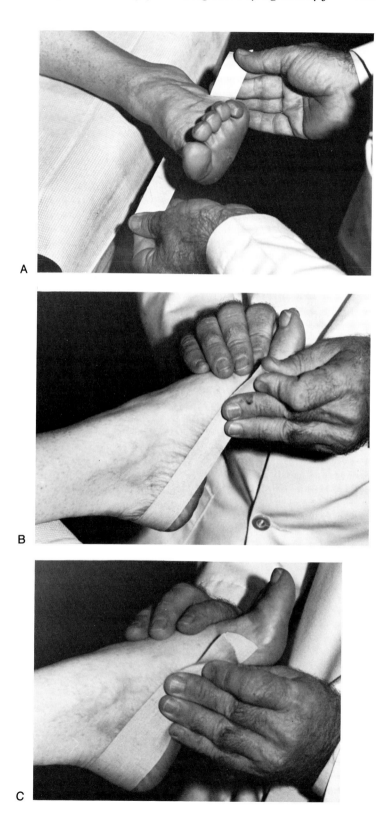

Fig. 28-21. Application of two 1-inch horizontal harness straps. **(A)** Alignment of strap on heel. **(B)** Application of strap. **(C)** Application of second strap.

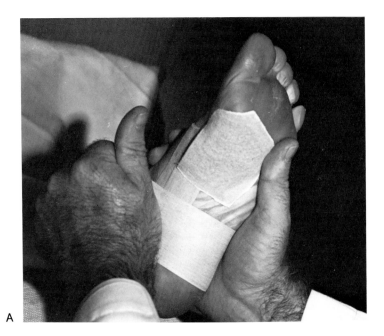

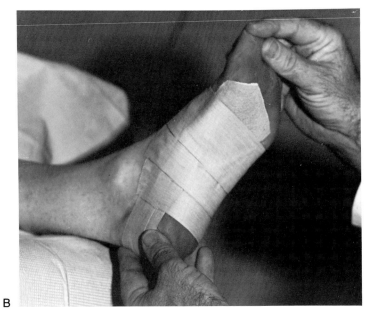

Fig. 28-22. **(A)** Application of three 2-inch short plantar straps. **(B)** Completed appearance.

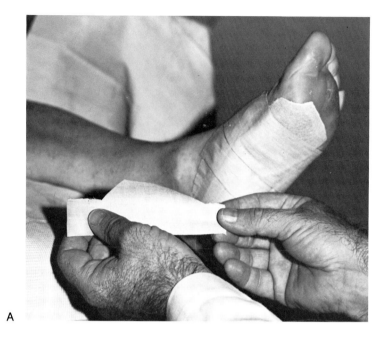

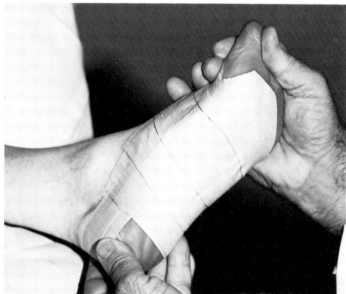

Fig. 28-23. (A) Application of the distal 2-inch plantar cover straps. **(B)** Completed appearance.

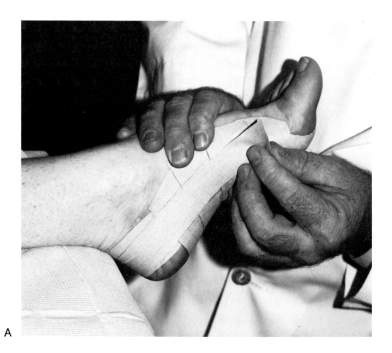

A

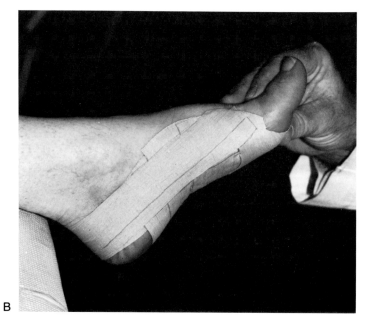

B

Fig. 28-24. (A) Application of two more 1-inch horizontal harness straps. **(B)** Completed appearance.

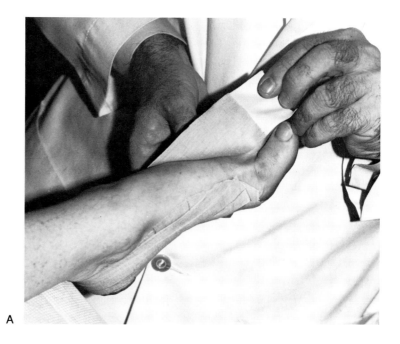

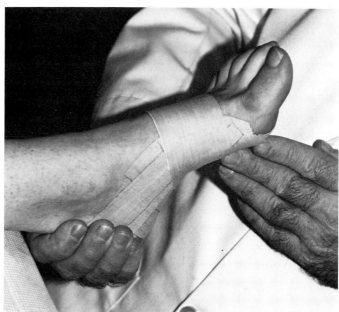

Fig. 28-25. (A) Application of 2-inch dorsum strap. **(B)** Completed appearance.

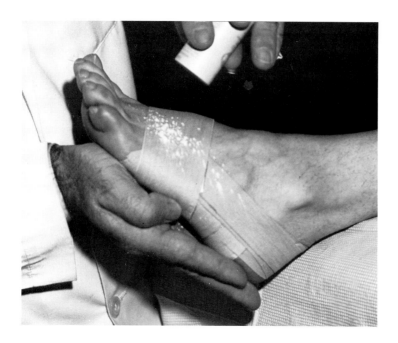

Fig. 28-26. Application of powder to the finished dressing.

3. Plantaris strapping (Fig. 28-35C)
4. Box heel strapping (Fig. 28-35D)

Midtarsal control variations[8]

1. Campbell "rest" strapping (Fig. 28-36A)
2. Lawson strapping (Fig. 28-36B)
3. Peroneal "crossdown" strapping (Fig. 28-36C)
4. Plantar fascial "V" strapping (Fig. 28-36D)

Forefoot control variations

1. Hallux retentive strapping (Turchin) (Fig. 28-37A)
2. Metatarsus latus strapping (Fig. 28-37B)

Instructions for Adhesive Taping Therapy

The following instructions should be given to the patient both verbally and as a printed take-home sheet for further reference. Additional instructions specific to each patient may be written onto the take-home sheet.

1. The tape on your feet is relatively water resistant but should not be vigorously scrubbed during bathing. Merely pat the tapes dry with a towel after bathing and the body heat will evaporate the remaining moisture.
2. The taping will feel somewhat tight at first but then loosens to comfortable tension within a short time. Do not expect complete comfort with this therapy because definite changes take place during correction that may produce temporary discomfort in the feet, legs, back, or even shoulders.
3. As your circulation improves with better foot function, a minor skin itching or irritation sometimes occurs under the tape. This is a reaction that can be alleviated by applying a dry cold pack over the affected area for 10 to 15 minutes. Repeat if desired.
4. Marked pain, itching, or other skin reaction should *not* be tolerated. In such an instance, please phone for specific instructions. If for any reason we cannot be reached immediately, carefully remove the strapping.
5. Unless otherwise instructed, leave the tape on until your next visit.
6. Each morning lightly powder the adhesive dressing. Avoid standing or walking without shoes because this greatly reduces the efficiency of the taping therapy.

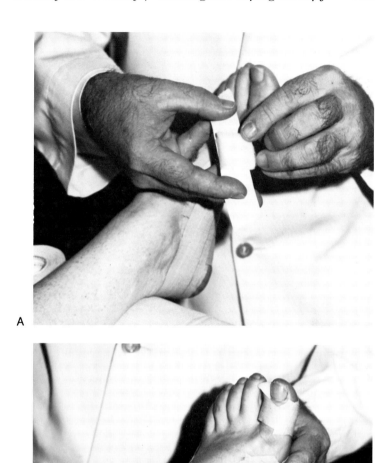

A

B

Fig. 28-27. (A) Application of the cushioned 1-inch hallux anchor strap. **(B)** Completed appearance.

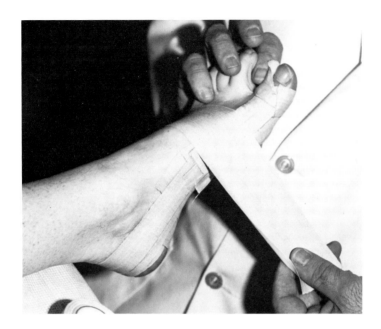

Fig. 28-28. Application of the 2-inch metatarsal anchor band.

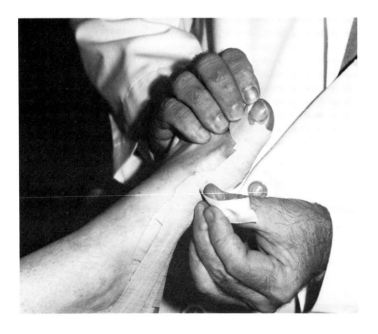

Fig. 28-29. Application of the medial 1-inch hallux tension strap.

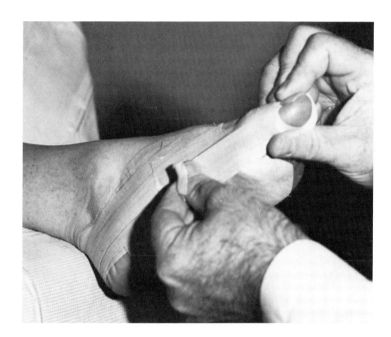

Fig. 28-30. Application of the plantar-medial 1-inch hallux tension strap.

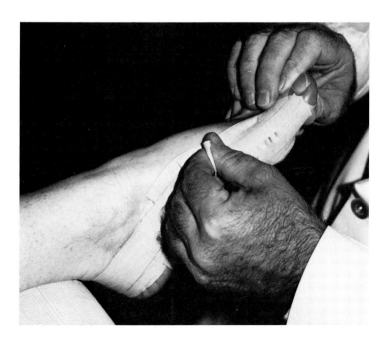

Fig. 28-31. Application of the dorsomedial 1-inch hallux tension strap.

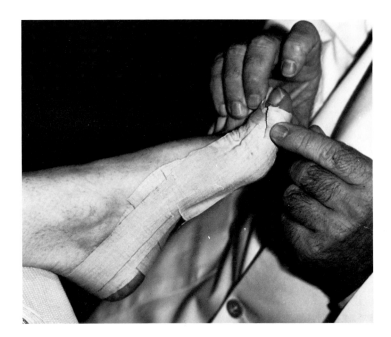

Fig. 28-32. Application of the top 1-inch hallux anchor strap.

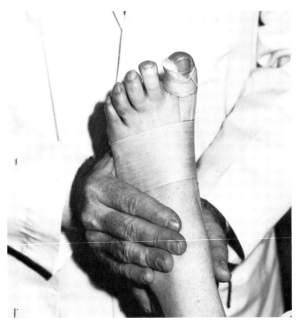

Fig. 28-33. Application of the top 2-inch metatarsal anchor strap.

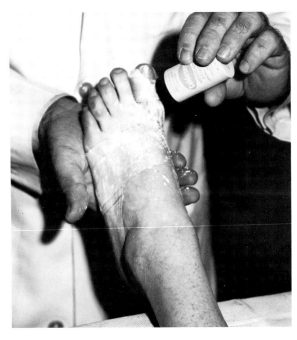

Fig. 28-34. Application of powder to the finished dressing.

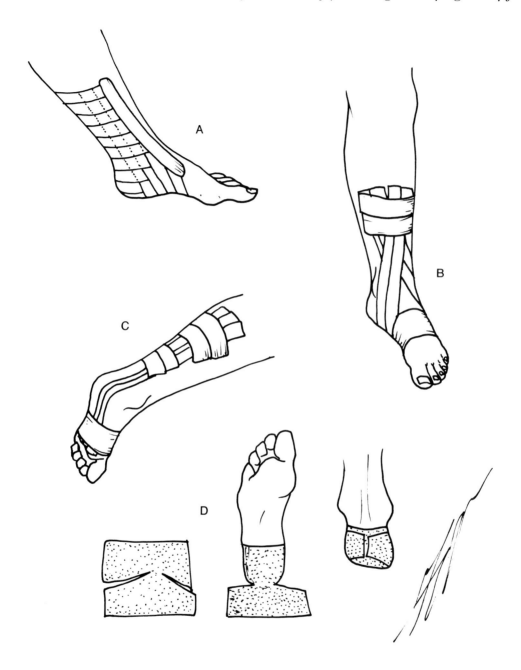

Fig. 28-35. Rearfoot control strapping pattern variations. **(A)** Gibney strapping. **(B)** High-dye strapping. **(C)** Plantaris strapping. **(D)** Box heel strapping.

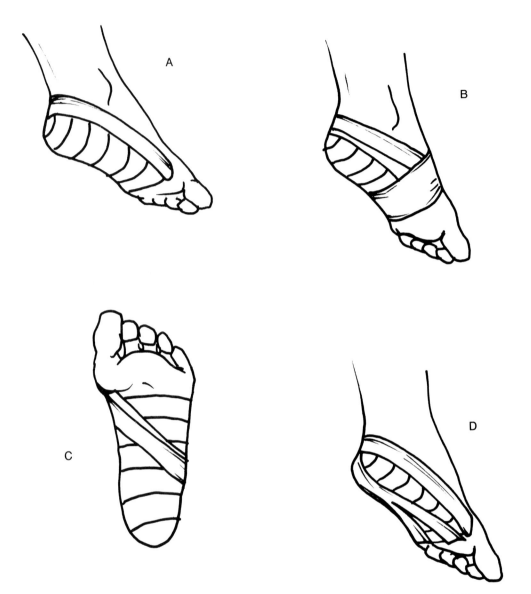

Fig. 28-36. Medtarsal control strapping pattern variations. **(A)** Campbell ''rest'' strapping. **(B)** Lawson strapping. **(C)** Peroneal ''crossdown'' strapping. **(D)** Plantar fascial ''V'' strapping.

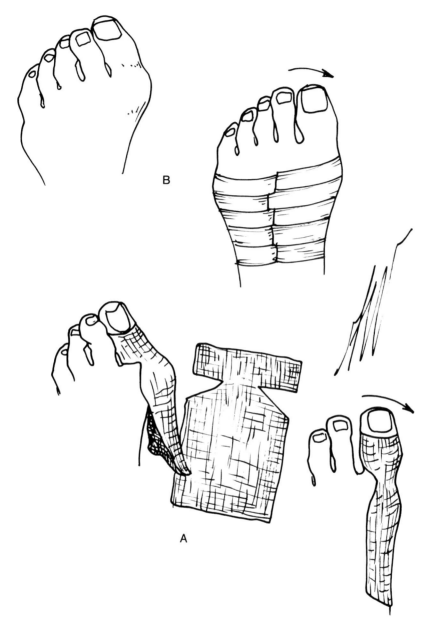

Fig. 28-37. Forefoot control strapping pattern variations. **(A)** Hallux retentive strapping (Turchin). **(B)** Metatarsus latus strapping.

7. Again, if you experience undue pain between visits, you should report it at once for our attention. Doing this can eliminate days of needless discomfort.

REFERENCES

1. Charlesworth F: Chiropodical Orthopedics. E. and S. Livingstone Ltd, Edinburgh, 1951
2. Donick II: Podiatry for the Assistant. Futura Publishing Co, Mt. Kisco, New York, 1977
3. Whitney AK: Biomechanical Footwear Balancing. Pennsylvania College of Podiatric Medicine, Philadelphia, 1979
4. Carleton FJ: Shoes and Feet. Printing Plate Craftsmen, Pennsylvania, 1946
5. Lantz FA: Taping and padding advocated in treating athletes' shin splints. Podiatry News, 12(2):00, 1974
6. Whitney AK: Adheso-Tensive Therapy (A Teaching Minicourse). Pennsylvania College of Podiatric Medicine, Philadelphia, 1971
7. Professional Uses of Adhesive Tape. Johnson and Johnson, New Brunswick, NJ, 1972
8. Sandler M: Treatment Procedure — Strapping Techniques (A Teaching Minicourse). Pennsylvania College of Podiatric Medicine, Philadelphia, 1968

Basic Concepts of Physical Medicine and Rehabilitation

29

Arthur E. Helfand, D.P.M.

The terms *physical medicine* and *rehabilitation,* in a broad sense, include the use of physical modalities and procedures and a total approach to patient care. They include such issues as social needs, the environment, and a need to consider the patient as a total entity. They include the primary objectives of relieving pain, restoring a maximum level of function, and maintaining that restored functional ability mentally, psychologically, spiritually, and vocationally. Evaluation of the patient's foot pain, ambulatory dysfunction, and functional disability, regardless of the etiology or related disease processes, must also consider the social implications of immobility and the limitations on the activities of daily living. Rehabilitation must also include a team approach to patient care that must be multidisciplinary in character.

Good foot health involves more than specific disease care. It must include education and prevention as well as therapeutic approaches. It needs to consider orthotics, special shoes or shoe modifications, preventing infections, and minimizing bed confinement and institutionalization. There is a need for the health care team members to utilize communication skills with each other, the patients, and their families to assure compliance and to maximize the care provided by professionals.

In a sense, the use of physical medicine has long been a part of podiatric clinical practice. It has been primarily modality focused and directed toward a disease process or condition and a specific outcome, many times measured by the utilization pattern for that spell of illness. Modalities have been utilized to augment other forms of therapy and, for the most part, directed toward the relief of pain in acute conditions or in the exacerbations of common chronic diseases that manifest in the foot as a primary focus for pain.

However, there is a need to examine a broader approach that considers foot care and podiatric procedures a part of the total rehabilitation of the patient. Foot problems in old, injured, and disabled persons are generally chronic in nature and provide some limitation of ambulation. It is also well accepted that once a patient begins to move about, he or she will comply with other forms of therapy and can be motivated toward self-care. However, because the foot and its problems are for the most part non–life threatening, consideration of care may be deferred. When one considers the goals that must be established for chronically ill and elderly patients, which emphasize comfort and not cure, the need for foot care becomes essential in the total management of the patient. For example, the ability to walk from the bed to a chair for the recent stroke patient may be most difficult if a local foot problem precipitates pain. In turn, the integration of podiatric care as part of total care is equally important if the patient's focus relates to foot pain, discomfort, disability, and/or dysfunction.

Practitioner attitudes and patient communication are also essential elements of a rehabilitation concept that utilizes physical medicine as part of the treatment program. The ability to communicate hope to the patient, demonstrate progress and improvement, and help establish attainable short-term goals are equally important as the treatment itself. One must consider the total needs of the patient and consider the team approach to care. There needs to be a knowledge of the community and its resources. There is a need to know the patient's resources. The attitude of all individuals involved in patient care is essential. Practitioners who are responsible for managing the problems of aging and chronic disease should become involved in rehabilitation programs. One also needs to remember the social, economic, and therapeutic needs of the patient to properly provide meaningful communication.

We need to talk to our patients so that they understand that they are real people with real problems and that we are concerned. We need to accept what the patient says, because it is the patient who experiences the pain and disability. Whether it is real pain or some other manifestation, it is pain to that particular patient. We need to touch our patients both physically and emotionally so that they know there is a feeling of caring and a belief that they are individuals and not a computerized diagnosis with cookbook program for care. We need to hold out hope and try to relieve pain and discomfort. We need to provide hope, for without hope there is no future and motivation for progress is lost. We need to support our patients when the cause is just and become advocates for the patient. This is especially true as reimbursement programs and utilization efforts place limits on care that are based not upon patient need but on a statistical norm. We need to be honest and not blame the patient for his or her misfortune. Most importantly, we need to make sure that the care provided does not make the patient worse.

We must remember to talk to the patient's family, which is especially important when treating elderly as well as very young patients. We need to provide an assurance that all of the components of the care program are met and maximized.

BASIC CONSIDERATIONS

Physical medicine can broadly be defined as that element of health care that utilizes physical agents (such as light, heat, cold, water, and electricity) and mechanical agents (such as exercises, aids to ambulation, gait training, tests and measurements) in the diagnosis and treatment of disease. The term *rehabilitation* in a global sense has been utilized to deal with patient restoration for handicapped conditions, be they physical, mental, social, or vocational, to maximize the patient's capabilities to a near-normal state. Given this concept, the examination of the patient should also consider the use of electromyography, nerve conduction studies, vascular evaluations, neuromuscular reviews, muscle testing, range of motion studies, and goniometry.

Because patient management is projected from a physical foundation, the vocational, psychiatric, and psychological aspects of care also need to be considered. Most conditions do present some psychosomatic overtones, and symptoms, real or perceived, can produce similar disabilities. The management of chronic disease and aging clearly demonstrates the relationship of body and mind. In many ways, ambulation is the catalyst to the management of many conditions, and foot health is a key element to that process. Foot problems that are acute in nature, chronic by neglect, or residuals of other disease processes deserve consideration for care. This concern might appear holistic but it is really part of a learning tree that involves total care and concern for the patient.

If one were to list those physical modalities that are usually utilized for the management of foot conditions as a part of the rehabilitation process, the list would include, ultrasound, short-wave diathermy, infrared lamps, radiant light bakers, hot packs, whirlpool baths, contrast baths, paraffin baths, massage, ultraviolet radiation, electrical stimulation (high-low galvanic current, faradic current, and sinusoidal current), transcutaneous electrical nerve stimulation (TENS), cold packs, lasors, traction, intermittent compression, exercise (passive, active assistive, voluntary active, active resistive, and coordinative), gait training (using crutches, walkers, canes, braces, parallel bars, prosthetics, and orthotics), training for activities of daily living, and various other diagnostic procedures and tests.

There are a wide variety of chronically disabling conditions that usually present with pedal manifestations. Examples include arthritis, burns, cerebral palsy, cerebral vascular accidents, congenital deformities, dermatomyositis, degenerative spinal cord disease, joint deformities, muscular contractures, muscular atrophy, paraplegia and quadraplegia, peripheral nerve injuries, peripheral vascular disease, poliomyelitis, polymositis, polyneuritis, residuals of severe trauma, scleroderma, spina bifida, spinal cord injuries, stasis dermatitis, ulcerations, chronic renal failure, alcohol abuse, drug abuse, and chemical dependency. Appropriate podiatric principles, coupled with the use of physical activities, can aid in ambulation, prevent excessive pressure and infection, and increase the patient's personal comfort.

PATIENT EVALUATION

The evaluation of the patient is essential to determine the needs of the patient in relation to the primary and secondary diagnosis. The statistical and demographic information forms the basic elements of the evaluative process. The chief complaint should be elicited in the patient's own words, particularly when the patient has been referred for care. This will provide a feeling of caring within the partnership involved in a doctor-patient relationship. The concerns identified by the patient as to his or her impression of the condition and how that problem relates to functional and occupational needs is a most important element of the evaluation. It permits the establishment of attainable goals that are reasonable and will demonstrate improvement.

The present condition, a historical review, a systems review, and all prior care should be fully explored and documented. The past medical and surgical history should include an occupational history as well as exposures, military service, geographic considerations, and the percentage of weightbearing during normal work activities. Flooring, foot-

wear, and stress (such as occupations involving weight lifting) are also important in projecting a prognosis. A social history is equally important in relation to drugs, alcohol, and interpersonal relationships in today's society. The patient's reaction to his or her own illness may well be a key factor in the prognosis of comfort, management, and/or cure. The patient's subjective symptoms should relate to the practitioner's objective findings.

The peripheral vascular elements of the evaluation should consider at least the following: pedal pulses and those proximal to the foot, color, temperature, trophic changes, edema, varicosities, stasis, induration, ulceration, night cramps, claudication, fatigue, burning, plantar ischemia, venous filling time, blood pressure, Doppler studies, plethysmography, and oscillometry.

Notation should be made of the structural changes and relationship present in the foot and its related structures. The prime considerations include foot type, gait, postural deformities, range of motion studies, goniometry, limitations of motion, and palpation of pain.

The basic elements of the neurologic evaluation, which augment the physical impressions, must be related to gait and include patellar, Achilles, and superficial plantar reflexes, ankle clonus, Romberg's sign, pallesthesia (vibratory sensation), reaction to temperature and pain, insensitivity, and joint position.

Additional components of the neuromuscular system that relate to the utilization of physical medicine and rehabilitation include muscle grading, contractions, atrophy, pain, spasticity, hysteria, muscle function (active, passive, active assistive, and active resistive), group muscle strength (fatigue and endurance), coordination, functional tasks, walking aids, and orthotics.

The drug history of the patient should be reviewed with particular attention to the use of hypertensives, antidiabetics, cortisone, sedatives, topical medications, antibiotics, anti-inflammatory drugs, muscle relaxants, and the use of chemically abusive substances. Sensitivities to therapeutic products, such as ultraviolet radiation and allergies to footwear elements, should be noted.

Footwear is an essential element in dealing with the rehabilitative process for conditions involving the foot and any condition that relates to gait. Some of the elements include the shoe last (inflare, straight, outflare, and special lasts), shoe material and components, sole, shank, counter, heel, quarter (high or low) in relation to foot type (flaccid, rigid, or spastic), and special modifications (pads, wedges, external bars, flares, and special heels, such as Thomas or reverse Thomas heels).

The use and type of orthotics also require consideration not only with regard to the foot or related conditions, but with regard to the footwear utilized for the patient at the time of therapy. Shoe and foot attachments, such as stirrups, should be noted as elements and components of bracing procedures.

Once the evaluative process is completed, augmenting the patient's total record, the treatment goals and aims should be developed so that the patient knows what to anticipate in outcome and time. The types and areas of treatment should be explained to the patient and should include the duration, frequency, precautions, and instructions to be followed during the therapeutic program. The patient must be made to recognize that physical medicine is the same as other forms of medicine so that the proper therapeutic levels are attained, in order to effect a positive result.

TREATMENT CONSIDERATIONS

As part of the diagnostic and prescriptive process, the types of treatment injuries possible should be identified. These include burns from heat lamps, warm compresses, hot packs, short-wave diathermy, galvanic current, and ultraviolet treatment. The dangerous effects of cold also need to be considered, particularly with the increasing age of patients seeking care. Electric shock should be considered with transformer breakdown, contacts with grounded objects, and low-frequency difficulties in cardiac patients. Mechanical injuries are a factor with improper modality support. Proper technique, knowledge of the modality, and maximizing patient and practitioner attention can minimize potential risks. Patient contributory negligence and rare idiosyncrasies are also elements of concern.

In general, most utilization procedures for physical modalities and rehabilitation procedures employ a 30-day time frame for initial treatment for a particular spell of illness, with review and evaluation at the end of that time to consider continuation, if indicated. It is not unusual for treatment in an acute care hospital to involve two encounters per day. However, one considers 15 treatments on a noninstitutionalized patient during a 30-day period as an initial approach to management.

Examples of conditions involving the foot that benefit from the use of physical medicine and rehabilitation include adhesive capsulitis, antalgic gait, arthritis (acute or severe, or with nerve root pressure), ataxic gait, atrophy, burns, bursitis, causalgia, capsulitis, cerebral vascular accidents, compression syndromes (entrapments), contractures, contusions, degenerative joint disease (acute or severe), dislocations, fasciitis, fibrositis, foot-drop (peroneal palsy), fractures, hemiplegia, inflammation (acute or subacute), multiple sclerosis, muscle spasm (acute or severe), muscular dysfunction, myositis, nerve palsy, neuralgia, neuritis, osteoarthritis (acute or severe), osteomyelitis, osteoporosis, pain, paralysis from nerve disease or injury, paraplegia or quadriplegia, Parkinson's disease, periostitis, peripheral neuritis (acute or severe), peripheral neuropathy, recuperation from joint surgery, radiculitis, residuals of spinal tumors, scleroderma, sclerosis, sesamoiditis, severe and generalized weakness, severe osteochrondritis dessicans, sprains, strains, Sudeck's atrophy, synovitis, tendonitis, tenosynovitis, trauma and recovery from trauma, and ulcerations.

With a proper diagnosis and therapeutic plan, the use of physical modalities, physical medicine, and rehabilitation will provide assistance to the patient. It will also help the patient regain a pain-free state, maximizing function and ambulation.

THERAPEUTIC MODALITIES AND PROCEDURES

Therapeutic Cold

Cryotherapy, or the use of cold for its therapeutic effects, has as a primary physical property a cooling of tissues. Based on the mode of application and the duration of exposure, the basic physiologic effects are sedation, refrigeration, and possible tissue destruction. An example of tissue destruction includes the utilization of dry ice for the surgical removal of skin lesions.

Cold decreases metabolism, induces vasoconstriction, creates a reactive hyperemia, decreases swelling, reduces hemorrhage and muscle efficiency, and provides a form of analgesia by impairing neuromuscular transmission. Collagen extensibility is also reduced at the site of local application. Pain is also reduced with the local application of cold, with a decrease of spasticity of muscle tissue.

The general indications for the localized use of cold applications for therapeutic purposes include:

Reducing swelling and edema following trauma
Reducing pain
Reducing muscle spasm
Creating a reactive hyperemia
Helping to reduce inflammatory reactions
Providing for local tissue destruction
Decreasing local tissue metabolism
Helping to facilitate muscle contraction in some forms of neurogenic weakness

The basic contraindications and precautions include:

Hypertension
Raynaud's disease or phenomenon
Vascular disease
A history of frostbite or perniosis
Rheumatoid arthritis
Cold hypersensitivity
Any condition that produces a cold pressor response

The primary methods of application of cold are immersion, cold packs, ice massage, cryokinetics, and contrast applications with heat. The application of cold for therapeutic purposes, except for tissue destruction, usually has a duration of between 5 and 20 minutes, followed by a 30-minute period of rest. Applications are repeated for a 24- to 48-hour period in usual circumstances. Longer periods of application require adequate evaluation and a careful determination as to outcome. The most common local applications include during the immediate post-trauma or surgical period, to help

reduce edema, hemorrhage, and the pain associated with trauma and muscle spasm. Another example in relation to pain and swelling is the use of cold in the management of acute bursitis and fibrositis, provided there are no general contraindications to its use. Cold for the relief of pain and spasm is often more beneficial than heat.

Therapeutic Heat

Therapeutic heat is usually applied for one of two primary physical effects: superficial and deep heating. The physical agents used for superficial heating generally include hot water, hot air, infrared radiation, radiant light, whirlpool baths, paraffin baths, and hot packs. The physical agents used for deep heating generally include short-wave diathermy, microwave diathermy, and ultrasound.

The basic physiologic effects for each segment are similar in character but vary in intensity, based on the modality, duration of application, and intensity factors. The primary physiologic effects include hyperemia, sedation, analgesia, increased regional vascularity, increased tissue temperature, increased metabolic rate, arterial dilatation, increased capillary flow and hydrostatic pressure, increased collagen extensibility, increased tissue inflammatory response, and increased edema.

The general indications for the utilization of therapeutic heat include:

Analgesia
Increasing local vascular cutaneous flow
Sedation
Hyperemia
Muscle spasm
Accelerating the suppurative process
Muscle spasticity
Joint stiffness
Contractures

The general contraindications and precautions include:

Tendency to hemorrhage, such as patients who are hemophiliacs or those patients on anticoagulants
Active hemorrhage
Impaired sensation to pain and temperature

Ischemia and vascular impairment
Noninflammatory edema
Recovery from trauma, during the immediate (24- to 48-hour) post-trauma period
Known malignancies
Patients with coma or paralysis

Also, extreme caution should be used if there is a threat of hemorrhage, in the very young, in the very old, and in those patients who have debilitated or insensitive conditions.

Superficial Heating

Most forms of application of superficial heating are by conduction, and include the use of baths, electric heating pads, hot packs, hot water bottles, compresses, paraffin baths, and radiant heat (lamps or bakers). The usual forms for the application of superficial heat by convection include the use of hot air baths, moist air baths, and agitated water baths or whirlpools.

Infrared Radiation. Infrared radiation is a form of superficial heat that is, for the most part, conductive in nature. Infrared radiation causes an increase in local tissue temperature at the treatment site and creates a reflex dilatation at parts distal to the site. The radiation penetrates the skin to a 2- to 3-mm depth. There is a transfer of heat from superficial tissue fluids to the deeper structures, which accounts for the feeling of heat. The patient experiences a cutaneous sensation of heat and erythema for as long as the treatment is in process; this rapidly resolves following therapy. A distinct advantage of infrared radiation is that the part can be observed during treatment.

The primary sources of infrared radiation include bulbs, bakers, heat lamps, heated carborundum rods, and glowing wire coils with proper reflectors. Care needs to be expressed when utilizing filament bulbs to avoid spotting and an uneven distribution of heat. In addition, reflectors can change the direction and amount of heat and, coupled with distance, heat to the part is consistent with Lamber's cosine and the inverse square laws.

The general application method is to position the heat source between 15 and 24 inches from the part to be treated. The part to be treated should be positioned so that continuing observation can occur, and drapes should not be utilized to increase heat. The intensity of heat is controlled by the source, the distance to the part being treated, the type and quality of the reflectors, and air movement. The usual treatment time is 20 to 30 minutes. However, it should be noted that the true guide is patient comfort, which must consider intensity, distance, and the modality. These can be varied to provide the same therapeutic effect and still maintain patient comfort.

The general indications for the use of infrared radiation include:

Subacute and chronic inflammation
Contusions, following the threat of hemorrhage
Rheumatoid arthritis
Early joint stiffness
Degenerative or osteoarthritis
Sprains and strains, following the initial post-trauma period
Neuritis
Myositis
Fasciitis
Tenosynovitis
Tendonitis
Preliminary to exercise
Reflex vasodilatation, with caution

In general, the following contraindications and precautions usually apply:

Acute inflammation
Malignancy
Impaired vascularity (ischemia)
Impaired sensation, particularly to pain and temperature
Special care for the very young and elderly, who are unable to respond to the effects of heat

Hot Packs. Moist hot packs usually consist of silica gel, enclosed in canvas, heated to temperatures between 120 and 160°F. The unit of application is a hydrocollator. When the hot pack is removed from the unit it needs to be wrapped in either plastic or some other form of protective material, prior to application to the part under treatment. In addition, cloth towels should be interposed between the pack and the part to minimize potential burns. This form of superficial heat is applied for a treatment time ranging between 20 and 30 minutes. Depending on the temperature of the pack, the application may need to be changed during the 30-minute period. It can be applied twice per day and can be utilized as home therapy. Once dry, the pack can be reheated and utilized over again.

The indications are similar to other forms of superficial heat, and include:

Reducing muscle spasm
Increasing local metabolism
Reduce pain
Muscle sedation
Neuritis
Fibrositis
Fasciitis
Myositis

Indications and contraindications are similar to other forms of superficial heat.

Electric Heating Pad. The electric heating pad is a good home modality when properly applied by the patient as indicated and under appropriate direction. Pain after the 24- to 48-hour post-trauma period and the possibility of hemorrhage can be relieved with this form of heat.

The indications and contraindications are the same as those listed for superficial heat. Comfort of the patient is of prime concern, and care should be taken to avoid thermal burns. Most units provide three levels of heat: low, medium, and high. The medium or low setting should be utilized by the patient for a treatment time of 20 to 30 minutes, every 4 to 12 hours. The heating pad should be placed over the anatomic part to avoid excessive pressure from the weight of the part. Because of the comforting effect of the heating pad, the time of treatment is essential; the patient must be prohibited from being lulled to sleep during treatment and creating a burn.

Hot Water Bottle. The clinical use of the hot water bottle permits the patient, under proper direction and with caution, to provide a program of superficial heat at home. The same basic indications and contraindications apply as those outlined for superficial heat in general.

Thermal burns from the hot rubber container and the potential for burns from scalding water are of primary concern.

Water of about 130°F should be the thermal limit for a hot water bottle. When filled, excess air should be carefully removed. Three to six layers of Turkish towels should be placed between the bottle and the skin to minimize the potential for burns. Applications can be made for 20 to 30 minutes two times per day. Again, the body part should be placed under the bottle to avoid pressure and the potential for bottle rupture.

Hot Wet Towels. Hot wet towels for compresses usually consist of cloth, gauze, or towels that are soaked in water, at various temperatures, wrung out, and utilized for physical and physiologic effects, depending on the temperature of the compress.

Their utilization as a heat modality for home care provides local dilatation of the vascular supply, relaxation of muscles, and relief of pain associated with sprains, strains, muscle spasms, and exacerbation of arthritic pain. The indications are similar to those outlined for superficial heat in general, and they provide an excellent home modality.

Paraffin Baths. The application of paraffin is a superficial thermal modality. The paraffin bath consists of a tank with a thermal element in the base/outer core. The tank is filled with solid paraffin, and a small amount of mineral oil is added to provide an emollient quality to the paraffin. The composition is usually about one part mineral oil to six or seven parts paraffin. The unit is then heated to 160°F to dissolve the wax and provide a mineral oil–paraffin mix. The heat is then reduced to 126°F for patient application.

This modality and its proper application provides a comfortable form of superficial heat that leaves the skin soft and supple. The suggested method is to apply a few layers of wax to the foot or part of the foot to act as an insulator, with a small brush. The foot can then be dipped in the paraffin bath for several more applications of the wax-oil mixture. After the final layer is applied, the foot can be wrapped in waxed paper to help retain the comfortable heat for 20 to 30 minutes. This is another modality that can be prescribed for use once or twice a day at home use with proper instruction, to augment other forms of treatment.

The basic indications include:

Subacute arthritis
Chronic arthritis
Joint pain
Limitation of motion
Rheumatoid arthritis
Degenerative arthritis
Bursitis
Tendonitis

The general contraindications that apply to other forms of superficial heat also apply to paraffin. In addition, new skin, scar tissue, denuded skin, severe vascular insufficiency, impaired sensation, and allergy to wax and/or oil also need to be considered.

As a caution, a thermometer should always be utilized to measure the temperature of the unit. Care should be taken to assure a clean foot to avoid unit contamination. Given the usual application of 10 to 12 layers of paraffin by the patient, particularly in home use, the wax can be reused, provided appropriate concerns are met.

Deep Heating

The current use of high-frequency alternating current for deep heating generally consists of the basic forms of short-wave and microwave diathermy and ultrasound, which comprises high-frequency acoustic vibrations above 17,000 cycles per second.

The primary physical effect is a deep heating of both the superficial and deeper structures. The diathermy units convert electromagnetic radiation to heat and the ultrasonic unit converts sonic energy to heat. Both are forms of nonionizing radiation utilized for therapeutic thermal effects.

Physiologic effects are noted at the site of application and also involve tissue distant from the target site. Temperature elevation occurs as a result of cellular elevated function and reflex vasodilatation. Capillary dilatation occurs with increased blood flow and permeability, which increases tissue metabolism. Pain thresholds may be altered with dermatome involvement. Skeletal muscle relaxation does reduce spasm.

The major factors that determine tissue reaction to deep heat include:

Level of tissue temperature change
Rate of temperature elevation
Area under direct treatment (target site)
Duration of temperature elevation and treatment time

The target site receives the greatest amount of temperature elevation, and comfort and patient tolerance are key indicators to temperature control. Heating may be vigorous, with significant and rapid temperature elevation, or mild, with moderate temperature elevation.

Short-Wave Diathermy.   Short-wave diathermy represents the most common method and modality for larger areas and those involving the foot as a whole. It produces deep heat with elements of hyperemia, sedation, and resultant analgesia. There is an associated increase in the vascular supply to the part being treated, with a resultant reduction of muscle spasm, followed by relaxation.

Dosimetry requires proper application and tuning of the unit. The patient's response should be one of comfortable heat. The term *hot* should not be utilized because it may suggest to the patient the need to tolerate excessive temperatures and ultimately result in thermal injury. Treatment time is usually 20 to 30 minutes. Continued observation and supervision of the patient is essential to avoid inappropriate reactions and responses. Metal tables and/or chairs should never be utilized with short-wave diathermy.

The basic techniques include the condenser or pad method, where the part is placed between two electrodes. The alternative method is inductive, utilizing the cable or drum to encompass the part. Patient movement can change the amplitude of the heating of the part, again indicating the need for proper patient positioning and monitoring during the entire treatment time. Athermal or pulsed diathermy is also available in a therapeutic form.

The indications for short-wave diathermy include:

Post trauma care, after the threat of hemorrhage
Analgesia

Pain and spasm
Inflammation, subacute or chronic, associated
    with bursitis, periostitis, arthritis, neuritis,
    neuralgia, myositis, and capsulitis
Postfracture care
Fibrositis
Tenosynovitis
Tendonitis
Sprains
Strains
Rheumatoid arthritis
Postdislocation care
Reflex vasodilitation

In general the following contraindications and/
or precautions apply to the use of short-wave diathermy for foot conditions:

Hemorrhage or suggestion of same
Sensory loss
Application over moist dressings
Malignancy
Tuberculosis
Areas of ischemia
Arteriosclerosis
Thromboangiitis obliterans
Phlebitis
Metallic implants
Foreign bodies
Pregnancy/menstruation
Suppuration
Special care for the geriatric or pediatric patient
Special care for cardiac patients and patients
    with pacemakers
Metal contact with skin or other tissues
Epiphyseal and developing bone

Care should also be taken to utilize absorbent
material to help absorb perspiration. Felt spacers
are also needed with the condenser method of application to minimize electrode contact. The unit
should be tuned and adjusted with each application
to patient tolerance, comfort, and position .

Burns must be avoided. They can result from inappropriate patient behavior, improper technique,
faulty equipment, and inadequate supervision.
Subtherapeutic doses should be avoided because
they will produce negative results and may do more
harm than good.

Microwave Diathermy. Microwave diathermy utilizes high-frequency electromagnetic radiation to
produce deep heat. The physiologic activities are
similar to short-wave diathermy (i.e., analgesia, sedation, and hyperemia). Its activity is increased in
tissues that have a high cellular water content.

Its application is easier than short-wave diathermy because the unit is aimed at the part under
treatment and observation of the part is possible
during application. In addition, by increasing the
distance between the director and the part, heat
can be reduced. The unit should be adjusted to
provide a comfortable form of heat, with the treatment time between 20 and 30 minutes. Care must
be taken to avoid beads of perspiration, which can
become a focus for increased heat and potential
burns.

The primary indications include:

Deep heating of subcutaneous tissue and super-
    ficial musculature
Musculoskeletal joint diseases, such as degener-
    ative joint disease, rheumatoid arthritis, bur-
    sitis, and tendonitis
Post-trauma care, after the threat of hemorrhage
Sprains
Strains
Neuritis

The precautions identified for the general use of
deep heat and those suggested for short-wave diathermy also apply to the clinical use of microwave
diathermy. The general contraindications and/or
precautions involve judgment factors, rather than
absolute issues, and include:

Ischemia
Hemorrhagic areas
Tumors
Impaired sensation
Debilitation
Edema
Use over wet dressings
Metallic implants
Pregnancy
Use over adhesive dressings
Special care over bony prominences
Peripheral vascular disease
Synovitis and excessive areas of synovial fluid

Systemic and local infections
Patients with pacemakers
Special care for the geriatric or pediatric patient

Ultrasound. Ultrasound is a form of deep heat that utilizes acoustic vibrations at frequencies above the human audible spectrum to produce thermal, mechanical, and chemical effects on tissue. Ultrasound physiologically produces hyperemia and sedation. It produces chemical effects within tissue as well as a phonophoretic effect, governed by the drug or chemical employed.

The transducer in the unit converts the electrical energy to sonic energy. Sound propagates through tissue and is absorbed and converted to a form of deep heat. In addition, with cavitation, fluids are reduced to their chemical states.

The dosage of ultrasound is computed by the total wattage, as developed by the unit, or by watts per square centimeter, which is based on the total unit output and the size of the ultrasonic head. The initial starting dose is usually 1 watt/cm^2. This is a guide, and actual dosage must be based on the goals for treatment, the indications, and clinical judgment. Intensity of the dose is also governed by the thickness of the part and the degree of soft tissue over bone. The patient should experience a comfortable warm feeling or no feeling at all, without excessive heat or pain. Proper and periodic tuning of the unit is essential to assure adequate power output between the unit and the registered elements of the unit meter.

The initial treatment time is approximately 5 minutes, with the range being between 3 and 10 minutes. The sonic head must be kept in motion and a coupling medium must be employed between the sound head and the part under treatment. Agents such as gels, creams, and water have all been utilized. Movement or stroking will avoid hot sports and potential harm to patients. When treatment is carried out with an underwater technique, the sound head should remain between 0.25 and 1 inch from the part.

The clinical use of ultrasound causes an increase in the peripheral flow, hyperemia, and an inflammatory response. There is increased cell membrane permeability. Phonophoresis takes place when a drug is utilized as a coupling medium and then penetrates the skin to produce its effects. The

size of the chemical particle and the cream base are also factors in phonophoresis.

The propagation of ultrasound in the tissues depends on factors such as transmission, absorption, refraction, and the reflection of sonic energy. These factors change with different tissues, producing different frequencies and times to achieve the desired therapeutic effect. Cavitation is also a factor. This breaking up of both chemical and cellular bonds provide assistance in the management of certain conditions such as fibrous tissue, scar tissue, and joint adhesions.

The basic indications for ultrasound include:

Joint contractures associated with immobilization, trauma, scarring, rheumatoid arthritis, and degenerative joint disease
Pain
Muscle spasm
Periarthritis
Tendonitis
Acute inflammation due to trauma
Adjunct to exercise therapy
Phonophoresis with indicated drugs
Subacute sprains and strains
Joint adhesions
Subacute and chronic bursitis
Calcific bursitis
Resolution of hematomas
Neuroma/neuritis

Additional indications in which ultrasound has limited value include:

Fibrosis from paralysis, burns, and scleroderma
Scarring
Tendonitis
With intra-articular and intralesional injections to aid in drug distribution in the tissues
Phantom limb pain
Soft tissue trauma
Nerve root pain
Reflex vasodilatation
Myofascial pain
As an aid in ulcer débridement
In combination with electrical stimulation

The primary contraindications and/or precautions include:

Basic contraindications for all forms of deep heat
Large fluid-filled areas
Hemorrhagic diseases
Decreased sensation and insensitivity
Vascular insufficiency
Tumors
Malignancies
Over epiphyses of growing bone
Pacemakers
With caution over implants, both from a thermal
    and mechanical concern

Ultrasound has become a most popular modality in managing foot problems with deep heat because of its target method of application, time, and safety, and the wide variety of conditions in the foot that respond to ultrasound.

Hydrotherapy

In broad terms, hydrotherapy implies the utilization of water for therapeutic purposes. Water absorbs and releases heat slowly so that it can be utilized for both heating and cooling for the foot and its related structures. Water is utilized in its three physical forms: liquid (water), solid (ice), and vapor (steam). Archimede's principle also permits water to essentially remove the forces of gravity, thus permitting motion and activity and permitting buoyancy to assist or resist activity. Other properties of water include cohesion and viscosity. Water is utilized in a mechanical sense for stimulation with sprays and whirlpools.

The therapeutic effects of water depend on the temperature range, which is given in Table 29-1. The physiologic effects of water are related to temperature. Cold to cool water is tonic or stimulative, and results in pallor, chilliness, increased muscle tone, increased pulse rate, increased respiratory rate, shivering, and increase in blood pressure. Warm to hot water is sedative, and results in relief from painful sensory conditions and spasm, increased temperature, increased circulatory rate, perspiration, loss of body fluids and salt, and lowering of blood pressure.

Decisions as to the methods of hydrotherapy should include the modality or application procedure, diagnosis, temperature to be utilized, dura-

Table 29-1. Temperature Ranges of Water

Very cold	33–55°F
Cold	56–65°F
Cool	66–80°F
Tepid	81–92°F
Neutral	93–96°F
Warm	97–98°F
Hot	99–104°F
Very hot	105–115°F

tion of the treatment period, and frequency of application. In addition, with the appropriate temperature, based on the diagnosis and proposed effects, hydrotherapy as a basic procedure can take the form of underwater exercise for the following conditions:

Muscle weakness
Postamputation care
Post–joint injury care
Paraplegia
Rheumatoid arthritis
Burns
Selected postsurgical débridement
Selected spastic palsy
Selected flaccid paralysis

Regardless of the modality, when water is utilized for its therapeutic effects, the preceding general rules apply.

Whirlpool Baths

The whirlpool unit is utilized as a major form of hydrotherapy and usually to provide superficial heat. In addition to temperatures that provide superficial heat, the mechanical agitation and the use of chemicals for antisepsis are also therapeutic goals. The basic units employed include the foot unit, the foot and leg unit, and, in institutions, the low-boy and full-body whirlpool or Hubbard tank. Mechanical agitation relaxes and massages muscles. Heat produces sedation and analgesia. Exercises can be utilized to increase range of motion. When properly adjusted, débridement can be assisted.

Temperature should always be properly measured with a thermometer and recorded at each clinical visit. The mechanical effects are controlled by the aerator and level throttle, to control the force and direction of the agitation. For the most part, the usual temperature for superficial heat is between 95 and 102°F. A good rule of thumb is to keep the temperature below body and skin temperature for those patients who demonstrate any vascular insufficiency. The usual treatment time is 20 minutes. In the presence of edema, dependent use should be avoided and, if indicated, the low-boy should be employed. Active flexion and extension in the unit will also help reduce swelling and aids the exercise potential.

The therapeutic effects of superficial heat and mild mechanical action are indicated for:

Chronic post-traumatic conditions
Inflammatory conditions
Early joint stiffness
Pain
Painful scars
Adhesions
Neuritis
Arthritis
Tenosynovitis
Strains
Sprains
Painful stumps
Preliminary to massage, exercise, and electrical stimulation
Burns
Post–cerebral vascular accident care
Postfracture care
Vascular insufficiency
Decubitus ulcers
Industrial medicine
Post–peripheral nerve injury care
Dermatologic débridement
Sports and dance medicine
Postsurgical rehabilitation

The general contraindications and/or precautions for the use of whirlpool for superficial heat include:

Acute phlebitis
Osteoporosis (caution)
Cardiac patients (caution)
Immediate trauma
Excessive edema
Vascular or neurologic impairment
Noninflammatory edema
Caution with the geriatric or pediatric patient

Water Baths

Water baths provide multiple therapeutic effects. Their physiologic effects are based on the temperature of the water. *Cold baths* generally produce vasoconstriction and a reduction of pain and swelling. The cold bath is generally utilized at 60 to 65°F for a period of 10 minutes twice a day, and usually following acute trauma. *Neutral baths* provide sedation, muscle relaxation, and a degree of vasodilatation. The temperature is between 93 and 96°F, which is about normal body skin temperature. *Hot baths* are utilized to provide analgesia and reduce stiffness in patients with chronic arthritis with multiple joint involvement, fibrositis, muscle spasm, neuritis, and tendonitis. The usual temperature is between 99 and 104°F.

The basic forms of water baths include compresses, pouring, and immersion. *Ablutions* consist of a sponge or towel bath. They are usually employed to reduce elevated temperature and fever. The direction of one or more streams of water against a part or the whole body is termed a *douche.* The basic types include fan, jet, Scotch, shower, needlepoint shower, and even rain. The shape of the water stream and the pressure and temperature of the water control the therapeutic effects.

Contrast baths are sudden and alternate immersion of the foot in first hot and then cold water to stimulate peripheral circulation in patients without the presence of occlusive or spastic vascular disease. The usual sequence is 4 minutes of heat followed by 1 minute of cold. The sequence is repeated five times, starting and ending with heat. Patients with sensory and neuropathic changes should not be considered for this form of therapy. It can be utilized following contusions, after the threat of hemorrhage has passed, and for some forms of arthritis. Patient tolerance and acceptance is needed as a guide, as it is for any therapeutic procedure.

Ultraviolet Radiation

Ultraviolet radiation is utilized for its actinic or photochemical effect. Physiologically, ultraviolet radiation produces erythema and pigmentation, activates ergosterol, and has both a bactericidal and fungicidal effect. The basic therapeutic device employs the use of electric currents to excite mercury vapors in a lamp. The resultant emission of energy is ultraviolet radiation.

Other therapeutic devices include the hot quartz lamp, the cold quartz lamp, the sun lamp with tungsten filament, the carbon arc unit, and the black light or Woods filter, which is utilized for diagnostic fluorescence.

Ultraviolet radiation in the range of the solar spectrum is absorbed or reflected, when it strikes a surface. When that reflection is converted into a higher wavelength, the phenomenon is termed *fluorescence*. The wavelengths usually fall between 3,100 and 3,400 Angstrom units. Utilizing a Woods' filter or black light, tissue fluorescence can be observed. This technique can aid in some diagnostic procedures, including those for tinea, pityriasis versicolor, monilial paronychia, verruca, psoriasis, and onychomycosis.

Erythema from exposure generally occurs between 2,500 and 2,970 Angstroms, utilizing both the mercury vapor and/or cold quartz method of application. The vasodilatation that produces the erythema results in pigmentation or a tanning effect. There is also an antirachitic effect from ultraviolet radiation.

Care must be exercised when utilizing ultraviolet radiation, as it is taken in avoiding exposure to sunlight, in the presence of those dermatologic diseases that produce an abnormal response to light. Examples include polymorphic light eruptions, squamous cell carcinoma, basal cell carcinoma, lymphogranuloma venereum, urticaria solaris, and hypersensitivity.

When indicated, exposure should include only the part under treatment, and other areas of the body should be protected from exposure. The eyes of both the patient and operator should also be protected to avoid direct exposure to the source. Disposable protection is best for the patient, particularly with the current concern for AIDS. In addition, the part to be tested and the part under treatment should be cleansed with alcohol or another appropriate solvent to enhance penetration and permit the minimal therapeutic dose to be employed.

There is a need to determine each patient's own tolerance to ultraviolet radiation and determine the minimal erythematous dose (MED). A technique most often employed is called the "sleeve test." A small area is exposed, at 30 inches, for 15, 30, 45, and then 60 seconds, with each area properly protected to provide a controlled response. A determination is then made as to which site produces a first-degree erythema. That level is known as the MED. This forms the basis for all treatment planning and determines the ultimate dose to achieve first-, second-, third-, and fourth-degree erythema.

First-degree erythema is known as a light dose and produces an erythema that can be compared to a mild sunburn. It aids healing. The second degree is usually computed at 2.5 times the MED and is known as the stimulative dose. Exfoliation and redness are longer lasting. The third degree is known as the reactive dose and is usually computed at five times the MED. It produces an ultraviolet burn and is germicidal. The fourth degree of ultraviolet radiation also produces a burn and is known as the destructive dose. Blistering and exfoliation do occur and it is utilized for small areas where destruction is indicated.

The frequency of treatment is usually daily for light doses, every two days for stimulative doses, every three days for a reactive dose, and every 10 to 14 days for a destructive dose.

The general indications for the use of ultraviolet radiation, with varying degrees of erythema, include:

Local ultraviolet radiation for its bactericidal and fungicidal effects for superficial infections, infected wounds, dermatophytosis, and sterilization for fresh wounds
Decubitus ulcers
Boils, carbuncles, and furunculosis
Burns
Dermatitis
Eczema
Contact dermatitis
Erysipelas
Felon
Granulating tissue
Infectious eczemoid dermatitis
Intertrigio
Leukoderma and vitiligo
Psoriasis
Varicose ulcerations

Urticaria
Diabetic ulcerations, with caution

The general contraindications and precautions include:

Photo-opthalmia of patient and operator
Hypersensitive areas, such as skin folds
Unusual skin sensitivities
Photosensitive drugs (e.g., sulfonamides, tetracyclines, green soap, dyes (eosin, fluorescein), coal tar preparations, oral hypoglycemics, chlorothiazide diuretics, and phenothiazines)
Excessive exposure
Encapsulated pus without drainage
Acute generalized dermatitis
Malignancies
Sarcoidosis
Lupus erythematosis (systemic and discoid)
Herpes simplex
Patients with cardiac, renal, or hepatic insufficiency, as a marked caution

Kinetic Procedures

There are a series of procedures that have been utilized for their kinetic effects, including massage, manipulation, vibration, traction, and exercise. Their collective primary physiologic effects include muscle stimulation; stimulation active exercise; increasing venous, arterial, capillary, and lymph flow; tissue stretching; and reflex stimulation.

These procedures have survived centuries of use and are effective in individuals with certain types of soft tissue ailments. A prime podiatric example is traction and crest therapy to help treat and manage deformities such as hammer toes and contracted tendons and to augment other forms of therapy. They are also utilized in the postoperative period to help restore a greater degree of function and ambulation.

Massage

Massage can broadly be defined as a manual procedure employing a group of systematic and specific manipulations of soft tissue to produce a therapeutic effect. Massage produces stimulation of

peripheral receptors, relaxation, and sedation. It provides a centripetal movement of blood and lymph and intramuscular motion or stretching of adhesions.

The primary techniques for therapeutic massage include (1) *effleurage,* or stroking, which includes both superficial and deep stroking; (2) *pétrissage,* or compression, which includes kneading and frictions (cross-fiber and digital kneading); and (3) *tapotement,* or percussion, which includes hacking, slapping, cupping, beating, vibration, and shaking. Stroking is performed in a distal-to-proximal direction and utilized to help enhance local circulation, lymph drainage, and relaxation. Compression helps enhance local circulation, reduces muscle tightness, and creates relaxation. Percussion helps enhance local blood flow and increase sensory stimulation.

The primary indications for massage include:

Relief of pain
Arthritis
Periarthritis
Bursitis
Neuritis
Fibrositis
Mobilization of contracted tissue
Reduction of swelling and induration following soft tissue trauma; associated with joint injuries, sprains, strains, and tendon and nerve injury; and associated with other therapeutic procedures for the above.

A significant factor in the prescription and utilization of massage is an assurance of a proper diagnosis, so that treatment does not produce complications. Some of the primary contraindications include:

Infection
Cutaneous inflammation
Tumors
Malignancies
Burns
Skin diseases, in relation to contamination and irritation
Clotting disorders
Fractures
Thrombophlebitis

Aneurysms
Thrombosis
Presence of fever
Acute systemic disease

Manipulation

Manipulation can broadly be defined as the passive movement of a joint for therapeutic purposes. It has been utilized in the peripheral joints, including those of the foot, to increase range of motion, stretch tight ligaments, and assist, in selected cases, the breaking up of adhesions.

The prime motions employed during manipulative procedures involving the foot include rotation, flexion, extension, and gliding motions.

Its primary indications include:

Loss of range of motion
Residuals of long periods of immobilization
Residuals of trauma and/or capsular inflammation

The primary contraindications include:

Immediate post-trauma care
Joint effusion
Acute inflammation
Ligamentous rupture
Dislocation (unless used for repositioning)
Fracture (unless used for repositioning)

The final decision regarding the use of manipulative procedures must be based on sound clinical judgment.

Therapeutic Exercise

Therapeutic exercise can be defined as a series of prescribed bodily movements designed to correct, restore, modify, or improve function and to maintain well-being.

The prescription of an exercise program for a patient needs to be preceded by an adequate history and physical examination, an evaluation of the patient's problems and concerns, the establishment of a working diagnosis and/or impression, the development of therapeutic goals and objectives, and a knowledge of kinesiology. Maintaining muscle tone and joint range of motion and the preven-tion of muscular atrophy are primary considerations in which therapeutic exercise can help the patient regain and retain his or her activities of daily living. Therapeutic exercise can and should be tailored to meet each individual patient's needs and changed to reflect current patient status. Secondary disabilities that cause inactivity, which leads to disuse, create additional impairment, disability, and disease, which can be reduced with appropriate exercise programs.

Some of the causes of disuse syndromes that relate to the foot and ambulation include immobilization and immobility associated with casts, braces, wheelchairs, and bed rest. Residual atrophy of muscle, contractures, and osteoporosis are also related to this complex set of circumstances. Intractable pain, psychological and emotional disturbances, and depression are factors that limit movement and activity and tend to remove purpose from life, which adds to functional disability and ambulatory dysfunction.

Exercises are generally prescribed to increase and maintain joint and soft tissue mobility, prevent adhesions and fibrosis, and aid in soft tissue healing. The techniques that are usually employed include passive exercises (manipulation and stretching), active assistive exercises, voluntary active exercises, active resistive exercises, and stimulation active exercise (electrical stimulation).

Some of the selective exercises that can be applied in the management of foot and related problems include heel stretching, with the toe in, using a wall, step, or book; digital contraction, with a towel, the edge of a step, or book; walking on the outer border of the feet; tiptoe inverted gait; rocking on toes and heels, or on a rocking chair (particularly for the geriatric patient); isometrics in casts; traction; and progressive resistive exercises.

The usual prescription includes at least one set of exercises daily. The minimum accepted activity should never fall below three days a week, and suggested activity would be directed to those procedures that can be done at home to assure a maximum degree of compliance. Care must be taken to explain the *why* of exercise for the patient. In addition, the patient should be asked to demonstrate his or her activity at each visit to demonstrate interest and to provide modifications as the patient progresses.

The general indications for the prescription of exercise include:

Preventing joint contractures.
Preventing joint adhesions.
Increasing joint range of motion after trauma or muscle spasm, or in disease states that limit function and mobility and prevent activity
Arthritis and related conditions
Postamputation care
Neuromuscular and collagen diseases that produce contractures and limited ranges of motion
Paresis due to multiple conditions, such as cerebral vascular accident
Weakness and atrophy due to disuse and/or after immobilization
Muscular weakness
To strengthen muscles

The general precautions, limitations, and/or contraindications for the use of exercise include:

Acute active inflammation
Acute post-trauma period
Severe cardiovascular disease
Severe pulmonary disease, such as chronic obstructive pulmonary disease
Metastatic malignancies
Nonunion fracture sites, with caution
Pain in the arthritidies, with caution
Severe joint and/or muscle pain, with caution
Infection

The final determination is based on patient need and clinical judgment and knowledge. Exercise is a controlled and graduated program and, when utilized therapeutically with full patient cooperation, can provide a means to maintain ambulation.

Tissue Destruction: Surgical Procedures

Physical modalities can be utilized for tissue destruction. These include high-frequency currents and galvanic current for tissue drying and tissue liquifaction, and the use of dry ice for surgical cryotherapy.

High-Frequency Current Electrosurgery

The clinical use of high-frequency currents for electrosurgical procedures utilize both monoterminal and biterminal techniques. With the monoterminal technique, the current is either sprayed on the lesion (fulgeration) or applied to the lesion by placing the needle electrode into the lesion (desiccation). In both cases, the effects are dehydrating or drying. The biterminal technique involves a cutting current and electrocoagulation. This produces a greater current release and is generally not employed for the destruction of superficial lesions.

The primary advantages of fulgeration and desiccation include a generally good cosmetic result with a minimal scar when properly utilized, sharp delineation between normal and abnormal tissue, a sterile wound, minimal blood loss, speed and simplicity of technique, little or minimal postoperative pain, and little or no anesthesia required for small areas. The anesthesia usually required is regional or local, with regional blocks preferred to infiltration to avoid excessive fluid in the tissues.

Postoperative care includes a dry sterile dressing, the use of alcohol compresses and dry sterile dressings by the patient, and continued observation to assure a healthy, granulating wound. Healing is by granulation followed by epithelialization in 10 to 20 days. The residual soft scar tends to fade rapidly. Proper care minimizes postoperative infection.

The general indications for electrosurgery include:

Xanthoma
Senile keratosis
Keloids
Molluscum contagiosum
Vascular nevi
Hemangioma
Moles, preceded by biopsy
Verruca
Fibroma
Papilloma
Granulation tissue

The following precautions should be employed with electrosurgical procedures:

Fire prevention
Avoidance of colored solutions
Proper patient management to prevent infection
Proper care to minimize scar formation
Biopsy as needed
Limited use on weight-bearing areas to minimize scar formation.

Galvanic Current Electrosurgery

The negative pole of the galvanic current can also be utilized for tissue destruction by liquifaction. The same precautions and indications generally apply to this procedure. In addition, the galvanic current has been utilized for onychial surgery for matrix destruction, certain skin lesions, and electrolysis.

Cryosurgery

The use of dry ice as a form of cryosurgery results in localized frostbite, bulla formation, and local tissue destruction. The primary indications include:

Angiomata
Granuloma pyogenicum
Keloids
Verruca

It should be noted that the contraindications and precautions for the use of cold apply, and adherence to them is critical when cold is utilized for tissue destruction.

Electrical Stimulation and Galvanic Currents

Galvanic, faradic, and sinusoidal currents produce an electrochemical effect. The faradic and sinusoidal currents produce their medical effects with stimulation of muscles. The primary physical effect of electrical stimulation is muscular contraction. It should be employed with specific therapeutic goals and a rational basis for treatment. The same principles and concerns exist for both low-voltage and high-voltage currents. The choice of current needs to be determined on an individual basis in relation to patient comfort and causing the least amount of skin irritation.

Galvanic Current

Galvanic current is a direct current that produces its medical effects without muscle stimulation and is utilized when polar effects are desired. The positive (anode) pole is acidic. Its physiologic effects are sedative, and include vasoconstriction, hardening of tissue, repellance of positive ions, and a mild thermal effect. The negative (cathode) pole is alkaline. Its physiologic effects are irritative, and include vasodilatation, softening (liquefication) of tissue, repellance of negative ions, and a mild thermal effect.

Other indications for the use of galvanic current include:

Reducing pain
Reducing swelling
Increasing local circulation
Aiding in nerve regeneration
Softening scar tissue so that it can be stretched

Iontophoresis includes the introduction of drugs and/or chemicals into the body by the use of the polar effects of the galvanic current. The principle of the law of magnetism indicates that like poles repel and unlike poles attract. Drugs and medications are introduced through intact skin by repelling the desired chemical with an electrode of the same polarity. Examples of such chemical activity are given in Table 29-2.

The usual treatment duration for medical galvanism, iontophoresis or ion transfer is 20 minutes, depending on the concentration of drug/chemical (usually 1 to 2 percent), the indications, and the individual patient. The usual dosage formula is 0.5 to 1 mA/in^2 of the *smallest* surface electrode. All other general precautions should be observed and a thorough knowledge of the patient is essential.

The basic contraindications and/or precautions include:

Denuded skin and over scar tissue
Allergy to drugs/chemicals by iontophoresis
Pacemakers
Special concerns for vascular and neurologic deficiences

Table 29-2. Chemical Treatment Utilizing Iontophoresis

Chemical	Source	Pole	Indications
Acetate	5–6% acetic acid	Neg	Calcium deposits; calcification of tendons, sheaths, etc.; bursitis
Calcium	Calcium chloride	Pos	Myospasm, frozen joints
Chloride	Sodium chloride	Neg	Scars, adhesions, bromidrosis
Copper	Copper sulfate	Pos	Fungus infections, indolent and varicose ulcers
Enzymes	Enzyme ointments	*a*	Dermatitis, psoriasis, decubitus and varicose ulcers
Histamine	Imidazoylethylamine	Pos	Myospasm, myositis, myofasciitis, myositis ossificans (traumatic), nerve injury, neuritis, fibrositis, vascular insufficiency (local effects), arthritis, varicose ulcerations
Hyaluronidase	Hyaluronidase	Pos	Edema, lymphedema, postsurgical adhesions, scleroderma, hemarthrosis, hematoma, bursitis, postfracture care sprains
Iodine	Iodex	Neg	Myositis, myofasciitis, fibrositis, tendonitis, adhesions, arthritis
Lithium	Lithium chloride	Pos	Gouty arthritis
Magnesium	Magnesium	Pos	Myositis, neuritis, osteoarthritis, rheumatoid arthritis, periarthritis, bromidrosis
Novocaine	2% Novocaine	Pos	Neuritis, bursitis, painful limitation of motion
Salicylate	Sodium salicylate	Neg	Rheumatoid arthritis, myalgias
Steroids	Steroid creams	*a*	Dermatitis, irritated joints
Zinc	Zinc	Pos	Dermatologic conditions, indolent and varicose ulcers

a Pole depends on the chemical composition of the chemical/drug and the indication of chemical/drug use.

Improper technique
Overt patient concern for the procedure

In addition, adequate electrode preparation, contact, electrode placement, and amplitude are essential, as is a proper diagnosis.

Galvanic current (as well as faradic current) may also be utilized for electrodiagnosis, which can encompass the following tests:

Galvanic tetanus ratio test
Reaction to degeneration
Myesthenic reaction
Myotonic reaction
Hysteria
Heald's subfaradic test for hyperesthesia
Psychogalvanic reflex response

Transcutaneous Electrical Nerve Stimulation

Transcutaneous electrical nerve stimulation (TENS) also utilizes a waveform of galvanic or direct current. When the current is interrupted, it becomes a kinetic current and may be utilized to contact denervated muscle directly. It helps retard atrophy and maintains contractility to enhance tissue response. A slow sinusoidal current can also be utilized to provide similar contractility effects. In general, the same precautions should be employed for the TENS unit as for any other direct or galvanic unit.

TENS is a current method that provides electrical stimulation on the skin overlying painful areas. It is developed by a battery-powered unit and, like other forms of electrical stimulation, is noninvasive. The control and moderation of pain is suggested by the gate control theory and the endorphin theory, which suggests that the stimulation of cutaneous sensory fibers may inhibit the perception of pain and/or may release a morphine-like substance that may inhibit the transmission of pain.

The electrodes of the TENS unit are applied to the dermatomes, which are sensory nerve root areas. The controls are adjusted to the patient's tolerance and comfort. The time of application can vary with each patient from seconds to minutes to hours.

The primary indications include:

Chronic pain
Acute pain associated with postoperative control
Arthritis
Bursitis
Strains and sprains
Tenosynovitis
Metatarsalgia and related foot pain
Painful motor and sensory nerve lesions

Postamputation pain, including phantom pain
Peripheral neuritis
Postoperative pain

Absolute contraindications include:

Individual patient reactions
Allergy
Insulin pump
Placement of electrodes over malignancies
Presence of electrical life-support systems
Severe inflammation
Placement of electrodes over the brain
Placement of electrodes over the cardiac area (e.g., carotid sinus)
Special concerns in the presence of vascular and/or neurologic deficiencies, denuded areas, and pacemakers

Stimulation Active Exercise

Electrical stimulation as stimulation active exercise (SAE) is defined as the electrical stimulation of nerve, muscle, or both by an electrical current that will cause a contraction of muscle, followed by a period of relaxation. SAE should produce the same chemical and physical phenomena connected with nonmuscular activity. Interrupted currents are better than those that create a continuous contraction or tetanize the part, to avoid localized vascular insufficiency.

Some of the nonchemical effects of muscular contraction include increased circulation (arterial, venous, lymphatic, and capillary), inhibition of fibrosis (inter- and intrafascicular), aid in relieving spasticity, aid in preventing postoperative phlebothromosis, aid in relieving postoperative pain and intractable pain (TENS), aid in retarding atrophy, sedation, stimulation, aid in reducing swelling, increased proprioceptive sensation, reduced fatigue, aid in muscle reeducation, and motivation of the patient.

The dosage factors or amplitude of current must demonstrate strength and initiate contraction, according to the individual patient's tolerance. The basic schedule for treatment should be daily, with three times per week as a minimum. Treatment should be followed by active voluntary exercise if feasible. The treatment time is usually 20 minutes.

The basic indications for the use of electrical stimulation by the utilization of alternating currents (surge, tetanizing, pulsating, reciprocal, automatic, and so on) include:

Injury to muscles, tendons, and joints
Paralysis
Sprains and strains
Postfracture and postdislocation care, to help retard atrophy and restore muscle function
To help restore muscle tone and strength
To help provide tissue contraction to milk tissues of excess fluids
To relieve muscle spasm from trauma and associated postural conditions
Muscle pain and spasm
Myositis
Metatarsalgia
Postpolio care
Muscle reeducation
Following surgery to help prevent clots and embolism
With ultrasound for trigger points and pain
Denervated muscles
To help retard muscle atrophy
Synovitis
Disuse
Fibrosis
Contractures
Pain with ankylosis
Stress and anxiety

CONCLUSION

The principles of physical medicine and rehabilitation and the associated physical modalities should be viewed and utilized as a vital and important link in the therapeutic management of foot problems.

SELECTED READINGS

Downer AH: Physical Therapy Procedures, Selected Techniques. 2nd Ed. Charles C Thomas, Springfield, IL, 1974

Finkelstein HB, Abraham MY, Crismali NC et al: Basic Concepts of Physical Therapy for the Lower Extremities. Dr. William M. Scholl College of Podiatric Medicine, Chicago, 1983

Helfand AE: Clinical Podogeriatrics. Williams & Wilkins, Baltimore, 1981

Helfand AE, Bruno J: A positive approach to rehabilitation. J Am Podiatry Assoc, 60:239, 1970

Helfand AE, Bruno J: Rehabilitation of the foot. Clin Podiatry, 1(2), 1984

Kottke FJ, Stillwell GK, Lehmann JF: Krusen's Handbook of Physical Medicine and Rehabilitation. 3rd Ed. WB Saunders, Philadelphia, 1982

Licht S: Therapeutic Electricity and Ultraviolet Radiation. 2nd Ed. Williams & Wilkins, Baltimore, 1967

Mennell J McM: Foot Pain. Little, Brown & Co, Boston, 1969

Neale D, Adams IM: Common Foot Disorders, Diagnosis and Management. 2nd Ed. Churchill Livingstone, New York, 1985

Okamoto GA: Physical Medicine and Rehabilitation. WB Saunders, Philadelphia, 1983

Rusk H: Rehabilitation Medicine. 3rd Ed. CV Mosby, St. Louis, 1971

Schriber WJ: A Manual of Electrotherapy. 4th Ed. Lea & Febiger, Philadelphia, 1977

Williams TF: Rehabilitation in the Aging. Raven Press, New York, 1984

Management of Wounds and Ulcerations

30

Kenneth G. Canter, D.P.M.
Gerit D. Mulder, D.P.M.

HISTORICAL OVERVIEW

Throughout the long history of wound dressings, from the first description in the Ebers and Edwin Smith papyri (1500 to 1600 B.C.) of dressing materials used in ancient Egypt (including bandages with grease) to the close-meshed cotton net impregnated with soft paraffin that Lumière introduced during World War I, little change has taken place. Many types of fabric have been used, including lint, muslin, and Gamgee tissue (pads of absorbent cotton wool with gauze).

The value of dressings to keep out bacteria has been well known, and the incorporation of antiseptics to enhance their protective value was shown to be effective by Lister. In 1937 Lister advocated using a damp lint over operative wounds at all times. In 1943 Owens used a wound model to demonstrate that bacteria could pass through 64 thicknesses of gauze, but that an outer layer of impervious material prevented this. Using an artificial wound, Colebrook and Hood (1948) showed that once a dressing became moist with serous exudate, many common pathogens could pass through to the underlying wound. This penetration was reduced by the inclusion of an impervious sheet, but tended to keep the wound moist, causing maceration and delayed healing. Their conclusion was that the ideal material would be permeable to water vapor but not to liquid or bacteria. Antibacterial agents have been incorporated into dressings for over 100 years. The use of carbolic acid was described by Pirie in 1867, and Maylard used mercuric chloride in 1892. Over the past 30 years the use of antibacterial creams in combination with absorbent dressings has been studied extensively.[1]

Occlusion as a means of treatment also has a century-old history. In 1864, Lawson Tait advocated treatment of burns by occlusive hard paraffin. The precursor to the use of polyurethane materials was the idea of Z.J. Lusk in 1892 to use skin blisters in wound dressings.[2] In 1963 Hinman and Maibach observed that the rate of reepithelialization was increased when experimental wounds were covered by occlusive dressings. More recently, useful vapor-permeable polyurethane film and a specially treated polyurethane foam have been developed.

767

PODIATRIC WOUNDS

The majority of wounds seen by the podiatric physician are of a chronic nature. These include lesions of diabetic, venous, and pressure etiology. Traumatic and iatrogenic wounds are usually surgically treated and allowed to heal by primary rather than secondary intention. Although specialized wound dressings and care may be used to treat surgical lesions, chronic wounds demand a more diversified and specialized form of treatment.

Greater than 2,000 wound-care products are presently available on the medical market, necessitating a basic knowledge of their capabilities by the physician in order to assist in selection of the appropriate modality. An understanding of the primary etiology of the specific wound is required prior to selection of the appropriate dressing material. Emphasis in this chapter is placed on diabetic, venous stasis, and pressure-related chronic wounds.

Diabetic lesions are, by nature of their location, perhaps the most common dermal ulcer seen by the podiatrist. Estimates for diabetes occurrence in the United States are between 1 and 5 percent.[3-5] Foot-related lesions are believed to account for over one-fifth of total hospitalizations.[6] Mortality associated with amputations resulting from limb lesions is as high as 20 percent.[7] Early attention to diabetic ulcers followed by appropriate care would reduce the high mortality and morbidity rates.

Primary causes of lesions have included vascular, neurologic, and endocrine abnormalities. Variables including age, length of disease state, glucose control, weight, diet, and smoking habits must all be considered.

Microvascular changes have been implicated as probable contributing factors, although their exact role in ulcer occurrence is unclear.[8-14] Neuropathy and its associated impairment appears to play a more important role. Both sensory deficit and compromised motor control with associated muscle weakness and osseous subluxation can contribute to tissue trauma and necrosis. Because of the pathophysiology of the disease, diabetics are more prone to ulceration. Occlusive disease and neuropathy, in association with tissue trauma and calluses in the diabetic, are more likely to result in ulceration.[15]

The most common cause of ulcers is untreated corns and calluses. These often conceal evidence of deeper damage to the dermis that has resulted from unrelieved pressure sources and associated subkeratotic ulcerations.

The major contributors to the development of diabetic foot ulcers were identified as micro/macrovascular occlusive disease, neuropathy, and infection.[11,16,17] Infection control is important in the prevention of ulcer control, gangrene, and subsequent limb loss.

Selection of an appropriate dressing is imperative if one is to reduce infection risk, protect the wound, and create an environment optimal for wound repair. Once the bacterial flora of the wound has been established and wound grade, location, and status have been evaluated, the appropriate material can be selected. Prior to use of any of the products discussed in this chapter, a wound should always be thoroughly cleansed and debrided of necrotic and nonviable tissue.

Venous stasis ulcers may vary in size and location. Since drainage of the greater saphenous vein is associated with the medial ankle, the most common presentation is on the medial aspect (malleolus) of the leg. Stasis ulcers may be foul smelling, with irregular borders and associated with induration, scaling, and liposclerosis. Differentiation must be made from ulcers of neuropathic, arterial, and bacterial etiology.

Venous ulcers may occur when edema and pericapillary fibrin deposition result from lower extremity pump failure. Poor venous return, venous stasis, excessive venous pressure, and prolonged edema are known to contribute to ulcer formation. The concept that anoxia results from prolonged edema and increased lower extremity venous pressure, thereby producing ulcers, is no longer in favor. It is currently believed that fibrinogen leakage results in precapillary fibrin layers that produce the tissue anoxia and damage.[18-20]

Nonsurgical treatment of venous lesions inevitably mandates use of appropriately selected external compression. Overall medical status, drugs, nutrition, and other systemic factors must also be addressed. Once the primary etiology has been treated, attention can then be addressed to selection of an appropriate wound dressing to enhance wound repair at the tissue level.

Pressure on the lower extremity is more preva-

Table 30-1. Shea Classification of Pressure Sores

Grade	Anatomic Limit
I	Dermis
II	Subcutaneous fat
III	Deep fascia
IV	Extensive

(From Kosiak,[27] with permission.)

lent than one would anticipate. Most ulcers (95 percent) are located in the lower half of the body.[21] The sacral, coccygeal, ischial tuberosities, greater trochanter, heels, and malleoli are the most common sites.[22] The geriatric bed-ridden patient is more likely to develop heel and malleolar lesions than are ambulatory individuals. Improperly applied casts are likely to cause lesions in the ambulatory patient. Patients with arterial obstruction are also at a higher risk for pressure ischemia ulcers.[23]

The cause of pressure ulcers is believed to be irreversible ischemia. Risk of development is compounded by friction, shear forces, moisture, and hospitalization. Minimum pressure values necessary for irreversible ischemia and tissue damage range from 45 to 70 mm Hg over a 1- to 3-hour period.[24-26]

Complications that can arise from pressure ulcers include sepsis, osteomyelitis, and extension of lesion to deep structures. Osteomyelitis is expected to be higher in grades III and IV ulcers based on a Shea scale[27] (see Table 30-1). Common organisms are as one would expect: *Bacteroides fragilis,* enteric gram-negatives, and occasionally staphylococcus.[22,28]

WOUND MANAGEMENT

The fact that skin is a complex organ and not just epithelial tissue is the basis for proper wound management. Since organs do not regenerate, skin will heal as basically all organs do by formation of a fibrous tissue scar.

Wound dressings are required to protect against additional trauma, shield against bacterial contamination, and provide partial immobilization of skin surrounding the wound. Simple adhesive strips ap-

plied in many different directions can be used to splint an injured area of skin. Since the active part of collagen synthesis and remodeling occurs between the 17th and 42nd days, it is necessary for the splint dressing to be maintained during this period (with caution taken to prevent adhesive irritation) to affect the final appearance of the scar.[29]

Epithelialization of a wound can be delayed by mechanical injury, chemical injury, or infection. Although a dressing will afford artificial protection, unskilled application or improper selection of dressing materials can retard epithelialization. The effect can adversely interfere with cell migration and promote bacterial proliferation.[30]

In considering the wound cover to expedite the rate of epithelial movement, the tightness of weave (as found in fine mesh) is extremely important. A larger mesh will cause interstitial cell growth, and when this dressing is removed there is detachment of the delicate epithelial cells and hemorrhage.

The length of time that dressings should cover the primarily closed wound is based on our knowledge of the period during which the wound is susceptible to bacterial penetration. In experimental studies performed by Edlich, surface contamination (wound swabbed with *Staphylococcus aureus*) on the third postoperative day did not produce gross infection in any sutured wound.[31] The susceptibility of the sutured wound to infection during the early postoperative period confirms the apparent value of dressings to protect fresh incisions. The experiments clearly indicate that wounds closed with tape have a greater capacity to resist infection than sutured wounds. The skin suture has the objectionable features of a drain.[31]

In order to make the usual dressing changes before wound healing is complete, measures should be taken to protect the new epithelium in an atraumatic fashion. Water-soluble creams and emollients impregnated on the gauze will prevent the coagulated exudate of the wound surface from sealing to the dressing. Although a few layers of gauze are frequently added for further protection, there is no biologic evidence for the application of a pressure dressing to a wound undergoing epithelialization. However, a bulky pressure dressing could cause circulatory impairment to the wound by means of occlusion.

If a natural dressing (scab) can be maintained long enough for epithelialization to occur, then there is no biologic reason for the application of an artificial dressing for a grade 1 wound.

Dressings have historically been utilized and selected on the basis of their physical properties. Their function has been to protect or cushion the wound, carry medicaments, and shield the patient from the sight of the wound. Much less consideration has been given to their role in the biologic process of wound healing. The role of dressings in cutaneous healing has been appreciated and recognized most fully on epithelial defects. The laboratories of Maibach, Winter, and Rovee have shown that occlusive dressings, through their role in preventing secondary dessication of viable tissue, promote a more rapid reepithelialization. This impact was measured on all three phases of epidermal repair: mitosis, migration, and differentiation.[32]

WET DRESSINGS AND OINTMENTS

The effectiveness of topical therapy derives from both physical and chemical actions of the applied medicaments on the damaged skin. The normal physiologic state of skin is regained and maintained by the physical actions of drying, wetting or hydration, softening, lubricating, cooling, warming, and protection from noxious external influences. The principal action of wet dressings is to cleanse the affected skin of crusts, scales, debris, microorganisms, and previously applied medications. The exact mechanism of action by which wet dressings accomplish drying of intact skin is unknown, but they provide symptomatic relief for the patient while the skin is healing. Wet dressings are indicated in vesicular, bullous, pustular, or ulcerative disorders.

Compresses are the main form of wet dressings, since they allow continuous evaporative cooling in contrast to soaks or baths. There is no evidence that hot solutions are more beneficial than are those of lower temperature. The compress pads may be cotton, soft toweling, sheeting, or gauze. Numerous preparations are used in wet dressings, ranging from plain water to aqueous solutions of various agents such as a 5 percent silver nitrate solution or neomycin solution. Isotonic or hypertonic saline, aluminum acetate (Burow's solution), aluminum sulfate, calcium acetate (Bluboro), and magnesium sulfate (Epsom salts) are among the most popular wet dressing preparations, and claim to have antibacterial and anti-inflammatory effects.

Lotions are liquid preparations in which medications are suspended or dissolved. The vehicles commonly used in lotions are water, alcohol, or propylene glycol. The prepared lotions are emulsion-type formulations and are classified as oil-in-water or water-in-oil emulsion, differing in their liquid consistency from counterpart ointment bases.

Powders are designed to absorb water and are best used in intertriginous areas. These sites, while moistened with perspiration, are subject to maceration and irritation by rubbing of opposing skin surfaces.

Ointments include the topical preparations of greasy bases, creams, pastes, and gels. All ointment bases (natural or synthetic) are either hydrophilic or hydrophobic, and are indicated in the treatment of chronic inflammatory and dry skin areas. Ointments are semisolid preparations that may be spread easily over the surface, providing a complete and protective cover with the added effect of lubrication. More importantly, they are excellent vehicles by which medicaments can be applied to the wound for the purpose of absorption. Petrolatum is the simplest natural hydrophobic ointment base and probably the most occlusive.

Creams (hydrophilic ointments) are a versatile oil in a water emulsion-type base. In all forms, the cream is water washable, penetrating, and not greasy. Among the most important ingredients of creams are the preservatives, which are potent contact sensitizers. The most widely used preservatives are the parabens or paraben esters. The parabens are not required in petrolatum bases or in propylene glycol creams. The latest class of topical formulations is the gel. With a clear, colorless thixotropic base, the gel is greaseless and water miscible. The active ingredients are completely in solution in the base.[33]

Semirigid dressings are bandages impregnated with material, such as zinc oxide, which hardens on drying to form a castlike dressing. They not only provide protection for the wound from scratching and irritants, but can afford support to the venous system in the treatment of stasis ulcers. The most popular form of this semirigid dressing is the Unna boot.

RIGID DRESSINGS

Rigid dressings, in the form of a below-the-knee total-contact cast, are being used to assist in the healing of neuropathic ulcers, most typically in diabetes, The cast, as described by Coleman and Brand, uses an inner shell of plaster conforming exactly to the contour of the foot and leg, but without the usual cotton padding. The outer shell of either plaster or fiberglass is capped plantarly by a ¼-inch plywood board (cut smaller than the patient's foot) and then a walking heel is placed just behind the middle of the foot.

The total-contact cast dressing has several functions. It permits molding under the foot, controls edema, alleviates body weight from the foot resulting from the conical contoured shape of the leg, and prevents spread of infectious exudate to unwounded tissue through immobilization.[34]

Healing will occur only if pressure is reduced, since the typical plantar neuropathic ulcer is not ischemic, but rather exhibits hyperemia as a result of the inflammation. The cast increases the surface area of contact, thereby reducing the pressure of walking to a negligible level. Because the foot is enveloped in the cast, shear forces are eliminated. This rigid-type dressing permits mobilization of the patient while immobilizing the wounded part.

TOPICAL ANTIMICROBIALS AND ENZYMES

The antibacterial qualities of the skin are both active and passive. The secretion of sebaceous glands, sebum, contains high levels of fatty acids, particularly oleic acid. In addition to lubricating the surface, sebum actively destroys streptococci and, less effectively, staphylococci. Any break in the skin or any inflammation, however, results in serum accumulation, which inactivates sebum, and in this situation streptococci may rapidly colonize.[35]

Many topical antimicrobials have been evaluated for their effect on wound healing. The presence of bacteria in a wound does not equal bacterial infection. The bacterial count should be 10^5 or less per gram of tissue in the granulating wound for successful closure of an ulcer.[36] The use of a topical antimicrobial may result in the presence of resistant bacteria. Topical antibiotics such as neomycin, effective against gram-positive bacteria, and polymyxin, active against gram-negative bacteria, have both been shown to promote reepithelialization; however, they are both frequent sensitizers. Two others, bacitracin, active against gram-positive, and gentamycin, active against gram-negative, have basically little effect on reepithelialization.[37]

The most widely used topical agent is currently silver sulfadiazine 1 percent aqueous cream. Silver sulfadiazine creams should not be used in pregnant women approaching term, premature infants, or neonates less than 2 months of age. Other topical agents include silver nitrate 5 percent aqueous solution, the iodophors, and bacitracin cream.

Where the topical antibiotic antimicrobial could enhance wound healing, four antiseptics were found to be cytotoxic: 1 percent povidone-iodine, 3 percent hydrogen peroxide, 0.5 percent sodium hypochlorite, and 0.25 percent acetic acid. For an antimicrobial agent to eliminate bacterial contamination, it must reach the bacteria in an active form.[38] Iodophors have activity against gram-positive and gram-negative organisms. However, iodine is inactivated by blood and body fluids. Results of a study by Rodeheaver et al. demonstrated that aqueous iodine and povidone-iodine surgical scrub solution significantly reduced the wound's ability to resist infection, which is likely due to the cytotoxicity.[39] Hydrogen peroxide is a weak germicide and its oxygen-producing effervescence may be of more value than its antimicrobial activity.

Numerous topical enzymatic agents have been used on wounds over the past 20 years for the purpose of débridement, but some fail to discriminate between necrotic and normal tissues. Granulation tissue will not develop until residual necrotic tissue is removed. Collagenase-type enzymes digest native and denatured fibrous collagen by peptide bond cleavage under physiologic conditions of pH and temperature. The collagenases are effective preparations because nearly 80 percent of the dry weight of necrotic tissue is collagenic, and that necrotic tissue may be bound to the wound surface by strands of undenatured collagen, which must be weakened or dissolved.[40] Another topical enzymatic debriding agent (Elase) contains fibrinolysin and deoxyribonuclease, which is effective against the denatured proteins found in devitalized tissue because of the fibrinolytic component.[41]

Débridement with dry, porous hydrophilic beads (Debrisan) is accomplished when they are applied to a wound by exerting a suction force that reduces the concentration of noxious agents, including bacteria, and lessens local inflammation and edema. These dextranomer beads require cellular exudate on which to act, and should be thoroughly cleansed from the wound following each application.[42]

SEMIOCCLUSIVE AND OCCLUSIVE MEMBRANES

An increasing number of synthetic membranes are being introduced on the market. The ever-increasing variety leaves the clinician bewildered by the choice she or he must make. The occlusive dressings can be considered those that are adherent with low to zero oxygen permeability and low vapor-moisture transmission. Semiocclusives would include those of higher oxygen permeability and vapor-moisture transmission, and generally decreased adherence. Synthetic membranes are more practically grouped into hydrocolloid, polyurethane/film, and biologic/gelatinous dressings. The slight variations that differentiate a dressing as occlusive or nonocclusive are not sufficiently supported in the literature to establish a significant difference in terms of properties. Noticeable differences in function and wound interaction are more accurately attributed to dressing composition (see Table 30-2).

The hydrocolloid dressing is made up of an adhe-sive side (to be applied to the wound surface) and a bacteria- and water-impermeable backing. It may contain varying amounts of gelatin, carboxymethylcellulose, isopropyl butylene, and pectin. A gel is usually produced from wound exudate–dressing interaction. The majority of hydrocolloids are indicated for more superficial grade I and II (Shea scale) ulcers that are not infected. The dressings can be left on for a maximum of 7 days. Contraindications include a diagnosed clinical soft tissue infection, osteomyelitis, bone or tendon exposure, and heavily draining wounds. These dressings are designed to create an environment optimal for wound repair while protecting the wound surface from outside contamination and disruptive influences.[43–50]

Polyurethane/film dressings are commonly transparent films with an adhesive or nonadhesive surface. These materials absorb minimal to no exudate, are often difficult to apply, and are easily disrupted from the wound surface. Polyurethane has been shown to adhere to newly formed epithelial cells.[49]

The gelatinous/biologic dressings may contain hydrogels of polyethylene oxide and water, silicon, nylon, and/or collagens. They are usually nonadhesive. The gels may readily desiccate and need to be rehydrated. Lower exudate wounds seem better suited for these materials.

Use of synthetic membranes on diabetic ulcers is best advised on more superficial, low-exudate lesions not located on weight-bearing areas. The aforementioned materials can be difficult and ineffective when used on plantar ulcers in diabetics. Plantar pressure and shear forces on weight-bearing areas may force the membranes into the wound or displace them, resulting in further damage. Excessive gel formation and moisture retention in high-exudate wounds may result in excessive maceration and increase in wound size. When used on higher exudate wounds, dressings should be changed at the first sign of exudate leakage from the dressing. Ideally the diabetic patient should not be bearing weight at the site. Synthetic membranes can be used in conjunction with windowed contact casts to provide an excellent combination of non-weightbearing and optimal wound environment. Whenever a synthetic membrane is applied to a wound in a diabetic, or to any wound, the lesion should first be debrided of excessive necrotic tissue

Table 30-2. Synthetic Membrane Application in Ulcer Management[a]

	Ulcer Etiology		
Dressing	Venous Stasis	Diabetic	Pressure
Hydrocolloid[b] and occlusive	Excellent on low- to moderate-exudate wounds. May be left on first 3–5 days. Good adherence, conformity, and retention. Excessive maceration and frequent (often daily) changes make these materials impractical on high-exudate wounds.	Good on all superficial wounds (not extending beyond dermis) with minimal drainage and without sinus tracts. Not recommended when sinus tracts are present. Tend to be ineffective when applied to weight-bearing areas.	Excellent on all pressure lesions except ones where high amounts of exudate or drainage are present. May be left on up to 7 days. Areas of irregular contour (heel) may make application difficult. Not recommended on weight-bearing surfaces.
Polyurethane and thin films	Good on low-exudate wounds. Dressing change required approximately every 2 days. Poor retention on moderate- and high-exudate wounds. Often difficult to apply.	Generally not useful except on superficial abrasion-type wounds located on the dorsal aspect of the foot.	Good on superficial wounds on non-weight-bearing surfaces. Easily displaced from pressure sites.
Hydrogels	Good when used in conjunction with compressive therapy on low-exudate wounds.	Generally good on superficial, low-exudate wounds *only*. Cannot be used on weight-bearing surfaces.	Generally of no use.

[a] The reader should be familiar with each type of dressing.
[b] Hydrocolloids especially may vary in their adhesive, gel-producing, and retention properties. No two hydrocolloids are identical.

and thoroughly cleansed. Since gel, which is often malodorous, is often produced by the dressing, the by-product is often confused with purulent exudate. The wound should be examined for any signs of infection (cellulitis, extensive erythema, sinus tracts with drainage) after wound cleansing. Contamination must be differentiated from infection. Although numerous data are documented on organisms cultured from chronic wounds,[46,51–53] little evidence is available to suggest occlusive dressings promote infection and sepsis.

Synthetic membranes, when used as indicated, may provide a useful supplement to treatment of diabetic ulcers (see Table 30-2).

Venous stasis ulcers are more easily and successfully treated with membranes than are diabetic lesions. The stasis ulcers are not located on weight-bearing or highly irregular surfaces. Dressings can be applied with relative ease and adequate retention. As is the case with diabetic ulcers, all venous stasis lesions should be appropriately debrided and cleansed prior to dressing application. Retention time will be relative to wound exudate, varying from 2 to 7 days.

Synthetic dressings may not be the most effective means of treating high-exudate lesions. Frequent changes no longer remain cost effective. Excessive exudate, when retained under a dressing, produces excessive maceration and additional wound damage.

The hydrocolloid dressings are the most easily used with stasis lesions. Polyurethane and gel dressings are difficult to maintain on the wound surface. The absorptive properties of the latter materials are also very poor. Caution must be taken in severe cases of stasis associated with dermatitis. Dressings contain adhesives to which patients may develop a contact dermatitis. Status of viable tissue must be determined prior to application of dressing materials.

Synthetic membranes contribute to optimization of wound environment. They do not address wound etiology. Appropriate modalities (e.g., compressive wraps, stockings) must still be used in conjunction with dressings so as to assist venous return.

Patients presenting with exceptionally large (greater than 10 by 10 cm) ulcers, fragile skin, and other dermatologic disorders are best treated with modalities other than adhesive occlusive dressings.

Pressure ulcers, when free of deep tissue infections, sinus tracts, and high amounts of exudate, are most easily treated with synthetic membranes. Grades I and II and occasionally grade III (Shea scale) lesions, once cleansed and debrided, may successfully heal when treated with hydrocolloid

Table 30-3. Contraindications for Occlusive and Semiocclusive Dressings

Osteomyelitis
Infection/cellulitis
Bone/tendon involvement
Purulent drainage
Sinus tracts
Lack of viable periwound tissue
Periwound dermatitis
Friable intact tissue
Extensive undebrided area
Necrotic tissue in wound

dressings. When possible, hydrocolloid dressings should be left on from 5 to 7 days. Once pressure sources (the primary etiology) are removed, these lesions will rapidly close, provided the wound environment is kept occluded, clean, and free from outside disruption. Heel or dorsal foot lesions occluded with hydrocolloid membranes need to be kept free from shoe pressure in ambulating patients because this may disrupt the dressing. Postoperative shoes with Velcro straps on the dorsum of the foot and with heel adjustments are most beneficial.

Polyurethane dressings are cost effective and useful when lesions do not extend below the dermis and have a clean, red, granulating base free of necrotic tissue. Gelatinous dressings should be selected for lesions that are of an abrasive or "burn" nature.

Occlusive dressings may reduce time spent with wound care while allowing normal wound repair.

Diabetic, stasis, and pressure ulcers can be successfully managed with synthetic membranes when the following general wound care principles are observed: (1) address primary etiology of wound; (2) remove necrotic tissue; (3) appropriately cleanse ulcer; (4) address general health care (e.g., correct edema, diabetes, dehydration); (5) avoid contraindications (see Table 30-3); and (6) use dressings as recommended.

BIOLOGIC WOUND MATERIALS

Current research is directed at the investigation of biologic materials that can be used to alter normal physiologic occurrences. The use of bovine-derived collagen that has been glutaraldehyde cross-linked is being investigated as a potential material for ulcer prophylaxis.[54] A pilot study with Keragen implant was conducted by Mulder et al.[55] Tyloma sites with a previous history of ulceration were injected with Keragen implant. Controls were treated with standard palliative care. padding, and special shoes. Of 16 patients, the ulceration rate was 100 percent for controls and 17.6 percent for treatment patients. These data suggest that Keragen implant can reduce the rate of reulceration in patients with diabetes.

Platelet-derived and other growth factors are known to have an effect on cell replication.[56] Growth factors have been investigated in preliminary studies of replication, but further investigation is still necessary to support the purported benefits.[57]

Presently no material is available that goes beyond altering cell environment to significantly affect wound repair at the cellular level. There is a need for a biologic material in the form of an applied dressing that will affect fibroblasts, macrophages, and other important components of the wound repair system. Current research indicates that such a modality may soon be available.[58]

REFERENCES

1. Lawrence J: What materials for dressings? Injury 13:500, 1982
2. Mulder G: Synthetic membranes used in diabetic ulcer. Clin Podiatric Med, 4:419, 1987
3. Penn, I, Kempczinski R: The impact of diabetes mellitus. p. 51. In The Ischemic Leg. Year Book Medical Publishers, Inc., Chicago, 1985
4. Stemmer EA: Vascular complications of diabetes mellitus. p. 415. In Moore WD (ed): Vascular Surgery: A Comprehensive Review. Grune & Stratton, New York, 1983
5. Brandman O, Redisch W: Incidence of peripheral vascular changes in diabetes mellitus. Diabetes, 2:194, 1953
6. Penn I: Management of the diabetic foot. Continuing Education for the Family Physician, 13:37, 1980
7. West KM: Epidemiology of Diabetes and Its Vascular Lesions. p. 351. Elsevier-North Holland, New York, 1978

8. Pederson J, Olson S: Small vessel disease of the lower extremity in diabetes mellitus. Acta Med Scand, 171:551, 1962

9. Goldenberg S, Alex M, Joski RA: et al: Nonatheromatous peripheral vascular disease of the lower extremities in diabetes mellitus. Diabetes, 8:261, 1959

10. Strandness DE Jr, Priest RE, Gibbons GI: Combined clinical and pathologic study of diabetic and nondiabetic peripheral arterial disease. Diabetes, 13:366, 1964

11. Towne JB: Management of foot lesions in the diabetic patient. p. 661. In Rutherford RB (ed): Vascular Surgery. Vol. 63. Publisher, City, 1984

12. Guggenheim W, Koch G, Adams AP et al: Femoral and popliteal occlusive vascular disease. Diabetes, 18:428, 1969

13. Ferrier RM: Comparative study of arterial disease in amputated lower limbs from diabetics and nondiabetics. Med J Aust, 1:5, 1967

14. Conrad MC: Large and small artery occlusion in diabetics and nondiabetics with severe vascular disease. Circulation, 36:83, 1967

15. Rudolph R: Pressure ulcers: decubitus ulcers. p. 75. In Rudolph R, Noe J (eds): Chronic Problem Wounds. Little, Brown and Co, Boston, 1983

16. Donovan JC, Rawbotham JL: Foot lesions in diabetic patients: cause, prevention, and treatment. p. 732. In Marble A, Krall LP, Bradley RF (eds): Joslin's Diabetes Mellitus. 12th Ed. Lea & Febiger, Philadelphia, 1982

17. Bessman AN: Foot problems in the diabetic. Comp Ther, 8:32, 1982

18. Falanga V, Eaglestein W: Management of venous ulcers. Am Fam Physician 33:274, 1986

19. Browse NL: Etiology of venous ulceration. World J Surg, 10:938, 1986

20. Burnand KG, Whinster I, Naidoo A, Browse NL: Pericapillary fibrin in the ulcer bearing skin of the leg. Br Med J, 285:1071, 1982

21. Anderson KE, Jensen O, Kvorning SA, Bach E: Prevention of pressure sores by identifying patients at risk. Br Med J, 284:1370, 1982

22. Cooney TJ, Reuler JB: Pressure sores. West J Med, 140:622, 1984

23. Seiler WO, Stahelin HB: Decubitus ulcers: preventive techniques for the elderly patient. Geriatrics, 40:53, 1985

24. Reuler JB, Cooney TG: The pressure sore: pathophysiology and principles of management. Ann Intern Med, 94:661, 1981

25. Dinsdale SM, Decubitus ulcer: role of pressure and friction in causation. Arch Phys Med Rehabil, 55:147, 1974

26. Kosiak M: Etiology of decubitus ulcer. Arch Phys Med Rehabil, 42:19, 1961

27. Shea JD: Pressure sores: classification and management. Clin Orthop Related Res, 112:100, 1975

28. Galpin JE: Sepsis associated with decubitus ulcers. Am J Med, 61:346, 1976

29. Peacock E: Repair of skin wounds. p. 141. In Peacock E: Wound Repair. 3rd Ed. WB Saunders, Philadelphia, 1984

30. Peacock E: Skin grafts, flaps and treatment of burns and other special wounds. p. 187. In Peacock E: Wound Repair. 3rd Ed. WB Saunders, Philadelphia, 1984

31. Edlich R: Technical considerations in closure of skin wounds. p. 4. In Sparkman R (ed): The Healing of Surgical Wounds. American Cyanamid Co, New York, 1985

32. Linsky C, Rovee D, Dow T: Effects of dressings on wound inflammation and scar tissue. p. 191. In Dineen P, Hildick-Smith GC (eds): The Surgical Wound. Lea & Febiger, Philadelphia, 1981

33. Hurley H: Dermatologic therapy. p. 1608. In Moscella S, Pillsbury D, Hurley H (eds): Dermatology. WB Saunders, Philadelphia, 1975

34. Coleman W, Brand P, Birke J: The total contact cast. J Am Podiatry Assoc, 74:548, 1984

35. Munster A, Chiccone T: Burns. p. 23. In Dagher J (ed): Cutaneous Wounds. Futura Publishing Co, New York, 1985

36. Kucan J, Robson M, Heggers J, et al: Comparison of silver sulfadiazene, povidone-iodine and physiologic saline in the treatment of chronic pressure ulcers. J Am Geriatr Soc 29:232, 1981

37. Reed B, Clark R: Cutaneous tissue repair: practical implications of current knowledge II. J Am Acad Dermatol, 13:919, 1985

38. Lineaweaver W, Howard R, Soucy D, et al: Topical antimicrobial toxicity. Arch Surg, 120:267, 1985

39. Rodeheaver G, Bellamy W, Kody M, et al: Bactericidal activity and toxicity of iodine-containing solutions in wounds. Arch Surg, 117:181, 1982

40. Scherer P: An assessment of collagenase therapy for dermal ulcerations of the foot. J Am Podiatry Assoc, 74:25, 1984

41. Lurie H: Enzymatic debridement with elase. J Am Podiatry Assoc, 58:345, 1968

42. Adhami Z: Surgical dressings. J Hosp Infect. 6:123, 1985

43. Friedman SJ, Daniel Su WP: Management of leg ulcers with hydrocolloid occlusive dressings. Arch Dermatol, 120:1329, 1984

44. Pruit BA, Levin NS: Characteristics and uses of biological dressings and skin substitutes. Arch Surg, 119:312, 1984

45. Mulder GD: Synthetic membranes: use in diabetic ulcers. Clin Podiatr Med Surg, 4:419, 1987

46. Alper JC: Recent advances in moist wound healing. South Med J, 79:1398, 1986

47. Eaglestein WH: Effect of occlusive dressings on wound healing. Clin Dermatol, 2:107, 1984

48. Alper JC, Welch EA, Ginsberg M et al: Moist wound healing under a vapor permeable membrane. J Am Acad Dermatol, 8:347, 1983

49. Alvarez OM, Mertz PM, Eaglestein WH: The effect of occlusive dressings on collagen synthesis and re-epithelialization in superficial wounds. J Surg Res, 35:142, 1983

50. Mulder GD, Albert S, Grimwood R: Clinical evaluation of a new occlusive hydrocolloid dressing. Cutis, 4:396, 1985

51. Mertz PM, Eaglestein WH: The effect of a semiocclusive dressing on the microbial population in superficial wounds. Arch Surg, 119:287, 1984

52. Lookingbill DP, Miller SH, Knowles RC: Bacteriology of chronic leg ulcers. Arch Dermatol, 114:1765, 1978

53. Aly R, Shirley C, Cumico B, Maiboch HI: Effect of prolonged occlusion on the microbial flora, pH, carbon dioxide and transepidermal ulcer loss on human skin. J Invest Dermatol, 71:378, 1978

54. Mulder GD, Jahnigen D, Vandepol CJ: Diabetic ulcers: etiology and pathophysiology. (In press)

55. Mulder GD, Vandepol W, Jahnigen D: Diabetic ulcer prophylaxis with injectable collagen. J Am Diabetic Assoc, (In press)

56. Knighton DR, Ciresi KF, Fiegel VD et al: Classification and treatment of chronic nonhealing wounds: successful treatment of autologous platelet-derived wound healing factors. Ann Surg, 204:322, 1986

57. Ross R: Platelet-derived growth factor. Annu Rev Med, 38:71, 1987

58. Ross R, Bowen-Pope DF, Raines EW: Platelet-derived growth factor: its potential roles in wound healing, atherosclerosis, neoplasia, and growth and development. CIBA Found Symp, 116:98, 1985

Section IV

PATIENT MANAGEMENT

B. Surgical Procedures

General Anesthesia

31

John P. McDonough, CRNA, Ed.D.
Steven R. Quam, D.O.

HISTORICAL REVIEW

Prior to 1842, an operative procedure was, to say the least, a struggle for the surgeon and an ordeal for the patient. The most prized attribute for a surgeon was not his skill, but his speed. Were a surgery to last too long, the patient would surely lapse into shock and die. Many agents had been used in an attempt to alleviate pain but with only limited success. The discovery of anesthesia was an American success. It has probably proved to be the major contribution that has come from the American health care professions.

Horace Wells, a dentist in Hartford, Connecticut, was the first to use nitrous oxide as an anesthetic. After he observed that a friend who had been given the gas at a popular science lecture felt no pain after injuring his leg, he reasoned that the gas could be used to relieve the pain of dental extraction. He experimented on himself and concluded that he was correct. Unfortunately, the demonstration that he had arranged in Boston at the Massachusetts General Hospital was not so successful. He attempted to extract a tooth from a volunteer medical student. During the extraction, the student cried out. All in attendance concluded as a result that the demonstration was an abject failure. As a result, nitrous oxide was discredited as a potential anesthetic. This was doubly unfortunate because when the volunteer was questioned after the procedure, he stated that although he had been told that he cried out in apparent pain, he had no recall of the tooth being extracted and had, in fact no pain at the time. But alas, the damage had already been done.

In Georgia, Crawford Long, in 1842, removed a lypoma from a patient painlessly after the administration of ether vapor. This application of ether was not reported at the time. On October 6, 1846, William Morton, a medical student and an associate of Wells the dentist, administered ether to a patient at Massachusetts General Hospital while John Collins Warren, the chief surgeon, removed a parotid growth from a patient. The patient did not struggle or vocalize during the surgery. At the conclusion of the operation, Dr. Warren pronounced the now-famous words: "Gentlemen, this is no humbug." With this was born the age of surgical anesthesia. The news was quickly spread in medical journals and the new discovery swept the world and rapidly increased in popularity.

James Simpson, an obstetrician in Scotland, discovered the anesthetic properties of chloroform in

1847. By this time, anesthesia had made surgeons quick to operate now that it was painless and seemed to be without consequence. In that same year, in an English country village, Hanna Greener, an unfortunate young woman, stubbed and injured her great toe while working in the garden. By the time she sought treatment, the toe and nail bed had apparently become septic. When she summoned the local surgeon to attend her, he concluded that the nail must be removed. She demanded a general anesthetic for the surgery, which was done at home. Since his meager living was dependent upon the number of cases he could do in a day, and an advantage of chloroform is that it has a much faster onset than does ether, the surgeon decided to administer chloroform to her and proceeded to perform an unguinectomy. That was a decision he lived to regret, but Ms. Greener, unfortunately, did not. She was the first patient to suffer a reported anesthetic mortality. This event cast a pall over the development of and excitement concerning anesthesia.

In spite of this, progress in anesthesia was made. Those who administered anesthetics at that time were hardly specialists. The person administering the anesthetic was often the most junior member of the medical team, who was not experienced enough to assist at the surgery. As a result of this, anesthesia mortality was astoundingly high. In fact, there were calls from the medical establishment to investigate the situation. Gradually, it became clear that the way to decrease the problem of anesthetic mortality was to have the anesthesia administered by a specialist in the field. In the late 1800s John Snow, a London physician, developed a great interest in anesthesia, and wrote several works on the subject. Snow is generally considered to be the first anesthesiologist. In the United States, William Halstead, a surgeon, developed nerve block anesthesia through the injection of cocaine. Shortly thereafter, August Bier, a German, reported the first spinal anesthesia. As luck would have it, in the same article he also reported the first post–spinal anesthesia headache! In this period of time, sufficient progress was made through specialization that in 1899, Alice McGaw, the chief nurse anesthetist at the Mayo Clinic, reported a series of over 14,000 administrations of general anesthetic without a single anesthesia-related mortality. Such an accomplishment was no small feat for that time.

As time passed new and better anesthesia agents and techniques were developed by anesthesiologists and nurse anesthetists. Today these two groups are the providers of anesthesia services to patients in the United States. Anesthesiologists are physicians who have received residency training in anesthesia. After their training they are certified by an appropriate speciality board. There are approximately 23,000 certified registered nurse anesthetists (CRNAs) practicing in the United States. CRNAs are registered nurses who have completed an approved postgraduate program in anesthesia and have successfully completed the certification examination and maintain continuing medical education in the speciality.

Because it is perfectly proper to describe the person who actually administers an anesthetic as the "anesthetist," that term is used throughout the remainder of this chapter. It should be understood that the term is intended to apply to both physician anesthesiologists and certified registered nurse anesthetists.

PREOPERATIVE EVALUATION

The preoperative evaluation is often the anesthetist's first contact with the patient prior to surgery. This is the opportunity for the anesthetist to interview the patient and question the patient about past medical history. It is during this time that the anesthetic plan is formulated that will best meet the needs of both the patient and the surgeon. In addition to serving as a vehicle for medical fact finding, the preanesthetic evaluation interview provides the opportunity for the anesthetist to establish a sense of rapport with the patient. Often, as medical professionals, we neglect to recall that although experiences such as surgery and anesthesia are very common to us, very often they are strange and frightening experiences for the patient. A calm, uninterrupted, and unhurried preanesthetic evaluation session between the anesthetist and the patient can often help the patient develop a sense of trust in the individual who will administer his or her anesthesia and allow the patient's fears to be allayed, thus causing the experience to be considerably less traumatic and anxiety provoking for the patient. It has been demonstrated that an effective preanesthetic interview has a calming effect that is equal to a preoperative sedative medication.

The preoperative evaluation has changed considerably over the last few years. This change is due in part to the rather dramatic increase in outpatient surgery. Prior to the advent of outpatient surgery, most patients were admitted to the hospital prior to surgery and the anesthetist had the opportunity to see them on the afternoon or evening prior to the scheduled day of surgery. Unfortunately, in this day of medical cost-containment concerns, this is a luxury that is seldom afforded to our patients. The advantage of seeing the patient at least a day before the scheduled surgery was that it provided an opportunity for the anesthetist to investigate areas that required further study based on the patient's medical history. Because we are no longer able to see most elective surgical patients within the hospital setting as inpatients prior to surgery, it is often advisable to have patients make an appointment to visit the anesthesiology department at the surgical facility at which the operation is to be performed a day or two prior to the scheduled surgery. At this time an anesthetist can obtain the patient's medical and anesthetic history and decide if further diagnostic intervention is required in order to provide the patient with the safest possible anesthetic experience.

The first and probably most important activity in the preanesthetic evaluation is obtaining the patient's history. The purpose of the preanesthetic history is to identify areas of potential medical concern and to glean the facts required to assign an appropriate American Society of Anesthesiologists (ASA) classification to the patient. The ASA classification system was developed in an effort to make an attempt to quantify relative anesthetic risks from patient to patient. After the history has been taken, the patient can be classified according to the following scheme:

Class I: The patient who is normal and healthy except for the surgical pathology.

Class II: The patient with mild systemic disease that is neither incapacitating nor a threat to life. (e.g., a patient with mild unsymptomatic chronic obstructive pulmonary disease or relatively mild untreated hypertension).

Class III: The patient who has severe systemic disease that limits activity, although is not incapacitating (e.g., a patient who has documented coronary artery disease or a proven myocardial infarction of any age).

Class IV: The patient with incapacitating disease that is a constant threat to life (e.g., a patient who either has a recent myocardial infarction or is currently suffering from unstable or crescendo angina).

Class V: The patient who is moribund and is not expected to survive past the next 24 hours whether or not surgery is performed (e.g., a patient who has sustained disastrous head injury, has a ruptured aortic aneurysm and is in moribund end-stage shock upon presentation, or has suffered any other circumstances that would render him or her near death).

Class VI: A patient who has been declared legally brain dead and is awaiting organ harvesting.

Systems Review

Obviously, the attempt to gain appropriate preanesthetic information on which to base your clinical assessment should follow an orderly review of systems. The nature of this review is not required to be as comprehensive as a complete medical history, but rather is designed to bring to light facts that will be of clinical importance in the anesthetic management of the patient's care.

Cardiovascular System

Since coronary artery disease is a fairly common occurrence in the adult population of the United States, questioning relative to the cardiovascular system is certainly of importance in determining preanesthetic risk factors. Although exact statistics vary from study to study, it can be stated conservatively that approximately 1.3 million persons sustain myocardial infarction in the United States yearly. This makes coronary artery disease a major health problem in our population. The risk of coronary artery disease associated with anesthesia is significant. Although patients who have never sustained a myocardial infarction in the past are not likely to do so during the perioperative period, those who have suffered myocardial infarction have a greatly increased tendency to reinfarct during the period of surgery, anesthesia, and the postoperative phase. Unfortunately this significant increase in reinfarction rate also carries a fairly high level of mortality. In view of these facts, it is certainly important for the anesthetist to understand the level of the patient's cardiovascular risk status.

One of the factors to keep in mind, in addition to actual questions directed toward the patient relative to cardiovascular symptoms, is what if any previous predisposing risk factors the patient has in relation to cardiovascular disease. One's index of clinical suspicion would certainly be increased if the patient has a history of hypertension, diabetes, familial hyperlipidemia, or prolonged exposure to stress in the occupational setting, or if the patient is a cigarette smoker. In addition to the mentioned risk factors, it is also noted that obese patients tend to suffer from coronary artery disease more so than the nonobese.

A careful history relative to the cardiovascular system can assist the anesthetist in assessing the probability of pathology. Obviously, the patient should be asked about history of chest pain. Unfortunately, it is not uncommon to stop with that particular question, namely about the presence of pain. Patients, however, sometimes do not identify the feeling of discomfort with the sensation of pain. It would certainly develop a false sense of security on the part of the anesthetist if a question relative to chest pain was answered negatively by the patient and was not pursued further. Very often patients with significant coronary artery disease, rather than talking about "pain," mention feeling of pressure, sensations of heaviness, or a perception that their chest is being squeezed by a vise. Although these patients will respond positively to questions relative to such discomforts, they often answer negatively when they are asked specifically about "pain." The pain and discomfort associated with coronary artery disease is not, of course, necessarily isolated to the chest. Patients with significant coronary artery disease have been known to complain of pain and discomfort, not only in the chest, but in the neck, jaw, and shoulder. If, in fact, the patient does present a positive history for chest discomfort, it is well to attempt to ascertain what, if anything, exacerbates or relieves the patient's sensation of discomfort. It would certainly be advisable, should a patient present with symptoms that

are consistent with angina, that the patient be seen and appropriately "worked up" for his complaints of chest discomfort in an effort to either confirm or rule out the presence of coronary artery disease.

Patients should be questioned about arrhythmias. Questions should be directed to the patient in an effort to determine if the patient ever senses periods of palpitations or other episodes in which they perceive their heart to be beating in an irregular fashion. Along with symptoms consistent with arrhythmias, the patient should be questioned relative to possible syncopal episodes. The origin of episodes involving either lightheadedness or syncope can well be abnormalities of the heart rhythm. The syncopal episode could well have resulted from the brain receiving inadequate oxygen secondary to either a tachyarrhythmia or profound bradycardia.

Included at this time should be general questions relative to the patient's level of vitality; questions relative to their fatigability, stamina, and sense of energy can indicate the level of cardiac reserve. The patient can also be questioned relative to the presence of edema in the extremities. In addition to the other potential causes of dependent edema, one cause is certainly right ventricular heart failure. In the United States, a common cause of right ventricular heart failure is, in fact, left ventricular heart failure. Since arteriosclerotic heart disease is a common cause of left ventricular failure in contemporary western culture, questions relative to the symptoms of right ventricular failure are certainly appropriate in an attempt to quantify pathology in the cardiovascular system.

Respiratory System

The patient should be questioned relative to recurrent, acute, or chronic lung diseases. The patient should be questioned as to whether or not he or she has a chronic cough. If so, it is well to note whether this cough is productive. An attempt should be made to determine whether the cough is as a result of a transient condition, such as a respiratory tract infection, or whether the cough is truly of a chronic nature and is associated with smoking and subsequent pulmonary disease. The presence of an acute respiratory infection is a relative contraindication to elective anesthesia and surgery. If chronic lung disease is suspected, it would be well to attempt to ascertain the level of disability that this causes the patient. For instance, is the patient's activity limited by dyspnea? If this is the case, it would certainly be advisable to obtain optimal bronchopulmonary toilet prior to elective anesthesia and surgery. Perhaps the patient would benefit from a period of prophylactic antibiotics and bronchodilator therapy prior to elective surgical intervention.

Especially worthy of note relative to the respiratory system is the fact that it is certainly unwise to electively anesthetize children with upper respiratory infections lest serious postoperative respiratory complications ensue. In children, it is best to delay surgery and anesthesia for at least 2 weeks after the cessation of symptoms associated with acute upper or lower respiratory infection. Children tend to have hyperreactive airways, and the presence of increased secretions and exudates associated with infection predisposes children to marked bronchospasm and ventilatory difficulties while under anesthesia.

Another respiratory topic of concern to the anesthetist is whether or not the patient has a history of asthma. Certain drugs have a tendency to cause the body to release endogenous stories of histamine, and as a result should be avoided in patients with significant asthma history. A common example of this problem in drugs used for induction is sodium thiopental. In asthmatic patients, sodium thiopental is best avoided. There are several other acceptable induction agents that can be used in lieu of sodium thiopental. Another example of a drug that could potentially cause problems in asthmatic patients is *d*-tubocurarine. Curare is a drug that is often used as a pretreating drug prior to the administration of succinylcholine, a depolarizing neuromuscular-blocking drug, that is frequently used to facilitate intubation of the trachea immediately after the induction of general anesthesia. Curare has been shown to release histamine and can cause significant bronchospasm in patients who are predisposed to bronchospastic episodes as a result of asthma. If the anesthetist is aware of this predisposition, appropriate changes in anesthetic management can be planned and implemented in an attempt to minimize adverse consequences associated with the induction of anesthesia and subsequent manipulation of the patient's airway.

Should the patient display significant history of pulmonary pathology or show abnormal physical examination results on auscultation and/or percussion of the chest, additional diagnostic intervention may be required. The state of the patient's disease may indicate that a pulmonary function test is required to quantify the patient's ability to properly ventilate during anesthesia and in the postoperative period. In addition to pulmonary function tests, posteroanterior and lateral radiographs of the chest may be indicated. It may also be advisable to obtain a sample of arterial blood for gas analysis.

Hepatorenal System

The majority of drugs that are administered to patients in the operating room setting are often detoxified by the liver. It is advisable to obtain a history relative to the patient's liver function prior to surgery. The patient should be questioned as to whether or not he or she has ever displayed the symptom of jaundice. If possible, the cause of this jaundice should be ascertained. If the patient has in the past suffered from hepatitis, it should be noted whether the hepatitis was type A, type B, or non-A/non-B, or resulted from another identifiable cause. Many believe that patients with significant hepatic history would be better not exposed to halogenated hydrocarbon vapors of the type that are commonly found in inhalation anesthetic agents. Should it be advisable to avoid halogenated hydrocarbons in a particular patient, many other anesthetic management options remain open. The patient could be given either a regional anesthetic or a general anesthetic utilizing dissociative, narcotic, or tranquilizing drugs used in conjunction with nitrous oxide.

The kidneys are the organ that will be primarily responsible for the maintenance of the patient's fluid and electrolyte balance and excretion of drugs during surgery. Questions should be asked of the patient relative to the possibility of preexisting kidney disease. The patient should be questioned relative to previous kidney infections, as well as indications of other renal pathology.

Neuromuscular System

There are several reasons why questions relative to the neuromuscular systems are important in elucidating potential anesthetic problems. It has been reported that the volatile inhalation anesthetic enflurane will produce spike-dome complexes in patients who are monitored electroencephalographically during surgery and anesthesia if the concentration of the drug becomes high at a time when arterial carbon dioxide tension is abnormally low. Although clinically this may have little practical significance to the management of the case, because there will seldom be any demonstrable muscle activity because the patient has received a paralyzing drug, the spike-dome complexes have been known to be epileptiform in nature. This suggests that people with preexisting seizure disorders might benefit from using an agent other than enflurane.

Patients who suffer from lower motor neuron disease are particularly susceptible to particularly abrupt and troublesome fluctuations in serum potassium should they be given succinylcholine to facilitate intubation. In such patients, the administration of intravenous succinylcholine will result in dramatic increases in serum potassium levels. There has been some concern that such a rapid increase in serum potassium levels can precipitate cardiac arrhythmias that result in untoward complications.

Endocrine and Hematologic Systems

By far the most common endocrine disorder seen in patients presenting for surgery and anesthesia is diabetes mellitus. It is essential that the patient's disease be under control and that the patient not display substantial variations in blood sugar prior to surgical intervention. This presents little problem if that patient's diabetes is well controlled with diet or a combination of diet and oral antihyperglycemic agents. In such patients, it would be wise to have the patient take nothing by mouth after midnight and avoid taking oral hypoglycemic agents the morning of surgery. Patients who are insulin dependent, however, present another problem. Caution must be exercised to preclude a patient taking nothing by mouth after the midnight prior to surgery and then taking the usual dose of insulin in the morning. The result of such an action could be profound hypoglycemia with disastrous consequences. It would be better to have such patients remain off oral intake and then refrain from taking their morning insulin. These patients can then be managed with appropriate doses of intravenous

glucose and insulin as required during the perioperative period. Of course, patients with diabetes should be evaluated for the presence of the sequelae normally associated with long-standing diabetes, Such patients commonly display symptoms associated with peripheral vascular disease as well as neuropathies.

Another common endocrine disorder in operative patients is thyroid disease. In an effort to maintain appropriate blood levels, it is recommended that the patient remain on thyroid supplementation if he or she is being treated for hypothyroidism. A more significant problem is presented by the patient who is hyperthyroid and not adequately controlled. Markedly hyperthyroid patients should be evaluated medically and their condition stabilized prior to elective surgery. Failure to do so can result in the possibility of precipitating a "thyroid storm" during the time of surgery.

Patients suffering from pulmonary diseases and rheumatic disorders are commonly treated with corticosteroids. The administration of these exogenous steroids can result in a markedly decreased ability of the patient's adrenal glands to appropriately respond to the expected stress of anesthesia and surgery. Those patients require supplemental doses of steroids prior to and immediately following the surgical episode.

In addition to laboratory study results, which are considered later, the preanesthesia history should include questions relative to anemias and other hematologic disorders. If the patient is chronically anemic but has hemoglobin within acceptable ranges, elective surgery and anesthesia can probably be undertaken with some margin of safety. Obviously, patients who display an acute anemia must be appropriately investigated to determine the cause of this abnormality. In patients who are potentially susceptible, screening should be carried out for sickle cell disease. Should these findings be positive, the use of a pneumatic tourniquet on the extremity would be contraindicated because of the potential complications associated with red cell sickling.

Previous Anesthesia

The patient should be questioned relative to what previous surgeries he or she has had and what type of anesthetic was administered. It should be determined if the patient had any untoward reaction to these anesthetics. Appropriate questions might include whether the patient had difficulties associated with a general anesthetic, such as protracted nausea or vomiting after surgery or experiencing a particularly prolonged emergence. If the patient's previous anesthetic experience was a regional or major conduction anesthetic, questions should be directed relative to the presence or absence of postoperative headache, pain, or neurologic sequelae.

A family history should also be obtained regarding experiences of relatives who have received anesthesia. Of particular concern is the potential of developing the syndrome of malignant hyperthermia, which results from a hereditary error of metabolism that, when triggered, results in a massive increase in the body's metabolic rate. This massive increase in metabolism results in tremendous increases in the utilization of oxygen by the cells. The end-product of this metabolic increase is a marked increase in the production of both carbon dioxide and lactic acid. The addition of these metabolic end-products to the body causes the patient to become tremendously acidotic. The pH of the blood drops tremendously and the patient will suffer life-threatening cardiac arrhythmias. Historically, this syndrome has resulted in a very high mortality rate. However, with the advent of dantrolene, a specific pharmacologic mode of therapy, combined with increased understanding of the problem and vigilance by anesthesia personnel, the mortality rate has decreased significantly over the past few years. In an effort to determine the possibility of the existence of the trait predisposing a person to malignant hyperthermia, the patient should be questioned relative to history of relatives dying suddenly on the operating table or others in the patient's family who have died suddenly for no apparent reason at a young age.

Drug Therapy

Many patients present for elective surgical intervention while they are receiving drug therapy for other conditions. In many circumstances, the patient can refrain from taking his or her medication from midnight prior to the surgery until after recovering from the anesthetic. There are, however,

certain situations in which withholding the patient's medication prior to surgery would not be advisable. Patients who have hypertension and/or coronary artery disease are often treated with nitrates, calcium channel blockers, and/or β blockers. It is best to have these patients continue their medication regime until the time of surgery. Patients who are being maintained on oral medication of this type can take this medication the morning of surgery with a small amount of clear liquid, just sufficient to permit them to swallow the drug. Other medications that should probably be continued up to the morning of surgery are anticonvulsant drugs and anti-infectives, in which maintaining a constant therapeutic blood level is of considerable importance.

Just as there are drugs that should be continued up to the time of surgery, there are also medications that would best be discontinued prior to elective surgery. The hallmark example of such drugs are monoamine oxidase (MAO) inhibitors. Because of the risk entailed, it would be best to discontinue MAO inhibitors, if at all possible, at least 14 days prior to elective anesthesia. The administration of MAO inhibitors has a desired effect that consists of increasing the patient's endogenous stores of norepinephrine. As a result of this increase in norepinephrine stores, the patient would be at considerable risk should a situation develop in which a vasopressor would be required to treat perioperative hypotension. Patients receiving MAO inhibitors have demonstrated dangerous levels of hypertension when treated with even small doses of vasopressor drugs.

Diagnostic Studies

The number and complexity of diagnostic studies required to properly evaluate a patient prior to anesthesia is determined primarily by the condition of the patient and the history with which the patient presents. Depending on the potential surgery considered, hematology studies consisting of at least a hemoglobin and hematocrit determination are required. If there is any indication of the potential of an infective process, a white blood cell count with differential should also be included. Depending on the patient's age, history, and condition, determination of serum electrolyte levels may also be indicated. Of particular import would be the determination of serum potassium level in patients who have been receiving thiazide diuretic therapy. Although there have been recent studies indicating that the serum potassium level has been historically granted an exaggerated importance, further study will probably be required before the practitioner can justifiably omit serum potassium determination in patients prone to potassium depletion.

In those patients who present with either a history of bleeding diathesis or anticoagulant therapy, determination of coagulation status is, of course, mandatory. Patients who have been receiving coumadin should have a prothrombin time measurement, and those who have been maintained on heparin should have a partial thromboplastin time measurement. A female of child-bearing age with a history of delayed menses or other signs consistent with possible pregnancy should have a β-human chorionic gonadotropin level measurement. Unless the surgery is of an urgent nature, it would probably be better to delay elective anesthesia and surgery until after the first trimester of pregnancy. Other particular blood studies might be indicated in certain patients depending upon the history and findings of physical examination.

Patients who are over the age of 45 or present symptoms consistent with cardiac disease should have a preanesthesia electrocardiogram (ECG). Although as a diagnostic technique the ECG is certainly not infallible, it can provide valuable evidence relative to the existence of coronary artery disease. This evidence can be shown by changes in the S-T segment or the presence of pathologic Q waves, indicating a previous transmural myocardial infarction. In any event, even if the ECG is not diagnostic of cardiac disease, it will serve as a useful baseline should the patient develop problems later in his or her hospital course. Those patients displaying a history or symptoms of pulmonary disease might be considered candidates for pulmonary function studies. If an inhalation anesthetic is planned, the pulmonary function studies can provide information relative to the patient's ability to ventilate during surgery and in the postoperative period. Of particular interest would be forced expiratory volume as a predictor of obstructive pulmonary disease.

Miscellaneous Information

In addition to the information gleaned from the review of systems and diagnostic tests performed, additional information should be noted on the patient's record. The patient's height and weight should be recorded. This information is important not only because most drug dosages are calculated on the basis of weight, but because general body structure might be a significant factor in such activities as patient positioning. The dentition should be examined and notations made relative to the condition of the teeth and gums. Such an examination will provide forewarning of potential damage to dentition or the presence of preexisting dental damage. Additionally, certain types of orofacial structures, such as a profound overbite, can make intubation difficult. The patient should also be questioned relative to allergies and this information documented on the patient's record.

Developing the Care Plan

Utilizing the information that the practitioner has gained through the review of systems, physical examination, and results of diagnostic studies, we may then assign the patient an appropriate ASA category rating. When the patient has been properly categorized, the total body of information can be used to construct an anesthesia management care plan. The proposed care plan should then be discussed with the patient and the risks and benefits of the anesthetic explained. In this way, the patient's informed consent can then be obtained and a plan will have been constructed that is agreeable to the anesthetist, the surgeon, and the patient.

PREANESTHESIA MEDICATIONS

In the past, preanesthesia medications were used more routinely than they are today. Occasionally, however, preanesthetic medications are still indicated even for patients undergoing surgery on an outpatient basis. The desired effect of preanesthesia medication is to allay apprehension, provide amnesia, give analgesia, decrease secretions and undesirable reflexes, and suppress nausea and vomiting. When received at the appropriate time and under appropriate conditions, the desired effects can be achieved. Numerous drugs are currently available to be used as preoperative medications. The selection of drug and dose will depend upon the desired results to be achieved. Some types of drugs that are used as preanesthetic medicants are short-acting barbiturates, benzodiazepines, butyrophenones, narcotics, and dissociative agents. Anticholinergic drugs such as atropine, scopolamine, and glycopyrrolate are often administered in addition to the above-named drugs to decrease both secretions and vagal tone. These drugs can be administered singly or in combination 1 to 2 hours preoperatively if given by the intramuscular route, or they may be given closer to the time of surgery through intravenous administration in a preoperative holding area. If these drugs are administered intravenously, the patient should be under the care of a professional member of the staff.

MONITORS AND EQUIPMENT

There is a certain risk of adverse reaction any time an anesthetic is administered. This risk is present whether the agent is administered as a local anesthetic, intramuscularly, intravenously, or by the inhalation route. As a result of these risks, there are certain minimum requirements for patient care that must be met prior to the administration of anesthetic drugs.

An area in which anesthesia is to be administered must contain an oxygen source, a means of controlling an airway, equipment required for laryngoscopy and intubation, intravenous drugs to treat cardiac arrest or other untoward complications, and the equipment required to monitor the patient's vital signs. As one enters an operating suite, all of the minimally required drugs and equipment are available. If anesthetic intervention is undertaken

outside the operating room, plans must be constructed in such a way that the required equipment and drugs will be immediately available.

Within the last few years, standards of practice relative to patient monitoring have changed. Currently it is accepted within the speciality that minimum standards of patient monitoring will include continuous electrocardiographic monitoring, blood pressure measurement, a precordial or esophageal stethoscope, continuous temperature monitoring, and the ability to monitor neuromuscular blockade if a neuromuscular blocking agent has been administered. These standards of monitoring apply to both general and regional anesthesia cases.

When one is administering a general anesthetic, the anesthesia machine must have an oxygen monitor in line, disconnect alarms, airway pressure alarms, respirometer, and an alarm to indicate ventilator malfunction. Some of the new technology that has recently been added to our armamentarium consists of pulse oxymetry and capnography. The pulse oxymeter is being used so frequently now that it, along with the expiratory capnograph, will soon be considered standards of care. It should also be noted that areas where anesthetic drugs are administered should be equipped with not only a cardiac monitor but a defibrillator as well, and a "crash cart" should be available that has been stocked with all medications needed to treat potential emergency situations. Additional types of monitoring may need to be undertaken, depending upon the patient's condition and the type of surgery being performed. Examples of such additional monitoring include direct arterial pressure monitoring, pulmonary artery catheter, electroencephalography, and evoked neuromuscular potentials.

ANESTHETIC METHODS

Although it is outside the scope of this chapter to engage in a detailed discussion of anesthetic agents and the rationale for choices between them, it would be helpful for the surgeon to have some understanding of the choices faced by the anesthesia specialist. Modern anesthesia is achieved most often by the use of a combination of drugs designed to produce specific results. If one examines what the patient who is to undergo surgery requires, it may be concluded that there is a need for hypnosis (sleep and amnesia), analgesia (pain relief), and, to a varying degree, muscle relaxation. How these patient needs are met will vary with each patient and type of surgery.

Volatile Inhalation Agents

The inhalation anesthetic agents in use today are capable of meeting all of the above patient requirements. The most common agents in use today are isoflurane, enflurane, and halothane. All are considered 100 per cent potent and, as a result, can produce surgical anesthesia without supplementation with other drugs or agents. Each of these agents have specific advantages and disadvantages that will be considered by the anesthetist in making the choice for a particular patient. All of the agents are administered through the use of an anesthesia machine with a vaporizer. The agent is administered to the patient by using a mixture of oxygen, nitrous oxide, and/or air to carry the agent vapor to the patient. Most anesthetists use a semiclosed breathing circuit that contains a device to absorb carbon dioxide that is produced by the patient's respiration. Because there are medications that may not be compatible with all of these agents, the surgeon would be well advised to discuss the administration of any drugs to be used during the surgery with the anesthetist prior to the case.

Narcotics

In cases in which it has been elected not to administer the anesthetic solely with a volatile agent, or where additional analgesia may be required during either the surgery or the postoperative period, the anesthetist may choose to administer a narcotic to the patient. Meperidine has been and continues to be used by anesthetists to treat pain parenterally. Today, its use is often confined to the postoperative period in the recovery room. There was a time when this drug and morphine were the drugs of choice. With recent advances in the pharmacology of synthetic narcotics, these older drugs are being replaced by newer synthetic narcotics such as fentanyl, sufentanil, and alfentanil. Each has specific indications that relate to their half-life and rates of excretion and metabolism.

Other Central Nervous System Depressants

Although it is certainly possible to induce general anesthesia exclusively through the inhalation of a volatile agent, this is seldom done. Because of considerations of patient safety, patient acceptance, and speed, induction is most often accomplished through the administration of intravenous sedatives.

Ultra-short-acting barbiturates are the most commonly used drugs for this purpose. Thiopental sodium, a thiobarbiturate has certainly stood the test of time and is still in common use today as an induction agent. Contrary to the belief generally held by the lay public, such drugs are not, in fact, anesthetics. They are used only to speed the induction process and make it more pleasant for the patient. It is for this reason that the patient seldom has to be anesthetized by breathing a less than pleasant-smelling "gas" from an anesthesia machine.

Other drugs can also be used to accomplish the same purpose. Benzodiazepines such as diazepam and midazolam can be used for this task as well. The advantages of these drugs are that these are less depressing to the cardiovascular system and also provide an increased level of perioperative amnesia. Although it may be tempting to use such drugs as an adjunct to local or regional anesthesia, it should be recalled that when such drugs are administered intravenously, the patient should be continuously monitored by an appropriate practitioner whose sole task is to render care to that patient and who has no other duties.

At certain times, the anesthetist may elect to use a dissociative agent. Ketamine is the drug used almost exclusively for such purposes. This drug provides certain unique advantages that include increases in the heart rate and blood pressure. Some patients have experienced postoperative dysphoria and hallucinations after the use of ketamine. These side effects can be minimized through the use of concurrent sedation with a benzodiazepine or a butyrophenone.

Muscle Relaxants

Although surgery of the foot seldom requires very profound levels of muscle relaxation, this class of drug will nearly always be used to facilitate intubation of the trachea by the anesthetist. In certain circumstances, such as when the anesthetist is using a "balanced" technique that consists of nitrous oxide and a narcotic, supplemental muscle relaxation may be required.

POSTANESTHESIA CARE

After the completion of the anesthesia and surgery, the patient should emerge from anesthesia in a special area designed, equipped, and staffed for this purpose. The patient will be kept in the postanesthesia recovery area until such time as he or she is capable of protecting his or her own airway and has awakened enough to be oriented to time, place, and person. Because of the effects that are caused by anesthetic drugs and their metabolites, patients must be cautioned not to drive, use machines that require eye-hand coordination, or even make any important decisions until at least the next day after surgery and anesthesia.

During the patient's stay in the recovery area, all drugs and equipment that might be needed to treat problems related to the airway and circulation must be available immediately. The postanesthesia recovery area is the location in which patients will make the transition from being "asleep" and under the constant care of the anesthetist and being "awake" enough to maintain their own safety.

CONCLUSION

The practice of anesthesia today is like the practice of surgery in that both should be done by specialists in the field. It is hoped that, through the jointly collaborative efforts of each of these specialists, patients can be guided through the perilous seas of their surgical experience to a safe and successful outcome.

SELECTED READINGS

Bartkowski RR: Incomplete reversal of pancronium neuromuscular blockade by neostigmine, pyridostigmine and edrophonium, Anesth Analg, 66:594, 1987

Beard K: Adverse respiratory events occurring in the recovery room after general anesthesia. Anesthesiology, 64:269, 1986

Carroll JB: Increased incidence of masseter spasm in children with strabismus anesthetized with halothane and succinylcholine. Anesthesiology 76:559, 1987

Carpenter RL: The extent of metabolism of inhaled anesthetics in humans. Anesthesiology 65:201, 1986

Chung F: General or spinal anesthesia: which is better in the elderly? Anesthesiology 67:422, 1987

Cousins MJ: Intrathecal and epidural administration of opioids. Anesthesiology, 61:276, 1984

Gelman D: Hepatic circulation during surgical stress and anesthesia with halothane, isoflurane and fentanyl. Anesth Analg, 66:936, 1987

Heindel D: Deep neck abscesses in adults: management of the difficult airway. Anesth Analg, 66:774, 1987

Hirsch IA: The overstated risk of preoperative hypokalemia. Anesth Analg, 67:131, 1988

Larach MG: Prediction of malignant hyperthermia susceptibility by clinical signs. Anesthesiology, 66:547, 1987

Lichtor JL: Preoperative anxiety level the afternoon before surgery predict anxiety level just before surgery? Anesthesiology 67:595, 1987

Loper K: Comparison of halothane and isoflurane for rapid anesthetic induction. Anesth Analg, 66:766, 1987

Mattby JR: Preoperative oral fluids: is five hour fast justified prior to elective surgery? Anesth Analg, 65:1112, 1986

Melnick BM: Effects of eliminating nitrous oxide in outpatient anesthesia. Anesth Analg, 67:982, 1987

Miller RD: Anesthesia. Churchill Livingstone, New York, 1981

Nusbaum LM: Intravenous regional anesthesia for surgery on the foot and ankle. Anesthesiology, 64:91, 1986

Pittinger CB: The anesthesia of Fanny Longfellow for childbirth on April 7, 1847. Anesth Analg, 66:368, 1987

Rusy BF: Anesthetic depression of myocardial contractility: a review of possible mechanisms. Anesthesiology 67:745, 1987

Slogoff D: Further observations on perioperative myocardial ischemia. Anesthesiology 65:539, 1986

Stanley TH: New routes of administration and new delivery systems of anesthesics. Anesthesiology 68:665, 1988

Stoelting RK: Basics of Anesthesia. Churchill Livingstone, New York, 1984

Tait AR: The effects of general anesthesia on upper respiratory tract infections in children. Anesthesiology 67:930, 1987

Weber S: Improvement in blood flow during lower extremity microsurgical free tissue transfer associated with epidural anesthesia. Anesth Analg, 67:303, 1988

White PF: Comparison of alfentanil with fentanyl for outpatient surgery. Anesthesiology 64:99, 1986

Regional and Local Anesthesia

32

Gregory S. Duncan, D.P.M.

Regional anesthesia uses local anesthetics to interrupt the conductivity of sensory fibers of nerves in various regions of the body. Motor function may be partially or totally altered depending upon the size of the nerve and the drug concentration used. Regional anesthesia includes various methods of blocking nerve conduction — topical, infiltration, peripheral nerve block, field block, subarachnoid or spinal block, and epidural or peridural block. Local anesthetics are agents that can reversibly block the conduction of nerve impulses and provide a temporary loss of sensation to a confined area of the body. All local anesthetics originated from cocaine, the alkaloid found in the South American shrub *Erythroxylon coca.* It was not until 1905 that procaine was developed as a synthetic substitute for cocaine and became the prototype for all future local anesthetic drugs.

CHEMISTRY

Most useful local anesthetics are composed of three structural elements: a carbocyclic or hetero-cyclic aromatic ring (lipophilic portion), an intermediate chain, and an amine group (hydrophilic portion) (Fig. 32-1). Alterations in any portion of the structure will modify the anesthetic's activity and affect such properties as molecular weight, potency, protein binding, lipid-water distribution, duration, and toxicity. Most local anesthetics can be classified chemically into two groups, ester and amide, depending on the linkage between the aromatic group and the intermediate chain. This difference in the aromatic group – intermediate chain link influences the metabolic pattern of the chemical structure. Thus, the ester-type agents are hydrolized in plasma by a pseudocholinesterase and the amide-type agents are metabolized in the liver.

The base of the local anesthetic is the active molecule. Because of the instability and poor water solubility of the base, its salts, of which hydrochloride is the most common, are stable and water soluble. The local anesthetics are aqueous solutions of the salt of the local anesthetic base. The base must be placed in the vicinity of the nerve membrane because the salt does not possess anesthetic activity. This dissociation reaction frees hydrogen ions, requiring adequate tissue buffering to obtain the maximal amount of free base. In an acid or poorly buffered medium, such as infection, little free base is formed from the salt and it is less effective.

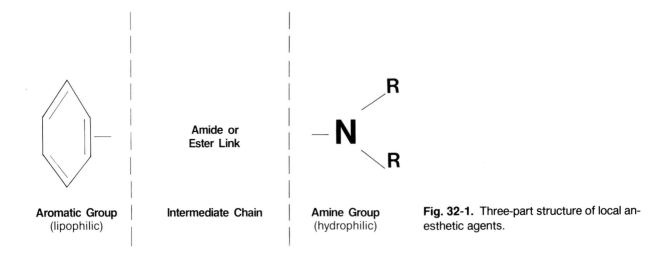

Aromatic Group | Intermediate Chain | Amine Group | **Fig. 32-1.** Three-part structure of local an-
(lipophilic) | | (hydrophilic) | esthetic agents.

MECHANISM OF ACTION

Local anesthetic agents exert their effect by altering the electronilogic excitation process of peripheral nerve fibers and nerve endings. Covino stated that this is caused by displacement of calcium ions from some binding sites in the cell membrane; decrease in permeability of the cell membrane to sodium ions; decrease in the rate of depolarization of the membrane action potential; failure of the action potential to reach the firing level required for complete depolarization; failure of a spike potential of adequate amplitude to develop; and failure of action potential propagation, resulting in conduction block.

Peripheral nerves are of three types, A, B, and C, depending on their fiber properties. A fibers are subdivided into A alpha, A beta, A delta, and A gamma. They decrease in diameter from alpha to gamma. The A fibers are myelinated somatic nerve fibers; A alpha and A beta are motor fibers. B fibers are myelinated, preganglionic nerve fibers. C fibers are unmyelinated, postganglionic nerve fibers. The nerve fibers vary in size from 0.5 to 2.0 μ. The larger the fiber, the more resistant it is to local anesthesia.[2] A delta, A gamma, and C fibers convey pain and temperature sensation; these are blocked first. Thus, the sensations lost from local anesthetics are pain, temperature, touch, proprioception, and skeletal muscle tone. Recovery usually proceeds in the reverse order.

TYPES OF LOCAL ANESTHETICS

There are a variety of local anesthetic agents available for clinical use (Table 32-1). They vary in potency and duration, which are determined by lipid solubility and protein binding, respectively. An example would be the addition of a butyl group to the aromatic end of procaine, resulting in a compound known as tetracaine, which is considerably more lipid soluble and potent. The addition of a butyl group to mepivacaine leads to formation of bupivacaine, which is 35 times more lipid soluble and four times more potent than mepivacaine.[3] The protein binding of bupivacaine and etidocaine exceeds 90 percent, whereas that of mepivacaine and lidocaine is 65 and 75 percent, respectively. The higher percentage of protein binding in bupivacaine and etidocaine makes them two to three times longer acting than mepivacaine or lidocaine.

The physical-chemical parameter pK_a indicates the pH at which the ionized and un-ionized forms of a specific substance are present in solution in equal amounts. This will affect the time of onset of the local anesthetic. Agents with a lower pK_a (7.6 to 7.8), such as lidocaine, mepivacaine, prilocaine, and etidocaine, tend to have a more rapid onset than bupivacaine, tetracaine, and procaine, whose pK_a values are 8.1 to 8.6.

The rate of absorption of local anesthetics is mainly influenced by pharmacologic characteristics of specific agent (degree of vasodilation), site of

Table 32-1. Types of Local Anesthetics Commonly Used

Generic (Trade Name)	Potency	Duration (hr)	Primary Use	Adult Max Dosage (mg)/ (with Epinephrine)
Para-aminobenzoic acid esters				
Procaine (Novocain)	Low	1–1.5	Infiltration	(1000)
Chloroprocaine (Nesacaine)	Low	0.5–1	Infiltration, peripheral nerve, OB/GYN epidural	800 (1000)
Tetracaine (Pontocaine)	High	3–10	Spinal	200
Amides				
Lidocaine (Xylocaine)	Intermediate	1.5–3.5	Topical, infiltration, peripheral nerve, epidural, spinal	300 (500)
Mepivacaine (Carbocaine)	Intermediate	2–4	Infiltration, peripheral nerve, epidural	400
Bupivacaine (Marcaine)	High	3–10	Infiltration, peripheral nerve, epidural	175 (225)
Prilocaine (Citanest)	Intermediate	2–4	Infiltration, peripheral nerve, epidural	600 within 2-hr period
Etidocaine (Duranest)	High	3–10	Peripheral nerve, epidural	300 (400)

injection, total dose administered, and presence of vasoconstrictor drug in the anesthetic.[1] All local anesthetics except cocaine cause peripheral vasodilation by a direct relaxation of vascular smooth muscle. Cocaine constricts blood vessels by potentiating the action of norepinephrine, thereby preventing its own absorption through vasoconstriction. Many local anesthetic solutions will contain a vasoconstrictor such as epinephrine (1 : 100,000 or 1 : 200,000), which results in a longer lasting block and reduces systemic toxicity by decreasing vascular absorption.

REGIONAL ANESTHESIA

Topical or *surface anesthesia* refers to the placement of local anesthetic agents to induce anesthesia in the eye, in various mucous membranes, and in the skin. Local anesthetics penetrate through the intact skin to some extent, but no significant quantities are absorbed. Rapid absorption occurs when the agent is applied to mucous membranes, and may result in possible adverse systemic reactions caused by high plasma levels of the absorbed drug. Topically active local anesthetics are of two types: the nitrogen-containing compounds and the alcohols. The nitrogen-containing compounds are all secondary or tertiary amines, whose names usually end with the suffixes *-caine* or *-ane.* The non-nitrogen-containing substances are less efficacious

and more cytotoxic than those containing nitrogen. Adriani and Zepernick found that dyclonine and ethyl aminobenzoate caused no systemic reactions, were least cytotoxic, and were relatively safe.[4] They also found vasoconstrictors to have no significant effect on duration of topical anesthetics.

Infiltrative anesthesia refers to injecting the anesthetic agent intradermally or subcutaneously at or around the area to be anesthetized. Lidocaine (0.5 to 1.0 percent) or mepivacaine (1.0 percent) are frequently used for infiltrative anesthesia in podiatric medicine. Placing a wheal under or around a lesion produces analgesia for many common procedures.

A *field block* is obtained by encircling local anesthetic agents around an operative field, covering various planes of the anatomic structure. This will block all the nerves crossing these planes on route to the operative site. The injection is given proximal to the area requiring surgery. An example would be the hallux, digital, and Mayo blocks.

Depositing the local anesthetic directly near a nerve, as in the common peroneal, deep peroneal, and posterior tibial nerve blocks, results in a *peripheral nerve block.*

Spinal anesthesia or *subarachnoid block* refers to the mixing of a local anesthetic solution with the cerebrospinal fluid in the subarachnoid space. It provides the most predictable anesthesia for the least amount of drug. This type of block is best suited for surgery below the umbilicus, and is used in podiatric surgery where general anesthesia is contraindicated secondary to metabolic, respiratory, or cardiovascular disease. Anesthetic localization at a specific level of the spinal cord can be obtained by using a solution with a particular specific gravity. Most solutions have a specific gravity greater than that of spinal fluid (1.004) and are hyperbaric. Hypobaric solutions have a specific gravity less than that of spinal fluid, and isobaric solutions are of equal density.

Epidural or *peridural anesthesia* is produced by injection of a local anesthetic into the space surrounding the dura mater, within the spinal canal. It accomplishes most of the objectives desired with spinal anesthesia. The advantage of epidural over spinal anesthesia is that it avoids penetration of the subarachnoid space and possible complications (i.e., post–spinal anesthesia headache, hypotension, urinary retention, and neurologic sequelae). It differs in the larger volume of local anesthetic needed, the slower onset of action, and a less predictable complete block. The contraindications to using spinal or epidural anesthesia are: when the patient is on anticoagulant therapy or has a clotting defect; hypovolemia; increased risk of contamination with skin organisms; raised intracranial pressure; active infections of the central nervous system; patient compliance problems; and chronic neuromuscular disease, peripheral neuropathy, poliomyelitis, and disseminated sclerosis.

Other options available for regional nerve block for lower extremity surgery are the sciatic and femoral nerve blocks.[5] They, along with spinal and epidural blocks, require a trained anesthesiologist or nurse anesthetist.

Intravenous Regional Anesthesia

Intravenous regional anesthesia was first described by Bier in 1908, hence the term *Bier block*.[6] Holmes improved the technique and described its usefulness in lower extremity surgery.[7] This procedure uses a double pneumatic tourniquet placed on the leg. An intravenous catheter is inserted into a dorsal vein on the foot. The lower leg is exsanguinated by elevation or elastic bandage, and the proximal tourniquet is inflated. The local anesthetic solution is injected through the catheter, which is then removed. Just prior to surgery, the distal tourniquet is inflated over the anesthetized tissue and the proximal tourniquet is deflated. Duncan et al. recommended 30 to 50 ml of 0.6 percent lidocaine (300 mg) with midcalf tourniquet pressures between 250 and 300 mm Hg for podiatric surgeries. Constant monitoring of the patient throughout the procedure is imperative because of the potential systemic complications from the intravenous anesthetic.

NERVE BLOCKS IN PODIATRY

The nerve supply to the foot is primarily from divisions of the sciatic nerve, its tibial, sural, and peroneal branches. The femoral nerve contributes

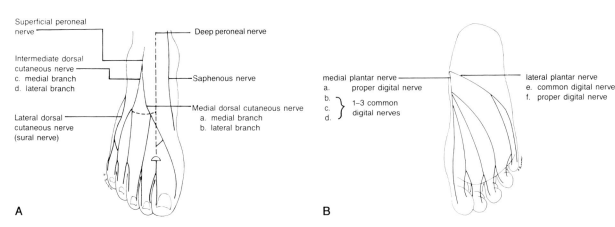

Fig. 32-2. (A) Dorsal aspect of foot with pattern of nerve innervation. **(B)** Plantar aspect of foot with branches of posterior tibial nerve, the medial and lateral plantar nerves, and their derivatives.

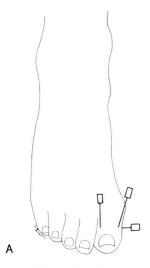

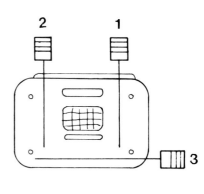

Fig. 32-3. Hallux block technique. **(A)** Injection site at base of hallux. **(B)** Cross section of area, showing three injections to block four digital nerves.

its terminal branch to the foot, the saphenous nerve. The common peroneal nerve divides into superficial and deep branches that supply the majority of the dorsum of the foot. The superficial peroneal nerve innervates all the skin on the dorsal aspect of the foot except for the first intermetatarsal interspace, which is supplied by the deep peroneal nerve; the dorsolateral aspect of the foot, which is supplied by the sural nerve and its extension, the lateral dorsal cutaneous nerve; and the medial aspect of the foot to the first metatarsophalangeal joint, which is supplied by the saphenous nerve (Fig. 32-2A). The plantar aspect of the foot is innervated by the terminal branches of the posterior tibial nerve, the medial and lateral plantar nerves (Fig. 32-2B).

Hallux Block (Fig. 32-3)

The hallux block is ideal for procedures distal to the first metatarsophalangeal joint. Inject the local anesthetic through the skin at the dorsomedial aspect of the base of the hallux and raise a wheal. Direct the needle inferiorly until the needle is palpated at the plantar aspect, then inject. Continue depositing anesthetic while removing the needle. Follow the same steps on the lateral aspect of the hallux and from medioplantar to lateroplantar. The

dorsal aspect does not usually need to be blocked because of absence of digital nerves and possible damage to the extensor tendon.

Digital Nerve Block (Fig. 32-4)

The digital nerve block is used for procedures distal to the second, third, and fourth metatarsophalangeal joints. Enter through the skin dorsally at the base of the digit, and raise a wheal. Direct the needle to the medioplantar side and inject. Deposit anesthesia while returning to the dorsal aspect. Without removing the needle, block the lateral side. This should resemble a "V" pattern. The fifth digit usually requires an additional plantar injection, similar to the hallux block, because of the common varus rotation of the toe.

Mayo Block (Fig. 32-5)

The Mayo block is used for procedures around the distal one-third of the metatarsal and metatarsophalangeal joint. It is more common for first and fifth metatarsal surgery. The goal is to deposit a ring of local anesthetic around the metatarsal, covering the nerve supply on all four quadrants. This may be done with three injections.

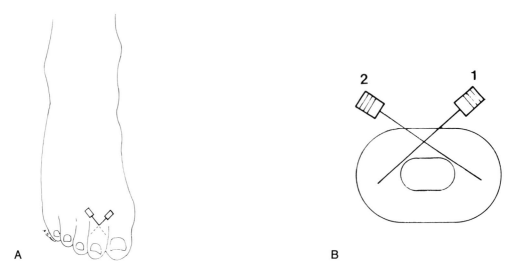

Fig. 32-4. Digital block technique. **(A)** Injection site at base of second digit. **(B)** Cross section of area, showing one injection for block.

Common Peroneal Nerve Block
(Fig. 32-6)

To produce a common peroneal nerve block, first identify the common peroneal nerve as it becomes more superficial at the proximal lateral fibular head. Usually the nerve can be palpated by rolling the fingers against the fibular head. Insert the needle through the skin at the proximal lateral fibular head. Manipulate the needle until a parethesia like a shooting, electric pain to some portion of the foot is described by the patient; this will assure a more accurate block. The anesthetic is deposited after aspiration. If the block is complete a temporary foot-drop is induced. It is important not to let the patient walk unassisted because of ankle instability.

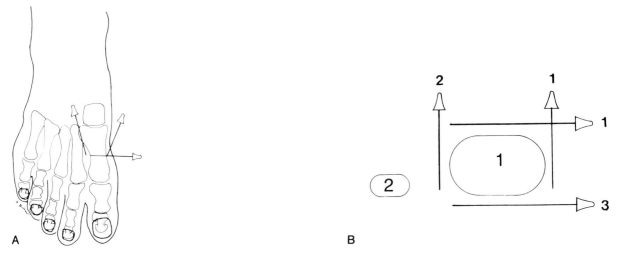

Fig. 32-5. Mayo block technique. **(A)** Injection site at midshaft of first metatarsal. **(B)** Cross section through midshaft of first and second metatarsals showing three injection sites.

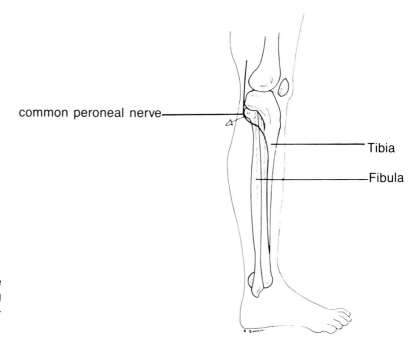

Fig. 32-6. Common peroneal nerve block. Lateral view of lower leg showing course of nerve as it becomes more superficial at proximal head of fibula.

Superficial and Deep Peroneal Nerve Block (Fig. 32-7)

Because of the variability in anatomy of the superficial peroneal nerve and its branches, the best way to assure a complete block is to raise a wheal of local anesthetic in a ringlike fashion across the dor- sum of the foot or more proximally at the ankle region. The deep peroneal nerve can be blocked after clinically identifying the tendon of the extensor hallucis longus, the extensor digitorum longus, and the dorsalis pedis artery at the level of the anterior ankle. The deep peroneal nerve runs along with the dorsalis pedis artery. The needle is in-

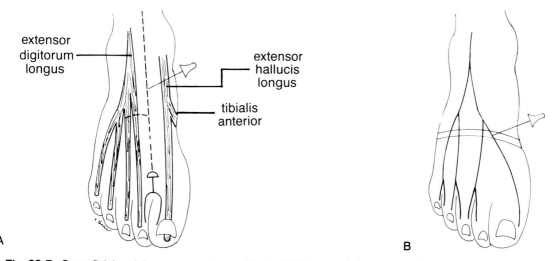

Fig. 32-7. Superficial and deep peroneal nerve block. **(A)** Course of deep peroneal nerve in between extensor hallucis and digitorium longus tendons. **(B)** Superficial peroneal block achieved by raising wheal across foot.

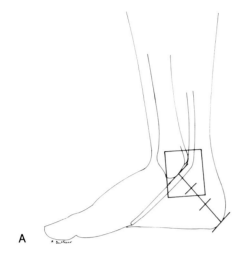
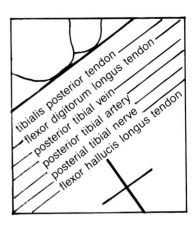

Fig. 32-8. Posterior tibial nerve block. **(A)** Medial ankle divided into thirds with vascular bundle located in first third. **(B)** Close-up of structures passing through area. Note that nerve is lateral and deep to posterior tibial artery.

serted in between the extensor hallucis longus and the most medial tendon of the extensor digitorum longus and, after aspiration, the local anesthetic is deposited.

Posterior Tibial Nerve Block
(Fig. 32-8)

The posterior tibial nerve is the largest terminal branch of the sciatic nerve. The sciatic nerve divides into the common peroneal nerve and the posterior tibial nerve at the distal one-third of the thigh. The tibial nerve courses between the two heads of the gastrocnemius muscle, medially along the Achilles tendon, and deep to the flexor retinaculum, dividing into medial and lateral plantar nerves. The technique is to clinically map out the area between the medial malleolus and the medial calcaneous, dividing it into thirds. Usually the posterior tibial nerve lies within the neurovascular bundle of the first third. The nerve is located lateral and deep to the posterior tibial artery. First, palpate for the arterial pulse and insert the needle at this level. Manipulate the needle until the patient describes a paresthesia, then aspirate and inject. With a complete block the plantar aspect of the foot should be anesthetized. The posterior tibial, superficial and deep peroneal nerve blocks together constitute an *ankle block.*

Sural and Saphenous Nerve Blocks

The sural nerve is formed by the union of the medial sural cutaneous branch of the tibial nerve and the peroneal anastomotic branch of the lateral sural cutaneous branch of the common peroneal nerve at the middle third of the leg. The sural nerve accompanies the small saphenous vein lateral to the Achilles tendon, passes inferior to the lateral malleolus, and continues on as the lateral dorsal cutaneous nerve. The saphenous nerve is the longest branch of the femoral nerve. It runs along the medial side of the leg with the great saphenous vein, passes superior to the medial malleolus, and extends to the medial aspect of the first metatarsophalangeal joint. Although the sural and saphenous nerves contribute to sensation on the medial and lateral aspects of the lower leg and foot, they are not usually addressed as single units for nerve block. A Mayo block or superficial peroneal nerve block may be used to include the area innervated by the sural or saphenous nerves.

HYPERSENSITIVITY AND TOXICITY

Hypersensitivity to local anesthetics is generally rare. The ester-type local anesthetic has a greater likelihood of reactions than do the amide agents. Multiple-dose vials of some amide agents contain preservatives, such as methylparaben in mepivacaine, that might be responsible for allergic reactions. Because of the similar chemical structure of certain antihistamines to local anesthetics, they have been used on patients who have shown hypersensitivity reactions to all the conventional local anesthetic agents.

Local anesthetic *toxicity* mainly affects three organ systems: the central nervous, cardiovascular, and respiratory systems. Most local anesthetics, when approaching their toxic dosages, manifest clinical symptoms of central nervous system stimulation: apprehension, disorientation, giddiness, lightheadedness, muscle twitching, tinnitus, and verbosity. Also, sleepiness, a sensation of cold, a feeling of pressure on the forehead, numbness of lips and tongue, and difficulty in talking are symptoms of local anesthetic toxicity.[9] Further increases in anesthetic level can lead to convulsions and respiratory distress. Most local anesthetics will cause arteriolar dilatation, but cardiovascular changes are seen at high systemic concentrations, and central nervous system symptoms precede them. The primary site of action is the myocardium, where decreases in electrical excitability, conduction rate, and force of contraction occur. Thus, it is important to be aware of the initial signs of approaching toxicity and prevent such serious consequences.

REFERENCES

1. Covino BG: Local anesthesia. N Engl J Med 286:975, 1972
2. DeJong RH, Wagman IH: Physiological mechanisms of peripheral nerve block by local anesthetics. Anesthesiology 24:684, 1963
3. Covino BG: Pharmacology of local anesthetics. Resident and Staff Physician 28:60, 1982
4. Adriani J, Zepernick R: Clinical effectiveness of drugs used for topical anesthesia. JAMA 188:711, 1964
5. Bridenbaugh LD: Regional anesthesia for surgery of the extremities. Clin Anesth 2:193, 1969
6. Bier A: Uber einen neuen weg localanasthesie en den gleidmassen zu erzeugen. Arch Klin Chir 86:1007, 1908
7. Holmes CMcK: Intravenous regional anesthesia. Lancet 1:245, 1963
8. Duncan GS, Quam S, Hetherington VJ: The use of intravenous regional anesthesia in podiatric surgery. J Foot Surg 25:411, 1986
9. Englesson S, Matousec M: Central nervous system effects of local anesthetic agents. Br J Anaesth 47:241, 1975

SELECTED READINGS

DiPalma JR: Basic Pharmacology in Medicine. 2nd Ed. Chap. 7. McGraw-Hill Book Company, New York, 1976
Ritchie JM, Greene NM: p. 302. In Gilman AG, Goodman LS (eds): The Pharmacological Basis of Therapeutics. Macmillan Publishing Company, New York, 1985

Digital Surgery

33

Rodney L. Tomczak, D.P.M.

ANATOMY AND BIOMECHANICS

In order to surgically approach digital deformities the pathophysiology must be understood along with the thorough knowledge of anatomy and the biomechanics of the lesser toes. The digits consist of the phalanges, the extrinsic muscles, an extensor apparatus, and the associated arteries, nerves, veins, and lymphatics.

Phalanges

The phalanges are the most distal part of the skeleton of the foot. Each digit consists of a proximal, middle (intermediate), and distal phalanx, except for the fifth toe, which may have a fusion of the middle and distal phalanges, and the first toe, which has only a proximal and distal phalanx. The phalanges are miniature long bones that have heads, shafts, and bases. The edges of the articular surfaces of the heads of the proximal and middle phalanges mark the sites for capsular attachments, and the small tubercles found on the sides of the heads serve for the attachments of the collateral ligaments. The capsule also attaches along a narrow grove that is just anterior to the articular surface of each base of the proximal, middle, and distal pha-

langes and is found on the medial and lateral sides of each base. Tubercles are present for the attachments of the collateral ligaments.[1]

Extrinsic Muscles

The extrinsic muscles of the lesser digits arise in the leg and insert into the phalanges. They are the extensor digitorum longus and flexor digitorum longus. The extensor digitorum longus muscle originates from the lateral edge of the tibia, medial surface of the fibula, and interosseous membrane in the anterior intramuscular system. As the muscle passes distally it becomes more tendinous and courses deep to the extensor retinaculum. At the level of the inferior extensor retinaculum the tendon splits into four tendons that at the metatarsophalangeal joint give off multiple lateral fibrous extensions that unite plantarly to encircle the proximal phalanx. The tendons pass distally to attach to the middle and distal phalanges. Each tendon splits into three slips at the dorsum of the shaft of the proximal phalanx. The central slip attaches to the base of the middle phalanx while the lateral slips reunite to form the terminal slips attaching to the base of the distal phalanx (Fig. 33-1). The extensor digitorum longus muscle functions in aiding dorsiflexion of the lesser toes during the swing phase of gait and at heel contact.[2]

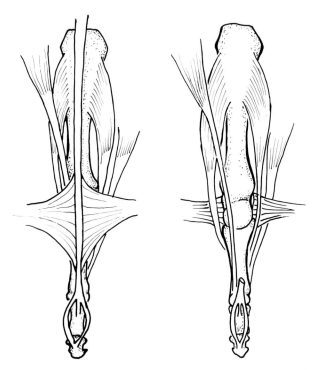

Fig. 33-1. Tendon splitting into three slips at the dorsum of the shaft of the proximal phalanx.

During the propulsive phase of gait the extensor digitorum longus acts to stabilize the proximal phalanx against the metatarsal heads to prepare for foot lift and dorsiflex the metatarsophalangeal joint.[3]

The flexor digitorum longus arises from the posterior surface of the tibia and the adjacent intramuscular septum. This muscle passes distally, narrowing to a tendon that slides in a groove of the medial malleolus under the medial inferior flexor retinaculum. It then passes anteriorly on the plantar aspect of the foot, where it splits into four tendons. Each tendon inserts into the base of the distal phalanx on the plantar surface. Here it functions to plantar flex the distal interphalangeal joint during the stance phase of gait. It is important to remember that the extrinsic muscles of the lesser digits also function across the ankle, subtalar, and midtarsal joints.

Intrinsic Muscles

The intrinsic muscles affecting the lesser digits are the extensor digitorum brevis, flexor digitorum brevis, the interosseous and lumbricale muscles, and the quadratus plantae. Also included is the flexor digiti quinti brevis and abductor digiti minimi muscles that act on the fifth digit.

The extensor digitorum brevis muscle is the only intrinsic muscle on the dorsum of the foot. This thin muscle mainly arises from the dorsal lateral aspect of the calcaneous. It passes distally and medially and splits into four smaller muscle bellies that give way to four tendons. The most medial of the tendons attaches to the base of the proximal phalanx of the hallux and therefore is named the extensor hallucis brevis. The other three insert into the lateral sides of the tendons of the extensor digitorum longus to the second, third, and fourth toes, usually just distal to the metatarsophalangeal joint of these digits (Fig. 33-2). There is no tendinous slip of the extensor digitorum brevis to the fifth digit. The extensor digitorum brevis muscle works in concert with the hood apparatus of the extensor expansion to create dorsiflexion of the proximal phalanx at the metatarsophalangeal joint via the sling mechanism.[1]

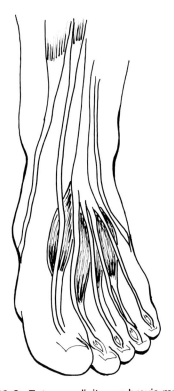

Fig. 33-2. Extensor digitorum brevis muscle.

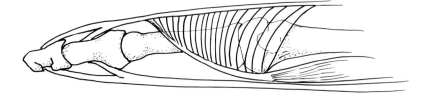

Fig. 33-3. The lumbricales.

The flexor digitorum brevis muscle is found in the first layer of the plantar surface of the foot. It originates from the medial process of the calcaneal tuberosity and splits into four muscle bellies that give way to the tendinous slips for insertion. At the level of the proximal phalanx of each of the lesser toes, each of the tendinous slips divides into two slips, allowing the flexor digitorum longus muscle to pass through on its way to the distal phalanx. The flexor digitorum brevis tendons reunite to insert on the shaft of the middle phalanx of each of the lesser toes.[1]

The flexor digitorum brevis along with the flexor digitorum longus create a significant plantar flexory force at the interphalangeal joints. However, the flexors primarily function during the stance phase of gait. This force during stance may be a retrograde force on the metatarsophalangeal joint to cause dorsiflexion. This occurs because the phalanges cannot be plantarflexed through the ground. When the flexor digitorum brevis is the primary plantar flexory force it creates a strong plantar flexion at the proximal interphalangeal joint in an absence of plantar flexion at the distal phalangeal joint; this may lead to a contracted toe with the distal interphalangeal joint hyperextended. When the flexor digitorum longus is the primary plantar-flexory force it may create plantar flexion of the distal interphalangeal joint and a strong secondary plantar-flexory force of the proximal interphalangeal joint.[4]

The word *lumbricus* means "earth worm" in Latin. The lumbricales are small wormlike muscles, of which there are four, and belong to the second layer of muscles in the plantar surface of the foot. The lumbricales arise from the tendons of the flexor digitorus longus and insert on the medial sides of the extensor wings of the extensor expansions of the lesser toes into the medial side of the base of the proximal phalanx. These smaller muscles function to flex the metatarsophalangeal joints

and extend the proximal and distal interphalangeal joints of the lesser digits (Fig. 33-3). These muscles have not as yet been accurately recorded electromyographically in gait. Therefore, their function in gait is theoretical. During the swing phase of gait the lumbricales probably function to stabilize and create an early end range of motion at the metatarsophalangeal joint. This allows the extensor digitorum longus force to be directed at the ankle joint at an early and effective time during gait. In theory, then, the lumbricales and extensor muscles function in unison.

These muscles then act during the swing phase and have a somewhat inhibitory force on contraction of the toes.

Dorsal and plantar interossei muscles are found in the fourth layer of muscles on the plantar aspect of the foot. Two heads from adjacent sides of adjacent metatarsal bones serve as the origins for the dorsal interossei, of which there are four. They are usually bipenate. The plantar aspect of the proximal phalanx and its extensor expansion serve as the insertion points of the central tendon that has been formed by the convergence of these two heads. This is somewhat controversial and some authors seem to disagree with the attachments.[4-6] The first dorsal interossei inserts medially, and the second, third, and fourth insert laterally into the second, third, and fourth digits, respectively. There are no dorsal interossei to the fifth digit. These muscles serve to abduct the toes from the midline of the foot. Since two dorsal interossei insert into the second toe, one medially and one laterally, they serve to move the second toe both medially and laterally. Each plantar interosseus has one site of origin. They are therefore termed unipennate muscles and originate from the shafts of the third, fourth, and fifth metatarsals on the medial aspect. The plantar interossei insert into the extensor expansion, metatarsophalangeal joint capsule, and proximal phalanx on the medial side of the digit from which the muscle originates on the metatarsal shaft, namely the third, fourth, and fifth metatarsals. Manter[5] did not find attachments into the extensor expansion; however, Sarrafian and Tuposian,[6] in a unique anatomic investigation of the extensor apparatus of the toes, did find insertion of the interossei into the extensor slings of the extensor expansion. The plantar interossei serve to adduct the third, fourth, and fifth toes toward the midline of the foot.

The flexor digiti quinti brevis is a small, fleshy muscle found in the third layer of the plantar aspect of the foot. This is on the lateral aspect of the forefoot. It arises from the base of the fifth metatarsal and the tendon of the sheath of the peroneus longus. It runs parallel to the fifth metatarsal and inserts on the plantar lateral aspect of the proximal phalanx of the fifth digit, where it serves to abduct and flex the fifth toe.

The reason the lumbricales and interossei muscles have been discussed is that as a group they function to stabilize the toe so that the actions of the flexor digitorum longus and flexor digitorum brevis muscles, when contracting in the stance phase of gait, do not serve to contract the lesser digits. When the interossei contract because there is force applied to both they serve to move the toes to adduct, plantar flex, and abduct and plantar flex so the toes become stabilized in the transverse plane. The weak lumbricales and interossei can certainly be a cause for hammering deformities of the lesser digits. When the intrinsic muscles are overpowered a hammer toe deformity, a claw toe deformity, or a mallet toe deformity may result (Fig. 33-4). In the hammer toe deformity the flexor digitorum brevis is contracted without contraction of the flexor digitorum longus past the proximal interphalangeal joint. When there is contraction of the flexor digitorum longus tendon past the proximal interphalangeal joint along with contraction of the flexor digitorum brevis the classic claw toe results. When there is strong unopposed contraction of the flexor digitorum longus without contraction of the flexor digitorum brevis the mallet toe deformity, in which there is only contracture of the distal interphalangeal joint, results.

The clinical picture presented in the classic hammer toe deformity is the proximal phalanx dorsiflexed on the metatarsal head with a plantarly prominent metatarsal head that may be painful, especially after the contracture has become fixed and

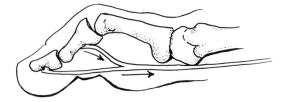

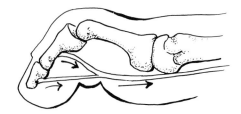

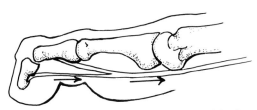

Fig. 33-4. Causes of hammering deformities of the lesser digits.

rigid. The middle phalanx of the hammer toe deformity is plantar flexed and when the distal phalanx becomes plantar flexed the hammer toe is then termed a claw toe deformity. In this deformity the associated findings of the hammer toe coexist with the severe plantar flexion of the distal phalanx. The picture of the mallet toe deformity is usually a straight toe with a plantar contracture of the distal phalanx at the distal interphalangeal joint.

SURGICAL CORRECTION OF LESSER TOE DEFORMITIES

Soft Tissue Procedures

When considering the soft tissue procedure for hammer toe correction it is appropriate to consider the terms *extensor substitution, flexor substitution,* and *flexor stabilization*. Extensor substitution refers to that phenomenon where the extensor digitorum longus muscle serves to dorsiflex the ankle. If the foot is of a cavus type, the extensor digitorum longus tendons are constantly pulling the metatarsophalangeal joint. During the swing phase of gait these extensors act to dorsiflex the foot and create even more pull on the metatarsophalangeal joint, causing a dorsal contracture of the proximal phalanx. This can also be caused by inadequate dorsiflexion of the ankle as a result of a short Achilles tendon or an osseous abnormality leading to ankle equinus. In extensor substitution the lumbricales have lost their ability to stabilize the metatarsophalangeal joints. In flexor substitution and flexor stabilization the interossei have lost their ability to stabilize the metatarsophalangeal joints. In flexor substitution there is usually evidence of a supinated foot, whereas in flexor stabilization the foot is generally pronated. Root et al. thought that the pronated foot caused the quadratus plantae to not pull the flexor apparatus laterally, resulting in hammering and varus rotations of the fourth and fifth toes.[3] They also believe that flexor substitution in the supinated foot is a result of the weak triceps surae and that the posterior muscle groups of the leg and the long extrinsic muscles are contracted longer during the gait cycle and cause contraction of the digits. These are extremely important considerations when contemplating a soft tissue procedure. It makes little sense to perform extensor tenotomies when flexor stabilization or flexor substitution is the primary cause of the hammer deformity.

Proper clinical examination and accurate problem-solving techniques to determine etiology are extremely important in the choice of proper procedures.

Flexor Tendon Transfers

In 1947, Girdlestone described treatment of flexible hammer toes by transfer of the flexor digitorum longus and flexor digitorum brevis tendons into the extensor hood over the proximal phalanx.[7] The purpose of the procedure was to allow the flexors to stabilize the metatarsophalangeal joint when there were weak intrinsic muscles. In 1951, Tailor described the tendon transfers along with

capsulotomy at the metatarsophalangeal joint and plantar capsulotomies at the proximal and distal interphalangeal joints.[8] He also suggested lengthening of the extensor digitorum longus tendons. In 1980, Kuwada and Dockery described a procedure where the flexor digitorum longus tendon is passed through the neck of the proximal phalanx from plantar to dorsal and sutured into the capsule at the proximal interphalangeal joint.[9]

This procedure can only be used in a dynamic or flexible hammer toe. This can be determined by the Kelikian pushup test, where pressure is applied to the metatarsal head plantarly and the foot loaded. A flexible hammer toe is one in which the toe then straightens. Not only is there reduction of the plantar flexion at the proximal interphalangeal joint, but there is also reduction of the dorsoflexion of the proximal phalanx at the metatarsophalangeal joint. It is the action of the long flexor that keeps the proximal phalanx from dorsiflexing.

The procedure for flexor tendon transfer is usually accomplished through two incisions. One incision is generally made on the plantar lateral or plantar medial aspect of the toe, where the long flexor is severed at the distal interphalangeal joint. The long flexor is then split into medial and lateral slips that are then transferred dorsally and are sewn into the dorsal aspect of the distal portion of the proximal phalanx at the extensor expansion.[10] Although this type of procedure works in flexible hammer toes, it appears to have no real advantage over arthrodesis of the digits and in fact may result in certain damage to the soft tissues because of the amount of soft tissue manipulation required to correctly perform the procedure.

Osseous Correction of Digital Deformities

The first popular recorded operation for a nonflexible hammer toe deformity was reported by Post.[11] His correction was essentially the removal of the head of the proximal phalanx without arthrodesis. Of course this is the most common procedure in use today. Six years later Terrier's procedure involved the resection of the head of the proximal phalanx as in the Post procedure, but he added resection of the base of the middle phalanx.[12] Again this was an arthroplasty with no attempt at arthrodesis. In 1910 Soule utilized the plantar approach with resection of the base of the middle phalanx and a partial resection of the head of the proximal phalanx.[13] Using plaster of Paris the toe was allowed to fuse. Between 1931 and 1938 three researchers introduced peg-in-hole operations. Tierney described an operation in which the hole was in the dorsal aspect of the head of the proximal phalanx.[14] The peg was fashioned from the shaft of the proximal phalanx. The head was then rotated proximally and plantarly and a new joint was formed for the proximal interphalangeal joint. Higgs, in 1931, described an operation in which the head of the proximal phalanx was fashioned into a sharp point and inserted into a hole in the base of the middle phalanx.[15] This fusion took place without any external fixation. Young's procedure was essentially the same as Higgs' procedure; however, the proximal phalanx was not sharpened into a point, but rounded to more approximate the shape of a bullet.[16] It was then inserted into the base of the middle phalanx. The first use of K wire to fuse the proximal interphalangeal joint was made by Taylor in 1940.[17] Taylor felt that in order to obtain a successful result from an operation on a hammer toe:

1. The flexion contracture of the proximal interphalangeal joint must be overcome and this was best done by an arthrodesis of this joint in good position.
2. The fixation of the arthrodesis must be maintained until bone union has occurred.
3. The toe must be plantar flexed at the metatarsophalangeal joint. This position can be obtained by tenotomizing the taut, distended tendons and by maintaining the toe in the plantar-flexed position by means of adhesive strapping for 3 weeks.

Reflection on the above principals by Taylor reveals that the goals of his operation still hold true today and that indeed, should all these be achieved, the correction would give outstanding results.

Osseous Correction of Hammer Toe Without Arthrodesis

By far the most popular osseous correction of hammer toe is simple head resection of the proxi-

mal phalanx. This procedure is generally effected by means of a linear incision over the proximal interphalangeal joint extending over the metatarsophalangeal joint, where release of soft tissue structures resulting in dorsiflexion of the proximal phalanx is often necessary. The procedure at the head of the proximal phalanx is often performed by surgeons utilizing two semi-elliptical incisions that are in a transverse plane over the head of the proximal phalanx and base of the middle phalanx. Over the years some have advocated that these two incisions not be used for fear that the neurovascular bundles on the medial and lateral aspects of the toes could be placed in jeopardy. In actuality there appears to be no substantial evidence that proper care and technique with the two semi-elliptical incisions will result in vascular compromise. The major problem, however, is that should the proximal phalanx not reduce on the metatarsal head a second incision is required over the metatarsophalangeal joint. The advantage of the semi-elliptical incisions is that this approach in effect removes the heloma over the proximal interphalangeal joint, and when the incision is closed it aids in dorsiflexing the distal toe and removing extra skin. Once the incision has been made through the skin the extensor tendon may then be tenotomized in a transverse fashion along with freeing of the medial and lateral collateral ligaments and plantar attachments. It is also possible to free the tendon from its attachments dorsally and retract the tendon medially or laterally without severing the tendon. Another approach is to incise the tendon in a linear fashion, thereby separating it into medial and lateral portions, but not transecting it and thereby exposing the joint area.

The head of the proximal phalanx is then delivered into the incision site and is usually resected with sharp bone cutters or power equipment. The amount of bone to be resected is a clinical judgment that is determined at the time of surgery; however, if too much bone is removed the digit may become flail and if too little is removed, inadequate reduction is achieved.

The tendon, if severed, is then repaired with an absorbable suture and the skin closed. At the conclusion of surgery the toe is bandaged in a plantar-flexed position at the metatarsophalangeal joint and in a straight manner at the proximal interphalangeal joint. This bandaging is often required for up to 6 weeks. It is not uncommon for the patient to notice edema for extended periods postoperatively.

The same procedure can generally be carried out at the distal interphalangeal joint should correction be required there.

Arthrodesis of the Interphalangeal Joints

By fusing the interphalangeal joints the digit becomes rigid, allowing the long flexor and long extensor to function where the intrinsic muscles stabilizing the metatarsophalangeal joint have ceased to work effectively.

Fusion of the toe allows for a toe that is not too short, since very little cartilage is removed as is done in arthroplasty, and assures that the toe is not "floppy." The major drawback in this procedure is a K wire protruding through the distal phalanx that may serve as a portal for infection even with the most conscientious care. Because there is no flexibility at the interphalangeal joints the patient may sometimes complain of stiffness.

The procedure itself is closely related to arthroplasty. The skin incision may again be two semielliptical incisions or a linear incision stretching from the base of the middle phalanx to the metatarsophalangeal joint if soft tissue release is necessary. Once the skin incision is made the surgeon must choose whether to transect the extensor tendon in a transverse fashion at the interphalangeal joint or to linearly incise the tendon or to free the tendon dorsally and retract it medially or laterally. Having accomplished this, the collateral ligaments and soft tissue attachments are released and the head of the proximal phalanx and the base of the middle phalanx are freed and delivered into the incision site. The articular cartilage on the head of the proximal phalanx is removed and the base of the middle phalanx is also removed. A minimum of cartilage is removed so that there is not substantial shortening of the digit and, when K wire placement has been accomplished, there will not be puckering of the skin medially and laterally. The dorsal aspects of the phalanges may have to be remodeled so that there are no bony prominences. Having accomplished this and exposing cancellous bone, a K wire is driven from the base of the middle phalanx distally out the distal phalanx and skin. Care should be taken that the K wire does not contact the nail plate or matrix. This can usually be accomplished by dorsiflexing the toe. Having driven the K wire through the distal end of the toe the tip, which is within the interphalangeal joint, is guided into the medullary canal of the proximal phalanx. The new base of the middle phalanx and head of the proximal phalanx are aligned when the K wire is driven into the proximal phalanx. Having accomplished stabilization of the toe, the wound is treated as in the arthroplasty procedure. The wire is bent to 90 degrees and cut at the distal aspect of the toe. This ensures easy removal and some area for swelling on the distal aspect of the toe. If the K wire crosses the metatarsophalangeal joint, in order to preserve soft tissue release at the metatarsophalangeal joint care must be taken that the patient does not ambulate without rigid support on the plantar aspect of the foot. This may result in bending or breaking of the K wire while weight is borne as the toes are dorsiflexed during propulsion. The patient must also be instructed in proper care of the pin track to lessen the chance of infection.

Lesser Toe Implants

Considerable experience has been gained during the past 5 or 6 years so that the use of lesser toe implants is not merely a passing fancy or anecdotal. Sgarlato et al. reported on 920 lesser toe implants.[18] Of these 920 only 7 were removed, and those because of infection. There appears to be great success in the use of these lesser toe implants.

The indications for the lesser toe implants include such conditions as flail or loose toes, failed arthroplasties, arthritic interphalangeal joints, shortened toes, digital clavei at the proximal phalangeal head, varus rotation of toes (especially fifth toes), and excessively long toes. An implant by itself does not correct all types of hammer toe deformities, and other surgical procedures, such as release of soft tissue at the metatarsophalangeal joint, may have to be included in the repair to ensure a straight toe.

The procedure for implantation does not appear to differ drastically from other arthroplasties or arthrodeses. Once the arthroplasty of the proximal interphalangeal joint is achieved the medullary

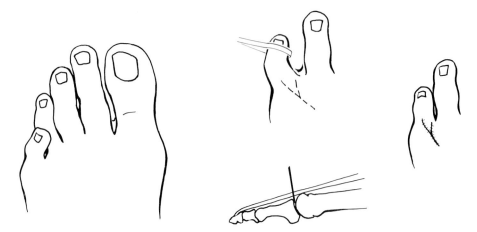

Fig. 33-5. VY procedure as described by Wilson.

canals are reamed to accept the implants. As in other implant surgery, the implants are sized and placed in the bone and the soft tissue is repaired. Aftercare, according to Sgarlato et al., appears to consist of wrapping the digit in an iodophore dressing for 2 to 3 weeks postoperatively.[18]

The advantages of the procedure are quite clear in that flexibility of the digit is better than fused toes. Also, the toe is not shortened since the implant acts as a spacer yet stabilizes the distal toe and the proximal phalanx.

Varus Deformity of the Fifth Toe

Varus deformity of the fifth toe is that condition in which the fifth toe generally overlaps the fourth toe. In an individual in whom this is manually reducible a soft tissue procedure is usually adequate. The correction most often used is the VY procedure described by Wilson.[19] The procedure is quite simple and consists of placing the fifth toe in an abducted and plantar-flexed position while a V incision is made at the base of the proximal phalanx of the fifth toe (Fig. 33-5). The extensor tendon and soft tissue of the metatarsophalangeal joint are released and as the toe is plantar flexed the skin will slide, leaving a new Y-shaped incision that is sutured in that position without repair of the capsule or tendons. This condition only works for flexible overlapping fifth toes that are manually reducible.

Should the fifth toe not be manually reducible it is usually necessary to treat this condition as a ham-

mer toe that is adducted, performing what usually appears to be a bicorrectional arthrodesis at the proximal interphalangeal joint with K wire fixation and release of soft tissue at the metatarsophalangeal joint. In extreme situations resection of the base of the proximal phalanx may be needed if there is dorsal dislocation of the proximal phalanx on the metatarsal head. Sgarlato et al., in their article on lesser toe implants, stated that they have had success in derotating varus fifth toes using the smallest implant available.[18]

REFERENCES

1. Draves D: Anatomy of the Lower Extremity. pp. 133–135. Williams & Wilkins, Baltimore, 1986
2. Close JR: Motor Function in the Lower Extremity: Analysis by Electronic Instrumentation. Charles C Thomas, Springfield, IL, 1964
3. Root M, Orien WP, Weed JH: Normal and Abnormal Function of the Foot: Clinical Biomechanics. Vol. II. Los Angeles Clinical Biomechanics Corp, Los Angeles, 1977
4. Jarret VA, Manzi JA, Green DR: Interossei in lumbracales muscles of the foot in anatomical and functional study. J Am Podiatry Assoc 70:1–13, 1980
5. Manter JT: Variations of the interosseous muscles of the human foot. Anat Rec 93:117–124, 1945
6. Sarrafian SK, Tuposian LK: Anatomy and physiology

of the extensor expansions of the toes. J Bone Joint Surg [Am] 51:669–680, 1960

7. Girdlestone GR: Charted Soc Physiother 32:167, 1947

8. Tailor RG: The treatment of claw toes by multiple transfers of flexor into extensor tendons. J Bone Joint Surg [Br] 33:4539, 1951

9. Kuwada GT, Dockery GL: Modification of the flexor tendon transfer procedure for the correction of flexible hammer toes. J Foot Surg 19:38–40, 1980

10. Sorto OA: J Am Podiatry Assoc 64:930–940, 1974

11. Post AC: Hallux valgus with displacement of the smaller toes. Med Rec 22:120–121, 1882

12. Terrier: Orteils en marteau avec durillons et bourses seremses sous-jacentes enflammes. Resection des deux Cotes, et dams la meme seance, de l'articulation phalango sha langienne. Bull Mem Soc Chir 14:624–626, 1888

13. Soule RE: Operation for the correction of hammer toe. NY Med J pp 649–650, 1910

14. Tierney A: Hammertoe, the cup and ball procedure. p. 265. In Pauchet V (ed): La Pratique Chirurgicale Illustree. 2nd Ed. Vol. 9. G. Doin and Co, Paris, 1937

15. Higgs SL: Hammer toe. Med Press 131:473–474, 1931

16. Young CS: An operation for the correction of hammer toe and claw toe. J Bone Joint Surg 20:715–719, 1938

17. Taylor RG: An operative procedure for the treatment of hammer-toe and claw toe. J Bone Joint Surg 22:608–609, 1940

18. Sgarlato TE, Carine TA, Andrews MC: Sutter lesser toe implant. J Am Podiatr Med Assoc 78:335–338, 1988

19. Wilson JN: Br J Surg 41:133–135, 1953

Lesser Metatarsal Surgery

34

Vincent J. Mandracchia, D.P.M.
Walter W. Strash, D.P.M.

Unlike hallux abductovalgus surgery, lessor metatarsal surgery does not have strict criteria with respect to various angles to determine the correct surgical procedure. Hallux valgus surgery, when proper preoperative protocol is adhered to, has predictable results. Lesser metatarsal surgery is "unpredictable surgery." The purpose of this chapter is to discuss the authors' preoperative criteria, the most common procedures utilized, and some of the more frequent complications encountered during lesser metatarsal surgery.

HISTORY OF METATARSAL SURGERY

In 1916 it was Meisenbach who treated lesions beneath the second, third, and fourth metatarsals in cavus feet by performing osteotomies 3 cm proximal to the metatarsophalangeal joint.[1] The distal fragment was displaced superiorly and the patient was casted, and Meisenbach noted that the toes "jumped in a more rectus position."

Davis[2] in 1917 performed metatarsal head resection to correct plantar protrusion, and in 1940,

Mau[3] reported the resection of trapezoidal portions of bone from the metatarsal for the correction of cavus foot deformities. One of the more radical approaches for the treatment of plantar warts occurred in 1949 when Dickson and Dively[4] performed entire digit and ray resection. DuVries[5] in 1953 advocated plantar condylectomy for the treatment of plantar verruca.[11]

McKeever[6] reported on shortening of the metatarsals for plantar keratotic lesions, and Giannestras[7] performed "step-down osteotomy," which he reported in 1958 to have excellent results in 82.5 percent of the patients in his study.[8]

In 1969, Davidson[9] performed osteoclasis on the second, third, and fourth metatarsals in a procedure very similar to Meisenbach's but at the distal metatarsal neck. The osteotomy is performed 90 degrees to the metatarsal shaft, completely through bone, and without the use of fixation. The rationale was to allow nature to determine the exact amount and degree of elevation by leaving the guesswork out of positioning. A fifth metatarsal procedure was described in this procedure on a single metatarsal or intervention. Addante[10] performed the same procedure by modifying the angle of the osteotomy from perpendicular to oblique (dorsal-proximal to plantar-distal) (Figs. 34–1 and 34–2).

811

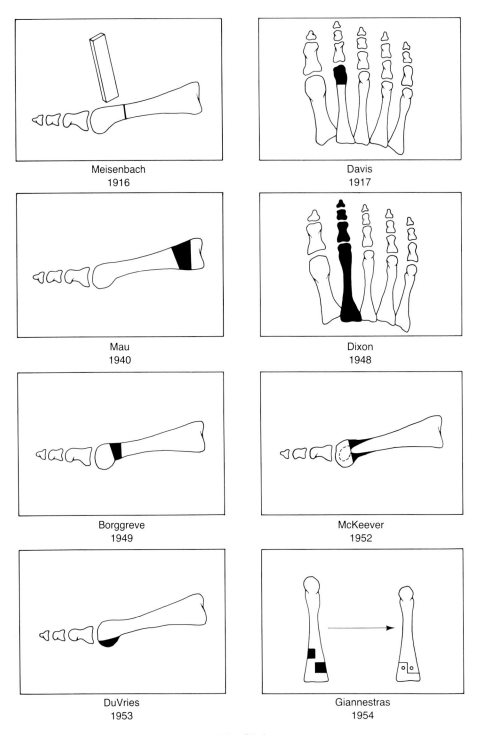

Fig. 34-1.

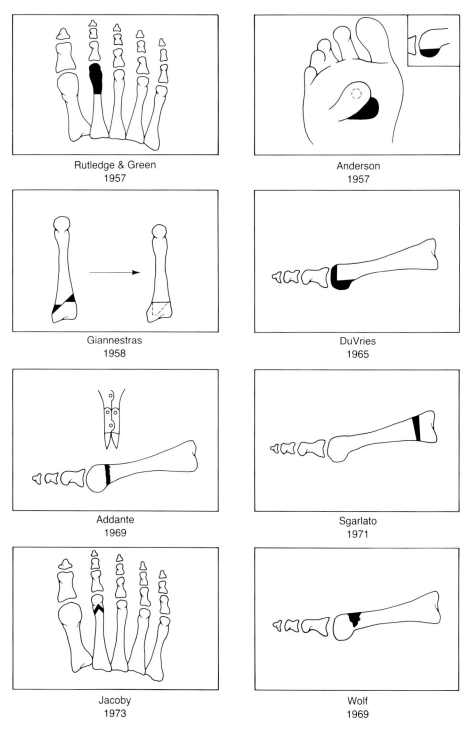

Fig. 34-2.

Jacoby,[11] in 1973, described a V-osteotomy for the correction of intractable plantar keratosis. The osteotomy is performed at the surgical neck with the apex just proximal to the articular cartilage and the arms projecting proximally 45 degrees from the apex.

Bartel[12] reported on removing a V-shaped wedge of bone from the metatarsal neck using a power roto-osteotome. He used increasing sizes of burrs to create the osteotomy.

Jimenez[13] in 1930 used a double oblique osteotomy at the surgical neck, leaving the plantar cortex intact. The osteotomy was performed with a sawblade, and closed and fixated with either a K wire or a 2.7-mm cortical screw.

INTRACTABLE PLANTAR KERATOSIS SURGERY

Because of the lack of strict surgical criteria, the success rate of intractable plantar keratosis (IPK) surgery approaches only 50 percent.

Weightbearing on the metatarsals is commonly thought to occur on the plantar condyles, usually the lateral condyle. However, the metatarsal shaft does not lie parallel to the plantar aspect of the foot, but descends at an angle of 30 to 40 degrees. Because of this angle of declination, even if the condyles were hypertrophic, they would be rotated out of the way. Therefore, weightbearing on the metatarsals occurs on the anterior one-third of the metatarsal head.

There are two basic plantar lesion types. *Discrete plantar keratosis* is usually present under the metatarsal head and is often described as a "corn inside a callus." This is the true IPK and is due to a *structural or osseous deformity.* (i.e., depressed metatarsals, abnormal metatarsal parabola, etc.). These lesions do benefit from surgical intervention.

The second type of lesion is a diffuse fibrous, shearing-type lesion. This is a diffuse tyloma and is due to an underlying positional deformity related to functional or biomechanical anomalies. This lesion does not benefit from surgery and is better remedied by biomechanical treatment.

The following underlying *structural deformities* lead to IPK formation:

1. Plantar-flexed metatarsals
2. Hypertrophied condyles – deformed metatarsal heads, as seen in degenerative joint disease
3. Abnormal metatarsal length or pattern
4. Iatrogenically induced lesions
5. Hallux abductovalgus (HAV) – causative lesions
6. Degenerative joint disease (DJD).

Management

Plantar-Flexed Metatarsals

For plantar-flexed metatarsals, the following procedures are possible management choices: (1) dorsiflexory wedge osteotomy (DFWO), (2) V-osteotomy, (3) cartilaginous articulation preservation procedure (CAPP), (4) osteoclasis, (5) condylectomy, and (6) DFWO (at head of metatarsal).

Three radiographic views of the foot should be taken. The dorsoplantar, lateral, and axial views are the most useful. The axial x-ray projection allows one to determine which metatarsal is plantar flexed very easily. It should be noted, however, that the first and fifth metatarsal heads should sit slightly higher than the second, third, and fourth metatarsals. This is because of the retrograde plantar flexory force being exerted on the first and fifth metatarsals while shooting an axial projection.

Hypertrophied Condyles

For hypertrophied condyles, the following procedures are possible management choices: (1) condylectomy (cheilectomy), and (2) partial metatarsal head section.

Deformed or malformed metatarsal heads are common. This is seen in Freiberg's disease, which is an osteochondrosis of the second metatarsal head. X-ray evaluation shows flattening of the metatarsal head with osteophytic lipping. The joint is narrowed and the metatarsal head is shortened.

Degenerative joint disease of the metatarso phalangeal joints can also cause hypertrophic bony growth above the head of the metatarsal and a resultant IPK plantarly.

Abnormal Metatarsal Length Pattern

For metatarsals with an abnormal length pattern, the following procedures are possible management choices: (1) chevron, (2) CAPP, and (3) peg and hole metatarsal shortening.

The normal length pattern is second>first >third>fourth>fifth; occasionally the second is equal to the first in length. The normal metatarsal protrusion angle of the first and second metatarsals should be approximately plus or minus 2 mm.

The metatarsal break angle is normally 142.5 degrees. This is determined by a line connecting distal points on the first and second metatarsal heads and a line connecting distal points on the second and fifth metatarsal heads.

When evaluating metatarsal length, systemic disorders such as pseudohypoparathyroidism must be considered when a short second or fourth metatarsal is encountered particularly the fourth metatarsal.

Iatrogenically Induced Lesions

For iatrogenically induced lesions, the following procedures are possible management choices: (1) biomechanical accommodation, and (2) second surgery (corrective).

Transfer lesions secondary to metatarsal osteotomies are the most frequent iatrogenically induced lesions. Lesions under the second metatarsal secondary to a first metatarsal head procedure can also occur if the capital fragment has been dorsiflexed on the metatarsal shaft intraoperatively. A similar lesion develops under the fourth metatarsal if the capital fragment on the head of the fifth metatarsal has been dorsiflexed during surgery for a Tailor's bunion.

HAV-Causative Lesions

For HAV-causative lesions, management consists of addressing the HAV with an appropriate surgical procedure, and then performing surgery on the second metatarsal (possible procedures include the V-osteotomy and condylectomy).

As the metatarsus adductus angle increases, more and more weight is borne by the second metatarsal and a lesion under the second metatarsal eventually develops. The same is also true of a hy-

permobile first ray. This causes an intermittent-type pressure that yields hypertrophy. The result is hypertrophy of the metatarsal condyles leading to a submetatarsal IPK lesion.

Degenerative Joint Disease

For degenerative joint disease, the following procedures are possible management choices: (1) metatarsal head resection, and (2) total joint implant.

Complaints of joint pain and pain upon range of motion during physical examination may be an indication of degenerative joint disease. Further evidence of this may be identified upon x-ray examination of the feet.

Choice of Procedure

According to a review of osteotomies for IPK at Northlake Hospital, the procedures most frequently performed were the percutaneous metaphyseal osteotomy, distal V-osteotomy, partial metatarsal head resection, total metatarsal head resection, osteoclasis, extension osteotomy, and extension osteoarthropathy.[14] Hatcher et al.[15] reported that the overall success rate for proximal osteotomy (extensor osteotomy, extensor osteoarthrotomy) was 46 percent, that for distal osteotomy (percutaneous metaphyseal osteotomy, distal metaphyseal osteotomy, V-osteotomy, and osteoclasis) was 61 percent, and that for joint arthroplasty (partial head, total head) was 53 percent. The above results emphasize to the surgeon that the proximal osteotomy is not recommended for IPK correction except in specific circumstances because of the increased surgical difficulty and the generally protracted postoperative healing period. It is also believed that joint arthroplasty procedures should not be performed unless pathology at the metatarsophalangeal joint is present. By choosing this procedure, the surgeon limits his or her surgical options should a second procedure be required for a transfer lesion or recurrence. The surgical procedures of choice, then, are the neck osteotomies.

Although single osteotomies are preferred by most surgeons, it is believed by these authors that the more lesser metatarsal osteotomies performed on a single foot the better the result. Single osteotomies appear to have a significantly lower percentage of acceptable results than a combination of procedures.[15] It is thought that three reasons exist for this:

1. Multiple lesions tend to be more diffuse, whereas isolated lesions are more likely discreet and intractable.
2. Isolated lesions are in all likelihood a structural problem, whereas diffuse ones are functional in nature. If the lesion is found to be functional in nature, the surgeon should consider the use of biomechanical devices as an adjunct to surgery.
3. The potential for transfer lesion is obviously decreased if the adjacent metatarsal, under which the transfer might take place, is also osteotomized. As a consequence prophylactic surgery of adjacent metatarsal heads is advocated if there is any evidence of another lesions starting at those locations.[15,16] We also advocate multiple osteomies in this case.

The most common or "in vogue" osteotomy being performed today is the V-osteotomy. What ever osteotomy is chosen, some basic principles must be considered, such as:

1. Osteotomy placement—metaphyseal bone is the best healing bone.
2. Adequate bone-to-bone contact.
3. Lever arm—procedures done at the base have a longer lever arm, thus creating a greater amount of motion at this point when compared to procedures done at the neck.

SURGICAL PROCEDURES

Head Osteotomies

CAP Procedure

The CAP procedures was described by Suppan for shortening the metatarsal while preserving the articular cartilage. The metatarsal is osteotomized at the condylar groove, just proximal to the articular set. The metatarsal stump is shortened as desired. Because of the distal metaphyseal location of this procedure, it is also necessary to resect the plantar condyles. The area is fixated with a K wire or left alone. The CAPP may also be slightly dorsally relocated to correct for a plantar-flexed metatarsal or a hypertrophied plantar condyle.

The most common postoperative complication with the CAPP is degenerative arthritis. The procedure is very difficult to accomplish and is only successful in the most skilled hands.

V-Osteotomy

Originally the V-osteotomy was devised because of the problems that existed with postoperative medial or lateral deviation of the capital fragment following an osteoclasis (transverse osteotomy) (Fig. 34–3). The "V" is performed at the surgical neck or slightly distally depending upon the surgeon's preference. The "V" is made with the two arms forming a 45 degree angle with the apex ex-

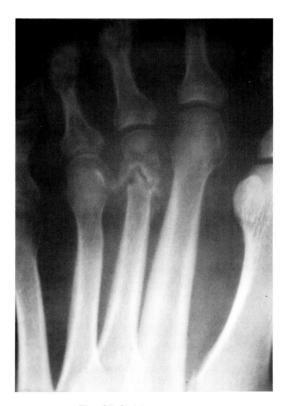

Fig. 34-3. V-osteotomy.

tending distally. Also, the cuts may be slightly angulated from dorsal-distal to plantar-proximal to control the amount of dorsal migration. Postoperatively the patient ambulates with a surgical shoe, allowing the capital fragment to relocate itself in a more dorsal attitude.

Modified Waterman Procedure

This procedure was originally described by Waterman for treatment of hallux limitus/hallux rigidus deformity due to metatarsus elevatus of the first metatarsal. The Waterman procedure, also known as the "tilt osteotomy," is actually a dorsiflexory wedge osteotomy just proximal to the cartilage of the first metatarsal head, leaving the plantar cortex intact. Then, the capital fragment is tilted up. This procedure could be done with a Bonnie-Kessel procedure, which is a dorsiflexory wedge osteotomy done at the base of the proximal phalanx.

At the head of the lesser metatarsals small, 2-mm width osteotomies are made with a Stryker blade. With gentle pressure the metatarsal head is tilted up until a greenstick fracture occurs at the plantar cortex. In a study at Northlake Hospital, multiple second, third, and fourth metatarsal osteotomies were done for diffuse plantar tyloma with excellent results being achieved.

Metarsal Head Resection

In total metatarsal head resection, the head of the metatarsal is completely removed, at a 15 degree angle in a dorsal-distal to plantar-proximal attitude ensuring that the plantar condyles are not remaining (Fig. 34–4 and 34–5).

A modified head resection is accomplished by removing only part of the metatarsal head; part of the articular cartilage is left dorsally and the plantar condyles are removed. The partial metatarsal head resection is done for subluxed metatarsophalangeal joints. The partial metatarsal head resection seems to produce better results than the removal of the base of the proximal phalanx. When the base of the proximal phalanx is removed, instability at the joint occurs. The hood ligament and the soft tissue structures should be left intact for more stability. Degenerative arthritis is already occurring at a subluxed joint, so the risk of causing it

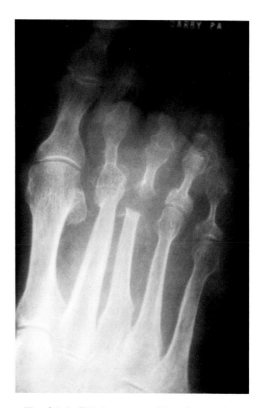

Fig. 34-4. Third metatarsal head resection.

by partial metatarsal head resection is not a consideration in this case.

It must be kept in mind that when the head is removed the weight-bearing surface distal to the remaining shaft is being taken away. This sets up the possibility of transfer lesions medial or lateral to the resected metatarsal head. The opportunity for proximal or distal toe contractures also exists. When a head resection is performed, soft tissue interposition of the capsule or hourglassing helps fill in the void. Total implant replacement is a viable option when metatarsal head resection are performed.

Plantar Condylectomy

DuVries described a "modified Mayo procedure" as a surgical correction for an IPK plantar to the metatarsal head, regardless of its etiology.[17] A hockey stick–shaped incision extending from the web space over the metatarsophalangeal joint to the distal one-third of the metatarsal shaft is made. The transverse metatarsal ligament, collateral ligaments, and capsule are incised, thereby freeing up

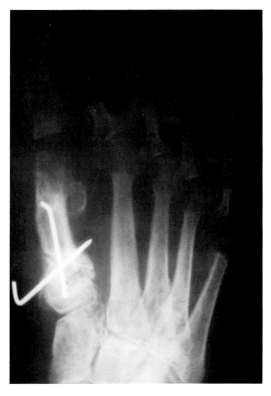

Fig. 34-5. Fifth metatarsal head resection.

will be satisfied with the first cut. The chevron is a double V-osteotomy performed by excising the wedge of bone between the two V-osteotomies. Ultimately, the bone is shorter by approximately 5 mm. Internal fixation and non weighbearing postoperately are necessary.

Transverse Osteotomy

After the V-osteotomy, this is the next most popular procedure (Fig. 34–6). This is a straight transverse osteotomy (similar to osteoclasis) through the anatomic neck from dorsal to plantar. Care should be taken to place the cut just proximal to the plantar condyles. Unlike the V-osteotomy, this procedure allows motion in all three planes. This procedure can be equated with the percutaneous metatarsal osteotomy (PMO) on the fifth metatarsal, in which a very small skin incision is followed by a through-and-through transverse osteotomy. Because of anatomic logistics, this is easily performed on the fifth metatarsal. PMO's can also be done on the lesser metatarsals by making a skin incision and then either cutting between the two tendons (ex-

the joint. The involved toe is plantar flexed, giving adequate exposure to the plantar condyles. Approximately 2 mm of the distal metatarsal head is removed along with at least one-half of the plantar condyles (the cut is angled to include most of the larger lateral condyle). Rasping, irrigation, and closure follows.

Bony regeneration or proliferation occurs in metatarsal head resection if the proximal phalanx has articular cartilage left undamaged. To prevent this from occurring Zang designed bone caps (Sutter Bone Caps) to prevent bony regrowth secondary to lesser metatarsal head resection.

Chevron

This procedure is mainly used for shortening a metatarsal. Even with the standard "V" procedure a considerable amount of shortening of bone is obtained. To begin with, the Stryker sawblade is 2 to 3 mm thick, and it is very unlikely that the surgeon

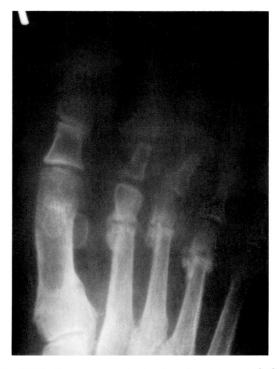

Fig. 34-6. Transverse osteotomies of metatarsals 2, 3, and 4.

tensor digitorum longus and extensor digitorum brevis) or moving the extensor digitorum longus laterally and then making a cut.

There are two benefits to performing the PMO on the lesser metatarsals. First, despite allowing motion in all three planes, PMO's offer stability because the collateral ligaments remain intact. Second, because of the minimal amount of periosteal dissection, the patient will experience less pain.

Transverse osteotomies are better suited for third and fourth metatarsals where stability is not as important as with the second metatarsal. A distal V-osteotomy is a better choice for second metatarsal surgery.

Midshaft Osteotomies

Giannestras[7] initially described the "step-down osteotomy" for surgery at the metatarsal base. Two square wedges of bone are removed, one medial and one lateral, and the bone is stepped down.

Duvries[17] modified the above procedure and made his cuts at an angle. A long oblique osteotomy in the anteroposterior plane through the metatarsal shaft is made. The distal segment of the metatarsal is then slid proximally and the osteotomy is fixed with the surgeon's choice of hardware.

A very important risk to consider when performing these procedures is violating the metatarsal nutrient artery with possible resultant non-union.

Base Osteotomy

The extension osteoarthrotomy (EOA) as described by Johnson is indicated for plantar-flexed metatarsals and is only performed on the second, third, and fourth metatarsals. This procedure is used much less frequently than distal osteotomies because it is more difficult to perform. The proximal cut of the osteotomy is made 1.0 cm distal to the metatarsal cuneiform joint. The osteotomy begins dorsally but does not cut the plantar aspect of the metatarsal. The distal cut is made first and is angulated to create a wedge-shaped osteotomy. The wedge of bone is resected and the plantar hinge is closed and fixed. Immobilization of the foot following this procedure is desirable.

Tailor's Bunion of the Fifth Metatarsal

An enlargement of the fibular side of the fifth metatarsophalangeal joint has been termed a Tailor's bunion. In days gone by, tailors would sit with their legs crossed as they sewed clothing, thereby placing abnormal pressure on the fifth metatarsal head, which often caused painful symptoms, and resultant bursitis.

Fifth metatarsal pathology is unique because there is a potential for three different types of lesions: plantar, lateral, and plantar-lateral. If the lesion is plantar, then any of the osteotomies described for the other metatarsals will work. For lateral lesions an osteotomy that will allow motion in the transverse plane is needed. A condylectomy to remove the hypertrophied dorsal lateral eminence (Fig. 34–7) along with an oblique osteotomy or a V-osteotomy (reverse Austin) in the transverse plane is recommended. To correct plantar-lateral lesions an osteotomy that allows the

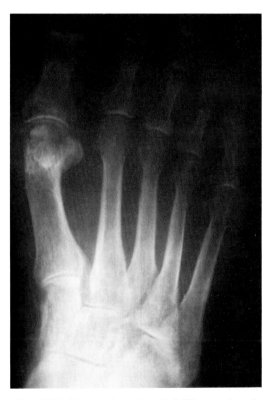

Fig. 34-7. Exostectomy head of fifth metatarsal.

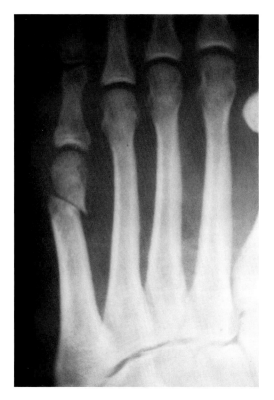

Fig. 34-8. Reverse Wilson osteotomy of fifth metatarsal.

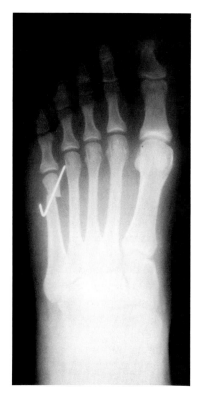

Fig. 37-9. Reverse Wilson osteotomy of fifth metatarsal with K-wire fixation.

head to move in at least two of the three planes (sagittal and transverse) is necessary (Fig. 34–8 and 34–9). For patients 45 years of age or older, a fifth metatarsal head resection is recommended.

Fallat and Buckholz proposed a means of measuring the intermetatarsal angle between the fourth and fifth metatarsals.[18] Their findings suggest that if the tailor's bunion is caused by a high intermetatarsal angle, the procedure of choice may be a base osteotomy. If the intermetatarsal angle approaches normal and the deviation angle is large, an osteotomy at the metatarsal neck may be indicated. If all measurements are normal, the procedure of choice may be resection of the lateral surface of the hypertrophied fifth metatarsal head (Fig. 34–7).

The closing base wedge osteotomy is indicated for a tailor's bunion when an increased intermetatarsal angle between the fourth and fifth metatarsals is present. At the base of the metatarsal (distal to its flare) the proximal cut is made perpendicular to the shaft, leaving the lateral cortex intact. The second cut is made distal to the first, forming a wedge of bone with the base medially. The wedge is resected, the lateral hinge is closed, and the osteotomy is fixed. Immobilization with a slipper or short leg cast is recommended for a period of 4 to 6 weeks.

SUMMARY AND CONCLUSIONS

This chapter has reviewed the more commonly performed procedures utilized for lesser metatarsal surgery. The idea that there are no definitive and easy-to-follow surgery criteria when dealing with the lesser metatarsals is only partially true. The second, third, and fourth metatarsals are dealt with in the same manner, but we believe the fifth metatarsal is a separate entity.

Since the fifth metatarsal functions with an independent range of motion as compared to the second, third, and fourth metatarsals, it is quite comparable to the first metatarsal. Therefore the surgery criteria that are used with reference to the first metatarsal and its associated intermetatarsal angle can also be utilized for the fifth metatarsal. In fact, all procedures that are performed in the way of bunion repair involving the first metatarsal head shaft and base can be applied in reverse to the fifth metatarsal. The most common procedure involving the fifth metatarsal, and one that these authors find to work quite well given associated deformity of the fifth metatarsal, is an oblique slide at the distal aspect of the head and fifth metatarsal head resection. Rarely does a fifth metatarsal head resection cause any transfer-type lesion to the associated fourth metatarsal; however, it does carry with it a shortened fifth toe unless an implant is utilized.

With reference to the second, third, and fourth metatarsals, we categorize the lesion on the plantar surface of the foot as either diffuse or discreet. We then proceed by treating diffuse lesions biomechanically and discreet lesions surgically. Unfortunately we have found that this is the only basic guideline that presents itself to the podiatric surgeon when dealing with these three metatarsals. We have been able to categorize the discrete lesions into five major types: elongated metatarsals, plantar-flexed metatarsals, dystrophic metatarsals (hypertrophied plantar condyles, Freiberg's disease), iatrogenically induced lesions, and those lesions seen secondary to a severe hallux abductovalgus deformity with associated metarsus primus adductus. We hope that the presentation of these categories of deformity will serve as a broad basis for identifying the need for surgery versus that of biomechanical control.

When considering surgery on the lesser metatarsals there are a great number of procedures that can be used and many variables come into play when trying to choose the correct procedure. However, in spite of careful planning all lesser metatarsal surgery is unpredictable. Therefore, the degree of difficulty in performing the procedure must be weighed against the probable success. It is the general consensus of the authors that, with all factors being equal, the "V"-type osteotomy of the surgical neck is the most popular and satisfactory procedure for lesser metatarsal surgery when no degenerative joint disease is present. When a dislocated lesser metatarsal phalangeal joint is present our procedure of choice is the partial metatarsal head resection.

Correct diagnosis, the understanding of the etiology, and the choice of the right surgical procedure will aid in achieving success in lesser metatarsal surgery.

REFERENCES

1. Meisenbach RO: Painful anterior arch of the foot: an operation for its relief by means of raising the arch. Am Trans Orthop Surg 14:206–211, 1916
2. Davis GF: Cure for hallux valgus: the interdigital incision. Surg Clin North Am 1:651–658, 1917
3. Mau C: Eine operation des kontrakten spreiztusses. Zentralbl Chir 67:667–670, 1940
4. Dickson FD, Dively RC: Surgical treatment of intractable plantar warts. J Bone Joint Surg 30:757–760, 1948
5. DuVries HL: New approach to the treatment of intractable verruca plantaris. JAMA 152:1202–1203, 1953
6. McKeever DC: Arthrodesis of the first metatarsal phalangeal joint for hallux valgus, hallux rigidus and metatarsus primus varus. J Bone Joint Surg [Am] 34:129, 1952
7. Giannestras NT: Shortening of the metatarsal shaft for the correction of plantar keratosis. Clin Orthop 4:225–231, 1954
8. Giannestras NT: Shortening of the metatarsal shaft in the treatment of plantar keratosis. J Bone Joint Surg 40:61–71, 1958
9. Davidson MR: A simple method for correcting second, third and fourth plantar metatarsal head pathology—especially intractable keratomas. J Foot Surg 8:23–26, 1969
10. Addante JB: Metatarsal osteotomy as an office procedure to eradicate intractable plantar keratosis. J Am Podiatr Med Assoc 60:397–399, 1970
11. Jacoby RP: "V"-osteoplasty for correction of intractable plantar keratoses. J Foot Surg 12:8–10, 1973
12. Bartel PF: Lesser metatarsal osteotomy. J Am Podiatry Assoc 67:358–360, 1977
13. Jimenez AL: Oblique "V"-lesser metatarsal osteotomy. In Schlefman N, (ed): Doctors Hospital Podiatric Education and Research Institute, 12 Surgical

Seminar Syllabus. Doctors Hospital Podiatry Institute, Tucker, GA, 1983

14. Gudas CJ: A review and results of osteotomies for plantar intractable keratoses. In: A Critical Review of Biomechanical Foot Surgery. Northlake Surgical Seminar, City, ST, 1973

15. Hatcher RM, Goller WL, Weil LS: Intractable plantar keratoses—a review of surgical corrections. J Am Podiatry Assoc, 68:377, 1978

16. Thomas WH: Metatarsal osteotomy. Surg Clin North Am 49:879, 1969

17. DuVries HL: Surgery of the Foot. 4th Ed. CV Mosby Co, St. Louis, 1978

18. Fallat LM, Buckholz J: An analysis of the tailor's bunion by radiographic and anatomical display. J Am Podiatry Assoc 70:597, 1980

SELECTED READINGS

Fielding MD: The Surgical Treatment of Hallux Abducto Valgus and Allied Deformities. Futura Publishing, Mount Kisco, NY, 1973

Jahss MH (ed): Disorders of the Foot. WB Saunders, Philadelphia, 1982

Kelikian H: Hallux Valgus, Allied Deformities of the Foot and Metatarsalgia. WB Saunders, Philadelphia, 1965

Mandracchia VJ: Lesser Metatarsal Surgery Lecture Notes. Pennsylvania College of Podiatric Medicine, Philadelphia, 1978–1984

McGlamry ED (Ed): Comprehensive Textbook of Foot Surgery. Williams & Wilkins, Baltimore, 1987

Root ML, Orien WP, Weed JH: Clinical Biomechanics. Vol. 2. Clinical Biomechanics Corp, Los Angeles, 1978

Hallux Abductovalgus and Surgery of the First Ray

35

Gary Peter Jolly, D.P.M.

FUNCTIONAL ANATOMY

The first ray, which includes the first cuneiform, the first metatarsal, the phalanges of the great toe, and the sesamoid apparatus, plays a pivotal role in human ambulation. The first ray anchors the medial column of the foot during the stance phase of gait and provides a lever for the conversion of vertical torque from the leg. In addition, it is the first metatarsophalangeal joint that helps to provide a smooth transition from midstance to toe-off by being passively dorsiflexed by the triceps surae.

Therefore, any condition that affects the function of the first ray is likely to exert a profound effect on the normal function of locomotion.

First Metatarsophalangeal Joint

The first metatarsophalangeal joint (MTPJ) consists of the base of the proximal phalanx of the hallux, the first metatarsal head, and the plantar plate, which contains the sesamoid bones. The joint is invested by a joint capsule, which is contiguous with the plantar plate, and contains medial and lateral collateral ligaments as well as the medial and lateral suspensory ligaments (metatarsal-sesamoid) (Fig. 35-1A).

The thickened portion of the plantar capsule known as the plantar plate provides, in conjunction with the base of the proximal phalanx, a deep receptacle for the metatarsal head during propulsive activities (Fig. 35-1B).

Intrinsic Muscles of the First Ray

Plantar Intrinsics

The plantar intrinsics include the abductor hallucis; the adductor hallucis (transverse and oblique heads); and the flexor hallucis brevis (medial and lateral heads). These muscles all insert into the plantar aspect of the sesamoid apparatus and ultimately the plantar aspect of the proximal phalanx. They serve to anchor the sesamoid apparatus and proximal phalanx to the weight-bearing surface during the later part of the stance phase.

When conditions arise that affect the function of the plantar intrinsics, then the ability of the hallux to stabilize normally will certainly be compromised.

Extensor Hallucis Brevis

The extensor hallucis brevis (EHB) is rather insignificant except when it is used to actively dorsiflex the hallux following a Jones tenosuspension.

823

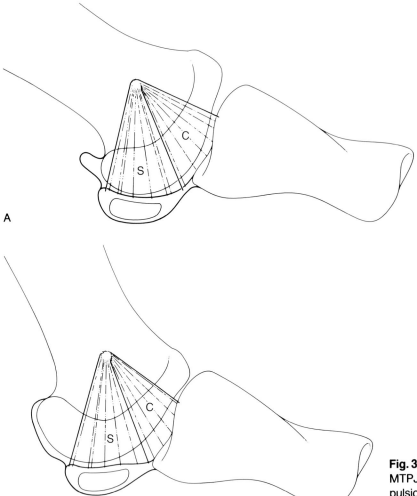

A

B

Fig. 35-1. Supporting structures of the first MTPJ depicted during stance **(A)** and propulsion **(B)**. *c*, collateral ligament; *s*, suspensory ligaments.

Extrinsic Muscles of the First Ray

Extensor Hallucis Longus

The extensor hallucis longus (EHL) inserts into the base of the distal phalanx dorsally, after passing through the extensor hood expansion. Because of the tethering effect of the hood, the primary action of this myotendinous unit is to actively extend the first MTPJ.

The EHL will frequently shorten as the result of a long-standing hallux abductovalgus deformity, and through a bowstring effect, become a deforming force on the great toe (Fig. 35-2). Shortening of the tendon will also occur in hallux hammer toe.

Flexor Hallucis Longus

The flexor hallucis longus (FHL) inserts into the plantar aspect of the distal phalanx of the great toe. Its action, in concert with the flexor hallucis brevis (FHB), is to stabilize the great toe during the second half of stance. Since the FHL tendon passes through a tunnel between the sesamoids, displacement of the sesamoids will significantly alter the angle of pull, and may contribute to a transverse plane deformity of the great toe.

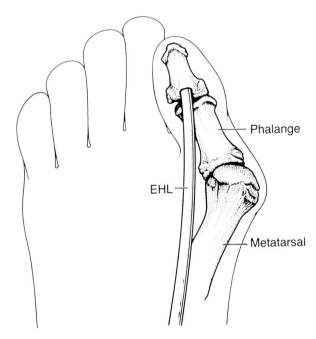

Phalange

EHL

Metatarsal

Fig. 35-2. Lateral deviation of the great toe allows the EHL to become a deforming force through its "bowstring effect."

Sensory Nerves

The skin overlying the first ray is innervated dorsally by branches from the medial dorsal cutaneous and deep peroneal nerves; medially by terminal branches of the saphenous nerve; and plantarly by terminal branches of the medial plantar nerves.

In the author's experience, the most clinically significant branch is the dorsomedial sensory nerve to the great toe, in that patients may present with complaints of pain and numbness in the hallux. It is this branch that becomes irritated by shoe pressure against a prominent bunion. Frequently, a Tinel's sign will be present.

Cuneiform Joints

The first navicular-cuneiform joint (NCJ) and the first cuneiform-metatarsal joint function together during weightbearing to provide the dorsiflexion-eversion/plantarflexion-inversion motion of the first ray.

Two conditions that affect the metatarsal-cuneiform joint of the first ray and are clinically significant are dorsal metatarsal-cuneiform exostosis, known alternatively as a tarsal boss or peak of Lamphier,[1] and degenerative arthritis of this joint. Degenerative disease can arise from direct trauma such as a Lisfranc fracture-dislocation or from more insidious microtrauma.

APPROACHES TO THE FIRST RAY

General Rules

The placement of an incision is crucial to the success of any surgical procedure. An incision must provide adequate exposure and yet not interfere with function once the wound is healed. This is particularly true in the hand and foot. An improperly placed incision near a digit or on the palm or sole can result in a significant loss of motion and sensation, or produce a scar that is painful to walk on or to grip with.

Interphalangeal Joint

Dorsal Approaches

The skin overlying the interphalangeal joint (IPJ) of the hallux is rather tightly bound and relatively inelastic. Therefore, adequate exposure can only be obtained if the incision is well placed and adequate in size. In addition, linear incisions through the extensor creases should be avoided since axial shortening of a linear incision will tend to produce a thickened, painful scar (Fig. 35-3). Linear incisions may be used proximal or distal to the extensor creases, but at the joint the incision should parallel the joint line (Fig. 35-4A).

Plantar Approaches

Access to the plantar aspect of the great toe's interphalangeal joint may be necessary in order to remove an ossicle, resect an exostosis, or advance the plantar plate in cases of hyperextensibility.

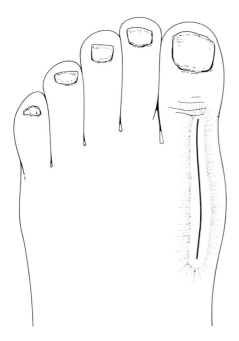

Fig. 35-3. Incisions that cross the extensor creases of joints are likely to result in painful, thick scars that interfere with function.

Linear scars must not be used on the flexor surface of a digit since this would most likely lead to scar contracture, which on a weight-bearing surface could prove disastrous. Double hockey stick incisions provide excellent exposure and yet rarely interfere with function (Fig. 35-4B). When utilizing a complex incision care must be taken to identify and protect the neurovascular elements to the toe.

First Metatarsophalangeal Joint

Surgical approaches to the first MTPJ have been classically described as medial, dorsomedial, and lateral (Fig. 35-5). The medial incision has been advocated for use in medial sesamoidectomy, in medial sesamoid planing, and for the Hiss bunion procedure, as well as for the osteochondral autograft of Regnauld[15] (Fig. 35-5A). The medial approach provides excellent medial exposure and its midaxial orientation avoids the medial neurovascular structures. Lateral exposure, however, is compromised.

Similarly, an incision in the first interspace will allow for direct visualization of the lateral structures, but, unless the first MTPJ is disarticulated, the medial eminence cannot be clearly seen[2] (Fig. 35-5B).

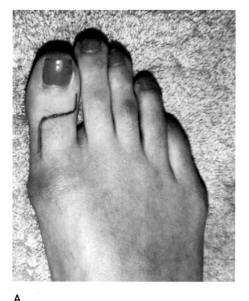

A

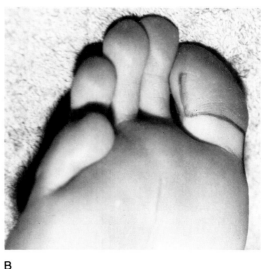

B

Fig. 35-4. Double hockey stick incision provides excellent exposure without violating surgical principles. **(A)** Dorsal view. **(B)** Plantar view.

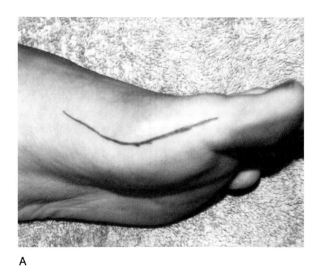

Fig. 35-5. Approaches to the first MTPJ. **(A)** Medial approach. **(B)** Lateral approach. **(C)** Dorsomedial approach.

A

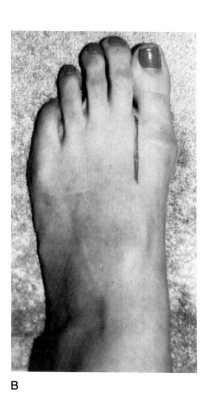

B

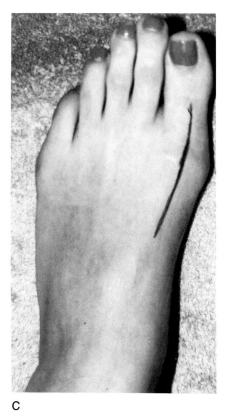

C

A dorsomedial incision affords a compromise, but may often lead to a scar that can be prominent, and, if medial and lateral exposure is desired, necessitates rather aggressive retraction (Fig. 35-5C).

Universal Incision of the First MTPJ

The author's preference is for a double hockey stick incision. The transverse component is located within an extensor crease and the linear segments

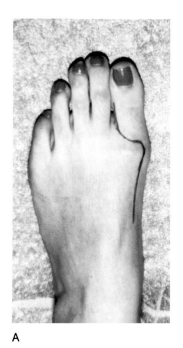

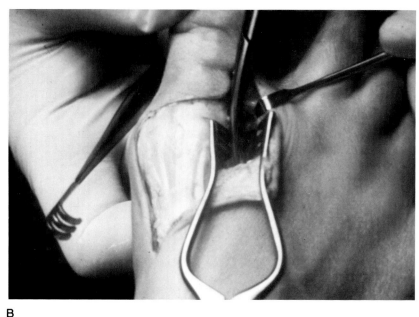

A   B

Fig. 35-6. (A) Universal approach to the first MTPJ. **(B)** Easy access to the medial and lateral aspects of the joint is provided by the universal incision.

are far enough medial and lateral to be well hidden. In addition, the exposure gained is much greater and facilitates dissection on either side, often without the need for retraction (Fig. 35-6).

First Metatarsal Osteotomies

Incisions for these procedures are usually medial to the EHL tendon. If a procedure is being planned concurrently on the first MTPJ, then one long incision can be made.

OBJECTIVES IN RECONSTRUCTIVE SURGERY OF THE FIRST RAY

When planning an operation on the first ray, it is crucial that consideration be given to the functional effects of that procedure. The first MTPJ plays an important role during the propulsive phase of gait. If that joint's ability to dorsiflex is

impaired, weight must be transferred laterally to the lesser metatarsal heads. This frequently produces severe metatarsalgia that is often more disabling than the original problem involving the great toe.

HALLUX ABDUCTOVALGUS

Hallux abductovalgus is a common deformity that involves a prominence of the medial aspect of the first metatarsal head and a lateral deviation of the great toe. In long-standing, severe cases the great toe may be seen to roll into valgus (Fig. 35-7).

Symptoms and Complaints

Pain and the inability to wear shoes comfortably are the usual presenting complaints. Occasionally, the patient will present because of associated metatarsalgia involving the second or third metatarsal

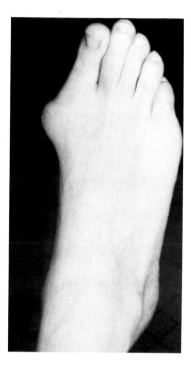

Fig. 35-7. Typical presentation of hallux abductovalgus.

head. In severe cases, the lateral drift of the hallux may be associated with hammering of the second toe, and that may be the patient's source of pain rather than the first ray deformity.

Women are far more likely to present with a painful hallux abductovalgus deformity than men, presumably because of the irritating effects of the narrower last shoes that they wear.

Physical Findings

The most consistent finding in hallux abductovalgus is an enlargement of the medial or dorsomedial surface of the first metatarsal head. In some instances there may be a palpable bursa over the bony eminence. Pain may be present on palpation, or it may not, if the patient has been off his or her feet and barefoot just prior to examination.

In older patients, or individuals with exceptional deformities, the range of first MTPJ motion may be painful or limited. For the most part, however, range of motion is usually normal with the toe held in the position of deformity. With the toe held in the corrected position, range and quality of motion may deteriorate dramatically.

Radiographic Findings

When evaluating a bunion deformity radiographically, it is necessary to obtain anteroposterior, lateral, and forefoot axial views in the angle and base of gait. Non-weight-bearing films are useless.

Radiographic analysis of hallux abductovalgus may be thought of in terms of qualitative and quantitative. Appreciation for the appearance of bone stock and the presence of accessory bones, intraosseous cysts, or evidence of joint disease within the foot may be thought of as the qualitative component of the x-ray evaluation. The measurement of clinically significant angles and distances comprise the quantitative component.

Although the quantitative findings, in large part, determine the procedure or procedures that are selected to correct the deformity, it may be that the qualitative findings mitigate against them. For example, the absence of adequate bone stock as a result of osteoporosis would certainly contraindicate the use of a basilar first metatarsal osteotomy. Similarly, gross evidence of degenerative changes in the first MTPJ would be at least a relative contraindication to a joint preservation procedure.

Quantitative Radiographic Assessment of Hallux Abductovalgus Deformities

Transverse Plane (Anteroposterior Projection). The intermetatarsal, hallux abductus, interphalangeal, and metatarsus adductus angles are the geometric expressions of the relationships within the skeletal architecture of the foot. The angles are determined by finding the longitudinal axes of the appropriate bones (refer to appropriate figures in Chapter 12).

The proximal and distal articular set angles express the relationship of the long axis of the first metatarsal with the position of the first metatarsal's articular cartilage and the longitudinal axis of the hallucial proximal phalanx and articular surface of its proximal end.

The tibial sesamoid position indicates the location of the intrinsic and the FHL tendons relative to the first metatarsal (Fig. 35-8). Generally the de-

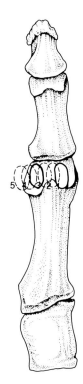

Fig. 35-8. Diagram indicating the positions of the tibial sesamoids. Generally, higher numbers are associated with greater clinical deformity.

gree of medial buckling is directly related to the degree of sesamoidal displacement.

When evaluating the anteroposterior radiograph of a bunion deformity it is also important to evaluate the length of the first ray relative to the second. This has been referred to as the relative metatarsal protrusion (refer to appropriate figure in Chapter 12). Failure to address a long first metatarsal during reconstruction may lead to a recurrence of the deformity. This occurs because the first metatarsal functions as a lever arm. Since the metatarsal head protrudes beyond that of the second, during the propulsive phase of gait a much greater load is brought to bear on the first metatarsal head than on the second. The base of the second metatarsal is locked tightly in a mortice and therefore cannot be moved. However, when the relative metatarsal protrusion is a positive value the increase in the reactive force of gravity acting on the first metatarsal head causes the first ray to dorsiflex and invert, thereby producing a medial buckling at the first MTPJ.

A positive relative metatarsal protrusion will also produce a clinically more severe hallux abductovalgus deformity than one would expect given the angular measurements alone. This occurs because a longer metatarsal will protrude more medially than will a shorter one (Fig. 35-9).

Pressman et al. believed that the intermetatarsal angle may be regarded as either a positional or a fixed component to a hallux abductovalgus deformity.[3] They relied on the metatarsal split distance to make that determination. The metatarsal split distance is determined by measuring the distance between the bases of the first and second metatarsals. Pressman et al. believed that, if the distance is 3 mm or greater, then the intermetatarsal angle is reducible by rebalancing the MTPJ.

Frontal Plane. A forefoot axial radiograph will yield valuable information about the metatarsal-

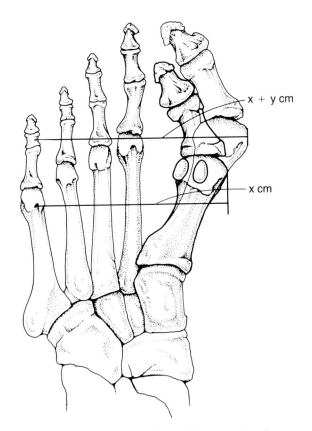

Fig. 35-9. Effects of a positive relative metatarsal protrusion. A longer first ray will produce a clinically more significant deformity than a ray with a negative relative metatarsal protrusion.

sesamoid articulation. It can indicate degenerative changes in the joint in the form of narrowing of the metatarsal-sesamoid joint spaces, as well as identify the condition of the crista. Pressman and Stanno believed that an intact crista is needed to prevent loss of correction following a soft tissue repair of a bunion deformity.[3]

Sagittal Plane. Lateral projection radiographs will provide information about the first metatarsal declination angle. This is particularly useful when evaluating a dorsal or dorsomedial bunion. If a first metatarsal is significantly elevated, consideration would have to be given to a plantarflexory osteotomy.

TREATMENT OF HALLUX ABDUCTOVALGUS

The primary concern of the physician treating hallux abductovalgus should be alleviating pain. In certain instances, this can be accomplished by using molded shoes, orthodigital devices, or even a wider last shoe. However, if surgery is to be the treatment of choice, then careful consideration must be given to the preoperative planning, the intraoperative technique, and the postoperative management of the patient. There is no such thing as a simple bunion, only simple surgeons.

A hallux abductovalgus deformity may be strictly a hyperostosis of the first metatarsal head, or it may be part of a more complex, compound deformity that can include clinically significant metatarsus adductus or a paralytic flatfoot. Repair should be thought of in terms of reconstructing the deformity with all coexisting problems in mind.

Joint Preservation

Over the years, there have been an abundance of arthroplasties of the first MTPJ described in the literature. Included among the joint preservation procedures are those of Silver, Hiss, and McBride, along with their subsequent modifications. While some authors have been characterized by the simplicity of their operations, others have been re-

membered for their ingenuity. The one thing that all arthroplasties for correction of hallux abductovalgus have in common is that the medial soft tissues of the first MTPJ are plicated while the lateral soft tissues are released. This allows for the proximal phalanx to assume a more anatomic relationship with the first metatarsal head. In addition, the medial eminence of the first metatarsal head is usually reduced concomitantly.

Indications

Rarely does one consider repair of a bunion without considering some form of arthroplasty. Even in those instances, such as in juvenile hallux abductovalgus, the first MTPJ is opened and the hyperostosis is remodeled.

For a first MTPJ arthroplasty to be used alone, certain conditions must exist in order for that arthroplasty to succeed. First, the intermetatarsal angle must be below 12 degrees and the relative metatarsal protrusion must have a negative value. If the intermetatarsal angle is between 8 and 12 degrees, the metatarsal split distance should be above 3 mm in order to allow reduction of the intermetatarsal angle by medial MTPJ capsular plication.

Also, the first ray should be free of structural abnormalities such as high proximal or distal articular set angles, and the metatarsus adductus angle should be below 20 degrees. From the standpoint of qualitative assessment, the first MTPJ should not show evidence of degenerative changes, beyond some mild cystic changes beneath the medial eminence.

In the successful performance of any bunion operation, but even to a greater extent in a tendon-capsule balance procedure, the first MTPJ must be prevented from undergoing medial buckling. The most common reason for this failure is that the sesamoid apparatus, which contains the plantar plate, the intrinsic tendons, and the FHL tendon, was never restored to its anatomic position beneath the metatarsal head. This can usually be avoided by completely releasing the conjoined tendon of the adductor hallucis, and sectioning the lateral suspensory ligament and the lateral collateral ligament.

The medial suspensory ligament can be sepa-

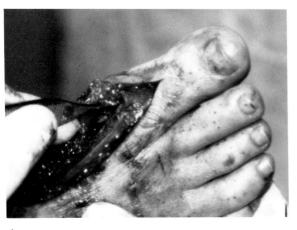
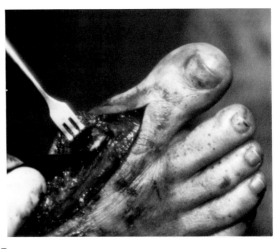

A   B

Fig. 35-10. (A) The medial suspensory ligament has been separated from the overlying capsule and has been grasped by the forceps. **(B)** The medial suspensory ligament has been pulled in a pure dorsal direction. Note the change in position of the great toe when compared with its position in A.

rated from the more superficial capsule and then used as a lead to reduce the sesamoid apparatus. When the medial ligament is pulled dorsally, the sesamoid apparatus moves medially and the great toe is seen to adduct and roll out of valgus (Fig. 35-10). The medial sesamoid–metatarsal ligament can then be anchored to the first metatarsal head in a more dorsal position as in a *desmopexy*, or the adductor hallucis tendon can be transferred me-

dially over the neck of the first metatarsal to the medial ligament[3] (Fig. 35-11).

Complications

The most commonly seen complications following joint preservation arthroplasties of the first MTPJ are recurrence of the hallux abductovalgus, hallux varus, and stiffness of the first MTPJ.

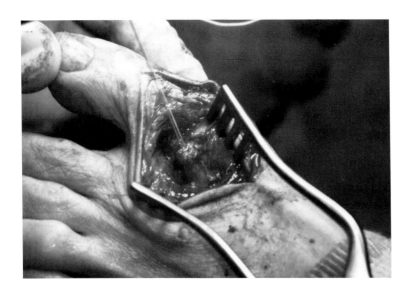

Fig. 35-11. The adductor hallucis tendon being rerouted over the first metatarsal to be sutured to the medial suspensory ligament as a tendoligamentous sling. (Courtesy of M. Pressman, D.P.M., Milford, CT.)

Recurrence is by far the most common complication, and in the author's experience is most commonly associated with failure to adequately mobilize and to reduce the sesamoid apparatus.

Hallux varus still occurs, although not as commonly as it once did. This condition, in which the great toe deviates medially from the longitudinal axis of the first metatarsal, has been associated with an overly aggressive medial correction of the first MTPJ and removal of the lateral sesamoid.

Acquired hallux varus is really a biplane deformity, when associated with lateral sesamoidectomy. Removal of this bone allows the abductor hallucis and medial head of the FHB to exert a mechanical advantage in the transverse plane and pull the great toe medially. However, of equal importance is the fact that the sesamoid enhances the ability of the plantar intrinsics to stabilize the proximal phalanx during stance. When that effect is weakened by sesamoidectomy, the great toe buckles dorsally at the MTPJ, allowing the FHL to plantarflex the interphalangeal joint and compound the dorsal buckling at the MTPJ (Fig. 35-12).

Postoperative *stiffness* following any arthrotomy is common, but with adequate physiotherapy it is usually transient. However, when large sections of capsule are removed, ostensibly to correct transverse plane great toe deformities, sagittal plane ex-

cursions of the great toe can become severely impaired. For this reason it is the author's preference to dorsally advance the medial suspensory ligament and merely repair the capsular defect without excising tissue.

Joint Destructive Procedures

Joint destructive procedures have been advocated for use in patients with bunion deformities that demonstrate evidence of degenerative changes. This group of techniques includes the Keller procedure, the Mayo procedure, the implant arthroplasties, and fusions of the first MTPJ. These procedures have been in use for many years, and have proven themselves useful.

Resection arthroplasties such as the Keller or Mayo procedure allow for removal of the bony prominence and the first MTPJ itself. The void created by the osseous resection is filled by fibrous tissue, which usually allows the great toe to bend in the sagittal plane. Although the Keller procedure is still commonly performed today, resection of the first metatarsal head is not.

Resection of the base of the proximal phalanx of the great toe has traditionally been a procedure that is reserved for older patients, since a number of problems have been associated with Keller's operation. While these problems in an older, less active patient may produce disability, in a younger, active patient, they can be disastrous.

Mann and Coughlin[4] and Kelekian[2] both cite metatarsalgia and cock-up deformity of the hallux as complications of the Keller procedure. It would appear that the loss of stability of the first MTPJ results in a lateral "dumping" of the body weight onto the lesser metatarsals, resulting in metatarsalgia and even stress fracture of the second and sometimes the third metatarsal.

Hallux hammer toe occurs as a result of loss of the intrinsic muscles' ability to stabilize the proximal phalanx against the reactive force of gravity. The frequency of occurrence of these complications can be reduced by tethering the FHL to the proximal phalanx. In addition, the EHL can be lengthened when there has been adaptive shortening.[5]

The technique of tethering the FHL described by Fuson involves drilling a 1.5-mm hole through

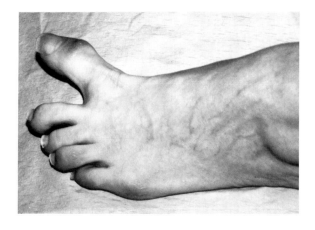

Fig. 35-12. Example of iatrogenic hallux varus. Note the hammering of the interphalangeal joint. This illustrates the biplane nature of the deformity when a lateral sesamoidectomy has been performed.

the plantar cortex of the proximal phalanx following resection of the base.[6] The periosteum and underlying bone is then roughened with a rasp. The FHL tendon sheath is identified and split lengthwise below the proximal phalanx. An absorbable 2-0 suture is then placed through the FHL tendon and passed through the drill hole in the proximal phalanx, where it is tied.

Phalangeal Osteotomies

Angulational osteotomies of the proximal phalanx of the great toe have been developed to treat structural deformities within the hallux, both real and imagined.[7-9] Most commonly, phalangeal osteotomies are used to reduce an abnormally high distal articular set angle (DASA) or interphalangeus and are performed in concert with an arthroplasty of the first MTPJ (Fig. 35-13).

Unfortunately, phalangeal osteotomies are often employed improperly as a means of realigning the toe in the face of a more complex type of deformity. When these osteotomies are utilized as a "cheater," they rarely are successful and the deformity that reoccurs is often worse than the original.

Phalangeal osteotomies, both proximal and distal, must be managed as phalangeal fractures. A minimum of 4 weeks of protection in the form of a wooden-soled surgical shoe is required. If rigid internal fixation is used, active range of motion exercises may begin immediately after surgery in order to minimize first MTPJ stiffness.

Complications may include nonunion, malunion, and avascular necrosis of the proximal fragment.

Metatarsal Osteotomies

Osteotomies of the first metatarsal have been described to effect changes in the length, transverse or sagittal plane position, and orientation of the

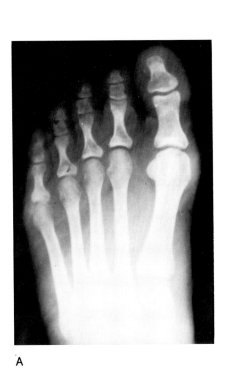
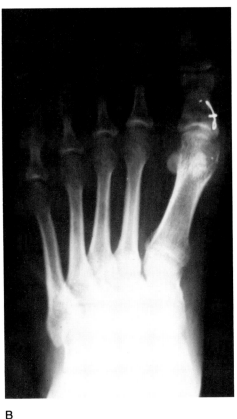

A   B

Fig. 35-13.   Pre- **(A)** and postoperative **(B)** radiographs demonstrating a phalangeal osteotomy.[8] A figure-of-eight fusion-bound wire has been applied for fixation.

articular cartilage of the head of the first metatarsal. Osteotomies may be grouped into two main categories: proximal or distal.

Proximal osteotomies are used to reduce significant abnormalities in the intermetatarsal angle, or to change the sagittal plane position of the first ray, and therefore are considered to be angulational. Distal osteotomies are used to effect changes in the proximal articular set angle (PASA) and to reduce intermetatarsal angles of modest proportions. These may be angulational, transpositional, rotational, or a combination of these types.

Proximal Metatarsal Osteotomies. Proximal osteotomies of the first metatarsal are generally indicated when the intermetatarsal angle is greater than 15 degrees in a rectus foot or 12 degrees in a foot with metatarsus adductus, and is associated with a symptomatic hallux abductovalgus. Proximal osteotomies should only be considered in cases in which the bone stock is good and the patient is capable of being compliant with his or her postoperative care.

When performing a proximal first metatarsal osteotomy it is important to avoid excessive soft tissue stripping of the osteotomy site in order to preserve extraosseous blood supply. The creation of an avascular osteotomy may result in an avascular nonunion.

Complications. In addition to the usual risks involved with surgery on the musculoskeletal system, there are a number of untoward results that can occur following proximal first metatarsal osteotomies.

Postoperative elevation of the first ray has been a well-recognized complication of proximal first metatarsal osteotomies. Many of these iatrogenic deformities occur at the time of surgery, and can be easily avoided. When an angulational osteotomy is performed, the distal fragment is rotated toward the second metatarsal. This rotation occurs, in fact, around a hinge. The orientation of this hinge axis relative to the cardinal planes of the body determines the position of the first ray. (refer to Figures in Chapter 12). It is therefore imperative that the axis be placed perpendicular to the transverse plane of the body, not to the long axis of the first metatarsal. The hinge axis applies equally to opening wedges, closing wedges, (transverse or oblique) and crescentic techniques.

The most common complication involves elevation of the first metatarsal and the subsequent development of lateral metatarsalgia as the first ray bears less weight. In addition, range of motion of the first MTPJ decreases with sagittal plane elevation of the first metatarsal head.

First ray elevatus may be seen as either an early or late complication. When it occurs early, it is either the result of faulty placement of the hinge axis or loss of reduction of the osteotomy. Faulty placement of the hinge axis may necessitate reoperation in the form of an osteotomy with dorsal autogenous bone graft, or a plantar flexory osteotomy of the first metatarsal.

The appearance of a first ray elevatus after 6 weeks may result from the phenomenon of plastic remodeling of bone callus. Plastic remodeling rarely occurs when rigid internal fixation is utilized and primary bone healing results, but it can occur when a large exocallus forms at the osteotomy site and the first ray is subjected to premature weight-bearing. The cyclical loading produced leads to dorsal resorption of the bone callus, which causes the distal fragment of the first metatarsal to be displaced dorsally (Fig. 35-14).

This phenomenon can be avoided by keeping patients with unstable osteotomies from bearing weight on the involved foot for longer than the usual 6 weeks. In addition, the use of a walking heel in conjunction with crutches will also spare the first ray from bearing a full load.

Distal Metatarsal Osteotomies. Osteotomies performed through the head and neck of the first metatarsal have been designed to correct several structural abnormalities.[10,11] As a rule, osteotomies of this type are effective in reducing intermetatarsal angles that are below 15 degrees. If an intermetatarsal angle is greater than 15 degrees, sufficient lateral displacement of the capital fragment would result in a very unstable osteotomy.

Many of the distal osteotomies have the ability to change the orientation of the articular cartilage, thereby reducing the PASA. This is particularly important in cases of juvenile hallux abductovalgus, where an abnormal PASA is a primary component rather than an adaptive change.

A third indication for a distal first metatarsal osteotomy is a positive relative metatarsal protrusion. Using any one of the through-and-through

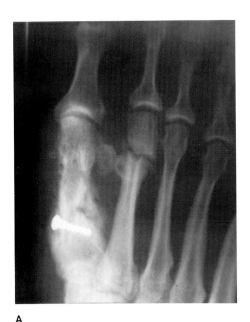

A

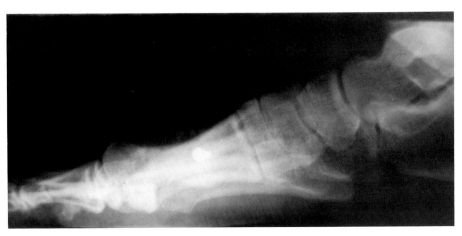

B

Fig. 35-14. (A) Radiograph demonstrating exuberant callus around a basilar osteotomy of the first metatarsal, the result of inadequate fixation. **(B)** Lateral radiograph of the same foot showing elevatus of the first metatarsal.

osteotomies, a section of the first metatarsal can be removed and the fragments reduced, thereby shortening the first metatarsal.

Complications. Although distal first metatarsal osteotomies have become popular procedures, due in part to the technical ease with which they are performed and in part to frequently good cosmesis, there are a number of pitfalls that can lead to failure.

Avascular necrosis of bone occurs when the normal vascular supply to a bone or section of bone is disrupted. This results in death of the osteocytes and a disruption in the normal turnover of matrix and calcium salts. As a result of this, the affected bone becomes weakened and, if subjected to stress, will undergo deformation.

Avascular necrosis of the first metatarsal head is a known risk of distal first metatarsal osteotomies.[12] Disruption of the bone's nutrient artery from interspace dissection or during osteotomy can result in an avascularity of part or all of the distal fragment. When the subchondral bone is affected it becomes structurally weakened and the stresses of weight-bearing and normal joint loading can produce sub-

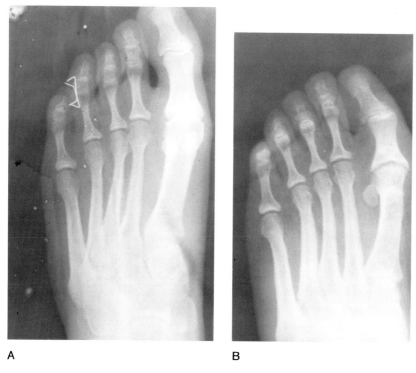

A   B

Fig. 35-15. (A) Anteroposterior radiograph of a foot with a moderate juvenile hallux abductovalgus. **(B)** The same foot approximately 5 years after a Mitchell procedure was performed. Note the irregularity of the articular surface of the metatarsal head and the trumpeting of the base of the proximal phalanx of the great toe. This patient had been functioning with a complete hallux rigidus since the original operation.

chondral collapse and therefore loss of joint congruity (Fig. 35-15).

Although avascular necrosis is not always disabling, it occurs far more commonly than was originally thought. The risk of developing avascular necrosis can be reduced by limiting the dissection in the interspace to precise tenotomy of the adductor hallucis tendon and release of the lateral collateral ligaments.

Hallux Hammer Toe is a subtle change that can occur following a distal first metatarsal osteotomy. It can be caused by dorsal displacement of the distal fragment, in which case the entire hallux loses its purchase. A loss of first MTPJ motion will frequently be seen with this condition.

When the development of hallux hammer toe is more insidious following distal osteotomy, the etiology would appear to be a loss of short flexor function. Distal osteotomies are located directly above the distal ends of the flexor hallucis brevis muscles

(Fig. 35-16). If excessive fibrosis develops between the bone and muscle postoperatively, the ability of these muscles to stabilize the proximal phalanx against the reactive force of gravity will be affected and dorsal buckling of the great toe will result.

When a distal first metatarsal osteotomy is performed rigid fixation is preferable to splintage or, even worse, no fixation at all. Rigid internal fixation will allow the patient to begin range of motion exercises immediately and, it is hoped, limit the amount of fibrosis in the plantar intrinsics.

Special Procedures

Implant Arthroplasty

Swanson first described the use of a silicone rubber spacer used in the first MTPJ.[13] Since 1972 there have been a number of implants developed to preserve length and function of the great toe fol-

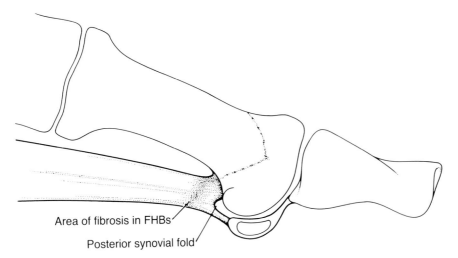

Area of fibrosis in FHBs

Posterior synovial fold

Fig. 35-16. Diagram depicting the relationship between the first metatarsal, the plantar plate, and the intrinsic muscles of the first ray. Fibrosis of the muscles at the surgical neck, the result of a metaphyseal osteotomy, weakens the pull of the short flexors and allows a hammer toe deformity of the great toe to develop.

lowing resection of the first MTPJ. Currently two general types of implant are in use. The first is a descendant of the original Swanson design. It is intended to replace the base of the proximal phalanx and allow the hallux to go through a more normal range of motion. The second type is a hinged bipolar prosthesis that allows for removal of the base of the proximal phalanx and the head of the first matatarsal. This design allows for sagittal plane motion of the great toe by pistoning of the stems within the medullary canals of the phalanx and metatarsal.

By the late 1970s implant arthroplasty of the first MTPJ had become a very popular procedure. It was thought that replacement of the joint with a spacer prevented degeneration of the joint and, in addition, correction of deformities could be accomplished by angular resection of joint surface. However, a number of reports have indicated that these silicone rubber implants have been experiencing material failure in the form of microsharding, and even gross fragmentation[14] (Fig. 35-17).

Osteochondral Autografts

An an alternative to joint destructive and implant arthroplasty, Regnauld described a procedure in 1968 that will correct a hallux valgus or limitus and yet retain joint function and adequate digital length.[15] This is accomplished by removing the proximal one-third of the proximal phalanx of the great toe, reshaping it, and then reinserting it.

Since the articular portion (including the subchondral plate) is preserved, yet the vascular supply is stripped, it is by definition an osteochondral autograft (Fig. 35-18).

Like the Keller procedure, the intrinsic muscular attachments are released during Regnauld's operation, thereby releasing transverse as well as sagittal plane contractures. (Fig. 35-19). Care must be exercised, however, in postmenopausale women, since osteoporosis may result in the loss of cancellous bone, creating a highly unstable graft recipient site. In these instances, fixation by internal splintage is indicated.

HALLUX RIGIDUS AND HALLUX LIMITUS

Arthritic changes within the first MTPJ that limit excursion of the great toe can be quite disabling. The inability of the hallux to passively dorsiflex during heel-off causes a profound disturbance in normal gait mechanics. Although patients with hallux limitus or rigidus may present with pain in the first MTPJ, their complaints frequently do not involve the first MTPJ and hallux, but rather the lateral metatarsal area. When first MTPJ pain is

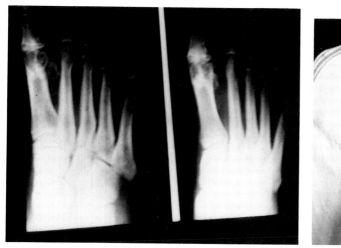

A

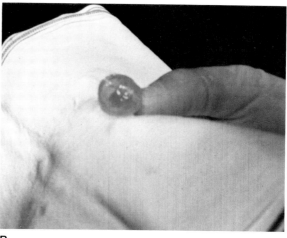

B

Fig. 35-17. (A) Radiographs of the foot of a 46-year-old male who underwent an implant arthroplasty 8 years prior. Note the cortical overgrowth on the proximal phalanx as well as the cystic degeneration within the metatarsal head and in the shaft of the proximal phalanx. This was the result of multiple giant cell foreign body reactions to shards of silicone rubber. **(B)** The great toe prosthesis removed from the same patient. Note the marginal tears and general irregularities.

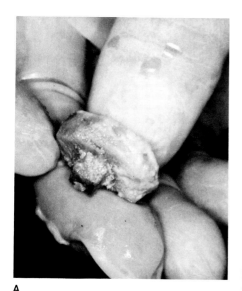

A

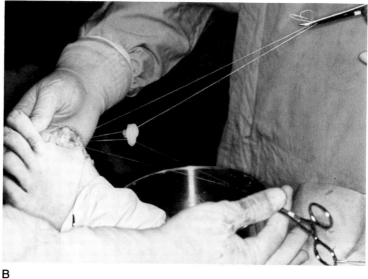

B

Fig. 35-18. (A) Base of the proximal phalanx of the hallux. The articular disc has been preserved, as has a medullary stem. **(B)** Intraoperative photograph demonstrating the technique of reinsertion of an osteochondral autograft.

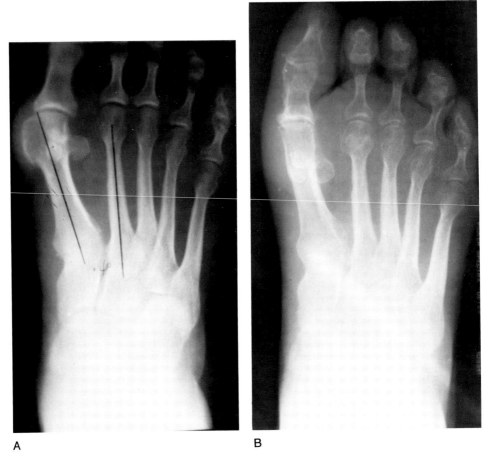

A   B

Fig. 35-19. (A) Preoperative radiograph demonstrating a hallux abductovalgus deformity. Note the absence of first MTPJ congruity. **(B)** Postoperative radiograph of the same foot 6 months after an osteochondral autograft. Note the apparent reduction in the intermetatarsal hallux abductus angles as well as the restoration of joint congruity.

present it is usually the result of shoe irritation of the exuberant juxtarticular bone.

Conservative treatment of hallux rigidus includes the use of metatarsal bars, orthoses, nonsteroidal anti-inflammatories, and intrarticular injections of corticosteroids. When these methods fail, surgery may be indicated. The objectives of surgery are to provide a painless first MTPJ and a foot that is capable of heel-toe progression with normal weight distribution across the forefoot. Traditional surgical treatment of hallux rigidus and hallux limitus includes arthrodesis of the first MTPJ or resection arthroplasty. Over the last 15 years, implant arthroplasty and chielectomy have been

added to the list. More recently, the osteochondral autograft of Regnauld is finding proponents in this country.[15]

When employing any of these procedures to correct a hallux rigidus, similar considerations must be given as when correcting hallux abductovalgus: restoration of motion and preservation of stability. Therefore, tethering of the flexor hallucis longus tendon should be considered as part of a Keller-type procedure, with or without implant arthroplasty, or with a Regnauld autograft. The use of silicone spacers should be reserved for older patients whose level and intensity of activity is minimal. Their use in younger patients, especially those below the age of 50, is contraindicated in most instances.

REFERENCES

1. Marcinko DE, McGlamry ED: The first cuneimetatarsal exostosis. J Am Podiatr Med Assoc 75:401, 1985
2. Kelekian H: The hallux. p. 575. In Jahss MH (ed): Disorders of the Foot. Vol. I. WB Saunders Co, Philadelphia, 1982
3. Pressman M, Stano G, Krantz M, Novicki D: Correction of hallux valgus with positionally increased intermetatarsal angle. J Am Podiatr Med Assoc 76:611, 1986
4. Mann RA, Coughlin MJ, Du Vries HL: Hallux rigidus, a review of the literature and a method of treatment. Clin Orthop Related Res 142:57, 1979
5. Ganley J, Lynch F, Darrigan R: Keller bunionectomy with fascia and tendon graft. J Am Podiatr Med Assoc 76:602, 1986
6. Fuson S: Modification of the Keller operation for increased functional capacity. J Foot Surg 21(4):292, 1982
7. Akin OF: The treatment of hallux valgus—a new operative procedure and its results. Med Sentinal 33:678, 1925
8. Allan FG: Hallux valgus and rigidus. Br Med J 1:579, 1940
9. Daw SW: An unusual type of hallux valgus. Br Med J 2:580, 1935
10. Hohman G: Symptomatische oder physiologische Behandlung des Hallux Dolgis. Münch Med Ohnschr 33:1042, 1921
11. Mitchell G, Hawkins A, Austin DW, Lerenten EO: A new osteotomy for hallux valgus: a horizontally directed "V" displacement osteotomy of the metatarsal head for hallux valgus and varus. Clin Orthoped 157:24, 1981
12. Meier DJ, Kenzora JE: The risks and benefits of distal first metatarsal osteotomies. Foot Ankle 6(1):7, 1985
13. Swanson AB: Implant arthroplasty for the great toe. Clin Orthop 86:74, 1972
14. Vanori J, O'Keefe R, Pikscher I: Silastic implant arthroplasty: complications and their classification. JAPMA 74(9):423, 1984
15. Regnauld B: The Foot. pp. 271-280. Springer-Verlag, Berlin, 1986

SELECTED READINGS

Bonney G, Mac Nab I: Hallux valgus and hallux rigidus. J Bone Joint Surg [Br] 34:366, 1952

Cohn I, Kanat IO: Functional limitation of motion of the first metatarsophalangeal joint. J Foot Surg 23:477, 1984

Dooley BJ, Berryman DB: Wilson's osteotomy of the first metatarsal for hallus valgus in the adolescent and the young adult. Aust NZ J Surg 43:255, 1973

Fitzgerald JAW, Wilkinson JM: Arthrodesis of the metatarsophalangeal joint of the great toe. Clin Orthop Related Res 157:70, 1981

Ford LT, Gilula LA: Stress fractures of the middle metatarsal following the Keller operation. J Bone Joint Surg [Am] 59:117, 1977

Gudas C, Schuberth J, Reilly C: The closing wedge osteotomy. J Am Podiatry Assoc 74:13, 1984

Hardy RH, Clapham JCR: London, England: observations on hallux valgus. J Bone Joint Surg [Br] 33:376, 1951

Harrison MHM, Harvey FJ: Arthrodesis of the first metatarsophalangeal joint for hallux valgus and rigidus. J Bone Joint Surg [Br] 45:471, 1963

Hawkins FB, Mitchell CL, Hedrick D: Correction of hallux valgus by metatarsal osteotomy. J Bone Joint Surg 27:387, 1945

Hiss JM: Hallux valgus: its cause and simplified treatment. Am J Surg 11:51, 1931

Inman VT: Hallux valgus: a review of etiologic factors. Orthop Clin North Am 5(1):59, 1974

Joplin R: Sling procedure for correction of splay-foot, metatarsus primus varus, and hallux valgus. J Bone Joint Surg 32A(4):779, 1950

Keller WL: The surgical treatment of bunions and hallux valgus. Med Record 80:741, 1904

Kempe S, Grapel D, Hovanec P: A mathematical approach to closing base wedge osteotomy. J Am Podiatry Assoc 74:601, 1984

Kessel L, Bonney G: Hallux rigidus in the adolescent. J Bone Joint Surg [Br] 40:668, 1958

Lahz JC: Metatarso-phalangeal arthrodesis for hallux valgus. J Bone Joint Surg [Br] 55:220, 1973

La Porta G, Melillo T, Olinsky D: X-ray evaluation of hallux abducto valgus deformity. J Am Podiatry Assoc 64:544, 1974

Mann R, Thompson F: Arthrodesis of the first metatarsophalangeal joint for hallux valgus in rheumatoid arthritis. J Bone Joint Surg [Am] 66:687, 1984

Mayo CH: The surgical treatment of bunions. Am Surg Assoc 48:300, 1908

McBride E: A conservative operation for bunions. J Int Coll Surg 21:99, 735, 1954

McBride E: The McBride bunion hallux valgus operation. J Bone Joint Surg [Am] 49:1075, 1667, 1967

McKeever D: Arthrodesis of the first metatarsophalangeal joint for hallux valgus. Hallux rigidus, and metatarsus primus varus. J Bone Joint Surg [Am] 34:129, 1952

Nayfa M, Sorto LA, Jr.: The incidence of hallux abductus following tibial sesamoidectomy. J Am Podiatry Assoc 72:617, 1982

Piggott H: The natural history of hallux valgus in adolescence and early adult life. J Bone Joint Surg [Br] 42:749, 1960

Stokes IAF, Hutton WC, Evans MJ: The effects of hallux valgus and Keller's operation on the load bearing function of the foot during walking. Acta Orthop Belg 41:695, 1975

Swanson AB, Lumsden RM, Swanson G, Braunhohler W: Silicone implant arthroplasty of the great toe (a review of single stem and flexible hinge implants). Paper presented at the annual meeting of the American Orthopedic Foot Society, Las Vegas, Nevada, Feb. 3, 1977

Wilson JN: Oblique displacement osteotomy for hallux valgus. J Bone Joint Surg [Br] 45:552, 1963

Rearfoot Surgery

36

Gunther Steinböck, M.D.

The heel represents a key position in human locomotion. It is the first part of the body to touch ground in walking, and in many individuals also in running. Taking over the load, the position of the rearfoot is responsible for the development of movements within the foot. Also, it is an area where structures running craniocaudal are turned around into a posteroanterior direction, passing through narrow channels that hold them in place.

It is the aim of the author to describe problems of the region that can be solved by surgery, following unsuccessful conservative measurements. Although certain surgical procedures, such as osteotomies and arthrodeses, will be discussed in other chapters of this book, this chapter describes surgical interventions that proved to be valuable measures in the author's hands.

TARSAL TUNNEL SYNDROME

In contrast to the upper extremity, nerve compression syndromes in the foot are rather rare[1] and seldom bilateral. Tissue constriction of the tibialis posterior nerve or its branches can occur within the tarsal canal and distal to it as it divides into the medial and lateral plantar nerve.

Etiology and Pathology

Etiologic factors are all space-reducing processes within the canal. In 80 percent of all tarsal tunnel syndromes a cause can be found, most commonly trauma. Distal tibial fractures, fractures of the ankle, calcaneous, or talus, or ankle sprains and contusions can lead to transient lesions of the posterior tibial nerve.[1]

Tarsal tunnel syndromes caused by trauma that evolve after a latency period are often created by scar formation around the tarsal tunnel. Osteophytes in post-traumatic or degenerative subtalar osteoarthritis; tenosynovitis of the posterior tibial, flexor digitorum longus, and flexor hallucis longus tendons; varikosis; and tumorous conditions such as lipomas, ganglioneuromas, and schwannomas can create compression of the nerve. Ehricht mentioned tarsal tunnel syndromes in decompensated cavus foot.[2] Increased tension at the adductor hallucis muscle in the plantar aponeurosis caused the compression in three of his 11 cases.

Heimkes et al. emphasized that a proximal and distal tarsal tunnel syndrome ought to be distinguished according to their anatomic findings.[1] The flexor retinaculum extends from the medial malleolus to the navicular tuberosity and to the medial calcaneal tuberosity. Proximally it extends to the crural fascia. Distally it splits at the superior margin of the abductor hallucis into a superficial and a deep fascial sheath for this muscle.[1]

In 55 of 60 preparations Heimkes et al. found a fibrous membrane between the medial and lateral plantar nerve.[1] It originates from the periosteum of the medial face of the calcaneus, extends to the deep fascia of the abductor hallucis, and forms a strap between two fibrous canals through which the plantar nerves find their way to their compartments. Thus the bottleneck for the two nerves is created under the abductor hallucis muscle. This has to be considered in the preoperative diagnosis and the planning of the operation.

Evaluation

According to Mann,[3] diagnosis ought to be established on the basis of the type of pain described by the patient, a positive Tinel's sign over the tarsal tunnel, and a positive electroneurodiagnostic study.

Heimkes[1] summarized the symptoms from the literature: rather diffuse pain at the medial malleolus, radiating into the plantar part of the foot, heel, and also calf; paresthesia, dysesthesia, and hypalgesia along the sensory innervation area of the posterior tibial nerve; increased pain by walking and extension of the foot; weakness in spreading the toes; and fatigue and atrophy of the intrinsic muscles of the foot. Sometimes reduction of sudomotor activity can be found. Electroneurography and electromyography will support the diagnosis.

To rule out damage of the tibialis posterior nerve before entering the tarsal canal electroneurographic studies should be done above as well as below the tunnel. The medial and lateral plantar nerve ought to be investigated separately.[4] According to Freising,[5] Mosimann,[6] and de Stoop,[4] a normal nerve conduction velocity and a normal electromyogram (EMG) do not rule out tarsal tunnel syndrome.

Kaplan and Kernahan found no significant differences of posterior tibial motor nerve conduction velocities from knee to ankle between a control group and a group of patients with tarsal tunnel syndrome, but there were significant differences between the two groups concerning amplitude and duration of evoked potentials.[7] This was independent of the distal electrode used for the recording (the one of the abductor digiti minimi or the one to the abductor hallucis). They measured significantly greater distal latencies from the ankle to the abductor digiti quinti in the group with tarsal tunnel syndrome (7.5 ± 0.6 ms) than in the control group (5.0 ± 0.5 ms) but the values measured from the ankle to the abductor hallucis (6.4 ± 0.8 ms) showed some overlap with those in the control group (4.4 ± 0.5 ms). However, even when the distal latencies from the ankle to the abductor hallucis were within normal ranges the evoked potentials had reduced amplitudes and prolonged durations in the tarsal tunnel syndrome patients.

Surgery (After Heimkes)

The skin incision starts about 1.5 cm behind the medial malleous and is carried distally. After passing the tip of the malleolus it is curved parallel to the tibialis posterior tendon. After freeing the flexor retinaculum from the subcutaneous tissue, it is carefully incised longitudinally. An incision perpendicular to this is made at the superior rim of the abductor hallucis.

The tarsal tunnel is now opened like the wings of a door. The vessels in this area are always found medial to the nerve. They must be clamped and pulled aside to allow a clear view of the division of the nerve into its terminal branches.

Fasciectomy under the abductor hallucis muscle is performed next. The superior rim of the abductor hallucis muscle is exposed in the operating field. The muscle belly is freed at its inferior contour and is retracted, so that the deep fascia of this muscle becomes visible. Now the deep fascia of the abductor hallucis muscle, including the fibrous strap that pulls from this fascia to the calcaneus, is resected. This frees both plantar nerves. The tourniquet is opened. After careful hemostasis and insertion of a small, calibrated closed suction drain, the subcutaneous tissue is sutured with a resorbable 3-0 thread, and the skin with 4-0 nonresorbable thread. Mann[3] recommended instillation of

1 ml of hydrocortisone before closure. A mild compression dressing is applied, and the foot is elevated in bed. Slow ankle movements are encouraged on the second day. The patient is mobilized with a bath chair until the third day. Then walking with crutches is initiated.

INFERIOR HEEL PAIN

Etiology and Pathology

Since different opinions can be found for the origin of pain that has traditionally been attributed to an inferior heel spur, a more differentiated approach to the problem of inferior heel pain appears appropriate.

According to Regnauld, pain at the area of the medial plantar tuberosity of the calcaneus results from an inflammatory tendopathy at the origin of the short flexor muscles of the foot and the plantar fascia, forming a degenerative osteophyte at the osteoperiosteal zone in this area.[8] It seems to be caused by repeated static microtrauma in combination with a loss of elasticity of the plantar myoaponeurotic system, supported by the "windlass mechanism" of Hicks.[9]

Dorsiflexion of the great toe winds the plantar aponeurosis, which is attached to the plantar pad of the metatarsolphalangeal joint, around the metatarsal head, thus contributing to the tension of the aponeurosis.[10] Mau mentioned the inflammation of the subcalcaneal bursa as an additional source of pain.[11] Baxter and Thigpen[12] came to the conclusion that the entrapment of the mixed nerve to the proximal portion of the abductor digiti quinti muscle between the deep fascia of the abductor hallucis and the inferior medial ridge of the calcaneus may cause recalcitrant pain (Fig. 36-1).

With respect to the etiologic significance of the heel spur itself, there is no relation between the size of the spur and the pain, indicating that the spur itself is not responsible for the pain.

Evaluation

The primary symptom is usually a circumscript pain at the medial side of the heel at the area of origin of the abductor hallucis muscle, or sometimes more laterally. Pain is often more intensive in the morning; stepping out of bed can be extremely painful. The character of the pain can be burning,

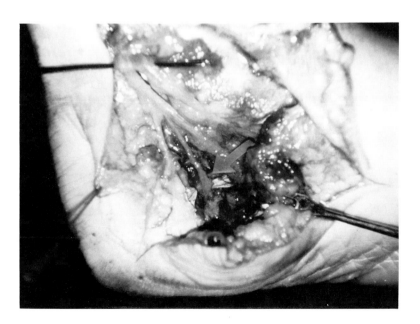

Fig. 36-1. Branches of the posterior tibial nerve.

stinging, tearing, or like the penetration of a nail or a needle through the heel.[8]

Inferior heel pain is found most frequently in females in their 50s when weight is gained, and in all types of feet, frequently with biomechanical disturbances.[8,13]

Management

Management of this syndrome is usually conservative. Before surgery an exact analysis of the structure at fault has to be made. Although rather painful, this can be achieved by injection of a local anesthetic to the point of maximum pain, that is, at the medial tuberosity of the calcaneus. If this does not lead to immediate relief, other structures must be tested. Considerations of differential diagnosis include tarsal tunnel syndrome; sinus tarsi syndrome[8]; entrapment of the branches of the posterior tibial nerve; tenosynovitis of the flexor hallucis longus, digitorum longus, and tibialis posterior tendons, and myofascial disorders at the short plantar muscles.

Referring to the heel spur diseases of the rheumatic group, rheumatoid arthritis, ankylosing spondylitis, Reiter's syndrome, and psoriasis can usually be ruled out clinically and by laboratory findings. Surgery is indicated in cases in which pro-

longed and skillful conservative measures do not lead to a lasting success. The objective of all surgical procedures is to achieve a pain-free foot with the least surgical intervention possible.

Surgery

Preoperative Criteria

In a lateral x-ray of the calcaneus a spur may or may not be seen. An axial x-ray helps to exclude other pathomorphologies of the calcaneus.

Technique

In the author's practice at the Orthopaedic Hospital of Vienna the following technique is used. After general anesthesia, or more recently infiltration anesthesia of the posterior tibial nerve at the ankle ("ankle block"), a 5- to 7-mm skin incision is made with a slender tenotome just over the medial tuberosity in a slightly oblique direction paralleling the cleavage lines of the skin. With the tip of the tenotome contact is made with the medial tuberosity. The forefoot is held in a dorsiflexed position to put the plantar fascia under tension (Fig. 36-2). Without breaking contact with bone, the plantar fascia and the origin of the abductor hallucis muscle are separated from the medial tuberosity (Fig.

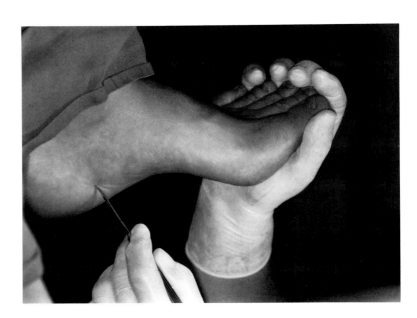

Fig. 36-2. Inferior heel pain. Tenotome points to site of stab incision.

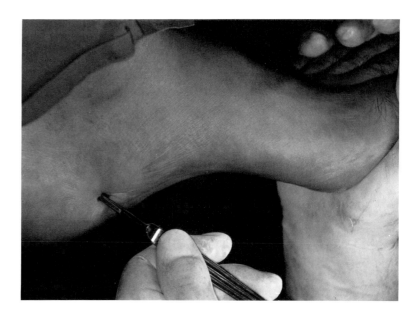

Fig. 36-3. Inferior heel pain. Tenotome inserted. With continuous bone contact the origin of the adductor hallucis muscle and the plantar fascia are severed.

36-3). Suture of the skin is not necessary; a butterfly closure device can be applied.

After dressing of the wound a split below-knee plaster cast is attached, holding the foot in a neutral position. The patient is allowed out of bed on the following day using crutches. On the third day he or she is encouraged to begin walking on the cast, gradually adding weight and eventually breaking it. The plaster is removed when it is broken. Usually a week after operation the patient is free of pain or has some minor pain that is different from the preoperative type.

Discussion. This author's experiences with this simple but effective procedure recommend it as a preferable first step in the operative treatment of the heel spur syndrome.

Removal of the spur or even more invasive procedures, such as the osteotomies recommended by Steindler and Smith[14] or the countersinking osteotomy of Michele and Krueger,[15] ought to be abandoned. If open surgery is preferred, the procedure of Baxter and Thigpen[12] appears to give good results. From a du Vries horizontal incision, the posterior tibial nerve is prepared (see Fig. 36-1). A probe is used to elevate the point at which the nerve branches into the medial (Fig. 36-1, right) and lateral (Fig. 36-1, left) plantar nerve. From the lateral plantar nerve a thicker medial calcaneal nerve and the mixed nerve (Fig. 36-1, arrow) to the abductor digiti quinti muscle separate. The abductor digiti quinti muscle is identified and followed to the plantar aspect of the heel. The inferior edge of the deep abductor hallucis fascia (Fig. 36-1, inferior to arrow) is crossed by the nerve on its extension toward the lateral side of the calcaneus. The deep fascia of the abductor hallucis muscle is released and a small portion of the medial plantar fascia can be incised if it is causing impingement. A complete plantar fascial release or a complete heel spur removal is not recommended by Baxter and Thigpen. They expect this to lengthen the postoperative recovery time and in athletes to cause problems in high performance.

SINUS TARSI SYNDROME

First described by O'Connor[16] in 1958, the sinus tarsi syndrome is characterized by pain over the lateral opening of the sinus tarsi. There is often also a feeling of instability of the ankle.[17]

Etiology and Pathology

According to Rosensky, a direct injury to the structures of the tarsal sinus can be created by an inversion as well as an eversion sprain.[18] Lesions of the ankle joint are often connected with lesions at the subtalar complex.[19] Sequelae of fractures of the calcaneus and the neck of the talus can be at fault.[20] Also, microtrauma to the subtalar joint caused by biochemical dysfunction can initiate the syndrome.[18]

According to Hauser, the lesions found at operation consist of laceration or rupture of the interosseous talocalcaneal ligament and capsular herniation.[21] Debrunner described degenerative hyaline lesions of the ligament and considerable hyalinization of the vessels in the sinus.[22] This was also found by Komprda.[23]

Meyer et al. found that subtalar and ankle sprains were frequently associated with sinus tarsi syndrome.[19] In an analysis of 40 patients using subtalar arthrograms and ankle stress films, they found 32 cases with lesions of both subtalar and ankle capsuloligamentous structures. Isolated subtalar sprains were diagnosed in six patients at arthrography. In chronic cases the obliteration of synovial recesses on posterior subtalar joint arthrography was explained by synovial hyperplasia and cicatricial remodeling of ligament tissue.[24]

Evaluation

Pain at the sinus tarsi augmented by palpation and by inversion of the calcaneus and adduction of the forefoot is the main feature at clinical evaluation. Pes valgoplanus or valgocavus leading to sinus tarsi syndrome often is associated with contracture of the peroneal muscles. Injection of a local anesthetic into the sinus resolves pain and can be used as a diagnostic aid. Lesions of the ankle joint must be ruled out by stress radiographs. Negative stress films after a clinically serious ankle injury should raise suspicion of an underlying subtalar sprain.[19]

Surgery

The operation is aimed at removal of the fatty tissue in the tarsal sinus containing vegetative nerves and vessels, and of lacerated and degenerative parts of the interosseous ligament.

Technique

With the patient under general anesthesia and after application of a tourniquet at the ankle, a Grice-type incision is made over the sinus tarsi that can be palpated well. The subcutaneous tissue and the fascia are divided taking care to avoid the lateral branch of the superficial peroneal nerve. Extensions of the extensor retinaculum are divided, aiming for the sinus. The fat pad is removed from the sinus with a knife and the remaining tissue is removed with a curette (Fig. 36-4). Lacerated fibers of the interosseous ligament are resected. Parts of the capsule of the subtalar joint are removed if altered by trauma or inflammation.[20] The integrity of the fibulotalar ligaments is verified.

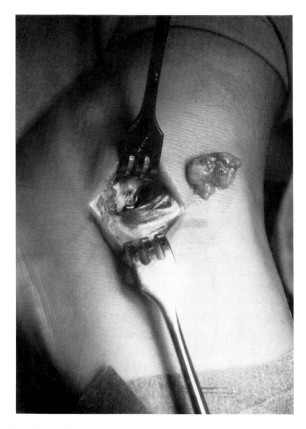

Fig. 36-4. Sinus tarsi syndrome. The fatty tissue is removed from the sinus tarsi. Fibers of the cervical ligament are seen in the depth of the wound.

After hemostasis a small, calibrated Redon suction drainage is installed and the fascia and subcutaneous tissue are closed by 3-0 resorbable sutures, and the skin with nonresorbable 4-0 sutures. A compression dressing is applied. Dressings are changed on the second postoperative day and an elastic adhesive bandage is put on. The drain is removed on the day following surgery and the patient is allowed out of bed with crutches. Weight-bearing is gradually increased with the abilities of the patient.

Discussion. The Key point of the operation is the removal of the fatty tissue containing the autonomous nerve fibers that create a proprioceptive reflexogenic zone, the "eye of the foot" according to Valenti.[20] Thus the main feature is a denervation of the sinus tarsi.

Complications

Complications are usually not expected in this rather simple intervention in the foot.

TENDON DISORDERS

Tendo Calcaneus (Achilles Tendon)

The calcaneal tendon is the conjoined tendon of the gastrocnemius and soleus muscles. It is the largest tendon of the human body, moving within the paratenon, a loose, gliding tissue in connection with the superficial crural fascia. Each muscle fiber continues into a tendon fiber.[25] They rotate from their origin to the insertion in a spiral manner in a varying degree.[26]

The arterial blood supply for the tendon is provided proximally by the sural arteries for both heads of the gastrocnemius muscle and the plantaris longus muscle, by the posterior tibial artery, and by the peroneal artery for the soleus muscle. Distally a subcutaneous arterial network between the posterior tibial and the peroneal artery cares for arterial blood supply. Between the two areas, about 5 cm proximal to the insertion of the tendon in the posterior tuberosity, there is a region of diminished blood supply,[27] coincident with the smallest diameter of the tendon.[28] This is an area of minor resistance and usually the site of ruptures. Reduction of capillary vessels and ongoing obliteration of vessels starting at the age of 30 years contribute to degenerative changes within the tendon.[28]

Chronic Calcaneal Paratenonitis

Etiology and Pathology. Pain at the Achilles tendon is one of the most frequent symptoms of sports injuries, not only in high-performance athletes but also in the increasing number of those participating in leisure activities. It is attributed to inflammatory reactions of the gliding tissue of the tendon and degenerative alterations of the tendon itself, whether localized or diffuse, nodular or plain.[29]

Pathologic changes around the insertion area of the tendon and the posterior protrusion of the calcaneus must be distinguished from chronic calcaneal paratenonitis. Mostly the cause is chronic overuse of the tendon in sports connected with running and jumping.

Evaluation. Histologic evaluations show that paratenonitis is characterized by edema of the network of elastic fibers, fibrinous exudate, hyperemia, augmentation of perivascular cells, and formation of granulation tissue partly infiltrated with lymphocytes.[30] In the adjacent parts of the tendon formations of necrosis can be noticed.

On physical examination in a standing position, preferably on a podoscope, the posterior aspect of the leg may be visualized. Often thickening of the area can be noticed. Functional and structural deformities of the foot are analyzed. The patient is asked to stand up on tip-toe and on the heels, and finally to squat, heels on the ground. The latter maneuver is always limited and painful in paratenonitis. In a supine position passive flexion and extension is compared with the contralateral side. In a prone position Thompsons's sign is tested. Painful resisted movements are symptomatic for paratenonitis and tenonitis. Palpation reveals thickening and eventually crepitus, and creates pain.

Lateral x-rays are made in a standing position at low voltage to delineate the contours of the soft tissues, especially in respect to thickening and the integrity of Kager's triangle.

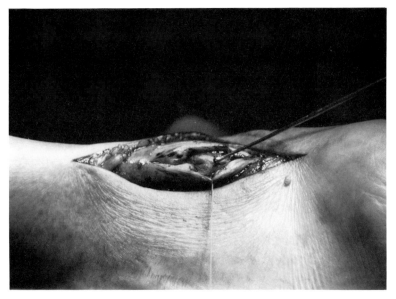

A

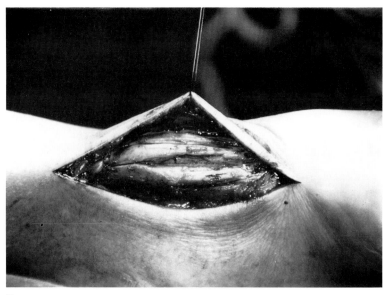

B

Fig. 36-5. Partial necrosis of Achilles tendon **(A)** After opening of the paratenon necrotic areas are exposed in the Achilles tendon at a location typically 4 to 5 cm above the posterior process of the calcaneus. Partial necrosis of Achilles tendon **(B)** Necrotic areas are excised and the Achilles tendon is divided into several bundles.

Recently ultrasound has been used to evaluate the quality of the paratenon and the underlying tendon tissue.[31,32]

Clinical findings can be documented. In paratenonitis a general or localized thickening of the tendon with a reduction of the echo pattern can be found. Distinction between the paratenon and the tendon and subcutaneous tissues can no longer be made. Also, progress in healing of the lesions following conservative therapy can be demonstrated.[31,32]

Management. Management is at first conservative. Treatment is aiming at the inflammatory reactions of the paratenon and at the cause of the condition.[29] Only if this fails after a selected period of time, preferably more than 6 months, is surgery indicated.

Surgery.   The objective of surgery is to create a pain-free condition by removing the altered peritendinous tissue, remove necrotic areas of the tendon, and trying to revascularize and augment the tendinous tissue by the formation of scars.

With the patient in a prone position under general anesthesia and after application of a tourniquet, a longitudinal incision at the medial aspect of the tendon is made from the calcaneus to the musculotendinous junction (Fig. 36-5A). Then the paratenon is incised and the thickened areas are removed by sharp dissection, except the anterior portion, which is retained to preserve the vascular supply. After removal of the thickened parts of the paratenon the tendon is palpated between two fingers to identify indurated areas. After that the tendon is separated longitudinally with a knive, respecting the direction of the fibers, from the musculotendinous junction down to the calcaneus. Any necrotic areas that become visible are excised (Fig. 36-5B). Depending on the thickness of the tendon more longitudinal incisions forming four to six cords are performed.[29] This helps to find intratendinous lesions such as fibrous nodules, cysts, and calcifications. These must be excised to reduce pain after the operation. It should be noted that this "combing through" the tendon creates scar tissue, reinforcing the tendon and providing for revascularization.[29] In cases of severe damage of the tendon Biehl and Harms recommended reinforcing the Achilles tendon by weaving through the plantaris longus and if necessary also the peroneus brevis tendon and muscle after removal of the necroses.[30]

After opening the tourniquet careful hemostasis is provided, a closed-suction drainage system installed, the subcutaneous tissue is sutured with resorbable 3-0 material, and the skin is closed with a 4-0 nonresorbable suture. Postoperatively a split, below-knee plaster cast is applied with the foot in a 15 degree equinus position. Dressings are changed on the first and sixth postoperative days. Ten days after the operation the sutures are removed from the skin and a below-knee walking cast in neutral position of the ankle joint is put on for 6 weeks. After removal of the cast physiotherapy is started to regain mobility of the ankle joint and strength in the calf muscles. Four weeks after removal of plaster slow running is allowed, but full sports activity should not be permitted before 4 months after surgery. Excellent results are reported with this method by Saillant et al.[29] and Biehl and Harms.[30] In this author's experience full recovery needs 6 months in more severe cases.

Discussion.   Criteria for acceptable results are pain-free full-range mobility of the ankle joint and the ability to take up competitive sports activities again.

Complications.   Complications, mostly consisting of disturbed wound healing, can be avoided by (1) atraumatic surgical technique, especially in respect to manipulations of the skin by retractors and at suturing; (2) careful hemostasis before closure of the wound; and (3) avoiding hematoma by closed-suction Redon drainage.

Rupture of the Achilles Tendon

Etiology and Pathology.   After the third decade a reduction of vascularization of the Achilles tendon takes place. This is especially true for an area about 5 cm proximal from the insertion of the tendon in the calcaneus, where the vascular supply is least[27] and the tendon has its smallest diameter.[28] Here degenerative changes take place that weaken the strength of the tendon tissue. Degenerative alterations also involve the paratenon. The elasticity of the tendon is reduced and it becomes prone to lesions at suddenly increasing tension, as in sprinting and jumping.

Injection of corticosteroids in the tendon or paratenon in the form of crystalline preparations leads to formation of necrosis within the tendon.[33] Also, systemic medication with corticosteroids can lead to ruptures of the tendon.[34] There is still some controversy as to whether degenerative changes are the prerequisite for ruptures.[28] It has been proved, however, that even a healthy tendon can rupture at extreme, sudden overload. Wilhelm found a maximum load capacity of the Achilles tendon of 400 to 600 kp in static experiments and 930 kp in dynamic studies.[35] He proved that resistance to rupture can also be overcome in healthy tendons by extreme actions, such as double backward somersaults or ski accidents.

According to Schwarz et al., 80 percent of patients are men and 20 percent are women, with an average age of 34 years.[36]

Dederich et al. found in 90 percent of their operated Achilles tendons degenerative alterations of various degrees.[28] Könn and Löbbecke, in 1975, described edema with fibrinoid warping of the tendon fibers in the early stages of degeneration.[37] The tendon bundles are separated by fresh and old resorbed hematomas and necrosis. At overuse microruptures with creation of connective tissue scars can develop and further reduce the carrying capacity of the tendon. In severe degeneration the texture of the tendon is altered by necrosis, microruptures of different age, and scar tissue with fibers that are already directed longitudinally again. Hemorrhages and deposits of hemosiderin are found.[37]

Evaluation. Although usually easy to diagnose, Achilles tendon ruptures are often overlooked or not searched for, resulting in a delay of treatment. Pain and swelling of the site of the rupture, a palpable ditch at the gap of the stumps, weak flexion at the ankle joint, a positive Thompson sign (at squeezing of the calf muscles by the hand of the investigator plantar flexion of the foot does not occur), and an absent Achilles tendon reflex, together with the history, will lead to the diagnosis. On radiographs Kager's triangle will show an interrupted hypotenuse.

Ruptures can also take place at the calcaneal insertion, usually with a bony fragment, or at the musculotendinous junction of the gastrocnemius muscle, the so-called tennis leg.[28]

Management. There is still some controversy as to whether the ruptured Achilles tendon ought to be treated conservatively or by operation. According to the review of Carden et al., the results in patients treated conservatively within 48 hours were very similar to those in patients treated by operation.[38] They found more complications in the patients treated by operation (17 percent) than in the group treated conservatively (3 percent). Conservative management yielded inferior results after treatment with a delay of more that 1 week after injury.

Wills et al., in their review of the literature, distilled a rerupture rate for surgically treated patients of 1.54 percent (12 of 777) and for nonsurgically managed patients of 17.7 percent (40 of 226),

and a 20 percent complication rate in the surgical group compared to 10 percent in the nonsurgical group.[39] It is pointed out, however, that in more recent publications the complication rate in surgery is low (3.1 percent in Shield et al.[40]) and also that complications tend to be minor and do not affect the final results.[39] Wills et al. concluded that surgical is superior to conservative treatment with respect to the incidence of rerupture and to functional strength. This is especially true for the active athletic patient. Wills et al. advocated nonsurgical treatment for high-risk and sedentary patients only. This is supported by Kelikian and Kelikian.[41]

Surgery. The objectives of surgery are to restore full strength and free mobility at the ankle joint. According to Wills et al. surgery seems to be indicated in all cases of ruptures with the aforementioned exceptions.[39]

Preoperative Criteria. Preoperative criteria are the clinical findings supplemented by radiographs and ultrasound investigations to document the lesion.

Technique. Schönbauer, in his review of the literature, found 80 different surgical methods and modifications for the treatment of Achilles tendon rupture.[34] Simple adaptive sutures can be combined with fibrin glue. Bunnel-type sutures with resorbable or nonresorbable material, fascia lata, lyophilized fascia lata and dura, cutis straps, plantaris or peroneus brevis tendon, wire, and carbon fibers have been used as suture or augmenting material. Turn-down plasties after Bosworth[42] are used by several authors in different modifications.[43] Slipping a healthy part of the proximal stump distally as a free graft, like a pencilbox, was advocated by Lange.[44] The method to restore function of a ruptured calcaneal tendon has to be as simple and efficient as possible. This author recommends the methods used by Schwarz et al.[36] and Dederich et al.[28]

Bleeding must be controlled from the beginning of the operation so subsequent hematoma formation will be avoided. A longitudinal, slightly curved incision is made at the medial aspect of the tendon, long enough to expose the fragments sufficiently for reconstruction (Fig. 36-6A). The paratenon is incised longitudinally at the medial side and the fragments of the tendon are exposed. In flexion of

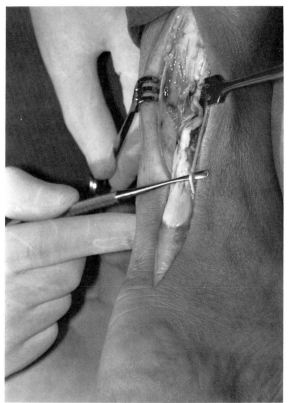

A

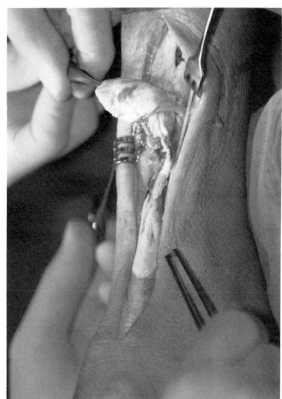

B

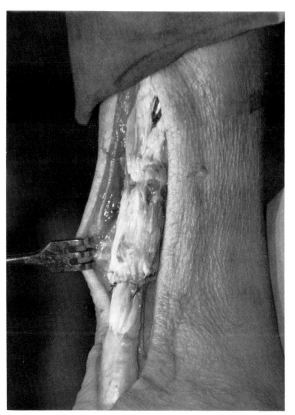

C

Fig. 36-6. Rupture of Achilles tendon. **(A)** Defect in the Achilles tendon is exposed and plantaris longus tendon prepared. **(B)** Pedunculated flap from proximal tendon fragment is reflected distally. **(C)** Pedunculated flap is sewn to distal tendon stump.

the ankle joint the tendon stumps are anastomosed by Dexon or Vicryl 4-0 sutures. If present, the plantaris longus tendon is severed proximally by a special stripper (after Schöttle), pulled out distally, and woven through the tendon stumps with a special needle (after Jungbluth). Then a distally pedunculated flap of 3 mm thickness is created in the frontal plane from the proximal fragment, reflected distally, and sutured over the site of the rupture (Fig. 36-6B). The edges of this flap are secured with 2-0 Dexon or Vicryl sutures (Fig. 36-6C). It might be difficult to suture the paratenon over the reconstruction. A Redon suction drain is inserted. The skin is closed by intracutaneous resorbable sutures (4-0 Dexon or Vicryl), and secured by adhesive strips. A split, below-knee plaster cast is applied and a dorsal window is cut on the day following surgery to enable changing the dressing. The leg is elevated on a Braun's frame to prevent edema.

After 10 days a below-knee walking cast with the foot in 20 degrees of plantar flexion is made and the patient is allowed to walk. The plaster is removed after 6 weeks. An elastic stocking is given until swelling ceases.

Discussion. Key points of the operation include the following. The slightly curved medial incision results in good cosmesis and allows access to the plantaris longus tendon. The direct suture, secured by the plantaris longus tendon, and the inversion plasty warrant good stability of the reconstruction. The wound must be handled very carefully to avoid disturbed healing. A soft wound dressing must be used and changed on the day following surgery.

A long leg cast is not necessary. Benum et al., in their electromyographic study, found that strain during weightbearing in a walking cast with the foot in 20 degrees of flexion will not exceed the strength of the sutured tendon.[45]

Criteria for acceptable results are full strength in the triceps surae muscle with pain-free full mobility in the ankle joint.

Complications. Complications are mostly created by disturbed wound healing, or by hematoma and necrosis at the site of repair with subsequent rerupture. This can be avoided by atraumatic handling of the tissues and careful hemostasis before closure of the wound. Postoperative surveillance of the wound is necessary.

Rupture of the Tibialis Anterior Tendon

The anterior tibial muscle gets tendinous at the border of the lower and the middle third of the tibia,[41] and below this develops its synovial sheath that reaches down to the level of the talonavicular joint.[46] It passes under the superior extensor retinaculum and under the supero- and inferomedial band of the inferior extensor retinaculum, winds around the medial border of the foot, and inserts on the base of the first metatarsal inferomedially and on the medial aspect of the first cuneiform. The site of rupture is usually between the superior extensor retinaculum and the superomedial band of the inferior extensor retinaculum.[47]

Etiology and Pathology

Rupture of the tibialis anterior tendon usually occurs in men between 50 and 60 years of age. The mechanism of trauma is a sudden plantar flexion of the dorsiflexed foot,[48,49] as occurs in missing a stair. In most cases an inadequate trauma is inflicted on an already damaged tendon.[50] According to Bengert, rheumatoid alterations and diabetic angiopathy seem to contribute to the degenerative lesions predisposing to the ruptures.[51] Kashyap and Prince described a case in a diabetic patient.[47] It is well known that corticosteroids can produce necrosis tendons.

The distal segment of the torn tendon retracts, becomes thickened, and protrudes between the superior and inferior retinaculum like a tumor. Frequently it is taken for a ganglion. Necrotic areas, microruptures, hemorrhages, and peritendinous apposition of fibrin are described.[50]

Evaluation

In the history there is often a trauma that leads to a sudden extension of the foot. Pain, swelling, and weakness of extension of the foot result, and a foot-drop gait develops. The patient often receives treatment similar to that for a sprained ankle, but a tumor-like formation develops proximal to the ankle joint that moves with the foot in flexion and extension (Fig. 36-7A). Power of extension is re-

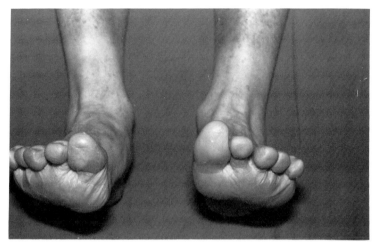

A

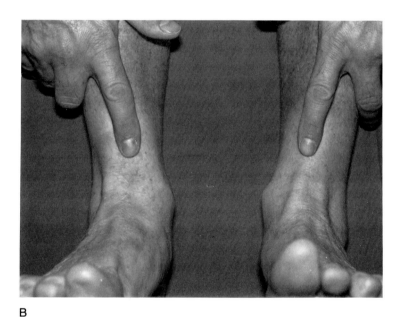

Fig. 36-7. (A) Clinical signs of rupture of tibialis anterior tendon. **(A)** Note depression of first ray at the right foot. **(B)** Clinical signs of rupture of tibialis anterior tendon. The contour of the tendon is missing on the right side. Investigator's finger "falls into a ditch." *(Figure continues.)*

B

duced, and the contour of the tibialis anterior tendon is missing (Fig. 36-7B). Atrophy of the tibialis anterior can be seen. At palpation the continuity of the tendon is absent.

Management

Management is surgical, and usually even after several weeks of delay primary suture can be accomplished.

Surgery

Objectives are to restore extension power of the foot and a normal gait pattern. The operation is indicated except in individuals in whom complications at surgery can be expected.

A longitudinal incision is made lateral to the tumor-like protrusion and the tendon sheath is divided (Fig. 36-7C). The wound is enlarged proximally, following the tendon sheath to the proximal

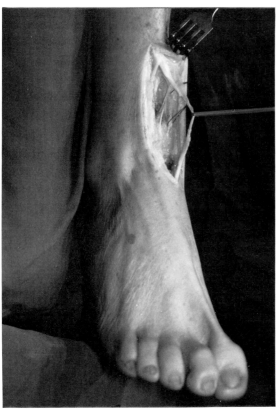

C

Fig. 36-7 *(Continued).* **(C)** Incomplete rupture of tibialis anterior tendon. Tendon exposed at operation. Thinned out connection of the degenerated tendon stumps.

fragment. Adhesions to the sheath are divided bluntly, altered synovium is excised, and the freshened fragments of the tendon are approximated with a Bunnel-type suture using a long-term resorbable material (PDS-1). The foot is held in extension. After closure of the tendon sheath with resorbable sutures (3-0 Dexon or Vicryl), the skin is closed with intracutaneous resorbable sutures. Adhesive straps are used to maintain approximation of the edges of the wound.

A split, padded, below-knee cast is made in easily attainable extension of the foot. After 10 days a new plaster cast is applied for 4 weeks from the day of operation. Then a walking device is added and full weightbearing is allowed. At 6 to 8 weeks after surgery the cast is removed and rehabilitation is started.

Rupture of the Tibialis Posterior Tendon

The tendon, retained in a fibrous tunnel, courses just posterior to the medial malleolus, crosses the medial aspect of the posterior talus and the medial aspect of the talar neck, passes through the tarsal tunnel, and is located above the sustentaculum tali.[52] Further distally it crosses the inferior surface of the inferior calcaneonavicular ligament. Here the flat tendon contains a fibrocartilaginous or bony sesamoid.[52] The tendon has widespread insertions at the plantar side of the foot. A navicular, plantar, and recurrent insertion are distinguished. The main insertions are at the navicular, at the first cuneiform, and a cuneometatarsal portion to the second and third cuneiform and bases of the second and third metatarsals.

The muscle is the main dynamic stabilizer of the hindfoot against valgus deformity, forming a strong support for the head of the talus. Ruptures of the tendon result in a severe flatfoot deformity.

Etiology and Pathology

Rupture usually occurs in a tendon being deranged by chronic tenosynovitis, necrosis resulting from decreased blood supply to the tendon, and steroid injections.[53] The rupture usually happens in an eversion injury,[54] but most patients cannot remember an inciting injury. Among Johnson's 11 cases there were only four patients who were able to recall an injury.[55] Accidental division near the medial malleolus is easily overlooked and also causes painful planovalgus deformity.[56,57]

Funk et al. distinguished between avulsions of the tendon from its insertion, midsubstance ruptures, and incontinuity tears.[58] A tear leads to loss of support of the rearfoot at the medial arch of the foot. Excessive stress is exerted on the ligamentous connections of the hindfoot. They gradually elongate, the head of the talus moves medially and downward, and a flatfoot deformity develops. This rather insidious progress of the deformity often leads to delayed diagnosis.[54] Tenosynovitis is frequently present in ruptures of the tibialis posterior. Johnson speculated that tenosynovitis may be a secondary reaction to a tendon tear, and also that the deformity may cause the tenosynovitis.[55] As in ruptures of other tendons, degenerative changes would appear soon after the trauma. In one of this author's cases necrosis of the tendon fibers, myxoid degeneration, and initial chondral metaplasia were found, as well as regeneration with proliferative fibroblasts and vascular formations. In the peritendinous tissue chronic inflammatory infiltration and vascularized granulations were described by the investigator.

Evaluation

Patients are mostly women over 40 years of age.[55] Since often a trauma is not noticed by a patient or is neglected because it seems inadequate to produce the resulting lesion, diagnosis is often delayed. The patient presents with a painful planovalgus deformity of the foot. Pain and tenderness are found from the medial malleolus to the infranavicular insertion area of the tendon. Later the lateral tarsal area also may become painful.[55] Swelling will be found at the medial side of the hindfoot. A planovalgus type of foot will be present. The forefoot abduction is best seen from a frontal view, and the rearfoot valgus from a posterior view. Johnson's "too many toes" sign (because of the abduction more toes are visible at the lateral side of the foot) also is of use in the estimation of the degree of deformity. A podoscope will be a helpful tool in evaluating the severity of the resulting flatfoot.

Functional evaluation sometimes is difficult because the inversion and supinating action of the tibialis posterior tendon can be mimicked by the long flexor tendons of the toes. With an intact tibialis posterior tendon the foot can be inverted and supinated and then plantarflexed and dorsiflexed while held in this position.[56] Johnson recommended the single heel raise test for evaluation of the tibialis posterior function.[55] The tibialis posterior brings the hindfoot into a locked, stable varus position. This is necessary before the patient can rise onto the ball of the foot by use of the triceps sural muscle.[55] The single heel raise test is positive if the hindfoot does not achieve a stable position and it becomes difficult to raise the heel from the ground. When the investigator holds the foot and asks the patient to invert and adduct it, weakness of this movement will be noticed and the palpating finger will not notice tension over the bed of the tendon.

Radiographs are taken with the patient in a standing position. In the dorsoplantar view the talocalcaneal angle will be increased, and subluxation of the talonavicular joint will be present. On lateral x-rays a break at the talonavicular articulation will be seen together with an increased calcaneometatarsal angle. Reactive periostitis of the distal tibia was seen by Rosenberg et al. in 71 percent of their cases.[59]

Management

Surgery is the treatment of choice and ought to be done as early as possible. Nonsurgical treatment is recommended only in decrepit individuals who are at high risk during surgery.

Surgery

In the most common tears, where longer parts of the degenerated tendons are involved, transfer of the flexor digitorum longus tendon is advocated.[55,58] Mann directly inserts the flexor digitorum longus tendon into the navicular.[60] Flexion of the lesser toes will be possible to a certain degree by the short flexors. The distal flexor digitorum longus stump can be anastomosed with the flexor hallucis longus tendon. When the area of tissue damage at the tendon stumps is short and the rupture rather clear cut, a direct end-to-end Bunnel-type suture will be possible.

If the insertion at the underside of the navicular is severed, the tendon will have to be reattached.[55]

Objectives of the operation are the reestablishment of a well-powered tendon inserting at the navicular tuberosity and the cuneiform to provide for dynamic support of the medial arch of the foot. The operation is indicated as soon as the diagnosis is established. Preoperative criteria are x-ray findings of flatfoot with a loss of function of the posterior tibial tendon. Ultrasound, computed tomography,[59] and magnetic resonance imaging[61] seem to be of rather academic value.

Technique. A curvilinear incision is made following the direction of the tibialis posterior tendon. Since the rupture is to be expected just distal to the malleolus, the incision is deepened there to the flexor retinaculum, which is split longitudinally.

The hypertrophied and inflamed synovium is removed and the incision is widened proximally and distally to identify the stumps of the tendon. Necrotic tissue is resected and the tendon is repaired with an end-to-end suture of Bunnel's type using long-term resorbable material (PDS-0).

If the ends of the fragments are separated too far by retraction, a reversion plasty can be used by dividing the proximal fragment longitudinally and leaving it in connection with the proximal stump (Fig. 36-8).

The edges of the area of reflection are secured by two sutures and the deflected part of the proximal stump is sutured to the distal fragment with PDS-0, holding the foot in inversion and slight flexion. If damage of the tendon is too serious, the tendon sheath of the flexor digitorum longus is opened and the tendon cut obliquely 3 cm distal to the proximal end of the peripherial part of the tibialis posterior tendon. A side-to-side suture unites the proximal stump of the flexor digitorum longus tendon to the distal stump of the tibialis posterior tendon. The proximal fragment of the tibialis posterior tendon is sutured to the flexor digitorum.

In the rather rare cases of avulsion at the insertion, the avulsed end of the tendon is pulled into an osseous canal from plantar to dorsal by means of a Bunnel-type suture. The ends of the suture are tightened in the periosteum.

After hemostasis and insertion of a Redon drain, the flexor retinaculum is sutured with resorbable 3-0 Dexon or Vicryl, and the skin closed by intracutaneous resorbable sutures. A padded, split, below-knee cast is applied. After 10 days a new cast is made. Four weeks after surgery a walking cast is given for 6 to 8 weeks following surgery. After that reeducation of mobility and strength is started.

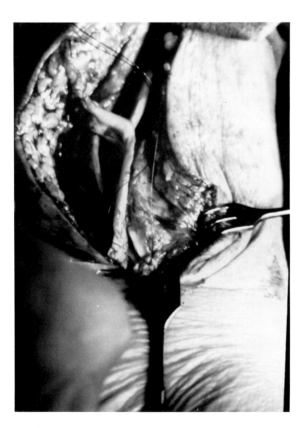

Fig. 36-8. Tibialis posterior tendon rupture. Proximal stump is divided longitudinally and half of proximal portion is reflected distally.

Rupture of the Peroneal Tendons

Traumatic rupture of the peroneal tendons is a rare event.[62,63] Abraham and Stirnaman[62] could not find any cases in the world literature at the time of their review. They suspected that the lesion might be common but rarely recognized.

Etiology and Pathology

Rupture of the peroneal tendons occurs at the site of the os peroneum by fracturing it,[64] at a point proximal to the superior peroneal retinaculum,[62] or at the musculotendinous junction, causing a hematoma and subsequently a peroneal compartment syndrome.

Tenosynovitis, degenerative alterations in diabetes, and injections of steroids at the site of the rupture, as well as systemic treatment with corticosteroids, have been discussed as causative factors for direct ruptures of the tendons.[62] In cases with rupture at the site of the os peroneum, which is present in 14 to 26 percent of feet,[65] and lesions at the musculotendinous junction, excessive sudden overload in an inverted position of the foot may be responsible even in a not previously damaged tendon.

Evaluation

In all cases with pain at the lateral side of the foot and ankle, lesions of the peroneal tendons, although rare, have to be taken in account.[63] Ruptures of the lateral collateral ligaments, subtalar instability, sinus tarsi syndrome, and contusions of this area should raise suspicion of a concomitant lesion of the peroneal tendons. Physical examination includes testing of extension and eversion power in movements of the foot. Ruptures at the musculotendinous junction will reveal more dramatic symptoms, especially if an anterolateral compartment syndrome develops. The tendons usually can be sutured.[62-64] In a peroneal compartment syndrome decompression must be carried out as soon as possible.[66]

Dislocation of the Peroneal Tendons

Etiology and Pathology

Elongation or rupture of the superior peroneal retinaculum is responsible for dislocation of the peroneal tendons. As a primary presupposition for the lesion, Muralt postulated a hypoplasia of the posterior groove of the lateral malleolus.[67] The mechanism of dislocation is usually movement of the foot as follows: supination — pronation — extension,[68] elicited by jumping down onto an oblique surface.

Evaluation

A lesion of lateral collateral ligaments has to be ruled out when pain, swelling, and hematoma about the lateral malleolus occur after an acute trauma. In chronic cases diagnosis is usually not difficult. Raising on tiptoe with a slight eversion sometimes leads to a snapping anterior dislocation of the tendons (Fig. 36-9). The tendon sheaths are often thickened by chronic irritation.

Management

Management of the condition is by surgery.

Surgery

The objectives are to definitely retain the tendons behind the lateral malleolus. Operation is indicated when dislocation and subluxing create painful inflammatory reactions and when instability of the ankle joint results. Preoperative criteria are the findings at a careful clinical examination.

Technique. Of the numerous operative techniques, a modification by Leitz[69] of Platzgummer's[70] transportation of the tendons under the calcaneofibular ligament has proved valuable in this author's experience. With the patient in a lateral position a tourniquet is placed at the thigh. A curved incision is made behind the lateral malleolus. The peroneal tendons are retracted dorsally with their usually thickened sheaths. The calcaneofibular ligament is prepared. A curved hemostatic forceps is passed under the ligament to evaluate its width in the frontal plane. A flat corticocancellous scale of bone is removed from the posterior two-thirds of the malleolus in connection with the origin of the calcaneofibular ligament.

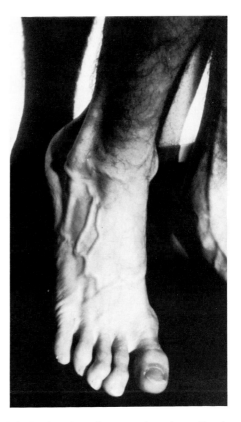

Fig. 36-9. Dislocation of peroneal tendons. Tendons displaced anteriorly by raising on tiptoe with slight eversion of the foot.

The piece of bone is pulled downward and backward under the peroneal tendons. The peroneal tendons are repositioned behind the malleolus with their sheaths. Sometimes because of the hypertrophic tissue the posterior part of the sheaths has to be removed to place the tendons behind the lateral ankle. The bone scale is replaced in its bed and fixed with a screw or two Kirschner wires. If there is no groove at the posterior face of the malleolus, the piece of bone can be moved dorsally some 2 to 3 mm to provide for better bony support of the tendons. The tourniquet is opened.

After hemostasis a small calibrated closed Redon suction drain is inserted and the wound is closed in layers. Size 3-0 resorbable material is used for subcutaneous sutures and 4-0 nonresorbable threads for the skin. A split plaster cast is put on. Dressings are changed on the second postoperative day, and the sutures are removed on the 10th day. A snugly fitting walking cast is applied for 6 weeks postoperatively. Physiotherapy is started after removal of the cast to regain mobility of the ankle joint.

Discussion.   The key points of the technique are as follows. Anatomically there is sufficient room for the tendons under the calcaneofibular ligament, because it is originating from the lateral cortex of the malleolus.[70] A redislocation of the tendons is not possible except with rupture of the ligament. The oblique direction of the ligament appears ideal to retain the tendons.

Criteria for acceptable results are a reliable rerouting of the tendons behind the lateral malleolus without any mechanical irritation. Disadvantages of this operation were not seen in Leitz's material with regard to function or possible peritendinitis.[69] This matches with this author's experiences.

Complications.   Since the operation is rather simple severe complications are not expected.

Pöll and Duifjes Modification.   An improvement of the operative technique was published by Pöll and Duifjes in 1984.[71] They mobilized the distal insertion of the calcaneofibular ligament with a rectangular bone block to transpose it to the lateral side of the peroneal tendons. The replaced bone block was then refixed with a cancellous screw. The authors think that, in contrast to Leitz's modification, the possibility of adhesions is avoided and that a safer refixation of the distal bone block is obtained.

HAGLUND'S HEEL

Prominence of the posterosuperior corner of the calcaneus causing painful symptoms in this area is commonly known as Haglund's heel (Fig. 36-10). Most authors do not, as did Mann,[72] distinguish be-

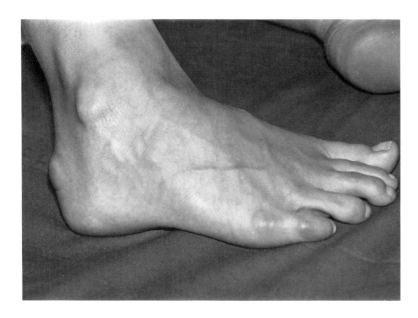

Fig. 36-10. Haglund's heel. Callosity at posterosuperior edge of calcaneus.

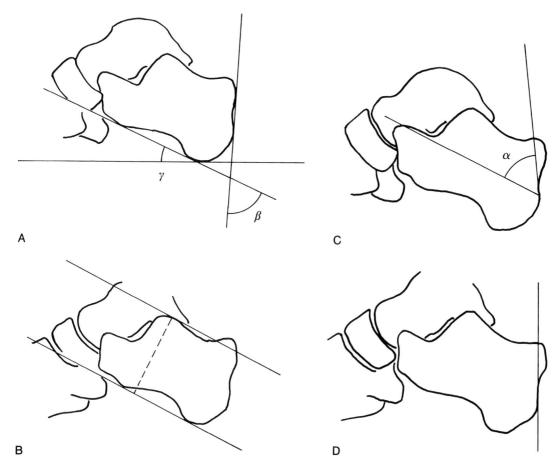

Fig. 36-11. Measurements for the definition of Haglund's heel. **(A)** Fowler and Philipp[75]: The angle β between the posterior and plantar surface of the calcaneus ranges between 44 and 69 degrees. To evaluate the importance of the prominence the calcaneal inclination angle γ must be added. According to Vega et al.[76] the prominence is likely to become symptomatic if the addition of these two angles exceeds 90 degrees. **(B)** Pavlov et al[77]: A tangent to the posterior lip of the talar articular facet paralleling the anterior and medial tubercle of the posterior tuberosity will touch the upper contour of the posterior process of the calcaneus or pass superior to it in normal feet. **(C)** Steffensen and Even[78]: The angle α between a line being drawn parallel to the longitudinal axis of the calcaneus through the superior margin of the insertion of the Achilles tendon and the most superior point of the calcaneal tuberosity measured on a standing lateral x-ray view must not exeed 60 degrees in normal feet. **(D)** Denis and Hubert-Levernieux[79]: A vertical tangent is drawn to the middle part of the tuberosity in a lateral standing x-ray view. The tangent is not supposed to cut the posterosuperior edge in normal feet.

tween the posterior protrusion of the calcaneus and a lateral ridge along the posterior aspect of the calcaneus that is observed even more frequently. Taylor described the site of the prominence as posterolateral.[73] In only 10 heels out of 61 was it found directly posterior.[73]

Evaluation

Symptoms are usually elicited by the upper margin of the shoe counter exerting mechanical irritation on the prominence.[74] Usually the patient presents with painful swelling at the upper lateral edge of the calcaneus. Superficial skin lesions such as blisters, hyperkeratosis, and deep irritation such as formation of a bursa and periostitis can be found. Several authors have attempted to establish measurements for an objective evaluation of the posterosuperior prominence.

Fowler and Philip described an angle between the posterior and the plantar surface of the calcaneus ranging between 44 and 69 degrees in normal feet (Fig. 36-11A).[75] Above 75 degrees abnormal pressures are to be expected. The extent of the prominence is also influenced by the calcaneal inclination angle. According to Vega et al., the calcaneal inclination angle has to be added to Fowler and Philip's angle to evaluate the importance of the prominence.[76] Above 90 degrees the prominence appears to become symptomatic.

Another objective method to depict the prominence has been given by Pavlov et al., using parallel pitch lines (Fig. 36-11B). The inferior line is a tangent to the anterior tubercle and medial to the tubercle of the posterior tuberosity. Parallel to this a superior line is drawn as a tangent to the posterior lip of the talar articular facet. In normal feet the posterior prominence is touching the line or below it.

Steffensen and Even measured an angle defined by the longitudinal axis of the calcaneus and the most superior point of the calcaneal tuberosity (Fig. 36-11C).[78] It must not exceed 60 degrees.

Denis and Huber-Levernieux traced a vertical tangent at the middle part of the tuberosity in a lateral standing x-ray view (Fig. 36-11D).[79] The contour of the upper edge of the tuberosity may touch the tangent or pass anterior to it. It is not supposed to be crossed by the tangent.

For the differential diagnosis of heel pain in this area rheumatoid arthritis, ankylosing spondylitis, psoriasis, Reiter's syndrome, and Behçet's syndrome must be taken into consideration. Metabolic disorders producing microcrystalline formations, such as gout, chondrocalcinosis, and hydroxyapatite-related reactions at or near the insertion of the Achilles tendon, can also cause inflammation in this area.

Management

Most of the time conservative measures fail or appear too complicated in the patient's opinion.

Surgery

At the time of surgery the calcaneal apophysis must be fused.[80] Otherwise regeneration of the prominence with recurrence of symptoms can occur.

The operation is aimed at removal of the protruding posterosuperior aspect of the calcaneus (Fig. 36-12). It is performed under general intubation anesthesia with the patient in a prone position if the condition is bilateral or in a lateral position if it is unilateral. A tourniquet is used. A lateral hockey stick–shaped 5-cm skin incision is made just anterior to the contour of the Achilles tendon. The subcutaneous tissue is separated and the tendo calcaneus is identified. The connections of the peritendinous sheath with the deep fascia are divided, the retrocalcaneal bursa is opened, and the posterosuperior calcaneal prominence is exposed. Resection of a superficial tendo calcaneus bursa is usually not necessary. A blunt, 1-cm wide bayonet-shaped Hohmann retractor is inserted around the dorsally exposed calcaneal tuberosity, and a second one is inserted perpendicular to it around the superior and medial circumference of the calcaneus.

It is necessary to sever the most superiorly inserting fibers of the tendo calcaneus, especially on the medial side where the insertion is reaching more proximally (Fig. 36-13), in order to be able to remove a sufficient piece of bone. The periosteum is incised with a scalpel, delineating the line of osteotomy at the lateral and superior aspect of the calcaneus. With a 3-cm wide sharp osteotome a

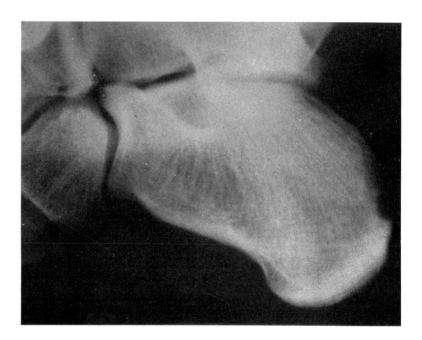

Fig. 36-12. Haglund's heel. Posterosuperior edge of calcaneus is removed.

wedge-shaped piece of bone with its base superior is resected transversely throughout the posterior tuberosity (Fig. 36-14). Care must be taken to make a clear cut that extends plantarward but not exceeding the insertion of the tendo calcaneus fibers, which are left intact. Cutting into the tendon fibers with the osteotome must be avoided because this will create little pieces of bone adhering to the fibers. If not removed they have a tendency to grow and cause irritations of the tendon. The sharp lateral edge created must be rounded by an osteotome and smoothed with a rasp or a prodder.

After opening the tourniquet hemostasis at soft tissues is performed. There will be some bleeding from the large cancellous surface of the calcaneus. Bone wax can be used to seal it. After inserting a closed-suction drainage tube the fascia is sutured to the paratenon with 3-0 absorbable sutures. Subcutaneous suturing is usually not performed; skin sutures with a nonresorbable 4-0 material and a compression dressing with a foam rubber are applied. Plaster fixation is usually not necessary. Patients are allowed out of bed on the third day after surgery with a bath chair to reach the toilet. After 4 days they take up walking with crutches depending on their ability with respect to pain.

Discussion

Although doubt has been expressed about the value of surgery for Haglund's disease,[73] this author believes that a thoroughly performed operation with sufficient and clear-cut resection of the prominence will give satisfying results. So-called recurrence of symptoms is usually due to insuffi-

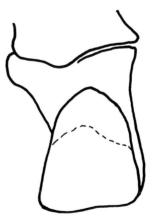

Fig. 36-13. Insertion of Achilles tendon at calcaneus (posterior view). Dotted line shows upper borderline of insertion of the tendon, reaching higher up at the medial side.

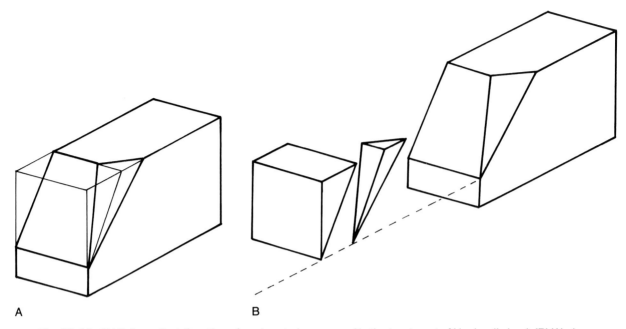

Fig. 36-14. (A) Schematic delineation of wedges to be removed in the treatment of Haglund's heel. **(B)** Wedges removed.

cient resection of bone (51 percent of cases in Taylor's[73] study) and osseous particles adherent to tendon fibres that are not removed. Rupture of the Achilles tendon following surgery remains a rare event in the literature.

THE ACCESSORY NAVICULAR

Etiology and Pathogenesis

An accessory navicular originates from a separate ossification center at the medial aspect of the navicular. The terms *os tibiale externum*, *accessory scaphoid*, *secondary scaphoid*, and *secondary navicular* are also used synonymously for this bone. Being a correlate to the navicular tuberosity, there is an extensive insertion of the posterior tibial tendon at its medial-plantar side. The tendon con-

tinues distally and also inserts at the plantar tuberosity of the first cuneiform bone and the base of the second and third metatarsal.

Three types of accessory naviculars have been distinguished.[81] Type I is considered a sesamoid in the substance of the posterior tibial tendon. Type II accessory naviculars are adherent to the navicular by a cartilaginous synchondrosis measuring 1 to 3 mm in width. Type III is in bony connection with the navicular forming a cornuate navicular.

When exposed to tensile and shearing forces of the posterior tibial tendon and to compression when the foot is pronated, synchondroses of type II accessory naviculars can become symptomatic.[81] Clinical symptoms can arise from lesions at the cartilaginous junction, especially when it is injured.

Sella et al., at histologic examination of surgically achieved specimens of synchondrosis and adjacent bone, found prolifarating vascular mesenchynal tissue, cartilage proliferation, increased fibrocartilage, osteoblastic and osteoclastic activity, and remodeling of bone.[81] They found this to be compatible with chronic repetitive injury and repair. Bone scans can reveal increased metabolism at the site of the lesions.[82,83]

Evaluation

Patients are usually children and young adults complaining of pain at the navicular tuberosity when walking or during sports activities. Sometimes swelling is present in the region. In adults pain often is elicited by trauma.

At physical examination a prominence at the medial side of the navicular can be seen. (Fig. 36-15). Palpation is usually painful. According to Giannestras, the accessory navicular is only occasionally associated with pes planovalgus.[84] Dorsoplantar radiographs will reveal the skeletal variant.

Management

Conservative therapy in cases following trauma consists of immobilization in a below-the-knee walking cast followed by use of an adequate arch support.[85] Injections of corticosteroids into the tender area will sometimes be beneficial.[85] When conservative measures fail to succeed, surgery is indicated.

Surgery

Objectives are the removal of the accessory navicular and the protruding medial part of the navicular itself. Special procedures to reroute the tibialis posterior tendon are not necessary.[81]

MacNicol and Voutsinas, comparing long-term results after simple excision of the ossicle and after the Kidner procedure, were not able to detect apparent advantages of the Kidner technique of operation.[86] The complex insertion of the tendon at the plantar side of the midfoot seems to tolerate the separation from the navicular. The procedure also apparently did not correct mobile flatfoot in MacNicol and Voutsinas' cases.

Technique

A longitudinal skin incision is made over the prominence at the medial side of the foot. The incision is carried down to the tibialis posterior tendon. The upper border of the tendon is followed to the navicular. Here the periosteum is incised and the tendon is carefully separated from the accessory navicular, keeping the knife in contact with the bone (Fig. 36-16). A small Hohmann elevator is inserted separating the tendon from the bone. The

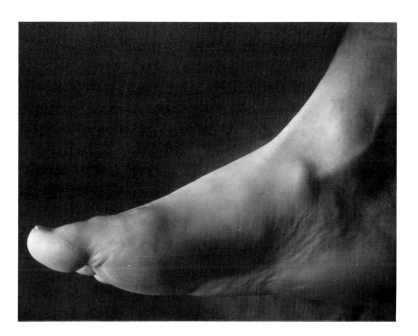

Fig. 36-15. Os tibiale externum. Tendon of tibialis posterior muscle leads to navicular protrusion.

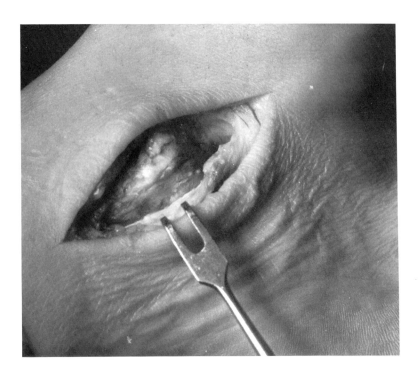

Fig. 36-16. Os tibiale externum. After exposure by a longitudinal skin incision dissection of the tendon from the accessory navicular is started dorsally and proceeds plantarward. The tendon remains intact.

synchondrosis is identified and the accessory navicular removed by sharp dissection. Any residual medial prominence is removed, improving the shape of the medial border of the foot. This also reduces the risk of recurrent symptoms.[86]

After hemostasis a closed-suction Redon drain is inserted. The upper border of the tendon is sutured to the periosteum with resorbable sutures. The fascia and subcutaneous tissue are closed with resorbable 3-0 sutures, and the skin with nonresorbable 4-0 material. A compression dressing is applied. The drain is removed the day following operation, and the dressings are changed on the second postoperative day and an adhesive-type bandage is applied. On the third postoperative day the patient is allowed to walk on his or her heel. The sutures are removed on the 10th day. Arch supports that were prepared preoperatively are used for the next 6 months.

Complications

Complications are usually not expected in this procedure.

TARSAL COALITIONS

A tarsal coalition is the union of two or more tarsal bones into a single structure. Fibrous, cartilaginous, or osseous connections between tarsal bones result from failure of segmentation of the tarsal bones during development.[87] The connection of bones progresses from cartilaginous to osseous at variable degrees. Ossification of talonavicular coalitions occurs at age 3 to 5, calcaneonavicular coalitions from 8 to 12, and talocalcaneal coalitions from 12 to 16 years.[87]

In 1769 Buffon described tarsal coalition.[88] Cruveilhier in 1829 first described calcaneonavicular and Zuckerkandl in 1877 talocalcaneal coalition anatomically. X-ray findings in calcaneonavicular fusions have been published, and in 1934 Korvin described the technique to visualize talocalcaneal connections.[89] Harris and Beath in 1948 showed that with their technique, an axial (so-called ski jump) view, it was possible to visualize alterations in the middle and posterior facets of the subtalar joint.[90] Inheritance in an autosomal dominant fashion was demonstrated by Wray and Herndon for calcaneonavicular coalitions.[91]

Etiology and Pathology

Tarsal coalition reduces mobility in the subtalar complex. Talocalcaneal motion is markedly reduced in calcaneonavicular coalition and is absent in talocalcaneal[87] and in talonavicular fusion. If movements are limited because of a biomechanically disadvantageous alignment of the tarsal components the coalition sooner or later will become symptomatic.

Often these painful conditions are found in pes planus or planovalgus type of feet and are described as peroneal spastic flatfoot. Cowell and Elener suggested the term *rigid flatfoot* instead.[87] They are of the opinion that the peroneal muscles have shortened to adapt to limited subtalar motion. The shortened peroneal muscles contract to protect the painful subtalar joint when inversion is provoked, resulting in a spasm of these muscles but not spasticity.[87]

Evaluation

Patients present with flatfoot and pain at walking, and sometimes at rest,[92] situated at the sinus tarsi and dorsum of the foot.[87] Subtalar motion is limited or absent in the subtalar joint and the midtarsal joint. Pain is triggered by passive inversion of the forefoot. Often spasm of the peroneal muscles is present. Occasionally an ankle sprain has initiated the symptoms.[93]

The diagnosis is made by radiographs. On suspecting a tarsal coalition, in addition to an anteroposterior and a lateral view the Isherwood lateral oblique projections at 45 and 60 degrees and the Harris and Beath ("ski jump") views should be taken.[94] These are produced with the patient standing on a film, heels toward the x-ray generator, knees bent with the ankle joint extended 10 degrees. Films are taken with the talar head set at 35, 40, and 45 degree angles.[94]

Lateral projections will reveal fusions between the talus and navicular as well as the calcaneus and cuboid. Secondary signs of coalitions in the subta-

lar joint, such as breaking of the talus (an exostosis on the dorsal aspect of the talarhead), broadening of the lateral process of the talus, and narrowing of the talocalcaneal joint, can be detected in the lateral view.[87] Sometimes a "halo" sign around the sinus tarsi can be observed.[94]

The 45 degree oblique view will reveal the relationship between the calcaneus and navicular, and the 60 degree oblique view makes observation of the anterior subtalar joint facets possible. The ski jump views serves to evaluate the middle and posterior subtalar joint surfaces. They are supposed to appear parallel to each other and to the ground and should be present and complete. If they are not parallel to each other a functional coalition will occur.[93,94]

A cartilaginous or fibrous coalition is sometimes difficult to diagnose. Signs in calcaneonavicular coalition are flattening of the calcaneus as it approaches the navicular.[87] Close proximity of these bones suggests a coalition. In fibrous or cartilaginous coalitions the dense cortical surfaces of the bones concerned will be flattened, indistinct, and irregular at their junction.[87] Lateral tomographs will confirm the diagnosis. Axial computed tomography may show the entity more clearly in size and location.[88]

Management

Most authors agree with trying conservative treatment first and move to surgery after its failure.

Surgery

The objective of an operation in tarsal coalitions is to establish a biomechanical situation that enables pain-free motion of the foot. Often this is achieved by resecting the bar. Sometimes, if pain persists or the coalition is too large in extent, arthrodesis will be necessary.

Indications

In talonavicular coalitions symptoms are rarely elicited. It is usually an incidental radiographic finding.[95] The operative treatment of calcaneonavicular coalitions usually gives good results; 75

percent satisfactory results were reported by Mitchell and Gibson,[96] 69 percent by Inglis et al.,[92] and 90 percent by Cowell (as noted by Inglis et al.[92]) with adding an interposition of the extensor digitorum brevis muscle. According to Scranton, in talocalcaneal coalitions surgery can be tried if less than one-half of the width of the joint surface between the talus and calcaneus is involved.[88]

Degenerative arthritic changes in joints of the rearfoot are supposed to be absent. Preoperative criteria are x-ray findings confirming the diagnosis. For evaluation of the extent of the coalition computed tomography scans are desirable. For cartilaginous and fibrous coalitions magnetic resonance imaging may be valuable.

Calcaneonavicular Coalition Surgery (After Cowell and Elener)

A Kocher-type incision is made from the proximal end of the sinus tarsi in the direction of the second cuneiform. The extensor digitorum brevis is separated from its origin and reflected distally. The coalition is identified. Cowell and Elener recommend identifying the adjacent joints, such as the subtalar, the calcaneocuboid, and the joint between the navicular and third cuneiform.[87] With Freer-type periosteal elevators that are inserted at either side of the coalition the surrounding joints are protected. Ligaments must not be injured. A rectangular piece of bone and cartilage is removed from the coalition to identify the bony portions of the navicular and the calcaneus. All the cartilage in the middle of the bone is resected with an osteotome; otherwise the coalition will reestablish.

The belly of the extensor brevis muscle is pulled down into the defect by using a 0 resorbable suture (Dexon, Vicryl). The ends of the suture are passed through the medial aspect of the foot and tied over a sponge and button. By this maneuver hematoma is minimized and new bone formation is prevented.[87] A small-caliber Redon suction drain is inserted.

After surgery a split below-knee cast is applied with the foot in neutral position. Passive motion exercises are started on the third postoperative day and the patient is allowed out of bed on crutches. Weightbearing is not allowed until subtalar motion equals the degree that was present during operation.[87]

Talocalcaneal Coalition Surgery (After Scranton)

Through a curvilinear incision plantar to and parallel to the tibialis posterior tendon, the flexor retinaculum is divided, and the flexor digitorum longus tendon, the flexor hallucis longus tendon, and the neurovascular bundle are retracted posteriorly. The talar attachment of the sheath of the flexor digitorum longus is sharply dissected in a proximal direction. This exposes the medial aspect of the coalition and the middle facet of the subtalar joint. The anterior and posterior borders of the coalition are visualized and the coalition is resected with a sharp osteotome. When the resection is complete motion of the subtalar joint must be possible. An autologous free fat graft taken from the fatty tissue at the posterosuperior aspect of the calcaneus is interposed. The sheath of the flexor digitorum longus tendon is sutured with absorbable material (Dexon, Vicryl 000), and the skin is closed with nonresorbable sutures. A non-weight-bearing below-knee cast is applied and left on for 3 weeks postoperatively. After removal a second cast is applied for another 3 weeks. After that physiotherapy is started. Supports may be helpful to maintain good results of the operation.

OSTEOCHONDRITIS DISSECANS OF THE TALUS

Etiology and Pathology

Since Berndt and Harty[97] were able to experimentally create lesions in cadaver specimens that syntopically and according to quality matched those found clinically following a special mechanism of trauma, it is agreed by the majority of authors that osteochondritis dissecans tali is of traumatic origin.[98] This is also expressed by the naming of the lesions: osteochondral, dome, flake, transchondral, and chip fracture of the talus.

Berndt and Harty stated that torsional impaction is the principal force creating the characteristic medial and lateral lesion of the talar trochlea.[97] Medial lesions were caused by strong inversion of the plantar-flexed foot with lateral rotation of the tibia on the talus, impacting the posteromedial edge of the talar dome against the posteromedial lip of the tibia. With increasing force the posterior fascicle of the deltoid or the anterior fascicle of the lateral collateral ligament are increasingly stressed and distorted.

Strong dorsiflexion and inversion, impacting the lateral talar margin against the medial articular surface of the fibula, creates a shearing and compressing force that is able to produce and displace an osteochondral fragment at the anterolateral surface of the trochlea. By increasing inversion force the medial and anterior fascicles of the lateral collateral ligaments are exposed to increased stress and distortion. These mechanisms also explain why lateral lesions are found rather anteriorly and medial lesions in the posterior area of the talar dome. In 1975 Zollinger and Dietschi,[99] in experimental cadaver studies, obtained results similar to those of Berndt and Harty. They stated that the mechanism creating the medial lesions is reinforced by insufficiency or rupture of the anterior fibulotalar ligament. Lambiris and Zilch found medial lesions in 80 percent and lateral lesions in 20 percent of the total number of cases.[100] Sometimes a medial and a lateral lesion will be found simultaneously. Also, isolated central lesions have been described.[101]

According to the mechanism of trauma the shape of the lateral lesions is generally thin and shallow, and that of the medial lesions more spherical and deep.[98] Bauer et al.,[102] as well as other authors, are of the opinion that the high incidence of bilateral lesions (in 7 of 30 patients in Bauer et al.'s study) also suggests other causes. Ischemic necrosis, abnormal patterns of vasculature, congenital factors, and spontaneous necrosis have been discussed as etiologic factors.[103]

Histologically the classical appearance of osteochondritis dissecans shows hyaline cartilage with living chondrocytes and necrotic subchondral bone.[97,98]

Evaluation

Following the classification of Berndt and Harty,[97] the fracture patterns are staged according to the degree of displacement of the osteochondral fragment:

Stage I: a small area of compression of subchondral bone

Stage II: beginning avulsion of the osteochondral fragment

Stage III: a completely detached osteochondral fragment remaining in place

Stage IV: a displaced osteochondral fragment (loose body)

Stages II and III cannot always be differentiated radiologically.[98]

In evaluating pain at the ankle joint the possibility of an osteochondral lesion must be kept in mind even if trauma is not remembered by the patient. The possibility of such lesions must be considered in every ankle injury, especially those with an inversion component.[98,104,105] Diagnosis is established by x-rays. It must be emphasized that the anteroposterior x-ray must be taken with an internal rotation of the leg of 20 percent (mortise view)[100] to present the contour of the trochlea of the talus without any overlaps.[98] Sometimes in a lateral radiograph the anteroposterior extent of the lesion can be seen. Anteroposterior radiographs in maximum flexion for medial localization and in neutral position or extension for lateral localization are useful.

Sometimes it is still hard to detect a lesion, especially in stage I. Tomographs, computed tomograms (Figs. 36-17 and 36-18), and bone scans will

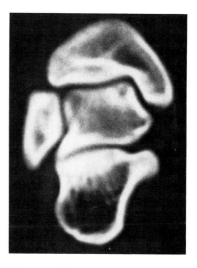

Fig. 36-17. Computed tomogram of osteochondritis dissecans of talus (frontal section). Lesion is at medial edge of talar dome.

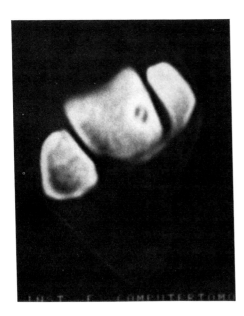

Fig. 36-18. Computed tomogram of osteochondritis dissecans of talus. Horizontal section shows increased density around the defect with dissecate in the center.

help in establishing the diagnosis. During the last few years arthroscopy has become more and more involved in diagnosis and treatment.

Management

In the literature the results of conservative management are rather poor. Berndt and Harty, in a review of the literature prior to 1958, found 74 percent poor, 9 percent fair, and 17 percent good results.[97] They thought plaster immobilization of 4 months would improve the outcoming. After a more recent review, Flick and Gould are of the opinion that poor results in their own conservatively treated cases were due to the failure to immobilize the ankle for a long enough period of time.[98]

In view of the fact that results after surgery are reported to be excellent or good in 75 to 79 percent of cases,[98] surgical procedures are usually chosen for the treatment of symptomatic osteochondritis dissecans. Long-lasting immobilization may or may not cure osteochondritic lesions, but certainly is not beneficial for the joint since damage to the otherwise healthy cartilage is to be expected.

Therefore only in stage I lesions does conservative treatment seem reasonable.

Surgery

Treatment is aimed at pain-free full range of motion at the ankle joint and at preventing osteoarthritis. Surgery is indicated with an established diagnosis of osteochondritis and clinical signs and symptoms such as ankle swelling, ecchymosis, and impaired function in the acute cases and stiffness, intermittent deep aching sensations, crepitus, and intermittent ankle swelling aggravated by increased activity but improved with rest in the chronic cases.[98]

Preoperative Criteria

To localize the lesion precisely radiographs must clearly show the position and size of the defect. Tomographs or computed tomograms may be necessary.

Open Surgery

Depending on the type of lesion, different methods of treatment will be chosen. Access to the defect will usually be more difficult in medial sites because of the more posterior location. If possible a medial malleolar osteotomy is avoided. Flick and Gould recommended grooving of the anteromedial corner of the distal tibia to allow treatment of medial talar dome lesions.[98] They did not find adverse effects of the procedure during 2 years' follow-up. To treat the lesion the following procedures are at the surgeon's disposal:

Stage II:
1. Drilling through lesion
2. Removal of dissecate
3. Curettage of bed, freshening the bony surface of the dissecate, bone grafting, and refixation of dissecate with fibrin glue

Stage III:
1. Simple removal of dissecate
2. Removal of dissecate and drilling and curetting of bed to provide formation of fibrous cartilage in the defect
3. Curettage and bone grafting using fibrin glue

Stage IV: search for loose body; treatment as in
stage III

With open surgery, especially when reconstructive measures are planned, the medial lesions often are barely accessible without removal of the medial malleolus.[103] Flick and Gould described a method to avoid this,[98] but their follow-up period of 2 years may be too short for a definite evaluation.

Technique for a Medial Lesion. Under general anesthesia using a tourniquet at the thigh a dorsally convex curved incision is made over the dorsal contour of the medial malleolus and a flap of skin is removed anteriorly to gain access to the anteromedial aspect of the ankle joint, preserving the saphenous vein and nerve. The fibrous and synovial capsule is divided and the joint is inspected. Usually a lesion cannot be detected from this access. The apex of the malleolus is identified. A 1.6-mm Kirschner wire is driven through the malleolus in an oblique direction from inferomedial to superolateral, avoiding the joint. This can be controlled by visualizing the joint space from the anterior capsular incision. Following the hole left by the wire, a 3.2-mm drill is used to create a canal to receive an AO cancellous malleolar screw. Perpendicular to the direction of the canal the malleolus is osteotomized incompletely to 3 to 4 mm below the superomedial edge of the joint space (Fig. 36-19A). The osteotomy is completed by cautiously breaking the malleolus off, moving the osteotome medially as a lever. This provides for better fitting of the fragment when it is repositioned. By pronating the foot the lesion now appears in the operating field in its entire extension.

Repair of Grade II Lesions. Grade II lesions are treated as follows. The flake, being still in connection with the cartilage, is carefully elevated and its bed is drilled and curetted with a burr, breaking the sclerotic bone layer that surrounds the bed of the lesion (Fig. 36-19B). If the flake is large enough and the cartilage in a good condition the bony part is freshened with a small burr. The defect in the trochlea of the talus is filled with autograft or allograft cancellous bone using fibrin glue to provide for better revascularization. Finally, the flake is also fixed to its new bed with fibrin glue. The malleolus is repositioned and a malleolar screw with a washer is inserted into the previously prepared drill canal.

Repair of Grades III and IV Lesions. If in a grade III lesion the fragment is large enough and the cartilage is in good condition, the procedure may be done as in grade II lesions. In a grade III lesion with a small bony fragment or poor appearance of cartilage and in grade IV lesions, the bed is also freshened with a burr and the defect filled with cancellous bone grafts using fibrin glue to secure them (Fig. 36-19C).

Completion of Surgery. After inserting a Redon suction drain the subcutaneous tissue is sutured with 3-0 resorbable threads and the skin with 4-0 nonresorbable material. A split plaster cast is replaced after removal of the sutures on the 10th postoperative day by a non-weight-bearing below-knee cast for 8 weeks after surgery. Then the cast is removed and the patient is allowed to walk with crutches for another 2 weeks without weightbearing. Physiotherapy is started after removal of the cast to regain mobility of the joint. Full weightbearing is gradually taken up after 10 weeks following the operation.

Arthroscopic Surgery

Arthroscopy has already become an important tool in evaluating articular lesions of the ankle joint. With arthroscopic techniques only removal of flakes and curetting and drilling have been described in osteochondritis dissecans of the talus.[106] The objectives of the operation are to drill a grade II lesion according to Berndt and Harty,[98] to curette grades III and IV lesions, and to remove loose bodies. The indications depend on the knowledge and experience of the surgeon.[101] The preoperative criteria are as in the open operation.

The operation is carried out with the patient under general anesthesia and using a tourniquet at the thigh. Because of the tightness of the ankle joint there is little opening of the joint space, even with distal pulling or manipulation of intact ligaments.[101] Therefore, in cases of posterior sites of lesions we apply distraction with an external fixator. One screw is inserted at the lateral side of the calcaneus 1.5 cm distal to the apex of the lateral malleolus. A proximal screw is applied just anterior to the fibula, penetrating into the distal third of the tibia. Setting the distractor under tension, the joint

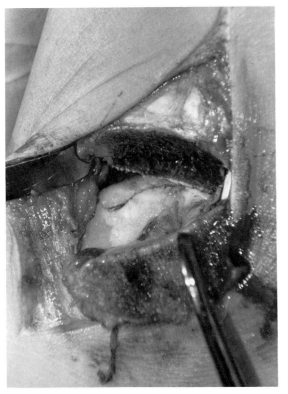

A

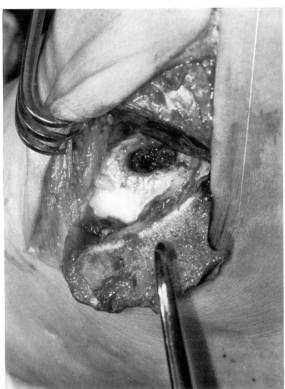

B

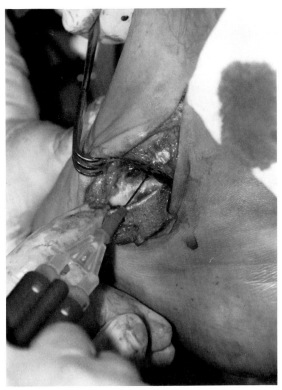

C

Fig. 36-19. Osteochondritis dissecans. **(A)** Medial malleolus is osteotomized and deflected. Dissecate is clearly delineated. **(B)** Dissecate is removed; the sclerosis was broken with a burr down to cancellous bone. **(C)** Defect has been filled with homologous cancellous bone using fibrin glue to secure the chips and to promote faster healing.

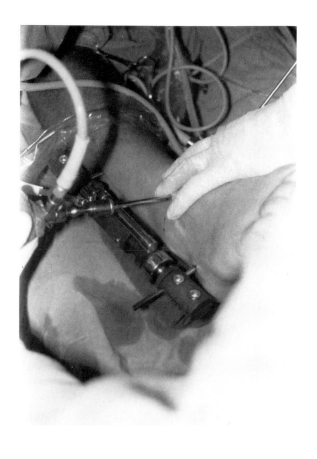

Fig. 36-20. Arthroscopy of the ankle joint. Distractor in place. Arthroscope inserted through central approach.

space is opened adequately to reach posterior areas and to flex the ankle joint. Before distraction the joint is distended with Ringer's solution by inserting a no. 18 needle after identifying the joint line by palpation moving the foot.

Two portals are used, one for the arthroscope and one for the instruments. The anterolateral portal is just anterior to the lateral malleolus and lateral to the common extensor tendon to the joint line level. The anteromedial portal is between the anterior margin of the medial malleolus and the tendon of the anterior tibial muscle.[106,107] Both are 0.5 to 1 cm distal to the joint line.[107] At operation the arthroscope is inserted from the contralateral side of the lesion and the instruments at the side of the defect.

For surgery Guhl recommends the anterocentral approach, especially in rather rigid joints in which distraction is limited. A 5-mm longitudinal incision is made over the common extensor tendon at the

level of the joint line. Skin and subcutaneous tissue are spread with a hemostat and the extensor tendon is pushed medially. By this means the neurovascular bundle is pushed away to the medial side of the joint, ahead of the extensors.[107] The joint is then entered from a central position (Fig. 36-20). An operating cannula is inserted to keep this access free for the passage of instruments. After inspection the anterolateral portal is incised and a probe is inserted to evaluate cartilaginous lesions. A stab incision is made at the anterolateral portal and the sheath of a 5-mm arthroscope with a sharp trocar is inserted at a rather small angle to the frontal plane. As soon as the capsule is penetrated, the sharp trocar is replaced by a blunt trocar and the joint is entered. The trocar is removed and the arthroscope is inserted.

According to recommendations of Pritsch et al. grade I lesions of Berndt and Harty's scale are treated by restrictions of sports activities only,

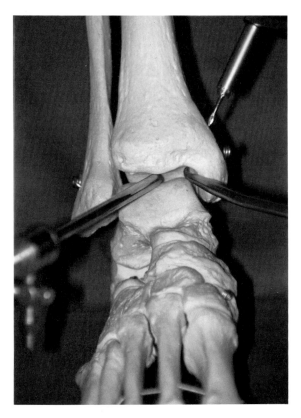

Fig. 36-21. Skeletal illustration of arthroscopic drilling of osteochondral defect. Arthroscope is inserted through a central approach, and drill guide through a medial approach.

grade II lesions with soft overlying cartilage are drilled (Fig. 36-21), and grade III lesions in which the overlying cartilage is frayed are treated by curettage and removal of the fragment. After a search for loose bodies, grade IV defects are also curetted, providing for formation of fibrous cartilage.[97] If curettage is difficult because of formation of sclerosis around the bed of the dissecate, drilling is also used to break it.

After rinsing the joint with Ringer's solution and inserting a Redon drain the stab wounds of the skin are closed with 4-0 nonresorbable sutures. Postoperatively physiotherapy is started to maintain mobility of the ankle joint on the day following operation. The patient is mobilized with crutches and gradually full weightbearing is taken up.

OSTEOTOMIES AT THE REARFOOT

Tarsal V-Osteotomy for the Treatment of Pes Cavus

Described by Japas[108] in 1968, this operation was designed to correct a simple anterior pes cavus with an equal plantar-flexion deformity of the forefoot in its medial and lateral columns.[109] A slight medial deviation of the forefoot can also be corrected by this method.

The operation is indicated in simple cavus feet with painful callositis over the metatarsal heads that cannot sufficiently be relieved by supports or metatarsal bars. Usually this occurs in a cavus with an angle of Hibbs[110] and Dennemann[111] below 130 degrees. According to Dennemann the angle ranges from 130 to 140 degrees, with an average of 139 degrees, in the normal foot.

Preoperative Criteria

Preoperative criteria are deducted from lateral radiographs in a standing position in which the angle is measured (Fig. 36-22). Baropedograms show the severity of the deformity to compare it with the postoperative result.

Technique (Modified after Japas)

The patient is in a supine position, and a tourniquet is used if preferred. Without a tourniquet the dorsalis pedis artery and its concomitant structures are more easily avoided. This author adds the Steindler procedure only when a very tight plantar fascia is found. A longitudinal incision is made over the third ray extending from the head of the talus distally to the proximal third of the metatarsals. The fascia of the foot is separated and the incision is carried down to the periosteum of the tarsal bones between the extensor tendons of the second and third toe, dividing the fatty tissue under the tendon sheath. By blunt dissection the tarsus is exposed. With the talonavicular joint as a landmark the navicular is identified and the cuneonavicular joint is opened with a scalpel. After inserting Chiari or

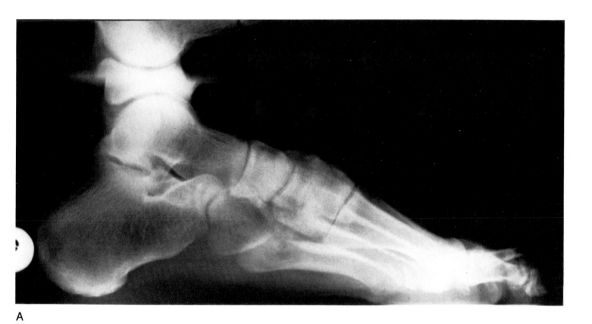

A

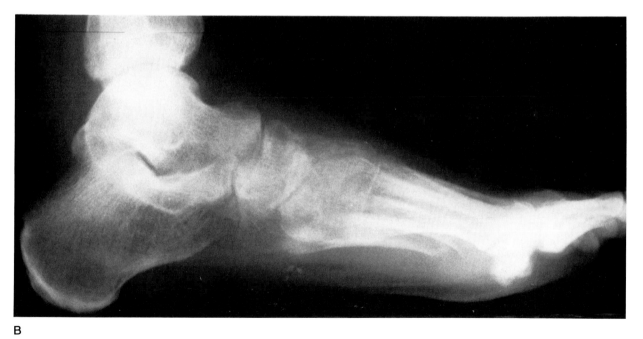

B

Fig. 36-22. The Japas operation for cavus foot. **(A)** Preoperative lateral view. Hibbs angel is 120 degrees. **(B)** Eight weeks after surgery, following removal of plaster. Patient apparently avoided full weightbearing when lateral x-rays were taken.

Hohmann elevators at the medial and lateral side of the tarsus or dorsoplantar hole is drilled through the center of the navicular and a Kirschner wire is inserted as a landmark to avoid extending the osteotomy too far proximally. Otherwise the navicular would be in danger of being fractured.

With an osteotome the V-shaped osteotomy is delineated. The angle is approximately 130 degrees. The medial branch runs through the navicular and a small part of the second and a larger part of the first cuneiform, ending just behind the first cuneometatarsal joint. The lateral branch passes through the third cuneiform and the cuboid, ending just behind the articulation of the cuboid with the fifth metatarsal. The osteotomy is completed with an oscillating saw. Since usually it has proved difficult to elevate the forefoot and impinge the apex of the "V" by depressing it, this author resects the dorsally based wedge with an opening angle necessary for correction of the deformity following the "V" that has been cut. The angle is usually 20 to 25 degrees. The wedge is taken from the distal fragment of the osteotomy. When precisely cut the osteotomy may now be snugly closed by elevating the forefoot. Because of the large angle of the "V" a medial or lateral deviation of the forefoot can also be accomplished by manipulating the foot into the desired direction. Care must be taken to hold the foot in a plantargrade direction before fixation with a K wire (Fig. 36-23). Japas recommended insertion of a Steinmann pin through the shaft of the first metatarsal into the cuboid and the calcaneus.

After inserting a Redon drain the wound is closed. Usually only the skin is sutured to avoid damage to the abundant cutaneous nerves running at the dorsum of the foot. A split plaster cast is applied after wound dressing; the dressings are changed on the second or third day after surgery. The stitches are removed on the 10th day and a below-knee plaster cast is given for 6 weeks following the operation. After that a walking plaster cast is applied for 4 weeks. Ten weeks after the operation the cast is removed, fusion is confirmed by x-rays, and physiotherapy is started to regain mobility and strength at the ankle joint and the foot.

Discussion. Key points of the intervention are a subtle atraumatic preparation of the structures on the dorsum of the foot and a precise osteotomy.

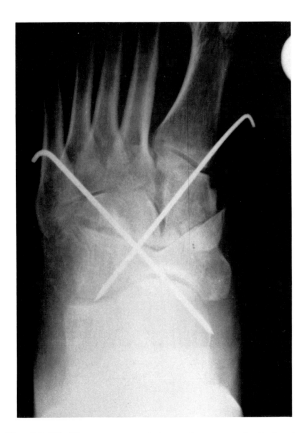

Fig. 36-23. V-osteotomy of Japas for cavus foot. Angle measures 135 degrees. K wires are removed 2 weeks after surgery.

With this procedure deformities in the sagittal and transversal plane (i.e., the cavus and adduction) can be corrected. In case of an additional varus of the heel a Dwyer osteotomy can be added. In contrast to midtarsal fusion, this would result in a corrected foot with free motion in the subtalar and midtarsal joint.

Criteria for acceptable results will be a normally shaped foot with a Hibbs angle larger than 140 degrees and a plantargrade forefoot. Usually mobile claw toes will stretch after the procedure; if not they can be manipulated. The method has proved a valuable tool in this author's experience to treat simple cavus deformities. In a moderate cavo varus deformity the operation can be combined with a Dwyer osteotomy to preserve the midtarsal joints.

Complications

The surgeon must avoid cutting into the tuberosity of the fifth metatarsal. Rude mobilization of the fragments of the osteotomy with various instruments can lead to fracture of the navicular. This will create damage to the talonavicular joint, resulting in painful osteoarthritis in this important connection between forefoot and rearfoot.

Osteotomy of the Calcaneus for Pes Cavus (After Dwyer)

In 1955 Dwyer published his "New approach to the treatment of pes cavus" that was read at the sixth Congress of Orthopaedic Surgery in Berne, Switzerland.[112] In 1959 a second publication followed in the *Journal of Bone and Joint Surgery* confirming the value of the procedure.[113] Dwyer noticed that, whatever the underlying etiology of cavus deformity, the deformity rapidly becomes worse with the onset of varus.[113]

The objectives of the operation are to counteract the disadvantages of the varus of the heel, consisting of the calcaneal tendon becoming an active invertor and contracture of the plantar fascia with the patient walking on the outer border of the foot, thus increasing the varus deformity.[113] Indications are cavus deformities with the heel in a varus position to prevent progression of the deformity, and furthermore to reestablish normal forefoot-hindfoot relations.

Preoperative Criteria

Determination of the necessary correction according to x-rays is not well established since it would be difficult to delineate the oblique wedge osteotomy on x-rays. Clinical measurement of the degree of varus serves to estimate the necessary correction.

Technique

The plantar fascia is divided subcutaneously. With the patient in a lateral position a straight incision is made at the lateral side of the calcaneus just behind the peroneal tendons and paralleling them, extending from the Achilles tendon to the inferior border of the calcaneus. The tendon sheath of the peroneus longus tendon is exposed. Just distal to it the periosteum is incised and elevated to the inferior border of the tendon sheath. At a distance of 8 to 12 mm distally and paralleling the first incision of the periosteum a second incision is made. A Hohmann elevator is moved around the posterior prominence of the calcaneus between the Achilles tendon and the subtalar joint. A second elevator is passed around the anterior process of the calcaneus. The osteotomy is delineated with an osteotome paralleling the peroneal tendons and completed with an oscillating saw. Leaving a saw blade in the first osteotomy, the second osteotomy is cut, removing a wedge tapering down to the medial cortex. By pressing the forefoot up against the pull of the calcaneal tendon the osteotomy is closed. At this stage of the operation the correction of the varus has to be controlled. The heel must be in a neutral or slight valgus position. A Redon suction drain is inserted, the periosteum, subcutaneous tissue, and skin sutured, and a split plaster cast applied. After 6 weeks full weightbearing in the cast is allowed, and after 8 weeks the cast is removed.

Discussion The osteotomy corrects the varus by abducting the posterior prominence of the calcaneus along an oblique medial axis. A slight elevation of the heel results, flattening the cavus. The mechanical axis of the leg now runs lateral to or through the center of the ankle joint. In addition to the fasciotomy this will also flatten the longitudinal arch and contribute to counteract the cavus deformity. If the heel is small, as often happens in relapsed clubfoot with a residual cavus, an opening wedge osteotomy at the medial side is recommended by Dwyer.[115]

Criteria for acceptable results are a heel in neutral or slight valgus position with subsequent improvement of the cavovarus deformity.

Complications

If the osteotomy cannot be closed this is usually because of a small piece of the apex left behind.[113] Care must be taken not to cut into the subtalar joint when performing the proximal osteotomy.

If sufficient correction is not achieved, more bone has to be resected. Care must be taken not to interpose soft tissue into the osteotomy. This would prevent direct contact of the surfaces of the osteotomy and thus early healing of the osteotomy.

Imhäuser's Osteotomy for Cavovarus Foot

Etiology of Cavovarus Foot

Cavus foot is an expression of an imbalance of muscle groups induced by neurologic dysfunction. A sagittal plane cavus deformity is seen at the beginning, but usually progression of development of rearfoot varus, forefoot adduction, depression of the first ray, and pronation are seen.

Evaluation

The distinction between forefoot and rearfoot cavus is rather academic when trying to analyze this complex deformity. The description of four different anterior pes cavus types depending on the apex of the deformity is of interest in a positional but not in a structural deformity.

To evaluate the deformity many different methods of measuring the forefoot-rearfoot angulation have been established. In this author's practice Dennemann's so-called instep angle, measured between a line paralleling the longitudinal axis of the calcaneus and passing the center of the navicular and a second line representing the longitudinal axis of the first metatarsal, has proved useful to express the severity of the deformity. The angle ranges between 130 and 140 degrees, averaging 139 degrees. It must be kept in mind, however, that depending on the degree of adduction of the first ray, the angle may appear slightly larger on a lateral x-ray than it is in reality.

Management

At the beginning treatment can be initiated by supports, technical alterations in normal shoes, and later custom-tailored orthopedic shoes. Gradually this will become more and more difficult. At this point surgery is necessary.

Surgery

The operation is supposed to definitely correct the varus of the heel; normalize the longitudinal arch and eliminate the forefoot equinus; correct the adduction of the forefoot (Fig. 36-24); correct pronation of the forefoot, especially the marked

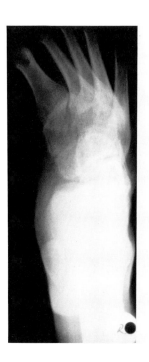 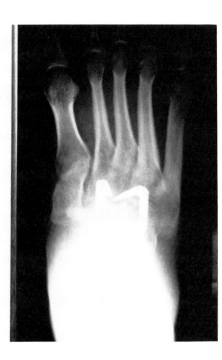

Fig. 36-24. Residual pes cavovarus after treatment of clubfoot by the Evans procedure. *Left,* Preoperative forefoot adduction. *Right,* Adduction is corrected after surgery.

plantar deviation of the first metatarsal; straighten the toes; and provide for plantargrade orientation of the foot in relation to the transverse axis of the ankle joint.

Technique. With the patient in a supine position with or without a tourniquet around the thigh, a skin incision is made at the lateral side of the foot, 1.5 cm above the sole, from the heel to the base of the fifth metatarsal. A nonresorbable thread is attached to the peroneus longus tendon and the tendon is separated distally to the attached thread. The first metatarsal is manipulated into extension. A longitudinal incision is made at the dorsum of the foot followed by subperiosteal preparation of the head of the talus and the cuneiforms. The cartilage-covered part of the talor head is resected and the osteotomy is carried through the anterior part of the calcaneus.

The second plane of the osteotomy starts in the proximal parts of the cuneiforms and proceeds into the cuboid. The severed bones, including the navicular, are removed. The forefoot is adapted to the rearfoot. More bone is resected to enlarge the wedge if necessary for correction. If necessary the plantar aponeurosis is separated form the lateral incision. The tourniquet is opened. After exact correction of the forefoot with respect to the rearfoot the talar head is united with the cuneiforms by means of two Blount clamps. The proximal end of the peroneus longus tendon is sutured under the insertion of the peroneus brevis tendon.

The wound is closed by layers. A split plaster cast is applied to the whole leg in 30 degrees of flexion of the knee and neutral position of the foot. After 4 weeks a below-knee walking cast is applied for an additional 6 weeks.

Discussion. The principles of this operation, used by Imhäuser[116] since 1954, are the following:

1. Separation of the peroneus longus tendon at the lateral border of the foot and insertion of the proximal stump at the base of the fifth metatarsal.
2. A dorsally based wedge osteotomy with removal of the cartilage-covered part of the talar head and a distal part of the calcaneus. The second plane of the osteotomy reaches through the proximal parts of the cuneiform bones into the cuboid. The following parts are removed: the navicular, proximal joint surfaces of the cuneiforms, part of the cuboid, and the distal joint surfaces of talus and calcaneus (Fig. 36-25). The arthrodesis will therefore unite the head of the talus with the cuneiforms and the calcaneus with the remaining part of the cuboid.
3. In severe cases plantar soft tissues are separated from the anterior surface of the calcaneal tuberosity. This was necessary in two-thirds of the 200 cases of Imhäuser.

By sectioning the peroneus longus tendon from the tuberosity of the first metatarsal its plantar-flexing and pronating effect on the first ray is eliminated. The dissection of the plantar aponeurosis facilitates the correction of the longitudinal arch and the toes. It must be emphasized, however, that the wedge osteotomy remains the main and most decisive step in the operation.

Operations on the toes are rarely necessary because the toes almost always stretch spontaneously by reduction of tension to the extensor tendons.

The advantages of this operation are that (1) it is a one-step procedure; (2) all degrees and shapes of severe cavus deformity, including paralytic deformities, if necessary combined with tendon transfers, can be corrected definitively; (3) a lateral stabilization is accomplished preventing any tilt of the foot; (4) the toes are straightened out to a remarkable degree; and, (5) there is no shortening of the foot (usually the foot is lengthened by 1 to 1.5 cm).

According to Trensz and coworkers, the mechanism of varus correction in Imhäuser's osteotomy has not yet been established precisely.[117] To accomplish this the biomechanics of the subtalar joint need attention. The movement of the talus on the calcaneus is defined by the medial pivot of the ligament of the canalis tarsi (talocalcaneal interosseous ligament) and the shape of the joint surfaces, especially in the posterior compartment. External rotation of the leg against the foot arrested on ground will rotate the head of the talus laterally. This forces the anterior process of the calcaneus anteriorly and medially, pushing the talar head upward. The posterior process of the calcaneus is approximating the lateral malleolus.[118] Following the shape of the surfaces of the posterior subtalar joint,

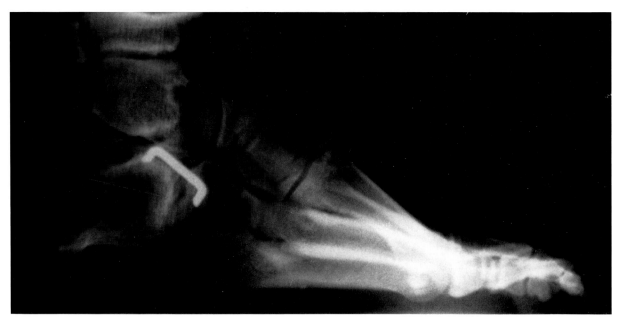

A

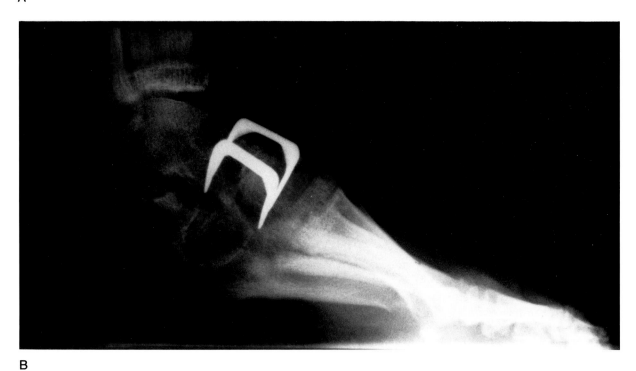

B

Fig. 36-25. (A) Residual cavovarus after clubfoot treated by the Evans procedure. **(B)** After Imhäuser's operation. Cavus is reduced, the heel touches ground.

the calcaneus is forced into a varus position. The talar head is pulling the navicular upward, resulting in a supination of the forefoot. The advancing anterior process of the calcaneus forces the forefoot into adduction. A compensatory pronation in the metatarsotarsal joints secures contact of the forefoot with the ground. Formally this is the mechanism creating cavovarus of the foot. The talus is in extension in relation to the leg, the calcaneus is in varus, and the forefoot flexed and in adduction.

By resecting the navicular and the calcaneocuboideal wedge the packing at Chopart's joint line is released and movement is free in the subtalar joint. The anterior process of the calcaneus can move backward and laterally, and the shape of the subtalar posterior joint surfaces moves the posterior tuberosity of the calcaneus into valgus. The correction of the deformity will depend on the relationship of the size and shape of wedges between talus and cuneiforms on the one, and between calcaneus and cuboid on the other hand.

Wagner's Transpositional Osteotomy of the Calcaneus

Etiology of Pes Valgoplanus

In the normal foot the point of the heel charging the ground lies lateral to the middle of the ankle joint so that from a dorsal view the rearfoot appears to be in a valgus position. However, the calcaneal tuberosity is in a medial position with respect to the "axis of movement" (compromise axis, after Fick[123]) of the subtalar joint, so that the pull of the Achilles tendon exerts a supinating effect on the hindfoot. In the stance phase and in static weight-bearing the load is distributed over the talus to the first and fifth ray and to the heel.

This equilibrium is lost when the point of charge of the heel is transposed laterally by a rearfoot valgus. The talus is now positioned medially with respect to the center of the three buttresses, and under weightbearing a movement in the form of a valgus is elicited. With increasing rearfoot valgus the forefoot deviates into abduction.[123] The talus now deviates further medially with respect to the three buttresses and the medial arch flattens. By this eccentric position of the talus the foot is put

into malposition with every step and by lateralization of the heel the Achilles tendon exerts a pronating force to the hindfoot. In such a severe deformity success cannot be expected from conservative treatment measures because the deformity cannot be counteracted by the muscles any longer. The key to treatment is a medial transposition of the tuber calcanei to establish the talus as a center of the three buttresses again.

The indication for the operation is any malposition involving the point of heel charge in the frontal plane. Although a supinated rearfoot also can be corrected with this method, clinical experiences show[119] that the unstable valgus foot is the most frequent indication for this intervention. The severe congenital pes valgus associated with hypo- or aplasia of the fibula shows the utility of the method.

In cases of severe unstable pes valgoplanus several methods have been applied to correct the valgus of the calcaneus and consequently the flatfoot deformity. The subtalar extra-articular arthrodesis (after Grice) has become most popular, and modifications of the technique have been published. The method is effective, but has the disadvantage of locking up the subtalar joint and also, by increasing the tension of the soft tissues at the lateral side of the foot creating a pronating pressure on the ankle joint.[119]

Extra-articular osteotomies have the advantage of preserving the movement in the subtalar joint, and thus providing for a better function of the foot. In 1893 Gleich described the first extra-articular osteotomy of the calcaneus for restoring the longitudinal arch in flatfeet of adults.[120] The principle is a plantarly based wedge osteotomy that shifts the tuber calcanei plantarward. Other osteotomies in this area that alter the direction of the heel have been described by Dwyer,[121] Silver,[122] and others.

Operative Technique According to Wagner

The calcaneus is exposed from the lateral side. Immediately dorsal to the peroneus longus tendon and paralleling it a straight skin incision of 4 cm is made reaching from the superior to the inferior edge of the calcaneum, as in Dwyer's operation. Care must be taken to avoid the sural nerve. After identification of this nerve the incision is carried down to bone without creating different layers of tissues to provide for better healing. If a mobilization of the rims of the wound is necessary this should be done in the epiperiosteal layer. Retractors ought to be avoided. The wound spreads sufficiently by shifting the skin. Occasionally it becomes necessary to open the tendon sheath of the peroneal muscles. The transverse osteotomy is executed with a slowly moving oscillating saw because smooth surfaces of the osteotomy are important for the displacement of the fragments.

The osteotomy runs from the dorsal border of the subtalar joint to the inferior border of the calcaneocuboid joint so that both joints remain intact and maximum length of the osteotomy is achieved.[119] In a subtly performed osteotomy the division of the opposite cortical bone can exactly be felt. The saw must not penetrate into the medial soft tissues. Here the flexor hallucis longus tendon, nerves, and vessels are at risk. After completion of the osteotomy the gap between the fragments is opened by two lamina spreaders. The fragments are gradually separated until good exposure is possible. With a small periosteal elevator the soft tissues at the medial edge of the distal fragment are separated to enable a sufficient medial displacement.

Now the extent of medialization is determined. Pushing the forefoot into extension under the third metatarsal head deviates the rearfoot into a valgus position. In a relaxed equinus position the distal fragment of the calcaneus can be shifted medially step by step. By forefoot extension it can be seen that the farther the distal fragment is moved medially the less valgus results in the rearfoot. Finally, an extent of displacement of the distal calcaneal fragment will be reached at which the rearfoot starts to move into the opposite (varus) direction. This is in accordance with the intended correction. To stabilize the osteotomy site two Kirschner wires are inserted diagonally through the fragments. It should be noted that tension of the skin and lateral soft tissues limits the medial displacement. Therefore, in severe deformities it is occasionally not possible to achieve full correction without jeopardizing the soft tissues. In such cases it is advisable to complete the correction in a second operation.[119]

The lateral edge of the proximal calcaneal fragment is rounded. After inserting a low-calibration drain the wound is closed. Because of the high risk of necrosis of the wound margins the skin is not sutured. With thin resorbable sutures the rims are adapted with superficial subcutaneous stitches and approximated with a fine self-adhesive veil. Thus necrosis can be prevented. A split, below-knee plaster cast is applied that is replaced by a walking cast after 2 weeks. Partial weightbearing is allowed using a crutch at the contralateral side. Six weeks after the operation bony fusion can be expected. The plaster is removed and x-rays are made to certify bony fusion. Full weightbearing with supports and physiotherapy is started.

If complete correction of the deformity is achieved 6 months after the operation all therapeutic measurements are terminated. The patients are controlled until the end of growth. If because of soft tissue problems a complete correction was not possible, a further correction is planned. In the meantime treatment is by supports and physiotherapy.

Discussion. Wagner reported excellent results in 37 of 45 feet with a one-step operation despite severe deformities.[119] The average age of patients was 10.7 years. The amount of transposition averaged 13 mm.

The advantages of this technique are that the subtalar joint and subsequently Chopart's joint line remain unimpaired and that with a relatively small transposition the point of charge of the heel is corrected more effectively than with a wedge osteotomy. Also the intervention is small and because of the large surfaces of cancellous bone the conditions for bone healing are excellent.

ARTHRODESES AT THE REARFOOT

Arthrodesis of the Ankle Joint

A great variety of methods to fuse the ankle joint have been published. After having collected experience with a sliding anterior tibial corticocancellous graft,[124] dowel techniques, and Boehler nails in fusing the ankle joint and the subtalar joint, this author has returned to and remained with a modified external compression technique after Charnley.

The dowel technique cannot be recommended in cases with marked subchondral sclerosis in severe osteoarthritis or in necrosis of the talus. In these cases sequesters are produced and fusion is not accomplished. Although the tools to perform the dowel technique according to Baciu[124] were used, it was not possible to remove the medial part of the lateral malleolus while leaving its lateral cortex intact. This must be a sophisticated technique which the author keeps a secret.

Objectives of ankle fusions are to establish a pain-free, stable ankle joint in a biomechanically most favorable position. This means a neutral position of the fused ankle in the sagittal plane,[125] a neutral or slight valgus position (up to 5 degrees depending on the forefoot-rearfoot relation), and an external rotation of the foot of 10 to 15 degrees.[125]

Indications are severe painful osteoarthritis of the ankle joint, most frequently following fractures of the ankle or fracture dislocations; avascular necrosis of the body of the talus after dislocation; infectious arthritis followed by destruction of the joint; rheumatoid arthritis; and failed total ankle arthroplasty.[126] Fortunately the latter is rather rare in this author's cases because I have not decided to perform total ankle arthroplasties, knowing that arthrodesis of the ankle usually gives good functional results.

Preoperative Criteria

Preoperative criteria are lateral radiographs taken in a standing position, anteroposterior radiographs of the ankle joint, and an evaluation of the mobility of the joints of the foot, deformities, and malpositions.

Technique

The patient is in a supine position, and the leg must be visible from the knee joint to the toes to avoid malpositions resulting from insufficient oversight. For external fixation a simple frame system is used (Fig. 36-26) consisting of two Steinmann pins and two axles with adjustable nuts to connect them with the pins. A tourniquet is used; however, if the operation lasts longer than 1.5 hours the tourniquet is opened, hemostasis is performed, and the operation is continued without a tourniquet. Major bleeding usually does not occur.

A longitudinal incision is made over the medial aspect of the tibia, passing curvilinearly over the medial malleolus and ending just above the tuber-

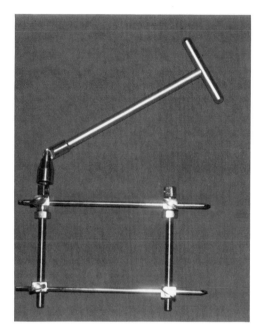

Fig. 36-26. Simple external fixator for ankle arthrodesis consisting of two Steinmann pins and two axles with adjustable nuts to connect them with the pins.

osity of the navicular. The skin is reflected anteriorly, including the saphenous vein and nerve. The anterior capsule of the ankle joint is opened and dissected from the distal tibia. The talar neck and the articular surface of the talus become visible. A 1.8-mm K wire is driven through the head of the talus perpendicular to the longitudinal axis of the tibia and to the longitudinal axis of the foot, provided the talus is in a normal position in the frontal plane. The position of the wire is controlled under the x-ray amplifier. Paralleling the K wire, a drill hole is made through the talus with a 3.8-mm drill at a position just anterior to the medial malleolus and just superior to the tibialis posterior tendon, avoiding the subtalar joint. With 2.5-cm osteotome the medial malleolus is removed, reflected downward, and discarded after separating it from the deltoid ligament. The articular cartilage is removed from the medial aspect of the talus down to cancellous bone.

A lateral incision is made along the posterior border of the fibula, curving anteriorly just below the tip of the fibula. The tendon sheath of the peroneal tendon is opened. The distal end of the fibula is exposed and a segment 1 cm in width is resected with an oscillating saw just proximal to the tibiofibular syndesmosis. The syndesmosis is incised and the lateral malleolus reflected downward, leaving the calcaneofibular ligament intact. With an oscillating saw the medial one-third of the lateral malleolus is resected in a sagittal plane. The lateral aspect of the tibia is decorticated at the level of the syndesmosis. The anterior dissection of the capsule of the ankle joint is now completed.

Retracting the peroneal tendons posteriorly after opening their tendon sheath, the posterior capsule of the joint is separated from the distal end of the tibia. The lateral articular surface of the talus is removed down to cancellous bone. After inserting an elevator between the articular surfaces of the tibia and the talus, they are prepared down to cancellous bone, trying to fit them snugly together in a correct position of the foot. Through a stab

incision in the skin a 4-mm Steinmann pin is driven through the previously drilled horizontal canal in the talus, holding the skin in the position it will be in after suturing it. Holding the foot in proper alignment, especially with respect to rotation, with the patella as a point of reference, a second drill canal is made through the tibia 8 cm above the joint line via a stab incision just anterior to the fibula (approaching from the lateral side and paralleling the Steinmann pin in the talus), penetrating both cortices of the tibia. This is a very important and decisive step in the operation, and proper alignment of bones and placement of the second stab incision are critical. A 4-mm Steinmann pin is inserted through the stab incision and driven through the tibia after preceding drilling. The ends of the pins are connected with the spindles and the arthrodesis is put under compression. The talus

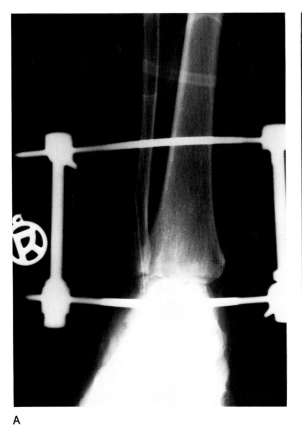

A

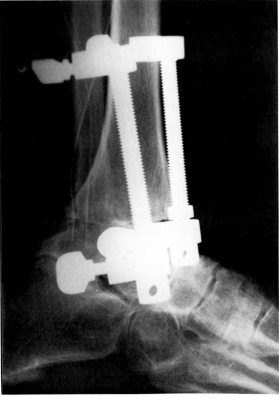

B

Fig. 36-27. (A) Postoperative anteroposterior x-ray after ankle fusion. Compression is exerted until the pins are slightly bent. **(B)** Postoperative lateral x-ray after ankle fusion. Distal Steinmann pin is anterior to longitudinal axis of tibia.

should be positioned rather posteriorly in relation to the tibia to preserve the prominence of the heel[127] and for biomechanical reasons. The screw clamps are tightened, and the position of the foot and the alignment of the osteotomy surfaces are controlled medially and laterally. Errors in rotation can be adjusted by releasing the compression.[127] If good alignment and position of the foot are achieved, compression is increased until the pins are slightly bent[127] (Fig. 36-27A). The stability of the arthrodesis is tested. The lateral malleolus is screwed to the talus with a malleolar screw after drilling a 3.2-mm drill canal.

A Redon suction drain is inserted medially and laterally, and the subcutaneous tissue is sutured with resorbable 3-0 material and the skin with 4-0 nonresorbable material. Dressings are applied and the leg rested on a Braun's frame. On the third day after surgery the patient is allowed out of bed with crutches. After 2 weeks the compression is controlled and eventually tightened. After 6 weeks the patient is allowed to touch ground. After 8 weeks the pins are removed, a plaster cast is applied for 4 weeks, and weightbearing is encouraged. If there is no inflamation or discharge from the pin sites the external fixator can be left in place until fusion is complete (Fig. 36-27B). This usually takes 3 months.

Discussion. Charnley[126] pointed out that compression arthrodesis of the ankle joint "perhaps demands a little more mechanical aptitude than is necessary in most orthopaedic procedures." To fit the osseous surfaces snugly together in the correct position of the foot sometimes demands much effort in accuracy and patience. We prefer osteotomes for the preparation of the surfaces because corrections can be performed more accurately than with a saw. Definite compression of the external fixator must not be performed before an ideal position of the foot is accomplished.

A varus position and excessive valgus positions of the heel must be avoided. The foot should be in a balanced forefoot-rearfoot relation according to pronation and suppination. This must also be tested before definitely applying compression. Any endfeeling close to the plantargrade position of the forefoot must be avoided. Some degree of forefoot movement into eversion must be guaranteed;

otherwise painful tarsal and metatarsal conditions can arise.

The criterion for acceptable results is a pain-free foot in a normal position, which is in a neutral position at the level of the ankle joint in the sagittal plane, has an external rotation of 10 to 15 degrees in a horizontal plane, and is in a neutral position in the frontal plane. The patient should be able to wear normal shoes. To protect the midtarsal joints from overload, a rocker-bottom application at the sole of the shoe is recommended. This can be used in compensating for the loss of leg length. A cushioned heel will reduce the initial thrust of the stance phase.

Complications

Malposition and pseudoarthrosis are the most unpleasant complications in ankle arthrodesis. Efforts must be taken to avoid this by meticulous adaptation of the decorticated osseous surfaces and with the foot in the proper position. The resections must be carried down to cancellous bone, removing all sclerotic bone. Only with bone of good quality at the resection surfaces will fusion take place. Hematomas disturbing healing of the wounds and providing fertile soil for infection must be avoided by careful hemostasis and suction drainage.

Talocalcaneal Arthrodesis (Modified After Demyson and Fulford)

Subtalar arthrodesis are used to correct deformities of the foot resulting from subtalar dysfunction or instability (e.g., in pes planovalgus) or to fuse an otherwise painful joint. The most frequent indication in adults in this author's experience was a painful subtalar joint after fractures of the calcaneus that led to osteoarthritis of the joint as a result of incongruency of the joint surfaces and their deviation from the axes of movement.

Technique

Following a Grice-type incision over the sinus tarsi the subcuntaneous tissue, the fascia, and the fibers of the distal extensor retinaculum covering the sinus tarsi are divided. The fat pad of the sinus is excised, the walls of the sinus are curreted, and the cortex of talus and calcaneus is removed within the sinus with a burr down to cancellous bone. A second longitudinal incision is made at the dorsomedial aspect of the tarsal neck just medial to the tendon of the tibialis anterior muscle. The fascia is incised, and the incision is deepened between the tibialis anterior and the extensor hallucis longus tendon down to the neck of the talus.

A 2-mm Kirschner wire is drilled through the neck of the talus just distal to the articular surface of the talus. The calcaneus is held in the desired position and the wire is driven into it in a direction that is oblique to medial-lateral, anterior-posterior, and dorsal-plantar. The position of the wire is checked under the x-ray amplifier. If the position of the talus relative to the calcaneus and of the K wire is satisfying a drill hole is made with a 3.2-mm drill in the same direction as the wire and in its immediate vicinity. The drill is driven through the inferolateral cortex of the calcaneous, the length of the canal is measured, and a cancellous bone screw of adequate length is inserted. (Fig. 36-28). It can be visualized in the sinus tarsi. The screw is tightened until the head bites into the superior surface of the talus. The K wire is removed. Allograft bone chips (from fresh frozen femoral heads harvested at total hip replacements) and packed into the sinus.

The wound is closed in layers with resorbable 3-0 sutures after inserting a Redon suction tube. A padded, split plaster cast is applied. After removal of the skin sutures an unpadded cast is made and non-weight-bearing ambulation with crutches is allowed. After 4 weeks a walking cast is applied. It is removed 10 weeks after surgery. After an x-ray check for bony fusion the patient is referred to physiotherapy to regain mobility and strength at the ankle joint.

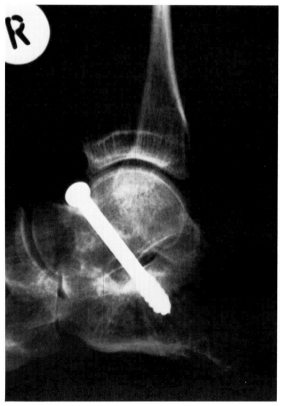

A

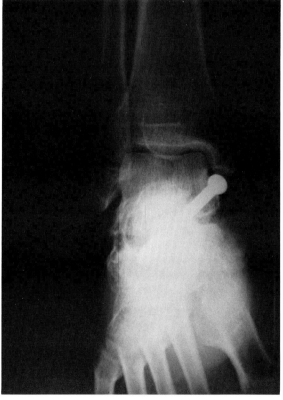

B

Fig. 36-28. Subtalar fusion after Dennyson and Fulford.[125] **(A)** Lateral view. Cancellous bone screw penetrating obliquely from the talar neck into the calcaneus, bridging the sinus tarsi. Head of screw ought to be more distal to avoid contact with anterior distal edge of tibia at extension of forefoot. **(B)** Anteroposterior view.

Discussion The K wire is an important aid in positioning the screw. It unites talus and calcaneus and acts as a guide for the screw. The use of human allograft bone eliminates the need for a second operation to remove cancellous bone from elsewhere in the patient's body and saves operating time.

The oblique direction of the screw tends to pull the talar neck and head laterally onto the anterior process of the talus, and also backward. This is especially useful in fusions aiming at correction of pes planovalgus since it counteracts the movement of the talar head medially and plantarward which is the main feature in this deformity.

Criteria for acceptable results are full correction of the deformity and a reliable fusion.

Complications

Major complications are not expected. It must be mentioned, however, that the talar neck must not be weakened by removing too much bone; otherwise a fracture might be possible when the screw is exerting a great deal of pressure on the neck of the talus.

Arthrodesis of the Navicular – First Cuneiform Joint

The objective of all operations correcting flatfoot is to reestablish a pain-free, stable foot with a normal longitudinal arch resistant to excessive pronation and to progression of the deformity.[124] The operation is indicated only after growth arrest; otherwise an adduction deformity will be created by destroying the epiphyses of the contiguous bones. In the young adult without osteoarthritis of the talonavicular joint a method saving the subtalar and midtarsal joint will be favored in comparison to fusion of the subtalar complex. There is widespread agreement that such operations should be performed only in unstable feet that cannot be controlled by conservative means.

The Hoke procedure for correction of extremely relaxed flatfoot consists of an arthrodesis between the first and second cuneiform and the navicular and a lengthening of the Achilles tendon.[128] Although the Hoke procedure has not found general approval, especially with respect to long-term re-

sults, this author has a better opinion of the method. Of 23 flexible flatfeet cases seen by this author, seven were operated on using the Hoke procedure. Eight to 33 years after surgery five patients showed excellent and two showed satisfying results.[129]

Preoperative Criteria

Preoperative criteria are deducted from lateral and dorsoplantar radiographs. The forefoot-rearfoot angle of Hibbs should exceed 140 degrees. Abduction of the forefoot is evaluated from the dorsoplantar radiographs.

Technique

With the patient supine, lengthening of the Achilles tendon is performed when extension at the ankle joint is less than 25 degrees. This can be done using various methods and is described elsewhere in this book.

A longitudinal incision is made at the medial side of the first cuneiform – navicular joint and the bones are exposed after reflecting the periosteum. The joint is opened and the articular surfaces of the first and second cuneonavicular joints are removed down to cancellous bone. At the medial face of the proximal metaphysis of the tibia a corticocancellous bone graft measuring 12 × 20 mm is removed. With the assistant pressing the anterior end of the first metatarsal forcibly into equinus, rectangular section of bone about 12 mm deep is cut from the scaphoid and internal cuneiform bones that is of a size to receive the bone graft.[130] A firm, carpentry-type connection ought to result. The gaps at the joint lines are filled with the bits of cancellous bone. The periosteal flaps are sutured.

A Redon suction drain is inserted and the skin is closed. Thin dressings are applied. A plaster splint is made for the foot up to the heel in equinus position and with the heel in varus. After hardening of the splint the foot is dorsiflexed and the cast is completed to the tibial tubercle. Precautions should be taken to enable splitting of the plaster dorsally after hardening in its entire length. Ten days after the operation the cast and sutures are removed and a new cast is applied in the corrected position of the foot. Weightbearing is allowed after 6 weeks and the cast is removed 8 to 10 weeks after surgery.

Physiotherapy is started to regain mobility and strength at the ankle joint and foot. Supports should be given for the first 6 months after surgery.

REFERENCES

1. Heimkes B, Stotz S, Wolf K, Posel P: Das tarsaltunnelsyndrom. Orthopäde 16:477–482, 1987
2. Ehricht HG: Das kompressionssyndrom doersal und distal vom tibialen malleolus. pp. 280–281. In Murri A (ed): Der Fuss. Medizinisch Literarische Verlagsgesellshaft m.b.H., Uelzen, 1981
3. Mann RA (ed): Surgery of the Foot. CV Mosby Co, St. Louis, 1986
4. De Stoop N: Tarsal tunnel syndrome: a series of 17 operated cases. Actual Med Chir Pied 16:159–164, 1986
5. Freising S: Das tarsaltunnelsyndrom. Chir Praxis 32:299–304, 1983
6. Mosimann W: Das tarsaltunnelsyndrom. Klinik und ergebnisse der operativen therapie an hand von 39 eigenen beobachtungen. Schweiz Arch Neurol Neurochir Psychiat 19:105, 1969
7. Kaplan PE, Kernahan WT: Tarsal tunnel syndrome. J Bone Joint Surg [Am] 63:96–99, 1981
8. Regnauld B: Le Pied. p. 328. Springer Verlag, Berlin, 1986
9. Hicks JH: The three weight bearing mechanisms of the foot. Cited by Sarrafian SK: Anatomy of the Foot and Ankle. p. 409. JB Lippincott Company, Philadelphia, 1983
10. Sarrafian SK: Anatomy of the Foot and Ankle. p. 404. JB Lippincott Co, Philadelphia, 1983
11. Mau, C: Ein Fall von ausgedehnter ossifizierender Periostitis des Calcaneus nach Operation eines Calcaneussporns, einer Bursa subcalcanea und Bursa achillea. Zbl Chr 53:2462–2465, 1926
12. Baxter DE, Thigpen MC: Heel pain — operative results. Foot Ankle 5:16–25, 1984
13. Shikoff MD, Figura MA, Figura MA, Postar SE: A retrospective study of 195 patients with heel pain. J Am Podiatr Med Assoc 76:71–75, 1986
14. Steindler A, Smith AR: Spurs of the os calcis. Surg Gynecol Obstet 66:663, 1938
15. Michele AA, Krueger FJ: Plantar heel pain treated by countersinking osteotomy. Milit Surg 109:26–29, 1950
16. O'Connor D: Sinus tarsi syndrome. A clinical entity. J Bone Joint Surg [Am] 40:720, 1958
17. Taillard W, Meyer JM, Garcia J, Blanc Y: The sinus tarsi syndrome. Int Orthop 5:117–130, 1981
18. Rosensky SL: Sinus tarsi syndrome. Curr Podiatr Med 35:24–26, 1986
19. Meyer JM, Garcia J, Hoffmeyer P, Fritschy D: The subtalar sprain. A roentgenographic study. Clin Orthop Related Res 226:169–173, 1988
20. Regnauld B: Le Pied. p. 547. Springer Verlag, Berlin, 1986
21. Hauser EDW: The sinus tarsi syndrome. Ann Podol 1:11–15, 1962
22. Debrunner H: Das sinus tarsi syndrom. Schweiz Med Wochenschr 93:47, 1960
23. Komprda J: Syndrome du sinus du tarse. Etude de 116 observations. Podologie 5:19, 1966
24. Meyer JM, Lagier R: Post-traumatic sinus tarsi syndrome. An anatomical and radiological study. Acta Orthop Scand 48:121–128, 1977
25. Schauwecker F, Weller S, Lenz B: Zur pathogenese des achillessehnenrisses. Dtsch Med Wochenschr 92:1758–1761, 1967
26. White JW: Torsion of the Achilles tendon: its surgical significance. Arch Surg 46:784–787, 1943
27. Lagergren C, Lindholm A: Vascular distribution in the Achilles tendon. Acta Chir Scand 116:491–495, 1958
28. Dederich R, Bonse H, Hild A et al: Achillessehnenrupturen. Unfallchirurg 91:259–269, 1988
29. Saillant G, Roy-Camille R, Thoreux P, Neves J: Clinical study and anatomo-pathology of chronic tendinous pathologies of the Achilles tendon. pp. 136–142. In Claustre J, Simon L (eds): Pathologie du Talon. Masson, Paris, 1986
30. Biehl G, Harms J: Operative behandlung der paratenonitis achillea bei hochleistungssportlern. Arch Orthop Unfall-Chir 87:309–315, 1977
31. Pfister A: Die ultraschalldiagnostik bei sportorthopädischen weichteilerkrankungen. Dtsch Z Sport Med 38:108–110, 1987
32. Graf R: Was leistet die sonographie in der sporttraumatologie? Dtsch Z Sport Med 38:82–86, 1987
33. Balasubramanian P, Prathap K: The effect of injection of hydrocortisone into rabbit calcaneal tendons. J Bone Joint Surg [Br] 54:729–734, 1972
34. Schönbauer HR: Erkrankungen der achillessehne. Wien Klin Wochenschr 98, Suppl 168, 1986
35. Wilhelm H: Die subcutane achillessehnenruptur. Unfallheilkunde 121:330, 1975
36. Schwarz B, Heisel J, Mittelmeier H: Achillessehnenrupturen. Ursache, prognose, therapie — spätergebnisse. Aktuel Traumatol 14:8–14, 1984
37. Könn G, Löbbecke F: Zur morphologie und den

ursachen der spontanen achillessehnenruptur. Hefte Unfallheilkd 121:297–301, 1975

38. Carden DG, Noble J, Chalmers J et al: Rupture of calcaneal tendon. The early and late management. J Bone Joint Surg [Br] 69:416–420, 1987

39. Wills CA, Washburn S, Caiozzo V, Prietto CA: Achilles tendon rupture. A review of the literature comparing surgical versus non surgical treatment. Clin Orthop Related Res 207:156–163, 1986

40. Shield CL, Kerlin RK, Jobe FW, Carter VS, Lombardo SJ: Cybex II evaluation of surgically repaired Achilles tendon ruptures. Am J Sports Med 6:369, 1978

41. Kelikian H, Kelikian AS: Disorders of the Ankle. WB Saunders Co, Philadelphia, 1985

42. Bosworth D: Repair of defects in the tendo Achillis. J Bone Joint Surg [Am] 38:111–114, 1956

43. Lindholm A: Cited by Justis EJ: Traumatic disorders. In Crenshaw AH (ed): Campbell's Operative Orthopaedics. 7th Ed. CV Mosby Co, St. Louis, 1987

44. Lange M: Orthopädisch Chir Operationslehre. 2. Auflage. p. 29. JF Bergmann Verlag, München, 1962

45. Benum B, Berg V, Fretheim OJ: The strain on sutured Achilles tendons in walking cast: an EMG analysis. Eur Surg Res, 16(Suppl 2):14–21, 1984

46. Saraffian KS: Anatomy of the Foot and Ankle. p. 199. JB Lippincott Co, Philadelphia, 1983

47. Kashyap S, Prince R: Spontaneous rupture of the tibialis anterior tendon. A case report. Clin Orthop Related Res 216:259–261, 1987

48. Hipp E, Weigert M: Subcutane Ruptur der Tibialis-articus Sehne. Z Orthop 101:398, 1966

49. Moberg E: Rupture of the tendon of tibialis anterior. Acta Chir Scand 95:455, 1947

50. Weissinger M, Landsiedl F: Die beidseitige subcutane ruptur der sehne des muskulus tibialis anterior und ihre differential-diagnose. Z Orthop 122:659–660, 1984

51. Bengert O: Spontane subcutane ruptur der sehne des vorderen schienbeinmuskels. Z Orthop 111:941, 1973

52. Sarrafian SK: Anatomy of the Foot and Ankle. pp. 216–217. JB Lippincott Co, Philadelphia, 1983

53. Simpson RR, Gudas CJ: Posterior tibial tendon rupture in a world class runner. J Foot Surg 22:74–77, 1983

54. Kerr HD: Posterior tibial tendon rupture. Ann Emerg Med 17:649–650, 1988

55. Johnson KA: Tibialis posterior tendon rupture. Clin Orthop Related Res 177:140–147, 1983

56. Citron N: Injury of the tibialis posterior tendon: a

cause of acquired valgus foot in childhood. Injury 16:610–612, 1985

57. Steinböck G, Polt E: Ergebnisse nach plattfussoperationenen. pp. 160–164. In Murri A (ed) Der Fuss. Medizinisch Literarische Verlags-gesellschaft m.b.H., Uelzen, 1981

58. Funk DA, Cass JR, Johnson KA: Aquired adult flatfoot secondary to posterior tibial tendon pathology. J Bone Joint Surg [Am], 68:95:102, 1986

59. Rosenberg ZS: Rupture of the posterior tibial tendon: CT and surgical findings. Radiology 167:489–493, 1988

60. Mann RA, Thompson FM: Rupture of the posterior tibial tendon causing flat foot. Surgical treatment. J Bone Joint Surg [Am] 67:556–561, 1985

61. Alexander JI, Johnson KA, Berquist TH: Magnetic resonance imaging in the diagnosis of disruption of the posterior tibial tendon. Foot Ankle 8:144–147, 1987

62. Abraham E, Stirnaman JE: Neglected rupture of the peroneal tendons causing recurrent sprains of the ankle. J Bone Joint Surg [Am] 61:1247–1248, 1979

63. Spontaneous rupture of the peroneus longus tendon with fracture of the os peroneum. J Foot Surg 27:328–333, 1988

64. Mains DB, Sullivan RC: Fracture of the os peroneum. J Bone Joint Surg [Am] 55:1529–1530, 1973

65. Burman MS, Lapidus PW: The functional disturbances caused by the inconstant bones and sesamoids of the foot. Arch Surg 22:936–975, 1931

66. Davis JA: Peroneal compartment syndrome secondary to rupture of the peroneus longus. J Bone Joint Surg [Am] 61:783–784, 1979

67. Muralt VRH: Luxation der peronealsehnen. Z Orthop 87:263, 1956

68. Folschweiller J: Abriss des retinaculum musculi fibularium proximale und seine folgen. Hefte Unfallheilk 92:98, 1967

69. Leitz G: Modifikation des von Platzgummer angegebenen Verfahrens zur operativen Behandlung der habituellen Peronealsehnenluxation. Arch Orthop Unfall-Chir 64:245–251, 1968

70. Platzgummer H: Über ein einfaches verfahren zur operativen behandlung der habituellen peroneussehnenluxation. Arch Orthop Unfallchir 61:144, 1967

71. Pöll RG, Duijfjes F: The treatment of recurrent dislocation of the peroneal tendons. J Bone Joint Surg (Br) 66:98–100, 1984

72. Mann RA: Miscellaneous afflictions of the foot. In

Mann RA (ed): Surgery of the Foot. 5th ed. CV Mosby Co, St. Louis, 1986

73. Taylor GJ: Prominence of the calcaneus: is operation justified? J Bone Joint Surg [Br] 68:467–470, 1986

74. Keck SW, Kelly PJ: Bursitis of the posterior part of the heel: evaluation of surgical treatment of eighteen patients. J Bone Joint Surg [Am] 47:267–273, 1965

75. Fowler A, Philip JR: Abnormality of the calcaneus as a cause of painful heel: its diagnosis and operative treatment. Br J Surg 32:494–498, 1945

76. Vega MR, Cavolo DJ, Green RM, Cohen RS: Haglund's deformity. J Am Podiatry Assoc 74:129–135, 1984

77. Pavlov H, Henegan MA, Hersh A et al: The Haglund syndrome: initial and differental diagnosis. Diagn Radiol 144:83–88, 1982

78. Steffensen and Even: cited in Denis A, Huber-Levernieux C: Tendinopathies mécaniques du tendon d'Achille. In Claustre J, Simon L (eds): Pathologie du Talon. Masson, Paris, 1986

79. Denis A, Huber-Levernieux C: Tendinopathies mécaniques du tendon d'Achille. In Claustre J, Simon L (eds): Pathologie du Talon. Masson, Paris, 1986

80. Ruch JA: Haglund's disease. J Am Podiatry Assoc 64:1000–1003, 1974

81. Sella EJ, Lawson JP, Ogden JA: The accessory navicular synchrondosis. Clin Orthop Related Res 209:280–285, 1986

82. Sella EJ, Lawson JP: Biomechanics of the accessory navicular synchondrosis. Foot Ankle 8:156–163, 1987

83. Lawson JP, Ogdon JA, Sella EJ, Barwick KW: The painful accessory navicular. Skeletal Radiol 12:250–262, 1984

84. Giannestras NJ: Foot Disorders. Medial and Surgical Management. 2nd Ed. Lea & Febiger, Philadelphia, 1973

85. Pfeffinger LL, Mann RA: Sesamoid and accessory bones. In Mann RE (ed): Surgery of the Foot. 5th edition. CV Mosby Company, St. Louis, 1986

86. MacNicol MF, Voutsinas S: Surgical treatment of the symptomatic accessory navicular. J Bone Joint Surg [Br] 66:218–226, 1984

87. Cowell RC, Elener V: Rigid painful flatfoot secondary to tarsal coalition. Clin Orthop 177:54–60, 1983

88. Scranton PE: Treatment of symptomatic talocalcaneal coalition. J Bone Joint Surg [Am] 69:533–539, 1987

89. Korvin H: Coalitio talocalcanea. Z Orthop Chir 60:105–110, 1934

90. Harris RI, Beath T: Etiology of peroneal spastic flatfoot. J Bone Joint Surg [Br] 30:624–634, 1948

91. Wray JB, Herndon CN: Hereditary transmission of congenital coalition of the calcaneus to the navicular. J Bone Joint Surg [Am] 45:365–372, 1963

92. Inglis G, Buxton RA, MacNicol MF: Symptomatic calcaneonavicular bars. J Bone Joint Surg [Br] 68:128–132, 1986

93. Olney BW, Asher MA: Excision of symptomatic coalition of the middle facet of the talocalcaneal joint. J Bone Joint Surg [Am] 69:539–544, 1987

94. In Weissmann SD (ed): Radiology of the Foot. Williams & Wilkins, Baltimore, 1983

95. Huurmann WW: Congenital foot deformities. p. 519. In Mann RA (ed): Surgery of the Foot. 5th ed. CV Mosby Co, St. Louis, 1986

96. Mitchell GP, Gibson JMC: Excision of calcaneonavicular bar for painful spasmodic flat foot. J Bone Joint Surg (Br) 49:281–287, 1967

97. Berndt AL, Harty M: Transchondral fractures (osteochondritis dissecans) of the talus. J Bone Joint Surg [Am] 41:988, 1959

98. Flick AB, Gould N: Osteochondritis dissecans of the talus (transchondral fractures of the talus): review of the literature and new surgical approach for medial bone lesions. Foot Ankle 5:165–185, 1985

99. Zollinger H, Dietschi C: Osteochondrosis dissecans des talus bei recidivierenden fussdistorsionen. Z Unfallmed 68:39–43, 1975

100. Lambiris E, Zilch H: Distorsion oder osteochondrosis dissecans der talusrolle nach einem trauma? Orthop Praxis 4:331–354, 1981

101. Johnson LL: Arthroscopic Surgery. CV Mosby Co, St. Louis, 1986

102. Bauer M, Jonsson K, Linden B: Osteochondritis dissecans of the ankle. J Bone Joint Surg (Br) 69:93–96, 1987

103. Pettine KA, Morrey BF: Osteochondral fractures of the talus. J Bone Joint Surg [Br] 69:89–92, 1987

104. Davidson AM, Steel HD, Mackenzie DA, Penny JA: A review of twenty one cases of tranchondral fracture of the talus. J Trauma 7:378, 1967

105. Huylebroek JF, Martens M, Simon JP: Transchondral talar dome fracture. Arch Orthop Trauma Surg 104:238, 1985

106. Pritsch M, Horoshovski H, Farine M: Arthroscopic treatment of osteochondral lesions of the talus. J Bone Joint Surg [Am] 68:862, 1986

107. Boe S: Arthroscopy of the ankle joint. Arch Orthop Trauma Surg 105:285–286, 1986

108. Japas LM: Surgical treatment of pes cavus by tarsal V-osteotomy. J Bone Joint Surg [Am] 50:927–944, 1968

109. Tachdjian MO: The Child's Foot. p. 514. WB Saunders Co, Philadelphia, 1985
110. Hibbs RA: An operation for "claw foot." JAMA 73:1583, 1919
111. Dennemann H: Möglichkeiten der röntgenologischen diagnostik von fussformen und fussdeformitäten. Verh Dtsch Orthop Ges 48:291–298, 1960
112. Dwyer FC: A new approach to the treatment of pes cavus. In: Sixième Congrès de Chirurgie Orthopédique, Berne, 30. aout–3. septembre 1954. p. 551. Société International de Chirurgie Orthopedique et de Traumatologie. Imprimerie Lielens, 1955
113. Dwyer FC: Osteotomy of the calcaneum for pes cavus. J Bone Joint Surg [Br] 41:80–86, 1959
114. Hoefinger J, Steinboeck G, Polt E: Ergebnisse der fersenbeinosteotomie nach Dwyer. pp. 45–47. In Murri A (ed): Der Fuss. Medizin Literarische Verlagsgesellschaft m.b.H., Uelzen, 1981
115. Dwyer FC: The treatment of relapsed clubfoot by the insertion of a wedge into the calcaneum. J Bone Joint Surg [Br] 45:67–75, 1963
116. Imhäuser G: Die operative behandlung des starken hohlfusses und des ballenhohlfusses. Z Orthop 106:488, 1969
117. Trensz JL, Lang G, Kehr P, Steib JP: La correction du varus calcananeen du pied creux par osteotomie mediotarsience. p. 86. In Claustre J, Simon L (eds): Pathologie du Talon. Masson, Paris, 1986
118. Bösch J: Die konservative klumpfuss behandlung des säuglings und kleinkindes. Med Orthop Technik 6:150–154, 1974
119. Wagner H: Calcaneus-verschiebeosteotomie beim kindlichen knickfuss. Orthopäde 15:233–241, 1986
120. Gleich A: Beitrag zur operativen plattfussbehandlung. Arch Klin Chir 46:358–362, 1893
121. Dwyer FC: Osteotomy of the calcaneum for pes cavus. J Bone Joint Surg [Br] 41:80–86, 1959
122. Silver CM, Simon SD, Spindell E et al: Calcaneal osteotomy for varus and valgus deformities of the foot in cerebral palsy. J Bone Joint Surg [Am] 49:232–246, 1967
123. Fick R: Handbuch der Anatomie und Mechanik der Gelenke. Vol. 3. p. 620. Teil Fischer, Jena, 1911
124. Baciu CC: A simple technique for arthrodesis of the ankle. J Bone Joint Surg [Br] 68:266–267, 1986
125. Dennyson WG, Fulford GE: Subtalar arthrodesis by cancellous grafts and metallic internal fixation. J Bone Joint Surg [Br] 58:507–510, 1976
126. Charnley J: Compression arthrodesis of the ankle and shoulder. J Bone Joint Surg [Br] 33:180–191, 1951
127. Hefti F: Die stellung des fusses bei arthrodesen des oberen sprunggelenkes. Bücherei des Orthopäden Vol 28. p. 67. Ferdinand Enke Verlag, Stuttgart, 1981
128. Hoke M: An operation for extremely relaxed flat feet. J Bone Joint Surg 13:373–383, 1931
129. Russel TA: Arthrodesis of lower extremity and hip. In Crenshaw AH (ed): Campbell's Operative Orthopaedics. 7th ed. CV Mosby Co, St. Louis, 1987
130. Blair HC: Comminuted fractures and fracture dislocations of the body of the astragalus: operative treatment. Am J Surg 59:37, 1943

Collapsing Pes Valgoplanus (Flexible Flatfoot)

37

Stephen J. Miller, D.P.M.

TERMINOLOGY AND DEFINITIONS

Contentious Issues

Although inaccurately referenced and attributed to Hoke, the following quote observes that: "The reason so little is known about the development of flatfoot is because these patients do not seek treatment until the condition is well developed and symptomatic."[1] Since the natural history of this common problem has never been investigated in any sort of ongoing or chronologic order, much of the information on which diagnosis and treatment are based comes from the observations of the many clinicians who have taken an interest in the subject. Even the differentiation between rigid and flexible flatfoot has been a relatively recent categorization.[2]

The pediatric flatfoot is often described as a benign and even normal condition, not worthy of treatment until significant symptoms are evident.[3] Yet, the experienced clinician is well aware of the stages in the pathologic deterioration of the flexible flatfoot, knowing full well that all such feet do not necessarily become symptomatic.

As the study of biomechanics and kinesiology has unveiled many of the inner workings of the foot-ankle complex it takes very little extrapolation to understand the pathology of the flexible flatfoot, well before symptoms arise. Yet, in spite of a fairly extensive digest of the literature on flatfoot, few authors agree on a consistent or even logical approach to its diagnosis and management. Why such contention?

McGlamry et al. identified three major issues that have prevented a unified approach to the flexible collapsed pes valgus foot.[4] First, the terminology is quite variable, leading to much confusion (Table 37-1). Second, the numerous theories as to the etiology have varied widely over the years, with little agreement among the writers as to the true nature of the deformity. Third, there is little agreement as to the indications, timing, and extent of surgery to correct the condition. I might add that there is little agreement in the literature as to the conservative approaches to treatment. Again, the source of such confusion is a lack of detailed study into the natural history of flexible flatfoot, with and without treatment.

Flexible Flatfoot

Flatfoot should first be divided into rigid and flexible deformities, both of which can be subdivided into congenital and acquired types (Table 37-2). Determining the flexibility is the first step

Table 37-1. Terminology for Flexible Flatfoot

Weakfoot
Relaxed foot
Relaxed flatfoot
Hypermobile flatfoot
Congenital hypermobile flatfoot
Flaccid flatfoot
Pronation syndrome
Developmental flatfoot
Talipes valgus
Talipes calcaneovalgus
Planovalgus foot
Compensated talipes equinus
Pes valgus planus
Pes valgo deformity
Pes valgoplanus
Collapsing pes valgoplanus

toward diagnosis of the hypermobile or flexible flatfoot. Observing weight-bearing and non-weight-bearing arch configuration, performing the Hubscher (or Jack) maneuver, and analyzing subtalar and midtarsal joint ranges of motion are investigative techniques that will help lead to an accurate conclusion.

Even though flexibility of the deformity has been determined, variations in flexibility may be seen. For example, a foot with ligamentous laxity will have much greater joint motion than a flatfoot with normal tissue laxity. The pediatric flexible flatfoot will certainly demonstrate a wider, more supple range of motion that the end-stage geriatric flexible

Table 37-2. Classification of Flatfoot

Rigid Flatfoot	Flexible Flatfoot
Congenital	Congenital
Congenital convex pes valgus (vertical talus)	Compensated forefoot varus
Tarsal coalition (peroneal spastic flatfoot)	Hypermobile flatfoot with short Achilles tendon (equinus)
Acquired	Talipes calcaneovalgus
Trauma induced (joint fracture)	Torsional flatfoot
Arthritis induced	Adducted flatfoot (Z-foot, skewfoot)
	Ligamentous laxity
	Accessory navicular
	Acquired
	Tendon laceration (posterior tibial)
	Arthritic condition
	Trauma
	Neuromuscular disorder
	Myelodysplasia
	Spasticity
	Poliomyelitis

flatfoot, which has a more restricted range of motion usually complicated by "tracking" — the functional malposition from years of weightbearing with the subtalar joint at its end range of motion.

Finally, one must differentiate between two types of flexible flatfeet.[4] One, designated the *pes planus foot,* is flexible yet has a perfectly normal low arch, both weight-bearing and non-weight-bearing. The foot shows few or no talocalcaneal signs of pronation physically or radiographically and the talonavicular joint is congruous. The second type of flexible flatfoot, termed *collapsing pes valgoplanus deformity,* demonstrates an arch in the non-weight-bearing position. The same arch collapses or flattens when full body weight is added. Multiple signs of pronation including sagittal plane breeches, can be observed by physical and radiologic examination.

Defining the Flexible Flatfoot

Flexible flatfoot is best defined as a supple pedal deformity that, through pronatory compensation, exhibits one or more of the following characteristics, best seen in the relaxed calcaneal stance position: eversion of the heel, abduction of the forefoot on the rearfoot, collapse of the medial column, medial talar bulge or ptosis, and flexibility of the foot with reducibility of the deformity. Through the gait cycle, the foot usually functions maximally pronated with little or no supination.

A posterior ankle equinus involving contracted gastrocnemius and/or soleus muscles usually accompanies flexible flatfoot as either a primary deforming force or a secondary adaptation. Many forms of compensation at the foot result from this powerful deforming force, including subtalar and midtarsal joint pronation, transverse plane abduction, medial column sag, tarsometatarsal breech, and early heel-off.[4]

Terminology

Since this is a dynamic deformity, it should be identified by a term that is not only descriptive of its static appearance but incorporates some indication of function as well. The term recommended is *collapsing pes valgoplanus* (CPVP).[4] The word *pes,* derived from Latin, means foot and has more of an acquired connotation.[5] *Valgo* describes the position of the heel in eversion and *planus* also has a Latin origin indicating plane or flat surface, to acknowledge the overall appearance of the longitudinal arch. The dynamic component of the term is "collapsing," which defines the loss of the arch contour as the foot accepts body weight.

For the sake of brevity, pes valgus deformity can be used as an acceptable designation of the collapsing pes valgoplanus condition.[4] Flexible flatfoot remains an appropriate term.

Incidence and Natural History

Many questions regarding the long-term history of pes valgus deformity with and without treatment remain unanswered. Besides a lack of information regarding the history, there have been no reliable large-number statistical studies that analyze the incidence of flexible flatfoot or the percentage of cases that become symptomatic, the exception being the Canadian Army Foot Survey by Harris and Beath (1947).[2] They found that 15 percent of the recruits had simple hypermobile flatfoot, 6 percent had the same with a tight heel cord, and 2 percent had a tarsal coalition.

Two important questions are often posed to the clinician. First, will a child outgrow a flexible flatfoot deformity? Giannestras stated that there is no spontaneous resolution to normal foot architecture.[6] This is in agreement with the opinions of most clinicians who are exposed to any large volume of foot disorders. However, it remains to be verified through long-term study.

The second question that has not adequately been answered by well-controlled studies is: What percentage of children with flatfeet will develop significant symptoms as they progress on through adolescence and adulthood?[7] Answers to this question are only speculative to date, although there are some clues to help in the prediction. If one or both parents have painful feet, it is much more likely that the child will. Although the flatfoot itself might not be inherited, the foot type that will compensate into a collapsing pes valgoplanus deformity very likely is transmitted genetically. To say that no flexible flatfeet should be treated in infancy or

childhood only demonstrates a poor understanding of the pathomechanics involved.

ETIOLOGY OF FLEXIBLE FLATFOOT

Historically, many authors' efforts at hypothesizing an etiology for flexible flatfoot have been expended largely to support their treatment. Others have applied basic anatomic and kinesiologic concepts to propose biomechanical theories. A brief review of some historic etiologies is found in Table 37-3.

Since flexible flatfoot is more of a compensatory problem, it is more important to identify the underlying condition that allows uncontrolled pronation to affect function through the subtalar and midtarsal joints. A pronating foot at maximum end range of motion becomes a flexible flatfoot. Treatment must then deal with the etiologic problem to neutralize the excessive pronation. These etiologies are seen in Table 37-4.

The biomechanics involved in pronation and compensation for other foot deformities are well covered in Chapter 3. It is critical to apply such principles to any treatment plan, whether conservative or surgical. Without such application treatment is doomed to fall short of consistent satisfactory results.

EVALUATING THE FLEXIBLE FLATFOOT

Planal Dominance and Range of Motion

Since pronation in the flexible flatfoot involves compensatory triplane motion about the subtalar and midtarsal joints, a determination of the range as well as the predominant plane of this motion is an essential part of the evaluation. The concept of planal dominance of both deformity and compensation, as developed by Green and Carol,[8] aids in a

Table 37-3. Historic Etiologies of Pes Valgus Deformity

Author	Proposed Etiology
Whitman (1888)	Inability of the muscles and ligaments to sustain the foot, a breakdown from overwork.
Lowman (1923)	Faults in leg alignment, faults in nutrition and lowered muscular and ligamentous tone, and faults in tarsal development (hereditary). Gradual loss of elasticity from plantar ligaments and muscles resulting in a "relaxed condition" (developmental).
Steindler (1929)	Compensation through the supinatory torsion of the forefoot.
Hoke (1931)	Inability of the medial muscles to support the flexible naviculocuneiform (first and second) joints as the ligaments stretch with weightbearing. Also recognized short Achilles tendon as component.
Kidner (1933)	Malposition of the posterior tibial tendon at its insertion and/or presence of an os tibiale externum causing a dynamic muscle imbalance with inability to support the arch.
Young (1939)	Collapse of the medial arch, correctible by realignment through tendon suspension. Also identified contracture of the tendocalcaneus muscles as a component.
Chambers (1946)	Abnormal abduction (of the foot) beneath the talus. Gleich (1893) and Lord (1923) also implicated the talocalcaneal alignment as a cause of flexible flatfoot by directing weight-bearing forces medial to the foot.
Harris (1948)	Excessive ligamentous laxity, weak support of anterior calcaneus, elongation of talar neck, absence of anterior calcaneal facet, often accompanied by short Achilles tendon.
Jack (1953)	Intrinsic structure of the bones and joints and integrity of the plantar ligaments.
Basmajian (1963)	Ruled out muscles in the primary support of the arch, except under high-stress loads.
Selakovich (1973)	The calcaneus does not support the talus, allowing for displacement of the latter. This promotes malalignment of the forefoot into abduction and supination.
Evans (1975)	Imbalance between the relative lengths of the medial and lateral columns of the foot, the lateral being excessively short.
Sarrafian (1987)	Untwisting of the foot plate placing tension on the plantar aponeurosis as the hindfoot and midfoot are pronated and the forefoot is supinated.

Table 37-4. Etiologies of Collapsing Pes Valgoplanus

Condition	Effect
Forefoot varus	Compensation for the forefoot to reach the supporting surface is through subtalar joint pronation, often to heel valgus, and unlocking of the midtarsal joint, causing hypermobility.
Flexible forefoot valgus	For the everted forefoot to reach the floor there is a certain amount of midtarsal joint instability achieved, especially when the flexible medial column gives way to allow subtalar joint pronation.
Ankle equinus	When there is less than the normal 10 degrees of dorsiflexion of the foot at the ankle, there must be compensation to allow the leg to come over the foot for toe-off. Subtalar and midtarsal joint pronation is one form of compensation. When there is no further motion left, the midfoot subluxes as a result of this powerful force.
Talipes calcaneovalgus	When this congenital deformity involving a dorsiflexion/valgus deformity of the whole foot is untreated, the pronated subtalar joint will remain so as weightbearing begins. With the force of body weight the foot cannot recover from pronation even with growth.
Torsional adduction	Any adducted position of the foot is compensated through pronation so it can better point in the direction of progression or even fit in the straight-last shoe.
Torsional abduction	Abduction deformities cause the foot to be positional more externally, bringing the central force of gravity medial to the center of the foot. As a result of this increased force on the sustentaculum tali over time, the foot will have a more difficult time recovering from prolonged pronation in the gait cycle.
Tibialis posterior loss	Weakness or loss of supinator power can allow the subtalar and midtarsal joints to rapidly pronate, unchecked. When the tibialis posterior is ruptured, or loses its mechanical advantage as a result of an accessory navicular, excessive pronation will then lead to a CPVP deformity.
Neuromuscular disorders	Any neurologic abnormality that creates an imbalance in the muscles controlling the foot can allow for development of flexible flatfoot. Primary examples are myelodysplasia, spastic disorders, and poliomyelitis.
Ligamentous laxity	Any tissue laxity syndrome (e.g., Marfan's, Ehlers-Danlos) or chronic arthritis (e.g., rheumatoid) can result in an acquired hypermobility. Loss of ligamentous stability will lead to unrestrained maximum pronation.
Neurotrophic feet	Lack of proprioception can lead to flexible flatfoot because muscle tone will provide insufficient support.
Medial weight shift	Any condition, anatomic or physiologic, that causes a medial shift in body weight can contribute to excess pronation. Once the calcaneus is everted to 5 or 6 degrees it becomes impossible for the supinator muscles to overcome the reactive force of gravity and the foot remains pronated.

(Adapted from McGlamry et al.,[4] with permission.)

greater measure of predictability and precision in the selection of treatment, especially when surgical procedures are indicated.[4]

The dominant plane of compensatory motion is a function of the position of the axis for the joint under examination. The location of the axis for the subtalar joint, as determined by Manter[9] and confirmed by Root et al.[10] was described as 42 degrees up from the transverse plane and 16 degrees from the sagittal plane. This measurement was an average, so that any individual's axis actually deviates from this norm.

Depending on the amount of deviation, the foot will function around the subtalar joint in a predominant plane. By examining the direction, quality, and range of motion about the subtalar joint, as well as the appearance of the foot when bearing weight, the examiner can estimate the primary plane of motion.

In order to determine the planal dominance of the midtarsal joint, examination must be made by observing forefoot movement and holding the calcaneus stationary. By combining the range and direction of the ankle joint[11] with the same information for the midtarsal and subtalar joints, the clinician can obtain the primary planal dominance for the entire foot.

The plane of motion is determined by the intersection of the axis of motion and the direction of motion. Three types of flexible flatfeet are identified by the predominant plane of motion:

Type I: Primary Frontal Plane Compensation — occurs when the joint axes lie close to the horizontal and sagittal planes (Fig. 37-1A).

Type II: Primary Sagittal Plane Compensation — occurs when the joint axes lie close to the horizontal and frontal planes (Fig. 37-1B).

Type III: Primary Transverse Plane Compensation — occurs when the joint axes lie close to the frontal and sagittal planes (Fig. 37-1C).

Clinical Presentation

Range of motion, quality of motion and planal dominance must be determined in the open kinetic, non-weight-bearing position. Palpation of the joints and sinus tarsi as well as the tendon sheaths might reveal areas of tenderness. These enthesopathies would provide further clues as to specific locations of jamming, subluxation, overuse, or traumatic inflammation from chronic joint function at the end range of motion.

The principle physical characteristics of CPVP have already been described. To observe these, the examination must be done with the foot in the relaxed calcaneal stance position (RCSP), which corresponds to the midstance phase of the gait cycle.

When calcaneal eversion is sufficient, Helbings' sign will be exhibited: lateral bowing of the Achilles tendon as observed from the posterior with the foot in RCSP (Fig. 37-2). Again, in the weight-bearing position, invoking the windlass principle as described by Hicks[12,13] the Hubscher maneuver or Jack test[14] can be performed to check for reducibility of the flatfoot deformity. When the great toe is passively extended in the flexible pes valgus deformity, tension is placed on the medial plantar fascia slip and the arch rises, with plantar flexion of the first ray, supination of the rearfoot, and external rotation of the leg (Fig. 37-3). This helps rule out rigid flatfoot deformity such as tarsal coalition. It also gives an idea of what the foot should look like in a more neutral functioning position.

Gait Analysis

Actual foot function should be evaluated. Using a corridor, treadmill, or gait observation platform, the patient can be observed walking. A logical approach is to observe from head to toes. Head tilt, shoulder drop, hip drop, and unilateral flatfoot are strong indicators for limb length discrepancy. Frontal plane deviation at the knees and legs will give some idea as to their contribution to any pronation that is present. Is there any genu recurvatum?

The angle and base of gait should be noted as well as any compensatory movements such as abductory twist at toe-off, early heel-off, or antalgia. Is there a midtarsal breech as weight is carried forward? Does the foot supinate at all or does it remain maximally pronated through the gait cycle?

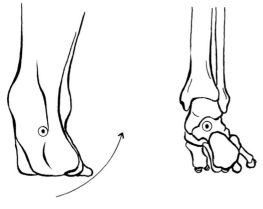

A

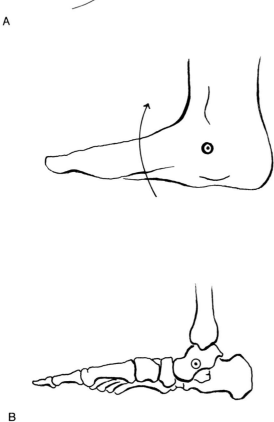

B

Fig. 37-1. **(A)** Type I flexible flatfoot—primary frontal plane compensation. **(B)** Type II flexible flatfoot—primary sagittal plane compensation. **(C)** Type III flexible flatfoot—primary transverse plane compensation. (Redrawn from Green and Carol,[8] with permission.)

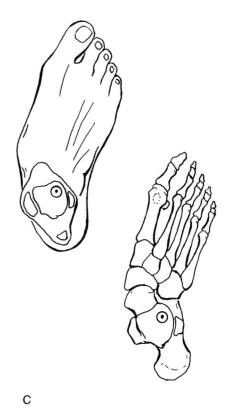

C

Stop the patient at midstance and run the foot through its full range of motion by having the patient actively raise and lower the arch. Palpate the head of the talus as it rotates back and forth. Is there any more motion left in the direction of pronation? Will the heel invert when the patient stands on the toes?

Radiographic Evaluation

Weight-bearing x-rays must be taken with the foot in angle and base of gait. The minimum views are anteroposterior or dorsoplantar, medial oblique, and lateral. They are indicated in evaluating the flexible flatfoot when certain measurable

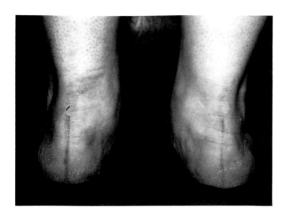

Fig. 37-2. Helbings' sign: lateral bowing of the Achilles tendon.

impingement. Harris and Beath (ski-jump) views and tomograms can reveal evidence of tarsal coalition if necessary. Computed tomography (CT) scanning is not indicated in evaluating the flexible flatfoot. This expensive modality is reserved for identifying more specific pathology such as tarsal coalitions and the extent of old osseous injuries.

Finally, neutral position weight-bearing dorsoplantar and lateral views can give an idea of what the foot would look like following surgical correction. They may also be used to observe the efficacy of biomechanical control when the foot is supported by an orthosis.

information is required, beyond that obtained by physical observation. They will also help rule out other painful flatfoot conditions, such as tarsal coalition, and evidence of old traumatic injuries. The radiographic signs of pronation can be found in Table 37-5.[15]

Radiographs can also provide much information as to the primary plane of compensation, including the direction of motion and the direction of subluxation[4] (Table 37-6).

Finally, special radiographic studies are available. Lateral views of the foot in "stress dorsiflexion" ("charger view") can exacerbate medial column faults and detect osseous ankle-talar

TREATMENT OF COLLAPSING PES VALGOPLANUS

Philosophy of Treatment

Throughout the medical literature, there has been little agreement not only on how to treat flexible flatfoot — conservatively or surgically — but whether to treat it at all. Some prefer to treat the majority of cases with information only or benign neglect.[3,16] Without substantial studies on the natural history of the disorder, the following information is based on a review of the literature, the vast

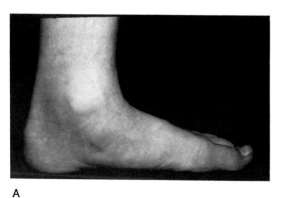

A

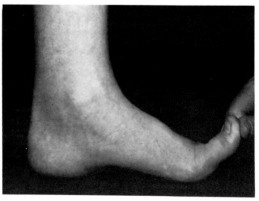

B

Fig. 37-3. The Hubscher maneuver **(A)** or Jack test **(B)** for determining the flexibility of the collapsed pes valgo planus deformity.

Table 37-5. Radiographic Signs of Pronation

Anteroposterior View	Lateral View
1. Increased talocalcaneal angle with broken cyma line	1. Anterior break in cyma line
2. Less than 75% articulation of the talar head in navicular acetabulum	2. Increased talar declination with midtalar line falling below the bisection of the first metatarsal
3. Abduction of the cuboid on the calcaneus greater than 11 degrees	3. Decreased talar declination angle below 20 degrees

	4. Medial column fault between:
	  —talus and navicular
	  —navicular and medial cuneiform
	  —medial cuneiform and first metatarsal

	5. Obliteration of the sinus tarsi
	6. Decreased first metatarsal declination angle

experience of clinicians exposed to pediatric foot problems, and personal clinical intuition observing the flexible flatfoot at various stages of development and deterioration, treated and untreated or neglected.

Experience has demonstrated that the majority of patients with flexible flatfoot can obtain successful relief of symptoms by means of conservative biomechanical control, which may even prevent progression of the deformity or associated sequelae.[4] The simple, nonpathologic pes planus foot usually requires no treatment. Overall, only a mi-

Table 37-6. Radiographic Signs of Planal Dominance in Flexible Flatfoot

Type I—Dominant Frontal Plan Compensation
  Widening of tarsal area, DP view
  Decrease in first metatarsal declination
  Decrease in height of sustentaculum tali
  Increased superimposition of lesser tarsus, lateral view
Type II—Dominant Sagittal Plane Compensation
  Increase in talar declination angle
  Naviculocuneiform (or other medial column) breach
  Increased talocalcaneal angle, lateral view
  Decreased calcaneal inclination angle
Type III—Dominant Transverse Plane Compensation
  Increased talocalcaneal angle, DP view
  Increased cuboid abduction angle
  Decrease in forefoot adductus angle (may be reversed)
  Loss of talonavicular congruency (<75%), DP view

(From McGlamry et al.,[4] with permission.)

nority of CPVP patients require surgical intervention.

It is the purpose of this section to present a detailed, logical approach to the management of collapsing pes valgoplanus.

Indications for Treatment

Some arguments have been made for no treatment in the infant and pediatric flatfoot. With careful evaluation and analysis not only of the patient but also of the blood relatives, indications for treatment become more precise.

McGlamry et al.[4] outlined several reasons why treatment can be important:

1. Pain: Although this is the most difficult symptom to elicit accurately in children, it is an important cause of reduced physical activity and perhaps social interaction as well. To say that all foot and leg pains are ''growing pains'' is totally ignoring the pathology present.
2. Fatigue: Symptoms of overuse include cramping, arch fatigue, and general discomfort, with resulting compensatory alteration in life-style, work, and recreation.
3. Joint degeneration: Rearfoot and midfoot degeneration occur over long periods of time, resulting in painful degenerative joint disease and deformity. Unfortunately, this is usually not evident until late in the natural course, by which time the joint damage is irreversible.
4. Associated deformities: The unstable rearfoot allows unlocking of the midtarsal joint and distal structures, resulting in or accelerating the development of hallux valgus, hammer toes, intermetatarsal neuromas, plantar fasciitis, and metatarsalgia.

Conservative Treatment

D'Amico compared the feet to the foundation footings of a building. Precise alignment is essential to withstand the stresses directed through them from above. Even a minor misalignment can result in a disastrous deforming force at a distant location.[17] So, to leave the developing foot in an unstable configuration invites deforming forces to incur

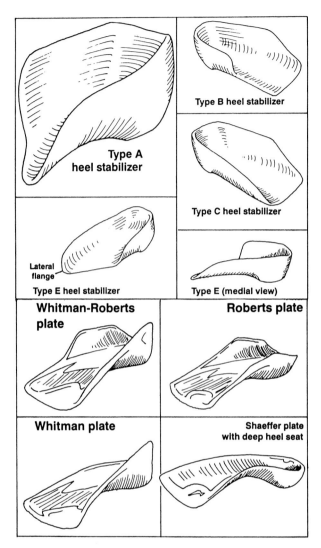

Type B heel stabilizer

Type A heel stabilizer

Type C heel stabilizer

Lateral flange

Type E heel stabilizer

Type E (medial view)

Whitman-Roberts plate

Roberts plate

Whitman plate

Shaeffer plate with deep heel seat

Fig. 37-4. Some rigid orthoses (orthotics) from functional support of the flexible flatfoot. (From McCrea JD: Pediatric Orthopedics of the Lower Extremity. Futura Publishing Company, Mt. Kisco, NY, 1985, p. 196, with permission.)

can be controlled biomechanically with orthoses (also described as "orthotics") (Fig. 37-4). Functional orthoses can only be fabricated from accurate non- or semi-weight-bearing cast impressions of the foot, usually in its neutral position unless contributing factors dictate otherwise (e.g., triceps equinus may require a pronated cast impression). This maneuver should only be done by or at the direction of a technically proficient clinician, well founded in the biomechanical kinesiology of the feet and lower extremities. A full biomechanical evaluation and gait analysis are necessary to provide the prescription for constructing such orthoses.

Other methods can be used alone or as adjunctive therapies: casts, splints, well-built shoes, shoe modifications, strappings, pads, physical therapy, anti-inflammatories and steroid injections. When these fail to resolve or control the problems, surgery can be considered.

Surgical Treatment

Basing the criteria for surgical intervention solely on subjective symptoms, as purported by many authors,[18-24] is unfair to the patient. "The difficulty with the symptomatic approach is that it most often allows the foot to sublux into increasing deformity while children or young adults adapt their activities, their life-styles, and indeed their very personalities and vocations to what their feet can accommodate."[4] Once the CPVP foot deformity is identified by definition, differentiated from the normal pes planus, and found to be unresponsive to conservative control, at least one of the following criteria should be met for it to qualify for surgical correction.

A. Subjective Criteria
　1. Pain unresponsive to conservative treatment.
　2. Inability to participate in running, walking or other activities requiring locomotion.
　3. Pain and/or disability from flatfoot deformity or its sequelae in genetic relatives.
B. Objective Criteria
　1. Increasing deformity in spite of attempts at mechanical control.

compensatory damage in the long term. By then, the damage is so painful and severe that conservative measures fail to relieve the frustrated patient.

Since the risk that worsening the situation with appropriate conservative treatment is minimal, the converse — that to neglect the pronated flexible flatfoot is the greater risk to the patient — might be closer to reality. The majority of flexible flatfeet

2. Deformity severe enough to anticipate disabling symptoms or deformity from stress transfer to neighboring joints.
3. Deformity of such magnitude or type that conservative control is impossible or impractical.

"The unpredictability of surgical results [has] lead many surgeons to the erroneous conclusion that surgical intervention is unwarranted except for the most severe cases, when triple arthrodesis is indicated."[4] Historically, the problem with many of the flatfoot procedures promulgated by numerous authors is that they were presented as a singular approach to a complex problem. The demonstration of more recent concepts, such as understanding the deformities that are compensated by pronation, the planal dominance of that compensation, the powerful influence of equinus, and the radiographic analysis available, allows surgeons to select in a more predictable manner the right combination of procedures appropriate to the individual foot.

Treatment of Ankle (Rearfoot) Equinus

The subject of ankle equinus has a special relevance to pes valgus deformity as a common contributing abnormality.[19-21,24-26] Regardless of the etiology, the inability to dorsiflex the foot on the leg at least 10 degrees past a right angle requires compensation for completion of the gait cycle. Early heel-off, abduction of the foot, or subluxatory pronation of the subtalar and midtarsal joints are the most common forms, the latter being the most destructive. It is a very powerful force.[27] Without attention to the equinus, treatment of the flexible flatfoot is doomed to failure.[4]

Stretching exercises can result in improvement if performed vigorously. Serial casting rarely causes sustained relief. Surgical lengthening is directed either at the Achilles tendon itself or via gastrocnemius recession, depending on whether one or both triceps surae muscles are involved. This surgery is the most frequent adjunctive procedure implemented in flexible flatfoot repair, regardless of the combination used.

Treatment of the Infant (Birth to 1 Year)

Prior to weightbearing, congenital calcaneovalgus deformity is identified as one of the most common precursors of the flexible flatfoot. It is diagnosed by observing the foot at birth positioned in full dorsiflexion, usually lying against the anterior aspect of the ankle. The creases on the dorsolateral aspect of the ankle transform into taut skin as the same tissues restrict forced plantar flexion of the foot.

The deformity is totally one of soft tissue and is best treated early with serial casts at weekly intervals until the foot maintains its correction after being shaken into relaxation.[25] Casts can be implemented as early as 1 to 2 weeks after birth. For correction, the foot should be positioned with the forefoot and ankle in equinus and the rearfoot neutral or slightly inverted.

Following casting, the Ganley splint should be used at night for several months as a retainer. It functions similar to casts in that it will tend to stretch the anterolateral soft tissue structures. Triplane positioning is the greatest asset of the splint, which should normally be set with the heel in inversion and the forefoot in eversion.[25] Without prompt conservative treatment, talipes calcaneovalgus will evolve into CPVP as soon as weightbearing is initiated.[1]

To say that all babies have flatfeet or a baby fat pad in the longitudinal arch is a misconception that can be rapidly dispelled by a thorough lower extremity examination of the infant. Ganley,[25] Giannestras,[6,28] and Tax[29] all encourage early recognition and prompt treatment of the flexible flatfoot and its precursors. This is an ideal time to mold the foot into proper alignment since the soft cartilagenous anlages are of pliable consistency and can adapt into proper functional alignment. Whether this will actually occur is only theoretical to date, and further exact research is needed.

Treatment of the Child Age 1 to 3 Years

When calcaneovalgus deformity is recognized late, beyond 1 year, casting the correction of the deformity becomes less tolerable to the walking child. The Ganley splint can be used at night even for several years. Although improvement is not a constant result, full correction of calcaneovalgus and pes valgus deformity has been reported.[4,25]

The ideal first shoe does not have to be rigid or high-topped to treat flexible flatfoot. It should consist of a stiff counter, a firm shank, and a flexible forefoot sole and have a well-molded arch on the inside. The last must not be pronated. The goal is to allow the cartilaginous foot to mold into an ideal neutral position rather than its own congenital neutral position.

For the child with more severe pronation at this age, a long medial counter and Thomas heel (distal extension of the medial heel to support the navicular cartilage) can be added for further support. Medial heel wedges will also help realign the calcaneus in this age group[30,31] (Table 37-7).

A semiflexible prefabricated orthosis can be fitted primarily to support the talonavicular joint. When the pronation needs more control a Helfet heel seat (heel stabilizer) is indicated. Control is directed at the rearfoot to allow reduction of any forefoot deformity that might be present. If the forefoot deformity is supported at this age it will most likely become fixed in that position.[4,29] As the

child outgrows the heel stabilizer a Shaffer plate without forefoot posting can be fabricated.

For the extremely severe, uncontrollable, and sometimes symptomatic pes valgus deformity in this age group surgery becomes an option. Arthrodesing operations such as medial column fusions are generally not indicated because of the lack of skeletal maturity. Combinations such as subtalar arthroereisis and medial arch reconstruction, usually with triceps lengthening, will realign the foot so that the bones will adapt in response to normal function. Severe transverse plane deformity may require an Evans calcaneal osteotomy.

Treatment of the Child Age 3 to Adolescence

Past 3 years of age, shoe therapy becomes more of an art than a science and is less effective. Up to about age 6 years, biomechanical control is aimed primarily at rigidly supporting the rearfoot and preventing subtalar joint pronation. Posting the forefoot should be avoided so as to not allow the foot to develop into a set forefoot varus deformity as it achieves osseous maturity.

Table 37-7. Treatment to Control Excessive Pronation in the Child

	7–18 Months			18 Months–3 Years		3–6 Years		
	Mild	Moderate	Severe	Mild	Moderate-Severe	Mild	Moderate-Severe	6+ Years
Shoe								
Rigid shank	X	X	X	X	X		X	
Long medial counter	X	X	X	X	X		X	
Thomas heel		X	X		X			
Medial heel wedge			X		X			
Orthotic								
Semiflexible prefabricated orthotic	X	X	X					
Navicular pad		X						
Arch cookie		X						
Shaffer plate				X	X	X		X
Schwartz heel meniscus						X		X
Helfet heel seat (heel stabilizer)							X	X
Silverman heel cup							X	X
UCBL insert							X	X
Whitman plate							X	X
Roberts plate							X	X

(From Spencer and Person,[30] with permission.)

For children from 6 to 10 years of age several devices are available (Table 37-7), since adult biomechanical casting techniques are difficult to accomplish on these pliable feet. Beyond 10 years, conventional biomechanical casting techniques can be used to control the compensating deformities causing the flexible flatfoot.

Ankle equinus is less responsive to conservative therapy in this period. Stretching should be attempted. If orthoses are prescribed the foot will not tolerate full correctional posting since the powerful triceps will attempt to drive or pronate the arch right through the device.[5] A partially or fully pronated orthosis can be fabricated. On occasion, a functional lengthening of the Achilles tendon has been observed with biomechanical therapy.

Symptoms commonly appear as children near adolescence and their athletic and recreational activities increase. The uncontrollable pes valgus deformity cannot meet such demands and the patient may be forced to avoid such activity.

Surgical procedures can be selected specifically from the variety available when indicated. Almost universally, a combination of procedures is necessary to achieve lasting correction. In addition, follow-up orthotic therapy is necessary for at least 2 years to support the correction.

Treatment of the Adolescent and Adult

By this stage the foot bones have reached skeletal maturity and any distorted alignment is the result of fixed deformities. Often, the unfortunate individual with CPVP, on entering the workplace, finds long-term standing and walking intolerable. Symptoms vary from arch fatigue to posterior tibial tendonitis.

Conservative therapy is directed at supporting the deformities and preventing uncontrolled pronatory compensation. No correction of deformity should be anticipated. Ankle equinus now becomes a persistent and pwerful force that when present, must be dealt with before any progress can be made in controlling pathologic pronation.

When surgical intervention is necessary, emphasis begins to shift away from soft tissue to osseous procedures as the pronated foot becomes more

fixed and joints begin to "track" near their end ranges of motion. The deformities actually become less reducible with time and adaptation. The Hubscher maneuver might simply result in the medial forefoot raising off the floor because the first ray can no longer plantar flex.

Sequelae of long-term pronation now start to appear: plantar fasciitis, intermetatarsal neuromata, hallux valgus deformities, and hammer toe syndromes. These must be dealt with individually and the patient should be made to understand their etiology.

Treatment of the Neuromuscular Flatfoot

When neuromuscular disorders result in an acquired flatfoot deformity, treatment approaches demand special considerations to ensure long-term success. Conservative therapy, including biomechanical control, is all but hopeless.

Whether the neuromuscular disorder is spastic or flaccid, arthrodesing operations are a necessary part of whatever treatment combination is selected, especially for spastic conditions. Tendon transfers can be effective adjunctive procedures to help alleviate the paralytic pes valgus deformity. They are selected depending upon the muscle imbalance present.[32]

Common recurrences in deformity were noted in one study of calcaneal osteotomies performed on patients with progressive central nervous system disease, as an example of the difficulties these disorders present.[33]

End-Stage Flatfoot

End-stage flatfoot is a tarsal enthesopathy that is the result of severe long-term pronation of the foot about the subtalar and other joints.[34] It usually becomes symptomatic following the fifth decade of life. After a lifetime of weightbearing on an unsupported flexible flatfoot, signs and symptoms will tend to show up within the foot at the points of greatest stress.

Here is a foot that has been functioning at its end range of subtalar joint motion, so it is that joint and its surrounding tissues that are most commonly affected. By way of further compensation, however, other joints and tissues can break down or become inflamed, usually in the rearfoot or midfoot. Again, the location depends on the dominant plane of compensation.

The most common pain is found in and about the sinus tarsi. This has been fairly well defined in the literature as sinus tarsitis or sinus tarsi syndrome.[35-39]

Although it can be caused by trauma, gout, rheumatoid arthritis, and other disorders, mechanical stress from end-range pronation is the common etiology. Besides local tenderness, aching on standing, and aggravation by walking on uneven surfaces, peroneal muscle spasm may be an initial presenting symptom.

Joint adaptation in end-stage flatfoot can cause "tracking" with a loss of reducibility of the deformity. On manual manipulation, the neutral position is almost impossible to maintain and the foot may not respond to the Hubscher maneuver.

Joint breakdown is seen at maximum compensatory stress points, especially in the sagittal plane. Loss of joint space and osteophytic proliferation might be seen at such locations as the navicular-cuneiform and first metatarsal–cuneiform joints. The complete midtarsal or tarsometatarsal joint can be affected in dominant transverse plane deformities. Talonavicular arthritis is common.

Long-term excessive abduction of the forefoot can cause chronic tenosynovitis of the posterior tibial tendon, which may eventually rupture.[40,41] Loss of this important muscle then leads to a complete collapse of the foot architecture, accelerating the progress toward end-stage flatfoot.[42-47]

Surgical Procedures for Management of Collapsing Pes Valgoplanus

Surgical procedures to correct flexible flatfoot are rarely performed independently. Careful evaluation usually leads to the conclusion that some combination of procedures is necessary not only to obtain structural realignment but to achieve long-term satisfactory results. The most common procedure to usually accompany pes valgoplanus corrections, when indicated, is a gastrocnemius recession or Achilles tendon lengthening.

Subtalar Joint Blocking Procedures

There are two major categories of subtalar joint blocking procedures: "extra-articular arthrodesis," which utilizes a bone graft in the sinus tarsi to fuse the talus to the calcaneus, and "arthroereisis," which limits pronation of the subtalar joint primarily in the frontal plane while allowing varus motion.[48]

Extra-articular Arthrodesis. This procedure, suggested by Green, was reported first by Grice in 1945.[49] A bone graft, preferrably autogenous, is wedged into the sinus tarsi to fuse the talus to the calcaneus in a more functional position, stopping pronatory motion completely. Various grafts can be harvested and fashioned (Fig. 37-5) for use

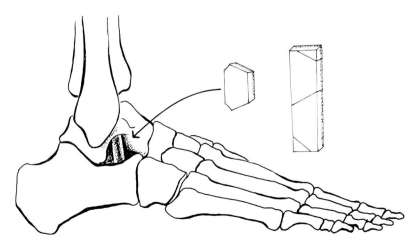

Fig. 37-5. Green-Grice extra-articular arthrodesis. The sinus tarsi is cleared and curretted to expose cancellous bone. Then a bone graft is fashioned and inserted to allow fusion to the talus and calcaneus, stopping motion between the two bones. (Redrawn from Grice,[49] with permission.)

Table 37-8. Indications for Green-Grice Extra-articular Subtalar Joint Arthrodesis

Table 37-8. Indications for Green-Grice
Extra-articular Subtalar Joint Arthrodesis

Paralytic instability and equinovalgus
Peroneal spastic flatfoot
Unresectable tarsal coalitions
Irreparable subtalar joint damage (trauma, postseptic arthrosis)

(From Vogler,[48] with permission.)

under appropriate indications (Table 37-8). Internal fixation is an option.[50,51] Results have been largely satisfactory as long as other deforming forces such as equinus have been dealt with.[48,51-56] Less success has been achieved when spasticity is present,[57-59] and complications have included resorption, slippage, and non-union.[59,60]

Arthroereisis of the Subtalar Joint. This concept, adapted by LeLievre,[24] was first described by Chambers in 1946,[61] the goal being to limit pronatory motion by blocking the lateral process of the talus and preventing its "approximation" with the floor of the sinus tarsi. Since then, various prostheses have been developed to block subtalar joint motion[48] (Table 37-9) (Fig. 37-6). Prior to implantation the talocalcaneal ligaments must be severed.

Indications for the procedure are found in Table 37-10. Although the technique was developed and found its success largely in young children, it has been used in much older individuals, over 69 years of age, with good results. Care must be taken when there is much joint adaptation present in the long-term pronated foot.

The goal of this flatfoot surgery is to realign the rearfoot and promote adaptation of the articular surfaces of the subtalar joint toward better function.[62] Similar long-term joint adaptation can be observed in the progressive hallux valgus deformity.

The extra-articular arthroereisis procedure has

obtained high success rates with almost no reactions to the implanted foreign materials, although only 13 years of use are available for follow-up. Up to 94 percent improvement in subjective symptoms has been reported,[63] and there is documented improvement in the calcaneal stance position, calcaneal inclination angle, talocalcaneal angle (dorsoplantar and lateral), and talar declination angle.[24,64,65]

The small number of complications have included extrusion of the implant, overcorrection, infection, prolonged pain, and biomaterial wear. Fortunately, removal of the implant is relatively simple and it can be performed under local anesthesia.[66-70] Whether the implant should be removed in later years when the patient is asymptomatic has not been determined.

Medial Column Procedures

Since it is well known now that the integrity of the longitudinal arch is not principally dependent upon the extrinsic or intrinsic muscles,[71] most medial column soft tissue balancing procedures are seldom done alone. Yet the importance of the muscles cannot be underestimated. This is readily seen when the foot rapidly collapses and abducts after rupture of the posterior tibial tendon.[40,42-47,72]

Medial column procedures consist of tendon transfers or transpositions, desmoplasties, arthrodeses, osteotomies, or some combination of these procedures with or without adjunctive surgeries.

Kidner Procedure. Kidner (1929)[73] thought this approach was important because the accessory navicular or os tibiale externum changed the leverage of the posterior tibial muscle, weakening its influence on the arch[18,73] (Fig. 37-7).

Alone, the procedure is usually done to relieve a

Table 37-9. Arthroereisis Devices by Anatomic Site Placement

Sinus Tarsi	Canalis Tarsi	Both
Valgus stop prosthesis	Valenti "threaded"	Johnson Free-Form
STA peg, both varieties	Viladot "umbrella"	
Addante sphere	Custom-carved plug (if desired)	
Sgarlato mushroom		
Pisani "composite"		
Custom-carved plug		

(From Vogler,[48] with permission.)

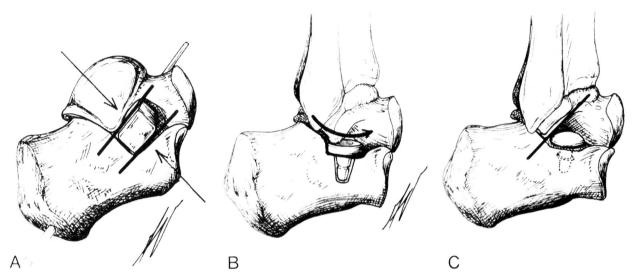

Fig. 37-6. The concept of arthroereisis is the insertion of a device in the sinus tarsi to block "contact" of the lateral talar process against the calcaneal sinus floor during maximum end-range pronation, which is prolonged in the flexible flatfoot. **(A)** Self-locking wedge. The self-locking wedge arthroereisis is a block of silicone plastic inserted in the sinus tarsi that functions to block pronatory motion by keeping the two bones apart. **(B)** Axis altering implant. The STA-Peg arthroereisis includes insertion of the stern by drilling a hole in the calcaneus for stable positioning. Cement is optional. The slope of the subtalar joint should determine the angle of the implant at placement. This will either block motion or alter the axis of the subtalar joint. **(C)** Direct impact implant. The Sgarlato mushroom "direct impact" device is also inserted using a drill hole. It simply blocks motion as the lateral talar process impacts on one side of the implant cap. (From Vogler,[48] with permission.)

symptomatic os tibiale externum.[74] For the flexible flatfoot, it is combined with other operations.

Satisfactory results have been reported when used to correct pes valgus deformity,[75] but symptoms at the accessory bone-tendon insertion have remained — in as many as 30 percent of the cases.[76] Augmentation of the transferred tibialis posterior tendon with the flexor hallucis longus tendon has been reported with pleasing results.[77]

Lowman Procedure. Reporting in 1923, Lowman ingeniously designed a multicomponent operation to correct several aspects of the flatfoot[19] (Fig. 37-8). Although there are almost no reports on results of the procedure itself, many of its component parts have been integrated into other operations. Variations described by Lowman himself included transfer of the peroneus longus to the underside of the navicular with suture into the spring ligament and sometimes transferring the extensor hallucis longus. He almost always included an Achilles tendon lengthening.

Young Procedure. In 1939 Young published his flatfoot procedure by which he rerouted the tibialis anterior tendon through a keyhole in the medial navicular bone as well as lengthened the Achilles tendon (Fig. 37-9). It was recommended for patients 10 years and older. His goal was to "balance the muscle power of the foot (so) that the weight of the body is sustained by the bones of the arch." [20,78]

Beck and McGlamry analyzed 20 of Young's tendosuspensions and found an improvement in the talocalcaneal relationships. They felt that the corrective influences would cause a "molding" of the subtalar joint by functional adaptation of bone.[79]

Krause reported on a similar procedure performed on 300 patients, of whom 82 were reexamined. He observed similar results as well as diminished heel valgus without Achilles tendon lengthening.[80] Schmied produced improvement in 90 percent of 55 patients with a tendosuspension similar to that of Krause, but performed additional procedures in 20 of his cases.[81]

Today, the rerouting of the tibialis anterior

Table 37-10. Clinical Indications for Arthroereisis of the Subtalar Joint

Uncontrollable and reducible hindfoot valgus
Eversion of the heel, at least 8° to 10°
Predominant frontal plane deformity of hindfoot with low subtalar joint axis
Flexible forefoot varus deformity above 10°
Midfoot collapse with ptosis of talonavicular joint
Dystonic and ligamentous laxity pathological flatfoot
Paralytic flatfoot (in combination with other procedures)
Chronic loss of tibialis posterior and hindfoot instability (in combination with other procedures)

(From Vogler,[48] with permission.)

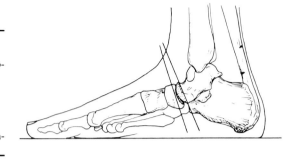

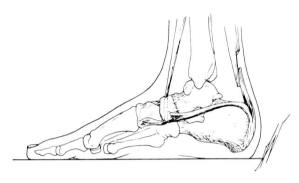

Fig. 37-8. Lowman procedure. Originally, this procedure included the following: Achilles tendon lengthening; talonavicular joint arthrodesis *(top)*; rerouting of the tibialis anterior tendon beneath the navicular with suturing to spring ligament *(bottom)*; folding the medial slip of the Achilles tendon to attach into the navicular *(bottom)*; and distal advancement of the talonavicular ligaments (desmoplasty). (From McGlamry et al.,[4] with permission.)

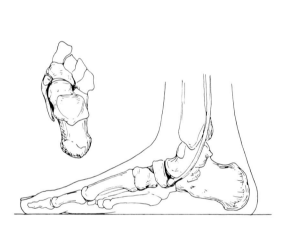

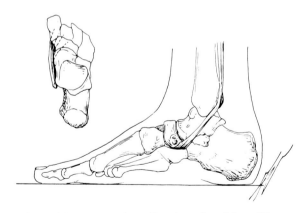

Fig. 37-7. Kidner procedure. Consists of excision of the os tibiale externum when present, resection of hypertrophic navicular tuberosity, and transposition of the tibialis posterior tendon to the plantar navicular bone. The lateral slip of tendon is left intact. *(Top)* Presurgical appearance. *(Bottom)* After Kidner procedure. (From McGlamry et al.,[4] with permission.)

through or near the navicular is rarely done alone. It has actually become part of the medial arch reconstruction procedure. In a patient under 10 years of age, the tendon is rerouted and attached to the underside of the navicular anlage as well as the spring ligament. In a patient over 10 years of age it is usually rerouted through a slot in the ossified navicular.[4]

Miller Procedure. Miller presented his "plastic flatfoot operation" in 1927 and included an Achilles tendon lengthening for the "pathologically shortened heel cord."[22] He reported satisfaction with the procedure in 16 feet over 2½ years (Fig. 37-10).

Variations in this combination technique have been described by Giannestras,[82] Lovell et al.,[83] and Coleman.[84] Lengthy immobilization was rec-

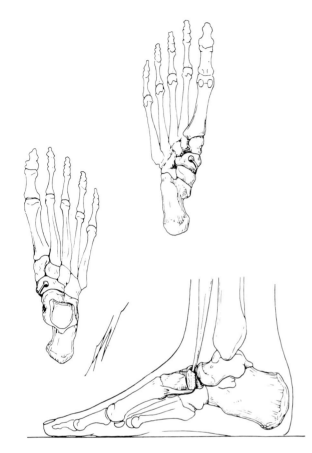

Fig. 37-9. Young procedure. The original procedure consisted of rerouting the tibialis anterior tendon through a slot made in the medial navicular bone *(top and middle)*, then advancing the tibialis posterior tendon over this to attach to the medial and plantar navicular *(bottom)*. It also included an Achilles tendon lengthening. (From McGlamry et al.,[4] with permission.)

ommended in the initial paper. Today, a modified version of this operation is seen as part of a multi-procedure approach to flatfoot on older pediatric patients and some adults. It is not appropriate for children with immature medial arch bones until there is satisfactory ossification. The age at which this is achieved is usually 10 to 12 years.

Durham Plasty Procedure. Caldwell, in 1953, described the "Durham plasty" for (flexible) flatfoot, although it was originally presented by its namesake in 1935.[84-86] It is similar to the Miller procedure and technically more difficult, although it in-

volves arthrodesis of the navicular – first cuneiform joint only (Fig. 37-11). It is not a procedure for immature bone. Caldwell reported on 76 feet with an average follow-up of 6 years, yielding excellent or good results in 91 percent of cases,[85] and Coleman presented the same results in 95 percent of 33 feet, with a maximum follow-up of 6 years.[84] Attention was paid to triceps contracture when present.

Hoke Procedure. Hoke believed that flexibility of the medial column is greatest at the first and second cuneonavicular joints and that loss of this lever arm interferes with the coordinated arch-lifting power of the tibialis posterior, tibialis anterior, and flexor hallucis longus muscles.[21] As a result the talus plantar flexes, the ligaments stretch, and the arch flattens. He recognized a short Achilles tendon as a component of the flatfoot syndrome as he presented his ideas in 1931.[87] (Fig. 37-12).

After analyzing naviculocuneiform fusions (72 patients) performed from 1927 to 1934, Butte found the end results to be excellent in 30, good in 40, fair in 34, and poor in 34 — 50 percent were less than satisfactory.[88] Jack reported 38 results as good or excellent out of 46 Hoke-type naviculo-cuneiform fusions followed from 15 months to 5 years.[14] He used a medial slot graft across the joint, neglected Achilles tendon lengthening, and casted the patients in plantar flexion. Using the same scale, Seymour later graded 32 of the feet from Jack's original series and found 50 percent unsatisfactory results 16 to 19 years after the operations.[89] Jack had failed to deal with the more powerful deforming force of equinus. The Hoke procedure alone was also condemned by Crego and Ford, who abandoned the procedure in 1934. They believed that additional attention must be paid to the subtalar joint.

Thus, the Hoke fusion is used as an adjunctive surgery to be combined with other procedures for flexible flatfoot. Its success when used in this manner has been proven (see "Hoke-Miller Procedure," later in this section). Additional procedures might include one or more of the following: Achilles tendon lengthening, arthroereisis, cuneiform osteotomy, desmoplasty, calcaneal osteotomy, and Miller osteoperiosteal flap transposition. Hoke fusion is generally reserved to stabilize the severe naviculocuneiform sag in patients with ma-

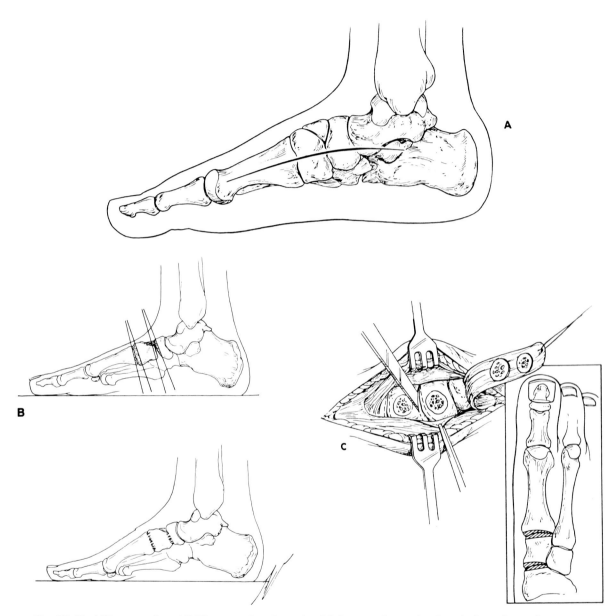

Fig. 37-10. Miller procedure. **(A)** The procedure frees the tibialis posterior tendon from its insertion and creates a flap from its distal attachments, including a thin slice of bone from the navicular and first cuneiform bones and the spring ligament. **(B)** Then there is resection of the articular surfaces of the first metatarsocuneiform and the first cuneonavicular joint for arthrodeses. **(C)** After internal fixation, the osteoperiosteal flap is transposed distally beneath the tibialis anterior tendon as far as the metatarsal base with the forefoot adducted. Miller also performed an Achilles tendon lengthening as an adjunctive procedure. (Parts A and C from Richardson,[86] with permission; part B from McGlamry et al.,[4] with permission.)

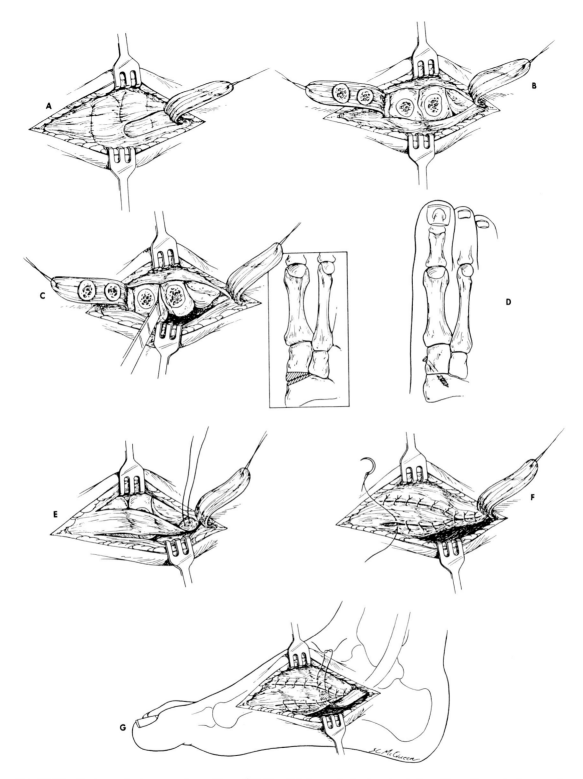

Fig. 37-11. Durham plasty procedure. **(A and B)** The tibialis posterior tendon is freed from its navicular attachment followed by elevation of a distally based osteoperiosteal flap from the navicular and medial cuneiform bones. **(C and D)** The navicular–first cuneiform joint is then prepared for arthrodesis and fixated. **(E and F)** The osteoperiosteal flap is layed down proximally with the foot supinated and is then sutured into drill holes in the sustentaculum tali. **(G)** The tibialis posterior tendon is finally sutured beneath the navicular. Caldwell lengthened the heel cord, when contracted, 4 to 6 weeks prior to performing the Durham plasty. (From Richardson,[86] with permission.)

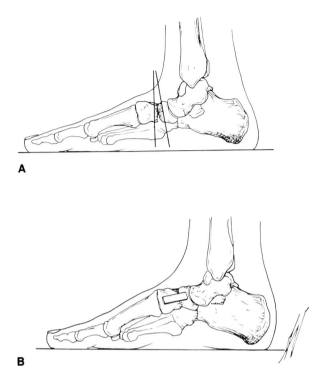

Fig. 37-12. Hoke procedure. **(A)** Originally, the Hoke procedure included resection of the articular surfaces of the distal navicular plus proximal first and second cuneiform bones. A rectangular section of bone is then removed from the medial cuneonavicular joint and broken into bits of bone. **(B)** The void is filled with an autogenous strut from the tibia and gaps packed with chips. Fusion is allowed by immobilization. (From McGlamry et al.,[4] with permission.)

ture ossified bones. Adequate internal fixation is essential with or without a bone graft.[4]

Talonavicular Desmoplasty. This combination procedure is all done on soft tissue as presented by Rodgveller in 1974.[90] It is recommended for young pediatric patients ages 3 to 7 years since, in Rodgveller's review of 14 procedures, poor results were seen in the older candidates. It has really become an adjunctive approach and is normally done in conjunction with an Achilles tendon lengthening (Fig. 37-13).

Jones Flatfoot Procedure. In 1975, this South African surgeon[91] described use of the medial Achilles tendon to reinforce the plantar fascia and raise the arch using the "windlass" principle as described by

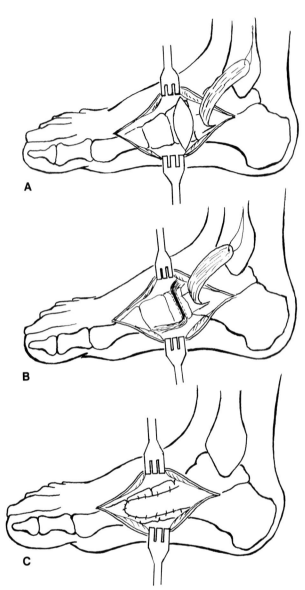

Fig. 37-13. Talonavicular desmoplasty. **(A)** The posterior tibial tendon is transected at its insertion and reflected. With the foot supinated a wedge of redundant capsule and spring ligament is removed from the medioplantar aspect of the talonavicular joint. **(B)** A notch is made in the medial navicular tuberosity to accept the rerouted one-half of the anterior tibial tendon. A sliver of the medial talar prominence is resected for capsulodesis effect and the gap sutured closed. **(C)** The posterior tibial tendon is finally advanced over the desmoplasty and sutured at the navicular plantarly under tension.

Hicks.[13] He presented three cases with satisfactory results, but there has been no further interest in the procedure.

Hoke-Miller Procedure. Sometimes called the Scottish Rite procedure,[84,86] it is combined with an Achilles tendon lengthening or gastrocnemius recession as indicated. It is used mainly in patients greater than 10 years old. The first metatarsocuneiform joint arthrodesis is omitted, and an opening wedge, dorsally based osteotomy of the cuneiform as described by Cotton[92] can be added if necessary to plantarflex the distal first ray (Fig. 37-14).

Marked improvement in bony realignment was observed in 10 patients operated on by Duncan and Lovell, with two non-unions and one deep infection.[93] Jacobs and Oloff performed this combina- tion procedure on 16 feet with 12 excellent and four satisfactory results.[94] Dockery proved the value of combination procedure flatfoot surgery by consistently adding gastrocnemius tendon reces- sion and subtalar joint arthroereisis to the Hoke- Miller procedure. He seldom included the cunei- form opening osteotomy. His report on the follow-up of 27 feet in 16 patients ages 7 to 15 years found 21 with excellent results and six with good results.[95]

Ruch-McGlamry Medial Arch Reconstruction. The most inclusive and thorough medial arch recon- struction was illustrated and described on motion picture film by Ruch et al.[96] and elaborated by McGlamry et al.[4] It can be applied at any age and, rarely performed alone, is best utilized as an ad-

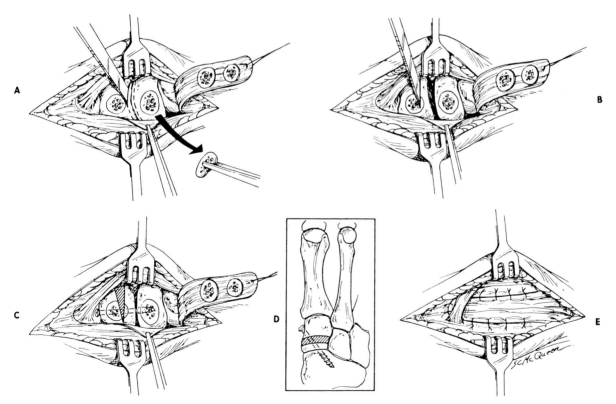

Fig. 37-14. Hoke-Miller procedure. **(A)** After the osteoperiosteal flap creation at the tibia's posterior insertion, the naviculocuneiform joint is prepared for arthrodesis and secured with internal fixation using staple, screw, or plate. **(B–D)** An opening wedge osteotomy is made in the medial cuneiform using a bone graft obtained by resecting the medial tuberosity of the navicular bone. **(E)** The osteoperiosteal flap from the navicular and cuneiform is advanced beneath the tibialis anterior tendon, placing the attached posterior tibial tendon under tension to adduct the foot. (From Richardson,[86] with permission.)

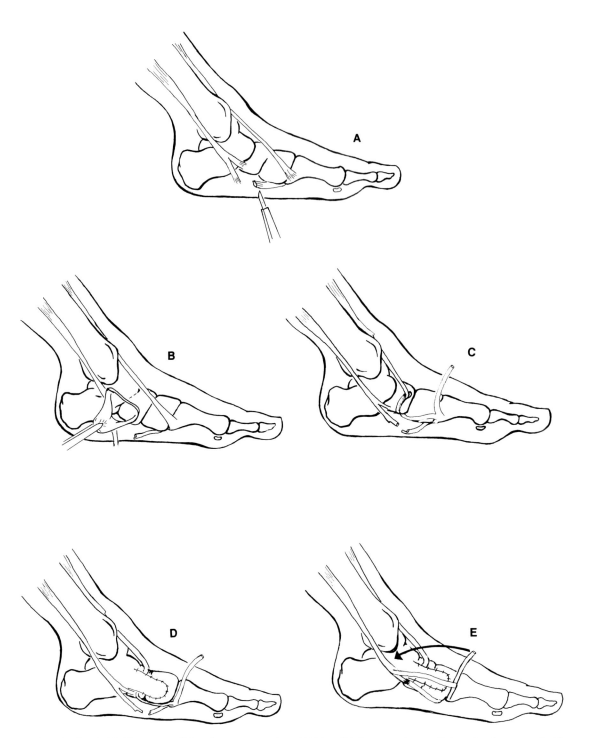

Fig. 37-15. Ruch-McGlamry medial arch reconstruction. **(A)** The tibialis posterior medial tendon is severed at its navicular attachment, leaving the lateral slip intact. **(B)** With tibialis posterior tendon reflected plantarly, the spring ligament is incised to create a distal flap. One-half of the distal tibialis anterior tendon is split off but left attached at its insertion. It will become a tenodesis ligament to reinforce this medial tendosuspension. **(C)** If the bone is mature, a "keyhole slot" is made in the navicular tuberosity medially. Then the remaining half of the tibialis anterior tendon is seated in the slot with the foot forcibly supinated. In young patients the tendon is simply sutured into the spring ligament. **(D)** The spring ligament flap is now advanced distally and sutured. The tibialis posterior tendon is advanced distally to overlap and, if possible, surpass its original insertion. **(E)** Finally, the tenodesis slip of tibialis anterior tendon is drawn proximally over the tendosuspension and sutured into the spring and/or deltoid ligaments prior to closure of the deep tissues. (Adapted from McGlamry et al.,[4] with permission.)

junct to most flexible flatfoot procedures (Fig. 37-15). The universal medial arch approach described by McGlamry et al.[4] allows access to the structures along the first ray and medial rearfoot. Although no long-term studies have been published to evaluate the efficacy of this procedure, this author has seen excellent results in over 100 patients. The best ages for implementation are 1 to 12.

Calcaneal Osteotomies

The large number of calcaneal osteotomies that have been used for pes valgus reconstruction can be confusing. One helpful approach to their understanding is the organization of the procedures into the Lindell classification as purported by Jacobs and associates[66] (Table 37-11).

Extra-articular Calcaneal Osteotomies. The purpose of these procedures is to realign the position of the talus on the calcaneus by altering some aspect of the subtalar joint complex with various periarticular opening calcaneal osteotomies. In general, these follow the arthroereisis principle. The idea is to preserve the joint anatomy and function, changing only the articular motion.

Chambers Procedure. After some anatomic experimentation, Chambers became the first to implement a procedure that would block the motion of the talus on the calcaneus.[61] This laid the foundation for the arthroereisis concept since it raised the floor of the sinus tarsi to abut against the lateral process of the talus, restricting its adduction and

plantar flexion on the calcaneus. Thus "postural collapse" of the foot is prevented (Fig. 37-16).

Miller, who recommended the procedure be performed on young patients preferably before age 8, reported on 82 Chambers procedures with an average follow-up of 6.5 years.[23] Of the 63 feet that demonstrated excellent results and the 14 feet with good results, 18 feet were noted to have arthrosis of the talonavicular joint. Narrowing of the subtalar joint was seen in four other feet studied. Overall, 70 feet underwent Achilles tendon lengthening as well.

Baker-Hill Procedure. Baker and Hill devised an opening wedge calcaneal osteotomy below the posterior subtalar joint facet used to realign the rearfoot in cerebral palsy patients[97] (Fig. 37-17). It was utilized with and without a variety of other procedures. By driving a wedge into the osteotomy the posterior calcaneus is driven plantarly while inverting and the subtalar joint is realigned somewhat, but without any bone block. Of the 31 feet in Baker and Hill's study treated by osteotomy alone, 21 had satisfactory alignment. No other studies have been published to date on this procedure.

Table 37-11. Lindell Classification of Calcaneal Osteotomies for Pes Valgus Reconstruction

Extra-articular
  Chambers (1946), Miller (1977)
  Baker-Hill (1964)
  Selakovich (1973)
  Garelli (1986)
Posterior
  Gleich (1893), Obalinski (1895), Lord (1923), Zadek (1935)
  Dwyer (1960)
  Silver (1967), Silver et al. (1973), Marcinko et al. (1984)
  Koutsogiannis (1971)
Anterior
  Evans (1975, 1961), Phillips (1983), Anderson and Fowler (1984)
  Mahan and McGlamry (1987)

(From Jacobs et al.,[66] with permission.)

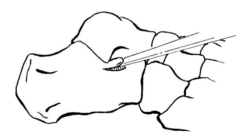

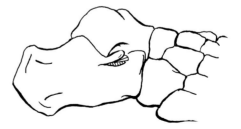

Fig. 37-16. Chambers procedure. An elevational osteotomy is made below the floor of the sinus tarsi to block the lateral process and leading edge of the posterior facet of the talus. (Redrawn from Chambers,[61] with permission.)

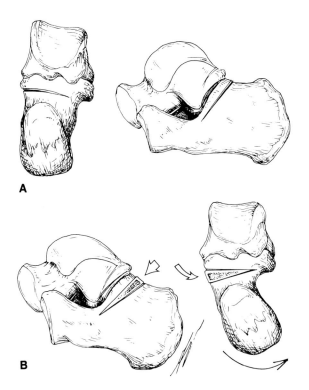

Fig. 37-17. Baker-Hill procedure. Through a vertical lateral approach **(A)**, a laterally and dorsally based wedge is driven into an essentially horizontal osteotomy in the calcaneus beneath the posterior subtalar joint facet **(B)**. The medial cortex is left intact to act as a hinge. (From McGlamry et al.,[4] with permission.)

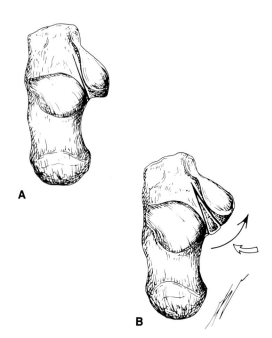

Fig. 37-18. Selakovich procedure. **(A)** After careful medial dissection an opening wedge osteotomy is performed just beneath the articular surface of the sustentaculum tali. **(B)** A wedge of bone is inserted to raise the anterior and middle subtalar joint facets. (From McGlamry et al.,[4] with permission.)

Selakovich Procedure. Selakovich based his surgery on the observation that the calcaneus does not adequately support the (head of the) talus in the flexible flatfoot.[98] This can be visualized in an axial calcaneal radiograph as medial and plantar sloping of the anterior facet of the subtalar joint. To correct this and thereby block adduction and plantar flexion of the talus at its head, Selakovich designed a delicate opening wedge osteotomy into the inferior portion of the sustentaculum tali (Fig. 37-18).

In addition to the osteotomy, Selakovich performed several other procedures, including: (1) temporarily fixating the realigned talonavicular joint with pins, (2) tightening the redundant spring ligament, (3) repositioning the tibialis posterior tendon, and (4) transferring one-half of the tibialis anterior tendon into the navicular area.

Johnson thought this procedure should be reserved for children 5½ to 9 years of age since the sustentaculum tali does not usually ossify until about 5½ years.[99]

Garelli Procedure. In attempting to preserve subtalar joint function Garelli devised a lateral opening wedge calcaneal osteotomy below the whole subtalar joint complex[100] (Fig. 37-19). With this "dynamic corrective osteotomy" the calcaneus is more vertically aligned beneath the talus and the Achilles tendon has its line of action shifted to a more physiologic axis.

Garelli recommended against Achilles tendon lengthening. He performed the operation on 11 feet with uniformly good results. When the correction produced supination of the forefoot he advised a closing wedge osteotomy in the plantar surface of the medial cuneiform bone.

Posterior Calcaneal Osteotomies. The purpose of retrotalar or posterior calcaneal osteotomies is to

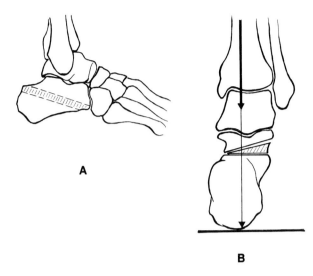

Fig. 37-19. Garelli procedure. **(A)** A laterally based opening wedge calcaneal osteotomy is made from just above the insertion of the Achilles tendon to the lower border of the calcaneocuboid joint. **(B)** This is maintained with a wedge of bone graft. (Redrawn from Garelli,[100] with permission.)

produce varus in the positionally everted calcaneus. The idea is to shift the weight center of gravity from its medial orientation (which aggravates and perpetuates pronation) to a more central location through the foot. These osteotomies are recommended for use in frontal plane–dominant flexible flatfoot and can be used in conjunction with medial column procedures.

The problem with varus-producing osteotomies is that, although they realign the calcaneus into a

more vertical position, sparing articular surfaces, the subtalar joint may continue to function maximally pronated. As a result, the same pathologies can develop in and around the subtalar joint over time as would develop in the uncorrected pes valgus.

Gleich Calcaneal Osteotomy. Lord[101] discovered the operation used by Gleich[102] in the German medical literature. However, Zadek[103] reported that the procedure was popularized by Obalinski in 1895 (Fig. 37-20).

Gleich used a medial "stirrup" approach, whereas Lord suggested a lateral approach would decrease tissue damage. The plantar-based closing wedge osteotomy through the body of the calcaneus is displaced plantarly (Gleich) and, if necessary, medially (Lord). This reduces the valgus position of the calcaneus while increasing the calcaneal inclination angle. Lord found excellent results in 14 cases through 7 years of experience, although all but one case involved supplementary procedures.

Dwyer Calcaneal Osteotomy. Originally, Dwyer advocated a laterally based closing wedge osteotomy through the body of the calcaneus to correct pes cavus deformities.[104,105] Later, he proposed the same closing wedge osteotomy from the medial side of the calcaneus for grossly everted feet, especially those seen with cerebral palsy.[106] Hence, his flatfoot procedure is sometimes alluded to as the "reverse Dwyer" (Fig. 37-21).

The procedure is recommended for patients over 3 years of age, aiming for slight overcorrection. The goal is to bring the heel into varus under the

Fig. 37-20. Gleich osteotomy. A plantar-based closing wedge of bone is removed through the body of the calcaneus and then the posterior fragment is displaced plantarly and, if desired, medially. (Redrawn from Gleich,[102] with permission.)

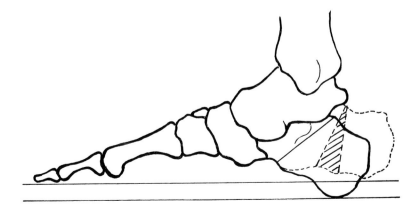

line of weightbearing and thereby support the head of the talus effectively. Thus, the balance of the foot is improved and the Achilles tendon is converted from an everting force to a neutral or inverting force.[107]

Dwyer's initial series study was on 46 grossly everted feet, 36 of which were on cerebral palsy patients.[106]

Silver Calcaneal Osteotomy. Silver and associates in 1967 presented a study of 20 cases of valgus feet realigned with a laterally based opening wedge osteotomy through the body of the calcaneus[108] (Fig. 37-22). With a 2- to 5½-year follow-up, 14 osteotomies produced excellent correction, four demonstrated mild residual valgus deformity, and two resulted in overcorrection with progressive varus deformity.

Supplementary soft tissue procedures were performed when necessary, including Achilles tendon lengthening. Homogeneous bone grafts were found to be as acceptable as autogenous bone with less morbidity to the patient. Fixation was unnecessary with 8 weeks of immobilization. The procedure was recommended for children ages 3 years and older.

A subsequent study by Silver and associates reviewed 82 calcaneal osteotomies used in cases of valgus deformities.[33] They obtained the following results: 68 good, eight fair with mild residual valgus, and six poor, in which four were overcorrected into varus and two recurred into marked valgus over the 2 to 11 years of follow-up. In the

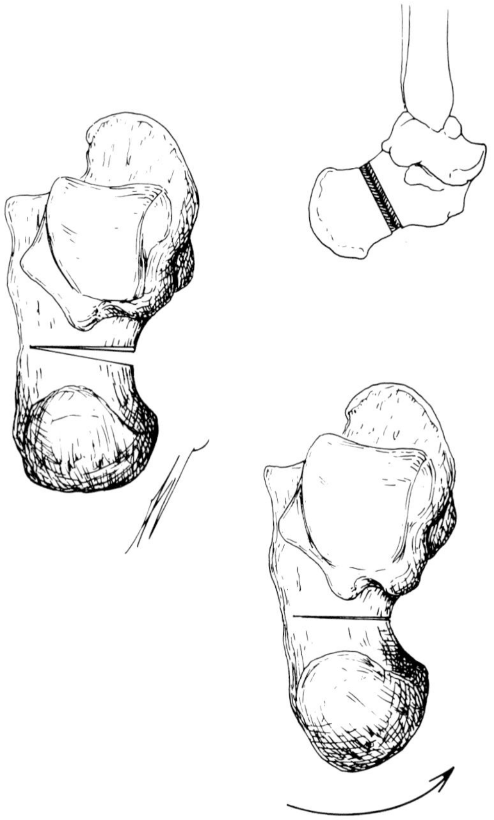

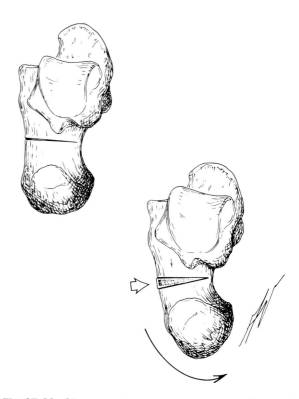

Fig. 37-21. Dwyer osteotomy ("reverse-Dwyer"). This procedure consists of a medial-based closing wedge osteotomy through the body of the calcaneus to bring the heel into varus. It is more commonly performed as a lateral opening wedge osteotomy as advocated by Silver. (From McGlamry et al.,[4] with permission.)

Fig. 37-22. Silver osteotomy. An autogenous or allogeneic bone graft is inserted into a laterally based opening wedge osteotomy through the body of the calcaneus to bring the heel into a more vertical configuration. The more anterior the osteotomy, the greater the correction. (From McGlamry et al.,[4] with permission.)

two recurrences, the authors recognized the cause as their failure to attend to the tight Achilles tendons. These were corrected satisfactorily at reoperation. Also noted, in spite of joint preservation, was a 50 percent reduction of motion at the subtalar joint.

Marcinko and associates analyzed the Silver procedure radiographically in 10 feet with "encouraging" results.[109] It has been reported that the more anterior the osteotomy the greater the correction that can be obtained, since this effectively provides a longer calcaneal arm.[4]

Koutsogiannis Calcaneal Osteotomy.   By means of an oblique osteotomy through the body of the calcaneus, Koutsogiannis described displacement of the posterior fragment medially to lie beneath the sustentaculum tali.[110] It can also be displaced inferiorly and anteriorly to help increase the height of the arch, but this may produce or aggravate an ankle equinus condition (Fig. 37-23).

In his analysis of 34 feet from 19 patients followed from a few months to 6 years, Koutsogiannis found that his procedure was effective in reducing the valgus alignment of the heel, arrested abnormal shoe wear, and relieved symptoms of fatigue in the majority of the patients (30/34). However, it met less success in improving the longitudinal arch or the abduction component of the deformity in general, especially in the more severely affected feet.

Anterior Calcaneal Osteotomies

Evans Calcaneal Osteotomy.   In 1961 Evans discovered, through revision of an error in overcorrecting the adduction component of a clubfoot, that the lateral column of the foot could be length-ened by executing an opening osteotomy through the distal calcaneus.[111] Applying this to his observation that in pes valgus the lateral column is shorter than the medial column, he performed this procedure on 56 feet affected by various forms of flatfoot.[112] He did not recommend it for spastic disorders because of the tendency to achieve overcorrection, nor for spina bifida, in which the bones are "soft and too yielding" (Fig. 37-24).

This procedure applies best to the type III flexible flatfoot, in which the close-to-vertical subtalar joint axis and resulting primary abduction component make nonsurgical care all but impossible. The same foot type has a high failure rate in response to medial column procedures. The main advantage of the procedure is that all joints are preserved.

Not only does the Evans procedure lengthen the lateral column to adduct the forefoot and realign the subtalar and midtarsal joints, but, as the author has observed with interest, it will often derotate the varus component in the forefoot. This is thought to be the result of reestablishing the windlass mechanism.[113] Sometimes, the Evans procedure can be augmented with medial column surgeries, such as the medial arch tendosuspension reconstruction, in addition to equinus correction.[4,114]

Nine cases were corrected and evaluated by Anderson and Fowler, with an average follow-up of 6 years and 8 months. Good to excellent results were noted in eight procedures, poor results in one.[115] They did note improved supination with the forced adduction and recommended the surgery be done at early ages (e.g., 6 to 10) to allow the tarsal joints to remodel as they functionally realigned.

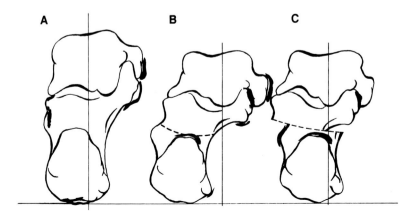

A   **B**   **C**

Fig. 37-23. Koutsogiannis osteotomy. This is an oblique displacement osteotomy from a lateral approach through the body of the calcaneus whereby the posterior fragment is moved medially to sit beneath the sustentaculum tali. It is then fixed with K wires. **(A)** Normal foot. **(B)** Flatfoot. **(C)** Corrected flatfoot. (Redrawn from McGlamry et al.,[4] with permission.)

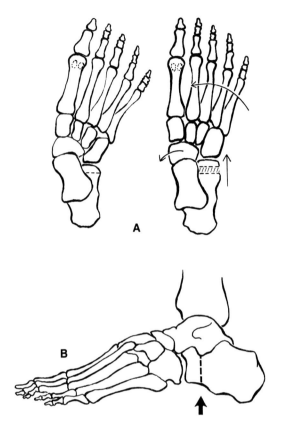

Fig. 37-24. Evans osteotomy. Through a lateral approach, a distal calcaneal osteotomy is made 1.0 to 1.5 cm. proximal to the calcaneocuboid joint. A trapezoid or T-shaped graft can be inserted to elongate the lateral column **(A)** or a wedge graft can be inserted in the hinged Evans procedure to elongate the lateral column and encourage adduction of the forefoot **(B)**. Care must be taken to not disturb the ligaments at the calcaneocuboid joints. Otherwise, the distal calcaneal fragment can be easily subluxed or dislocated. Fixation is optional. (Redrawn from Dollard et al.,[113] with permission.)

Phillips studied 23 feet to which Evans himself had applied his osteotomy. Follow-up of 7 to 20 years revealed 17 feet with good to excellent results, three feet with fair results, and three feet outright failures.[116]

Finally, Mahan and McGlamry reviewed the Evans procedure in 35 feet with an average clinical follow-up of 11.3 months.[117] Ancillary procedures were performed at the same time. They found dramatic improvements in the bony relationships radiographically (Table 37-12). Subjective patient satisfaction was achieved in 95.3 percent of the cases.

Generally, unsatisfactory results have been found when: (1) the deformity is primarily in a plane other than transverse, (2) there is failure to reduce the forefoot varus, and (3) the graft size is inadequate or there is excess graft resorption.[4] Since the procedure can markedly adduct the foot, careful preoperative evaluation is necessary to make sure there is little or no metatarsus adductus present in the foot initially, since it most likely will be greatly exaggerated by the surgery.

Other Tarsal Osteotomies

Cuneiform Osteotomy. A plantar-based closing wedge osteotomy of the cuneiform has been suggested by Anderson and Fowler[115] as well as Garelli[100] to reduce residual forefoot supination (varus) as an adjunct to calcaneal osteotomies (Fig. 37-25). Although it will plantar flex the medial column, it should be understood that a cuneiform osteotomy is performed distal to the usual talonavicular or naviculocuneiform sag. Cotton described a dorsally based opening wedge osteotomy of the cuneiform to achieve the same correction.[92] This

Table 37-12. Mean Radiographic Values Before and After the Evans Procedure to Correct Flexible Pes Valgus Deformity

	Preoperative	Postoperative	Change
AP talocalcaneal	29.9	18.8	−11.1
AP talus–2nd metatarsal	27.0	13.2	−13.8
Lateral talocalcaneal	42.0	40.8	−1.2
Lateral calcaneal inclination	15.2	22.3	+7.1
Lateral index	14.3	19.5	+5.2
First metatarsal declination	17.3	23.4	+6.1
Lang score	52.7	81.1	+28.4

(From Mahan and McGlamry,[117] with permission.)
N = 35.

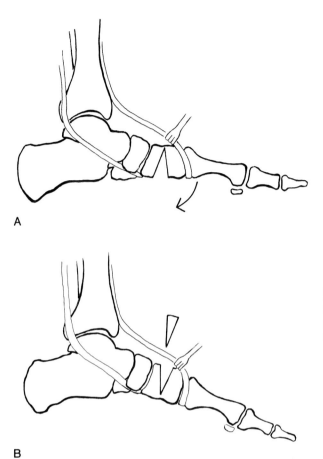

A

B

Fig. 37-25. Cuneiform osteotomy. Plantar closing wedge osteotomy **(A)** or dorsal opening wedge osteotomy with bone graft **(B)** are adjunctive procedures used to plantar flex the medial column.

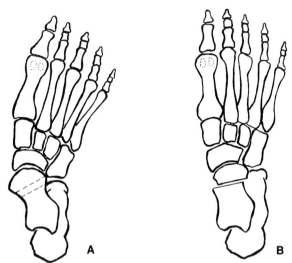

A

B

Fig. 37-26. Talar osteotomy. A cylindrical section of the neck is removed **(A)** and the capital portion displaced laterally **(B)** or otherwise to achieve correction. Fixation is via K wires.

latter technique is part of the combination "Scottish Rite procedure" advocated by Lovell and associates[83] and Coleman.[84]

Talar Osteotomy. In cases of severe flatfoot, uncontrollable by conservative care, where there is a high Kite's angle, talar ptosis (medial bulging of the head), and elongated talar neck, Miller[22] and Grumbine[118] have advocated a talar neck osteotomy. A portion of the neck is removed and the head transposed laterally or as necessary to reduce the deformity (Fig. 37-26).

Grumbine emphasized the need for adjunctive Kidner and other procedures as indicated. He evaluated 47 feet in 27 patients with an average follow-up of 33 months after the talar procedure. Overall, there was marked measurable improvement in the forefoot varus while radiographically there was an increased calcaneal inclination angle and decreased talocalcaneal and talar declination angles. Subjectively, 70.2 percent of the patients achieved good to excellent results, and 21.3 percent had fair results where there was substantial improvement but some significant residual deformity or restriction of motion. There were no failures, and 8.5 percent had poor results. Since a variety of other procedures were done in conjunction with the talar osteotomy in this study, it is difficult to evaluate the talar osteotomy alone in flatfoot correction.

Tarsal Arthrodeses

Talonavicular Arthrodesis. As originally advocated by Lowman,[19] fusion of the talonavicular joint can be executed as an adjunct to one or more other procedures. McGlamry et al. found it useful in several situations: (1) degenerative changes and/or severe collapse at the talonavicular joint, (2) as part of a repair for a ruptured tibialis posterior, and (3) in paralytic deformity.[4] They recommended fixation with a large interfragmentary compression screw.

Subtalar Arthrodesis. This procedure is indicated when the subtalar joint demonstrates severe degenerative changes or marked adaptive changes over time, as seen in the painful end-stage flatfoot[34] unresponsive to other forms of treatment. It is also used to stabilize paralytic valgus feet.

The procedure, when properly executed so the heel is vertical or in slight valgus, will restore the talocalcaneal alignment yet preserve midtarsal motion. Since the subtalar joint will no longer function, surrounding joints may develop arthrosis in response to the added stress.

Judet and Judet reported good results in using the procedure to "resaddle" the talus on the calcaneus.[119] Dennyson and Fulford applied subtalar arthrodesis to 44 valgus feet of mostly neurologic origin.[50] There have been no long-term studies to analyze the effect of subtalar arthrodesis on the function and possible degeneration of surrounding joints.

Triple Arthrodesis. In the past, triple arthrodesis was widely recommended and utilized in the treatment of otherwise unmanageable flexible flatfoot, either for functional stabilization or to eliminate pain. Today, indications are more specific. They include marked adaptive changes in the subtalar and midtarsal joints, severe degenerative changes in these joints, or need for stabilization of the pes valgus deformity in the presence of paralysis or spasticity. Painful end-stage flatfoot unresponsive to conservative care meets these criteria.

Many studies have been done on the short- and long-term results of triple arthrodesis as well as its complications. By eliminating the subtalar and midtarsal joints' function as a pronating mobile adaptor, compensatory stress will be taken up by joints proximally and distally, where arthrosis can develop. In consideration of known long-term changes, the benefits of triple arthrodesis should be weighted carefully against the effects of any possible functional limitation on the patient's future life-style.[4]

FUTURE OF FLEXIBLE FLATFOOT MANAGEMENT

Management of this common foot deformity requires a profound understanding of foot function. Future treatment must be based on long-term, statistically sound results of studies on its natural history with and without treatment. Ongoing investigations of large patient populations are much more possible in this age of computers. The challenge will be best met by the educational clinical institutions who accept the responsibility.

REFERENCES

1. Ferciot CF: The etiology of developmental flatfoot. Clin Orthop 85:7, 1972
2. Harris RI, Beath T: Army Foot Survey: An Investigation of Foot Ailments in Canadian Soldiers. National Research Council of Canada, Ottawa, 1947
3. Staheli LT: Evaluation of planovalgus foot deformities with special reference to natural history. J Am Podiatr Med Assoc 77:2, 1987
4. McGlamry ED, Mahan KT, Green DR: Pes valgo planus deformity. p. 403. In McGlamry ED, McGlamry R (eds): Comprehensive Textbook on Foot Surgery. Vol. I. Williams & Wilkins, Baltimore, 1987
5. Subotnick SI: The flexible flatfoot: diagnosis, conservative and surgical treatment. Arch Podiatr Med Foot Surg 1:7, 1973
6. Giannestras NJ: Recognition and treatment of flatfeet in infancy. Clin Orthop 70:10, 1970
7. Page JC: Symptomatic flatfoot: etiology and diagnosis. J Am Podiatry Assoc 73:393, 1983
8. Green DR, Carol A: Planal dominance. J Am Podiatry Assoc 74:98, 1984
9. Manter JT: Movements of the subtalar and transverse tarsal joints. Anat Rec 80:397, 1941
10. Root ML, Weed JH, Sgarlato TE: Axis of motion of the subtalar joint. J Am Podiatry Assoc 56:149, 1966

11. Inman V: The Joints of the Ankle. Williams & Wilkins, Baltimore, 1976

12. Hicks JH: Mechanics of the foot: joints. J Anat 87:345, 1953

13. Hicks JH: Mechanics of the foot: plantar aponeurosis and the arch. J Anat 88:25, 1954

14. Jack EA: Naviculocuneiform fusion in treatment of flatfoot. J Bone Joint Surg [Br] 35:75, 1953

15. Oloff-Solomon J: Radiographic evaluation of the pediatric patient. Clin Podiatr Med Surg 4:21, 1987

16. Barry RJ, Scranton PE: Flatfeet in children. Clin Orthop Related Res 181:68, 1983

17. D'Amico JC: Developmental flatfoot. Clin Podiatry 1:535, 1984

18. Kidner FC: The prehallux in relation to flatfoot. JAMA 101:1539, 1933

19. Lowman CL: An operative method for correction of certain forms of flatfoot. JAMA 81:1500, 1923

20. Young CS: Operative treatment of pes planus. Surg Gynecol Obstet 68:1099, 1939

21. Hoke M: An operation for the correction of extremely relaxed flatfeet. J Bone Joint Surg 13:773, 1931

22. Miller OL: A plastic flatfoot operation. J Bone Joint Surg 9:84, 1927

23. Miller GR: The operative treatment of hypermobile flatfeet in the young child. Clin Orthop Related Res 122:95, 1977

24. LeLievre J: The valgus foot: current concepts and correction. Clin Orthop 70:43, 1970

25. Ganley JV: Calcaneo valgus deformity in infants. J Am Podiatry Assoc 65:405, 1975

26. Rogers WA, Joplin RJ: Hallux valgus, weak foot and the Keller operation: an end-result study. Surg Clin North Am 27:1295, 1947

27. Subotnick SI: Equinus deformity as it affects the forefoot. J Am Podiatry Assoc 61:423, 1971

28. Giannestras NJ: The pronated foot in infancy and childhood. p. 97. In Foot Disorders: Medical and Surgical Management. Lea & Febiger, Philadelphia, 1973

29. Tax HR: Flexible flatfoot in children. J Am Podiatry Assoc 67:616, 1977

30. Spencer AM, Person VA: Casting and orthotics for children. Clin Podiatry 1:631, 1984

31. Valmassey R, Terrafranca N: The triplane wedge: an adjunctive treatment modality in pediatric biomechanics. J Am Podiatr Med Assoc 76:672, 1986

32. Miller SJ: Principles of muscle-tendon surgery and tendon transfers. p. 714. In McGlamry ED, McGlamry R (eds): Comprehensive Textbook of Foot Surgery. Vol. II. Williams & Wilkins, Baltimore, 1987

33. Silver CM, Simon SD, Litchman HM: Long-term follow-up observations on calcaneal osteotomy. Clin Orthop 99:181, 1974

34. Miller SJ: End-stage flatfoot: diagnosis and conservative and surgical management. J Am Podiatr Med Assoc 77:42, 1987

35. O'Connor D: Sinus tarsi syndrome: a clinical entity. J Bone Joint Surg [Am] 40:720, 1958

36. Brown JE: The sinus tarsi syndrome. Clin Orthop 18:231, 1960

37. Hauser EDW: The sinus tarsi syndrome. Podologie 1:11, 1962

38. Debrunner HV: Das sinus tarsi syndrom. Schweiz Med Wochenschr 93:1660, 1963

39. Taillard W, Meyer JM, Garcia J, Blanc Y: The sinus tarsi syndrome. Int Orthop 5:117, 1981

40. Banks AS, McGlamry ED: Tibialis posterior tendon rupture. J Am Podiatr Med Assoc 77:170, 1987

41. Mueller TJ: Ruptures and lacerations of the tibialis posterior tendon. J Am Podiatry Assoc 74:109, 1984

42. Mann RA: Rupture of the tibialis posterior tendon. A.A.V.S. International Course Lectures 33:302, 1984

43. Mann RA, Thompson FM: Rupture of the posterior tibial tendon causing flatfoot. J Bone Joint Surg [Am] 67:556, 1985

44. Lipsman S, Frankel JP, Count GW: Spontaneous rupture of the tibialis posterior tendon. J Am Podiatry Assoc 70:34, 1980

45. Funk DA, Cass JR, Johnson KA: Acquired adult flatfoot secondary to posterior tibial tendon pathology. J Bone Joint Surg [Am] 68:95, 1986

46. Goldner JL, Keats PK, Bassett FH, Clippinger FW: Progressive talipes equinovalgus due to trauma or degeneration of the posterior tibial tendon and medial plantar ligaments. Orthop Clin North Am 5(1):39, 1974

47. Mann RA: Acquired flatfoot in adults. Clin Orthop Related Res 181:46, 1983

48. Vogler HW: Subtalar joint blocking operations for pathological pronation syndromes. p. 447. In McGlamry ED, McGlamry R (eds): Comprehensive Textbook on Foot Surgery. Vol. I. Williams & Wilkins, Baltimore, 1987

49. Grice DS: An extra-articular arthrodesis of the subastragalar joint for correction of paralytic flatfeet in children. J Bone Joint Surg [Am] 34:927, 1952

50. Dennyson W, Fulford G: Subtalar arthrodesis by

cancellous grafts and metallic internal fixation. J Bone Joint Surg [Br] 58:507, 1976

51. Barrasso J, Wile PB, Gage JR: Extraarticular subtalar arthrodesis with internal fixation. J Pediatr Orthop 4:555, 1984

52. Grice DS: Further experience with extra-articular arthrodesis of the subtalar joint. J Bone Joint Surg [Am] 37:246, 1955

53. Grice DS: The role of subtalar fusion in the treatment of valgus deformities of the feet. p. 127. In American Academy of Orthopedic Surgeons Instructional Course Lectures. Vol. 16. JJ Edwards, Ann Arbor, MI, 1959

54. Ross PM, Lyne DE: The Grice procedure. Clin Orthop 153:194, 1980

55. Hunt JC, Brooks AL: Subtalar extra-articular arthrodesis for correction of paralytic valgus deformity of the foot. J Bone Joint Surg [Am] 47:1310, 1965

56. Malverez O: Arthrodesis subastragalina en el pie valgo pronado paralitico. Arthrodesis minima. Estudio de 87 casos. Rev Ortop Traum (B Aires) 2:251, 1957

57. Engstrom A, Erikson U, Hjelmstedt A: The results of extra-articular subtalar arthrodesis according to the Green-Grice method in cerebral palsy. Acta Orthop Scand 45:945, 1974

58. Keats S: Operative Orthopaedics in Cerebral Palsy. Charles C Thomas, Springfield, IL, 1970

59. McCall RE, Lillich JS, Harris JR, Johnston EA: The Grice extraarticular subtalar arthrodesis: a clinical review. J Pediatr Orthop 5:442, 1985

60. Hsu LCS, Jaffray D, Leong JCY: The Batchelor-Grice extra-articular subtalar arthrodesis. J Bone Joint Surg [Br] 68:125, 1986

61. Chambers EF: An operation for the correction of flexible flatfoot of adolescents. West J Surg Obstet Gynecol 54:77, 1946

62. Smith SD, Millar EA: Arthroereisis by means of a subtalar polyethylene peg implant for correction of hindfoot pronation in children. Clin Orthop Related Res 181:15, 1983

63. Smith RD, Rappaport MJ: Subtalar arthroereisis: a four-year follow-up study. J Am Podiatry Assoc 73:356, 1983

64. Lanham RH: Indications and complications of arthroereisis in hypermobile flatfoot. J Am Podiatry Assoc 69:178, 1979

65. Smith SD, Wagreich CR: Review of postoperative results of the subtalar arthroereisis operation: a preliminary study. J Foot Surg 23:253, 1984

66. Jacobs AM, Oloff LM, Visser HJ: Calcaneal osteotomy in the management of flexible and nonflexible flatfoot deformity: a preliminary report. J Foot Surg 20:57, 1981

67. Lundeen RO: The Smith STA-Peg operation for hypermobile pes planovalgus in children. J Am Podiatr Med Assoc 75:177, 1985

68. Lichtblau S: Section of the abductor hallucis tendon for correction of metatarsus varus deformity. Clin Orthop 110:227, 1975

69. Addante JB, Ioli JP, Chin MW: Silastic sphere arthroereisis for surgical treatment of flexible flatfoot: a preliminary report. J Foot Surg 21:91, 1982

70. Oloff LM, Naylor BL, Jacobs AM: Complications of subtalar arthroereisis. J Foot Surg 26:136, 1987

71. Basmajian JV, Stecko G: The role of muscles in arch support of the foot: electromyographic study. J Bone Joint Surg [Am] 45:1184, 1963

72. Johnson KA: Tibialis posterior tendon rupture. Clin Orthop 177:145, 1983

73. Kidner FC: The prehallux (accessory scaphoid) in its relationship to flatfoot. J Bone Joint Surg 11:831, 1929

74. Fenton CF, Gilman RD, Jassen M et al: Criteria for selected major tendon transfers in podiatric surgery. J Am Podiatry Assoc 73:561, 1983

75. Leonard MH, Gonzales S, Breck LW et al: Lateral transfer of the posterior tibial tendon in certain selected cases of pes valgo planus (Kidner operation). Clin Orthop 40:139, 1965

76. Howey TD, Hoversten DL: Evaluation of the Kidner procedure for prehallux. South Dakota J Med 38:21, 1985

77. Hansen ST, Jr., Clark W: Tendon transfer to augment the weakened tibialis posterior mechanism. J Am Podiatr Med Assoc 78:399, 1988

78. Beck EL, McGlamry ED: Modified Young tendo-suspension technique for flexible flatfoot. p. 305. In McGlamry ED (ed): Reconstructive Surgery of the Foot and Leg. International Medical Book Corp, New York, 1974

79. Beck EL, McGlamry ED: Modified Young tendo-suspension technique for flexible flatfoot. J Am Podiatry Assoc 63:582, 1973

80. Krause W: The operative treatment of juvenile flatfeet and abducted feet. Am Digest Foreign Orthop Lit First Quarter, p. 32, 1971

81. Schmied HR: Late results of translocation of the anterior tibial tendon around the navicular bone in plano-valgus feet. Z Orthop 104:309, 1968 (Am Digest Foreign Orthop Lit First Quarter, p. 34, 1971)

82. Giannestras NJ: Foot Disorders—Medical and

Surgical Management. 2nd Ed. p. 139. Lea & Febiger, Philadelphia, 1973

83. Lovell WW, Price CT, Meehan PL: The foot. In Lovell WW, Winter RB (eds): Pediatric Orthopedics. p. 946. JB Lippincott, Philadelphia, 1978

84. Coleman SS: Severe, flexible planovalgus foot (flatfoot). p. 193. In Complex Foot Deformities in Children. Lea & Febiger, Philadelphia, 1983

85. Caldwell GD: Surgical correction of relaxed flatfoot by the Durham flatfoot plasty. Clin Orthop 2:221, 1953

86. Richardson EG: The foot in adolescents and adults. p. 891. In Crenshaw AH (ed): Campbell's Operative Orthopaedics. 7th Ed. Vol. II. CV Mosby Co, St. Louis 1987

87. Beck EL: Naviculocuneiform arthrodesis for flexible flatfoot. p. 335. In McGlamry ED (ed): Reconstructive Surgery of the Foot and Leg. Intercontinental Medical Book Corp, New York, 1974

88. Butte FL: Naviculocuneiform arthrodesis for flatfoot. J Bone Joint Surg 19:496, 1937

89. Seymour N: The late results of naviculocuneiform fusion. J Bone Joint Surg [Br] 49:558, 1967

90. Rodgveller BN: Talonavicular desmoplasty: a preliminary report. p. 109. In Smith SD, DiGiovanni JE (eds): Decision Making in Foot Surgery. Symposia Specialists, Miami, 1976

91. Jones BS: Flatfoot: a preliminary report of an operation for severe cases. J Bone Joint Surg [Br] 57:279, 1975

92. Cotton FJ: Foot statistics and surgery. N Engl J Med 214:353, 1936

93. Duncan JW, Lovell WW: Modified Hoke-Miller flatfoot procedure. Clin Orthop Related Res 181:24, 1983

94. Jacobs AM, Oloff LM: Surgical management of forefoot supinatus in flexible flatfoot deformity. J Foot Surg 23:410, 1984

95. Dockery GL: Surgical treatment of the symptomatic juvenile flexible flatfoot condition. Clin Podiatric Med Surg 4:99, 1987

96. Ruch JA, Mahan KT, McGlamry ED: Anatomic Dissection of the Medial Arch. Doctors Hospital Podiatric Education and Research Institute, Tucker, GA, 1986

97. Baker LD, Hill LM: Foot alignment in the cerebral palsy patient. J Bone Joint Surg [Am] 46:1, 1964

98. Selakovich W: Medial arch support by operation: sustentaculum tali procedure. Orthop Clin North Am 4:117, 1973

99. Johnson JB: Sustentaculum tali procedure for medial arch support. p. 117. In Smith SD, DiGiovanni

JE (eds): Decision Making in Foot Surgery. Symposia Specialists, Miami, 1976

100. Garelli R: Osteotomy of the calcaneum in the treatment of idiopathic valgus foot. Ital J Orthop Traumatol 12:53, 1986

101. Lord JP: Correction of extreme flatfoot. Value of osteotomy of os calcis and inward displacement of posterior fragment (Gleich operation). JAMA 81:1502, 1923

102. Gleich A: Beitzagzur operativen plattsfussbehandlung. Arch Klin Chir 46:358, 1893

103. Zadek I: Transverse wedge arthrodesis for the relief of pain in rigid flatfoot. J Bone Joint Surg 17:453, 1935

104. Dwyer FC: A new approach to the treatment of pes cavus. p. 551. In: Sixieme Congres International de Chirurgie Orthopedique, Berne, 30 Aout–3 Septembre, 1954. Societe Internationale de Chirurgie Orthopedique et de Traumatologie. Imprimerie Lielens, Bruxelles, 1955

105. Dwyer FC: Osteotomy of the calcaneum for pes cavus. J Bone Joint Surg [Br] 41:80, 1959

106. Dwyer FC: Osteotomy of the calcaneum in the treatment of grossly everted feet with special reference to cerebral palsy. p. 892. In Huitieme Congres Internationale de Chirurgie Orthopedique, New York, 4–9 September, 1960. Societe Internationale de Chirurgie Orthopedique et de Traumatologie. Imprimerie des Sciences, Brussels, 1961

107. Dwyer FC: The relationship of variations in the size and inclination cancaneus to the shape and function of the whole foot. Ann R Coll Surg Engl 34:120, 1964

108. Silver CM, Simon SD, Spindall E et al: Calcaneal osteotomy for valgus and varus deformities of the foot in cerebral palsy: a preliminary report on 27 operations. J Bone Joint Surg [Am] 49:232, 1967

109. Marcinko DE, Lazerson A, Elleby DH: Silver calcaneal osteotomy for flexible flatfoot: a retrospective preliminary report. J Foot Surg 23:191, 1984

110. Koutsogiannis E: Treatment of mobile flatfoot by displacement osteotomy of the calcaneus. J Bone Joint Surg [Br] 53:96, 1971

111. Evans D: Relapsed clubfoot. J Bone Joint Surg [Br] 43:722, 1961

112. Evans D: Calcaneo-valgus deformity. J Bone Joint Surg [Br] 57:270, 1975

113. Dollard MD, Marcinko DE, Lazerson A, Elleby D: The Evans calcaneal osteotomy for correction of flexible flatfoot syndrome. J Foot Surg 23:291, 1984

114. McCrea JD: The Evans procedure for treatment of

severe pes valgo planus. J Am Podiatr Med Assoc 77:35, 1987

115. Anderson AF, Fowler SB: Anterior calcaneal osteotomy for symptomatic juvenile pes planus. Foot Ankle 4:274, 1984

116. Phillips GE: A review of elongation of os calcis for flatfeet. J Bone Joint Surg [Br] 65:15, 1983

117. Mahan KT, McGlamry ED: Evans calcaneal osteotomy for flexible pes valgus deformity: a preliminary study. Clin Podiatr Med Surg 4:136, 1987

118. Grumbine NA: Talar neck osteotomy for the treatment of severe structural flatfoot deformities. Clin Podiatr Med Surg 4:119, 1987

119. Judet J, Judet H: Pied plat: traitment par arthrodese sous-astragalienne avec reposition astragale calcaneum. Nouv Presse Med 8:3969, 1979

SELECTED READINGS

Allen FG: Treatment of flatfoot in children. Med Pres Circ, 212:248, 1966

Baker LD: Triceps surae syndrome in cerebral palsy. Surgery, 68:216, 1954

Baker LD: A rational approach to the surgical needs of the cerebral palsy patient. J Bone Joint Surg [Am], 38:313, 1954

Baker LD, Dodelin RA: Extra-articular arthrodesis of the subtalar joint (Grice procedure). JAMA, 168:1105, 1958

Basmajian JV: Functional and anatomical considerations in major muscle tendon imbalance. J Am Podiatry Assoc, 65:723, 1975

Beck EL, McGlamry ED, Kitting RW: The Young weak-foot suspension. J Am Podiatry Assoc, 63:528, 1973

Berg EE: A reappraisal of metatarsus adductus and skew-foot. J Bone Joint Surg [Am], 68:1185, 1986

Bernstein RH, Bartholomei FJ, McCarthy DJ: Sinus tarsi syndrome. Anatomical, clinical and surgical considerations. J Am Podiatr Med Assoc, 75:475, 1985

Bettman E: The treatment of flatfoot by means of exercise. J Bone Joint Surg, 19:821, 1937

Bleck EE, Berzins UJ: Conservative management of pes valgus with plantarflexed talus, flexible. Clin Orthop Related Res, 122:85, 1977

Bonnet WL, Baker WL, Baker DR: Diagnosis of pes planus by x-ray. Radiology, 46:36, 1946

Bordelon RL: Hypermobile flatfoot in children. Comprehension, evaluation and treatment. Clin Orthop Related Res, 181:7, 1983

Borelli AH, Arenson DJ: Sinus tarsi syndrome and its relationship to hallux abducto valgus. J Am Podiatr Med Assoc, 77:495, 1987

Brown PB: Rheumatoid flatfoot. J Am Podiatr Med Assoc, 77:39, 1987

Cahill DR: The anatomy and function of the contents of the human tarsal sinus and canal. Anat Rec, 153:1, 1965

Caldwell GA: Arthrodeses of the feet. p. 174. In: American Academy of Orthopaedic Surgeons, Instructional Course Lectures, Vol. 4. JW Edwards, Ann Arbor, MI, 1947

Chater EH: Foot pain and the accessory navicular bone. Ir J Med Sci, 442:471, 1962

Clark W: A rebalancing operation for pronated feet. J Bone Joint Surg, 13:876, 1931

Cooke AG, Stern WG, Ryerson EW: Report of the commission appointed by the American Orthopedic Association for the study of stabilizing operations on the foot. Orthop Surg, 3:437, 1921

Crego CH, Ford LT: An end-result study of various operative procedures for corrective flatfoot in children. J Bone Joint Surg [Am], 34:183, 1952

Davy R: An excision of the scaphoid bone for relief of confirmed flatfoot. Lancet, 1:675, 1889

Diamond LS: Dowel-type sub-talar arthrodesis in children. J Bone Joint Surg [Am], 58:725, 1976

Dickson FD, Dively RL: Functional Disorders of the Foot. JB Lippincott, Philadelphia, 1944

Dockery GL: Perioperative management of the infant and child. Clin Podiatry, 2:645, 1984

Duncan JW, Lovell WW: Hoke triple arthrodesis. J Bone Joint Surg [Am], 61:695, 1978

Dwyer FC: The treatment of relapsed club foot by the insertion of a wedge into the calcaneum. J Bone Joint Surg [Br], 45:67, 1963

Fisher RL, Shaffer SR: An evaluation of calcaneal osteotomy in congenital clubfoot and other disorders. Clin Orthop Related Res, 70:141, 1970

Fitch RR, King BB: The operative treatment of relaxed weak feet. J Bone Joint Surg, 24:574, 1942

Freid A, Dobbs B: Sinus tarsi synovectomy. A possible alternative to a subtalar joint fusion. J Am Podiatr Med Assoc, 75:494, 1985

Freid A, Hendel C: Paralytic valgus deformity of the ankle. J Bone Joint Surg [Am], 39:921, 1957

Fulp MJ, McGlamry ED: Gastrocnemius tendon recession. J Am Podiatry Assoc, 64:163, 1974

Gamble F, Yale I: Acquired foot fault syndromes associated with functional foot disorders. p. 214. In: Clinical Foot Roentgenology. 2nd Ed. Robert E. Krieger, Huntington, NY, 1975

Geist ES: The accessory scaphoid bone. J Bone Joint Surg, 7:570, 1925

Giannini S, Girolami M, Ceccarelli F: The surgical treatment of infantile flatfoot: a new expanding endo-orthotic implant. Ital J Orthop Traumatol, 11:315, 1985

Golding Bird CH: Operations on the tarsus in confirmed flatfoot. Lancet, 71:677, 1889

Gould N: Evaluation of hyperpronation and pes planus in adults. Clin Orthop Related Res, 181:37, 1983

Gray EG, Basmajian JV: Electromyography and cinematography of leg and foot ("normal" and flat) during walking. Anat Rec, 161:1, 1968

Green WT, Grice DS: The management of calcaneus deformity. p. 135. In: American Academy of Orthopaedic Surgeons, Instructional Course Lecture, Vol. 13. JJ Edwards, Ann Arbor, MI, 1956

Grumbine NA: The varus components of the forefoot in flatfoot deformities. J Am Podiatr Med Assoc, 77:14, 1987

Hall JE, Salter RB, Bhalla SK: Congenital short tendo calcaneus. J Bone Joint Surg [Br], 49:695, 1967

Hallgrimsson S: Studies on reconstructive and stabilizing operations on the skeleton of the foot. Acta Chir Scand, 88(Suppl 78):5, 1943

Hallock H: The surgical treatment of common mechanical and functional disabilities of the feet. Am Acad Orthop Surgeons Lect, 6:160, 1949

Haraldsson S: Operative treatment of pes planovalgus staticus juvenilis. Preliminary communication. Acta Orthop Scand, 32:492, 1962

Haraldsson S: Pes planovalgus. Svenska Lakäntidn, 60:2687, 1963

Haraldsson S: Pes planovalgus staticus juvenilis and its operative treatment. Acta Orthop Scand, 35:234, 1965

Haraldsson S: Arthroereisis procedure for the correction of flexible flatfoot in childhood. p. 123. In Smith SD, DiGiovanni JE (eds): Decision Making in Foot Surgery. Stratton Medical Book Corp, New York, 1976

Hare AW: Extreme flatfoot: operation; recovery; remarks. Lancet, 1:953, 1889

Harris R, Beath T: Hypermobile flatfoot with short tendo Achillis. J Bone Joint Surg [Am], 30:116, 1948

Helfet AJ: A new way of treating flatfeet in children. Lancet, 1:262, 1956

Herndon CH: Tendon transplantation at the knee and foot. p. 145. In: American Academy of Orthopaedic Surgeons, Instructional Course Lectures, Vol. 18. JJ Edwards, Ann Arbor, MI, 1961

Herzmark MD: Flatfeet in children. An ounce of prevention. Med Times, 12:23, 1963

Hibbs R: Muscle bound feet. New York Med J, 100:798, 1914

Hsu LC, O'Brien BS, Yau ACMC, Hodgson AR: Valgus deformity of the ankle in children with fibular pseudarthrosis. J Bone Joint Surg [Am], 56:503, 1974

Humphry J: Flatfoot and the construction of the plantar arch. Lancet, 1:529, 1886

Inman V, Ralston H, Todd F: Human Walking. Williams & Wilkins, Baltimore, 1981

Ireland ML, Hoffer M: Triple arthrodesis for children with spastic cerebral palsy. Dev Med Child Neurol, 27:623, 1985

Jensen JK: Ball and socket ankle joints. Clin Orthop Related Res, 85:28, 1972

Johanning K: Exochleatio ossis cuboidei in the treatment of pes equinovarus. Acta Orthop Scand, 27:310, 1958

Jones RL: The human foot, an experimental study of its mechanics and the role of its muscles and ligaments in the support of the arch. Am J Anat, 68:1, 1941

Jones RL: The functional significance of the declination of the axis of the subtalar joint. Anat Rec, 93:151, 1945

Joplin RJ: Some common foot disorders amenable to surgery. In: American Academy of Orthopaedic Surgeons, Instructional Course Lectures, Vol. 15. JJ Edwards, Ann Arbor, MI, 1958

Judet J: New concepts in the corrective surgery of congenital talipes equinovarus and congenital and neurologic flatfeet. Clin Orthop, 70:56, 1970

Kaplan EB: Some principles of anatomy and kinesiology in stabilization operations of the foot. Clin Orthop, 34:7, 1964

Kein HA, Ritchie GW: Weight-bearing roentgenograms in the evaluation of foot deformities. Clin Orthop, 70:133, 1970

Kirk JF, Hecker RL: Sinus tarsi pain: case history. J Foot Surg, 15:120, 1976

Kite JH: Treatment of flatfeet in children. Med Ann Dist Columbia, 21:316, 1952

Kite JH: Flatfeet and lateral rotation of legs in young children. Post-Grad Med, 15:75, 1954

Kleinberg S, Roth FB: The operative correction of flatfeet in children. Bull Hosp Joint Dis, 8:160, 1947

Kolker LD: A biomechanical analysis of flatfoot surgery. J Am Podiatry Assoc, 63:217, 1973

Lang G, Kehr P, Sejourne P, Pointer J: Notre experience due traitement chirurgical dupied plat valgus par remise en selle de l'astragale sur le calcaneum. Chirugie, 5:261, 1979

Langford JH, Bozof H, Horowitz BD: Subtalar arthroereisis: Valente procedure. Clin Podiatr Med Surg, 4:153, 1987

Lapidus PW: Misconceptions about the "Springiness of the longitudinal arch of the foot." Arch Surg 46:410, 1943

Leavitt DG: Subastragaloid arthrodesis for the os calcis type of flatfoot. Am J Surg, NS 49:501, 1941

Leeds WD: The recognition and treatment of congenital flatfoot in infancy. J Bone Joint Surg [Br], 49:872, 1967

Levitt RJ, Canale SJ, Gartland JJ: Surgical correction of foot deformity in the older patient with myelomeningocoele. Orthop Clin North Am, 5:19, 1974

Lovett RA, Cotton FJ: Pronation of the foot, considered from an anatomical standpoint. J Boston Soc Med Sci, II(9):155, 1898

Lowman CL: The treatment of flatfoot. Orthop Correspondence Club Lett, 1:12, 1941

Lowy A, Schilers J, Kanat IO: Sinus tarsi syndrome: a postoperative analysis. J Foot Surg, 24:108, 1985

Mann R, Inman F: Phasic activity of the intrinsic muscles of the foot. J Bone Joint Surg [Am], 46:469, 1964

McCrea JD: Flatfeet deformities. p. 159. In: Pediatric Orthopedics of the Lower Extremity: An Instructional Handbook. Futura Publishing Company, Mt. Kisco, NY, 1985

McGlamry ED, Kitting RW: Equinus foot: an analysis of the etiology, pathology and treatment techniques. J Am Podiatry Assoc, 63:165, 1973

Mereday CM, Dolan C, Lusskin R: Evaluation of the University of California Biomechanics Laboratory shoe insert in "flexible" pes planus. Clin Orthop, 82:45, 1972

Meyer JM, Lagier R: Post-traumatic sinus tarsi syndrome, an anatomical and radiological study. Acta Orthop Scand, 48:122, 1977

Meyer JM, Taillard W: L'arthrographic de l'articulation sousastragalienne dans les syndromes douloureux post-traumatiques de tarsi-posterieur. Rev Chir Orthop, 60:321, 1974

Meyer W: Operative treatment of flatfoot by supramalleolar osteotomy. NY Med J, 51:566, 1890

Milch H: Reinforcement of the deltoid ligament for pronated flatfoot. Inversion fasciodesis of the os calcis. Surg Gynecol Obstet, 74:876, 1942

Miller AG: Clinical lecture on flatfoot. Edinburgh Med J, 36:221, 1890

Minns RJ, Craxford AD, Park C: A study of foot shape, underfoot pressure patterns, lower limb rotations and gait of children. Chiropodist, 41:89, 1986

Navarre M: A propos du syndrome du sinus du tarse. Acta Orthop Belg, 32:743, 1966

Ogilvy C: An operation for the permanent correction of weak feet in children. J Orthop Surg, 1:343, 1919

Ogston A: On flatfoot and its cure by operation. Br Med J, 1:110, 1884

Paluska DJ, Blount WP: Ankle valgus after the Grice subtalar stabilization. Am Orthop, 59:137, 1968

Patterson RL, Jr., Parrish FF, Hathaway EN: Stabilizing operations on the foot; a study of the indications, techniques used, and end results. J Bone Joint Surg [Am], 32:1, 1950

Powell HDW, Cantab MB: Pes planovalgus in children. Clin Orthop Related Res, 177:133, 1983

Pressman MM: Biomechanics and surgical criteria for flexible pes valgus. J Am Podiatr Med Assoc, 77:7, 1987

Purvis D: Surgery of the relaxed flatfoot. Clin Orthop Related Res, 57:221, 1968

Riddell JS: Flatfoot: its pathology, causation and treatment. Int Clin, 1:244, 1893

Root M, Orien W, Weed J: Normal and Abnormal Functions of the Foot. Clinical Biomechanics Corp, Los Angeles, 1977

Rose GK: Correction of the pronated foot, 1. J Bone Joint Surg [Br], 40:674, 1958

Rose GK: Correction of the pronated foot, 2. J Bone Joint Surg [Br], 44:642, 1962

Rose GK, Welton EA, Marshall T: The diagnosis of flatfoot in the child. J Bone Joint Surg [Br], 67:71, 1985

Rosensky SL: Sinus tarsi syndrome. Curr Podiatr Med, 35:24, 1986

Rugtveit A: Extra-articular subtalar arthrodesis, according to Green-Grice in flatfeet. Acta Orthop Scand, 34:367, 1964

Ryerson EW: Tendon transplantation in flatfoot. Am J Orthop Surg, 7:505, 1910

Ryerson EW: Discussion of paper by RE Soule. JAMA, 77:1874, 1921

Ryerson EW: Arthrodesing operations of the feet. J Bone Joint Surg, 5:543, 1923

Samuelson KM, Tuke MA, Freeman MAR: A new reconstructive procedure to correct hindfoot valgus. Orthop Trans, 3:149, 1978

Samuelson KM, Tuke MA, Freeman MAR: A study of hindfoot mechanics with relation to valgus deformity. J Bone Joint Surg [Br], 60:282, 1978

Sarrafian SK: Functional characteristics of the foot and plantar aponeurosis under tibiotalar loading. Foot Ankle, 8:4, 1987

Schoolfeld BL: An original operation, shortening of the deltoid ligament. Dallas Med J, 14:17, 1928

Schoolfeld BL: Operative treatment of flatfoot. Surg Gynecol Obstet, 94:136, 1952

Schuster R, Otto F, Lewi MJ: Foot Orthopaedics. First Institute of Podiatry, New York, 1927

Schuster RO: Flexible flatfoot in childhood and adolescence. In Smith SD, DiGiovanni JE (eds): Decision Making in Foot Surgery. Symposia Specialists, Miami, FL, 1976

Schwartz RP, Heath DL: Conservative treatment of functional disorders of the feet in adolescents and adults. J Bone Joint Surg [Br], 44:642, 1949

Seymour N, Evans DK: A modification of the Grice subtalar arthrodesis. J Bone Joint Surg [Br], 50:372, 1968

Sgarlato TE: A Compendium of Podiatric Biomechanics. California College of Podiatric Medicine, San Francisco, 1971

Sgarlato TE: Pediatric foot surgery. Clin Podiatry, 2:709, 1984

Silfverskiold N: Reduction of the uncrossed two-joint muscles of the leg to one-joint muscles in spastic conditions. Acta Chir Scand, 56:315, 1923–1924

Silver CM et al: Calcaneal osteotomy for valgus and varus deformities of the foot: further experience. Int Surg, 58:24, 1973

Smith JW: Muscular control of the arches of the foot in standing: an electromyographic assessment. J Anat, 88:152, 1954

Smith SD, Weil LS: The Hoke procedure. In Smith SD, DiGiovanni JE (eds): Decision Making in Foot Surgery. Symposia Specialists, Miami, FL, 1976

Soule RE: Value of bone pin arthrodesis in the treatment of flatfoot. JAMA, 77:1871, 1921

Stephens R: An operation for the correction of pronated feet. J Bone Joint Surg, 17:424, 1935

Subotnick SI: The subtalar joint lateral extra-articular arthroereisis: a follow-up report. J Am Podiatry Assoc, 67:157, 1977

Subotnick SI: The subtalar joint lateral extra-articular arthroereisis: a preliminary report. J Am Podiatry Assoc, 64:701, 1974

Sullivan RW: Correction of the hypermobile flatfoot by the subtalar arthroerisis procedure. Milit Med, 150:546, 1985

Tachdjian MO: Pediatric Orthopedics. WB Saunders Co, Philadelphia, 1972

Tachdjian MO: The Child's Foot. WB Saunders Co, Philadelphia, 1985

Tax HR: Excessive pronation. p. 221. In: Podopediatrics. Williams & Wilkins, Baltimore, 1980

Thompson TC: Astragalectomy and the treatment of calcaneovalgus. J Bone Joint Surg, 21:627, 1939

Thomson SA: Hallux varus and metatarsus varus: a five-year study (1954–1959). Clin Orthop, 16:109, 1960

Vogler HW: Biomechanics of talipes equinovalgus. J Am Podiatr Med Assoc, 77:21, 1987

Vogler HW: Surgical reconstruction of talipes equinovalgus. J Am Podiatr Med Assoc, 77:134, 1987

Vogler HW, Buckholz JH: Arthroereisis: concepts and principles. p. 448. In Clark T (ed): Yearbook of Podiatric Medicine and Surgery. Futura Publishing Company, Mt. Kisco, NY, 1981

Von Volkmann R: Overlooked and unappreciated anatomical facts with regard to the development of pes planus. Z Orthop, 113:229, 1975

Wesley MS, Barenfeld PA: Mechanism of the Dwyer calcaneal osteotomy. Clin Orthop Related Res, 70:136, 1970

Westin FW, Hall CB: Subtalar extra-articular arthrodesis. J Bone Joint Surg [Am], 39:501, 1957

Wetzenstein H: Prognosis of pes cancaneo-valgus congenitus. Acta Orthop Scand, 41:122, 1970

White JW: Surgery of the foot. p. 218. In: American Academy of Orthopaedic Surgeons, Instructional Course Lecture. Vol. 1. Edwards Bros, Ann Arbor, MI, 1943

White JW: Surgical procedures on the foot—their indications and end results. In: American Academy of Orthopaedic Surgeons, Instructional Course Lectures. Vol. 1. Edwards Bros Inc, Ann Arbor, MI, 1943

White JW: Disorders of the foot—their treatment. In: American Academy of Orthopaedic Surgeons, Instructional Course Lectures. Vol. 4. JW Edwards, Ann Arbor, MI, 1947

Whitman R: Observations of forty-five cases of flatfoot with particular reference to etiology and treatment. Boston Medi Surg J, 118:598, 1888

Whitman R: The radical cure of confirmed flatfoot. NY Med J, 55:227, 1892

Whitman R: A review of the inception and development of a type of reparative surgery adapted to bodily mechanics. J Bone Joint Surg, 28:374, 1946

Wilson FC, Gardner FF, Lamotte P, Williams JC: Triple arthrodesis: a study of the factors affecting fusion after three hundred and one procedures. J Bone Joint Surg [Am], 47:340, 1965

Wilson HA, Patterson RV: The combined operation of arthrodesis and transplantation of the tendon of the extensor proprius hallucis for relief of flatfoot. Am Med, 9:725, 1905

Wood WA, Spencer AM: Incidence of os tibiale externum in clinical pes planus. J Am Podiatry Assoc, 60:276, 1970

Zachariae L: The Grice operation for paralytic flatfeet in children. Acta Orthop Scand, 33:80, 1963

Zadek I: The significance of the accessory tarsal scaphoid. J Bone Joint Surg, 8:618, 1926

Zadek I, Gold AM: Accessory tarsal scaphoid. J Bone Joint Surg [Am], 30:957, 1948

Pes Cavus

38

Allan M. Boike, D.P.M.
Bonnie Johng, D.P.M.
Vincent J. Hetherington, D.P.M. , M.S.

Some primitive mammals are thought to have been partly arboreal. Life in the trees for early primates required the development of many features that were important precursors to an upright position. Adaptation to an arboreal existence included increased body agility, development of the hand, stereotaxic vision, and a more complex brain.[1]

Anatomic differences between higher primates are few. Distinctive human features include the unique vertebral posture and hind leg structure associated with upright gait. With special significance is the foot, in which a particular architectural feature differentiates the human foot from all other primates. This special feature is the arch.

The arch of the foot developed 10 to 20 million years ago and is a phenomenon peculiar to homo sapiens.[2] It provides for suitable contact with the ground for bipedal locomotion and functions as a lever during ambulation.[3] During the gait cycle, the weight of the body is distributed between the calcaneus and the metatarsal heads. The actual shape and configuration of the arch is determined by alignment of individual tarsal and metatarsal bones, not by size or weight of the individual.

Pes cavus is defined as a foot with an abnormally high arch. Pes cavus was first identified as a specific deformity by Little in 1853.[4] Historically it has been referred to as hollow foot, clawfoot, bolt foot, pes arcuatus, talipes plantaris, griffe pied creux, Holfuss, and nondeforming clubfoot.[5] Clinical presentation and symptomology are quite variable. Pes cavus ranges from mild to severely crippling. It may be an isolated entity, the result of neuromuscular disease, or the result of multiple etiologic factors.

This chapter describes the anatomy of the pes cavus deformity, as well as the etiology, pathomechanics, classification, clinical and radiographic presentation, and surgical procedures utilized for correction.

ANATOMY OF THE LONGITUDINAL ARCH

The longitudial arch extends from the calcaneus to the metatarsal heads and includes all tarsal bones

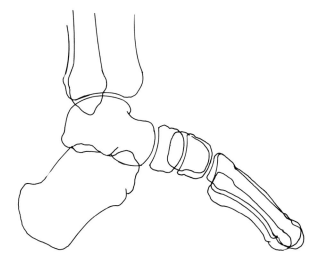

Fig. 38-1. Medial longitudinal arch.

1. Spring (C-N) ligament—connects sustentaculum tali and inferior surface of the navicular bones.
2. Short plantar ligament (C-C)—connects the anterior tubercle of the calcaneus and posterior groove of the cuboid bone.
3. Long plantar ligament—connects the plantar surface of the calcaneus and both the base of the lateral metatarsals and ridge of the cuboid.
4. Superficial plantar fascia—extends from the calcaneus to the metatarsal heads.

that lie therein. More specifically, the medial longitudinal arch consists of the calcaneus, the talus, the navicular, the three cuneiforms, and the first metatarsal bones[6] (Fig. 38-1). The lateral longitudinal arch consists of the calcaneus, the cuboid, and the fourth and fifth metatarsal bones (Fig. 38-2).

The ligaments maintain the anatomic alignment, particularly the position of the tarsal bones. There are four ligaments of particular importance in maintaining the integrity of the longitudinal arch[7] (Fig. 38-3):

PATHOMECHANICS/MECHANISMS OF PES CAVUS

Muscular

The etiology of pes cavus may include a variety of factors—contracted plantar ligaments, muscular or neuromuscular imbalance, and inherent structure of the foot—or may be idiopathic in nature.

Duchenne described the actions of the muscles of the body as elicited by faradic stimulation, and their correlation, with astute clinical observation in "The physiology of Motion."[8] Pertinent to this discussion is his demonstration of the actions of the triceps surae, peroneus longus, extensor digitorum longus, extensor digitorum brevis, flexor digitorum longus, and the intrinsic muscles of the foot. Muscle weakness is commonly associated with cavus foot. In examining normal function of each of these muscles, or muscle groups, its contribution to development of pes cavus becomes apparent.

Triceps Surae

The triceps surae forcefully plantar flexes the hindfoot and the lateral border of the forefoot and rotates the foot, carrying the anterior end medially.[3] Hence, it acts as a plantar flexor, adductor, and lateral rotator. Weakness of the triceps surae muscles will result in a decreased ability for heel-off in late stance. When this occurs, extrinsic muscles that pass behind the ankle mortice (flexor hallucis longus, flexor digitorum longus, tibialis

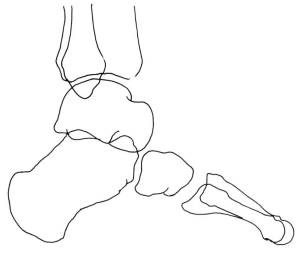

Fig. 38-2. Lateral longitudinal arch.

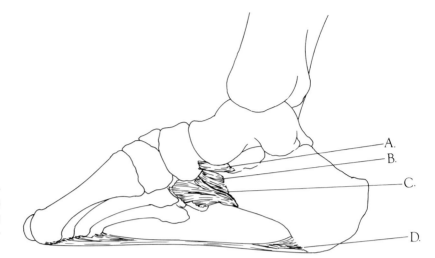

Fig. 38-3. Ligaments of the longitudinal arch. **(A)** Spring ligament. **(B)** Short plantar ligament. **(C)** Long plantar ligament. **(D)** Superficial plantar fascia.

Table 38-1. Abnormal Muscle Function and Development of Cavus Foot Deformity[a]

Muscle Status	Result	Overall Effect on Foot
A. Triceps surae (weak)	PL—plantar flexes first metatarsal ↓ Supination TP—Supinates foot FHL, FDL—Supinate foot, contract digits PB—Attempts to pronate STJ, plantar flexes outer foot	1) Supinated foot 2) ↑ Anterior cavus 3) Posterior cavus
B. Tibialis posterior (spasm)	TP—Overpowers ↓ Supination	↑ Anterior cavus
C. EHL (weak) EDL (weak) TA (strong)	TA—Overpowers ↓ Inverted foot-drop	↑ Anterior cavus
D. EHL (weak) EDL (weak) TA (weak)	Peroneals—Overpower ↓ Plantar flexed first ray	↑ Anterior cavus
E. EHL (strong) TA (weak)	EHL—Overpowers ↓ Hallux malleus	Hallux malleus, plantar flexed first ray
F. All anterior muscles (weak)	TP—Overpowers ↓ Supination	↑ Anterior cavus
G. PL (spastic)	PL—Overpowers Plantar declination of first metatarsal	↑ Anterior cavus
H. Intrinsics (weak)	Early function of extrinsics ↓ Extensor substitution	↑ Anterior cavus

[a] EDL, extensor digitorum longus; EHL, extensor hallucis longus; FDL, flexor digitorum longus; FHL, flexor hallucis longus; PB, peroneus brevis; PL, peroneus longus; STJ, subtalar joint; TA, tibialis anterior, TP, tibialis posterior.

posterior, peroneus longus, and peroneus brevis) will attempt to assist in plantar flexion of the foot for heel lift.[4] The result is a supinated foot type with increased plantar flexion of the anterior aspect (i.e., an anterior cavus foot type) (Table 38-1A).

The Tibialis Posterior

The tibialis posterior is a stance-phase muscle that begins to contract very early in the contact period, at about the time the forefoot first touches the ground.[9] Primary functions are to decelerate subtalar joint pronation and internal leg rotation at contact and accelerate subtalar joint supination and external leg rotation at midstance. Spasticity rather than weakness of this muscle would contribute to formation of the cavus foot deformity (Table 38-1B).

Anterior Muscle Group

The functions of the extensor hallucis longus muscle include stabilization, aceleration, and deceleration of the joints of the foot.[9] During propulsion, it provides extension stability to the first metatarsophalangeal joint (MPJ) and interphalangeal joint. During swing, the extensor hallucis longus accelerates the foot by neutral ankle dorsiflexion.

The functions of the extensor digitorum longus include stabilization of the phalanges at the MPJ and assisting in dorsiflexion of the foot (i.e., stabilization and acceleration).[9]

The primary functions of the tibialis anterior are acceleration and deceleration of the foot. The accelerating functions include dorsiflexion of the foot at toe-off and the first ray at swing, as well as supination of the foot just prior to heel strike. The decelerating functions include prevention of excessive pronation of the foot, supination of the midtarsal joint, and the resisting of plantar flexion of the foot at heel strike.

If the extensor hallucis longus and extensor digitorum longus are weak, the tibialis anterior will overpower them, resulting in a inverted foot-drop (Table 38-1C).

Weakness of the anterior muscle group will result in overpowering by the posterior muscle group, creating a plantar-flexed attitude of the foot at the ankle and the forefoot on the rearfoot. A form of foot-drop may result (Table 38-1D).

If the tibialis anterior muscle is weak in the presence of normal extensor hallucis longus, a "cocked hallux" develops placing additional retrograde plantar-flexory force on the first metatarsal (Table 38-1E). If all anterior muscles are weak, overpowering of the posterior group occurs with increased plantar declination of the anterior portion of the foot and increased cavus deformity[4] (Table 38-1F).

Peroneals

The peroneus longus is a stance-phase muscle. Its primary function is stabilization of the first ray transversely and posteriorly.[9] The peroneus longus forcefully lowers the medial border of the forefoot, and by turning the medial border laterally and carrying the anterior end laterally, it narrows and curves the plantar arch.[3] With spasticity the plantar declination of the first metatarsal increases, leading to an anterior cavus foot (Table 38-1G). Isolated weakness of the peroneus longus would most likely result in metatarsus primus elevatus with overpowering of the tibialis anterior.[4] Weakness of the triceps surae combined with weakness of the peroneus longus would allow the foot to follow the long flexion of the toes, resulting in a cavovarus deformity.[10]

Intrinsics

The interossei are stance-phase muscles that begin to contract late in midstance and continue to function until late propulsion.[9] Their function is to stabilize the proximal phalanges of the lesser toes at the MTJ. Weakness of the intrinsic muscles of the foot allows for early function of the extrinsic muscles, leading to the phenomenon of extensor substitution[11] (Table 38-1H).

Once the imbalance is present, a vicious cycle is established in which excessive dorsiflexion of the digits at the MTJ creates a "reverse buckling effect." Consequently, the digits force the metatarsal heads down, creating excessive plantar flexion of the forefoot and causing the extensors to work harder to dorseflex the ankle (Figure 38-4).

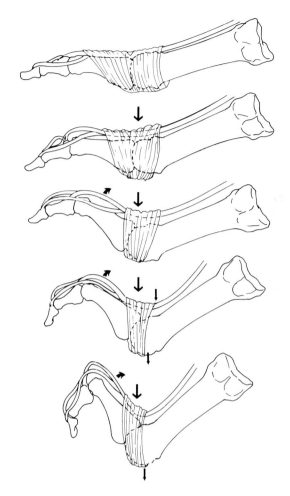

Fig. 38-4. Pathomechanics of extensor substitution.

Ligamentous

Although not the primary deforming force, contraction and shortening of the ligaments that support the longitudinal arch may contribute to the nonflexible nature of the cavus foot deformity. It has been suggested that contracture of the ligaments would act to draw the forefoot toward the rearfoot, shortening the foot and exaggerating the high arch formation.

Neurologic

Manifestations of pathology involving the spinal cord and cauda equina, such as herniated discs, tumors, or avulsed nerve roots, are frequently found in the lower extremities.[12] Pes cavus may result from lesions throughout the nervous system. There exists a high correlation between neuromuscular disease and pes cavus. In fact, pes cavus may be an early manifestation of a neuromuscular disease. It may be congenital or posttraumatic or may exist without an identifiable cause. Brewerton et al. demonstrated that a careful neurologic examination lowers the percentage of patients with reported "idiopathic pes cavus" from 81 to 31 percent.[13]

Because of the significant correlation between nervous system lesions at every level, it is imperative that a thorough history and physical examination of the patient, and if indicated the family, be performed (Table 38-2). A thorough examination may include evaluation of motor and sensory function, reflexes, and coordination; electromyographic and nerve conduction studies; and footprint recording.

Identifiable neurologic etiologies of pes cavus may be congenital or acquired (Table 38-3). There also exist many reported cases of cavus foot that are idiopathic in etiology.

Charcot-Marie-Tooth Disease

Hereditary neuropathies are commonly associated with "high arch" foot deformities.[14] Charcot-Marie-Tooth disease, (hereditary motor sensory neuropathy) is a disease of peripheral nerves, motor nerve roots, and often the spinal cord.[15] The presence of foot deformity in other family members is often used to help determine the type of inheritance. The disease may be latent, with only the foot deformity apparent. Clinically, these patients exhibit weakness about the ankles, resulting in a restless stance and a constant shifting of their weight from side to side.[16-18] As a result of difficulty with position sense and foot extension, these patients often develop a wide-based, high-stepping gait. The disease progresses slowly, and is characterized by atrophy of the muscle groups in the hands, feet, and calves, with the atrophy beginning distally. It was previously believed that the peroneal muscles were affected early, but more recent studies indicate that the peroneus longus is rarely

Table 38-2. Clinical Evaluation (Workup) of the Patient with Cavus Foot Deformity

I. Thorough history
  A. Patient
  B. Patient's family
II. Thorough physical examination
  A. Eyes, ears, nose, throat
  B. Cardiovascular electrodiagnostic studies — electrocardiogram
  C. Dermatologic — check lower back
  D. Upper and lower extremities
    1. Biomechanical
    2. Musculoskeletal — isolated muscle testing, joint range of motion, orthopedic evaluation
    3. Neurologic — deep tendon reflexes and sensation
  E. Neurologic — get consult
    1. Vestibular/auditory testing
    2. Mental status, cognitive function, amnesic evaluation
    3. Cranial nerves — tongue and gag reflex, dysarthria
    4. Visual exam — nystagmus, acuity, fundus, fields, night blindness
    5. Romberg's test
    6. Finger-to-nose, heel-to-shin tests
III. Gait analysis
  A. Base — wide or narrow
  B. Steps — high, slap or foot-drop, short, steppage gait
  C. Propulsive vs. apropulsive
  D. Antalgic or nonantalgic
  E. Digital deformities — extensor substitution, clawtoes, hammer toes
  F. Stability — foot or ankle instability, ataxia; heel in varus or valgus
IV. Roentgenographic evaluation
  A. Dorsoposterior view — looking for metatarsus adductus, forefoot adductus or abductus
  B. Lateral view — looking at calcaneal inclination angle, Meary's angle, Hibbs' angle, metatarsal declination angle, calcaneal sinus, tarsi ("bullet hole" sign)
  C. Axial view — looking for varus heel
V. Roentgenographic findings
  A. Increased calcaneal inclination angle (35–40 degrees on lateral view)
  B. Increased metatarsal declination angle (25–35 degrees on lateral view)
  C. Hammer toe, clawtoe deformities (lateral view)
  D. Calcaneus in varus (caloaxial view)
VI. Important angles:
  A. *Meary's angle* (drawn on lateral radiograph): formed by the bisection of the talus and the bisection of the first metatarsal; the intersection of the two lines occurs at the apex of the deformity.
  B. *Hibbs' angle* (drawn on lateral radiograph): formed by the long axis of the calcaneus and the bisection of the first metatarsal; the intersection of the two lines occurs at the apex of the deformity.
VII. Other diagnostic studies
  A. Complete blood count with differential, serum enzyme levels
  B. Electromyography and nerve conduction velocity studies, muscle and nerve biopsy in selected cases

Table 38-3. Etiology of Cavus Foot Deformity

Congenital
Myelodysplasia, myelomeningocele, spina bifida
Familial degenerative nerve disease
  Charcot-Marie-Tooth disease
  Friedreich's ataxia
  Roussy-Lévy disease
Cerebral palsy (spastic monoplegia and paraplegia)
Muscular dystrophy
Hypertrophic interstitial neuropathy
Congenital syphilis
Congenital clubfoot
Congenital lymphedema
Arthrogryposis
Acquired
Poliomyelitis
Dystonia musculorum deformans
Angioma of the medulla (other spinal cord tumors)
Syringomyelia
Trauma
Infection
Lederhosen disease (plantar fibromatosis)
Hysteria (cerebral level)
Polyneuritis

involved at an early stage, and in fact it has been successfully used in dorsal transfers.[19]

Lower lumbar muscular atrophy gives the apperance of "stork leg" or an inverted champagne bottle. Atrophy of muscles of the hand is demonstrated by weakness first in positioning of the thumb and fingers and then in all manipulative functions. The patient may develop clawtoes and clawhand. Deep tendon reflexes are absent at the ankles, Babinksi's signs are absent, and there is often little or no digital movement. The patient exhibits diminished vibratory sense. Charcot-Marie-Tooth disease is clinically distinguished from spinocerebellar degenerations (e.g., Friedreich's ataxia) by the absence of central signs and the presence of marked distal atrophy.[3]

Friedreich's Ataxia

The spinocerebellar degnerations are a heterogeneous group of disorders demonstrating symmetric, slowly progressive ataxia and motor symptoms with an inheritable tendency.[4] Friedreich's ataxia is the most common of the cerebella ataxias, involving both cerebellar and spinal cord pathways.[3] Onset is generally prior to 20 years of age.

The primary signs of Friedreich's ataxia include progressive ataxia, weakness, and sensory loss, and usually present before the end of puberty[3] (Table 38-4). The patient may demonstrate structural abnormalities such as symmetrical cavovarus foot and kyphoscoliosis, as well as endocrinologic or cardiac disorders. Pathologic abnormalities are primarily centered in the spinal cord, with degeneration of the posterior columns, cortical spinal tracts, and spinocerebellar tracts.[3]

Clinically, the patient exhibits muscle weakness and ataxia of gait. The lower extemities are flexive for deep tendon reflexes. There is a decreased vibratory and position sense apparent. Other neurologic symptoms include decreased visual acuity, nystagmus, paresthesias, partial deafness, and vertigo.

Table 38-4. Signs and Symptoms of Friedreich's Ataxia

PRIMARY SYMPTOMS AND SIGNS (100% constant; obligatory for diagnosis)

1. Onset before end of puberty and never after age 20
2. Ataxia of gait
3. Progression of ataxia within last two years preceeding examination to all extremities, without remission
4. Dysarthria
5. Decrease in position and/or vibratory sense in lower limbs
6. Muscle weakness
7. Deep tendon areflexia in lower limbs

SECONDARY (PROGRESSIVE) SYMPTOMS AND SIGNS (present in more than 90% of cases, eventually 100%; not obligatory for diagnosis)

1. Babinski's sign (extensor plantar response)
2. Pes cavus
3. Scoliosis
4. Cardiomyopathy

ACCESSORY SYMPTOMS AND SIGNS (present in less than 50% of cases)

1. Decrease in visual acuity (usually optic atrophy)
2. Nystagmus
3. Paresthesias
4. Partial deafness
5. Essential type tremor
6. Vertigo
7. Spasticity
8. Pain
9. Decrease in intelligence quotient (I.Q.)

(Based on Geoffrey G et al: Clinical description and roentgenologic evaluation of patients with Friedreich's ataxia. Can J Neurol Sci, 3:279–286, 1976, with permission.)

Poliomyelitis

Poliomyelitis causes paralysis and has historically been the frequent cause of cavus foot.[20] Poliomyelitis is an acute viral infectious disease that may inflict temporary or permanent destructive changes in motor function.[12] Specifically, it is due to destruction of the anterior horn cells of the spinal cord. Usually attacking younger patients, poliomyelitis causes motor paralysis and eventual muscle atrophy with no apparent loss of sensation. Reflexes, although diminished, are usually present, because reflex arcs remain intact unless all of the anterior horn cells are destroyed.[12] Lower extremity involvement generally includes weakness of the dorsiflexors and plantar flexors of the ankle, leading to claw toe deformities through extensor substitution. A weak triceps surae may be compensated for by flexor substitution of the long toe flexors. Poliomyelitis, until midcentury, was the most common acquired condition resulting in the development of pes cavus; it is also the most frequent cause of posterior cavus.[4]

TYPES OF PES CAVUS (TABLE 38-5)

Anterior Pes Cavus

Anterior pes cavus can be defined as excessive plantar flexion attitude of the forefoot or any of its component parts. Anterior pes cavus is primarily a sagittal plane deformity. There are four basic types, which are distinguished from one another

Table 38-5. Classification of Cavus Foot

I.	Anterior cavus foot		
	A.	Type of involvement	
		1.	Local
		2.	Global
	B.	Level of involvement	
		1.	Metatarsal cavus
		2.	Lesser tarsus cavus
		3.	Forefoot cavus
		4.	Combined anterior cavus
II.	Posterior cavus foot		
III.	Combined cavus foot—posterior cavus foot with anterior compensation		

Table 38-6. Anterior Pes Cavus Deformities

Types	"also known as"	Effect on the Foot
Metatarsus cavus	Metatarsus equinus	Excessive plantar flexion at Lisfranc's joint
Lesser tarsus cavus	Lesser tarsus equinus	Excessive plantar flexion over lesser tarsal bones
Forefoot cavus	Forefoot equinus	Excessive plantar flexion at Chopart's joint
Combined cavus	—	Excessive plantar flexion at two or more of the above areas

based on the apex of the deformity (i.e., the plantar angulation) (Table 38-6; Fig 38-5). Determination of the apex is through clinical examination, including both off-weight-bearing and weight-bearing positions and radiographic evaluation.

Sagittal plane deformity is dominant in this type of deformity; however, pure sagittal plane involvement is rare. Most often deformities in the two other body planes can be and often are associated with the cavus foot. Herein the complexity of the cavus foot deformity is appreciated. When the various planes of deformity are subdivided and individually considered, it will help one to understand

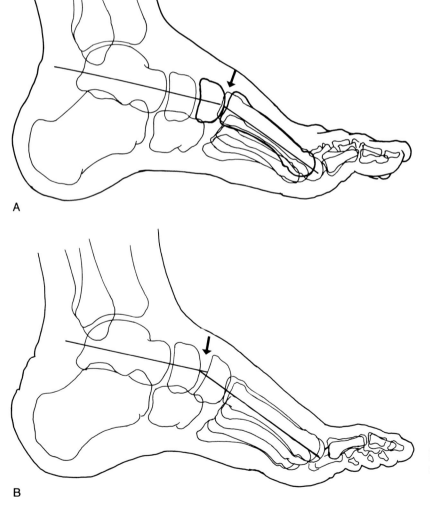

A

B

Fig. 38-5. Anterior pes cavus deformity. **(A)** Metatarsus cavus. **(B)** Lesser tarsus cavus.

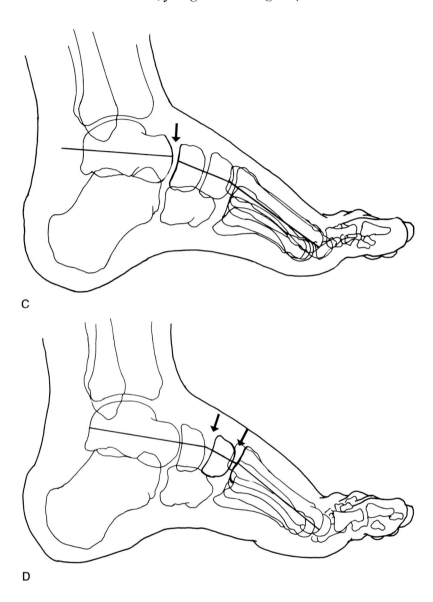

C

D

Fig. 38-5 *(continued)*. **(C)** Forefoot cavus. **(D)** Combined anterior cavus.

the function and compensation of the foot as a whole when the concomitant plane deformities are combined.

Compensation of Anterior Pes Cavus

Retraction of Digits at MPJ. This phenomenon can occur when there is an unopposed pull on the extensor digitorum longus tendon and the proximal phalanx dorsiflexes excessively at the MPJ via the sling mechanism.[11] This can occur during static non-weight-bearing position and is often exaggerated during the swing phase of gait and at heel contact. This phenomenon resultant from the active pull of the long extensors is known as extensor substitution.

Reverse Buckling at the MPJ. This occurs secondary to retraction of the digits at the MPJ whereby the metatarsal heads are depressed, allowing for increased retraction of digits, which causes more plantar flexion of metatarsal heads, and so on. Consequently, as the plantar flexion of the metatarsal heads increases, so does the anterior cavus deformity. These activities repeat themselves in cyclical fashion.

Forefoot Reduction of the Flexible Anterior Cavus. This occurs when the foot is bearing weight secondary to the ground-reactive forces. At this time, if the lesser tarsal sagittal plane flexibility is adequate, the forefoot may assume a normal position and realignment of the digits. Because this is purely sagittal plane reduction, no subtalar joint supination or pronation occur. However, in the non-weight-bearing and swing phases of gait, the retraction of the toes (extensor substitution) and reverse buckling of the MPJ continue to occur.[4] Initially flexible, these deformities often become rigid with the passage of time.

Dorsiflexion of the Foot at the Level of the Ankle. This will allow the foot to compensate more proximally for a rigid anterior cavus deformity. Because the entire foot is dorsiflexed at the ankle, the calcaneal inclination angle will be increased. If, with maximum available ankle joint dorsiflexion, there remains a need for more dorsiflexion in order to meet the demands of normal gait, a situation called "pseudoequinus" exists. Pseudoequinus is defined as a functional limitation of ankle joint dorsiflexion caused by premature utilization of ankle joint motion to compensate for structural (rigid) anterior pes cavus deformity.[4] Because this describes a true anterior pes cavus deformity, the subtalar joint is neither pronated nor supinated during the compensatory motion of ankle joint dorsiflexion.

Posterior Pes Cavus

Posterior cavus foot deformity is caused by flaccid paralysis of the calf musculature, either congenital or acquired.[21] In most situations, this results from a specific paralytic muscle imbalance in which the triceps surae is partially or completely paralyzed, with the remaining dorsiflexors and forefoot plantar flexors varying in strength. The paralysis can have many causes; however, poliomyelitis remains the most common cause throughout the world. With the decreased incidence of poliomyelitis in the United States, the problems posed by this foot deformity have significantly decreased.

The loss of normal strength of the triceps surae allows the gradual development of a "vertical calcaneus," which in the adult results in a "pistol grip deformity."[21] This shortens the lever arm upon which the triceps surae acts, thus creating the origin of a vicious cycle. Weaker calf muscles will result in a weaker pull on the calcaneal apophysis. This, when applied to a growing calcaneus, will lead to a shorter lever arm and weaker pull-off. The verticality of the calcaneus elevates the longitudinal arch, and the forefoot assumes a plantarflexed position.

Combined Pes Cavus Deformity

Etiology is most likely primarily a compensation for rigid anterior cavus deformity (i.e., the pseudoequinus foot type). It is caused by dorsiflexion of the entire foot on the ankle. Posterior pes cavus may be reduced or eliminated by ankle joint plantar flexion if no corresponding anterior pes cavus is present to resist this motion. Posterior cavus, if present, rarely occurs without an anterior cavus component.

CORRECTION OF PES CAVUS

Soft Tissue Correction

Soft tissue surgical procedures have been utilized in the treatment of pes cavus since the end of the last century.[22,23] For the most part these procedures have utilized the sectioning or transfer of the major tendinous structures of the foot. They are generally performed in combination with osseous correction of the cavus foot. Other soft tissue corrections have directed their attention to the neuromuscular imbalance frequently associated with cavus foot deformity by selectively denervating the plantar intrinsic musculature as advocated by Garceau and Brahms.[20] This procedure is mentioned only for historical purposes, because it has largely been abandoned in deference to the more frequently performed tendon transfers, which yield more predictable and reproducible results.[3]

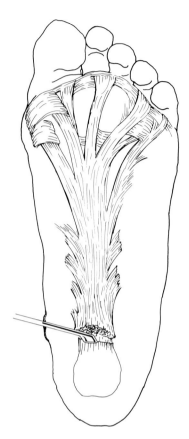

Fig. 38-6. Steindler stripping: release of the abductor digiti minimi, flexor digitorum brevis, abductor hallucis, and plantar fascia.

Plantar Release

Plantar fasciotomy has been advocated in the treatment of pes cavus since 1893.[1] Its use has been popularized by Steindler, who first described his procedure, which is a more extensive plantar release than the plantar fasciotomy, in 1917.[24,25] In his description of the procedure the plantar fascia, abductor of the fifth toe, short flexor, and abductor hallucis are released from the plantar aspect of the calcaneus (Fig. 38-6). The plantar release is utilized to release longstanding plantar contractures and is not designed to correct osseous deformity.[5]

Forefoot Tendon Transfers

Several tendon transfers have been described for the correction of the digital deformities that predominate in the cavus foot. One of the earliest de-

scriptions was Hibbs transfer of the long extensor tendon of the lesser digits to the lateral cuneiform (Fig. 38-7), with subsequent reduction of the claw-toe deformities.[26] Heyman[27] described a similar procedure with the extensor tendons being transferred to the surgical neck area of all five metatarsals, and a modification of this procedure was also performed by Frank and Johnson[28] in which the extensor tendons were combined in an "extensor shift procedure" to allow for gradation in the amount of eversion of the forefoot by shifting the majority of the tendons laterally or inversion by shifting one or more tendons medially. Jones, in the early 1900s, described his classic procedure for correction of a hammered hallux in which the extensor hallucis longus tendon is sectioned from its insertion and transferred to the head of the first metatarsal.[29,30] All of these procedures have a common feature in that they attempt to decrease dynamic force muscular imbalances that lead to the clawing of the digits and subsequent plantar flexion of the metatarsals on the midfoot. It must be kept in mind that these procedures should be utilized for the flexible forefoot cavus deformity and that in general they will be combined with osseous cor-

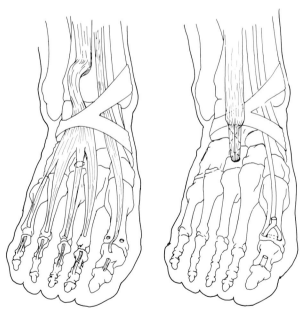

Fig. 38-7. Hibbs' procedure: release of the extensor digitorum longus tendons to all lesser digits. Transfer of combined tendons into the lateral cuneiform.

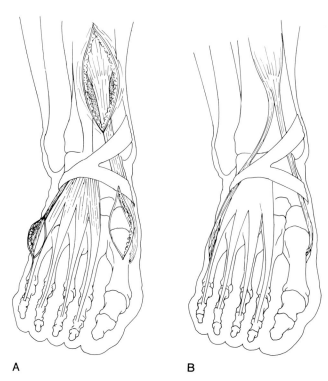

Fig. 38-8. Split tibialis anterior tendon transfer (STATT). **(A)** Tibialis anterior isolated for transfer. **(B)** Modification of STATT with lateral half of the tibialis anterior tendon transferred and anastomosed into the peroneus tertius tendon.

rection, such as fusion of the proximal interphalangeal joints of the lesser digits or interphalangeal fusion of the hallux, if the deformities have become rigid or there is significant musculotendinous imbalance at the metatarophalangeal joints.[3,4]

Rearfoot Tendon Transfers

Transfers of major tendons of the rearfoot have also been utilized in the treatment of cavus foot. Again it must be stressed that these transfers are intended for correction of the dynamic force acting to create the cavus foot and must be combined with osseous procedures if structural deformity exists.

In patients with weakness of the gastrocnemius-soleus complex, Peabody advocated transfer of the tibialis anterior tendon to the calcaneus.[31] This procedure was described for the postpoliomyelitis patient or patients with L4 and L5 myelomeningocele with an overpowering of the tibialis anterior leading to cavus foot deformity.[3,32,33]

Another more frequently utilized transfer of the tibialis anterior involves splitting it and either transferring the lateral half of the tendon into the cuboid[33] (Fig. 38-8) or anastomosing it to the peroneus tertius at the level of the fifth metatarsal base.[4] This allows for a decrease in the supinating effect that the tibialis anterior generally exerts at the longitudinal midtarsal joint axis and also aids in direct dorsiflexion of the ankle joint since the vector forces of its pull are now more perpendicular to the axis of the ankle joints.[4]

Transfer of the tibialis posterior has also been described for treatment of cavus foot deformities. Two of the main functions of the tibialis posterior are to (1) accelerate subtalar joint supination and external rotation of the leg during midstance, and (2) maintain stability of the midtarsal joint in the direction of supination around its oblique axis.[9] Because of this, Royle in 1927 proposed transfer of the tibialis posterior to the heel in patients in whom he believed the tibialis posterior was the primary deformity force and who demonstrated weakness of the gastrocnemius-soleus group.[35] Transfer of

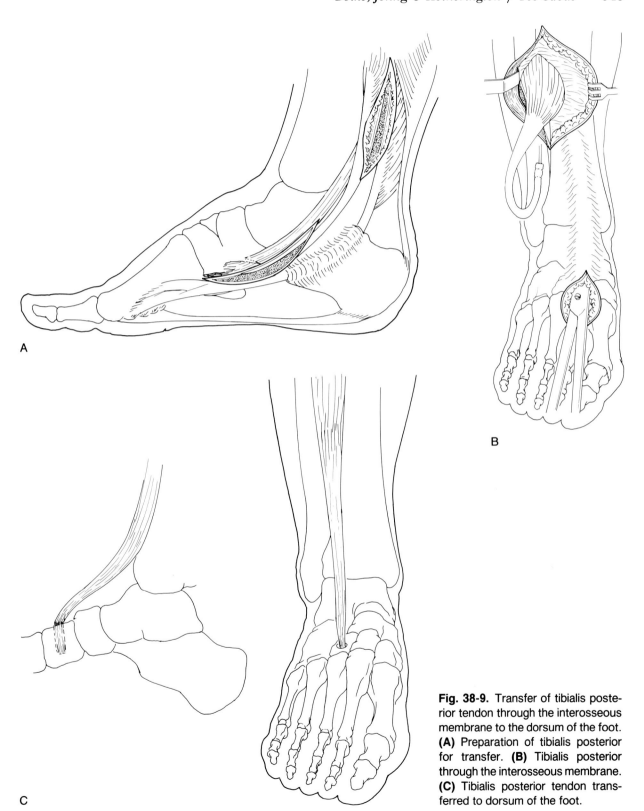

A

B

C

Fig. 38-9. Transfer of tibialis posterior tendon through the interosseous membrane to the dorsum of the foot. **(A)** Preparation of tibialis posterior for transfer. **(B)** Tibialis posterior through the interosseous membrane. **(C)** Tibialis posterior tendon transferred to dorsum of the foot.

the tibialis posterior is more frequently performed in the combined deformity of cavus foot with concomitant foot-drop [i.e., those patients with anterior (extensor) weakness]. In this situation the tibialis posterior is sectioned at its insertion on the navicular and is transferred through the interosseous membrane to the dorsum of the foot at the level of the third cuneiform[37] (Fig. 38-9). Because of the previously mentioned functions of the tibialis posterior, one must take into account the stability of the rearfoot complex, realizing that severe pes planus deformity may occur if stability is not achieved via rearfoot fusion.[4,38]

Peroneus longus transfers have been utilized to decrease plantar flexion of the first ray and also to aid in dorsiflexion of the ankle joint in patients with weak extensors (especially tibialis anterior function). The peroneus longus is sectioned deep to the lateral aspect of the cuboid and transferred through the intermuscular septum of the lateral and anterior compartment of the leg into the dorsum of the foot (Fig. 38–10). The tendon may be transferred as a unit into the lateral cuneiform area or may be split and anastomosed with the peroneus brevis tendon laterally and the tibialis anterior tendon medially.[4,39] The peroneus longus may also be sectioned deep to the lateral aspect of the cuboid and subsequently transferred or anastomosed to the peroneus brevis tendon insertion, thereby increasing the function of the peroneus brevis as a pronator of the subtalar joint with subsequent reduction of the cavus deformity. As with all tendon transfers for cavus foot, this transfer is dependent on the foot having a flexible deformity.[3,40]

It would seem appropriate at this time to mention the concomitant use of lengthening of the gastrocnemius or gastrocnemius-soleus complex in the treatment of cavus foot. Prior to any Achilles tendon lengthening or gastrocnemius recession it is of the utmost importance to rule out the presence of pseudoequinus [i.e., preutilization of ankle joint dorsiflexion secondary to a structural forefoot cavus (forefoot equinus)]. If a posterior lengthening is performed in these patients, an actual increase in calcaneal inclination may be seen with subsequent worsening of the deformity. It would be appropriate in these cases to perform procedures that would decrease the calcaneal inclination angle or forefoot equinus and thereby procedure a relative lengthening of the posterior group.[41]

Osseous Procedures in the Management of Cavus Foot

Osseous procedures used in the management of cavus foot are outlined in Table 38-7.

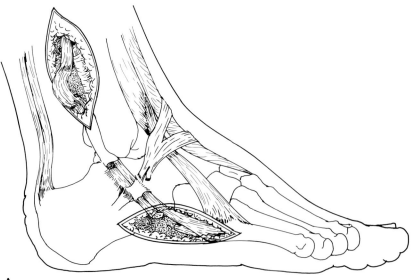

A

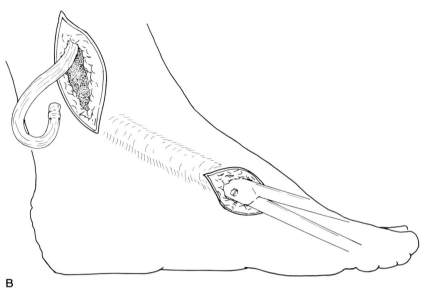

B

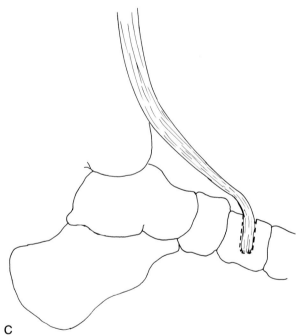

Fig. 38-10. Peroneus longus tendon transferred into the dorsum of the foot. **(A)** Preparation of peroneus longus tendon for transfer. **(B)** Peroneus longus transfer subcutaneously. **(C)** Peroneus longus transferred to dorsum of the foot.

C

Table 38-7. Osseous Procedures Used in the Management of Pes Cavus

Midfoot osteotomy	
Steindler[42]	1921
Cole[43]	1940
Imhauser[44]	1952
Japas[45]	1968
Akron midtarsal dome[47]	1985
Calcaneal osteotomy	
Dwyer[48]	1955
Silver[55]	1967
"T" osteotomy[56]	1980
Curvilinear osteotomy[57]	1981
Metatarsal osteotomy	
Japas (first metatarsal)[45]	1940
Swanson (metatarsal base)[58]	1966
Arthrodesis	
McElvenny and Caldwell[59]	1958
Jahss (tarsometatarsal arthrodesis)[60]	1980
Triple arthrodesis[61]	
Digital arthrodesis including the hallux	

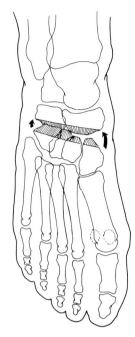

Fig. 38-11. Cole midfoot osteotomy.

Midfoot Osteotomy

Osteotomy of the midfoot for management of rigid pes cavus has been advocated by several authors. Steindler, in 1921,[42] discussed a cuneiform osteotomy involving the talar neck, cuboid, and anterior process of the calcaneus in cavus foot with marked skeletal deformity. Steindler reported satisfactory results in 31 cases using the osteotomy and the Steindler stripping procedure.

Cole,[43] in 1940, described a "so-called anterior-tarsal-wedge osteotomy." Cole did not believe that destruction of the midtarsal joint was justified and thought that function could be maintained using the anterior-tarsal wedge osteotomy (Fig. 38-11). Using a dorsolinear approach a wedge of bone is resected from the tarsus in the following manner. The first osteotomy, which is almost vertical, is made near the center of the navicular and cuboid, extending plantarly; the second osteotomy, beginning anterior to the first, is angled to form a wedge with the first osteotomy. The apex of the wedge is plantar, and the base dorsal. The size of the wedge required is relative to degree of deformity. The wedge of bone is removed and the forefoot placed in better alignment. In addition to the osteotomy, plantar fascial release may also be required. Hammer and claw digit deformity must be addressed

separately, and the wedge resection may be performed in conjunction with a tendon transfer such as the Hibbs procedure.

Imhauser in 1952 described a more extensive midfoot osteotomy for pes cavus. This osteotomy is a dorsally based wedge in which the proximal cut resects the talus and the calcaneus joint while the distal cut removes the entire navicular, the proximal joint surfaces of the cuneiforms, and part of the cuboid. After alignment osseous union will occur between the navicular, cuneiforms, and calcaneus and the cuboid (Fig. 38-12). This procedure allows for reduction of even severe deformity in multiple planes but sacrifices the midtarsal joint.[44] Tarsal "V" osteotomy for pes cavus was described and evaluated by Japas in 1968.[45] This osteotomy is performed between the midtarsal and tarsometatarsal joints (Fig. 38-13). The point of the "V" proximally is located ideally at the apex of the deformity. The limbs of the osteotomy extend to the cuboid laterally and the first cuneiform medially; a plantar fasciotomy is performed in conjunction with the osteotomy. The midtarsal joint line is determined prior to performance of the osteotomy so as to avoid compromise of this joint. After perform-

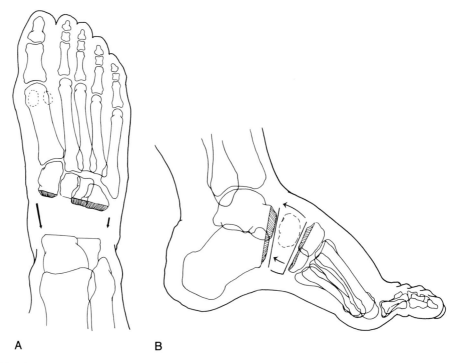

Fig. 38-12. Imhauser osteotomy. **(A)** Dorsal view. **(B)** Lateral view.

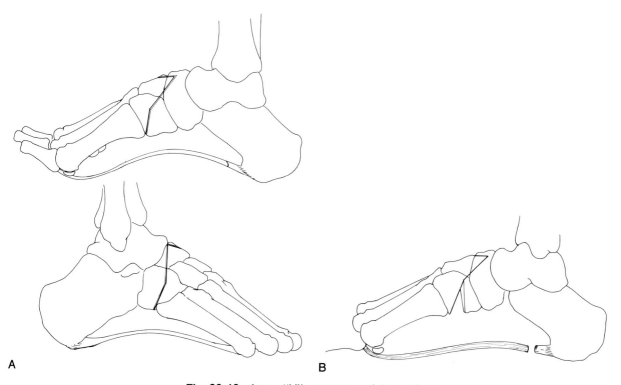

Fig. 38-13. Japas ''V'' osteotomy of the midfoot.

ance of the osteotomy the anterior portion of the osteotomy and the forefoot are dorsiflexed by displacement of the osteotomy, reducing the cavus. Japas recommended that transverse plane deviation of the forefoot be accomplished by simple manipulation of the forefoot. Once satisfactory alignment is obtained fixation may be by one or two pins. Japas reported subtalar joint range of motion to be unaffected or slightly limited following osteotomy. Midtarsal motion was reduced in all patients. He also reported a widening of the midfoot postoperatively. As pointed out by Japas, this osteotomy is indicated for anterior pes cavus in unilateral cases in which other resections or arthrodesis would result in unequal foot length. He advised against performance of the osteotomy in patients under 7 years of age.

Of the 17 feet treated by Japas 12 showed complete correction of the cavus, described as painlessness with good subtalar and midtarsal joint motion. Five feet were reported to have incomplete correction of the deformity with residual discomfort beneath the metatarsal heads on weightbearing.

Altehhuber and Grill[46] reported complete correction of pes cavus in 12 of 16 feet in 11 patients. They also reported, as did Japas, inadequate correction of the deformity with the "V" osteotomy. This may be a result of insufficient displacement of the osteotomy or other problems, such as a posterior component of the deformity not addressed with the "V" osteotomy or plantar flexion of the first metatarsal.

A midtarsal "dome" procedure for the management of rigid pes cavus or pes cavovarus was described by Wilcox and Weiner.[47] This is most commonly performed through the cuneiforms, cuboid, and base of the fifth metatarsal (Fig. 38-14). A 1-cm lateral curved wedge of bone is removed. The osteotomy has the potential for three-dimensional correction and is performed in conjunction with a plantar fascial release. The overall success rate reported was 67 percent. A 94 percent satisfactory result level was attained in patients greater than 8 years of age; all of the patients with unsatisfactory results were less than 8 years of age. Wilcox and Weiner attributed this failure rate in the younger age group as being due to considerable growth potential and therefore greater potential for continued deformity.

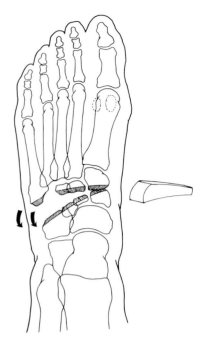

Fig. 38-14. Akron midtarsal dome osteotomy as described by Wilcox and Weiner.

Calcaneal Osteotomies

The best known of the calcaneal osteotomies for the management of cavus foot is that described by Dwyer.[48,49] This procedure is essentially a closing wedge osteotomy of the body of calcaneus performed through a lateral approach (Fig. 38-15). The apex of the wedge is located medially and the base laterally. Dwyer recommended a wedge of 8 to 12 mm of bone be resected; failure to completely correct the varus position of the heel will result in recurrence. Dwyer noted "In a few cases it has been necessary to repeat the operation either because incomplete correction was not obtained at the first operation or because of real recurrence." As did Cole and Japas, Dwyer recommended preservation of subtalar and midtarsal mobility. He also recommended that, in adults with fixed osseous deformity of the forefoot, an "appropriate wedge" be taken from the tarsometatarsal region[8] or osteotomy of the first metatarsal be performed for plantar flexion of the first metatarsal.[2] Dwyer[50] further modified this calcaneal osteotomy for the management of the varus heel secondary to relapsed clubfoot. This procedure consists of a medially based

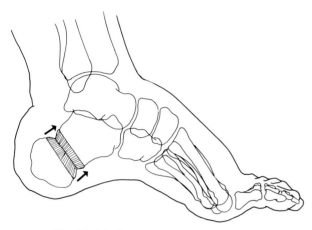

Fig. 38-15. Dwyer calcaneal osteotomy.

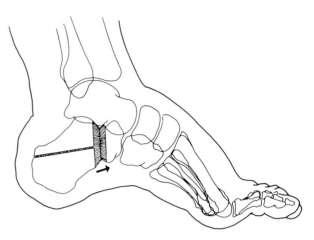

Fig. 38-16. "T" osteotomy of the calcaneus as described by Pandey et al.

opening wedge of the calcaneus with insertion of a bone graft.

Fisher and Shaffer,[51] in a review of calcaneal osteotomies of the Dwyer type, found calcaneal osteotomies to be effective in the correction of heel varus and recommended the procedure in children with clubfoot deformity requiring osseous correction but who are too young for triple arthrodesis. They were less than optimistic regarding the correction obtained for cavus foot and forefoot adduction. These findings were also confirmed by Dekel and Weissman.[52]

Calcaneal osteotomy of the Dwyer type is usually reserved for patients with a fixed calcaneal varus. Varus of the heel may be a reflection of a forefoot valgus or plantar flexion of the first metatarsal. To distinguish between a fixed varus or varus of the rearfoot secondary to a structurally plantar flexed first ray, the lateral block test[53,54] may be utilized. As described by Coleman and Chestnut,[53] the heel and lateral border of the foot are placed on a block so that full weightbearing can occur. The first metatarsal is allowed to hang free. A flexible rearfoot will assume a normal position, demonstrating a reduction in rearfoot varus. If the heel remains in varus, a rigid deformity is present. Calcaneal osteotomy was also advocated by Silver et al. for the management of the varus position of the rearfoot in pes cavus.[55]

A complex "T" osteotomy of the calcaneus is used for the management of resistant cavovarus with adduction of the forefoot[56] (Fig. 38-16). The osteotomy can also be described as a closing wedge osteotomy of the calcaneus performed 1.0 to 1.5 cm behind and parallel to the calcaneocuboid joint. The amount of wedge removed is relative to the degree of forefoot adduction present. The second portion of the osteotomy is performed horizontally in the remaining body of the calcaneus, beginning at the halfway point of the vertical osteotomy. The osteotomy may be modified to include a wedge resection. The posterior-inferior fragment with the attachment of the Achilles tendon is then displaced laterally. Pandey et al. reported, however, that complete reduction of forefoot adduction may not be accomplished by "T" osteotomy and may require additional correction via a separate procedure.

Bradley and Coleman[57] described a curvilinear displacement osteotomy for the management of calcaneocavus (Fig. 38-17).

Metatarsal Osteotomies

Japas[45] recommended osteotomy of the first metatarsal only in anterior cavus deformity resulting from plantar flexion of the first metatarsal. Proximal wedge resection osteotomy of the metatarsals for pes cavus has also been described by Swanson et al.[58]

Arthrodesis

Arthrodesis plays an important role in the management of the deformity and instability that may be associated with cavus foot. McElvenny and Caldwell[59] described fusion of the first

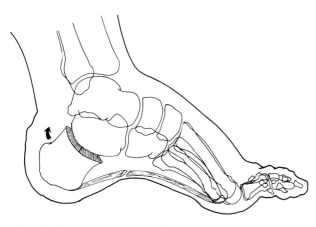

Fig. 38-17. Cresentic or curvilinear osteotomy of the calcaneus as described by Bradley and Coleman.

metatarsal – cuneiform joint and naviculocuneiform joint for the management of both flexible and rigid cavus deformity.

Jahss[60] recommended a tarsometatarsal truncated-wedge arthrodesis for pes cavus and forefoot equinus deformity and reported uniformly good results. It was pointed out that in severe cases of pes cavus correction was incomplete; however, the pa-

tients were satisfied. Excellent results were reported for relief of metatarsal pain, calluses, and deformity in mild to moderate forefoot equinus, pes cavus, and equinovarus agulation with normal metatarsal padding. Contraindications to the procedure as reported by Jahss include painful subtalar joint motion, varus deformity of the heel, plantar hyperkeratosis proximal to Lisfranc's joint, pes cavus associated with muscular imbalance, and performance of the procedure prior to skeletal maturity.

Triple arthrodesis is utilized in the management of cavus foot structural deformity of the rearfoot, instability, and in deformity associated with progressive neuromuscular disease. Reduction of deformity can be accomplished in several body planes at one time by careful preoperative planning and resection of bone of the appropriate size and angular configuration (Fig. 38-18). In a review of the surgical management of progressive neuromuscular disease in children, Levitt et al.[61] found triple arthrodesis to played a significant role. Triple arthrodesis should not be performed before the age of skeletal maturity. Prior to skeletal maturity the sequence of procedures used to manage deformity

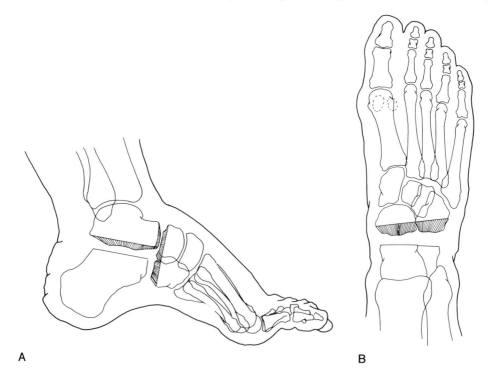

A   B

Fig. 38-18. Triple arthrodesis. **(A)** Lateral view. **(B)** Dorsal view.

and maintain function must be individualized. This includes the use of osseous as well as soft tissue procedures, including tendon transfers. After stabilization of the foot by triple arthrodesis, foot function may be augmented by subsequent tendon transfers. Complications associated with triple arthrodesis include degenerative changes of the ankle and midfoot, pseudoarthrosis, avascular necrosis of the talus, and residual deformity.[62]

Arthrodesis of the lesser digits is performed for clawtoe and hammer toe deformity and instability of the digits. Digital arthrodesis may also be performed as an adjunct procedure with tendon transfers such as the Hibbs procedure. Arthrodesis of the interphalangeal joint of the great toe is utilized for hallux hammer toe and in conjunction with the Jones tenosuspension of the first metatarsal.

REFERENCES

1. Romer AS: The Vertebrate Body, 4th Ed. p.68. WB Saunders, Philadelphia, 1971
2. Mayer PJ: Pes cavus: a diagnostic and therapeutic challenge. Orthop Rev 7:105–116, 1978
3. Hsu JD, Imbus CE: Pes cavus. p. 464. In Jahss MH (ed): Disorders of the Foot, Vol. I. WB Saunders, Philadelphia, 1982
4. Green DR, Lepow GM, Smith TF: Pes cavus. In Comprehensive Textbook of Foot Surgery, Vol. I. p. 287. Williams & Wilkins, Baltimore, 1987
5. Andry N: Orthopedia (Facsimile Reproduction of the First Edition in English, London 1943.) JB Lippincott, Philadelphia, 1961
6. Snell RS: Clinical Anatomy for Medical Students. p. 584. Little, Brown and Co., Boston, 1973
7. Giannestras NJ: Foot Disorders, Medical and Surgical Management, 2nd Ed. p. 35. Lea & Febiger, Philadelphia, 1973.
8. Duchenne GB: The Physiology of Motion (Translated by EB Kaplan.) WB Saunders, Philadelphia, 1959
9. Root ML, Orien WP, Weed JH: Normal and Abnormal Function of the Foot, Vol. II. p. 204. Clinical Biomechanics Corp, Los Angeles, CA, 1977
10. Basmajian JB, Steco G: The role of muscles in arch support of the foot. J Bone Joint Surg [Am] 45a:1184–1190, 1963
11. Jarret BA, Manzi JA, Green DR: Interossei and lumbricales muscles of the foot. J Am Podiatry Assoc 70:1–13, 1980
12. Hoppenfeld S: Evaluation of nerve root lesions involving the trunk and lower extremity. pp. 45–47, 72–74. In Orthopaedic Neurology. JB Lippincott, Philadelphia, 1974
13. Brewerton DA, Sandifer PH, Sweetman DR: Idiopathic pes cavus. Br Med J 1:659–661, 1963
14. McNutt W, Klingman W, Lynch H et al: Pes cavus and hereditary ataxia. Tex Rep Biol Med 18:222–232, 1960
15. Crenshaw AH (ed): Campbells Operative Orthopedics, 5th Ed., Vol. II. CV Mosby, St. Louis 1971
16. McGlamry ED, Kitting RW: Equinus foot — analysis of the etiology, pathology and treatment techniques. J Am Podiatry Assoc 63:165–184, 1973
17. Whitney AK, Green DR: Pseudoequinus. J Am Podiatry Assoc 72:365–371, 1982
18. Green DR, Ruch JA, McGlamry ED: Correction of equinus related forefoot deformities. J Am Podiatry Assoc 66:768–780, 1976
19. Cavuoto JW: Foot surgery in Charcot-Marie-Tooth disease. J Foot Surg 19:130–133, 1980
20. Garceau GJ, Brahms MA: A preliminary study of selective plantar muscle denervation for pes cavus. J Bone Joint Surg [Am], 38a:553–562, 1956
21. Coleman SS: Complex Foot Deformities in Children. pp. 147–149, 167–172. Lea & Febiger, Philadelphia, 1983
22. Thomas W: On the treatment of talipes cavus. Birmingham Med Rev 34:1–5, 1893
23. Barawell G: Pes planus and pes cavus; an anatomical and clinical study. Edinburgh Med J 3:113–124, 1898
24. Steindler A: Operative treatment of pes cavus. Surg Gynecol Obstet 24:612–615, 1917
25. Steindler A: Stripping of the os calcis. Am J Orthop Surg 2:8–12, 1920
26. Hibbs RA: An operation for "claw foot." J Am Podiatry Assoc 73:1583–1585, 1983
27. Heyman CH: The operative treatment of claw foot. J Bone Joint Surg 14:335–338, 1932
28. Frank GR, Johnson WM: The extensor shift procedure in the correction of clawfoot deformities in children. South Med J 59:889–896, 1966
29. Jones R: Note on Military Orthopedics. Cassel and Co, London, 1917
30. Jones R: The soldier's foot and the treatment of common deformities of the foot. Part II. Claw foot. Br Med J 1:749, 1916
31. Peabody CW: Tendon transposition. J Bone Joint Surg 20:193–205, 1938
32. Turner JW, Cooper RR: Posterior transposition of

tibialis anterior through the interosseous membrane. Clin Orthop 79:71–74, 1971

33. Feiwell E: Paralytic calcaneus in myelomeningocele. In McLaurin RL (ed): Myelomeningocele, Grune & Stratton, New York, 1977

34. Hoffer MM et al: The split anterior tibial tendon transfer is the treatment of spastic varus, third foot of childhood. Orthop Clin North Am 5:31, 1974

35. Royle ND: A new concept in the etiology of claw foot and associated talipes equinus. J Bone Joint Surg 9:465–468, 1927

36. Hsu JD, Hoffer MM: Posterior tibial tendon transfer anteriorum through the interosseous membrane. Clin Orthop 131:202–204, 1978

37. Turner JW, Cooper RR: Anterior Transfer of tibialis posterior through the interosseous membrane. Clin Orthop 83:241, 1972

38. Schneider M, Balon K: Deformity of the foot following anterior transfer of the posterior tibial tendon and lengthening of the Achilles tendon for spactic equino-varus. Clin Orthop 125:113, 1977

39. McGlamry ED (ed): Reconstructive Surgery of the Foot and Leg. p. 347. Symposium Specialists, Miami, 1974

40. Bentzon PGK: Pes cavus and the muscle peroneus longus. Acta Orthop Scand 4:50, 1933

41. Fenton CF, McGlamry ED, Perane M: Severe cavus deformity secondary to Charcot-Marie-Tooth disease. J Am Podiatry Assoc 72(4):171–175, 1982

42. Steindler A: The treatment of pes cavus (hollow claw foot). Arch Surg 2:225–237, 1921

43. Cole WH: The treatment of claw-foot. J Bone Joint Surg 22:895–908, 1940

44. Steinhaeuser J: Die Arthrodesen der Chopart' Schen Gelenklinie. Buckerei des Orthopaden 20. p. 78. Ferdinamd Euke Verlag, Stuttgart, 1978

45. Japas LM: Surgical treatment of pes cavus by tarsal V osteotomy. J Bone Joint Surg [Am], 927–944, 1968

46. Altehhuber J, Grill F: Treatment of pes cavus with the V-osteotomy according to Japas. Chir Piede 8(5):341–344, 1984

47. Wilcox PG, Weiner DS: The Akron midtarsal osteotomy in the treatment of rigid pes cavus: a preliminary review. J Pediatr Orthop 5:333–338, 1985

48. Dwyer FC: Osteotomy of the calcaneum for pes cavus. J Bone Joint Surg [Br] 41:80–86, 1959

49. Dwyer FC: The present status of the problem of pes cavus. Clin Orthop Related Res 106:254–274, 1975

50. Dwyer FC: The treatment of relapsed clubfoot by insertion of a wedge into the calcaneum. J Bone Joint Surg [Br] 45:67–75, 1963

51. Fisher RL, Shaffer SR: An evaluation of calcaneal osteotomy in cogential clubfoot and other disorders. Clin Orthop Related Res 70:141–147, 1970

52. Dekel S, Weissman SL: Osteotomy of the calcaneus and concomitant plantar stripping in children with talipes cavo-varus. J Bone Joint Surg [Br] 55:802–808, 1973

53. Coleman SS, Chestnut WJ: A simple test for hindfoot flexibility in the cavovarus foot. Clin Orthop Related Res 123:60–62, 1977

54. Paulos L, Coleman SS, Samuelson KM: Pes cavovarus. J Bone Joint Surg [Am] 62:942–953, 1980

55. Silver CM, Simon SD, Spindel E, Litchman NM, Scala M: Calcaneal osteotomy for valgus and varus deformities of the foot in cerebral palsy: a preliminary report on twenty-seven operations. J Bone Joint Surg [Am] 49:232, 1967

56. Pandey S, Jha SS, Pandey AK: "T" osteotomy of the calcaneum. Int Orthop 4:219–224, 1980

57. Bradley GW, Coleman SS: Treatment of the calcaneocavus foot deformity. J Bone Joint Surg [Am] 63:1159–1166, 1981

58. Swanson AB, Browne HS, Coleman JD: The cavus foot—concepts of production and treatment by metatarsal osteotomy. J Bone Joint Surg [Am] 48:1019, 1966

59. McElvenny RT, Caldwell GD: A new operation for correction of cavus foot: fusion of the metatarsocuneiform navicular joints. Clin Orthop Related Res 11:85–92, 1958

60. Janss MH: Tarsometatarsal truncated-wedge arthrodesis for pes cavus and equinovarus deformity of the fore part of the foot. J Bone Joint Surg [Am] 62:713–722, 1980

61. Levitt RL, Canale ST, Cooke AJ, Garland JJ: The role of foot surgery in progressive neuromuscular disorders in children. J Bone Joint Surg [Am] 55:1396–1409, 1973

62. Angus PD, Cowell HR: Triple arthrodesis. J Bone Joint Surg [Br] 68:260–265, 1986

Complex Deformations: Paralytic and Nonparalytic

39

Harold W. Vogler, D.P.M.

Major deformity of the foot can be divided into two main categories: paralytic and nonparalytic. The nature of the deformity and its process is relatively predictable in the various paralytic states. As an underlying tenet the surgeon must, whenever possible, define the underlying paralytic process. Nonparalytic deformations can present as equally challenging conditions. The basic principles of management differ, however. Thus, it becomes paramount for the physician to define the contributing etiology prior to designing a treatment regimen, surgical or nonsurgical.

PARALYTIC DEFORMITY OF THE FOOT AND ANKLE

Assessment of major deformity of the foot and ankle in paralytic states is dependent upon the level and extent of paralytic involvement.[1,2] Spastic deformities have a different natural course than flaccid conditions. Surgical and nonsurgical management is based upon principles that are specific for either entity.[2-4]

Spastic Deformities

Cerebral palsies comprise the largest single group of congenital neurodeformities contributing to recalcitrant foot and ankle deformity.[2,4,5] Such involvement can be apparent at birth or manifest itself in subtle forms insidiously over the early years of life of the child[2,6] (Fig. 39-1).

Extensive spastic involvement is usually diagnosed early—often at the time of birth. Birth "scoring" can provide early assistance in the prognosis of paralytic conditions, but this information must be correlated with other assessment and evaluation yardsticks. Unfortunately, the full impact of spastic paralytic involvement does not manifest itself initially but rather later, as growth proceeds and ancillary system involvement becomes apparent.[2]

Acquired spastic conditions such as those resulting from cerebral vascular accidents, brain-damaged states, or spinal cord injury or neoplasms, and amyotrophic lateral sclerosis, can also cause a variety of spastic lower limb deformities that are quite difficult to manage.[7] Each entity has typical hallmarks in terms of neurologic findings at examination as well as specific foot deformities produced as a result of the process.[2,3,7,8]

Spastic foot and ankle deformity will usually de-

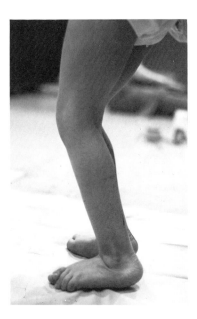

Fig. 39-1. "Crouch" stance position in a 5-year-old child with spastic cerebral palsy and compensated spastic equinovalgus bilaterally.

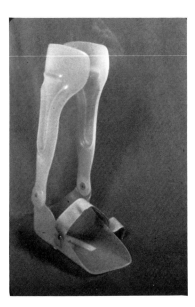

Fig. 39-2. Molded polypropylene orthoses are lightweight and can be made in a variety of forms to control spastic and flaccid deformity. Flaccid deformities are easier to accommodate than spastic deformities, which often require surgery in order to be properly placed in an orthotic.

velop from any upper motor neuron lesion regardless of the etiology.[1,2,7] Etiologic determination will facilitate the approach and solidify the treatment regimen. The age of encounter provides another aspect of consideration that will ultimately help determine which type of surgical or nonsurgical management is in the best interest of the patient.[2] In general, the longer the deformity is allowed to persist without treatment (splinting, bracing, or surgery) the greater the tendency for rigidity.[9] Bracing without benefit of surgical consideration is generally limited to those patients who are not candidates for surgery because of anesthesia risks or severity of involvement.[7,8] The decision regarding soft tissue surgery versus bone surgery will depend on whether or not the deformity is reducible passively, and the severity of the paralytic process. It should be noted that braces are important adjuncts in the management of spastic conditions, but they are much less able to control position and function than they are in states of flaccid paralysis[1,2] (Fig. 39-2).

Complex Spastic Foot and Ankle Deformities

All complex deformities of the foot and ankle are reflective of the distribution of the paralytic process at its level of origin. The most difficult aspect of these deformities to control is the spastic elements. The "acerebral" flaccid muscles that develop are typically under control of the motor area as opposed to the spastic muscles, which are controlled by the premotor area. The "acerebral" musculature plays an important role in assessment and management since it can be the companion of spastic paralysis, especially in cerebral palsy. Ultimately, the surgeon must recognize that spastic muscles will always remain spastic regardless of surgical or nonsurgical care. With this in mind, it becomes apparent that the results of motor redistribution surgery are difficult to predict yet valuable in achieving stabilization and permanence of correction.[1,2]

Spastic Equinus

Pure spastic equinus gait can occur in cerebral palsy, stroke, and multiple sclerosis. These condi-

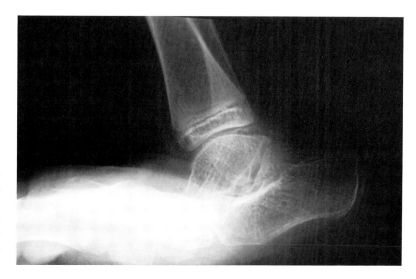

Fig. 39-3. Compensated spastic equinovalgus. This deformity is almost impossible to control with orthotics or braces, and Green-Grice extra-articular arthrodesis of the subtalar joint is usually indicated, with some form of equinus release.

tions must be differentiated from congenital nonspastic contracture of the triceps muscle group as well as psychomotor toe walking.[1] Thorough neurologic examination will ultimately yield the differential diagnosis. Persistence of this dynamic deformity is inconsistent with a functional gait, and it requires surgical treatment in younger patients. If this condition is allowed to persist, tarsal compensation in the form of midfoot collapse eventually develops and adds another complicating factor to the surgical regimen.[2,10] Severe equinovalgus develops by the time the patient reaches adolescence or earlier (Fig. 39-3). This compound deformity is more difficult to deal with than pure spastic equinus.

The triceps surae is the strongest muscle group of the musculoskeletal system. It has two major components: the gastrocnemius and the soleus. Electromyography (EMG) dynamics have demonstrated difficulty in separating the prime contributing role of each of these muscles in the production of phasic distortion.[11,12] Likewise, the Silfverskiold test (knee-flexed versus knee-extended position for determination of ankle dorsiflexion) has been determined to be unreliable in diagnosing selective contracture of the gastrocnemius.[11,12] Therefore, operative intervention is aimed at reconciling both major components of this muscle mass. The only operative concept that addresses this principle is transfer of the entire triceps anteriorly behind the

subtalar joint[13] (Fig. 39-4). This operation accomplishes this objective by shortening the lever arm of the muscle mass, reducing its mechanical advantage by 48 percent in the swing phase while only reducing its push-off effect by 15 percent in the propulsive phase.[2,14,15] Alternatively, lengthening of the gastrocnemius aponeurosis is said to reduce the tendency for recurrence more than regular

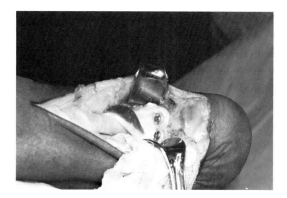

Fig. 39-4. Intraoperative scenario of Murphy triceps advancement. The Achilles tendon is passed anterior to the flexor hallucis longus to retard its tendency to return to its original anatomic site. It is inserted as posterior as possible behind the subtalar joint and fixated with serrated washers and cancellous screws to avoid pull-out sutures or other suture fixations.

Achilles tendon lengthening.[4,16] Selective lengthening of the gastrocnemius aponeurosis reduces the myotatic reflex by desensitizing the stretch reflex of the biarticular gastrocnemius.[16] The remaining pretibial musculature is then given the opportunity to overcome the phasic distortion of the triceps during swing phase function.[2] This operation can be augmented by the utilization of the Babinski response to facilitate firing of the acerebral tibialis anterior.[17] This is accomplished by weaving extensor hallucis longus through tibialis anterior, encouraging the later to fire spontaneously as the Babinski response engages.[2,17] Ankle foot orthotic (AFO) devices should be continued following these operations.

Spastic Equinovalgus

Equinovalgus of the foot develops when compensation occurs in cases of pure spastic equinus or when there is concurrent spastic involvement of the peroneus brevis.[4,10] The deformity is progressive and results in deterioration of the tarsus during the early years of ambulation. Pain develops from tarsal collapse and impingement of the talar head and navicular plantar as well as from collapse and impingement along the lateral column under the cuboid.[10] Early surgery is very beneficial in altering the disabling course of spastic equinovalgus. In childhood and adolescence, equinus release combined with Green-Grice extra-articular arthrodesis produces good tarsal stability and correction.[2,14,18] One should be very cautious in performing classic Achilles tendon elongations concurrently with Green-Grice fusions and anterior tendon transfers

for fear of producing reversal of deformity into calcaneus.[2] When augmentation of dorsiflexion is being considered (tendon transfers from the posterior deep compartment or lateral crural compartment to the anterior compartment), a two-stage operation is safe and predictable, following rehabilitation of the equinus release procedure.

Passively reducible spastic equinovalgus can be controlled with a combination of a valgus blocking procedure such as subtalar joint arthroereisis[19] and concurrent transfer of the offending spastic muscles to restorative positions[2,4] (Fig. 39-5). This usually takes the form of Murphy anterior advancement of the heel cord and into-talus transfer of the peroneus brevis.[2] Another option for elimination of the deforming force of the spastic peroneus brevis is retromalleolar transfer into the posterior tibial, which is usually "acerebral" or unable to function because of mechanical tarsal dysplasia. These augmentative transfers accomplish removal of the deforming forces while utilizing the power of these muscles to reverse the mechanogenesis of the valgus thrust of the talus. Tibialis anterior is usually "acerebral" in this condition and of little primary transfer use.

End-stage spastic equinovalgus with major collapse and rigidity will ultimately require correctional triple arthrodesis with equinus release. Failure to release the equinus component in young adults or late adolescents will make tarsal repositioning difficult and force the fusion to be accomplished in severe valgus.[2,4] In adults or older patients having the operation primarily for control of degenerative arthritic pain, fusion alone will be satisfactory. Varusation osteotomy of the heel by in-

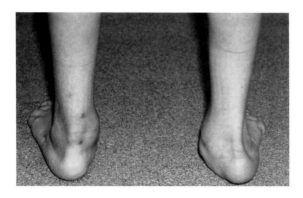

Fig. 39-5. Spastic equinovalgus controlled on the left with into-talus transfer of the spastic peroneus brevis, STA-Peg arthroeresis, percutaneous Achilles tendon lengthening, and split translocation of the tibialis anterior into the cartilage of a 5-year-old.

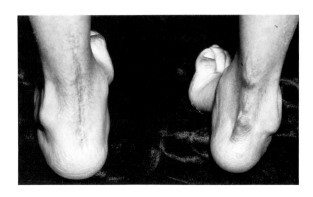

Fig. 39-6. Bilateral spastic clubfoot, worse on the right, in an 8-year-old child. The patient had undergone eight prior operations, none of which addressed the spastic posterior tibial. Reconstruction was performed with revisional radical posterior, medial, and lateral release with lateral column Evans calcaneal cuboid fusion and transfer of the posterior tibial through the interosseous membrane to the midfoot.

sertion of a bone implant into the lateral wall of the os calcis can centralize the heel back under the leg and be of benefit in this condition also.[2,4,20]

Spastic Equinovarus

Spastic clubfoot is a common deformity in cerebral palsy (Fig. 39-6). If the deformity is entirely dynamic without fixation, then selective tendon transfer can play an important role in producing stability.[2] More often than not major tarsal fusion is required for permanent correction. The most sound approach is the combination of major tarsal fusion with selective tendon transfers. One must determine whether or not the deformity is fixated and reducible.[21] This may require examination under general anesthesia to eliminate the influence of the higher brain centers. Such examination is usually performed at the time of surgery, with the surgeon prepared to perform the indicated procedure. Dynamic EMG may be of some aid in planning surgery; however, the appearance of the foot under the influence of general anesthesia ultimately provides the most reliable information as to the degree of rigidity of the condition.

Skeletal fusion may take the form of Green-Grice extra-articular arthrodesis if the child's bones are not ossified adequately for triple arthrodesis.[2,21] If the triceps is an offending factor it is lengthened or transferred anteriorly. Typically, the posterior tibial and the long digital flexors are the most spastic muscles in this deformity. They are preferably transferred into corrective positions. There are several alternatives. Most commonly the posterior tibial is transferred through the interosseous space to the middorsum of the foot. Interestingly, following forward transfer, the spastic posterior tibial may not fire in either phase of gait. This transfer nonetheless still performs an important function by removing a major deforming force in the mechanogenesis of the deformity. The digital flexors can be included in this transfer if they are offenders producing chronic digital flexion.

The digital flexors should also be considered for transfer on the basis that they augment the hindfoot varus component since they function medial to the subtalar axis. Alternatively, both the posterior tibial and flexor digitorum longus can be delivered to the middorsum by the circumtibial route subcutaneously.[2] This is a lesser known method of transfer that remains useful depending on the nature of multiple simultaneous procedures required in any given situation.

Other methods of altering the deforming spastic torque of the posterior tibial or digital flexors are intramuscular lengthening or transfer retromalleolarly into the peroneus brevis.[22] Split transfer of the posterior tibial (retromalleolarly) into peroneus brevis has been described and can be considered when the objective is reduction in the exorotatory torque of the posterior tibial on the leg.[2,22] This transfer is utilized most commonly in passively reducible hindfoot varus caused by inappropriate spastic firing of the tibialis posterior. Split transfer of the posterior tibial into the medial talar head is currently being assessed in a small series of patients. This operation utilizes the concept of direct talar control in reducing and altering the pathologic lateral rotation of the leg produced by tibialis posterior in closed kinetic chain mechanics.

Spastic Calcaneus

Spastic paralysis of the pretibial muscles results in a progressive calcaneus deformity[1,2] (Fig. 39-7). The posterior group muscles are reciprocally inhibited, allowing a severe dorsiflexory deformity to develop. The most severe forms of this condition appear in neurospinal dysraphisms causing the heel to be very prominent and subject to ulceration. Occasionally, participation by the lateral crural group will allow a calcanovalgus subgroup to develop.

Surgical reconstruction of this deformity is aimed at bringing the heel upward. This is usually accomplished with a combination of tendon transfers and fusions of the hindfoot complex.[2] The Elmslie triple arthrodesis has been designed specifically for this condition. This procedure also involves the use of the medial and lateral stabilizers as transfers into the heel as a second-stage operation. In a child or adolescent, rotation osteotomy of the os calcis to a more cephalad position[2,23] or Green-Grice extra-articular fusion combined with the previously mentioned tendon transfers offer the best chance of success.[18,23] The tibialis anterior is usually the most powerful offender and is therefore transferred posteriorly through the interosseous membrane to the heel. An adjunctive tenodesis of the paralyzed heel cord can be entertained either by total or split tenodesis into the fibula with the foot forced in plantar flexion.[1] When subgroup calcanovalgus presents, the offending peroneus brevis should be transferred into the heel cord or os calcis in conjunction with the other mentioned bone procedures.[22,24]

Spastic Cavovarus

Spastic cavovarus in its pure form is unusual. It is managed in accordance with the principles of spastic muscle surgery in general combined with the principles of surgical reconstruction of the cavovarus foot. It is seen most commonly in cases of stroke wherein the spastic digital flexors contribute to the multiple hammer toes and flexion deformity of the forefoot in combination with a spastic tibialis posterior. The long flexors and plantar intrinsics draw the forefoot and hindfoot together, maintaining the deformity.

Elimination of the deforming force of the spastic muscles contributing to the deformity is basic. The posterior tibial and digital flexors are transferred either to the heel or the dorsum of the foot. Achilles tendon lengthening procedures should not be considered in this condition and are contraindicated. Bone procedures are similar to those for the nonspastic cavus foot and include primary triple arthrodesis, valgusation osteotomies of the heel, Cole osteotomy of the midtarsus,[25] or elevational osteotomy of the metatarsals and digital interphalangeal fusions.

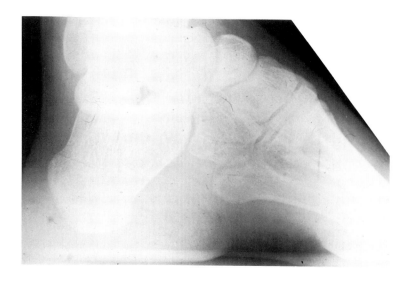

Fig. 39-7. Spastic calcanocavus. Primary triple arthrodesis followed by posterior transfer of the tibialis anterior or transfer of the long flexors into the heel is indicated.

Spastic Varus Hindfoot

Spastic heel varus is seen most commonly in stroke patients. Gait efforts are difficult and brace stabilization almost impossible since the foot slips out of the orthotic.[8] The prime offender in this condition is the spastic tibialis anterior muscle, usually by itself. The problem can be reconciled nicely by a split transfer to the cuboid or peroneus tertius.[8] Spastic digital flexion deformities commonly accompany this condition and require circumtibial transfer of the flexor digitorum longus to the middorsum of the foot.[2] Bone implantation is preferred over tendon-to-tendon anastomosis whenever possible. These simple procedures often have the ability to completely eliminate the need for bracing in these patients.

Total transfer of the tibialis anterior to the midfoot can balance this type of foot condition; however, because of the spasticity, the response is not as predictable as split transfer since the legs of the split spontaneously resolve their vectoral pull.

Flaccid Paralysis Deformities

Lower motor neuron lesions (including neuropathies) produce paralytic deformities that are static and reasonably well controlled by bracing.[9,24,26,27] The most classic of these conditions is represented by anterior poliomyelitis. The present principles of management of flaccid paralysis, by and large, have been developed through experience with polio patients.[26] It is not uncommon to encounter polio residuals in current practice. The denervating processes share many similarities with poliomyelitis, and hence the deformations they produce are managed in similar surgical fashion. In general, any phenomenon that results in loss of innervation to the muscle unit will deprive that unit of its function and allow a deformation to develop over the distribution served by that muscle-nerve unit. The neuropathic processes have a tendency to be slowly progressive depending on the disease in question. This usually results in slowly progressive foot and ankle deformity that requires redress at the time of reconstruction in order to arrest the deforming process.[2] Primary muscle disease (dystrophies) are believed to have their origin within the muscle unit itself and can simulate a slowly progressive neuro-pathic process. Some of the more commonly implicated processes include Charcot-Marie-Tooth disease and its variants (Roussy-Lévy disease), the entire group of spinocerebellar dysfunctions, posterior tract derangements, discogenic syndromes, traumatic and toxic neuropathies, and the entire category of muscular dystrophy.[1,2]

Talipes Equinus

Paralysis of the pretibials by way of a lower motor neuron process will cause a paralytic footdrop. If the paralysis is balanced and does not involve the medial or lateral stabilizers, then a relative pure sagittal plane equinus will develop in gait. In open kinetic chain mechanics (swing phase) the foot will automatically drop into gravity equinovarus. This makes the foot unstable at the time of contact phase initiation since heel contact is eliminated from the cycle. There is a natural tendency for lateral ankle sprains and recurrent falls in these patients. A standard ankle spring-loaded brace is functional and will work well in these patients. Molded polypropylene braces/splints are also available to allow a right-angle positioning of the foot and leg.

Surgical reconstructions are aimed at eliminating any fixed positional equinus due to myostatic contracture. This is accomplished by Achilles tendon or gastrocnemius lengthening if the equinus is selectively originating from that muscle.[1,2,15,22] If the foot is stable medially-laterally and no fixed equinus has developed, then a hemigastroc-soleus transfer (Caldwell) procedure can be considered.[2,28,29] This operation is essentially a tenodesis in which the medial one-half of the gastrocsoleus complex is split and passed subcutaneously around the medial aspect of the tibia. It is then transplanted into the midfoot. This operation functions on the basis of forcing a transfer to act against itself and lock the foot in a stable and functional sagittal position.

When fixed equinus is present, it must be released prior to further consideration of tendon transfer.[2,30,31] The alternatives available will depend on whether or not there are additional paralyzed muscles medially or laterally in conjunction with the pretibials. When the entire pretibial group has been lost, then usually a tarsal stabilization such as the Lambrinudi "forced equinus" triple arthrodesis is required to "free up," or make available, the medial and lateral stabilizers for transfer to the dorsum of the foot. This can result in a stable functional foot with adequate dorsiflexion. When the paralysis is more severe, including some of the medial or lateral musculature, then pantalar arthrodesis may be required to afford the necessary stability to carry out activities of daily living.

Talipes equinus as a result of Duchenne's dystrophy will respond to simple percutaneous Achilles tendon lengthening followed by bracing and immediate ambulation. Arthrodesis is rarely indicated in this condition since the ultimate objective is to keep the patient mobilized.

Bone blocks behind the ankle have limited application and can be considered when patients are reasonably well balanced in the sagittal plane in stance phase. The block will maintain the foot in a near-neutral position in swing phase and permit some heel contact to occur. The ankle arthroereisis bone blocks available for consideration are essentially two: the Gill subchondral talar block[32] and the posterior Campbell-type block. All bone blocks at the posterior ankle require the additional support of an anterior Gallie-type pretibial suspension using one or two of the paralyzed anterior tendons imbedded into the anterior tibial surface; this author prefers the use of tibialis anterior medially and peroneus brevis laterally (assuming both are paralyzed) to allow a balanced tenodesis.[2,22]

Talipes Equinovalgus

Lower motor neuron loss of the tibialis anterior or tibialis posterior will result in severe equinovalgus,[2,9] but the mechanism of production is different. Paralysis of both tibials results in the most severe form of talipes equinovalgus possible.

Loss of the posterior tibial will deprive the talus of its chief restraint for medial deceleration. The talus continues its drive medially and downward in midstance, like a cam shaft driving a machine.[33] This sets up a vicious cycle of events contributing to accommodative equinus, which eventually fixates itself and maintains the deformity in both valgus and equinus. There is no situation in which the tibialis posterior is lost and a pathologic flatfoot does not develop (Fig. 39-8).

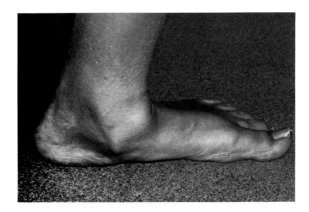

Fig. 39-8. Tarsal collapse and progressive equinovalgus from loss of the posterior tibial as a result of discopathy disease. In adults, triple arthrodesis is the ultimate salvage procedure.

Selective loss of the tibialis anterior also produces equinovalgus but through a different compensatory mechanism. Initially a foot-drop deformity develops. This allows a fixed equinus to develop. Gradually the fixed equinus compensates through the mechanism of tarsal collapse at the level of the midfoot. Additionally, there is a valgus overpull of the remaining pretibials, especially the extensor digitorum longus, that further aggravates the deforming process. This results in a vicious cycle of events that continually reinforces itself.

Surgical reconstruction in cases of paralytic equinovalgus will depend on age of encounter and severity of the condition.[10] In the child and adolescent, Green-Grice subtalar fusion is ideal combined with an equinus release procedure.[1,2,33] In children, simple percutaneous Achilles tendon lengthening is preferred since it is fast, simple, and effective.[2] Following recovery of the triceps strength, secondary forward transfer of the peroneus longus to the middorsum is effective in controlling foot-drop. The distal stump of the peroneus longus must be anastomosed to the peroneus brevis following its release at the base of the fifth metatarsal.[2,24] Thus, the peroneus brevis now functions as the peroneus longus, maintaining stability of the first ray and medial column of the foot.

Older patients and adults will require triple arthrodesis to stabilize the foot. Peroneus longus transfer to the dorsum may still be required if foot-drop is resultant from loss of the tibialis anterior. In

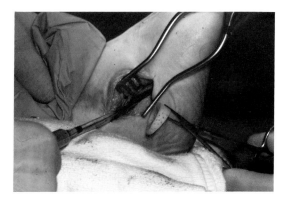

Fig. 39-9. Varusation osteotomy of the heel with freeze-dried femur bone implant is effective in placing the heel back under the leg in hindfoot valgus. It often requires additional soft tissue procedures such as equinus release and medial column arthrodesis or tendon transfer.

the event that the equinovalgus is caused by loss of the tibialis posterior, as in discopathy or traumatic loss/rupture, replacement of the tibialis posterior with the flexor hallucis longus soon after the loss can be an adequate substitute. This can be augmented with a self-locking wedge-type arthroereisis of the subtalar joint and into-talus transfer of the peroneus brevis to act as a decelerator of medial-downward talar excursion. When end-stage equinovalgus has been reached, with considerable arthrosis in the major tarsal complex, only triple arthrodesis can solve the problem.[10,15]

Paralytic equinovalgus resultant from loss of the tibialis anterior will usually require some transfer to the dorsum to reduce the foot-drop tendency, in addition to tarsal stabilization. If the deformity is caused by loss of the tibialis posterior alone, then tarsal stabilization can deal with the problem. Depending on the severity of tarsal midfoot collapse, there may be a role for varusation osteotomy of the heel combined with into-talus transfer of the peroneus brevis (Fig. 39-9). This is a less morbid alternative for older patients who do not manifest pain from severe tarsal joint arthrosis.

Talipes Calcaneus

Paralytic calcaneus has been discussed under the spastic paralysis section, and the principles of management are the same. The main difference be-

tween the spastic and flaccid varieties is the distribution of paralysis. The spastic variety is caused by spastic paralysis of the pretibial group, whereas in the flaccid variety the muscle loss is selectively the triceps surae. Flaccid calcaneus deformity is most commonly seen in myelodysplastics.[34]

Paralytic Calcanocavus

Calcanocavus is a pure sagittal plane deformity. It develops when there is paresis of the triceps surae.[1,2] Flexor substitution begins to draw the forefoot and hindfoot together, allowing the plantar intrinsics to contract and further maintain the deformity.[9,21] The heel and ball of the foot are prominent in this condition. It is seen in polio residuals as well as other lower motor neuron dysfunctions. When symptomatic and severe, reconstruction will require a combination of bone and soft tissue surgery. The Steindler release will liberate the forefoot from the hindfoot and allow skeletal or tendon transfer procedures to act independently of these two segments.[35] The objective is to flatten the arch and make the foot plantar grade. If it is determined that the flexor digitorum longus is contributing to the problem at the forefoot and rearfoot level, then transfer posteriorly into the heel is indicated. When the pitch of the heel is excessive, rotation osteotomy is also considered in conjunction with the Steindler release. This maneuver releases the windlass mechanism and permits the passive force of gravity to facilitate arch flattening.[2]

Cavovarus Deformity

Cavovarus is one of the most difficult progressive deformities of the foot and ankle to control and correct surgically (Fig. 39-10). Maintenance of correction has also been a well-recognized problem. Currently, the consensus of opinion regarding the underlying nature of this deformity is that it is of neuromuscular origin until proven otherwise.[2,36] The means that any reconstructive concept should employ a combination of hard and soft tissue surgery to achieve a lasting reduction and arrest the progress of the deformity. When the deformity appears early in childhood, the physician should be alerted to neuromuscular overlay. Appropriate

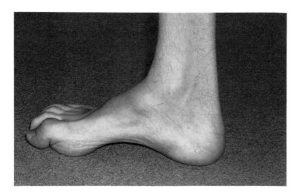

Fig. 39-10. Progressive pes cavovarus resultant from Charcot-Marie-Tooth disease. This condition often requires major reconstruction in the form of Cole midfoot osteotomy, Dwyer heel osteotomy, and a variety of soft tissue releases and tendon transfers, especially of the posterior tibial to the dorsum.

workup should be performed, including muscle biopsy and electrodiagnostic studies.

The pathomechanics of this deformity are obscure and varied. There is usually clinical or subclinical paresis of the triceps surae, which allows the remaining flexors to draw the forefoot against the mid- and hindfoot. The peroneus brevis is extremely weak or entirely lost in the neuropathic process. The tibialis anterior can be weak, permitting extensor substitution that cocks the hallux, which drives the first metatarsal plantar. The lesser digital extensors attempt to further compensate for paresis of the tibialis anterior, with substitutional hammer toe formation contributing to global forefoot equinus. The peroneus longus gains considerable mechanical advantage, aggravating the forefoot valgus, and synergizes with the extensor hallucis longus, compounding the problem of forefoot valgus. This process sets up a vicious cycle allowing the posterior tibial to also gain mechanical advantage and aggressively act upon the midfoot and hindfoot segments, producing heel varus.[1,2,36]

Surgery in early childhood can help reduce the tendency for more severe deformity with careful planning and evaluation. Steindler myofascial release is an important early procedure that can alter the natural course of the deforming process in the foot.[1,2,35,37] It releases the windlass mechanism and permits activity of the child (gravity) to facilitate arch flattening. It is uncommon for fixed-heel varus to develop prior to the age of 9 in cavovarus, and

hence soft tissue surgery is most effective during this period of life. The forefoot valgus (plantarflexed first metatarsal) may appear early and actually be the precursor of subsequent heel varus. Early correction of either flexible or rigid forefoot valgus is important to arrest progression of the deformity.[1,2]

Subsequent to early childhood and entering early adolescence, the condition fixates itself and bone surgery will be required. Bone surgery is aimed at the apex of the deformity in the sagittal plane. This may mean osteotomy-arthrodesis at the naviculocuneiform level or panbasal metatarsal elevational osteotomy. Correction through Lisfranc's joint is not recommended and is fraught with complications of non-union at the resectional fusion sites. The first metatarsal will require elevation in most cases that are severe enough to warrant midfoot osteotomy (Cole or Japas type) because the medial column depression cannot be entirely corrected through the midfoot osteotomy.[2] Valgus-producing osteotomy of the calcaneus by lateral wedge removal is effective but must be aggressive.[2,21] The tendency for undercorrection by inadequate wedge resection is common. Osteotomy placement should be as far anterior as possible inasmuch as the principle is to place as much of the posterior tuber lateral to the subtalar axis as possible.

Severe cases with end-stage muscle paresis may require triple arthrodesis for stabilization.[1,2,9,15] Carefully planned reconstructive osteotomies and selected midfoot surgery combined with the proper tendon transfers can avoid the more destructive triple arthrodesis in most cases. When deformity is extremely severe, muscle weakness advanced, and degenerative arthrosis present, triple arthrodesis then becomes the premier selection.[2]

Operative procedures commonly indicated and performed for this severe foot type include: triple arthrodesis, Dwyer-type valgus-producing heel osteotomies, first metatarsal osteotomy, Jones suspension with compression fusion of the interphalangeal joint of the hallux, Cole midfoot osteotomy, tendon transfer of the tibialis posterior through the interosseous membrane to the dorsum of the midfoot, Hibb's recession of the extensor digitorum longus to the midfoot, split transfer of the posterior tibial into the talar head, peroneus longus transfer to the dorsum, Steindler release, and peroneal switch, transferring the peroneus longus into the peroneus brevis or simply transferring the peroneus longus into the cuboid (leaving it retromalleolar).

The selection of any given regimen of procedures will depend on the specific situation and subtlety of deformity. Procedures aimed at lengthening the triceps mechanism are not indicated and in fact aggravate the deforming process by providing a greater range of excursion for the posterior heel to migrate further downward.[2] The exception to this rule is the older patient who suffers primarily from metatarsalgia due to accommodative positional equinus. This occurs as a result of external rotation of the tibiofibular-talar unit, which prevents adequate dorsiflexion. Selective gastrocne-mius lengthening may improve the forefoot symptoms in these patients if that is the only objective.

Idiopathic Clubfoot

Talipes equinovarus of congenital origin without evidence of neuromuscular involvement is handled primarily conservatively initially.[1] The major components are reduced serially — first the metatarsus adductus and varus of the forefoot and hindfoot followed last by equinus reduction. The latter is always the most recalcitrant component and often requires selective posterior surgical release. Failure to reduce the varus of the hindfoot will not permit equinus resolution. Adequate ankle dorsiflexion will never be achieved in lieu of a persistent

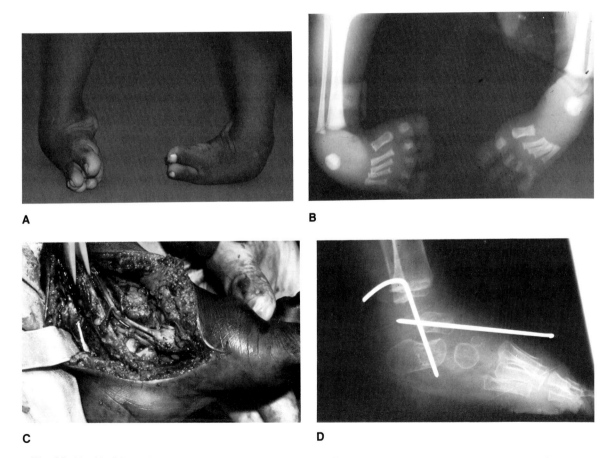

A

B

C

D

Fig. 39-11. **(A)** Bilateral congenital talipes equinovarus in a 3-year-old. **(B)** Radiographic appearance of classic talipes equinovarus. **(C)** Intraoperative situation of classic Turco release. **(D)** Postoperative radiographic appearance demonstrating proper alignment with talonavicular fixation and subtalar joint fixation. Both joints are recommended to be stabilized with smooth pins.

varus of the hindfoot. This is commonly seen in radiographs as a spurious correction causing an iatrogenic flatfoot. Careful examination of the radiographs will demonstrate an abnormal Kite's angle; the fibula will remain retrograde in relation to the normal ankle and the dome of the talus as well as the navicular typically are dysmorphic in appearance.

Soft tissue release is most effective as early as age 1 year. The classic posteromedial release of the Turco variety is effective if performed correctly.[1,15] The staged release must be complete in one operation (Fig. 39-11). The Cincinnati incision around the back of the ankle is available for consideration and is claimed to provide superior exposure, although it would seem that severe equinus conditions might present a difficult primary closure problem. Postoperative fixation of the talonavicular and subtalar joint is critical. The navicular must be placed in front of the talar head and Kite's angle restored at the end of the operation. Casting is continued for at least 3 months.

Once bony deformity is established, osseous surgery will be required. Depending on the residual deformity, various procedures are available addressing the different levels of deformity. For end-stage deformity, triple arthrodesis can be a solution especially if there is degenerative arthritis in the major tarsal complex. Dwyer osteotomy to restore heel position is effective if a large enough wedge is removed from the lateral wall of the os calcis. Cuboid wedge resection can help provide some abductory midfoot correction. Osteotomies of the metatarsals sometimes have a role if the main complaint is residual forefoot adduction. Tibiofibular rotation osteotomy is not indicated under usual circumstances of idiopathic clubfoot. Primary tendon transfers likewise are not appropriate, and are only considered following multiple relapses of conservative casting or operative regimens.

"Z" Foot

The combination of metatarsus adductus and hindfoot valgus presents a major challenge to any surgeon. This deformity can be severe and disabling, causing knee jamming pain and gait dysfunction. When the condition progresses to the point that tarsal collapse and deterioration is developing, surgical redress should be considered. The presenting appearance of this compound deformity is typically a valgus heel and arch bulge with a rectus-appearing forefoot. This should always alert the clinician to masked forefoot or metatarsus adductus. Surgical restoration is best accomplished in early adolescence when the deformity is severe enough to warrant surgery.

Surgery aimed at the hindfoot will ultimately "unmask" the forefoot adduction and make it appear worse following surgery if only rearfoot restoration is accomplished.[10,15] Thus, since the deformity is compound, correction at the forefoot and rearfoot segment is required. There are a variety of techniques available for rearfoot restoration and they are carefully selected based on the individual situation. If the rearfoot deformity is reducible an arthroereisis can be considered. Varus-producing heel osteotomies are effective in placing the hindfoot back under the vertical weight-bearing trajectory of the leg. Equinus is usually present in these feet and will require release by the method of one's choice. Percutaneous Achilles tendon lengthening is preferred up to age 12. Subsequent to this age, selective gastrocnemius lengthening will produce less morbidity in recuperation. Into-talus transfer of the peroneus brevis is a common accompaniment in this author's regimen.[2,38] Panbasal abductory metatarsal osteotomy will restore the forefoot alignment. This complex deformity may require a two-stage operation for those not experienced with a one-stage reconstruction.

Medial column fusions such as the Miller-Hoke type are not usually effective since they address sagittal plane breach for the greater part. Once operative reduction is decided upon, correction of both the hindfoot and forefoot components will be necessary.

PATHOLOGIC NONPARALYTIC EQUINOVALGUS

Pathologic hyperpronation syndromes often progress to serious tarsal collapse and pain. These feet do not display a paralysis but would almost imply such because of their severity! The condition is disabling and interferes with activities of daily living in adolescent and adult patients. The clinical appearance is that of total midfoot collapse with breach at the talonavicular and navicular cuneiform levels. The talus has escaped the navicular acetabulum and the cuboid has escaped its natural block at the overhang of the os calcis anteriorly, resulting in significant abduction deformity of the midfoot.[33] Subluxation is insidious, and equinus — either primary or secondary — is always present and requires recognition in any surgical reconstruction effort. Failure to release the equinus will not allow resumption of normal tarsal relationships.[4,10,15] Thus, the deformity will not be able to resolve itself regardless of any other procedures performed, including triple arthrodesis! Triple arthrodesis performed without benefit of equinus release will force the foot to be fused in severe valgus. This is a common error.

This deformity is usually rigid and displays varying degrees of heel valgus and midfoot-forefoot abduction. The navicular fills the arch area upon medial weight-bearing viewing. The talar head is prominent, with the classic bulge. The medial column is rotated into forefoot varus with the first metatarsal elevated. Conservative orthotic control does little or nothing to relieve the pain of the patient.

The adolescent age group require a combined approach of soft and hard tissue surgery. In a series of over 65 feet, an operation that has been designated as a "reverse Cole" has been found effective in correcting this difficult deformity. As its name would imply, the operation is an upside-down Cole operation through the level of the navicular-cuneiform joints and cuboid. The idea was developed based on the belief by the author that cavovarus and equinovalgus are mirror-opposite deformities![2,10] The wedge resection is aggressive and biplane to address the valgus hindfoot and abducted midfoot segment. The apex of the osteotomy-fusion resides in the cuboid laterally, with the base of the wedge facing medial and plantar. Upon completion of the osteotomy, the midfoot and hindfoot are hinged together on the axis of the osteotomy, correcting the deformity at both segmental levels. Fixation is usually with one or two heavy Steinman pins. The restoration of the "arch" is immediate and impressive. The typical wedge resection along the medial column is about 2.0 cm in width, both medially and plantarly. Equinus is always released,

as stated earlier. Into-talus tendon transfers of the peroneus brevis have been helpful in maintaining correction. Sometimes a split portion of tibialis anterior is translocated into a slot in the navicular.[2,10] If additional talar support is required, a talonavicular suspension is performed to provide additional direct talar control.

The "reverse Cole" with the described into-talus transfers has the potential to avoid triple arthrodesis, which would otherwise be required in the foot type under discussion. It has been designed as an alternative to triple arthrodesis and has in fact performed well for this purpose.

Varus-producing heel osteotomies and into-talus transfers of peroneus brevis and tibialis anterior suspensions provide the surgeon with latitude to avoid the more destructive triple arthrodesis. When severe heel valgus is not a major problem, open osteotomy of the medial cuneiform is useful in reducing the medial column varus rotation and gaining purchase of this portion of the foot back to the supporting surface.

Arthroereisis has no role in these foot types because of their rigidity. Ultimately, if deformity and disability are severe, triple arthrodesis will remain the only alternative.

SUMMARY

Paralytic and nonparalytic deformity of the foot and ankle can be serious and disabling. Recognition of the underlying factors and the natural course of the various deformities is important. The appropriate patient selection for any given operation is dependent upon this knowledge. The surgeon should be able to tailor the required operative regimen to any given set of circumstances.

REFERENCES

1. Tachdjian MO: The Child's Foot. WB Saunders Co, Philadelphia, 1985
2. Vogler HW: Surgical management of neuromuscu-

lar deformities of the foot and ankle in children and adolescents. Clin Podiatr Med Surg 4:175, 1987

3. Sharrard JW: Paralytic deformity in the lower limb. J Bone Joint Surg 2:374, 1972

4. Baker LD, Hill LM: Foot alignment in the cerebral palsy patient. J Bone Joint Surg [Am] 46:1, 1964

5. Sharrard JW, Bernstein S: Equinus deformity in cerebral palsy. J Bone Joint Surg [Br] 54:272, 1972

6. Sharrard WJW: The mechanism of paralytic deformity in spina bifida. Dev Med Child Neurol 4:310, 1962

7. Perry J: Orthopedic management of the lower extremity in the hemiplegic patient. J Am Phys Assoc 46:345, 1966

8. Mooney V, Perry J, Nickel V: Surgical and non-surgical orthopedic care of stroke. J Bone Joint Surg [Am] 49:989, 1967

9. Goldner JR, Irwin CE: The surgical treatment of poliomyelitis. Paralytic deformities of the foot. p. 190. In: American Academy of Orthopaedic Surgeons Instructional Course Lectures. Vol. 5. JJ Edwards, Ann Arbor, MI, 1948

10. Vogler HW: Surgical reconstruction of talipes equinovalgus. J Am Podiatr Med Assoc 77:134, 1987

11. Perry J, Hoffer M: Preoperative and postoperative dynamic electromyography as an aid in planning tendon transfers in children with cerebral palsy. J Bone Joint Surg [Am] 59:531, 1977

12. Perry J, Hoffer M, Giovan P et al: Giat analysis of the triceps surae in cerebral palsy: a preoperative and postoperative clinical electromyographic study. J Bone Joint Surg [Am] 54:511, 1974

13. Pierrot AH, Murphy OB: Heel cord advancement. Orthop Clin North Am 5:117, 1974

14. Smith SD, Weil LS: Anterior advancement of the tendo Achilles for spastic equinus deformity. J Am Podiatry Assoc 64:1016, 1974

15. McGlamry ED: Comprehensive Textbook of Foot Surgery. Williams & Wilkins, Baltimore, 1987

16. Baker LD: Triceps surae syndrome in cerebral palsy. Arch Surg 68:216, 1954

17. Tohen A, Carmona J, Berrera J: Utilization of abnormal reflexes in the treatment of spastic foot deformities. Clin Orthop 47:77, 1966

18. Grice DS: An extra-articular arthrodesis of the subastragalar joint for correction of paralytic flat feet in children. J Bone Joint Surg [Am] 34:927, 1952

19. Smith SD, Miller EA: Arthroereisis by means of a sub-talar polyethylene peg implant for correction of hindfoot pronation in children. Clin Orthop 181:15, 1983

20. Silver CM, Simon SD, Spindall E et al: Calcaneal osteotomy for valgus and varus deformities of the foot in cerebral palsy: a preliminary report on twenty-seven operations. J Bone Joint Surg [Am] 49:232, 1967

21. Coleman SC: Complex Foot Deformities in Children. Lea & Febiger, Philadelphia, 1983

22. Vogler HW, Bauer GR: Myotenoplastic maneuvers about the foot and ankle. In Jay R (ed): Current Therapy in Podiatric Surgery. CV Mosby Co, St. Louis, 1988

23. Samilson RL: Crescentic osteotomy of the os calcis for calcanocavus feet. In Bateman JE (ed): Foot Science. WB Saunders Co, Philadelphia, 1976

24. Herndon CH: Tendon transplantation at the knee and foot. p. 145. In: American Academy of Orthopaedic Surgeons Instructional Course Lectures. Vol. 18. JJ Edwards, Ann Arbor, MI, 1961

25. Cole W: The treatment of clawfoot. J Bone Joint Surg 22:895, 1940

26. Dunn N: Stabilizing operations in paralytic deformities of feet. Proc Soc Med (Sec Orthop) 15:15, 1922

27. Gill AB: Surgery of the foot in infantile paralysis. Am J Surg 44:252, 1939

28. Caldwell GD: Correction of paralytic footdrop by hemigastrosoleus transplantation. Clin Orthop 11:81, 1958

29. Gunn DR, Pillay VK: Transplantation of the medial head of gastrocnemius. Indian J Orthop 1:15, 1967

30. Mortens J, Pilcher MF: Tendon transplantation in the prevention of foot deformities after poliomyelitis in children. J Bone Joint Surg [Br] 38:633, 1956

31. Mollerud A: Tendon transference in poliomyelitis. Acta Orthop Scand 26:222, 1957

32. Gill AB: An operation to make a posterior bone block at the ankle to limit foot drop. J Bone Joint Surg 15:166, 1933

33. Vogler HW: Biomechanics of talipes equinovalgus. J Am Podiatr Med Assoc 77:21, 1987

34. Batna J, Sutherland DH, Wyatt M: Anterior tibialis transfer to os calcis with Achilles tenodesis for calcaneal deformity in myelomeningocele. J Pediatr Orthop 1:125, 1981

35. Steindler A: The treatment of pes cavus. Arch Surg 2:225, 1921

36. Gudas C: Mechanism and reconstruction of pes cavus. J Foot Surg 16:1, 1977

37. Dwyer FC: Osteotomy of the calcaneum for pes cavus. J Bone Joint Surg [Br] 41:80, 1959

38. Vogler HW: Transfer of the posterior tibial tendon. In Jay R (ed): Current Therapy in Podiatric Surgery. CV Mosby Co, St. Louis, 1988

Soft Tissue Injuries of the Lower Extremities

40

Eric Goldenberg D.P.M., M.S.

Nonosseous injuries to the foot and leg are an often-neglected topic in discussions of lower extremity trauma. The topics presented in this chapter review the injuries the practitioner may encounter in the office and emergency room. Management of soft tissue trauma will vary according to individual preference and training, and the techniques presented are those that are currently supported by the literature.

CLOSED WOUNDS

Contusions and hematomas, considered by many to be minor traumatic incidents, can often lead to more severe complications. *Contusions* (or bruises) result from blunt trauma that does not penetrate the skin. The patient will present with pain, tenderness, and ecchymoses. Erythema and hypesthesia or hypoesthesia may result. Symptomatic relief can be administered in the form of ice, elevation, and compression with appropriate analgesia as indicated.[1] When subdermal bleeding of the underlying muscle groups becomes severe the contusion can go on to become an acute compartment syndrome of the lower extremity. Compartment syndrome occurs when swelling of the muscle contents of one or more compartments of the leg attempts to extend beyond the surrounding fascia. The fascia prevents the expansion, resulting in increased intracompartmental pressure. Eventually the pressure will increase to a level that will constrict circulation and result in structural and functional damage to nerve and muscle. If not treated promptly the long-term sclerosis will lead to permanent damage.[2] Symptoms and signs will include pulselessness and decrease in sensation and pain. Management should be initiated as soon as possible and includes fasciotomy with release of intracompartmental pressure.

Hematoma formation can occur from blunt or sharp trauma or from idiopathic causes. Defined as an abnormal, ectopic collection of blood, symptoms usually include ecchymoses, blanching, pain, tenderness, and possible displacement of the normal anatomy.[1] Hematomas usually resolve without sequelae. However, depending on size, site of injury, and time of treatment following injury, more aggressive intervention may be warranted to relieve discomfort and symptoms. Acute or late-expanding hematomas can be evacuated by needle aspiration or incision and drainage.[3]

It should be noted that a chronic expanding hematoma of the lower extremity can be difficult to differentiate from soft tissue sarcoma before biopsy.[3] If no history of trauma presents with clinical signs of a slowly expanding mass, biopsy should be performed before excision or incision and drainage is attempted. Subungal hematomas are discussed under nail and nail bed trauma.

OPEN WOUNDS

Abrasions are the superficial removal of the epidermal layers of the skin resulting from scraping or rubbing trauma. Signs and symptoms usually include bleeding, weeping, pain, and loss of superficial skin layers with embedded debris. These wounds are similar to burns and can be detrimental to the diabetic patient, who may be vascularly compromised, because a resultant infection may occur. Treatment of the clean abrasion is by gently cleansing the wound and allowing reepithelization to occur. Abrasions with embedded debris require removal of the foreign matter. This can be facilitated by washing the wound and gently scrubbing with a soft sterile cloth or brush. Prevention of infection should be foremost in your mind. Depending on the clinical presentation of the abrasion, prophylactic systemic antibiotics may be warranted as well as a topical antibiotic dressing.

Lacerations are traumatically induced incisions that can be superficial (epidermis and upper dermis) or through all the layers of the skin and possibly the underlying tissues and structures.[1] These wounds usually have jagged edges and bleeding, and gaping of the wound edges may be observed. Treatment of lacerations will depend on whether the wound is considered clean or contaminated. Depending on the size and location of the wound, hemostasis can be achieved using either a pneumatic cuff or epinephrine in the local anesthetic block. Delay in treatment of the wound of over 3 hours will increase the chance of developing an infection, and jagged wound edges will reduce the number of bacteria per gram of tissue necessary to cause infection. For a clean-appearing wound that presents soon after the inflicting trauma, treatment includes irrigation with either sterile saline or dilute povidine-iodine followed by surgical débridement to remove necrotic-appearing tissue or jagged edges and surgical closure utilizing sterile technique. A sterile dressing is applied and appropriate tetanus and/or antibiotic prophylaxis is administered.

A contaminated wound or one that presents 8 hours after trauma should not be closed primarily. A good lavage and irrigation should be performed, followed by resection of any necrotic tissue and any jagged edges. This wound should be kept open and packed with sterile gauze. The packing of the wound allows for drainage and the wound will also be allowed to granulate in from the bottom so that an abscess cannot form. In addition, the packing aids in the débridement of the wound because necrotic tissue is removed each time the packing is changed. Delayed primary closure is performed at a later date or the wound can be allowed to granulate when free of infection.

PUNCTURE WOUNDS

Nonosseous puncture wounds of the foot are extremely common problems that confront the physician. One study showed that 0.8 percent of emergency room visits of children age 15 or younger were for puncture wounds of the foot.[4] Puncture wounds can be divided into superficial and deep. Superficial wounds may only require mild cleansing and a light dressing followed by appropriate tetanus prophylaxis. Deep puncture wounds should be explored for any foreign substances. Deep cleansing of the wound with removal of any necrotic tissue and tetanus and antibiotic prophylaxis should be administered.[5] A high percentage of infections of puncture wounds of the foot are caused by *Pseudomonas aeruginosa*.[6] Until recently, outpatient management of *Pseudomonas* infection was difficult because there were no adequate oral agents effective against *Pseudomonas*. However, the advent of a new class of antibiotics, 4-quinalones, including the antibiotic ciprofloxacin (which has anti-pseudomonal activity as an oral preparation), expands the armament of the office-based practitioner. Ciprofloxacin allows for the treatment and/or prophylaxis of pseudomonal infections on an outpatient basis. However, it should be noted that appropriate culture and sensitivity tests along with Gram's stain should be performed to determine the optimal effective antibiotic for the infection being treated.

GUNSHOT WOUNDS

For all practical purposes, gunshot wounds should be treated as any deep, contaminated, puncture-type of wound. The entrance and exit site (if present) should be explored for any clothing debris, metal fragments, and dirt and oil. Most people who die from small-caliber (i.e., .22) gunshots usually die from the infectious complication and not the gunshot wound itself. Radiographs should be taken even if one is quite sure that there is no bone involvement, because they will help determine the location of any radiopaque debris.

Depending on the distance the bullet traveled to hit the foot, the amount of powder burn will vary. Débridement of powder burn areas should be performed to prevent necrosis of the wound edges. When probing the wound, minimal enlargement of the wound is desired to facilitate healing and delayed closure. Any remaining bullets or shot material should be removed if they are adjacent to the skin, joints, nerves, or arteries.[7] Complete lavage of the wound should be performed and tetanus and antibiotic prophylaxis initiated. Simple or compressive dressing is applied, and repeat débridement and delayed closure are performed as necessary. Avoidance of tightly packing the wound will prevent any occurrence of a toxic shock–type staphylococcus infection, as reported in the literature.[8] Legal obligations preclude the notification of the police in *ALL* gunshot wounds, even those claimed to be a result of a hunting accident.

BURNS

Burns are a quite common injury seen in this country. Between 12,000 and 15,000 people die annually from burns and their sequelae. Over 300,000 people sustain burns that require some professional care, and over 60,000 people require hospitalization for their burns. Initially, when se-

vere heat is applied to the skin, a hyperemia and vasodilation of the skin capillaries result. Eventually, with continued severe heat application, the capillary permeability will increase and coagulation, thrombosis, and stasis will result. Coagulation necrosis of the skin follows, with surface loss of water, protein, and sodium. Once the skin is lost there is no barrier to fluid loss and the patient will dehydrate. If the burns are severe and widespread enough, acidosis and shock results. The more severe the burn the more aggressive the treatment warranted.

For review, burns are staged as first, second, and third degree. First-degree burns are exemplified by a sunburn. There is reactive hyperemia of the skin and some pain and blanching upon pressure. Second-degree burns are partial-thickness burns that may extend down to the dermis or part way through the dermis. Usually the skin may regenerate itself if any dermal component remains. Shallow second-degree burns usually will not scar, although deeper second-degree burns (into the dermis) may leave a hypertrophic scar, a keloid, or a painful scar. Eventually revision and skin grafting may have to be performed. Third-degree burns are those that result in a total-thickness skin loss and will not heal on their own. Skin grafting will be needed because the burnt skin cannot regenerate. Second-degree burns, if not treated correctly, may become third degree.

Types of burns include thermal (hot or cold), chemical, and electrical. These are discussed on an individual basis.

Thermal Burns

A thermal burn to the skin is a result of either too much heat to the skin or too little heat to the skin (frostbite). Those that are a result of too much heat should be graded as to their degree of damage. Second- and third-degree burns should be debrided as necessary, with the application of an appropriate topical dressing to help prevent infections and encourage healing. Topical medications for this purpose include silver nitrate (0.5 percent), silver sulfadiazine, and sodium mafenide. Surgical débridement of developing eschars is necessary as often as needed. Skin grafting is performed when and if skin is available from a donor site on the patient. Biologic dressings such as porcine skin can be used after débridement to help reduce the bacterial count and to keep the wound clean.[9]

Frostbite is a result of prolonged exposure to cold temperatures. Freezing of the tissues with ice crystal formation of the cells and intracellular dehydration results. The burn can be compounded by moisture along with the cold temperatures. The severity of the frostbite injury is usually proportionate to the duration of exposure and how low the temperature is. Cold temperatures also result in an increase in low blood viscosity, which leads to a decreased blood flow and thrombosis of the small vessels of the digits and foot. Frostbite may appear as a simple hyperemia of the skin, progress to blister formation, and then result in dry gangrene as ischemia results. When the patient presents with acute freezing of the tissue, gentle warming should be applied and supportive measures initiated.[10] Débridement of necrotic tissue should be performed until healthy, bleeding tissue is obtained. Skin grafts may be necessary to cover any skin defects present. Appropriate tetanus and antibiotic prophylaxis should be administered. When the patient presents with acute freezing of the tissue, gentle warming should be applied and supportive measures initiated.

Chemical Burns

Chemical burns result from exposure to strong acids, strong bases, or other chemicals, including bromine.[11,12] A large majority of chemical burns are of the lower extremity because they are usually the result of the dropping or spilling of the chemical from the work area. Acids and alkalis usually cause prompt, obvious injury to the skin. However, burns from compounds such as bromine will not demonstrate an immediate visible skin reaction. Bromine burns are not always initially noted and may result in a much deeper burn if treatment is delayed or no first aid is administered at the time of exposure. Prompt first aid for any chemical exposure includes removing the source of the burn, removing any contaminated coverings or clothing, and diluting the exposed area with copious amounts of water. When first aid is not administered coagulation necrosis of the skin and soft tissues will result, with thrombosis of the vessels in the involved area. These burns should be treated as any other burn, with adequate débridement, grafting, and antibiotic prophylaxis.[13]

Electrical Burns

Electrical trauma may be the result of exposure to a wide range of electric fields, from lightning injuries to exposure to common household currents. Skeletal muscle and nerve tissue are the most susceptible to electrical injury.[14] Muscle and nerve cell membranes may rupture upon electrical exposure. If severe muscle necrosis occurs amputation may be required.[15,16] Neurologic sequelae of electrical injury may range from localized hypoesthesia to spinal neuropathy to paralysis.[17] Skin damage may be a result of charring at the contact point or exit point for an electrical lightning bolt. Electrical energy is dissipated as heat, and skin and tissue burns will result. Again, adequate débridement and grafting along with antibiotic prophylaxis are necessary.

NAIL AND NAIL BED INJURIES

Nail trauma is one of the most common causes of nail deformity. Nail trauma may be self-inflicted or a result of occupational insults or external influences. The nail plate function is to protect the distal phalanx, to aid in tactile discrimination, and to assist in manipulating small objects.[1] Nail dystrophy may be the result of acute or chronic injury and may lead to reversible or irreversible damage. Acute traumatic insults include splinter hemorrhage, subungual hematoma, nail shedding, and laceration of the nail plate and bed. Delayed manifestations of acute injury include splits and ridges, pterygium, and ectopic nail spicules.[18]

Splinter hemorrhages are usually discussed as a sign of subacute bacterial endocarditis. However, splinter hemorrhages can result from traumatic insults to the dermal ridges of the nail bed. Eventually, with increased trauma, the splinter hemorrhages will coalesce into ecchymoses of the nail bed. When the trauma is severe and acute a resultant subungual hematoma appears. Hemorrhage into the matrix will eventually be incorporated into the nail plate, and hemorrhage into the nail bed results in the painful subungual condition. Usually release of the subungual pressure will relieve the symptoms. Various techniques, ranging from drilling, burring, or burning a small hole into the nail plate to total avulsion of the nail plate, have been described as treatment modalities for acute subungual hematomas.[14]

The shedding of the nails (termed *onychoptosis defluvium*) may occur when the nail plate is traumatically separated from the nail bed or indirectly separated by a subungual hematoma. Traumatic separation has been demonstrated to be the result of sports injuries or from catching a portion of the nail on bed clothes or clothing when the patient tripped or fell.[18,19] The force created in a fall will partially or totally avulse the nail plate. In a partial avulsion any loosely attached nail plate should be removed and the nail bed should be treated with a topical antibiotic and bandage to keep the area clean. A new nail plate will eventually grow; however, the patient should be advised that a deformed nail may result if injury to the matrix occurred during the traumatic episode.

Lacerations of the nail plate and nail bed may occur secondary to domestic or occupational injuries. These lacerations may range from the simple split of the nail plate to total avulsion of the plate and laceration of the nail bed. When there is severe damage a radiograph should be considered to rule out any phalangeal fracture. If there is damage to the matrix, scarring may result. There may be permanent longitudinal deformities in the nail plate, such as a median nail plate dystrophy (termed *dystrophia unguium mediana canaliformis*).[20] This condition can also be induced iatrogenically when performing a nail matrix biopsy. Longitudinal nail plate ridges may result instead of nail plate splits as a result of trauma or laceration to the matrix. Laceration to the nail bed should be treated by cleansing the area and suturing or steri-stripping the wound for closure.

Pterygium result when there is a fusion of the epidermis of the proximal nail fold to nail bed and matrix. This may happen when damage is so extensive that the nail plate is avulsed and laceration of the proximal nail fold and nail bed occur, allowing the tissues to contact one another. These small masses may also be seen in patients without trauma history, such as those with lichen planus and those with impaired circulation. Self-induced trauma to the nails may resemble lichen planus and present with atrophy and pterygium. An extensive history should be obtained to identify whether the pterygium are due to a disease entity or to self-induced trauma.[20]

Ectopic nail spicules may result from any trauma that displaces a portion of the nail matrix from its normal location. This displaced matrix will produce nail spicules that grow outside the usual proximal nail fold. Incomplete or unsuccessful matricectomy, either surgical or chemical, may result in ectopic nail spicule formation. This can be remedied by reperforming the matricectomy procedure to remove the spicule and matrix.

FOREIGN BODIES

The soft tissue of the foot is prone to the introduction of various foreign bodies. The incidence of foreign body penetration increases during the warm months when people are more apt to walk barefoot. Various methods of foreign body localization and removal and been described, and include radiopaque grid systems, cross needles of varying gauges in different planes, and computed tomography localization.[21–24] Computed tomography localization provides a precise three-dimensional localization of the foreign body and also allows for the detection of a wide variety of foreign bodies of different radiolucency.

A foreign body can cause an inflammatory response and should be removed if symptomatic. If the foreign body is asymptomatic and located in a non-weight-bearing area of the foot it should not present any problems. Tetanus prophylaxis should be administered if warranted. Shotgun wounds that leave a large number of lead pellets should be addressed by the removal of as many of the foreign bodies as possible to avoid any lead toxicity.[7]

BITE WOUNDS AND STINGS

Human Bites

The majority of human bite wounds happen to the hand, and a great portion of those are of the clenched-fist type. Actual bite wounds are less serious than clenched-fist injuries.[25] However, because human bites are more detrimental than animal bites a few comments are warranted in this chapter. Furthermore, with the changes in society and morality over the last few decades, human bite wounds to the foot and leg may not be all that uncommon. In addition, with the growing numbers of children being cared for in child care centers, the incidence of bite wounds from nonsibling children will increase.

Complications of human bites include osteomyelitis, septic arthritis, tenosynovitis, and amputation. In addition, other diseases may be transmitted through human bite wounds. These include hepatitis B, scarlet fever, tuberculosis, syphilis, and actinomycosis.

The normal human oral flora reflects the organisms usually seen in human bite wounds. The bacteria often cultured include group A streptococcus, *S. viridans*, *Staphylococcus aureus*, *Eikenella corrodens*, and mixed anaerobes, including *Bacteroides* and *Peptococcus*.[25]

Management of human bite injuries depends on the seriousness of the wound. Cultures and Gram's stain are warranted in infected wounds. Incision and drainage with irrigation should be performed as needed. Avoid primary closure in infected wounds and wounds that may be contaminated. Antimicrobial therapy would be used for prophylaxis within 12 hours of injury or as empirical therapy of established infection. Amoxicillin with clavulanic acid is the antibiotic of choice for prophylaxis or outpatient therapy. For more serious infections that require in-hospital intravenous antibiotics, cefoxitin has been shown to be quite effective. Hyperbaric oxygen therapy has been utilized for anaerobic infections secondary to human bites.[26]

Dog Bites

The majority of patients who present with bite injuries present with dog bite wounds.[25] Dog bite injuries to the lower extremity should be evaluated the same as any laceration or puncture wound. Copious irrigation and débridement should be performed to remove contaminated material and reduce bacterial inoculation.[27] Dog bite wounds can be injected with a wide spectrum of aerobic and anaerobic bacteria, including *Pasteurella multocida*, α-, β-, and γ- hemolytic streptococci, and *Bacteroides*. Gram's stain and culture should be performed and prophylaxis for tetanus and infection administered. Amoxicillin with clavulanic acid is adequate for antimicrobial prophylaxis. Tetracycline or erythromycin can be used in penicillin-allergic patients.

Rabies is rare in domestic dog bites; however, each dog bite case that presents should be evaluated for rabies exposure. When rabies transmission is suspected the wound can be irrigated with 1 percent benzalkonium chloride solution. This will kill the rabies virus; however, the wound should then be copiously flushed with saline solution because the benzalkonium chloride may destroy viable tissue. Rabies prophylaxis should be administered if appropriate. For domestic dog bites in which the dog is observed to be healthy for 10 days, no prophylaxis is necessary unless the dog develops rabies. In rabid or suspected rabid dogs bites human rabies immune globulin (HRIG) and human diploid-cell vaccine (HDCV) are administered. If the animal is unknown or escaped, consult public health officials. HRIG dosage is 20 IU/kg (9 IU/lb). Give one-half of dose intramuscularly and infiltrate one-half of dose into the wound. HDCV is administered as five 1-ml doses intramuscularly on days 0, 3, 7, 14, and 28 of therapy.[25,27]

Cat Bites

Cat bites are similar to dog bites in presentation, treatment, and prophylaxis. However, there is a lack of information regarding incidence and infection rates in the literature. *Pasteurella multocida* is the organism most often identified in cat bites and has been isolated from both bites and scratches.[25] Puncture wounds from cats are more likely to become infected than dog bite punctures since cats' teeth are long and narrow. Antibiotic therapy for prophylaxis and empirical treatment of infection is described as amoxicillin with clavulanic as the drug of first choice. Second-choice drugs are ceftriaxone and tetracycline.

Snakebite

Twenty-four percent of occurring snakebites involve the foot or ankle. Of the approximately 45,000 reported U.S. snakebites each year, 8,000 are from venomous snakes. Less than 1 percent lead to mortality.[28] Death as result of venomous snakebite occurs in patients who were mistreated or untreated or in children. The Crotalidae group (rattlesnakes and copperheads) and Elapidae group (coral snakes) are the two classes of venomous snakes present in the United States. Rattlesnakes are identified by retractable fangs, elliptical pupils, a triangular-shaped head, and a single row of subcaudal scales. Coral snakes always have a black-tipped head and lack retractable fangs. They gnaw on the flesh with retroverted teeth long enough to deposit the venom into the wound.

Envenomation by rattlesnakes (also known as pit vipers) results in both local and systemic reactions. Locally, venom will cause a necrotizing effect on the lymphatic vessels and tissue and small blood vessels. Pain and swelling are seen early, followed by ecchymoses, pectechiae, and hemorrhagic blebs. Systemic involvement is characterized by shock, renal failure, respiratory disorders, bleeding, and disseminated intravascular coagulation.[28]

Envenomation by coral snakes is less efficient than that by rattlesnakes because the mechanism of envenomation is by depositing venom during gnawing versus the direct injection through the fangs as seen with rattlesnakes. Local manifestations are less noticeable because minimal swelling, pain, or necrosis is seen. The systemic reaction of coral snake bite envenomation includes major neurologic dysfunction with cranial nerve and respiratory paralysis.

Treatment of venomous snakebites is quite controversial. The most important factor in treatment is to get the victim to a medical facility as quickly as possible. Treatment of venomous snakebites in the field is inadequate and delays more effective treatment. Cryotherapy, incision and suction, and tourniquet application are not as effective as the intravenous administration of antivenom. Antivenom is still the definitive therapy of value. The number of vials of antivenom to administer is dependant on the amount of envenomation and signs and symptoms, but could range from 3 to 15+ vials. Antivenom dosage is not weight or age dependent and needs to be individualized. It is not in the scope of this chapter to present a lengthy discussion on the administration of antivenom; however, it should be noted that this is the treatment of choice when confronted by a snakebitten patient.[29]

Some surgeons in the United States believe that wound excision and fasciotomy is the primary treatment of snake envenomation. They believe that excisional therapy provides a means of removing injected venom, thereby decreasing the systemic absorption, tissue necrosis, and infection.[30] This may only be effective if the excision is done less than 2 hours after envenomation. This seems unlikely considering that the time it takes to transport a person from the snakebite site to the operating room with adequate preoperative workup usually is greater than 2 hours. Fasciotomy may be necessary if swelling results in a compartment syndrome.

The use of antibiotics for prophylactic purposes is probably unnecessary because snake venom is sterile. Tetanus prophylaxis is routinely recommended with puncture-type snakebites. The potential for infection comes from the environment that the wound is exposed to after snakebite.

Bee and Wasp Stings

Bee stings and wasp stings are very similar except that because wasps are scavengers the wound is more likely to become infected. Wasp stings should then be prophylaxed for tetanus if the patient is not current on his or her immunizations. Most bee and wasp stings will result in a local reaction of erythema and swelling. Systemically the patient may experience a toxic reaction, which requires a large number of stinging incidents, or an anaphylactic reaction, which may only require a single stinging insult.

Local treatment consists of removal of any stinger component left and cleansing of the wound. Ice can be applied to reduce inflammation, and an antihistamine such as diphenhydramine hydrochloride can be administered to reduce local inflammation. If the wound becomes infected then débridement, culture and sensitivity tests, and appropriate antibiotic coverage are indicated. When anaphylaxis results, epinephrine, an antihistamine, and oxygen should be administered.

Blister Beetles

A few genera of blister beetles are found in the southwestern portions of the United States. These beetles are found in grasslands, in flower beds, along fences, and in other locales where they may come in contact with the exposed human foot or leg. They release cantharidin, which will slowly cause blistering of the outer layers of the skin. Systemic manifestations of absorption of cantharidin may include diarrhea, abdominal pain, muscle fasciolation, pulmonary collapse, renal necrosis, coma, and death.

Local treatment of skin lesions require cleansing with acetone, ether, fatty soaps, or alcohol to dissolve or dilute the cantharidin. Calamine lotion application may help decrease skin reaction and irritation.[31]

Spider Bites

Approximately 50 to 60 spider species in the United States have been documented to bite human beings. Few of these species cause any local or systemic reaction and most bites are considered clinically and medically insignificant. Spider bites are often difficult to identify without recovering the spider at the time of the bite. Many suspected spider bites may in fact be due to ticks, kissing bugs, scorpions, or snakes.

The black widow *(Latrodectus)* and brown recluse *(Loxoscles reclusa)* spiders have been known to cause a few rare deaths in humans, but the cutaneous manifestations of these and other spider bites are more common. Almost all spiders produce venom, but only a few can penetrate the human skin. These include, but are not limited to, the aforementioned brown recluse and black widow spiders, plus tarantulas *(Digesiella)* and sac spiders *(chircanthium)*.

Tarantulas

Tarantulas are the largest of all spiders; however, their reputation as being harmful is overexaggerated. Tarantulas bite only when being roughly handled or when agitated. The bite may be only slightly painful and transient. Systemic analgesics and local care consisting of immobilization and elevation will relieve any symptoms. More importantly, some tarantula species have hairs on their dorsal surface that they can propel into the skin of a threatening enemy. These hairs will produce pruritus and wheals on skin and mucous membrane that can remain for many weeks. Treatment of the edema and pruritus is with topical corticosteroids and oral antihistamine.[32]

Brown Recluse Spider

The brown recluse spider *(Loxoscles reclusa)* is perhaps one of the most dangerous spiders in North America. It can be identified by its light to dark brown color and a fiddle-shaped marking on the dorsum of the cephalothorax. Its habitat is beneath rocks and boards outside or in closets, storage boxes, clothes, bed linens, and dark dry areas inside houses and buildings. The spider is by nature quite timid and will only bite when forced to come in contact with human skin. Results of brown recluse spider bites may range from a transient stinging and burning sensation at the bite site to a severe systemic reaction that, if not treated, may result in the death of the patient. Approximately 50 percent of reported bites occur on the buttocks, thigh, or foot and therefore necrotic arachnoidism should be a part of the physician's differential diagnosis when a patient presents with the identifying symptoms of a brown recluse spider bite. These symptoms include an increasingly painful solitary plaque with a central ischemic area surrounded by erythema. As the necrotic area increases in size, systemic signs may manifest, including urticaria, arthralgias, myalgias, hemolysis, febrile episodes, vomiting, shock, coma, and death. Systemic signs usually present within 3 days of the bite or they may not become evident at all.[32]

The treatment of brown recluse spider bites is varied and includes intralesional and oral steroids, hydroxyzine hydrochloride, surgical excision of the bite wound and venom, and administration of dapsone. Tetanus prophylaxis should be instituted because these wounds may become secondarily infected. Mild bites with less than 2 cm of necrosis require only supportive measures such as pain medication, clean dressings, and follow-up. More severe bites with necrotic centers over 2 cm in diameter should be treated. Excision of the dermis is controversial since the venom may rapidly dissipate further than the necrotic area, making identification of surgical margins difficult. Steroids do not inactivate the venom, but may stabilize the cell wall and decrease hemolysis. Dapsone has been described as decreasing the necrotic ulceration. Antivenom is not available in the United States at this time, and will only prevent dermal necrosis if administered within 30 minutes of the inflicting bite. Local management of the ulceration includes daily dressings and débridement as necessary. These wounds are resistant to skin grafts and may take many months to granulate and heal.

Black Widow Spider

The black widow spider *(Lactodectus)* bite results in neurotoxic symptoms. Envenomation may result in necrosis affecting epithelial tissue and blood vessels of the liver, kidney, spleen, lungs, pericardium, lymph nodes, thymus, adrenals, and neural tissue. The neurotoxic symptoms are a result of a block in neuromuscular transmission caused by a depletion of acetylcholine and catecholamine at motor nerve endings. Symptoms include headaches, dizziness, speech disturbances, chest tightness, respiratory distress, tremors, hyperactive deep tendon reflexes, and peripheral parasthesis with abdominal and leg pain. Muscular spasm of the flexor groups of the extremities may result in a contracted fetal position. The plantar surface of the foot may exhibit burning sensations.[32]

The use of antivenom is effective if administered

early. Symptoms should resolve within 1 or 2 hours. In healthy people symptoms will resolve in 2 or 3 days without treatment. The antivenom should be used in those people who are at risk for the severe complications. These include the very young, the very old, or those who already have some underlying systemic illness such as hypertension or cardiac dysfunction. For these individuals, death is more likely if the bite is not treated.

Sac Spider

The sac spider *(Chirocanthium)* may inflict relatively mild to severe bites. Its venom is similar to that of the brown recluse spider. Early signs include stinging pain, urticaria, erythema, and pruritus. A crust may form at the bite site and the tissue beneath the crust undergoes necrosis.[34]

These spiders are numerous and indigenous in the United States and are found almost year-round within dwellings. The sac spider bites when disturbed, and reports have shown that they will bite sleeping individuals.[32] Symptomatic relief is adequate because the severity of the bite does not usually compare with those of the brown recluse spider since less venom is injected with the sac spider bite. Usually an oral antihistamine or topical antipruritic is enough to give a reduction of the symptoms. The lesion usually heals in about 4 weeks without sequelae.

Marine Animal Stings and Infections

Soft tissue infections to the lower extremity can be seen as a result of trauma inflicted while the patient is immersed in seawater. Infection results because seawater contains a wide variety of bacteria that can penetrate the human skin after injury. The penetrating trauma can be the result of coral or rock cuts, injuries from marine equipment, or injuries from handling fish or shellfish. The noncholera *Vibrios* have been described as causing invasive wound infection that leads to necrotizing tissue destruction and septicemia.[35] *Vibrio* wound infections present as an intense acute cellulitis with bullae formation.

Treatment of seawater-induced wound infection is the same as for any bacteria-induced wound infection. Culture and sensitivity tests should be performed with adequate débridement of devitalized tissue. Local wound care and systemic antibiotics should be initiated. Although coral will not grow in human tissue, a foreign body granuloma can result. Therefore, any particulate matter should be flushed from the wound early in order to prevent granuloma and infection.

Skin exposure to the stings of salt water sponges may result in dermatitis. The liquid (slime) on the surface of the sponge acts as an irritant or toxin to the skin. Dermatitis is the only symptom seen as a result of human contact with a sponge. Reaction to stings from the sponge may be delayed up to several hours. A burning or pruritic sensation with cutaneous paresthesia will increase in severity for a few days and persist for several weeks. Papules, vesicles, or bullae may result that then desquamate, leaving a postinflammatory hyperpigmentation after healing.[36] Antihistamines and topical steroids may alleviate symptoms, and local application of cold may be effective.

Lionfish and scorpion fish envenomation may result from contact with the fin spines of these tropical fish. When the fin is compressed against the skin of the victim, the venom is injected. The venom from these fish contains a toxic, heat-labile protein that can result in intense pain, cyanosis, erythema, and ecchymoses around the injection site. Necrosis and skin sloughing may result in the area of penetration. Severe envenomation may lead to hypotension, vasodilation, and muscle weakness.

The recommended treatment is the immediate immersion of the injured foot into hot water. The water should be as hot as can be tolerated by the patient because heat will inactivate the toxin. Immersion should continue for 30 to 40 minutes or until the pain subsides. Local wound care consisting of irrigation, débridement, and removal of foreign debris should be initiated.[37]

REFERENCES

1. Grossman JA: Contusions, hematomas and abrasions. Ch. 13. In Grossman J (ed): Minor Injuries and Disorders: Surgical and Medical Care. JB Lippincott Co, Philadelphia, 1984

2. Whiteside T Jr.: Compartment syndrome. pp. 1201–1203. In Jahss M (ed): Disorders of the Foot. WB Saunders Co., Philadelphia, 1982.

3. Lewis VL Jr., Johnson PE: Chronic expanding hematoma. Plast Reconstr Surg, 79:465–467, 1987

4. Fitzgerald RH Jr., Cowan JDE: Puncture wounds of the foot. Orthop Clin North Am, 6:965–972, 1975

5. Edlich RF, Rodeheaver GT, Horowitz JH, Morgan RF: Emergency department management of puncture wounds and needlestick exposure. Emerg Med Clin North Am 4:581–592, 1986

6. Johanson PH: *Pseudomonas* infections of the foot following puncture wounds. JAMA 204:170–172, 1968

7. Manton WI, Thal ER: Lead poisoning from retained missiles. Ann Surg 204:594–599, 1986

8. Kaminsky HH: Toxic shock and a gunshot wound. Milit Med 151:52–53, 1986

9. Luterman A, Dacso CC, Curreri PW: Infections in burn patients. Am J Med 81:45–52, 1986

10. Kyosola K: Clinical experiences in the management of cold injuries: a study of 110 cases. J Trauma 14:32–35, 1974

11. Mager TG, Gross PL: Fatal systemic fluorosis due to hydrofluoric acid burns. Ann Emerg Med 14:149–153, 1985

12. Sagi A, Baruchin AM, Ben-Yakar Y et al: Burns caused by bromine and some of its compounds. Burns 11:343–350, 1985

13. Jarowenko DG, Moncusi-Ungaro HR Jr.: The care of burns from methyl bromide. J Burn Care Rehab 6:114–123, 1985

14. Torre C, Varetto L: The ultrastructure of the electric burn in man: a transmission electron microscopy–scanning electron microscopy study. J Forensic Sci 30:448–455, 1985

15. Lee RC, Kolodney MS: Electrical injury mechanisms: dynamics of the thermal response. Plast Reconstr Surg 80:663–671, 1987

16. Lee RC, Kolodney MS: Electrical injury mechanisms: electrical breakdown of cell membranes. Plast Reconstr Surg 80:672–679, 1987

17. Ten Dvis HJ, Klasen HJ, Reenalda PE: Keraunoparalysis, a 'specific' lightening injury. Burns 12:54–57, 1988

18. Mortimer PS, Dawber RP: Trauma to the nail unit including occupational sports injuries. Dermatol Clin 3:415–420, 1985

19. Scott DA, Scher RK: Exogenous factors affecting the nails: cosmetics, trauma and occupational influence. Dermatol Clin 3:409–413, 1985

20. Norton LA: Self induced trauma to the nails. Cutis 40:223–227, 1987

21. Rutherford RL, Dinteho AS: Grid method for the location of foreign body: a care report. J Foot Surg 7:29, 1968

22. Weinstock RE: Non invasive technique for the localization of radiopaque foreign bodies. J Foot Surg 20:73–75, 1981

23. Rickoff SE, Bauder T, Kerman BL: Foreign body localization and retrieval in the foot. J Foot Surg 20:33–34, 1981

24. Goldenberg RA, Goldenberg EM, Estersohn HS: Needle localization of foreign bodies using computed tomography. J Am Podiatr Med Assoc 78:629–631, 1988

25. Rest JG, Goldstein EJC: Management of human and animal bite wounds. Emerg Med Clin North Am 3:117–126, 1985

26. Lehman WL Jr., Allo MD, Jones WW, Johnston RM: Human bite infections of the hand: adjunct treatment with hyperbaric oxygen. Infect Surg 6:460–465, 1985

27. Dire DJ, Quick G: Dog-bite wounds. Emerg Decision, Nov/Dec, pp. 38–46, 1986

28. Kurecki BA III, Brownlee HJ Jr.: Venomous snakebites in the United States. J Fam Pract 25:386–392, 1987

29. Kitchens CS, Van Mierop LHS: Envenomation by the Eastern coral snake *(Micrurus fulvius fulvius)*. JAMA 258:1615–1618, 1987

30. Huang TT: Surgical management of poisonous snakebite. J Miss State Med Assoc March, pp. 65–71, 1987

31. Burnett JW, Caton GJ, Morgan RJ: Blister beetles: "spanish fly," Cutis 41:22, 1988

32. Wong RC, Hughes SE, Voorhess JJ: Spider bites: review in depth. Arch Dermatol 123:98–105, 1987

33. Alario A, Price G, Stahl R, Bancroft P: Cutaneous necrosis following a spider bite: a care report and review. Pediatrics 79:618–621, 1987

34. Krinsky WL: Envenomation by the sac spider *Chiracanthium mildei*. Cutis 40:127–129, 1987

35. Chang WJ, Pien FD: Marine acquired infections: hazards of the ocean environment. Postgrad Med 80:30–41, 1986

36. Burnett JW, Calton GJ, Morgan RJ: Dermatitus due to stinging sponges. Cutis 41:476, 1988

37. Kasdan ML, Kasdan AS, Hamilton DL: Lionfish envenomation. Plast Reconstr Surg 80:613–614, 1987

Foot Fractures[✸]

41

George S. Gumann, Jr., D.P.M.

FOREFOOT FRACTURES

Metatarsal Fractures

Mechanism

Metatarsal fractures are a common injury sustained by the forefoot.[1] They can be the result of direct trauma, such as striking the foot against an immovable object or crushing the foot by dropping an object onto it.[2] Crush injuries can also occur by rolling a heavy object over the forefoot. An indirect force can produce fractures of the metatarsals by having the forefoot fixed on the ground as the patient rotates.[3] These mechanisms of injury can produce isolated or multiple metatarsal fractures. The fifth metatarsal is the most commonly fractured. Conversely, the first metatarsal is the least likely to be fractured because of its size.[4] When lesser metatarsals are involved, especially with crush injuries, it is more common to have multiple metatarsal fractures.

Anatomy

The metatarsals are long bones with a head, neck, shaft, and base proximally. The bases of the metatarsals articulate with the cuneiforms and cuboid. The shape of the metatarsal bases and their strong interosseous ligaments produce a very stable articulation between the metatarsals and the tarsus. Very little motion occurs at this level. The first and fifth metatarsals have the largest individual ranges of motion. Along the shafts, the metatarsals are stabilized by the interossei muscles. Distally, the metatarsal heads are connected by the transverse intermetatarsal ligaments. Finally, the metatarsal heads are connected to their associated phalangeal bases by the metatarsophalangeal joint capsule, collateral ligaments, and expansions of the extensor apparatus. The first metatarsophalangeal joint is further reinforced plantarly by the short flexor apparatus.

Diagnosis

A good history may give a clue to the possible mechanism of injury and the force of the initial trauma. Metatarsal fractures are often overlooked, especially in the severely traumatized patient.[5] Clinical examination generally reveals edema, per-

✸ The views presented are those of the author and are not to be considered as reflecting official Department of Defense or U.S.A. Medical Department policy.

haps ecchymosis, but generally no gross deformity of the forefoot. Palpation will demonstrate tenderness over the involved metatarsal or metatarsals, as will attempted flexion and extension of the associated digit or digits. Also, attempted motion of the forefoot will elicit pain. Crepitation at the fracture site may be palpated if there is not too much edema. The amount of edema is related to the force of the injury, the number of fractures produced, the time elapsed since the injury, and the individual characteristics of the patient. The greater the time interval from the injury to examination, the greater will be the amount of edema and ecchymosis. Also, because of the close proximity of the metatarsals, it may be difficult to isolate a particular metatarsal as being fractured from clinical examination alone. It is always important to evaluate the neurovascular status distal to the site of injury and the associated soft tissue damage.

Radiologic Evaluation

Metatarsal fractures are readily visualized on routine radiographs. The dorsoplantar, medial oblique, and lateral views are utilized. However, the lateral view may superimpose the metatarsals unless the forefoot is inverted. A lateral view taken at an oblique angle can be useful in delineating the metatarsals. The sesamoidal view can be helpful in detecting plantarflexion deformities but is difficult to obtain in the traumatized foot. Sometimes, tomograms or a computed tomography (CT) scan can be employed to better define fractures, especially of the metatarsal bases.

Metatarsal fractures can present on radiographs as transverse, oblique, spiral, segmental, or comminuted.[2] Depending on the direction of the injury, metatarsal fractures can be displaced or angulated in any plane. When evaluating the radiographs,

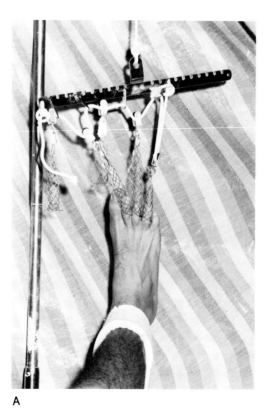
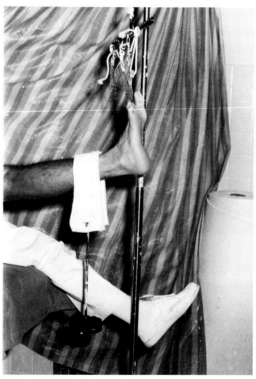

A   B

Fig. 41-1. Closed reduction of metatarsal fractures with Chinese finger-traps. The toes are placed in the finger-traps **(A)** and suspended with countertraction about the ankle **(B)**

two considerations are of paramount importance. First, is the metatarsal length changed, resulting in a distortion of the metatarsal parabola? Second, is there any displacement or angulational deformity present? Remember, when dealing with trauma, a minimum of three views are required for proper evaluation. Also, look for intra-articular involvement, either distally or proximally, which makes the prognosis more guarded because of the possibility of traumatic arthritis.

Closed Reduction Technique

Closed reduction should always be attempted first with metatarsal fractures. Chinese finger-traps are a very useful instrument in reducing metatarsal fractures (Fig. 41-1). The foot is anesthetized with a local anesthetic infiltrated as an ankle block. If the patient is apprehensive, some sedation can be employed either intravenously or intramuscularly. The digit of the fractured metatarsal, or digits in multiple metatarsal fractures, are placed in the finger-traps and countertraction is placed about the ankle. Usually 5 to 10 lbs is enough weight to produce distraction. The foot is suspended in the Chinese finger-traps for about 20 minutes. The principle employed is ligamentotaxis. The Chinese finger-traps apply a distraction force through the digits to the distal metatarsal fragment by the intact metatarsophalangeal joint capsule and collateral ligaments. The fractured metatarsal is pulled to length and straightened. If an angulational deformity is present, then a force opposite to that which produced the fracture can be applied to further manipulate the metatarsal position. Radiographs are then obtained with the foot still suspended in the finger-traps and the postreduction position evaluated. If further manipulation is required, it can be performed. If not, then a non-weight-bearing short leg cast (SLC) is applied with the foot still in traction but with the countertraction removed. After the cast has been applied, the digits are released and a second set of radiographs are taken to check for loss of reduction (Fig. 41-2).

Although an anatomic reduction is always the goal, small amounts of displacement of nonarticular fractures appear to be well tolerated if in a medial or lateral direction. However, dorsal or especially plantar angulation is not well tolerated.[6] A plantar-flexed metatarsal malunion will result in increased weight-bearing pressure, producing a hyperkeratotic lesion. A dorsiflexed malunion can result in a digital contracture, limited motion at the metatarsophalangeal joint, or a hyperkeratotic lesion under adjacent metatarsals. If a satisfactory reduction is obtained, then the patient is treated without bearing weight on the foot for 2 weeks, with radiographs taken weekly to check the fracture position. Then the cast is converted to a walker for the following 2 to 4 weeks. If the metatarsal fractures are reducible but unstable, then considerations can be given to percutaneous pinning. If an acceptable position cannot be obtained by closed reduction, then open reduction with internal fixation (ORIF) is indicated. This author prefers open reduction over percutaneous pinning.

Treatment

First Metatarsal. If the fracture is nondisplaced and stable, treatment consists of a weight-bearing SLC for 4 to 6 weeks. If the fracture is nondisplaced but unstable or potentially unstable, then a non-weight-bearing SLC is applied for 6 weeks. Because of the important weight-bearing function of the first metatarsal, an anatomic reduction is essential. No angulational deformity can be accepted, nor any shortening. If an anatomic reduction cannot be accomplished by closed reduction, then ORIF should be performed (Fig. 41-3). Intra-articular fractures of the first metatarsal head require anatomic reduction if possible.

Fifth Metatarsal. This is the most common metatarsal to be fractured. Fractures of the distal shaft occur most commonly by kicking an object with the foot. This usually produces an oblique or spiral fracture (Fig. 41-4). If mildly displaced, it can easily be treated by a weight-bearing SLC for 4 to 6 weeks. If significantly displaced with angulation and shortening, consideration should be given to ORIF. This fracture can be difficult to reduce as well as maintain in a reduced position. This author's preferred fixation is multiple 2.7-mm cortical lag screws. However, if only one lag screw can be employed, then a ¼ tubular plate should be

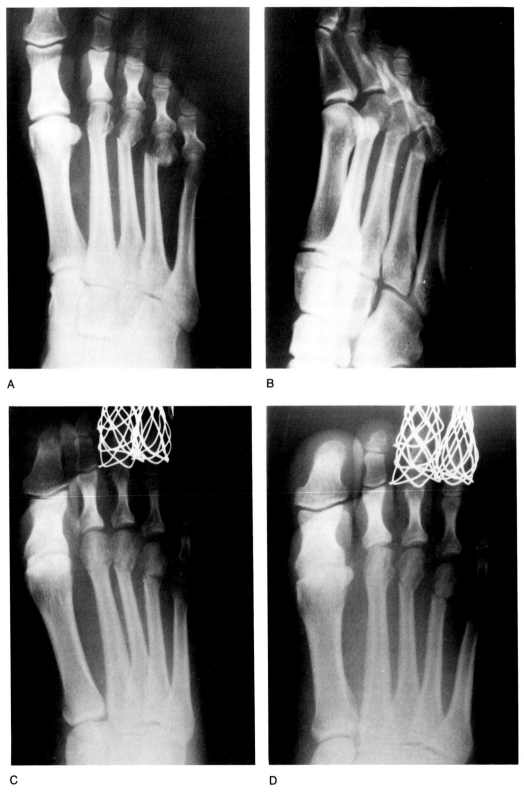

Fig. 41-2. Dorsoplantar **(A)** and oblique **(B)** views of multiple fractures involving the second, third, and fourth metatarsals sustained in a parachute jump. Dorsoplantar **(C)** and oblique **(D)** views of the closed reduction in Chinese finger-traps. *(Figure continues.)*

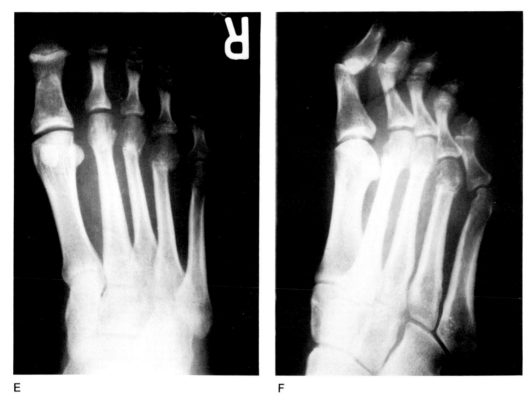

E

F

Fig. 41-2 *(continued).* Dorsoplantar **(E)** and oblique **(F)** views of the metatarsal fractures 2 months after injury showing signs of union.

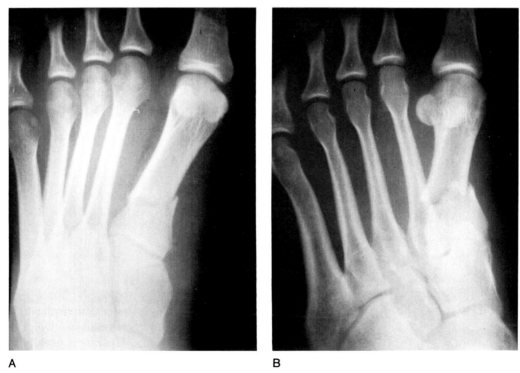

A

B

Fig. 41-3. Dorsoplantar **(A)** and oblique **(B)** views of a fracture of the first metatarsal caused by an object falling on the foot. *(Figure continues.)*

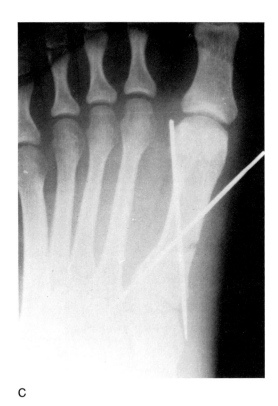

C

Fig. 41-3 *(continued)*. Dorsoplantar **(C)** and lateral **(D)** views of the open reduction with the fracture fixated with crossed K-wires.

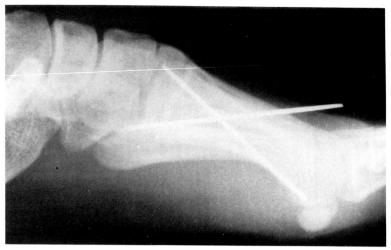

D

applied for neutralization. On occasion, severe comminution may require the use of cerclage wires with or without an intramedullary K-wire.

The most common fracture of the fifth metatarsal is the fracture at the tuberosity (Fig. 41-5). This fracture occurs with a forced inversion of the foot or ankle resulting in an avulsion force by the peroneus brevis. It is usually nondisplaced or minimally displaced and is treated in a weight-bearing SLC for 4 to 6 weeks. Healing is usually excellent and nonunion uncommon. Consequently, other authors have advocated noncasting treatment such as

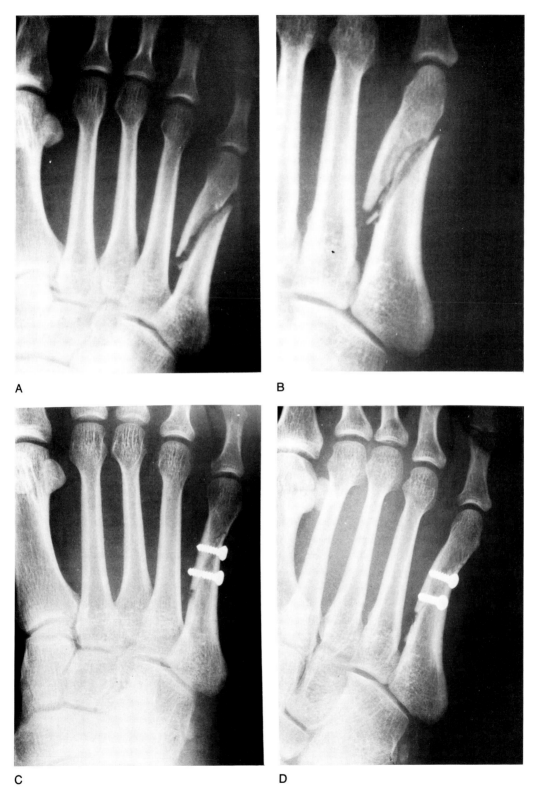

A

B

C

D

Fig. 41-4. Dorsoplantar **(A)** and oblique **(B)** views of the fracture of the distal fifth metatarsal. Dorsoplantar **(C)** and oblique **(D)** views of surgical reduction fixated by 2.7-mm cortical lag screws.

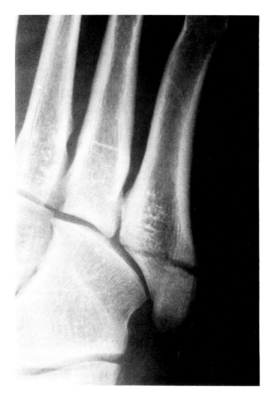

Fig. 41-5. Fracture of fifth metatarsal tuberosity.

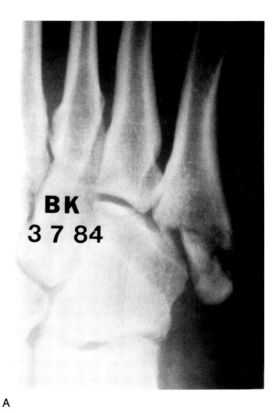

A

Fig. 41-6. Oblique **(A)** and lateral **(B)** views of displaced tuberosity fracture. *(Figure continues.)*

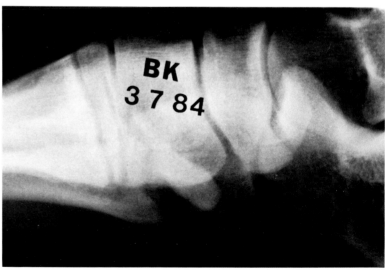

B

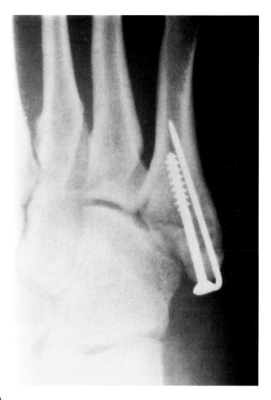

C

Fig. 41-6 *(continued)*. Oblique **(C)** and lateral **(D)** views of open reduction with internal fixation.

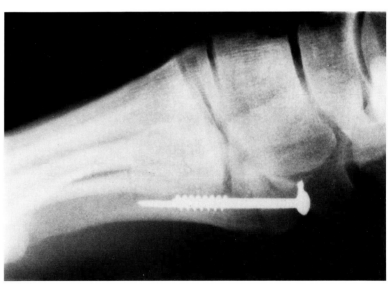

D

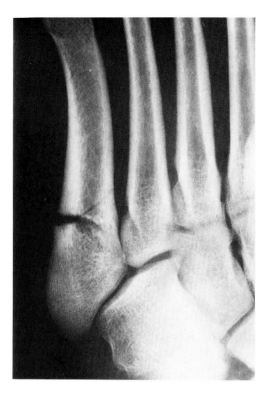

Unna boots, wooden shoes, or just weightbearing to tolerance with crutches or cane.[7] Occasionally, a patient has continued to engage in athletic activity after the injury and has presented with a significantly displaced fracture. If it is large and intra-articular, then it is surgically reduced and fixated. Fixation with a 4.0-mm cancellous screw and K-wire has been very successful (Fig. 41-6). An alternative technique is the use of a tension band wire.

The most troublesome fracture of the fifth metatarsal is the fracture of the proximal diaphysis, or Jones fracture (Fig. 41-7). This particular fracture is located within 1.5 cm of the tuberosity and has been reported to have a high nonunion rate.[8] In 1902, Jones first described the fracture, which he himself had sustained while dancing.[9] It can be caused by direct or indirect trauma and has also been reported to occur as a stress fracture.[10] Zelko et al. reported a nonunion rate of 50 percent and concluded that the type of treatment did not influence the outcome.[11] They used the term *intramed-*

Fig. 41-7. Type I fracture of the proximal diaphysis of the fifth metatarsal, or Jone's fracture.

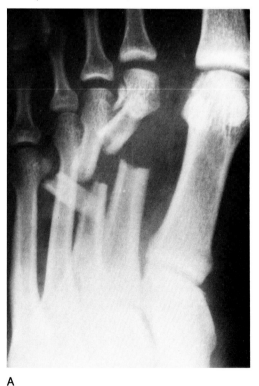

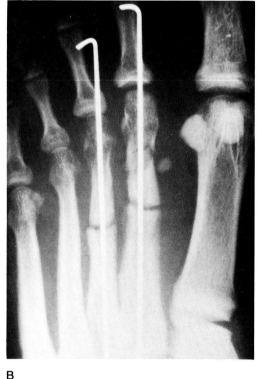

A   B

Fig. 41-8. (A) Multiple metatarsal fractures secondary to a motorcycle accident. **(B)** Open reduction of second and third metatarsals with intramedullary K wires for fixation.

ullary sclerosis to describe the cause of nonunion. However, Torg et al., in 1984, reported a 93 percent union rate in acute fractures without evidence of intramedullary sclerosis by utilizing a non-weight-bearing SLC for 6 to 8 weeks.[12] Lehman et al. have developed a standardized classification and treatment plan for Jones fractures.[13] Type I fractures are acute and have a well-delineated fracture line without previous history of pain, no intramedullary sclerosis, and minimal cortical hypertrophy. The recommended treatment is a non-weight-bearing SLC for 6 to 8 weeks. Type II fractures have a history of previous fracture with widened fracture line, some periosteal reaction, and evidence of intramedullary sclerosis. Treatment needs to be tailored to the patient. Fracture union can occur with a non-weight-bearing SLC but may be prolonged. However, in competitive atheletes, surgical intervention should be considered, using either intramedullary curettage and bone grafting or closed intramedullary screw fixation with a 4.5-mm malleolar screw. A type II fracture is essentially a delayed union. Type III fractures have a history of previous injury, widened fracture line, periosteal reaction complete intramedullary sclerosis and are essentially nonunions. Treatment requires surgical intervention with one of the two techniques described above.

Multiple Lesser (Internal) Metatarsal Fractures. Although isolated lesser metatarsal fractures do occur, it is more common to have multiple metatarsal fractures. If there is a stable, nondisplaced fracture of either an isolated lesser metatarsal or multiple metatarsals, treatment consists of a weight-bearing SLC for 4 to 6 weeks. Treatment can also be noncasting, with an Unna boot, a wooden shoe, or just guarded weightbearing. Impacted fractures of the metatarsal heads are well treated in this noncasting manner. However, multiple metatarsal fractures are more commonly displaced and angulated. Treatment consists of closed reduction with Chinese finger-traps and, if an acceptable position is obtained, wearing a SLC for 4 to 6 weeks. As described previously, in the first 2 weeks the patient does not bear weight on the foot, and radiographs are taken weekly to check for loss of reduction. Then the cast is converted to a walker for 2 to 4 weeks. Weightbearing is an important factor in fracture healing. If the fractures can be

aligned but are unstable, this author prefers ORIF, although closed percutaneous pinning is acceptable. Percutaneous pinning may have its best application with comminuted fractures of the metatarsal heads. If a satisfactory position cannot be accomplished by closed manipulation, then ORIF is indicated (Fig. 41-8). Depending on the fracture configuration and location, fixation can be obtained by intramedullary K-wires, crossed K-wires, lag screws (usually 2.7-mm cortical), or a combination of screws and a plate. In rare circumstances, an external fixator may need to be utilized in cases of severe comminution or segmental bone loss. After internal fixation, the patient is usually treated in a weight-bearing SLC for 4 to 6 weeks. An exception to weightbearing usually occurs with the use of an external fixator.

Open Metatarsal Fractures

Open fractures of the metatarsals are less common than closed fractures. In this type of injury, the trauma to the soft tissues is extremely important. This author grades open fractures based on the work of Gustilo and Anderson.[14] Grade I is an open fracture with a skin wound less than 1 cm, with little soft tissue damage and no bony comminution. The bone usually pierces the skin from inside to outside. Grade II is an open fracture with a skin wound greater than 1 cm but with little soft tissue loss, no extensive flaps, and minimal bony comminution. Grade III is an open fracture with gross contamination, extensive soft tissue loss, skin flaps, muscle damage or loss, injury to tendons, nerves, and blood vessels, and extensive bony comminution. A detailed description of the treatment of open fractures is too complex for this chapter, but this author adheres to the following principles. All open fractures are surgical emergencies and undergo débridement and copious irrigation as quickly as possible. After cultures the patient is placed on therapeutic antibiotics, usually a cephalosporin supplemented with an aminoglycoside in Grade III injuries. The antibiotics are continued for 72 hours and then discontinued unless the patient becomes septic. If septic, the antibiotics are adjusted according to the culture and sensitivity. In Grade III injuries the patient is returned to the operating room in 48 hours for a second débridement and dressing change. Internal fixation is performed primarily in grades I and II open fractures.

In grade III open fractures, internal fixation may be performed on a delayed basis in 5 to 7 days or when the soft tissue will allow. Grade III open fractures may require the use of an external fixator at the initial débridement to stabilize fractures and allow for wound care. Wound closure is performed by delayed primary closure in 5 to 7 days or obtained by split-thickness skin graft when the recipient site is ready. Extensive loss of soft tissue coverage of the forefoot, such as degloving injuries, may require plastic surgery consultation for a free flap transfer. The ultimate result of a severe open fracture to the forefoot can be amputation.

Lisfranc Fracture-Dislocations

Mechanism

Lisfranc fracture-dislocations are not common injuries. Aitken and Poulson, in reviewing 82,000 fractures, found only 16 such injuries.[15] The difficulty is that this injury may be misdiagnosed or even overlooked, especially in the polytrauma patient.[16] The mechanism of injury can be either direct or indirect. Motor vehicle accidents are now the most common cause of injury.[17] A direct blow to the foot can displace the metatarsal bases in any direction. Indirect trauma usually produces a hyperflexion of the forefoot, which ruptures the weaker dorsal tarsometatarsal ligaments. Additional abduction or adduction forces can then displace the metatarsals laterally or medially. The most common direction of displacement is in a dorsal and lateral direction.

Anatomy

An understanding of the anatomy will help to explain some patterns of Lisfranc injuries. The second metatarsal base, which is locked into a mortise between the three cuneiforms, is considered the key supporting structure.[18] It is common to sustain a fracture to the base of the second metatarsal while the other metatarsals dislocate. The bases of the second and third metatarsals are also wedge shaped, with the dorsal aspect being wider, which aids stability and resists dislocation in a plantar direction. The metatarsal bases have strong ligamentous attachments not only to the tarsal bones but also among themselves, with the exception of the first metatarsal. The strongest ligament is Lisfranc's ligament, which extends obliquely from the first cuneiform to the base of the second metatarsal. Additionally, the ligaments are stronger plantarly than dorsally and there are more secondary stabilizers plantarly, including the intrinsic muscles.

Clinical Examination

As with any injury a good history is important. Lisfranc fracture-dislocations can produce gross deformity of the forefoot. There will be diffuse tenderness over the metatarsal-tarsal articulation. One of the most consistent findings of this injury has been the presence of significant edema. Ecchymosis is usually present with time. Care must be exercised to evaluate the soft tissues as well as the neurovascular status of the distal forefoot. There will be tenderness on range of motion of the digits and foot.

Radiologic Evaluation

The routine radiographic examination includes the dorsoplantar, the medial oblique, and lateral views. A lateral oblique can help to evaluate fractures of the first metatarsal base. Most Lisfranc injuries are easily viewed and recognized on these films. It is rare to require special studies such as tomograms or a CT scan. One must be careful to closely scrutinize the other tarsal bones for fractures or dislocations as well as the metatarsophalangeal joints for dislocation. Nevertheless, there is a percentage of Lisfranc injuries that are very subtle. Stress radiography of the foot, especially with abduction of the forefoot, can reveal subtle subluxations of one or more of the metatarsal bases. A good clue to the Lisfranc fracture-dislocation is a small bony fragment between the first and second metatarsal bases. This represents an avulsion of the base of either the second metatarsal or first cuneiform and is called the fleck sign by Myerson et al., who found it present in 90 percent of their patients.[19]

Classification

The classic classification was described in 1909 by Quenu and Kuss.[20] They divided Lisfranc injuries into three categories: isolated, homo, and divergent. Isolated injuries involved one metatarsal

TYPE A: TOTAL INCONGRUITY

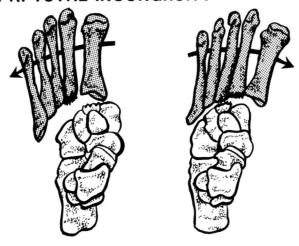

TYPE B: PARTIAL INCONGRUITY

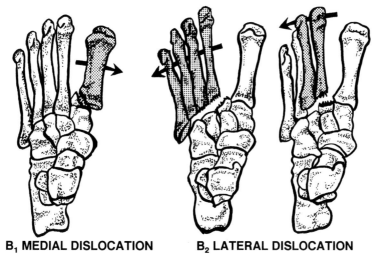

B₁ MEDIAL DISLOCATION   B₂ LATERAL DISLOCATION

TYPE C: DIVERGENT

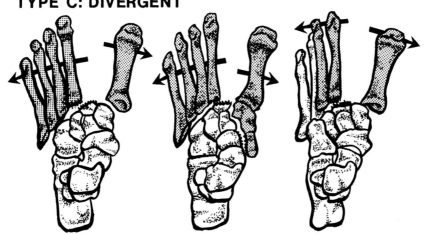

C₂ TOTAL DISPLACEMENT   C₁ PARTIAL DISPLACEMENT

Fig. 41-9. Classification of Lisfranc fracture-dislocations by Hardcastle. (Redrawn from Hardcastle et al.[21])

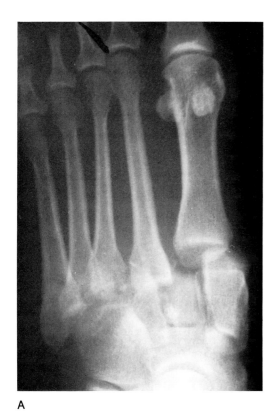

A

Fig. 41-10. Dorsoplantar **(A)** and lateral **(B)** views of type A Lisfranc injury with total incongruity in a lateral dorsal direction caused by slipping on a wet sidewalk.

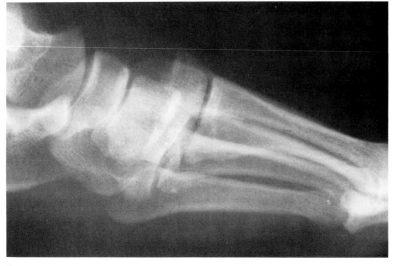

B

base. A homo injury was when all the metatarsals dislocated in the same direction. The most common was a homolateral fracture-dislocation. The divergent injury was one that split the forefoot, with the first metatarsal dislocating medially while the lesser metatarsals dislocated laterally.

Hardcastle et al. modified the above classification scheme into type A, type B, and type C[21] (Fig. 41-9). Type A represents total incongruity of the tarsometatarsal joint in any direction (Fig. 41-10). Type B is partial incongruity and is subdivided into B_1 and B_2. Type B_1 is partial incongruity affecting

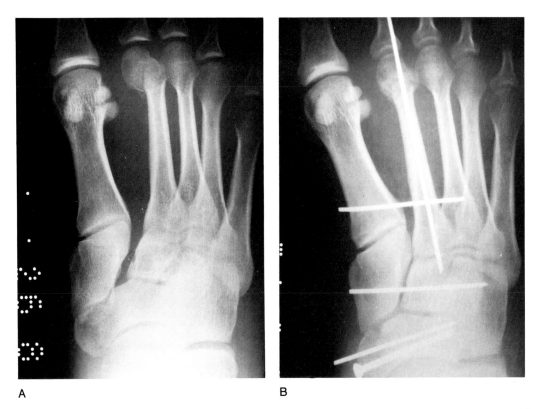

A

B

Fig. 41-11. (A) Type B₁ Lisfranc fracture-dislocation sustained while playing basketball. Note additional fractures of navicular, fibular sesamoid, and second and third metatarsals. **(B)** ORIF.

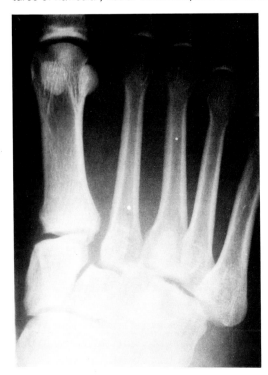

Fig. 41-12. Type B₂ Lisfranc injury with involvement of all lesser metatarsals.

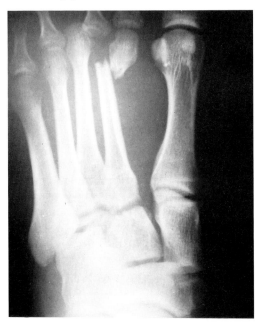

Fig. 41-13. Type C₁ Lisfranc fracture-dislocation sustained in a parachute jump. Base of second metatarsal is subluxed, differentiating this injury from a Type B₁. Again, note additional fractures to the navicular and second metatarsal with dislocation of the third metatarsophalangeal joint.

only the first ray (Fig. 41-11) and type B_2 is partial incongruity affecting one or more of the lesser metatarsals (Fig. 41-12). Type C represents a divergent pattern of injury and is subdivided into C_1 and C_2. Type C_1 has displacement of the first metatarsal medially and the lesser metatarsals laterally but with only partial incongruity (Fig. 41-13). Type C_2 is the same divergent pattern but with total incongruity.

Treatment

Treatment recommendations have been closed reduction with plaster immobilization, closed reduction with percutaneous pinning, and ORIF. Chinese finger-traps are utilized for closed manipulation. Many authors have pointed out the ease of reduction of Lisfranc dislocations that have no associated fractures. However, they indicate that gross instability exists and that loss of reduction is a significant problem.[17,19,21] Thus, if closed reduction without fixation is to be the method of treatment, the patient is maintained in a non-weight-bearing SLC with radiographic evaluation weekly to rule out loss of reduction. Patients are immobilized for 6 to 8 weeks with an initial period of non-weight-bearing of approximately 4 to 6 weeks, but there is no universal agreement on this point. At the end of the casting period, the patient is x-rayed and, if nontender, allowed to start bearing weight to tolerance. If there is a loss of reduction, then treatment should change to either a second closed reduction with pinning or ORIF. The further from the time of the injury, the more difficult it will be to remanipulate by closed means.

Closed reduction with percutaneous pinning has been advocated by several authors.[17,21] However, if a satisfactory position cannot be achieved with closed means, with or without fixation, then ORIF should be performed. In fact, this author's preferred method of treatment for Lisfranc injuries is ORIF, and multiple K wires are the usual choice for fixation (Fig. 41-14). It is critical that if the second metatarsal is involved, either fractured or dislocated, it be stabilized with a K-wire.[19] Depending on the pattern of the injury, stabilization may be obtained with as few as two K-wires. This is because the third, fourth, and fifth metatarsal bases may be dislocated from their corresponding tarsal bones,

but the intermetatarsal interosseous ligaments may be intact so that these three metatarsals act as one unit. Consequently, they can be fixated with a single K-wire. Other times, each individual metatarsal is unstable and needs to be fixated with a K-wire. Type B and certain type C injuries may lend themselves to screw fixation or a combination of screws and K-wires. The K-wires are allowed to remain for 6 to 8 weeks and the patient can be immobilized in either a weight-bearing or a non-weight-bearing SLC. After the K-wires are removed, weightbearing is begun to tolerance.

As with any intra-articular injury, traumatic arthritis is a long-term potential sequela. It has been emphasized that the major determinant for long-term acceptable results is the quality and maintenance of the initial reduction. Myerson et al. have reported that a satisfactory reduction has been accomplished if the distance between the first metatarsal–first cuneiform and the second metatarsal base is less than 2 mm on the dorsoplantar radiograph.[19] The talometatarsal angle as measured on the weight-bearing lateral should be less than 15 degrees. Nevertheless, this author prefers to use radiographs of the uninvolved foot as a guide to reduction along with the above guidelines.

At operation, it is unusual not to have some degree of osteochondral damage present on at least one of the metatarsal bases. Wilson has indicated that with time all Lisfranc fracture-dislocations will progress to degenerative arthritis.[17] If arthritis does develop, fusion is indicated if the pain is not alleviated by conservative modalities. Fusion can be accomplished in the traditional manner of resecting the involved articular surfaces with the application of some type of internal fixation. Johnson and Johnson have published their technique of dowel arthrodesis, which uses a percutaneous bone graft from the iliac crest supplemented by crossed K-wire fixation.[22]

Lesser Tarsus Fractures

Cuneiform Fractures

Mechanism. Fractures and dislocations of the cuneiforms are quite rare.[6] The mechanism of injury is usually direct trauma. When they do occur, they are usually associated with fractures and disloca-

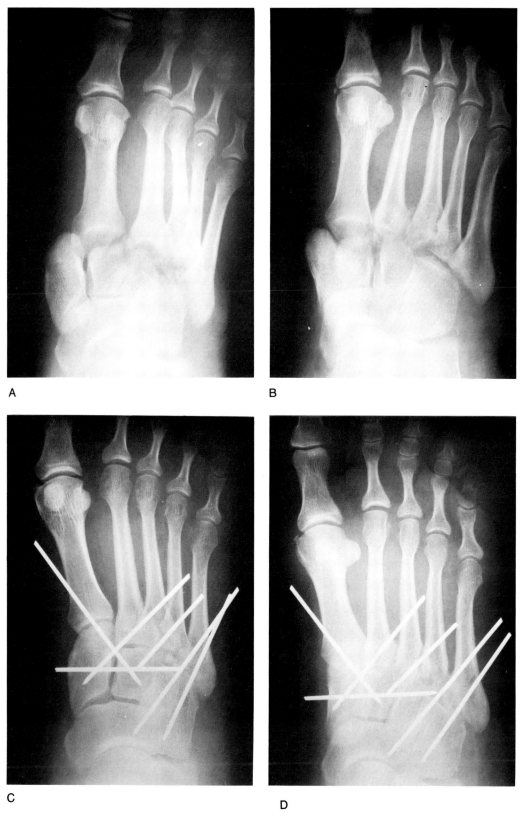

A

B

C

D

Fig. 41-14. *Top,* Dorsoplantar **(A)** and Oblique **(B)** views of a type A Lisfranc fracture-dislocation secondary to a motor vehicle accident. *Bottom,* Dorsoplantar **(C)** and oblique **(D)** views of anatomic reduction obtained by ORIF.

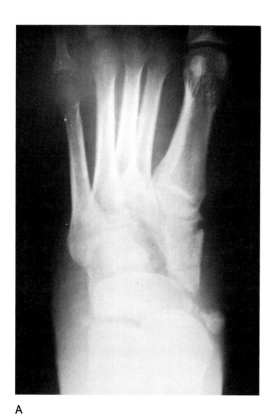

A

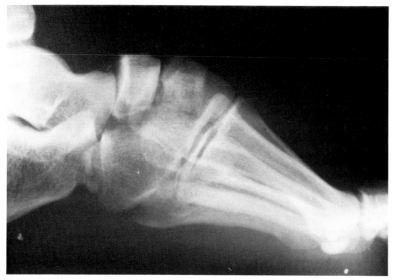

B

Fig. 41-15. Dorsoplantar **(A)** and lateral **(B)** views of fracture of the first cuneiform, which is highly comminuted. Injury was caused by a motorcycle accident, and associated osseous damage is common.

tions to other bones in the forefoot. Since crush injuries are a frequent cause of direct trauma, careful attention must be directed to the soft tissue.

Clinical and Radiographic Evaluation. The foot will usually be swollen and may be ecchymotic. Tenderness will be present over the midfoot but will become more diffuse with time. It may be difficult to isolate an individual cuneiform as having been fractured by clinical examination. There will be tenderness on attempted range of motion of the forefoot.

Dorsoplantar, oblique, and lateral views of the foot will usually delineate cuneiform fractures. Again, be careful to scrutinize the radiograph closely for associated forefoot fractures and dislocations (Fig. 41-15). Tomograms or CT scan might be useful in identifying a fracture not obvious on routine films or in evaluating the degree of comminution if surgery is contemplated.

Treatment. Heck reported that displacement of cuneiform fractures is uncommon.[23] In this case, a weight-bearing SLC is indicated for 4 to 6 weeks. However, if displaced, cuneiform fractures require operative reduction with fixation by K wires or lag screws (Fig. 41-15). Even with severely comminuted fractures, long-term complications are not common because of the limited motion occurring at the midtarsus.[24] If there is persistent pain from traumatic arthritis, then fusion can be performed.

Cuboid Fractures

Mechanism. Like cuneiform fractures, isolated cuboid fractures are rare.[25] Hillegass reported two types of cuboid fractures.[26] The most common is a cortical avulsion of the lateral aspect of the cuboid. The other type involves the entire body, and has been described by Hermel[27] as a "nutcracker fracture." Cuboid fractures can be caused by direct or indirect trauma. A direct injury can be caused by a crush injury or a direct blow. Indirect injury is produced either by abducting or inverting the forefoot.

Clinical and Radiographic Evaluation. There will be tenderness over the lateral aspect of the midfoot with edema and ecchymosis. There will be tenderness on inversion and eversion of the forefoot.

Routine foot radiographs will easily demonstrate cuboid fractures but the medial oblique view is

usually the best. Also, if the foot is supinated when the lateral view is taken, the cuboid will be more visible instead of being superimposed on the cuneiforms and navicular. In the case of a "nutcracker fracture," care must be exercised not to overlook an avulsion fracture of the navicular tuberosity or other osseous injuries.

Treatment. With a simple cortical avulsion, treatment can be related to the degree of symptoms. If not very symptomatic, the patient can be immobilized with an elastic bandage or Unna boot and a wooden shoe. Weightbearing to tolerance can be accomplished with the use of a cane or crutches if needed. However, if the pain is intense and ambulation difficult, then a walking SLC can be applied for 3 to 4 weeks.

Fractures of the cuboid body (Fig. 41-16) that are nondisplaced are treated with a weight-bearing SLC for 5 to 6 weeks. If the fracture is displaced, then ORIF is indicated (Fig. 41-17). DeLee indicated that a corticocancellous bone graft used as a

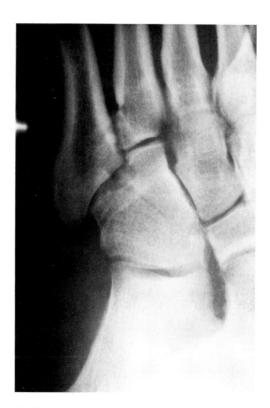

Fig. 41-16. Fracture of the cuboid sustained in a parachute jump.

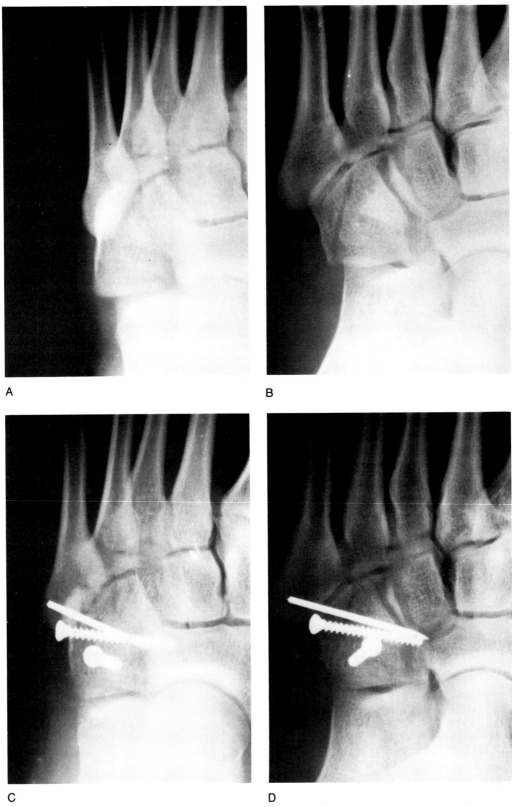

Fig. 41-17. Dorsoplantar **(A)** and oblique **(B)** views of a displaced fracture of the cuboid sustained in a parachute jump. Dorsoplantar **(C)** and oblique **(D)** views of ORIF.

strut may be necessary because of the compression to the cancellous bone that results from the "nutcracker" mechanism.[24] If the cuboid is severely comminuted, then a solution is a walking SLC for 5 to 6 weeks. Another solution is to use a corticocancellous graft and apply an external fixator in a distraction mode to prevent late collapse.

Navicular Fractures

Classification.   Fractures of the navicular are rare, but are more common than cuneiform or cuboid fractures.[28] Watson-Jones has divided navicular fractures into three types: chip fractures of the dorsal lip, fractures of the tuberosity, and fractures of the body.[29] The navicular is one of the key bones in the foot as it articulates with the talus to form part of the midtarsal joint. If the navicular is damaged, the motion of the midtarsal as well as the subtalar joint can be affected. Also, it has been demonstrated that the medial and lateral thirds of the navicular body have a good blood supply, while the central one-third is relatively avascular.[30] This can lead to problems with fracture union.

Clinical and Radiographic Evaluation.   With navicular fractures, there will be tenderness to palpation over the dorsal and medial aspects of the midfoot. There will be edema and usually ecchymosis. Tenderness will occur on attempted motion of the midtarsal and subtalar joints.

The routine dorsoplantar, oblique, and lateral radiographs are usually adequate to diagnose navicular fractures. Confusion can occur in regard to the tuberosity fracture if an accessory navicular (os tibiale externum) is present. An oblique film shot from the medial side will help to visualize the medial aspect of the navicular. Tomograms and CT scan can also be useful.

Dorsal Lip Fractures.   The dorsal lip fracture is the most common type, accounting for 47 percent of navicular fractures.[31] The mechanism is usually a plantarflexion–inversion of the foot. The talonavicular ligament avulses a piece of the dorsal aspect of the navicular at its attachment. It is best visualized in the lateral radiograph, and tenderness would be mostly over the dorsal aspect of the talonavicular joint. Since these fragments are usually small, treatment can be determined by the severity of symptoms. If only mild symptoms are present, then immobilization can consist of an elastic ban-

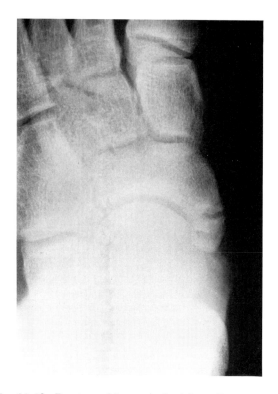

Fig. 41-18. Fracture of the navicular tuberosity versus accessory ossicle (tibiale externum).

dage or Unna boot with weightbearing to tolerance. However, if the pain is severe, then a walking SLC is applied for 3 to 4 weeks. Many times, these fragments do not unite and a delayed excision is recommended if symptomatic.

Tuberosity Fractures.   The navicular tuberosity fracture is an avulsion fracture caused by the posterior tibial tendon resulting from a forced eversion of the foot (Fig. 41-18). Significant displacement is uncommon because of the diffuse insertion of the posterior tibial tendon. The dorsoplantar and lateral oblique views best visualize this fracture radiographically. Care must be exercised to distinguish between a fracture and an accessory navicular. Radiographs of the opposite foot may help in the diagnosis, because the accessory navicular occurs bilaterally 90 percent of the time.[32] Again, the recommendation is individualized treatment of the patient according to symptoms. However, this author prefers a walking SLC for 4 to 6 weeks. If a painful nonunion develops, delayed excision with resuturing of the posterior tibial tendon through drill holes in the raw bone and immobilization in a SLC is

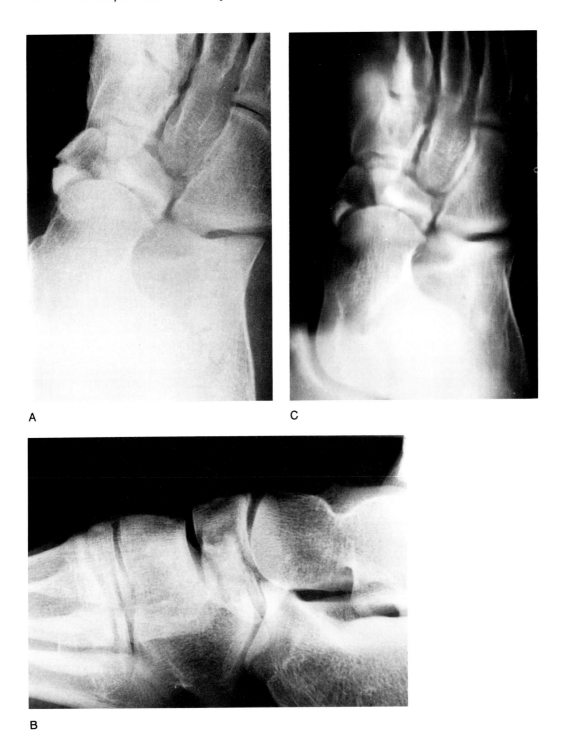

A

C

B

Fig. 41-19. Oblique **(A)** and lateral **(B)** views of comminuted navicular fracture. **(C)** Tomogram. **(D)** Dorsoplantar view of ORIF. *(Figure continues.)*

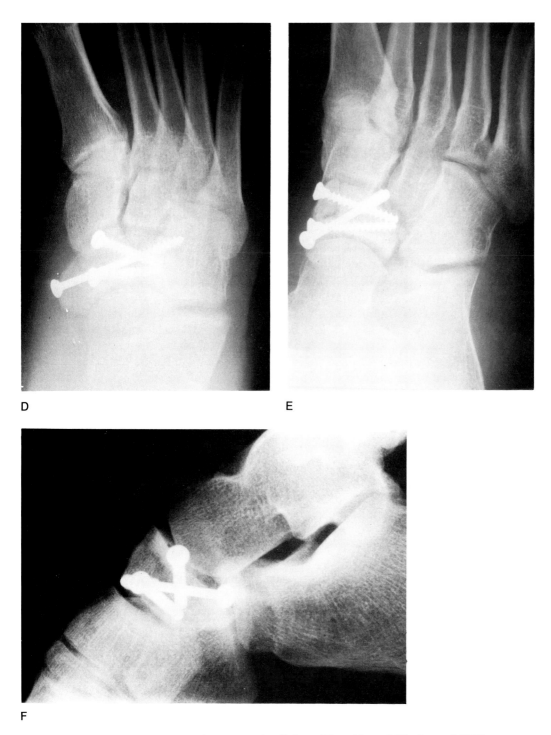

D

E

F

Fig. 41-19 *(continued)*. Oblique **(E)** and lateral **(F)** views of ORIF.

recommended. If significant displacement occurs, ORIF with 4.0 cancellous screws is utilized.

Fractures of the Navicular Body. Fractures of the navicular body can be caused by a direct blow or indirectly by a fall landing on a plantarflexed foot. Routine foot radiographs usually demonstrate the fracture. A nondisplaced fracture of the body is treated in a non-weight-bearing SLC for 6 to 8 weeks. Nonweightbearing is favored to prevent compressive forces from further damaging or displacing the navicular fracture. If displaced but not severely comminuted, then ORIF is performed with lag screw fixation. This author believes there is no indication for closed reduction in displaced fractures. If the decision is made for surgical intervention, then tomograms and/or CT scan can be helpful in determining the size and number of fragments. They can also help determine the type of fixation that can best be employed. While rigid internal fixation with lag screws is preferred (Fig. 41-19), highly comminuted fractures may require K-wires or a combination of K-wires and screws. If rigid internal fixation is obtained, then postoperative range of motion exercises can be used as with any intra-articular fracture. If fixation is not rigid and there is a fear of compressing a comminuted segment of the body, then an external fixator is applied in a distraction mode for 6 weeks. If the body is severely comminuted, then an external fixator is applied in addition to a corticocancellous graft to prevent additional collapse. If collapse occurs, this will adduct the forefoot. Obviously, traumatic arthritis is a potential complication of body fractures. Primary arthrodesis of the talonavicular joint is not recommended and is reserved as a secondary procedure if arthritis develops.

REARFOOT FRACTURES

Talar Fractures

Anatomy

The talus is a very unique bone, and this fact contributes in part to the significance of any major injury. Talar fractures were first reported in 1608 by Fibricius.[33] In 1919, Anderson coined the term *aviator's astragalus* from his experience during World War I with talar fractures resulting from airplane crash landings.[34,35]

The talus consists of a head, neck, and body. There are no muscular attachments. It articulates with the tibia, fibula, calcaneus, and navicular. There are multiple ligamentous attachments between the talus and the bones with which it articulates. Boyd and Knight stated that more weight is borne per square inch by the superior surface of the talar dome than by any other joint.[36] The two unique aspects of the talus that contribute to long-term complications after injury are its vascular supply and its biomechanical requirements. Disruption of the vascular supply can result in avascular necrosis and damage to the articular surfaces can lead to traumatic arthritis.

The blood supply to the talus has been reported to be poor.[37] New investigations have revealed an extensive blood supply to the talus but a limited area to enter the bone, resulting in easy disruption with injury.[38] The blood supply has been divided into extraosseous and intraosseous. The extraosseous blood supply comes from three arteries: (1) the artery of the superior neck, (2) the artery of the sinus tarsi, and (3) the artery of the tarsal canal. The artery of the superior neck of the talus is derived from the dorsalis pedis and is responsible for vascularization of the superior and medial aspects of the talar head. The artery of the sinus tarsi is an anastomosis of vessels from the dorsalis pedis, anterior tibial, perforating peroneal, and lateral malleolar arteries. This artery vascularizes the lateral two-thirds of the talar body as well as the inferior and lateral aspects of the head of the talus. The artery of the tarsal canal is a branch from the posterior tibial artery that pierces the deltoid ligament and supplies the medial one-third of the talar body.[39] The intraosseous vascular supply results from anastomosis of intraosseous vessels, which is highly variable and occurs in 60 percent of patients.[40] Depending on the pattern of disruption of the blood supply, various rates of avascular necrosis will ensue. The literature reports an avascular necrosis rate of between 16 and 71 percent.[41] Avascular necrosis can lead to collapse of the body of the talus, resulting in arthritis of the ankle and subtalar joint.

The unique biomechanical properties of the talus are the amount of weight that is supported by this relatively small bone and the fact that 60 percent of the talus is covered by articular cartilage. Consequently, any major fracture of the talus has an excellent probability of involving an articular surface and any incongruity is magnified by the increased amount of weight supported per square inch. Thus traumatic arthritis is also a possible long-term complication even if the talus does not undergo avascular necrosis and collapse. The rate of traumatic arthritis seems variable and has been reported to range from a low of 40 to 45 percent to a high of 90 to 95 percent.[42,43]

Clinical and Radiographic Evaluation

With major fractures of the talar neck and body, there will be tenderness about the entire ankle and rearfoot. If there is a fracture with dislocation of the subtalar joint or ankle joint, then a discernible deformity of the foot and ankle will be present. Edema and ecchymosis are present and can increase significantly with time. This can manifest itself as fracture blisters and skin necrosis. If a portion of the talar body is extruded from the ankle joint, it may be palpable as a bony deformity under the skin. There will be tenderness and limitation of motion of the foot and ankle. A percentage of fractures of the talar neck and body will present as open injuries. However, with the less severe fractures such as cortical avulsions of the talar head or fractures of the posterior process, the tenderness will be more pinpointed to the area of injury. Also, the amount of edema and ecchymosis will be smaller. There will be a greater range of motion available and there should be less tenderness on motion.

In evaluating fractures of the talus, one needs to have dorsoplantar and oblique radiographs of the foot, anteroposterior and mortise views of the ankle, and a lateral view encompassing both the foot and ankle. Additional information can be obtained with tomograms and CT scans as necessary.

Fractures of the Talar Neck/Body

In 1970, Hawkins presented a classification for fractures involving the talar neck and described groups I through III.[44] This classification is important since fractures and fracture-dislocations of the talar neck comprise 50 percent of all major talar injuries. Canale and Kelly described an additional fracture-dislocation of the neck of the talus that they called group IV.[45] The mechanism for these fractures is a forced dorsiflexion of the foot, so that the neck of the talus impinges on the anterior aspect of the tibial plafond.

Group I Talar Neck/Body Fracture. This is a vertical fracture of the neck of the talus without subluxation or dislocation of the subtalar or ankle joint (Fig. 41-20). There is some difference of opinion as to whether only nondisplaced talar neck fractures should be included in group I injuries. Penny and Davis stated that any displacement of the talar neck results in some degree of subluxation of the subtalar joint and should be a group II injury.[46] In this fracture only one source of the blood supply is lost, and the rate of avascular necrosis has been reported to be 13 percent.[45]

Group II Talar Neck/Body Fracture. This is a vertical fracture of the neck of the talus with subluxation or dislocation of either the subtalar or ankle joint, but not both (Fig. 41-21). With this type of fracture two sources of the blood supply are lost and the incidence of avascular necrosis increases to 40 to 50 percent.[44] This type of injury may present as an open fracture.

Group III Talar Neck/Body Fracture. This is a vertical fracture of the neck of the talus with dislocation of the body from both the subtalar and ankle joints (Fig. 41-22). The body of the talus is most commonly dislocated posteriorly and medially out of the ankle joint, resting on the superior surface of the calcaneus. The talar body can also be dislocated anteriorly out of the ankle joint. If fractures of the malleoli occur, the talar body could move medially or laterally. All three sources of the blood supply are lost in this type of fracture, and the incidence of avascular necrosis is 90 to 100 percent.[44] This injury presents as an open fracture approximately 50 percent of the time.[47]

Group IV Talar Neck/Body Fracture. This is a vertical fracture of the neck of the talus with subluxation or dislocation of either the subtalar or ankle joint or both with an associated subluxation or dislocation of the talonavicular joint (Fig. 41-23).[45]

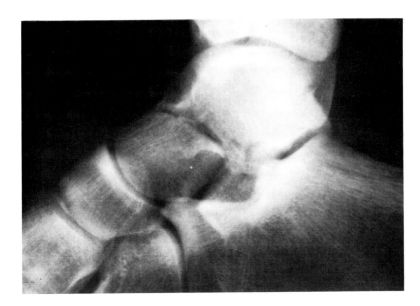

Fig. 41-20. Group I talar neck fracture that is nondisplaced and does not involve the subtalar or ankle joint.

Treatment. In group I (nondisplaced) talar neck fractures, treatment consists of closed reduction in a non-weight-bearing SLC cast. If the fracture is potentially unstable, then the cast is applied with the foot in plantarflexion. If the fracture is impacted and stable, then the cast is applied with the foot in a neutral position. Casting time is initially 8 weeks. However, if the plantarflexed cast is used, it is changed at 5 to 6 weeks and reapplied with the foot in less plantarflexion. This is done several times so that by the eighth week the foot will be close to a neutral position. Being casted in a plantarflexed position for 8 weeks can present difficulties when attempting to regain ankle motion.

The closed reduction of any displaced talar neck fractures requires plantarflexion with perhaps some inversion or eversion of the foot. Many have advocated the closed reduction of this fracture,[6,48] but this author feels that a displaced talar neck fracture is an indication for immediate ORIF, as-

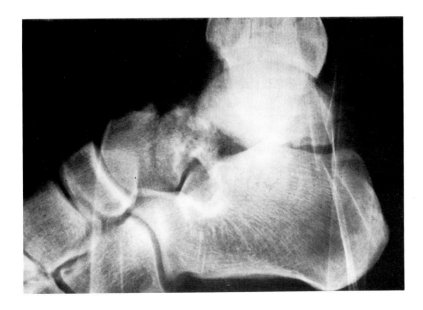

Fig. 41-21. Group II talar neck fracture with subluxation of the subtalar joint.

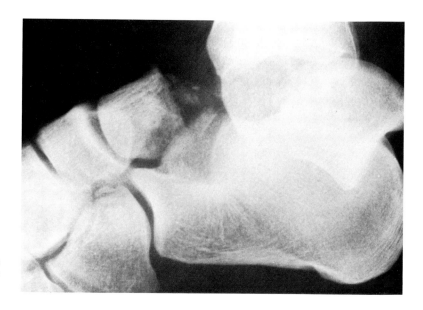

Fig. 41-22. Group III talar neck fracture with posterior dislocation of the talar body.

suming the patient is a surgical candidate and that the fracture is not highly comminuted (Fig. 41-24). Recent articles support this approach and indicate that this gives the best chance for the talus to reestablish its blood supply.[41,49] Fixation should be accomplished by cancellous screws (usually 4.0 mm) employed either from anterior to posterior or in the opposite direction (may use 6.5-mm screw in this case). An interesting technique recommended by Trillat et al. for group II fractures combines closed reduction under fluoroscopic control with a lag screw inserted from the posterior tubercle of the talus.[49] To attempt to close reduce a group III fracture is futile and definitely requires immediate ORIF. One can use a calcaneal pin for distraction in order to help reduce the talar body back into the ankle joint, or, as this author prefers, perform a medial malleolar osteotomy in an attempt to preserve any possible blood supply through the deltoid ligament. With rigid internal fixation, the post-

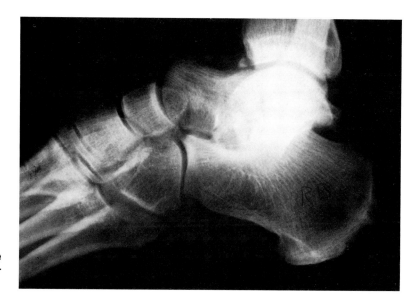

Fig. 41-23. Group IV talar neck fracture with involvement of both the subtalar and talonavicular joints.

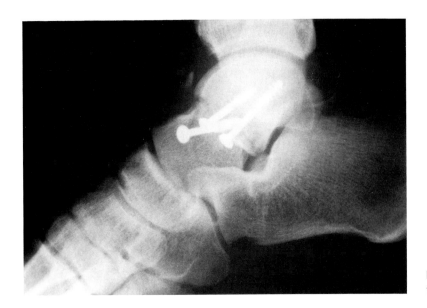

Fig. 41-24. ORIF of Hawkins' group II talar fracture seen in Fig. 41-22.

operative rehabilitation involves range-of-motion exercises of the foot and ankle while keeping the extremity from bearing weight. Nonweightbearing continues until fracture union has occurred and there is no evidence of avascular necrosis.

Since a percentage of talar fractures present as open injuries, it is even more important to be aggressive with this situation because of the added complications of infection and osteomyelitis. This author follows the same guidelines as described

with open fractures of the metatarsals except that rigid internal fixation is attempted at the initial débridement regardless of grade of injury. The most difficult question to answer is whether to replace a talar body that is devoid of soft tissue and contaminated. If at all possible, the talar body is saved. The complications of talar neck fractures include skin necrosis, infection, delayed union and nonunion, malunion, avascular necrosis, and traumatic arthritis.

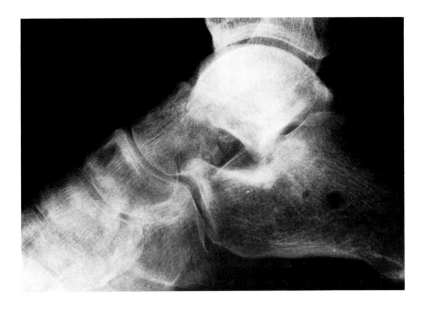

Fig. 41-25. Avascular necrosis of the talus.

Skin necrosis can be prevented by early, accurate reduction with atraumatic handling of the soft tissue during surgery. Skin breakdown increases the risk of infection, which can occur in the soft tissue or the bone. Osteomyelitis of the talus, especially in the presence of avascular necrosis, is very difficult to eradicate.[48]

Peterson et al.[50] reported a 10 percent incidence of delayed union, and Lorentzen et al.[42] noted a nonunion rate of less than 5 percent. To this author, these rates seem very low for such difficult injuries, and the three group III talar fractures I have seen within the last 15 months have all gone to nonunion. Malunion of talar neck fractures will lead to traumatic arthritis because of incongruity, and can affect the ankle, subtalar, and midtarsal joints. Malunion occurs from a lack of an anatomic reduction or by the loss of an anatomic reduction. Canale and Kelly reported that malunion occurs in a dorsal or varus position.[45] A dorsal malunion prevents ankle dorsiflexion and a varus malunion causes subtalar arthritis and an inverted foot. With ORIF, malunion can be mostly eliminated as a complication. Traumatic arthritis can occur from malunion, osteochondral damage to the articular surfaces at the time of the injury, or collapse of the avascular talar body, resulting in joint incongruity.

Avascular necrosis is primarily determined by the type of fracture and the disruption of the vascular supply to the talus. The rates of avascular necrosis have been previously stated and increase with the severity of the injury. A diagnosis is made on the basis of the radiograph if the talus appears dense and sclerotic (Fig. 41-25). There may be total or only partial involvement of the talar body, and revascularization may take up to 2 years through a process of creeping substitution. When one sees evidence of subchondral lucency along the talar dome on the anteroposterior ankle radiograph at about 8 to 12 weeks (Hawkins' sign[44]), this is a good indication that vascularity is present. If avascular necrosis develops, the treatment is nonweightbearing but there is little agreement on the length of time. Also, the presence of avascular necrosis does not mean that the patient will have a poor result.

What is interesting is the fact that there is little agreement in the literature on what to do with the patient with nonunion, avascular necrosis, and traumatic arthritis. Surgical options recommended have included subtalar fusion, triple arthrodesis, ankle fusion, pantalar arthrodesis, tibiocalcaneal fusion, and talectomy. The most commonly described type of ankle fusion is the modified Blair fusion.[51] This procedure excises the avascular talar body and fuses the tibia to the remaining head and neck portion by sliding a cortical graft downward from the anterior aspect of the tibia (Fig. 41-26). This author has experience with both ankle fusion and tibiocalcaneal fusion (Fig. 41-27), but is now using a modified tibiocalcaneal fusion. The talar body is excised, leaving the head and neck. The articular surfaces of the fibula, tibia, and posterior facet of the calcaneus are excised. A tricortical graft from the posterior iliac crest is used to wedge open the fusion site, which is also packed with cancellous bone and fixated with cancellous screws. This procedure maintains length of the extremity and preserves midtarsal joint function. The only surgical procedure listed that does not enjoy favor today is talectomy.[41]

Other Talar Fractures

Avulsion of the Dorsal Talar Head. This fracture is quite similar to the avulsion fracture of the dorsal aspect of the navicular. The findings and mechanism of injury are identical. The result is a cortical avulsion either from the attachment of the talonavicular ligament or the anterior ankle capsule. It would be best visualized on the lateral radiograph and treatment would be symptomatic, as previously described for the navicular.

Posterior Process Fracture (Shepherd's Fracture). The posterolateral tubercle of the talus can be fractured (Fig. 41-28) by either a forced dorsiflexion or forced plantarflexion injury. If the foot is dorsiflexed, the posterior process can either abut against the calcaneus or be avulsed by the posterior talofibular ligament. If the foot is plantarflexed, the posterior process impinges on the posterior aspect of the tibia.[52]

Clinically, there will be tenderness along the posterior aspect of the ankle. There may also be corresponding tenderness about the ankle ligaments. There will be edema and maybe some ecchymosis. Tenderness on range of motion of the ankle will occur. Forced dorsiflexion of the hallux

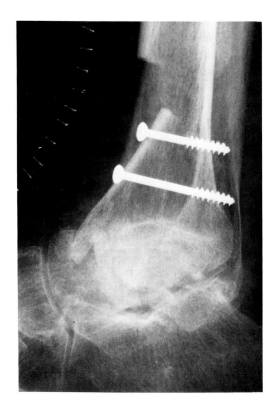

Fig. 41-26. Blair fusion.

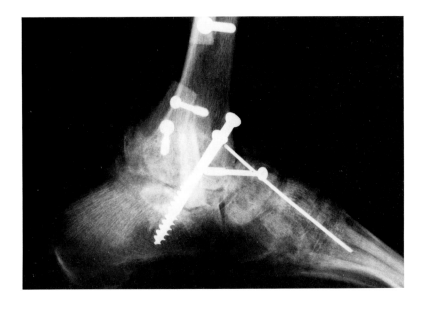

Fig. 41-27. Tibiocalcaneal fusion.

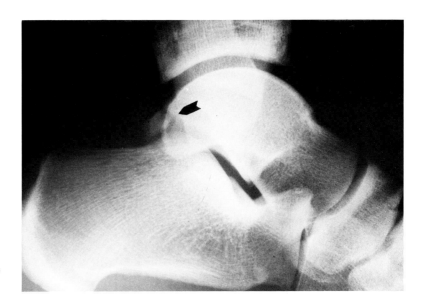

Fig. 41-28. Fracture of the posterior talar process *(arrowhead)*.

should elicit tenderness along the posterior aspect of the ankle as the flexor hallucis longus tendon courses next to the posterior process. There is usually no acute ligamentous instability of the ankle. The lateral radiograph will reveal an osseous fragment separated from the posterior aspect of the talus. However, one must ask if this represents a true fracture of the posterior process or a secondary ossification center (the os trigonum) that never fused. Supposedly, the os trigonum has a round contour with smooth edges while a fractured posterior process has a rough, irregular surface. This author has always found this distinction difficult to make and relies on the clinical examination to make the diagnosis. This is because it is possible to have an injury that disrupts the fibrous or cartilaginous attachment of the os trigonum to the talus. Paulos et al.[53] have demonstrated that a technetium bone scan will be positive for a fractured posterior process or a disruption of the os trigonum, but will be negative for an asymptomatic one.

Treatment consists of a weight-bearing SLC for 4 to 6 weeks. Radiographs at that time may or may not show osseous union, so the decision to begin unguarded weightbearing is based on clinical assessment. If pain persists in the posterolateral aspect of the ankle for about 6 months, then surgical excision of the fragment is indicated. There are two ways to help determine whether the pain is related to the osseous fragment. One way is to inject a local anesthetic into the area and see if it eliminates the pain. The second way is to take forced dorsiflexion and plantarflexion lateral radiographs looking for any movement of the fragment.

Fracture of the Lateral Talar Process. Fractures of the lateral process of the talus was first described by Dimon in 1961.[54] Hawkins[55] in 1965 and Mukherjee et al.[56] in 1974 have reported the largest series of this fracture. The mechanism of injury has been described as either an acute dorsiflexion and inversion of the foot or a direct blow.[57] The patient will present with all the same findings as seen with an acute ankle sprain. There will be tenderness over the lateral aspect of the ankle, especially inferior to the lateral malleolus. There will be edema and ecchymosis. Tenderness will be elicited on range of motion of the ankle and particularly inversion of the foot. Acute ligamentous instability has not been reported as associated with this injury. Routine ankle radiographs, including anteroposterior, mortise, and lateral views, will demonstrate the fracture. The most important thing is to know that this fracture exists and should be looked for on the radiograph. DeLee pointed out that this frac-

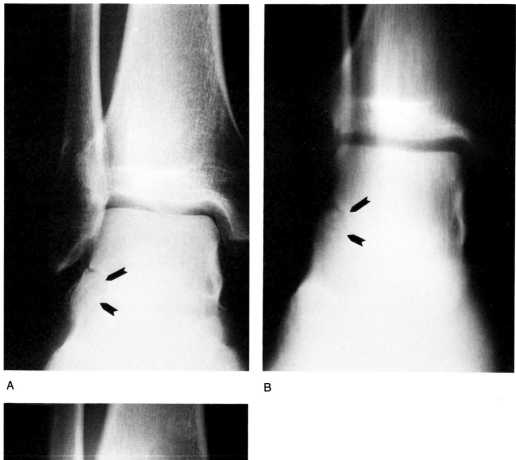

A

B

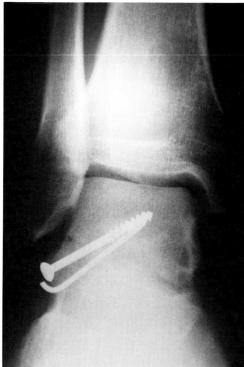

C

Fig. 41-29. (A) Fracture of the lateral talar process *(arrow-heads).* **(B)** Tomogram. **(C)** ORIF.

ture has a high incidence of disability if the diagnosis is missed or delayed.[24] He uses an additional oblique view with the ankle internally rotated 45 degrees and the foot plantarflexed 30 degrees as initially described by Dimon.[54] In addition, anteroposterior tomograms and CT scans are especially valuable in evaluating lateral process fractures (Fig. 41-29). Heckman and McLean have reported an accessory ossicle in this region that could be confused with a fracture.[58]

Treatment for a nondisplaced fracture involves a non-weight-bearing SLC for 4 weeks followed by a walking SLC for an additional 2 weeks. If the fracture is large and displaced, then ORIF is indicated. An anatomic reduction is essential because this fracture involves not only the talofibular articulation but also the subtalar joint. If the fracture is comminuted or its size does not allow internal fixation, it is excised. It has been stated that it is critical to mobilize this injury as soon as possible after surgery to prevent restriction of motion. If the fracture is discovered late, an attempt should be made to surgically reduce and fixate it. This becomes more difficult the further it is from the time of the injury. If the fracture cannot be anatomically reduced, it is excised. Late excision is indicated for a small ununited fragment that is symptomatic.

Calcaneal Fractures

Calcaneal fractures are a common injury comprising 60 percent of all rearfoot fractures.[59] They are usually produced by a fall from a height. When the fracture is intra-articular, it can be a source of great disability. The fracture tends to be complex and there is no consensus on the best way to treat it.

The calcaneus is composed of cancellous bone surrounded by a thin cortical shell. It has three articular facets for the talus and one for the cuboid. Consequently, the calcaneus contributes to both the subtalar and midtarsal joints. It is a bone designed to support the stresses of weightbearing, including running.

Clinical and Radiographic Evaluation

Most extra-articular fractures of the calcaneus produce only mild edema and localized tenderness over the area of the fracture. However, intra-artic-

ular fractures, being major injuries, result in severe tenderness and can produce significant edema. Ecchymosis will usually be present both medially and laterally. Ecchymosis along the plantar aspect of the foot has been referred to as Mondor's sign. If seen within a short time after the injury and prior to edema formation, the bony contour of the heel will feel widened. There will be tenderness to palpation about the rearfoot and ankle. Tenderness will be present on range of motion of the foot and ankle. Because the injury is produced from a fall, the soft tissue about the heel will also be severely traumatized. This fact, along with the severe edema, can produce fracture blisters and skin necrosis. Bilateral calcaneal fractures present in 9 percent of patients.[60] It is especially important to examine for proximal fractures, especially of the lumbar spine, which occur in 10 percent of cases.

This author obtains routine radiographic views of both the foot and ankle in evaluating calcaneal fractures. These include the dorsoplantar and oblique views of the foot, which can demonstrate involvement of the calcaneocuboid joint. An anteroposterior and mortise view of the ankle will reveal malleolar fractures. A lateral view of both the foot and ankle will demonstrate the collapse of the calcaneal body as well as involvement of the subtalar joint. The lateral view will be useful to evaluate two measures of calcaneal depression; Bohler's angle[60] and the crucial angle of Gissane.[24] Bohler's angle (Fig. 41-30A) is the intersection of a line drawn along the superior aspect of the calcaneal body and a line drawn from the superior aspect of the anterior portion of the calcaneus to the highest part of the posterior facet of the subtalar joint. The normal range is considered 25 to 40 degrees and is decreased in calcaneal fractures. The crucial angle of Gissane (Fig. 41-30B) is the intersection of a line drawn parallel to the posterior facet of the subtalar joint and a line drawn along the floor of the sinus tarsi. The normal values are 120 to 145 degrees and it is increased in calcaneal fractures. An axial view of the calcaneus will show widening of the calcaneal body as well as involvement of the posterior facet of the subtalar joint. An anteroposterior and lateral view of the lumbosacral spine are taken even in the absence of tenderness.

Special radiographs that can be taken are Broden's projections I and II, which demonstrate the

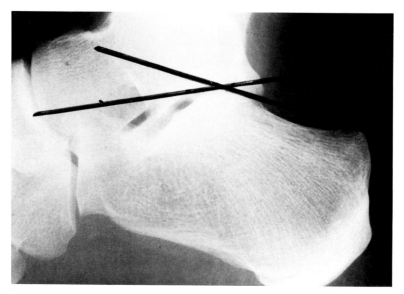

A

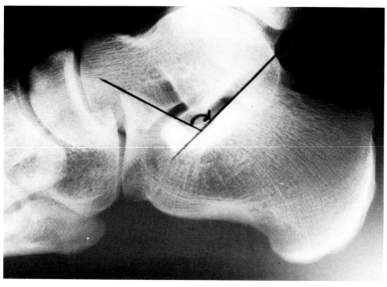

B

Fig. 41-30. (A) Bohler's angle measures from 25 to 40 degrees. **(B)** Crucial angle of Gissane measures from 120 to 145 degrees.

subtalar joint. The foot is held at a right angle with the leg internally rotated 45 degrees. In Broden I projections, the x-ray beam is directed from inferior to superior, aimed at the sinus tarsi and taken at 10, 20, 30, and 40 degrees (Fig. 41-31). The anterior aspect of the subtalar joint is seen with the 40-degree view and the posterior aspect is seen in the 10-degree view. These views will show the posterior facet involvement as well as the sustentaculum tali. This author uses these views routinely. Broden's II views are taken with the same position of the extremity, but the x-ray is directed 2 cm anterior to the medial malleolus and shot at 15 degrees in a superior direction in three radiographs differing by 3 to 4 degrees. This author has not utilized these views. Also, tomograms have not been found to be useful, but CT scans have delineated the fractures very well.

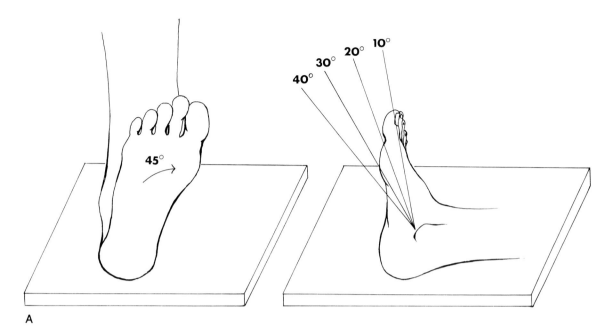

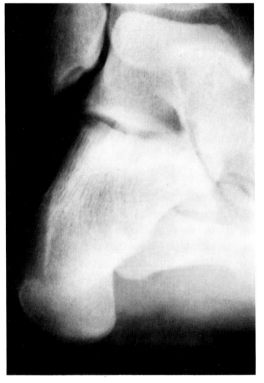

Fig. 41-31. (A) Foot position and x-ray beam directions for Broden's projection I. **(B)** Sample Broden I projection.

Table 41-1. Rowe Classification of Calcaneal Fractures

Type I
  Fracture of calcaneal tuberosity (Ia)
  Fracture of sustentaculum tali (Ib)
  Fracture of anterior process (Ic)
Type II
  Beak fracture
  Avulsion fracture involving achilles tendon
Type III — fracture of body not involving subtalar joint
Type IV — fracture involving subtalar joint
Type V — central depression fracture into subtalar joint

Mechanism

Cave indicated that many extra-articular fractures are the result of twisting injuries.[61] Calcaneal fractures can also result from a direct blow. However, most intra-articular fractures result from a fall from a height.

Classification

There are two commonly used classification schemes: the Rowe (Table 41-1) and Essex-Lopresti (Table 41-2) Schemes. Rowe et al. described a classification that ranged from type I to type V[62] (Fig. 41-32). Type I includes fractures of the calcaneal tuberosity (Ia), sustentaculum tali (Ib), or anterior process of the calcaneus (Ic). Type II includes beak fractures or avulsion fractures of the Achilles tendon. Type III includes fractures of the body not involving the subtalar joint. Type IV includes fractures of the body extending into the subtalar joint. Type V includes severe central depression fractures with subtalar involvement.

Table 41-2. Essex-Lopresti Classification of Calcaneal Fractures

I. Fractures not involving the subtalar joint
  A. Tuberosity fractures
    1. Beak type
    2. Avulsion of the medial border
    3. Vertical fracture
    4. Horizontal fracture
  B. Fractures involving only the calcaneocuboid joint
    1. Parrot-nose type
    2. Various types
II. Fractures involving the subtalar joint
  A. Without displacement
  B. With displacement
    1. Tongue type
    2. Joint depression
    3. Sustentaculum tali
    4. Combination with comminution

Essex-Lopresti divided his classification into fractures not involving the subtalar joint and those that did involve the subtalar joint.[63] This author believes that the category of extra-articular fractures offers no advantage over the Rowe classification. However, Essex-Lopresti identified two patterns of intra-articular fractures that are useful: tongue and joint depression (Fig. 41-33). The difference between these two fractures is found by evaluation of the lateral radiograph. Essex-Lopresti thought that the fall from a height caused the lateral process of the talus to impact on the relatively weak area of the crucial angle in the calcaneus. This produced a primary fracture line that went downward, exiting the inferior aspect of the calcaneus. Also, a secondary fracture line was produced that went posteriorly. The difference is that in the tongue type the fracture line proceeds posteriorly, exiting the posterior aspect of the calcaneus (Fig. 41-34A). In a joint depression fracture the secondary fracture line initially proceeds posteriorly but then turns upward and exits the superior aspect of the calcaneus just behind the subtalar joint (Fig. 41-34B).

Treatment

Fractures of the calcaneal tuberosities (type Ia) are treated conservatively. If small, a period of nonweightbearing followed by walking to tolerance is usually adequate. If the fragment is large and symptoms warrant, then a SLC is used. Even with a cast, a period of nonweightbearing may be required. Isolated fractures of the sustentaculum tali (type Ib) are very rare, comprising only 1 percent of all calcaneal fractures, and are rarely displaced.[64] Treatment consists of a weight-bearing SLC for 6 weeks. If displaced, then closed reduction is attempted by inverting the foot and pushing against the sustentaculum tali. A non-weight-bearing cast is applied for 3 to 4 weeks, followed by an additional 2 weeks in a walking SLC. If a symptomatic nonunion develops, excision is recommended. DeLee stated that, in his opinion, there is no indication for ORIF of isolated sustentaculum tali fractures.[24] This author believes a large displaced fracture could be easily treated by ORIF. With fractures of the anterior process of the calcaneus (type Ic), treatment is symptomatic. If the

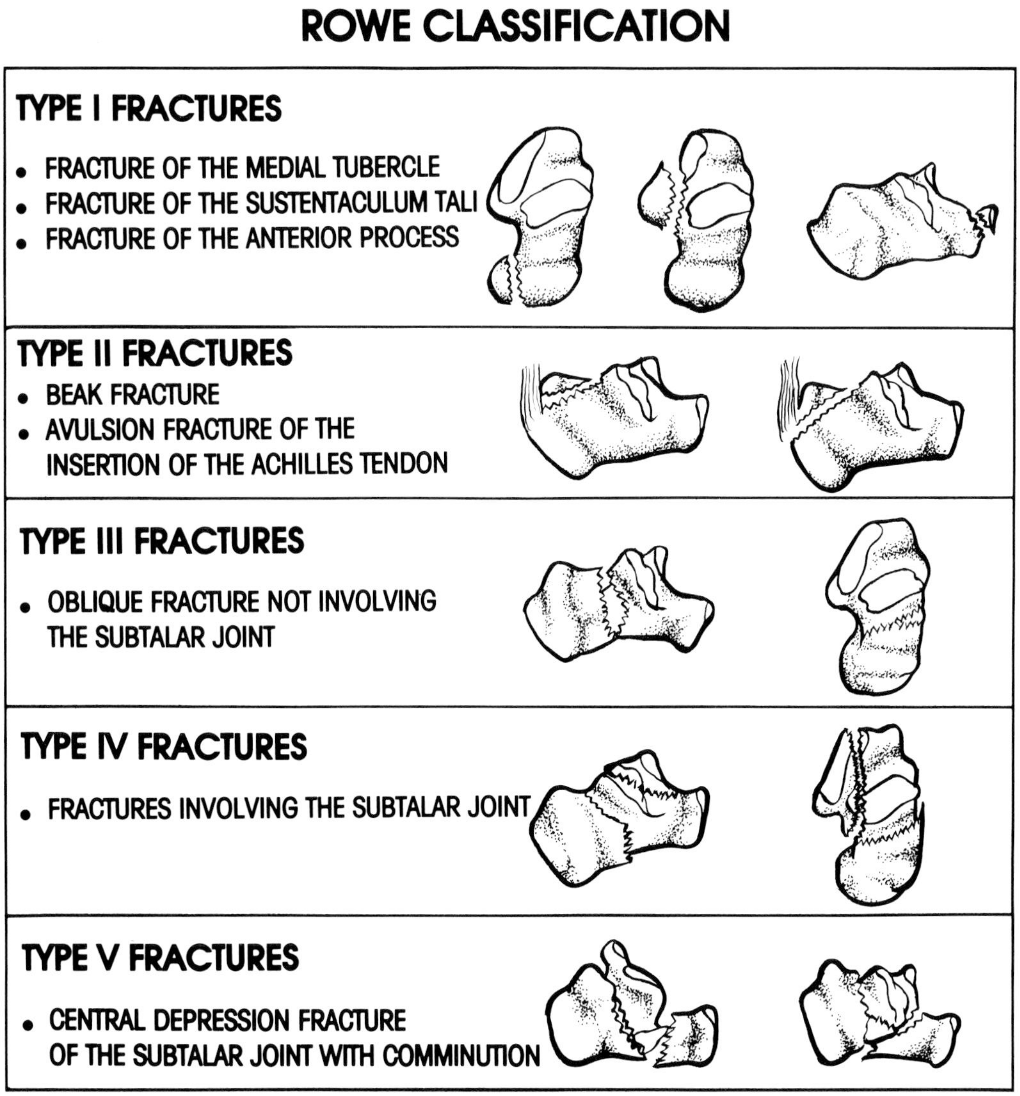

ROWE CLASSIFICATION

TYPE I FRACTURES

- FRACTURE OF THE MEDIAL TUBERCLE
- FRACTURE OF THE SUSTENTACULUM TALI
- FRACTURE OF THE ANTERIOR PROCESS

TYPE II FRACTURES

- BEAK FRACTURE
- AVULSION FRACTURE OF THE INSERTION OF THE ACHILLES TENDON

TYPE III FRACTURES

- OBLIQUE FRACTURE NOT INVOLVING THE SUBTALAR JOINT

TYPE IV FRACTURES

- FRACTURES INVOLVING THE SUBTALAR JOINT

TYPE V FRACTURES

- CENTRAL DEPRESSION FRACTURE OF THE SUBTALAR JOINT WITH COMMINUTION

Fig. 41-32. Rowe classification of calcaneal fractures. (Redrawn from DeLee.[24])

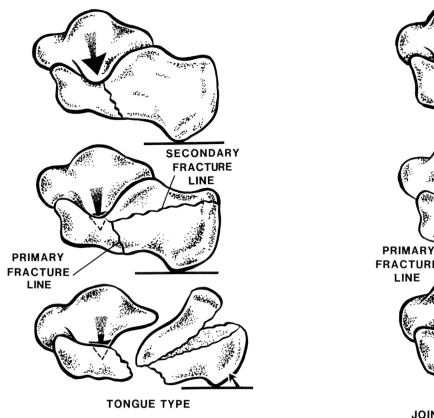

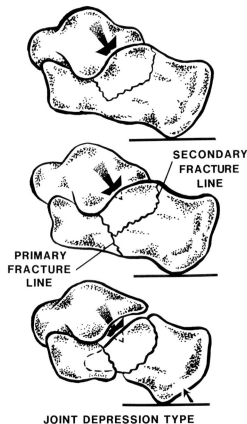

Fig. 41-33. Diagram representing the difference between the tongue-type and joint depression–type fractures as drawn by Essex-Lopresti. (Redrawn Cavaliere RG: Calcaneal fractures. p. 879. In McGlamry ED (ed): Foot Surgery. Baltimore, Williams & Wilkins, 1987.)

fracture is small, then progressive weightbearing is initiated with an elastic bandage or Unna boot. If the fragment is larger, then a weight-bearing SLC is applied for 4 to 6 weeks. If a symptomatic nonunion develops, then late excision is performed. If a large intra-articular fracture is present, then ORIF may be indicated.

Beak fractures of the calcaneus involve the posterior superior portion of the calcaneal body without involving the Achilles tendon. If the fracture is large enough, it can enter the posterior facet of the subtalar joint. With beak fractures, closed reduction can be performed by applying pressure to the superior aspect of the calcaneus and immobilization in a plantarflexed cast. If this is unsuccessful, then an ORIF can be performed. Avulsion fractures involve the calcaneal attachment of the Achilles tendon. With avulsion fractures, it is more critical to reduce and fixate the fracture to maintain the function of the Achilles tendon.

Fractures of the calcaneal body can be extra-articular or intra-articular, and there is great controversy with regard to treatment, especially when the subtalar joint is involved, which occurs 80 percent of the time.[65] If the fracture is nondisplaced, even with intra-articular extension, a reliable patient is treated in a splint with range-of-motion exercises and kept from bearing weight on the foot for 8 to 12 weeks. If the patient is unreliable, then a non-weight-bearing SLC is applied for the same amount of time. If the fracture is displaced, especially with subtalar joint involvement, many different treatment plans have been proposed.

As previously stated, Essex-Lopresti categorized

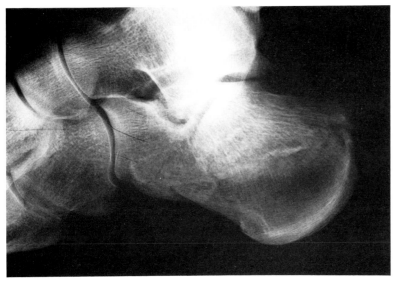

A

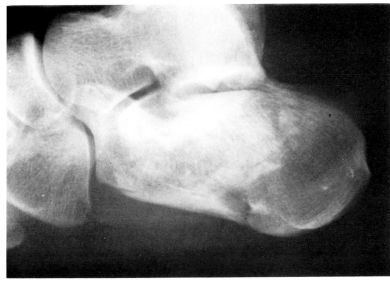

B

Fig. 41-34. (A) Tongue-type fracture. Primary fracture line goes inferiorly while the secondary fracture line exists posteriorly. **(B)** Joint depression–type fracture. Primary fracture line goes inferiorly while the secondary fracture line exists superiorly behind the subtalar joint.

intra-articular fractures into the tongue type and the joint depression type. He thought that the primary fracture line went downward and the secondary fracture line went posteriorly on the lateral radiograph. McReynolds[66] and Burdeaux[67] believe that the primary fracture line goes from medial to lateral on the calcaneal axial view. They pointed out that the fracture is produced not only by a downward force but also by a shearing force. This is because the midpoint of the talus is positioned me-

dial to the midpoint of the calcaneus. Consequently, the primary fracture line starts medially, extending distally and laterally and entering the posterior facet of the subtalar joint (Fig. 41-35). This produces a sustentacular fragment, also called the superomedial fragment by Stephenson,[68] and a tuberosity fragment. This pattern is seen in both the tongue and joint depression fractures. The sustentacular fragment moves downward, medially, and posteriorly. The tuberosity fragment moves

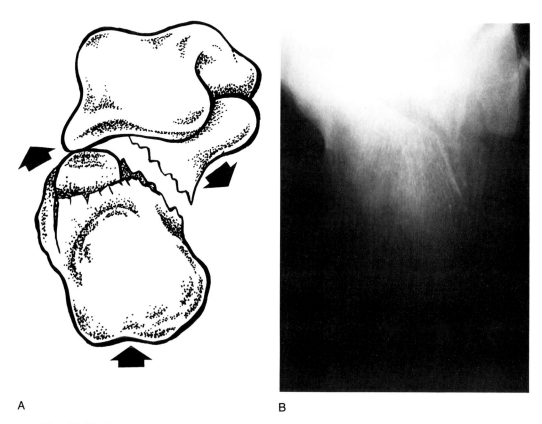

A   B

Fig. 41-35. Primary fracture line as described by McReynolds starting medially but extending distally and laterally while entering the posterior facet. This produces the sustentacular fragment and the tuberosity fragment. The sustentacular fragment is firmly attached to the talus. **(A)** Diagram showing motion of involved bones. **(B)** Radiograph of fracture.

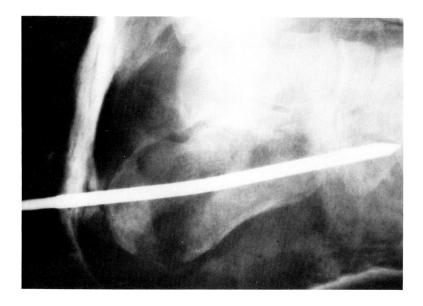

Fig. 41-36. Essex-Lopresti pin technique.

upward, laterally, and anteriorly. Consequently, the fracture produces deformities of the calcaneus including widening, shortening, a decrease in height, and involvement of the posterior facet of the subtalar joint. These deformities cause the long-term sequelae of difficulty in wearing shoegear, impingement of the tendons about the ankle (especially the peroneals), Achilles tendon weakness, and traumatic arthritis of the subtalar joint. When attempting to surgically fixate a calcaneal fracture, it is the sustentacular fragment that is the most stable because of its ligamentous attachment to the talus. Consequently, one attempts to reduce the tuberosity fragment to the sustentacular fragment.

McLaughlin recommended closed treatment without reduction and early range of motion while keeping the extremity from bearing weight.[69] This treatment does not address the fracture deformity, but aims for motion to mold the joints and prevent the stiffness of casting. Closed reduction with plaster immobilization was advocated by Bohler,[60] who utilized a clamp to reduce the calcaneal body. Omoto et al. recommended closed manipulation by molding the calcaneus with the palms of the hands followed by motion exercises and delayed weightbearing.[70] This author prefers this method in severely comminuted calcaneal fractures, which would defy fixation. Gissane[71] and Essex-Lopresti[63] recommended inserting a Steinmann pin into the posterior aspect of the calcaneal body and using the pin to reduce the fracture, followed by cast immobilization (Fig. 41-36). Essex-Lopresti performed the pinning closed for tongue-type fractures and by open reduction with the pin holding the reduction for joint depression types.

Palmer, in 1948, reported an open reduction of calcaneal fractures with elevation of the depressed posterior facet buttressed by bone grafting and a non-weight-bearing SLC for 12 weeks.[72] Stephenson performed ORIF with reduction of the depressed posterior facet and lateral cortical wall blow-out by a lateral approach.[68] McReynolds also recommended ORIF, but through a medial approach.[66] From the medial aspect, he reduced the posterior facet through the fracture, reduced displacement of the body by reconstructing the medial wall, reduced the lateral wall by manual pressure, and stabilized the fracture with a staple or K

wire. This author combines both philosophies by utilizing a lateral and a medial approach to reduce the deformities. The reduction is fixated with lag screws, K-wires, staples, or a plate depending on the fracture configuration (Fig. 41-37). A bone graft may or may not be required depending on the fracture. Postoperative treatment includes range-of-motion exercises and nonweightbearing protected by a splint for 8 to 12 weeks. Weightbearing depends on the radiographic evidence of bony consolidation. The final treatment option is primary fusion. Pennel and Yadau[73] advocated primary subtalar fusion, and Bankhart[59] recommended triple arthrodesis. This author does not favor this approach and reserves fusions as secondary procedures for traumatic arthritis. This author favors subtalar fusion if the midtarsal joint shows no signs of arthritic changes.

DIGITAL FRACTURES AND DISLOCATIONS

Digital Fractures

Digital fractures are a very common form of injury. They usually result from the toe striking against an object or by having it crushed by either dropping something on it or rolling something over it. Yet, there is no useful classification for digital fractures. Instead, one should simply observe the fracture configuration, which can be transverse, oblique, spiral, or comminuted, on the radiograph. Also, one should consider the amount of displacement and the degree of angulation. While the majority of digital fractures are simple and closed, severe trauma can occur from crush injuries or devices like lawn mowers. Crush injuries and complex open fractures can result in the loss of the digit. Digital fractures usually involve the shafts of the phalanges but can also be intra-articular, involving the distal interphalangeal, proximal interphalangeal, and metatarsophalangeal joints. The fifth digit is the most commonly fractured and, like the other lesser digits, is easily treated conserva-

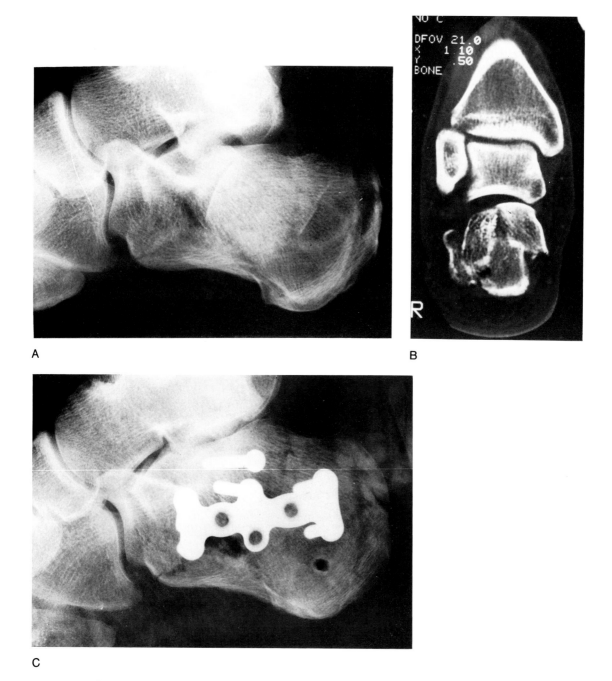

A

B

C

Fig. 41-37. (A) Joint depression fracture. **(B)** CT scan. **(C)** ORIF by both medial and lateral approach with fixation by lag screws and plate.

tively. However, the hallux requires a greater degree of skill and aggressiveness in treatment.

With injury there will be edema, ecchymosis, and tenderness to some degree. Inspection will detect whether the fracture is open or closed. Also, gross deformity is usually obvious in cases of severe displacement or dislocation. Look for an associated subungual hematoma. Carefully palpate each one of the phalanges and the digital joints for tenderness. Check for tenderness and limitation of motion of the digital joints. Finally, check the neurovascular status of the digits.

After a thorough clinical evaluation, scrutinize the radiographs. Standard views should include the anteroposterior, oblique, and lateral views. For the lesser digits a lateral view is many times useless because of superimposition. However, the hallux can be raised so as to obtain a good lateral image. Special radiographic studies such as tomograms and CT scan are usually not necessary for digital fractures.

Fractures of the Distal Phalanges

Tuft fractures of the distal phalanx are usually the result of crush injuries. They may be open or closed. There may, or may not, be a subungual hematoma present. A subungual hematoma many times has a nail bed laceration that communicates with the fracture site, making it an open fracture. The radiographs will reveal a comminuted irregular border of the tip of the distal phalanx. In severe cases the entire distal phalanx may be comminuted, with the fracture extending into the distal interphalangeal joint. The treatment is usually just a wooden shoe until regular shoes can be tolerated. It is difficult to stabilize these injuries with tape splinting.

Large subungual hematomas will require incision and evacuation or avulsion of the nail. The nail plate can be opened by using a heated paper clip, nail drill, or battery-powered electric cautery. If the nail is avulsed and there is a nail bed laceration, it should be debrided and irrigated. This author does not suture the nail bed because this is an open fracture. However, local soaks are instituted along with application of a topical antibiotic. The patient is not placed on systemic antibiotics. Also, the tetanus status of the patient is ascertained and treated

as indicated. The nail bed or open fleshy part of the toe can be allowed to heal by secondary intention. A delayed primary repair may also be possible. These types of injuries, including closed crush injuries, can lead to chronic pain at the tip of the digit. A distal Symes amputation may be indicated to obtain delayed primary closure of the wound or in eliminating a tender distal toe. Finally, if the nail matrix is damaged at the time of the injury, then deformity of the nail can result.

Fractures of the Proximal Phalanges of the Lesser Digits

Fractures of the shafts of the proximal phalanges of the lesser digits are the most frequent type of digital fracture. Spiral fractures are the most common pattern, usually being nondisplaced or minimally displaced (Fig. 41-38). These can be easily treated by tape splinting to the adjacent digits. Cast padding between the digits should be included to prevent maceration. The digit should be splinted for 3 to 4 weeks with periodic changes until the tenderness decreases. The patient should ambulate in a wooden shoe until symptoms decrease enough to allow normal shoegear. This can also take from 3 to 4 weeks, depending on the patient.

These fractures can be significantly displaced and angulated, especially when involving the fifth digit (Fig. 41-39). Fortunately, closed manipulation is usually successful. First, attempt to determine the mechanism of injury from the radiographs. After performing a digital block with local anesthetic, the fracture deformity is increased, followed by longitudinal traction and reversing the mechanism of injury. After reduction, check the position of the digit clinically and tape splint as discussed previously. Obtain postreduction radiographs to check the fracture position. In this case, do not change the tape for 2 weeks to allow the fracture to begin consolidating. If the tape is changed too early, there is the potential for loss of reduction. Also, weekly radiographs should be taken if there is a risk of the fracture slipping. If the fracture cannot be adequately reduced, then ORIF may be required (Fig. 41-40). This is more likely if the fracture enters the metatarsophalangeal joint. Small intra-articular fractures can be treated conservatively. If ORIF is undertaken, the form of fixa-

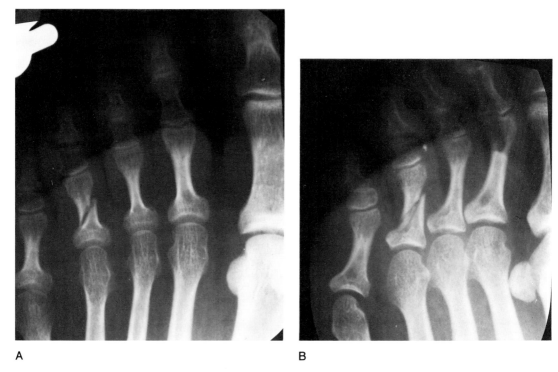

A   B

Fig. 41-38. Anteroposterior **(A)** and oblique **(B)** views of a minimally displaced spinal fracture of the proximal phalanx of the fourth digit.

tion is usually K-wires. However, occasionally mini-fragment (2.0-mm and 1.5-mm) screws can be utilized. One can also utilize closed reduction with percutaneous pinning to obtain a satisfactory reduction.[74]

Fractures of the Hallux

Fractures of the hallux are more complex, especially if they enter a joint. Nondisplaced or stable minimally displaced fractures can be treated with tape splinting and a wooden shoe. Fractures that are potentially unstable or require reduction should be immobilized in a forefoot cast with hallux spica and a wooden shoe or a SLC. If the hallux fracture needs to be reduced, the same principles apply as discussed previously. If a satisfactory position cannot be achieved, then ORIF is a viable option (Fig. 41-41). The phalanges of the hallux are larger than those of the lesser digits, making them easier to repair surgically. One can use K-wires or mini-fragment screws with or without a mini-fragment plate. An additional technique is percutaneous pinning, but this requires the use of an image

intensifier. Small intra-articular fractures can be treated conservatively. Many times they do not unite but usually they are not symptomatic. If they become symptomatic, then surgical excision is indicated. However, large displaced intra-articular fractures should have ORIF.

An anatomic reduction involving the interphalangeal joint or the first metatarsophalangeal joint is important to reduce the risk of traumatic arthritis, because the hallux plays a significant role in propulsion. Fusion of the interphalangeal joint is well tolerated. Traumatic arthritis of the first metatarsophalangeal joint can be successfully corrected with implant arthroplasty. However, traumatic arthritis in a young active individual can be a difficult problem, with the choice between implant arthroplasty or fusion.

Digital Dislocations

Dislocations can occur at any of the digital joints. Theoretically they can dislocate in any direction, but the most common direction in this author's ex-

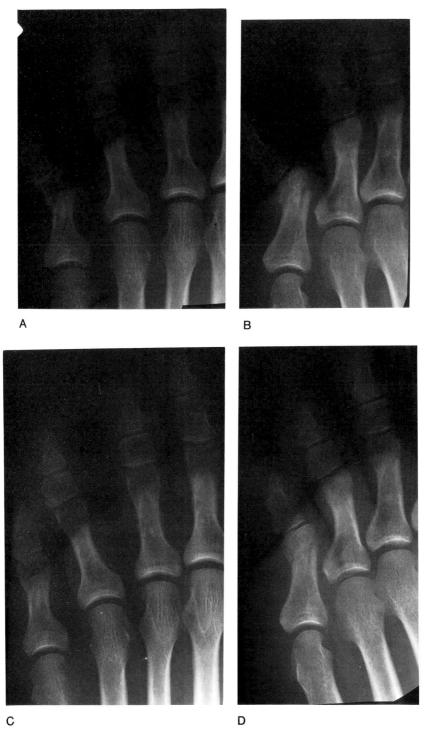

A

B

C

D

Fig. 41-39. Anteroposterior **(A)** and oblique **(B)** views of angulated fracture of the proximal phalanx of the fifth digit. Anterioposterior **(C)** and oblique **(D)** views of closed reduction.

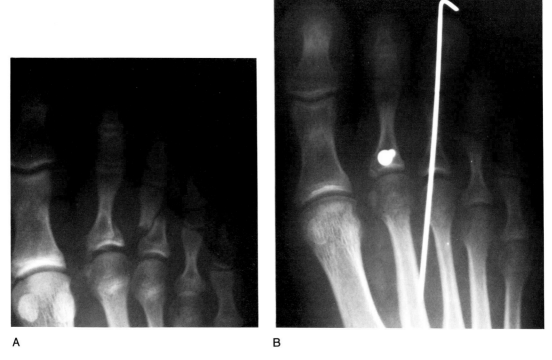

A   B

Fig. 41-40. (A) Transverse fracture of the proximal phalanx of the third digit, an intra-articular fracture of the base of the proximal phalanx of the second digit, and a small cortical avulsion of the base of the proximal phalanx of the hallux. **(B)** ORIF shows K-wire fixation of the third digit and fixation of the second digit with a 2.7-mm cortical lag screw.

perience is dorsally. Dislocations are usually obvious clinically. There will be tenderness with varying degrees of edema and ecchymosis. Range of motion of the involved joint will be tender and limited. Dislocations are usually obvious on radiographs. Immediate reduction is necessary. Anesthesia can be accomplished either by performing a digital block or by infiltrating the dislocated joint. A dorsal dislocation of the metatarsophalangeal joint would be reduced as follows. The dorsal dislocation would be increased by further dorsiflexing the digit. Next, traction would be applied while plantarflexing the digit and simultaneously pushing up on the head of the metatarsal with the other hand.

Most dislocations are reduced easily by closed manipulation. The metatarsophalangeal joints are quite stable after reduction because of their bony architecture. The interphalangeal joints are less stable. Nonetheless, the reduction should be stabi-

lized with tape splinting. Always obtain a postreduction radiograph to confirm the reduction position. With metatarsophalangeal dislocations, this author recommends gentle range-of-motion exercises after reduction when tenderness decreases. One must remember that with dislocations a significant disruption of the capsule and collateral ligaments has taken place. This will require about 6 weeks to repair. While most dislocations are easy to reduce, occasionally some will not be. This author has experienced a dislocation of the interphalangeal joint of the hallux that was not reducible because of an entrapped accessory ossicle. Excision of the ossicle was necessary to accomplish the rearticulation.

Dislocations of the first metatarsophalangeal joint are both unique and rare (Fig. 41-42). Jahss reported seeing only two cases in approximately 25,000 patients.[75] He described several types of dorsal dislocations involving rupture of the plantar

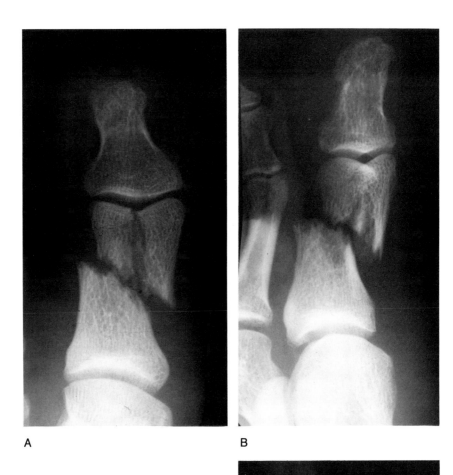

A   B

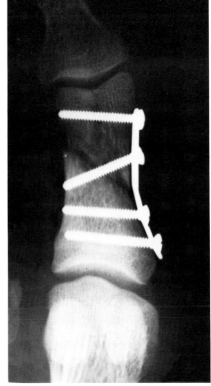

Fig. 41-41. Anteroposterior **(A)** and oblique **(B)** views of
intra-articular fracture of the hallux caused by dropping a
tire on it. **(C)** ORIF of hallux with mini-plate and 2.0-mm
cortical screws, with the two distal most screws using AO
lac technique for interfragmental compression.

C

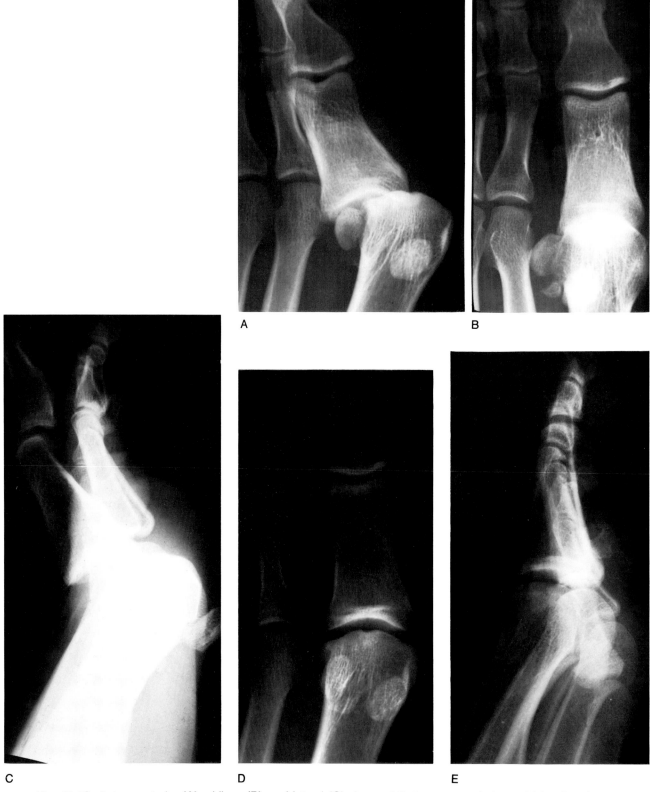

Fig. 41-42. Anteroposterior **(A)**, oblique **(B)**, and lateral **(C)** views of first metatarsophalangeal joint dorsal dislocation. Note fracture of the fibular sesamoid. Anteroposterior **(D)** and lateral **(E)** views of closed reduction.

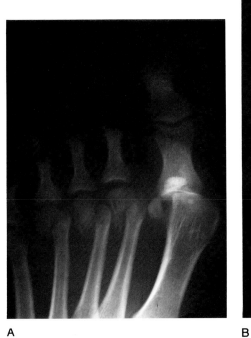 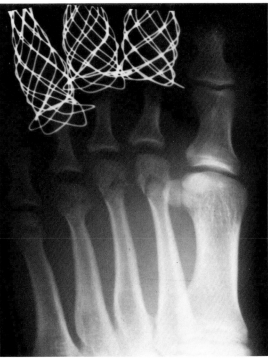

A   B

Fig. 41-43. (A) Anteroposterior view of dislocation of first metatarsophalangeal joint with multiple lesser metatarsal fractures. **(B)** Oblique view of closed reduction.

capsule and the sesamoids. Type I involved dorsal dislocation with the sesamoids still attached to the proximal phalanx of the hallux. This results in the sesamoids being displaced on the superior aspect of the metatarsal head, producing an irreducible dislocation. It requires surgical release. Type IIA is a dorsal dislocation with rupture of the intersesamoidal ligaments with separation from the proximal phallanx. Type IIB is a dorsal dislocation with a transverse fracture of one or both sesamoids. Both type II dislocations are easily reducible by closed means.

Final Comments

Two additional comments need to be made regarding fractures and dislocations of the digits. The first is that digital injuries may be associated with other fractures of the foot (Fig. 41-43). Therefore the radiographs should be evaluated closely. The second comment refers to the treatment of open fractures of the digits. These are treated more aggressively because of the risk of infection. The principles of treatment of open fractures are detailed previously under the section on metatarsal fractures.

ACKNOWLEDGMENTS

I would like to thank Mrs. Linda Dawson for the typing of this manuscript. Also, I would like to thank Mr. John Barbaccia and Ms. Rosa Iglesias for photographing the radiographs and Mr. Julio Rivera for the accompanying diagrams.

REFERENCES

1. Morrissey EJ: Metatarsal fractures. J Bone Joint Surg 28:594, 1946
2. Garcia A, Parkes JC: Fractures of the foot. In Giannestras NJ (ed): Foot Disorders: Medical and Surgical Management. 2nd Ed. Lea & Febiger, Philadelphia, 1973
3. Giannestras NJ: Shortening of the metatarsal shaft in the treatment of plantar keratosis. J Bone Joint Surg [Am] 40:61, 1958
4. Irwin CG: Fractures of the metatarsals. Proc R Soc Med 31 (pt. 2):789, 1938
5. Anderson LD: Injuries of the foot. Clin Orthop 122:18, 1977
6. Giannestras NJ, Sammarco GJ: Fractures and dislocations of the foot. In Rockwood CA, Jr., Green DP (eds): Fractures. Vol. 2. JB Lippicott Co, Philadelphia, 1975
7. Stewart IM: Jones fracture: fracture of the base of fifth metatarsal. Clin Orthop 16:190, 1960
8. Arango GA: Proximal displaced fractures of the fifth metatarsal (Jones fracture): two cases treated by cross pinning with review of 100 cases. Foot Ankle 3:293, 1983
9. Jones R: Fractures of the fifth metatarsal bone. Liverpool Med Surg J 42:103, 1902
10. Kavanaugh JH, Brower TD, Mann RA: The Jones fracture revisited. J Bone Joint Surg [Am] 60:776, 1978
11. Zelko RR, Torg JS, Rachun A: Proximal diaphyseal fractures of the fifth metatarsal: treatment of the fractures and their complications in athletes. Am J Sports Med 7:95, 1979
12. Torg JS, Balduini FC, Zelko RR et al: Fractures of the base of the fifth metatarsal distal to the tuberosity: Classification and guidelines for nonsurgical and surgical management. J Bone Joint Surg [Am] 66:209, 1984
13. Lehman RC, Torg JS, Pavlov H, DeLee JC: Fractures of the base of the fifth metatarsal distal to the tuberosity: a review. Foot Ankle 7:245, 1987
14. Gustilo RB, Anderson JT: Prevention of infection in the treatment of one thousand and twenty-five open fractures of long bones. J Bone Joint Surg [Am] 58:453, 1976
15. Aitken AT, Poulson D: Dislocations of the tarsometatarsal joint. J Bone Joint Surg [Am] 45:246, 1963
16. Leczner EM, Waddell JP, Graham JD: Tarsal-metatarsal (Lisfranc) dislocation. J Trauma 14:1012, 1974
17. Wilson DW: Injuries of the tarso-metatarsal joints: etiology, classification, and results of treatment. J Bone Joint Surg [Br] 54:677, 1972
18. Wiley J: The mechanism of tarsometatarsal joint injuries. J Bone Joint Surg [Br] 53:474, 1971
19. Myerson MS, Fisher RT, Burgess AR, Johnson JE: Fracture dislocations of the tarsometatarsal joints: end results correlated with pathology and treatment. Food Ankle 5:225, 1982
20. Quenu E, Kuss G: Etude sur les luxations du metatarse. Rev Chir 39:281, 1909
21. Hardcastle PH, Reschauer R, Kutscha-Lissberg E, Schoffman W: Injuries to the tarsometatarsal joint: incidence, classification and treatment. J Bone Joint Surg [Br] 64:349, 1982
22. Johnson JE, Johnson KA: Dowel arthrodesis for degenerative arthritis of the tarsometatarsal (Lisfranc) joint. Foot Ankle 5:243, 1986
23. Heck CV: Fractures of the bones of the foot (except talus). Surg Clin North Am 45:103, 1965
24. DeLee JC: Fractures and dislocations of the foot. In Mann RA (ed): Surgery of the Foot. 5th Ed. CV Mosby Co, St. Louis, 1986
25. Chapman MW: Fractures and dislocations of the foot and ankle. In Mann RA (ed): DuVries' Surgery of the Foot. 2nd Ed. CV Mosby Co, St. Louis, 1978
26. Hillegass RC: Injuries to the midfoot: a major cause of industrial morbidity. In Bateman JE (ed): Foot Science. WB Saunders Co, Philadelphia, 1976
27. Hermel MB, Gershon-Cohen J: The nutcracker fracture of the cuboid by indirect violence. Radiology 60:856, 1953
28. Wilson PD: Fractures and dislocations of the tarsal bones. South Med J 26:837, 1933
29. Watson-Jones R: Fractures and joint injuries. 4th Ed. Vol. 2. Williams & Wilkins Co, Baltimore, 1955
30. Torg JS, Pavlov H, Cooley LH et al: Stress fractures of the tarsal navicular. J Bone Joint Surg [Am] 64:700, 1982
31. Eichenholz SN, Levine DB: Fractures of the tarsal navicular bone. Clin Orthop 34:142, 1969
32. Mygind HB: The accessory tarsal scaphoid. Acta Orthop Scand 23:142, 1954
33. Fibricius, Hildanus: Observationum et curationum chirurgicarum centuriae, report quoted in Opera quae Extant Omnia (1646). p. 140. Francofurti ad Moneum Bever, 1608

34. Anderson HG: The Medical and Surgical Aspects of Aviation. Hodder & Co, London, 1919

35. Coltart WD: Aviator's astragalus. J Bone Joint Surg [Br] 34:545, 1952

36. Boyd HB, Knight RA: Fractures of the astragalus. South Med J 35:166, 1942

37. Sneed WL: The astragalus. A case of dislocations, excision, and replacement. An attempt to demonstrate the circulation of this bone. J Bone Joint Surg 7:384, 1985

38. Haliburton RA, Sullivan CR, Kelly PJ, Peterson LFA: The extra-osseous and intra-osseous blood supply of the talus, J Bone Joint Surg [Am] 40:1115, 1958

39. Sarrafian S: Anatomy of the Foot and Ankle. p. 47, 295. JB Lippincott Co, Philadelphia, 1983

40. Mulfinger GL, Trueta J: The blood supply of the talus. J Bone Joint Surg [Br] 52:160, 1970

41. Grob D, Simpsom LA, Weber BG, Bray T: Operative treatment of displaced talus fractures. Clin Orthop 199:88, 1985

42. Lorentzen JE, Christensen SB, Krogsoe O, Sneppen O: Fractures of the neck of the talus. Acta Orthop Scand 48:115, 1977

43. McKeever FM: Treatment of complications of fractures and dislocations of the talus. Clin Orthop 30:45, 1963

44. Hawkins LG: Fractures of the neck of the talus. J Bone Joint Surg [Am] 52:991, 1970

45. Canale ST, Kelly FB, Jr.: Fractures of the neck of the talus. J Bone Joint Surg [Am] 60:143, 1978

46. Penny JN, Davis LA: Fractures and fracture-dislocations of the neck of the talus. J Trauma 20:1029, 1980

47. O'Brien ET: Injuries of the talus. Am Fam Physician 12:95, 1975

48. Pennel GF: Fractures of the talus. Clin Orthop 30:53, 1963

49. Trillat A, Bousquet C, Lapeyre B: Les fractures-separations totales du col ou du corps de l'astragale: interet du visage par voie posterieure. Rev Chir Orthop 56:529, 1970

50. Peterson L, Goldie IF, Instram L: Fracture of the neck of the talus: a clinical study. Acta Orthop Scand 48:696, 1977

51. Blair HC: Comminuted fractures and fracture-dislocations of the body of the astragalus. Am J Surg 59:37, 1943

52. Hamilton WG: Stenosing tenosynovitis of the flexor hallucis longus tendon and posterior impingement upon the os trigonum in ballet dancers. Foot Ankle 3:74, 1982

53. Paulos LE, Johnson CL, Noyes FR: Posterior compartment fractures of the ankle: a commonly missed athletic injury. Am J Sports Med 11:429, 1983

54. Dimon JH: Isolated displaced fracture of the posterior facet of the talus. J Bone Joint Surg [Am] 43:375, 1961

55. Hawkins LG: Fractures of the lateral process of the talus. J Bone Joint Surg [Am] 47:1170, 1965

56. Mukherjee SK, Pringle RM, Baxter AD: Fracture of the lateral process of the talus: a report of thirteen cases. J Bone Joint Surg [Br] 56:263, 1974

57. Meisenbach R: Fracture of the os trigonum: report of two cases. JAMA 89:199, 1927

58. Heckman JD, McLean MR: Fracture of the lateral process of the talus. Clin Orthop 199:108, 1985

59. Bankhart ASB: Fractures of the os calcis, Lancet 2:175, 1942

60. Bohler L: Diagnosis, pathology, and treatment of fractures of the os calcis. J Bone Joint Surg 13:75, 1931

61. Cace EF: Fractures of the os calcis: the problem in general. Clin Orthop 30:64, 1963

62. Rowe CR, Sakellarides HT, Freeman PA, Sorbie C: Fractures of the os calcis: a long-term follow-up study of 146 patients. JAMA 184:920, 1963

63. Essex-Lopresti P: The mechanism, reduction technique, and results in fractures of the os calcis. Br J Surg 39:395, 1952

64. Lance EM, Cary ElJ, Wade PA: Fractures of the os calcis: treatment by early mobilization. Clin Orthop 30:64, 1963

65. Garcia A, Parkes JC, II: Fractures of the foot. In Giannestras NJ (ed): Foot Disorders: Medical and Surgical Management. 2nd Ed. Lea & Febiger, Philadelphia, 1973

66. McReynolds IS: Trauma to the os calcis and heel cord. In Jahss MH (ed): Disorders of the Foot. Vol. 2. WB Saunders Co, Philadelphia, 1982

67. Burdeaux BD: Reduction of calcaneal fractures by the McReynolds medial approach technique and its experimental basis. Clin Orthop 177:87, 1983

68. Stephenson JR: Displaced fractures of the calcaneus involving the subtalar joint: the key role of the superomedial fragment. Foot Ankle 4:91, 1983

69. McLaughlin HL: Treatment of late complications after os calcis fractures. Clin Orthop 30:111, 1962

70. Omoto H, Sakurada K, Sugi M, Nakamura K: A new method of manual reduction of intra-articular fracture of the calcaneus. Clin Orthop 177:104, 1983

71. Gissane W: News notes: the British Orthopaedic Association. J Bone Joint Surg 29:254, 1947

72. Palmer I: The mechanism and treatment of fractures

of the calcaneus: open reduction with the use of cancellous grafts. J Bone Joint Surg [Am] 30:2, 1948

73. Pennal GF, Yadav MP: Operative treatment of comminuted fractures of the os calcis. Orthop Clin North Am 4:197, 1973

74. Green DP, Anderson JR: Closed reduction and percutaneous pin fixation of fractured phalanges. J Bone Joint Surg [Am] 55:1651, 1973

75. Jahss MH: Traumatic dislocations of the first metatarsophalangeal joint. Foot Ankle 1:15, 1980

Ankle Fractures

42

William Sprague, D.P.M.

Ankle injuries have greatly increased with the advent of aerobics, running, and other sports in relation to the health craze that has spread throughout the world. These injuries cause soft tissue as well as bony structural injuries. With the ankle acting as a fulcrum between the floor and the leg during walking and exercise, the ankle joint is very vulnerable to increased stress. This stress can cause injury to the ankle joint, resulting in an unstable ligamentous ankle or a fracture of the ankle.

HISTORICAL REVIEW

In the past many authors have contributed to the understanding and treatment of ankle injuries. One of the first, Sir Percivall Pott, described a mechanism of injury involving ankle trauma. In 1768, he described a fracture involving the fibula proximal to the lateral malleolus.[1] He described a rupture of the deltoid ligament and lateral displacement of the talus. This injury, he believed, was one of the most common injuries involving the ankle, and he did not think there was any involvement of the tibiofibular syndesmosis. The use of Pott's name to

designate a bimalleolar fracture is a misnomer because the fracture he described does not exist. Pott, however, did contribute to the first understanding of reduction of fractures by understanding the forces being applied to the fracture. He accomplished this by bending the knee during the reduction process (Fig. 42-1).

Dupuytren's contribution was one of confusion because he mixed clinical observation and opinion with cadaver findings. Dupuytren, however, did understand the importance of the syndesmosis in relation to ankle fractures.[2] He believed that the fibular fracture occurred after a tear in the deltoid ligament, thereby allowing the talus to laterally displace, impinging on the fibula and causing a fracture of the fibula to occur (Fig. 42-2).

Maisonneuve, in 1840, reported on a series of cadaver studies in which he applied external rotation to the foot, causing oblique fractures to the fibula.[3] His contention was that an external force would cause rupture of the deltoid ligament or a fracture of the medial malleolus. If the force continued, the tibiofibular ligament would rupture, thereby causing force to be transmitted proximally, producing a fracture of the proximal fibula (Fig. 42-3).

Cotten, in 1915,[4] described a fracture of the posterior aspect of the tibia that he labeled "a new type of ankle fracture." Cotten's new fracture was

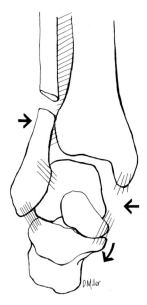

Fig. 42-1. Pott's fracture—a tear of the deltoid ligament with lateral displacement of the talus, forcing the fibula medially and the fracture focal point toward the tibia.

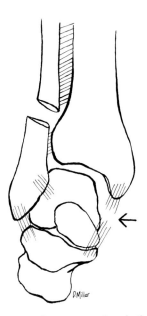

Fig. 42-2. Dupuytren fracture—a tear in the syndesmosis and lateral displacement of the fibula.

a fracture of the posterior articulating surface of the tibia.[5,6] The trimalleolar fracture has become known as a "Cotten fracture." In 1932 Henderson[7] described a "trimalleolar fracture of the ankle" but the trimalleolar fracture has continued to be identified as a Cotten fracture (Fig. 42-4).

The first real study with classifications was completed in 1922 by Ashhurst and Bromer.[8] In 1950, Lauge-Hansen did a study of classificaation that is used extensively today in describing the mechanism of injury and the treatment of those injuries.[9–13]

ANATOMY OF THE ANKLE

The ankle joint is a very complicated joint involving three osseous structures, multiple ligaments, and soft tissue that are found adjacent to the joint. The osseous structures include several joints. The first, the tibiofibular joint, is a syndesmosis type. There is a triangular facet on the lateral surface of the tibia and a corresponding facet on the medial aspect of the fibula. The ligaments involved and the interosseous ligament hold the distal ends of the fibula and tibia together. The anterior inferior tibiofibular ligament is found anterior to the syndesmosis between the fibula and the tibia. The posterior inferior tibiofibular ligament is found posterior to the syndesmosis and is the strongest of the two ligaments. The inferior transverse tibiofibular ligament is located deeper and more distally to the posterior inferior tibiofibular ligament. The inferior transverse tibiofibular ligament articulates with the talus and builds the posterior border of the ankle joint. When the talus moves into dorsiflexion, the fibula rotates slightly laterally and upward to a small extent. The ankle joint, per se, is the articulation between the lower leg and the foot. The tibia makes up the dorsal and medial surface; the fibula makes up the lateral surface; and the dome of talus makes up the distal surface. The concavity of the ankle joint is built by the dorsal dome of the distal tibia. The facet on the body of the talus laterally is triangular in shape. Medially, the facet is teardrop in shape. Posteriorly, the ankle joint is formed by the inferior transverse tibiofibula ligament.

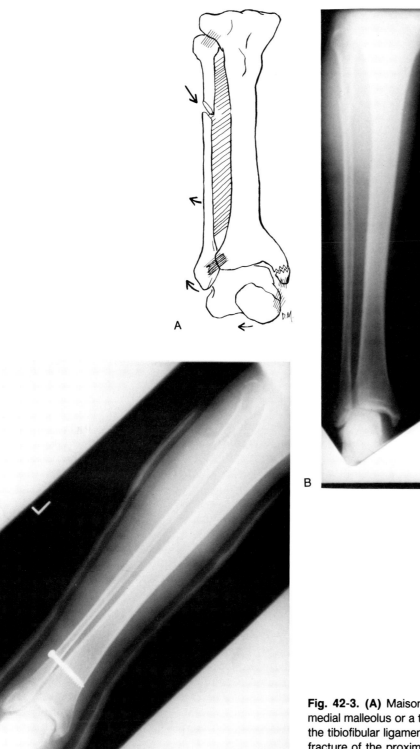

Fig. 42-3. (A) Maisonneuve fracture—a fracture of the medial malleolus or a tear in the deltoid ligament, a tear of the tibiofibular ligament, a tear of the syndesmosis, and a fracture of the proximal fibula. **(B)** Proximal fracture with lateral displacement of the talus. **(C)** Reduction with syndesmotic screw.

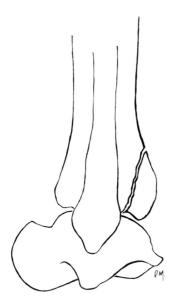

Fig. 42-4. Cotten described a fracture of the posterior aspect of the tibia, "a new type of ankle fracture."

Collateral ligaments of the ankle consist of two ligaments. The deltoid ligament is found on the medial surface of the ankle and is made up of three superficial and one deep slips. The superficial layer consists of the anterior tibionavicular and calcaneotibial and the posterior talotibial ligament slips. The posterior ligament of the lateral collateral ligament is more horizontal. The medial or deltoid ligament is the strongest of the collateral ligaments (Fig. 42-5).

The ankle joint forms an axis of 20 to 25 degrees to the frontal plane. The ankle joint axis is perpendicular to the third metatarsal and the movement of the ankle joint is of a ginglymus type. The distal tibial area is relatively horizontal as it articulates with the talus. This distal aspect, including the articular surface, is called the tibial plafond.

CLASSIFICATION OF ANKLE INJURIES BY MECHANISM OF INJURY

In the past, several different classifications of ankle injuries have been proposed formulated on the position of the ankle at the time of injury, the deforming force applied to the ankle, or the deformity present. All of these classifications were used to try to find the original deformity so that the deforming force could be reapplied and, it was hoped, an adequate reduction could be accomplished.

Ashurst and Bromer, in 1922, reviewed 300 ankle fractures and proposed a classification system based on what they considered to be the mechanism of injury.[8] In their article, the most significant force was external rotation. However, this classification did not take into account the combination of forces applied to the ankle joint during trauma.

In 1949, Lauge-Hansen published his classification based on the concept that fractures are accomplished by the force applied to the bone and soft tissue.[9] The failure of these structures causes injuries that can be interpreted from the fracture as seen on the radiographs. These failures usually follow a certain sequence that is pathognomonic of the force induced into the ankle. In 1952, Lauge-Hansen stated that in certain stages one fracture could be replaced by another.[11] Therefore, a traumatic progression exists that may terminate in a minor injury or a more severe one.

Lauge-Hansen used cadaver studies to produce four major injury types. The first word of the classification refers to the position of the foot at the time of injury; the second refers to the direction of the force imparted into the ankle and foot at the time of injury:

1. Supination-adduction (SA)
2. Supination-eversion (SE)
3. Pronation-abduction (PA)
4. Pronation-eversion (PE)

Three-fourths of the fractures that Lauge-Hansen classified in his study fit into the first two groups, SA and SE. The most prevalent fractures were found in the SA classification.

There have been other classifications made, including one by Danis in 1949[14] and a modification by Weber in 1966.[15] Yde, in 1980, modified the Lauge-Hansen classification.[16]

The Lauge-Hansen and Weber classifications overlap in some areas but are totally different in the mechanism of injury of other fractures. For example, PA and PE fractures, subclass 1, in the Lauge-

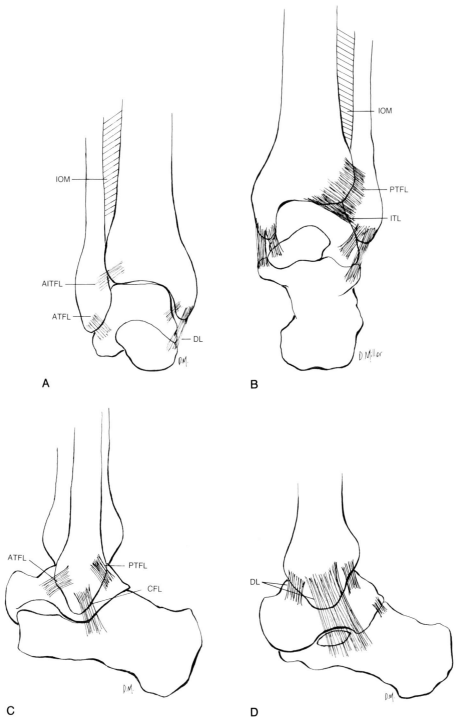

Fig. 42-5. **(A)** Anterior view of the ankle. *ATFL,* anterior talofibular ligament; *DL,* deltoid ligament, superficial and deep; *AITFL,* anterior inferior tibiofibular ligament; *IOM,* interosseous membrane. **(B)** Posterior view of the ankle. *IOM,* interosseous membrane; *PFTL,* posterior talofibular ligament; *ITL,* inferior transverse ligament; *DL,* deltoid ligament, superficial and deep. **(C)** Lateral view of the ankle. *ATFL,* anterior talofibular ligament; *CFL,* calcaneofibular ligament; *PTFL,* posterior talofibular ligament. **(D)** Medial view of the ankle. *DL,* deltoid ligament.

Hansen classification are described as having been caused by a supination in the Weber classification.

The Lauge-Hansen classification is the most helpful in evaluating fractures for closed reduction. The Weber classification is more appropriate for open internal fixation treatment. However, there is a shortage of studies in the literature using the Weber classification. The Lauge-Hansen classification is used in this chapter because it is the best classification to learn from and can be used by those who desire to use open or closed treatment. By understanding the Lauge-Hansen classification, one may easily convert to another classification as needed.

In all four types of injuries in the Lauge-Hansen classification, stage 1 is, or may be, a ligamentous detachment (i.e., a ligamentous ankle fracture).

Lauge-Hansen Classification Scheme

Supination-Adduction (Fig. 42-6)

Stage 1: A transverse fracture of the fibular malleolus at varying heights or a tear of the lateral collateral ligaments.

Stage 2: A spiral fracture of the fibula above the anterior tubercle plus stage 1.

Supination-Eversion (Fig. 42-7)

Stage 1: A tear of the anterior tibiofibular ligament, sometimes with a piece off the anterior aspect of the tibia.
Stage 2: A spiral fracture of the fibula above the anterior tubercle plus stage 1.
Stage 3: A posterior inferior tibiofibular stress pulling off the posterior position.
Stage 4: A fracture of the medial malleolus or a tear of the deltoid ligament plus stage 3, producing a trimalleolar fracture.

Pronation-Abduction (Fig. 42-8)

Stage 1: A fracture of the medial malleolus or a tear in the deltoid ligament, sometimes seen as an avulsion fracture of the medial malleolus.
Stage 2: a tear disruption of the anterior and posterior inferior tibiofibular ligament and the

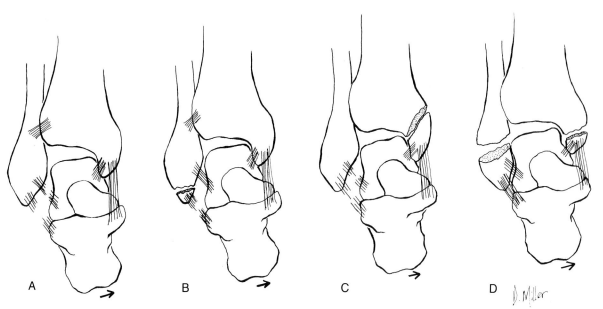

Fig. 42-6. Supination-adduction injury. **(A)** Tear of the fibular ligaments with a medial shift of the talus. **(B)** Avulsion fracture of the fibula with a medial shift of the talus. **(C)** Tear of the fibular ligaments, medial shift of the talus, and a fracture of the tibia. **(D)** Transverse fracture of the fibular malleolus, medial shift of the talus, and fracture of the tibial malleolus.

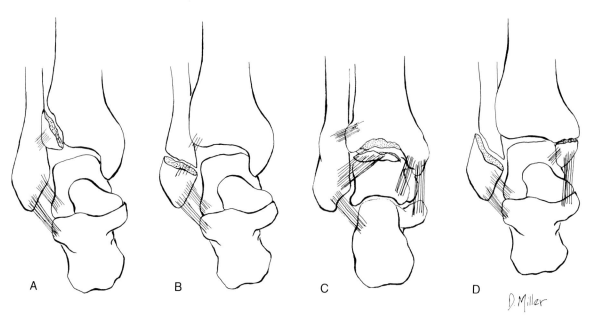

Fig. 42-7. Supination-eversion injury. **(A)** Tear of anterior tibiofibular ligament, sometimes with an avulsion fracture off of the anterior aspect of the talus. **(B)** Spiral fracture of the fibula at the ankle joint and tear of the anterior tibiofibular ligament. **(C)** Tear or avulsion of the posterior inferior aspect of the tibia. **(D)** Transvers fracture of the medial malleolus and spiral fracture of the fibula malleolus.

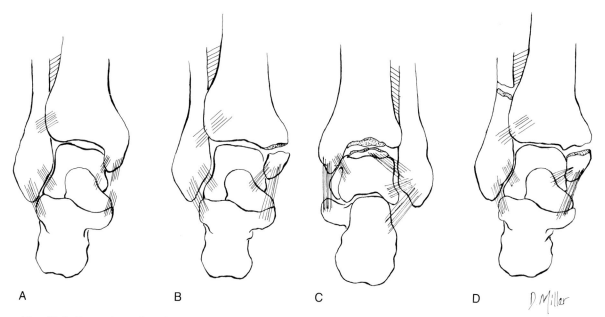

Fig. 42-8. Pronation-adbuction injury. **(A)** Tear of the deltoid ligament with medial shift of the talus. **(B)** Transverse fracture of the medial malleolus with medial shift of the talus and tear of the tibiofibular ligament. **(C)** Fracture of the posterior aspect of the tibia and tear of the posterior talofibular ligament. **(D)** Supramalleolar fracture of the fibula, tear of the tibiofibular ligament, and transverse fracture of the medial malleolus.

transverse ligament with a small or large fragment from the posterior lip of the tibia, an interosseous ligament tear, plus stage 1.

Stage 3: A supramalleolar fracture of the fibula ("straight-lined fracture") above the plafond of the tibia, plus stage 2.

Pronation-Eversion (Fig. 42-9)

Stage 1: A rupture of the deltoid ligament or an avulsion of the medial malleolus.

Stage 2: A disruption of the anterior inferior tibiofibular and interosseous ligaments.

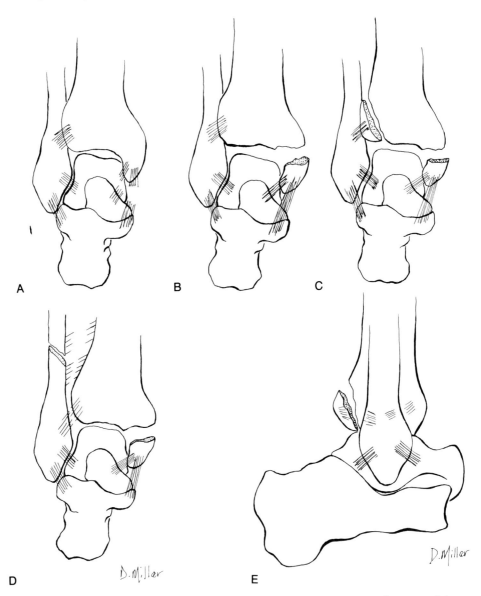

Fig. 42-9. Pronation-eversion injury. **(A)** Tear of the deltoid ligament. **(B)** Avulsion fracture of the medial malleolus with a lateral shift of the talus. **(C)** Avulsion fracture of the medial malleolus and avulsion of the anterior lateral aspect of the tibia at the talofibular ligament. **(D)** Avulsion fracture of the medial malleolus, tear of the anterior talofibular ligament, tear of the interosseous membrane, and spiral fracture of the fibula. **(E)** Fracture of the posterior aspect of the tibia, tear of the transverse posterior tibiofibular ligament, and tear of the anterior tibiofibular ligament.

Stage 3: A 7- to 8-cm proximal fracture of the fibula in a spiral pattern, the fibula rotated outward ("the door is open"), plus stage 2.

Stage 4: Stage 3 plus a posterior tibiofibular ligament tear, an inferior transverse ligament tear, and a fracture of the posterior tibia where the inferior transverse ligament attaches.

EVALUATION AND TREATMENT

The treatment of ankle fractures was first accomplished by closed reduction and, if that failed, internal fixation was considered. It was found that closed treatment did not work with unstable fractures. Kristensen noted that about 10 percent of the unstable ankle fractures were displaced with decreased edema.[17] Braunstein and Wade wrote that they found 70 percent of their cases had some loss of position in the cast after closed reduction.[18]

The most recent literature shows a shift from conservative therapy to surgical therapy with internal fixation. However, the use of internal fixation increases the possibility of complications. The use of general anesthetics is safer today than ever before, but there are still risks to consider, especially in poor-surgical-risk patients. Infection is always a possibility, especially when metal is used within the body and with the tissue compromised secondary to trauma. These considerations must be weighed in respect to the final outcome. Internal fixation allows for early range of motion, and therefore a better result and faster rehabilitation for the patient. Active motion of the ankle joint seems to increase the nutrient supply to the cartilage, thereby increasing the healing of the joint cartilage. This healing consequently decreases the chance of arthritis within the joint. As physicians, we must evaluate the patient and the fracture and then decide if closed reduction or internal fixation is the best treatment. The major goal of internal fixation is to obtain anatomic reduction with adequate internal fixation.

The ankle is a weight-bearing joint taking between one and a half to three or more times the body weight during different activities. Therefore, this author recommends that open reduction with internal fixation be accomplished in most cases. Closed reduction can be accomplished if needed in the experienced physician's hands. Even then, closed reduction must be carefully watched with frequent x-rays and cast changes to maintain the reduction. If this is not done, the chances of traumatic arthritis increase considerably. In all Salter-Harris fractures, closed reduction should be tried first.

The first consideration of closed treatment is the time since injury. A posterior splint or a cast that is bivalved should be used for the first 48 hours. After the first 24 to 48 hours, the ankle may be placed in a cast using three-point reduction and molding. This is better accomplished with plaster than with the new synthetic casting material. The patient should be followed with weekly radiographs for a minimum of 6 weeks. If radiographs do not show adequate bone healing at 6 weeks, the patient should be followed with x-rays until bone healing occurs. As stated before, with a decrease in edema, the cast will become loose and the reduction will be lost; therefore, it is imperative to check the cast weekly.

Since the ankle is a weight-bearing joint sustaining a tremendous amount of stress during its function, internal fixation should be considered as the primary reduction technique. This technique will greatly increase the probability of a functional joint and increase the chances of traumatic arthritis. The Swiss Association for the study of Internal Fixation technique should be used for internal fixation of the ankle.

Radiography

Radiographs of the ankle include anteroposterior, lateral, and mortise views. (Stress films are not covered in this chapter.) The anteroposterior radiograph is useful in evaluating fractures that might have occurred to the malleoli. This view is also helpful in determining if the ankle mortise is intact.

The anteroposterior radiograph, taken with the heel against the film, will help determine if the talus is out of the mortise. This view is also useful in observing the periosteal disruption of the fibula when there has been a fracture of the fibula that has reduced.

The lateral radiograph shows superimposition of the fibula on the posterior portion of the tibia. As in the normal physical examination, the lateral malleolus will be posterior to the medial malleolus. This view is useful in seeing posterior fractures of the tibia (third malleolus), butterfly fragments of the fibula, and any rotational deformity of the fibula. This view is also useful in visualizing any fractures of the anterior or posterior tibia. Because of the superimposition of the fibula and the tibia, it is difficult to visualize the entire anterior-posterior aspect of the fibula.

The most useful is the mortise view, which helps the physician examine the entire mortise to determine if all sides of the joint have equal joint space. The foot should be internally rotated by 15 to 20 degrees so the malleoli are parallel to the film. On a radiograph, a 3-mm increase in the distance between the medial malleolus and talus indicates a diastasis of the syndesmosis. This view will illuminate fractures of the tibia and malleoli that are missed in the other radiographic views.

Supination-Adduction Injury

Mechanism (Fig. 42-10)

The foot is usually found in a supinated position when adductory force is applied. This type of injury is found in two stages.

Stage 1 injury involves a rupture of the talofibular ligament or a fracture of the distal fibula at or below the level of the ankle joint. Stage 2 injury involves a fracture of the medial malleolus and is usually a vertical fracture.

Physical Examination

In stage 1 injury pain can be elicited over the lateral and anterolateral ankle joint with edema present. The patient will experience pain with inversion. In stage 2 the pain can be elicited over the medial ankle along the tibial fracture. There is usually pain elicited anteriorly across the entire ankle.

Treatment

A stage 1 injury is usually stable and may be treated with casting in a short leg walking cast. If the fibula is shortened a Rush rod or a semitubular plate, six holes or more, is used to return the fibula to full length. Most patients can be treated with touch-down to light weightbearing for the first 2 to 4 weeks. After 4 weeks, the patient may be allowed to put full weight on the ankle. The patient should be kept in a cast for 6 to 8 weeks total.

Stage 2 fractures are very unstable and should have internal fixation with a Rush rod or semitubular plate, six holes or more, placed in the fibula. The medial malleolus should be fixated with a compression malleolar screw. The fracture can be overdrilled if a malleolar screw is not available to obtain a compression-type fixation.

Supination-Eversion Injury

Mechanism (Fig. 42-11)

The foot is found in a supinated position at the time of injury when an eversion force is applied to the ankle and produces four stages of injury.

Stage 1 injury occurs when there is a tear in the anterior tibiofibular ligament. Continuation of the deforming force produces the next stage, which includes stage 1 plus a fracture of the fibula. Stage 3 injury is stage 2 plus a rupture of the posterior tibiofibular ligament or a fracture at the insertion of that ligament. Stage 4 injury produces a tear of the deltoid ligament or fracture of the medial malleolus ("straight line fracture"), producing a trimalleolar fracture.

Physical Examination

Stage 1–injured patients usually have pain over the anterior ankle. These patients will also have some pain with dorsiflexion of the ankle. Stage 2 injuries produce pain in the area of stage 1 plus pain at the height of the fracture of the fibula. Stage 3 injuries include the painful area of stage 2 plus pain with deep palpation of the posterior ankle at the level of the posterior inferior tibiofibular ligament. Stage 4 injuries will be painful at the same areas found in stage 3 as well as being painful over the distal tibial malleolus.

All the above-mentioned symptoms may be found, but if the patient is having much pain and guards against unnecessary movement, soft tissue examination will be very difficult.

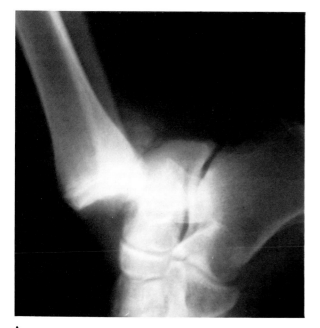

A

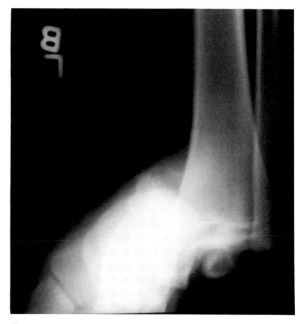

B

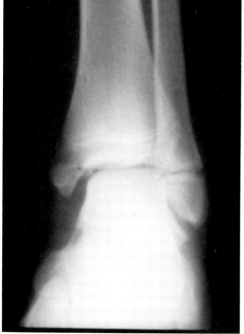

C

Fig. 42-10. Evaluation and treatment of supination-adduction injury. **(A)** Posterior dislocation of the talus. **(B)** Medial dislocation with fracture of the fibula, and medial displacement of the tibial malleolus. **(C)** Closed reduction. *(Figure continues.)*

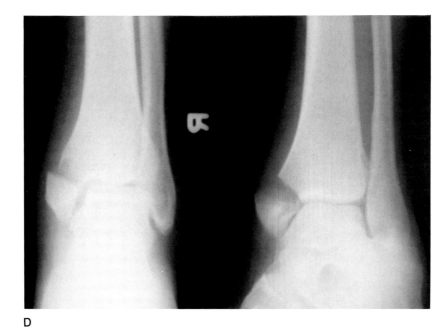

D

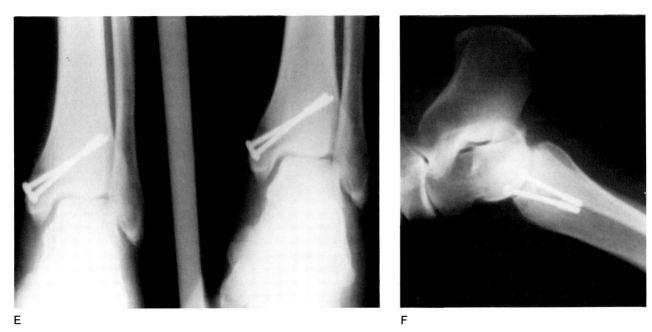

E

F

Fig. 42-10. *(continued).* **(D)** Medial fracture of tibial malleolus and a tear of the fibular ligament. **(E)** Open reduction with malleolar screws. **(F)** Lateral view.

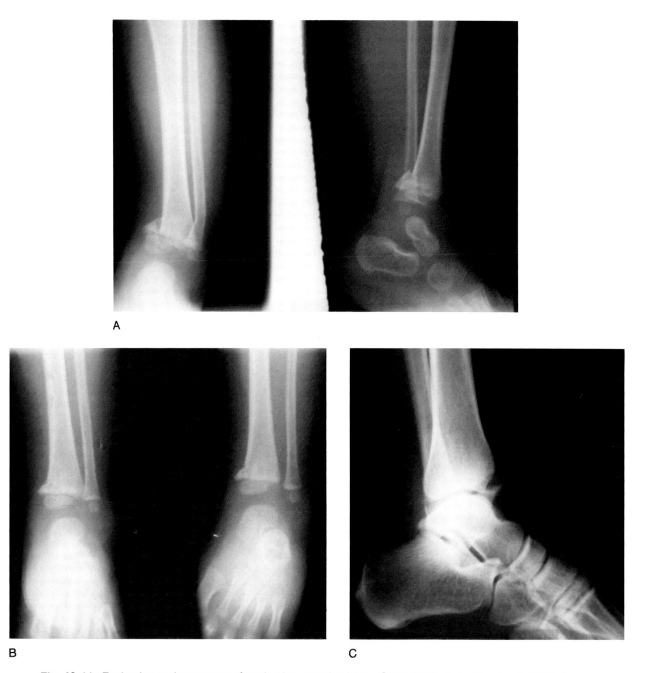

A

B

C

Fig. 42-11. Evaluation and treatment of supination-eversion injury (Salter-Harris type II fracture). **(A)** Eighteen-month-old child with fracture of the fibula, medial dislocation of the talus, and fracture of the medial malleolus. **(B)** Closed reduction. **(C)** Fracture of fibula and avulsion fracture of medial malleolus (lateral view). *(Figure continues.)*

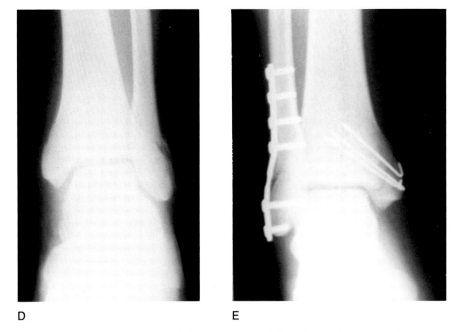

D

E

Fig. 42-11. *(continued).* **(D)** Mortise view of fibula fracture and avulsion of medial malleolus. **(E)** Open reduction internal fixation.

Treatment

Stage 1 injuries are usually stable and may be treated by casting in a short leg walking cast for 6 weeks. The first 3 to 4 weeks should involve no weightbearing.

Stage 2 injuries should be treated in a short leg walking cast for 6 to 8 weeks. This cast should be molded since there will be a tear in the anterior tibiofibular ligament as well as a tear in the syndesmosis and a fracture of the fibula. Some widening of the ankle mortise may occur upon weightbearing. This widening can be controlled with the molded cast. Radiographs should be taken weekly for 3 to 4 weeks to make sure that there is no movement of the fibula away from the tibia. If this occurs, internal fixation across the syndesmosis with a cortical screw that bites into the two cortices of the fibula and the lateral cortex of the tibia is indicated.

Stage 3 injuries become unstable because of the loss of the anterior and posterior tibiofibular ligaments, and fracture of the fibula. In the past, many authors recommend casting as the treatment of choice. However, because this injury is very unstable, I recommend internal fixation. The patient can then start early range-of-motion exercises in a patella weight-bearing cast, which should be in place for 6 weeks.

Stage 4 injuries are totally unstable; therefore, internal fixation is indicated. Early range of motion determination is indicated prior to casting. Partial weightbearing in a short leg walking cast at 4 weeks is allowed, followed by full weightbearing by 6 weeks. This type of injury has to be approached from the medial and lateral surface of the ankle. Yablon et al. showed that the fibula needed to be fixated.[19] Early investigators stated that when the medial repair was done first, the fibula would follow. This theory has not proven to be true. In fact, just the opposite was found. The fibula needs to be repaired to obtain good reduction of the ankle fracture.

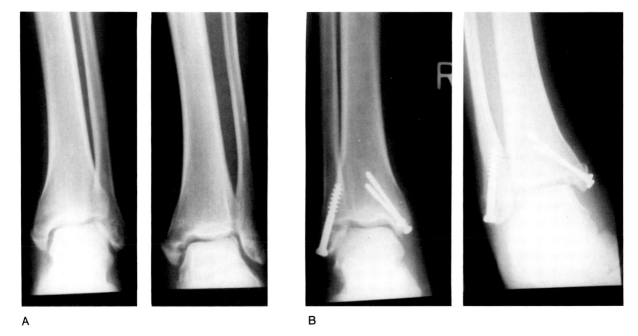

A   B

Fig. 42-12. Evaluation and treatment of pronation-abduction injury. **(A)** Fracture of medial malleolus, with transverse fracture of the fibula. **(B)** Reduction with short cancellous screw placed in the lateral fibula and malleolar screw placed in the medial malleolus.

Pronation-Abduction Injury

Mechanism

This injury occurs when the foot is held in a pronated position and an abductory force is applied. It produces three stages of injury.

Stage 1 injury includes a superficial or superficial and deep tear of the deltoid ligament. If the deltoid remains intact, there will be a fracture of the medial malleolus at or below the ankle. Stage 2 injury is a stage 1 injury plus a rupture of the anterior and posterior tibiofibular ligament and rupture of the syndesmosis. Stage 3 injury is a stage 2 plus a fracture of the fibula proximally at the syndesmosis (Fig. 42-12).

Physical Examination

Stage 1 injury patients have pain over the medial aspect of the ankle at the level of the deltoid liga-

ment or at the fracture. Stage 2 injury patients have pain over the medial aspect of the ankle and over the anterior and posterior lateral ankle. This pain will radiate proximal along the syndesmosis. Stage 3 injury patients have pain over the medial and anterior and posterior lateral aspects of the ankle, and over the fibula at the level of the fracture. This is a very unstable injury.

Treatment

Stage 1 injuries may be treated with a short leg walking cast for 6 weeks with partial weightbearing 2 to 4 weeks prior to full weightbearing.

Stage 2 injuries should be repaired with internal fixation. The medial deltoid ligament or medial malleolus fracture needs to be repaired and a syndesmotic screw placed across the syndesmosis. No weightbearing is allowed until the syndesmotic screw is removed. The patient can be started on early range-of-motion exercises with a patella weight-bearing cast. Such a cast can be made with a

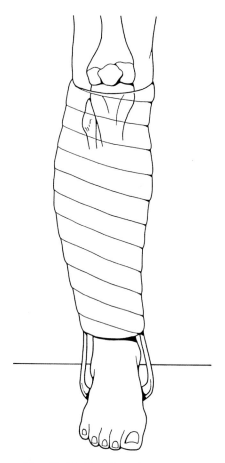

Fig. 42-13. Patella weight-bearing cast.

2-inch wide steel strip bent at 90 degrees in two spots, then run up the side of the cast and wrapped into the cast, thereby allowing the weight to be placed on the upper leg (Fig. 42-13). In this cast, the foot does not need to be incorporated into the cast therapy, allowing range of motion of the ankle.

Pronation-Eversion Injury

Mechanism

The foot is in a pronated position when an eversion force is applied to the foot, producing four stages of injury.

The first stage results in a tear of the deltoid ligament or a fracture of the medial malleolus. A stage 2 injury includes a stage 1 injury plus a rupture of the anterior tibiofibular ligament and

disruption of the syndesmosis. A stage 3 injury is a stage 2 injury plus a fracture of the fibula above the syndesmosis. Stage 4 injury is a stage 3 plus a rupture of the posterior tibiofibular ligament or a fracture of the posterior tibia, producing a trimalleolar fracture (Fig. 42-14).

Physical Examination

With a stage 1 injury, the patient will present with edema and pain over the medial malleolus or deltoid ligament. With a stage 2 injury, the patient will present with edema and pain over the medial surface of the ankle plus pain over the anterior ankle at the level of the anterior tibiofibular ligament and the syndesmosis area. Stage 3 injuries will present with the same physical evidence as the stage 2 injury and will have pain over the fibula at the fracture site. Stage 4 injuries will give all the same symptoms and pain may be elicited at the area of the posterior tibiofibular ligament.

Treatment

Stages 1, 2, and 3 injuries may be treated in a short leg walking cast if the medial malleolus is in good alignment. Upon x-ray, if in young, active individuals the medial malleolus is not in good position, internal fixation is indicated with a malleolar compression screw. The patient is then casted after early range of motion determination. Semiweightbearing is started, then full weightbearing after 4 weeks.

Stage 4 injuries are treated with internal fixation with a semitubular plate, medial malleolar compression screw, and syndesmotic screw. Treatment includes early range of motion determination then a short leg walking cast or patella weight-bearing cast. Weightbearing is not allowed until the syndesmotic screw is removed.

Vertical Compression Injury

Mechanism

The ankle joint will withstand up to three times the body weight before vertical force will cause injury. Several things may happen upon injury: (1) a fracture of the talus into several sections may occur; (2) a fracture of the tibial plafond—

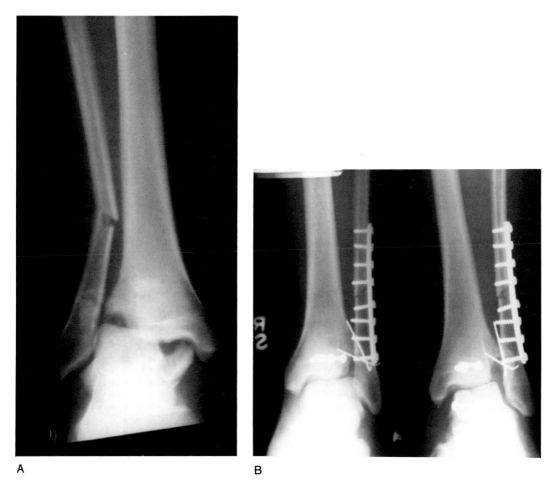

Fig. 42-14. Evaluation and treatment of pronation-eversion injury. **(A)** Spiral fracture of the fibula 7 to 8 cm proximal, fracture of lateral aspect of tibia, lateral displacement of talus with fracture of talus, tear of deltoid ligament. **(B)** Open reduction with internal fixation.

anterior, posterior, or both — may occur; or (3) the syndesmosis may rupture and the fibula fracture, usually proximal to the syndesmosis. A posterior fracture is usually an indication that the foot was in an equinus position at the time of injury.

Treatment

Because of the severity of these fractures, internal fixation is indicated with full knowledge that in the future fusion may well be indicated. The fibula and tibia must be brought back to length, then the joint surface as well as the medial malleolus must be placed back into position and held with screws and K wires. Early range of motion determination is a must in these fractures, with partial weightbearing allowed in a cast at 6 weeks. Full weightbearing is allowed in 8 weeks.

REFERENCES

1. Pott P: Some Few General Remarks on Fracture and Dislocations. Hawes, Clarke, Collins, London, 1768

2. Dupuytren G: Of fractures of the lower extremity of the fibula, & luxations of the foot. (reprinted in) Med Classics 4:151, 1939

3. Maisonneuve JG: Recherches sur la fracture du péroné. Arch Gen Med 1:165, 433, 1840

4. Cotten FJ: A new type of ankle fracture. JAMA 64:318, 1915

5. Cotten FJ: Injuries about the ankle. p. 603. In Dislocations and Joint Fracture. 2nd Ed. WB Saunders Co, Philadelphia, 1924

6. Cotton FJ: Ankle fractures, a new classification and a new class. N Engl J Med 201:753, 1929

7. Henderson MS: Trimalleolar fractures of the ankle. Surg Clin North Am 12:867, 1932

8. Ashhurst APC, Bromer RS: Classification and mechanism of fractures of the leg bones involving the ankle. Arch Surg 4:51, 1922

9. Lauge-Hansen N: "Ligamentous" ankle fractures: diagnosis and treatment. Acta Chir Scand 97:544, 1949

10. Lauge-Hansen N: Fractures of the Ankle II. Combined experimental-surgical and experimental-surgical and experimental-roentgenologic investigations. Arch Surg 60:957, 1950

11. Lauge-Hansen N: Fractures of the ankle IV. Clinical use of genetic reduction. Arch Surg 64:488, 1952

12. Lauge-Hansen N: Fractures of the ankle V. Pronation-dorsiflexion fracture. Arch Surg 67:813, 1953

13. Lauge-Hansen N: Fracture of the Ankle III. Genetic roentgenologic diagnosis of fractures of the ankle. Am J Roentgenol 71:456, 1954

14. Danis R: Théorie et Pratique de l'Ostéosynthese. p. 142. Paris, Masson, 1949

15. Weber BC: Klassifikation und operations indikation der oberen spruggelenks. p. 51. Verleg Hans Huber, Bern, 1966

16. Yde J: The Lauge-Hansen classification of malleolar fractures. Acta Orthop Scand 57:181, 1980

17. Kristensen TB: Fractures of the ankle. Follow up studies. Arch Surg 73:112, 1956

18. Braustein PW, Wade PA: Treatment of unstable fractures of the ankle. Ann Surg 149:217, 1956

19. Yablon IG, Heller FG, Shouse L: The key role of the lateral malleolus in the displaced fractures of the ankle. J Bone Joint Surg 57:169, 1977

Biomaterials

43

Joon B. Park, Ph.D.

Biomaterials can be thought of as materials that are brought into contact with living body tissues. One has to study not only the reaction between the tissues and the *bio*materials but also the changes in the structures and properties of the biomaterials caused by the tissues. The biomaterials should be compatible with tissues chemically, mechanically, and pharmacologically. Specifically, biomaterials should have adequate strength, fatigue, wear, and other physical properties (mechanical compatibility), be chemically inert and stable (chemical compatibility), and not elicit allergenic, carcinogenic, and toxic reactions (pharmacologic compatibility). Moreover, sound engineering design and cost should be considered for a particular application.

Biomaterials can be classified in many ways, according to the source (man-made or synthetic, and nature-made or natural), duration inside the body (permanent and transient), tissues (soft and hard tissues and blood), and medical disciplines (podiatry, orthopaedics, otolaryngology, neurosurgery, cardiology, dentistry, etc.).

Development of biomaterials as implants could not be advanced systematically until Lister's aseptic surgical technique was devised during the American Civil War. The various metal wires and pins made of iron, gold, copper, silver, platinum, and the like could not be evaluated properly since all implants failed as a result of infection. Development of metal alloys in the beginning of the 20th century and understanding the modes of failures of the implants made possible for continued improvements.

One of the early uses of synthetic plastics was the Judet femoral head prosthesis of the hip joint, made of polymethylmethacrylate. The same acrylic polymer, used to fabricate corneal implants, is noted for its high refractive index and good biocompatibility. Advent of open heart surgical techniques made possible the development of artificial blood vessels (1950s) and heart valves (1960s). Soon after, total heart implants had been developed, and they were tested in a human patient (1982). The first successful direct simulation of the heart was made in the late 1950s.

This chapter is not devoted to the structure-property relationship of biologic materials such as bones and skin because of space limitations. Table 43-1 gives some comparison of mechanical properties of various tissues and implant materials for a quick reference. As one might expect, metals and ceramics are primarily used for constructing implants that bear a large load, whereas elastomers (rubbers), plastics, and carbons are used largely for soft tissue replacements and for blood-interfacing implant fabrication. However, one should be care-

Table 43-1. Comparison of Mechanical Properties of Tissues and Biomaterials

Materials	Modulus (MPa)	Fracture Strength (MPa)	Fracture Strain (%)	Density (g/cm^3)
Polymers				
Silicone rubber	1–10	6–7	350–600	1.12–1.23
Polyamide (nylon 6/6)	2,800	76	90	1.14
UHMW polyethylene[a]	1,500	34	200–250	0.93–0.94
Acrylic (PMMA[b])	3,000	60	1–3	1.10–1.23
Metals				
316L stainless steel	200,000	540–620	55–60	7.9
Cobalt-chromium alloy (wrought)	230,000	900	60	9.2
Titanium-6/aluminum-4 alloy	110,000	900	10	4.5
Ceramics and carbons				
Al$_2$O$_3$ (single crystal)	363,000	490	<1	3.9
Pyrolytic carbon	280,000	517	<1	1.5–2.0
Hydroxyapatite	120,000	150	<1	3.2
Tissues				
Skin	0.34/38[c]	7.6	60	1.0
Aorta (transverse)	0.1/2[c]	1.1	77	1.0
Bone (femur)	17,200	121	1	2.0
Tooth (dentin)	13,800	138[d]	<1	1.9

[a]UHMW, ultra-high molecular weight.
[b]PMMA, polymethylmethacrylate.
[c]The initial portion and final portion of the stress-strain curve are distinctly different for most soft tissues, and the modulus is expressed for the two positions.
[d]Compressive strength.

ful not to generalize since oftentimes soft materials are used for the hard tissue applications (e.g., silicone rubber for toe and finger joint replacements).

METALS

Most metals employed to manufacture implants, such as iron, chromium, cobalt, nickel, titanium, carbon, molybdenum, and tungsten, can be tolerated by the body in minute quantities, and some of them are essential for many tissue functions, such as red blood cells (iron) or synthesis of vitamin B_{12} (cobalt).

Metals tend to oxidize or corrode, since oxide states are more stable than the pure form. This process poses two problems. One is weakening of the implant per se and the other is tissue reactions to the corrosion products locally as well as systemically. The ban on the use of stainless steels for implant fabrications in Scandinavian countries is due to the metal sensitivity (mainly to nickel) developed by many patients. These problems limit the number of metallic biomaterials to a few, such as 316L stainless steel, cobalt-chromium-molybdenum alloys and titanium alloys.

Stainless Steels

The first *stainless steel* used for implant fabrication was type 18-8 (18 percent nickel and 8 percent chromium), or type 302 in modern classification of the stainless steels. Later, a small amount of molybdenum (2 to 4 percent) was added to make it more corrosion resistant in salt water. This alloy is the predecessor of type 316L stainless steel, which limits the amount of carbon content to 0.03 percent instead of the 0.08 percent in type 316 for even better corrosion resistance in vivo. Only 316L stainless steel is suitable for making implants. Table 43-2 shows the composition of 316L stainless steel.

The most important structural feature of any stainless steel is to maintain the austenitic (gamma) phase, which has face-centered cubic (fcc) struc-

Table 43-2. Chemical Composition of Surgical Implant Metal Alloys[a]

	Co-Cr Alloys		316 Stainless Steel	Co-Ni-Cr-Mo Alloy (MP35N)	Wrought Co-Ni-Cr-Mo-W-Fe Alloy
	Cast	Wrought			
Chromium (Cr)	27.0–30.0	19.0–21.0	17.0–20.0	19.0–21.0	18.0–22.0
Molybdenum (Mo)	5.0–7.0	—	2.0–4.0	9.0–10.5	3.0–4.0
Nickel (Ni)	2.5	9.0–11.0	10.0–14.0	33.0–37.0	15.0–25.0
Tungsten (W)	—	14.0–16.0	—	—	3.0–4.0
Carbon (C)	max	0.05–0.15	0.08 max	0.025 max	0.05 max
Silicon (Si)	1.0	1.0	0.75 max	0.15 max	0.50 max
Manganese (Mn)	1.0	2.0	2.00 max	0.15 max	1.00 max
Iron (Fe)	0.75 max	3.0 max	remainder	1.0	4.0–6.0
Cobalt (Co)	remainder	remainder	—	remainder	remainder
Phosphorus (P)	—	—	0.03 max	0.015 max	—
Sulfur (S)	—	—	0.03 max	0.010 max	0.010 max

[a]Values are in weight percent.

ture. This can be achieved by controlling the relative amount of alloying elements. The usual way of hardening the stainless steel is *cold-working*. The cold-working is carried out by reducing the cross-sectional area by drawing the metal through a die or imposing other means of mechanical deformation (wrought metal). The cold-working does not increase the modulus of elasticity, although it produces a substantial increase in yield strength and a marginal increase in fracture strength. The trade-off of increasing hardness is made by the decreased fracture strain, as shown in Table 43-3.

Cobalt-Chromium Alloys

The cobalt-chromium alloys can be manufactured into final products by either the cast or the wrought process. The compositions of these alloys are quite different, as shown in Table 43-2. The

Table 43-3. Mechanical Properties of Surgical Implant Alloys

	Yield Strength (MPa)	Tensile Strength (MPa)	Ductility (Elongation %)	Young's Modulus (GPa)	Hardness (V.P.N.)	Fatigue Limit (MPa)
Stainless steels						
18 Chromium–8 nickel, fully softened	200–230	540–700	50–65	200	175–200	230–250
Extra-low carbon 18 chromium–8 nickel	200–250	540–620	55–60	200	170–200	—
Type 316, fully softened	240–300	600–700	35–55	200	170–200	260–280
Type 316, cold worked	700–800	1,000	7–10	200	300–350	300
Co-Cr-Mo alloys						
Cast alloy	450	655	8	200	300	—
Wrought alloy, solution annealed	380	900	60	230	240	—
Wrought alloy, cold worked	1,050	1,540	9	230	450	—
Co-Ni-Cr-Mo alloy (MP35N)						
Annealed	240–655	795–1,000	50.0	228	—	—
Cold worked and aged	1,585	1,790	8.0	—	—	—
Wrought Co-Ni-Cr-Mo-Fe-alloy						
Fully annealed	276	600	50	—	—	—
Cold worked and aged hard	1,172	1,310	12	—	—	—
Titanium						
Grade 3 pure	380	50	18	—	—	—
Grade 4 pure	485	550	15	—	—	—
Ti-6/Al-4V alloy	830	896	10	110	—	—

small amount of molybdenum in the casting alloy is readily work-hardened because of its lack of plastic deformability. Therefore, when one produces an implant by cold-working it has to be annealed. The mechanical properties of the cobalt-chromium alloys are better than those of the stainless steels, as shown in Table 43-3. Furthermore, they have excellent corrosion and fatigue resistance.

The cast alloys are frequently used in dental work for their excellent reproducibility of details. The casting procedure for this alloy is the "lost wax" technique. In this procedure one has to control the grain size and distribution by controlling solidification temperature, mold surface, and the presence of other elements (e.g., molybdenum) in order to achieve a homogeneous solid solution, which results in superior physical properties.

Titanium and Its Alloys

Titanium and its alloys are used as implant materials because of their high corrosion resistance and relatively low density (4.5 g/cm^3 compared with 7.9, 8.3, and 9.2 g/cm^3 for stainless steel and cast and wrought cobalt-chrome alloys, respectively). The excellent corrosion resistance of pure titanium is due to the tenacious oxide film (TiO_2) on the surface, as is the case of aluminum oxide (Al_2O_3), that protects the surface from further oxidation. However, unlike aluminum, the titanium oxide film is very stable in saline solution at room temperature.

Because of the inferior mechanical properties in the pure form, titanium is often used by alloying it with other elements such as aluminum, vanadium, manganese, silicon, molybdenum, and tin. The mechanical properties of two grades of titanium and an alloy are given in Table 43-3.

Another interesting alloy, Nitinol (titanium-nickel alloy; 50 percent each by atomic weight) is being considered for implant application. This alloy has "memory," which permits design of an implant that can be deformed structurally and then restored to its original form in the body by heating. The temperatures necessary for transformation can be controlled by altering the relative amount of titanium or a small amount of additives such as cobalt.

Other Metals

Another corrosion-resistant metal used for implant manufacture is tantalum. It forms an oxide film similar to that of titanium. The mechanical properties are similar to those of stainless steels, but it has much higher density (16.6 g/cm^3), making the metal less attractive to use. This metal is mostly used to fabricate sutures for neural and plastic surgery.

Platinum series metals (platinum, ruthenium, rhodium, palladium, osmium, and iridium) and their alloys have been utilized from time to time for surgical implants, although the high cost combined with relatively poor mechanical properties restricts their use in special cases such as dental bridges and electrodes for special circumstances (e.g. pacemaker tips).

POLYMERS

Polymers (*poly* = many, *mer* = unit) are linked together by the *primary* covalent bonding in the main *backbone* chain with carbon, nitrogen, oxygen, silicone and like atoms. The simplest example is polyethylene, which is made from ethylene (CH_2=CH_2) where the carbon (C) atoms share electrons with two other hydrogen (H) and carbon atoms: $-CH_2-(CH_2-CH_2)_n-CH_2-$, where n indicates number of repeating units in an average-length chain.

In order to make a strong solid the repeating unit, n, should be well over 1,000, making the molecular weight (m.w.) of the polymer over 28,000 g/mol. This is why the polymers are made of giant molecules. At low molecular weight the material behaves as a wax (e.g., paraffin wax used for household candles) and at still lower molecular weight as an oil or gas.

The main backbone chain can be of entirely different atoms; for example, polydimethyl siloxane (silicone rubber) has silicone (Si) and oxygen(0) as its backbone atoms: $-Si(CH_3)_2[O-Si(CH_3)_2]_nO-$. The side group atoms can be changed; thus if we substitute the hydrogen atoms of polyethylene with fluorine (F), the resulting material is the well-known Teflon (polytetrafluoroethylene).

In order to link the small molecules (monomers) one has to force them to lose electrons by the processes of condensation and addition. By controlling the reaction temperature, pressure, and time in the presence of catalyst(s), the degree to which monomers are linked into a chain can be manipulated.

During *condensation polymerization* a small molecule such as water will be condensed out of the chemical reaction:

$$R-NH_2 + R'-COOH \longrightarrow$$
(amine)   (carboxylic acid)

$$R'-CONH-R + H_2O \quad (43\text{-}1)$$
(amide)   (water)

This particular process is used to make polyamide (nylon), which was the first commercial polymer, made in the 1930s.

Typical condensation polymers are polyester (Dacron), polyurethane, and polydimethylsiloxane (Silastic rubber). Natural polymers, polysaccharides and proteins, are also made by condensation polymerization. The condensing molecule of natural polymers is always water (H_2O).

Addition polymerization can be achieved by rearranging the bond within each monomer. Since each "mer" has to share at least two covalent electrons with other mers the monomers have to have at least one double bond. For example, in the case of vinyl polymers:

$$
\begin{array}{ccc}
H & H \\
| & | \\
C & = C \\
| & | \\
H & H
\end{array}
\longrightarrow
\left(
\begin{array}{ccc}
H & H \\
| & | \\
-C & -C- \\
| & | \\
H & R
\end{array}
\right)_n
\quad (43\text{-}2)
$$

The breaking of a double bond can be done with an *initiator*, or free radical. Benzoyl and hydrogen peroxides are commonly used as initiators. The initiation process can be triggered by heat, ultraviolet light, and other chemicals. The free radical can react with monomer, which in turn becomes a free radical, and this free radical can react with another monomer and the process can continue on. This process is called *propagation*, and can be *terminated* by combining two free radicals, or transfer

Table 43-4. Monomers for Addition Polymerization

Vinyl chloride	$(CH_2{=}CHCl)$
Styrene	$(CH_2{=}CH-C_6H_5)$
Methylacrylate	$(CH_2{=}CH-COOCH_3)$
Acrylonitrile	$(CH_2{=}CH-CN)$
Vinyl acetate	$(CH_3COOCH{=}CH_2)$
Vinylidene chloride	$(CH_2{=}CCl_2)$
Methylmethacrylate	$\left(CH_2{=}C\overset{\displaystyle CH_3}{\underset{\displaystyle COOCH_3}{|}}\right)$

and disproportionate processes. Some of the commercially important vinyl monomers for addition polymers are given in Table 43-4.

Polymeric materials have a wide variety of applications for implantation since they can be easily fabricated into many forms: fibers, textiles, films, gels, sols, and solids. Almost all commercial polymers can be used for making implants provided that each polymer has undergone extensive in vitro and in vivo tests, including clinical trials. Because of the cost and time involved not all the polymers have been tested for possible use for implants. Polymers bear a close resemblance to natural tissue components such as collagen, which allows direct bonding with other substances (e.g., herapin coating on the surface of polymers for the prevention of blood clotting). Adhesive polymers can be used to close wounds or lute orthopaedic implants in place.

Polyolefins

Polyethylene and polypropylene and their copolymers are called polyolefins. These are linear *thermoplastics* that can be remelted and reused. *Polyethylene* is available commercially in three major grades: low and high density and ultra-high molecular weight (UHMWPE). Polyethylene is one of the vinyl polymers that contains a repeating unit structure with $R{=}H$.

The first polyethylene was made by reacting ethylene gas at high pressure (100 to 300 MPa) in the presence of a catalyst (peroxide) to initiate polymerization. This process yields *low*-density polyethylene. By using a *Ziegler catalyst*, high-density polyethylene can be produced at low pressure (10 MPa). Unlike the low-density type, high-density polyethylene does not contain branches. The result

Table 43-5. Properties of Polypropylene and Polyethylenes

Properties	Polypropylene	High-Density	UHMWPE
Molecular weight (g/mol)	—	5×10^5	2×10^6
Density (g/cm³)	0.90–0.91	0.92–0.96	0.93–0.944
Tensile strength (MPa)	28–36	23–40	34
Elongation (%)	400–900	400–500	200–250
Modulus of elasticity (MPa)	1.11–1.55	410–1,240	—
Crystallinity (%)	—	70–80	—

is better packing of the chains, which increases density and crystallinity.

The ultra-high molecular weight polyethylene (m.w. greater than 2×10^6 g/mol) has been used extensively for orthopaedic implant fabrications, especially for load-bearing surfaces such as total hip and knee joints. This material has no known solvent at room temperature; therefore, only high temperature and pressure sintering may be used to produce desired products. Conventional extrusion or molding processes are difficult to use. Some important physical properties for high-density and UHMW polyethylene, which are currently used for implants fabrication, are given in Table 43-5.

Polypropylene is another olefin polymer with an $R=CH_3$ repeating unit. Polypropylene can be synthesized by using a Ziegler-type stereospecific catalyst that controls the position of each monomer unit as it is being polymerized to allow the formation of a regular chain structure from the asymmetric repeating unit.

Three types of structure can exist, depending on the position of the methyl (CH_3) group along the polymer chain. The random distribution of methyl groups in the *atactic* polymer prevents close packing of chains and results in largely amorphous polypropylene. In comparison the *isotactic* and *syndiotactic* structures have regular positioning of the methyl side groups on the same side and on alternate sides, respectively. They usually crystallize. However, the presence of the methyl side groups restricts the movement of the polymer chains, and crystallization rarely exceeds 50 to 70 percent for material with isotacticity over 95 percent. Table 43-5 lists typical properties of commercial polypropylene.

Polypropylene has an exceptionally high flex life, hence it is used to make integrally molded hinges for finger joint prostheses. It also has excellent environmental stress-cracking resistance.

Polyamides (Nylons)

The polyamides are known as nylons and are designated by the number of carbon atoms in the parent diamine and diacid. Nylons can be polymerized by step-reaction (or condensation) and ring scission polymerization. They have excellent fiber-forming abilities because of their interchain hydrogen bonding, and a high degree of crystallinity, which increases strength in the fiber direction.

The basic chemical structure of the repeating unit of polyamides can be written in two ways, $-[NH(CH_2)_x NHCO(CH_2)_y CO]_n-$ and $-[NH(CH_2)_x CO]_n-$. The former equation represents polymers made from diamines and diacids such as types 66 and 610. The latter polyamides are made from ω amino acids and are designated as nylon 6 ($x = 5$), 11 ($x = 10$), and 12 ($x = 11$).

The presence of $-CONH-$ groups in polyamides attracts the chains strongly to one another through hydrogen bonding. Since the hydrogen bond plays a major role in determining properties, the number and distribution of $-CONH-$ groups are important factors. For example, the glass transition temperature (T_g) can be decreased by decreasing the number of $-CONH-$ groups, as given in Table 43-6. Conversely, an increase in the number of $-CONH-$ groups improves physical properties such as strength: 66 is stronger than 610 and 6 is stronger than 11.

As mentioned previously, the nylons are hygro-

Table 43-6. Properties of Polyamides

Properties	Type			
	66	1610	11	6
Density (g/cm³)	1.14	1.09	1.05	1.13
Tensile strength (MPa)	76	55	59	83
Elongation (%)	90	100	120	300
Modulus of elasticity (GPa)	2.8	1.8	1.2	2.1
Softening temperature (°C)	265	220	185	215

scopic (absorb water) and lose their strength in vivo when implanted. The water molecules serve as *plasticizers* that attack the amorphous region, which is less densely packed than the crystalline region. Proteolytic enzymes may also aid hydrolysis by attacking the amide groups.

Acrylic Polymers

Acrylic polymers are used extensively in medical applications such as (hard) contact lenses, implantable ocular lenses, and bone cement for joint fixation. Dentures and maxillofacial prostheses are also made from acrylics because they have excellent physical and coloring properties and they are easy to fabricate.

Structure and Properties of Acrylics and Hydrogels

The basic chemical structure of repeating units of acrylics can be represented by:

$$\left(-CH_2-\underset{\underset{COOR_2}{|}}{\overset{\overset{R_1}{|}}{C}}-\right)_n \qquad (43\text{-}3)$$

The only difference between polymethylacrylate (PMA) and polymethylmethacrylate (PMMA) is the R groups. The R_1 and R_2 groups for PMA are H and CH_3, respectively. These polymers are addition (or free radical) polymerized. These polymers can be obtained in liquid monomer or fully polymerized beads, sheets, rods, and the like. Because of the bulky side groups, these polymers are usually obtained in a clear, amorphous state. For the same reason, PMMA has higher tensile strength (60 MPa) and softening temperature (125°C) than PMA (7 MPa and 33°C, respectively). PMMA has an excellent light transparency (92 percent transmission) and a high index of refraction (1.49), and also has excellent weathering properties. This material can be cast, molded, or machined with conventional tools. It has an excellent chemical resistivity and is highly biocompatible in pure form. The material is brittle in comparison with other polymers.

The first *hydrogel* polymer developed that can absorb water to more than 30 percent of its weight, for soft contact lens applications, is poly(hydroxyethylmethacrylate) or polyHEMA. The chemical formula is similar to the previous one, with $R_1 = CH_3$ and $R_2 = CH_2OH$.

The OH group ($COOCH_2OH$) is the hydrophilic group responsible for hydration of the polymer. Generally, hydrogels for contact lenses are made by the polymerization or copolymerization of certain hydrophilic monomers with small amounts of a cross-linking agent such as ethylene glycol dimethacrylate (EGDM). The water content of the copolymer can be increased to over 60 percent, whereas the normal water content for polyHEMA is about 40 percent.

The hydrogels have a relatively low oxygen permeability in comparison to silicone rubber (see Table 43-7). However, the permeability can be increased with increased hydration (water content) or decreased (lens) thickness. Silicone rubber is not a hydrophilic material, but its high oxygen permeability and transparency make it an attractive lens material. It is usually used after coating with hydrophilic hydrogels by grafting.

Acrylic Bone Cement (PMMA)

Recently, bone cement has been used in greater numbers of clinical application to secure a firm fixation of joint prostheses such as hip and knee joints. Bone cement is primarily made of PMMA powder and monomer methylmethacrylate liquid. One commercial product, Surgical Simplex Radiopaque bone cement, is produced by mixing two components. One is an ampule containing a colorless, flammable liquid monomer that has a sweet, slightly acrid odor and has the following composition:

Methylmethacrylate (monomer)	97.4 v/o (volume percent)
N,N-dimethyl-*p*-toluidine	2.6 v/o
Hydroquinone	75 + 15 ppm

The hydroquinone is added to prevent premature polymerization, which may occur under certain conditions (e.g., exposure to light, elevated temperatures, radiation). *N,N*-dimethyl-*p*-toluidine is

Table 43-7. Oxygen Permeability Coefficients of Contact Lens Materials

Polymers	Pg $\times$ 10^4 (μl-cm/cm^2-h/kPa)	Comments
Poly(methylmethacrylate)	0.27	Hard contact lens
Poly(dimethylsiloxane)	1750	Flexible
Poly(hydroxyethylmethacrylate)	24	39% H$_2$O, soft lens

At standard temperature and pressure, to convert μl-cm/cm^2-h/kPa to μl-cm/cm^{2}h/mmHg, divide by 7.5.

added to promote or accelerate "cold-curing" of the finished compound. ("cold-curing" is the manner in which the polymerization process occurs at room temperature as opposed that in to some acrylics polymerized under high temperature and pressure.) The liquid component is sterilized by membrane filtration.

The other component is a packet of 40 g of finely ground white powder (a mixture of PMMA, methylmethacrylate-styrene copolymer, and barium sulfate, U.S.P.) of the following composition:

Poly(methylmethacrylate)	15.0 w/o (weight percent)
Methylmethacrylate-styrene copolymer	75.0 w/o
Barium sulfate (BaSO$_4$)	10.0 w/o

When the two components are mixed together, the monomer liquid is polymerized by the free-radical (addition) polymerization process. A minute amount of an initiator, dibenzoyl peroxide (see Equation 43-2), present in the powder will react with the monomer to initiate free radical generations. The propagation process will continue until long-chain molecules are produced. The monomer liquid will wet the polymer powder particle surfaces and link them together after being polymerized. The properties of cured bone cement are compared with those of commercial acrylic resins in Table 43-8.

Fluorocarbon Polymers

The best known fluorocarbon polymer is polytetrafluoroethylene (PTFE), commonly known as Teflon (DuPont). Other polymers containing fluorine are polytrifluorochloroethylene (PTFCE), polyvinylfluoride (PVF), and fluorinated ethylene propylene (FEP). Only PTFE is discussed here since the others have rather inferior chemical and physical properties and are seldom used for implant fabrication.

PTFE is made by placing tetrafluoroethylene under pressure with a peroxide catalyst in the present of excess water for removal of heat. The repeating unit is similar to that of polyethylene, except that the hydrogen atoms are replaced by fluorine atoms.

The polymer is highly crystalline (over 94 per-

Table 43-8. Physical Properties of Bone Cement and Commercial Acrylic Resins

Properties	Radiopaque Bone Cement	Commercial Acrylic Resins
Tensile strength (MPa)	28.9 $\pm$ 1.6	55–76
Compressive strength (MPa)	91.7 $\pm$ 2.5	76–131
Elongation (%)	1–3	3–7
Young's modulus (compressive loading, MPa)	2,200 $\pm$ 60	2,960–3,280
Endurance limit	0.3 uts[a]	0.3 uts
Density (g/cm^3)	1.10–1.23	1.18
Water sorption (%)	0.5	0.3–0.4
Shrinkage after setting (%)	2.75–5	—

Ultimate tensile strength.

Table 43-9. Properties of Polytetrafluoroethylene

Properties	Values
Tensile strength (MPa)	14
Modulus (MPa)	500
Elongation (%)	200–400
Density (g/cm^3)	2.15–2.20
Melting temp. (°C)	327

cent crystallinity), with an average molecular weight of 0.5 to 5×10^6 g/mol. This polymer has a very high density and a low modulus of elasticity and tensile strength, as given in Table 43-9. It also has a very low surface tension (18.5 erg/cm^2) and a low friction coefficient (0.1). This material is used to fabricate artificial blood vessels in knitted or (porous) expanded form. PTFE cannot be injection molded or melt extruded because of its very high melt viscosity, and it cannot be plasticized. Usually the powers are sintered to above 327°C under pressure to produce solids.

Rubbers

Three types of rubber — silicone, natural, and synthetic — have been used to fabricate implants. Rubbers are defined by the American Society for Testing and Materials (ASTM) as "a material which at room temperature can be stretched repeatedly to at least twice its original length and upon release of the stress, returns immediately with force to its approximate original length." Rubbers are stretchable because of the kinks of the individual chains, as seen in *cis*-1,4-polyisoprene:

$$\left(\begin{array}{c} \overset{\displaystyle CH_3 \quad H}{\underset{\displaystyle}{}} \\ H \diagup \overset{|}{C} = \overset{|}{C} \diagdown H \\ -\overset{|}{\underset{H}{C}} \qquad \overset{|}{\underset{H}{C}}- \end{array} \right)_n \qquad (43\text{-}4)$$

The *trans-* form of the isoprene isomer cannot be stretched since the chains cannot be kinked. Instead they crystallize, resulting in brittle *gutta percha:*

$$\left(\begin{array}{c} \overset{\displaystyle CH_3 \qquad H}{} \\ H \qquad | \qquad | \\ \diagdown \overset{|}{C} \diagup \overset{|}{C} = \overset{|}{C} \diagdown \overset{|}{C} \diagup \\ \overset{|}{\underset{H}{}} \qquad \overset{|}{\underset{H}{}} \qquad H \end{array} \right)_n \qquad (43\text{-}5)$$

The *repeated* stretchability is due to the cross links between chains that hold the chains together. The amount of cross linking for natural rubber controls the flexibility of the rubber: the addition of 2 to 3 percent sulfur results in a flexible rubber, while adding as much as 30 percent sulfur makes it a hard rubber.

Rubbers contain *antioxidants* to protect them against decomposition by oxidation, hence improving aging properties. *Fillers* such as carbon black or silica powers are also used to improve their physical properties.

Natural and Synthetic Rubbers

Natural rubber is made mostly from the latex of the *Hevea brasiliensis* tree, and the chemical formula is the same as that of polyisoprene. Natural rubber was found to be compatible with blood in its pure form. Also, cross linking by x-ray and organic peroxides produces rubber with superior blood compatibility compared to rubbers made by conventional sulfur vulcanization.

Synthetic rubbers were developed to substitute for natural rubber. The Natta and Ziegler types of stereospecific polymerization techniques have made this development possible. The synthetic rubbers rarely have been used to make implants. One of these rubbers, neoprene (polychloroprene), is listed in Table 43-10 for comparison.

Silicone Rubbers

Silicone rubber, developed by Dow Corning company, is one of the few polymers developed for medical use. The repeating unit is dimethylsiloxane

$$\left(\begin{array}{c} CH_3 \\ | \\ -Si-O- \\ | \\ CH_3 \end{array} \right)_n$$

which is polymerized by a condensation polymerization.

Low molecular weight polymers have low viscosity and can be cross linked to make a rubber-like material. Medical-grade silicone rubbers use stannous octate as a catalyst and can be mixed with base polymer at the time of implant fabrications.

Table 43-10. Properties of Rubbers

Properties	Types of Rubber			
	Natural	Neoprene	Silicone	Urethane
Tensile strength (MPa)	7–30	20	6–7	35
Elongation (%)	100–700	—	350–600	650
Hardness (Shore A Durometer)	30–90	40–95	—	65
Density (g/cm³)	0.92	1.23	1.12–1.23	1.1–1.23

Silicone rubbers use silica (SiO_2) powder as fillers to improve their mechanical properties. The more fillers are used the higher the density and the harder the rubber, since silica has higher density and hardness.

CERAMICS AND CARBON

Ceramics are inorganic, nonconductive compounds that are formed by some type of firing process at high temperatures. They may contain silicates, oxides, carbides, or various refractory hydrides, sulfides, and nitrides. The oxides, covalent compounds such as Al_2O_3, MgO, and SiO_2, contain *metallic* and *nonmetallic* elements, whereas other components are ionic salts ($NaCl$, $CsCl$, ZnS, etc.). Carbons, such as diamond, and carbonaceous structures such as graphite and pyrolized carbons, are covalently bonded.

Recently ceramic materials have been given a lot of attention as candidates for implant materials since they possess some highly desirable characteristics for some applications. Ceramics have been used for some time in dentistry as crowns because of their inertness of the body fluids, high compressive strength, and good esthetic appearance.

Carbons have been used as artificial heart valve disks, percutaneous buttons, and lead and dental implants. Although the black color can be a drawback in some dental applications, if used as implants, carbons have desirable qualities such as good biocompatibility and ease of fabrication.

Ceramics

Ceramics are generally hard. Measure of hardness is calibrated using *Moh's scale.* Diamond is the hardest, with a Moh's scale value of 10, and talc [$Mg_3Si_4O_{10}(OH)_2$] is the softest (1); others, such as alumina (Al_2O_3; 9), quartz (SiO_2; 8), and apatite ($Ca_5P_3O_{12}F$; 5), are in between.) Another characteristic of ceramic materials is their high melting temperatures, due to the high bonding energy.

Unlike metals and polymers, ceramics are hard to shear because of the ionic nature of their bonding. In order to shear, the planes of atoms should *slip* past each other as a result of attractive forces between neighboring atoms. However, for ceramic materials neighboring ions with the same electric charge repel each other; hence moving the planes of atoms is very difficult. This makes ceramics nonductile, and creep at room temperature is almost nonexistent. Ceramics are also very sensitive to notching or microcracks, since instead of undergoing plastic deformation (or yield) they will fracture elastically once the crack propagates. This is also the reason ceramics have low tensile strength compared to their compressive strength. In compression any cracks or pores tend to be closed, but in tension the opposite is true. In the case of compression the cross-sectional area of the narrowest section does not decrease, whereas in tension it becomes smaller. Since the area becomes smaller by the applied force the actual stress becomes larger, hence worsening the *stress concentration* effect, which is, in fact, a much more important factor than the changes in cross-sectional area. If the ceramic is made flawless then it becomes very strong even in tension. Glass fibers made this way have tensile strengths twice that of steel.

Although the use of ceramic materials is well known in dentistry, their use in medicine as implants is relatively new. The main advantage of ceramics over others types of implants is their "inertness" or "biocompatibility," which is due to their low chemical reactivity. However, some ceramics are made reactive to induce direct bonding between implant and hard tissues.

Aluminum Oxides

The main source of high-purity alumina is bauxite and native corundum. The commonly available α-alumina can be prepared by calcining alumina trihydrate, resulting in calcined alumina. The ASTM specifies 99.5 percent pure alumina and less than 0.1 percent of combined SiO_2 and alkali oxides (mostly Na_2O) for implant use.

The α-alumina has a rhombohedral crystal structure (a = 4.758 Å and c = 12.991 Å). Single crystals of alumina known as synthetic sapphire and synthetic ruby (depending on the types of impurities) have been used successfully to make implants. These large single crystals can be made by feeding fine alumina powders onto the surface of a seed crystal that is slowly withdrawn from an electric arc or oxy-hydrogen flame as the fused powder builds up. Alumina crystals up to 10 cm in diameter have been grown by this method.

The strength of polycrystalline alumina depends on the porosity and grain sizes. Generally the smaller the grains and porosity the higher the resulting strength. ASTM standards (F603-78) require a flexural strength of greater than 400 MPa and an elastic modulus of 380 GPa, as given in Table 43-11. Alumina in general is a quite hard material, varying from 2,000 to 3,000 kg/mm² (19.6 to 29.4 GPa) Vicker's hardness. This high hardness is responsible for the use of alumina as an abrasive (emery) and as a bearing for watch movements. The high hardness is accompanied by low friction and wear, which are major advantages of using the alumina as joint replacement material in spite of its brittleness.

Hydroxyapatite

The use of hydroxyapatite as an implant has been tried many times in the form of artificial bone. Recently this material has been synthesized and used for manufacturing various forms of implants (solid or porous) and as coatings on other implants.

The mineral part of bone and teeth is made of apatites of calcium (Ca) and phosphate (PO_4) that are similar to hydroxyapatite crystals $[Ca_{10}(PO_4)_6(OH)_2]$. The apatite family of minerals, $A_{10}(BO_4)_6X_2$, crystallize into hexagonal rhombic prisms and have unit cell dimensions of a = 9.432 Å and c = 6.881 Å. The ideal Ca:P ratio of hydroxyapatite is 10:6 and the calculated density is 3.219 g/cm³. It is interesting to note that the substitution of OH with F will give a greater chemical stability because of the closer coordination of fluorine as compared to the hydroxyl by the nearest calcium. This is one of the reasons for the better caries resistance of teeth treated by fluoridation.

There seem to be a wide variation of the mechanical properties of hydroxyapatite, due largely to differences in manufacturing methods and testing procedures. Some groups reported that the hydroxyapatite synthesized by them had an average compressive strength of 917 MPa and an average tensile strength of 196 MPa for fully densified polycrystalline specimens. Others reported compressive strength of 3,000 kg/cm² (294 MPa), bending strength of 1,500 kg/cm² (147 MPa), and Vicker's hardness of 350 kg/mm³ (3.43 GPa).

The elastic modulus of hydroxyapatite ranges from 40 to 117 GPa depending on the measurement techniques. Hydroxyapatite has a higher elastic modulus than those of the hard tissues, which range from 12 to 74 GPa. Along this line of thought, it is also interesting to note that the lesser organic material (mainly collagen) containing enamel has a higher elastic modulus (74 GPa) than bone (12 to 14.6 GPa) and dentin (21 GPa), which is indirect evidence that the mineral portion of the hard tissues is made of hydroxyapatite. The Poisson's ration for the mineral or synthetic hydroxyapatite is about 0.27, which is somewhat close to that of ($\sim$0.3). The properties of hydroxyapatite are summarized in Table 43-11.

The most interesting property of hydroxyapatite is its excellent biocompatibility, to the extent that it appears to form a direct chemical bond with hard tissues.

Many different methods have been developed to make precipitates of hydroxyapatite from aqueous solution of $Ca(NO_3)_2$ and NaH_2PO_4. The precipitates are filtered and dried to form fine powders.

Table 43-11. Properties of Alumina and Hydroxyapatite

Properties	Alumina	Hydroxyapatite
Density (g/cm³)	3.8–3.9	3.219
Elastic modulus (GPa)	380	40–117
Bending strength (MPa)	400	147
Hardness (Vicker's, GPa)	19.6	3.43
Poisson's ratio	0.25	0.27

After calcination for about 3 hours at 900°C to promote crystallization, the powder can be pressed into a final form and sintered at about 1050 to 1450°C for 3 hours.

Glass Ceramics

Glass ceramics are polycrystalline ceramics made by controlled crystallization of glasses, a process developed by S.D. Stookey of Corning Glass Works in the early 1960s. They were first utilized in photosensitive glasses in which small amounts of copper, silver, and gold are precipitated by ultraviolet light irradiation. These metallic precipitates help to nucleate and crystallize the glass into a fine-grained ceramic that possesses excellent mechanical and thermal properties. Bioglass and Ceravital are two glass ceramics developed for implants.

An important factor in forming glass ceramics is the nucleation and growth of crystals in small (less than 1 μm diameter) and uniform size. It is estimated that about 10^{12} to 10^{15} nuclei/cm^3 are required to achieve such small crystals. In addition to the metallic agents mentioned (copper, gold, and silver), platinum groups, TiO_2, ZrO_2, and P_2O_5 are widely used for this purpose. The nucleation of glass is carried out at temperatures much lower than the melting temperature when the melt viscosity is in the range of 10^{11} to 10^{12} poise for 1 to 2 hours. In order to obtain a higher crystalline phase it is further heated to a temperature for maximum crystal growth without deformation of the product, phase transformation within the crystalline phases, or redissolution of some of the phases. The crystallization is usually more than 90 percent complete, with grain sizes of 0.1 to 1 μm, which is much smaller than in conventional ceramics.

The glass ceramics developed for implantation are the SiO_2-CaO-Na_2O-P_2O_5 and Li_2O-ZnO-SiO_2 systems. There are two different groups experimenting with the SiO_2-CaO-Na_2)-P_2O_5 glass ceramic. Hench's group varied the compositions (except P_2O_5) in order to obtain the best composition to induce direct bonding with bone. The bonding is related to the simultaneous formation of calcium phosphate and a SiO_2-rich film layer on the surface, as exhibited by the 46S5.2 variant. If a SiO_2-rich layer forms first and a calcium phosphate film develops later as for 46 to 55 mol % SiO_2 samples, then direct bonding with bone is observed. When no phosphate film is formed (60 mol % SiO_2) then no direct bonding with bone is observed.

The composition of Ceravital is similar to that of Bioglass in SiO_2 content but differs somewhat in other components, as given in Table 43-12. Also, Al_2O_3, and Ta_2O_5 are used for Ceravital glass ceramic in order to control the dissolution rate. The mixtures were melted in a platinum crucible at 1500°C for 3 hours and annealed, then cooled. The nucleation and crystallization temperatures were 680 and 750°C, respectively, for 24 hours each. When the size of the crystallites was about 4 Å without exhibiting characteristic needle structure, the process was stopped.

Glass ceramics have several desirable properties compared to glasses and ceramics. The thermal coefficient of expansion is very low, typically 10^{-7} to 10^{-5} per degree (c.f. 8.8×10^{-6} for Al_2O_3, 11.5×10^{-6} for SiO_2), and in some cases it can even be made negative. Because of the controlled grain size and improved resistance to surface damage,

Table 43-12. Compositions of Bioglass and Ceravital Glass-Ceramics

Type	Code	SiO$_2$	CaO	Na$_2$O	P$_2$O$_5$	MgO	K$_2$O
Bioglass[a]	42S5.6	42.1	29.0	26.3	2.6	—	—
	46S5.2						
	(45S5)	46.1	26.9	24.4	2.6	—	—
	49S4.9	49.1	25.3	23.0	2.6	—	—
	52S4.6	52.1	23.8	21.5	2.6	—	—
	55S4.3	55.1	22.2	20.1	2.6	—	—
	60S3.8	60.1	19.6	17.7	2.6	—	—
Ceravital[a]							
Bioactive		40.0–50.0	30.0–35.0	5.0–10.0	10.0–15.0	2.5–5.0	0.5–3.0
Nonbioactive[b]		30.0–35.0	25.0–30.0	3.5–7.5	7.5–12.0	1.0–2.5	0.5–2.0

[a]The Bioglass compositions are in mol % and the Cervital composition is in weight %.
[b]In addition, Al_2O_3 (5.0–15.0), TiO_2 (1.0–5.0), and Ta_2O_5 (5.0–15.0) are added.

their mechanical strength can be increased by at least a factor of two, from about 100 to 200 MPa for tensile strength, and the resistance to scratching and abrasion is close to that of sapphire.

The main drawback of glass ceramic is its brittleness, similar to other glasses and ceramics. Also, because of the restrictions on composition needed to achieve biocompatibility (or osteogenicity), the mechanical strength cannot be substantially improved as for other glass-ceramics. Therefore, glass ceramics cannot be used for making major load-bearing implants such as joint implants. It is also doubtful that the direct bonding with hard tissues can be maintained for a long time, since old cells are replaced by new ones, constantly destroying the initial bonding. Glass ceramics can be used as fillers for bone cement, dental restorative composites, and coating material.

Other Ceramics

In addition to the ceramic materials mentioned so far there have been experiments on many other ceramics, notably titanium oxide (TiO_2), barium titanate ($BaTiO_2$), tricalcium phosphate ($Ca_3(PO_4)O_2$), and calcium aluminate ($CaOAl_2O_3$). Calcium aluminate was used to induce tissue ingrowth by making it porous for better attachment of implants. However, this material loses considerable strength after in vivo and in vitro aging. Tricalcium phosphate together with calcium aluminate was tested as biodegradable implants in the hopes of regenerating new bone. Barium titanate was tested for use in attaching an implant by providing textured surfaces and making it piezoelectric after the implant was polarized. Whenever the piezoelectric compound was loaded the implant was polarized, which resulted in stimulation of the adjacent tissues.

Carbons

Carbons can be made in many forms: allotropic, crystalline diamond and graphite, quasicrystalline glassy, and pyrolytic carbon. Among these only pyrolytic carbon is widely utilized for implant fabrication.

The crystalline structure of carbon is similar to that of graphite. The planar hexagonal arrays are formed by strong covalent bonds in which one valence electron per atom is free to move, resulting in high but anisotropic electric and thermal conductivity. The bonding between layers is stronger than the van der Waals force; therefore *cross links* between them were suggested. Indeed the remarkable lubricating property of graphite cannot be realized unless the cross links are eliminated.

The poorly crystalline carbons are thought to contain unassociated or unoriented carbons. The strong bonding within layers and the weaker bonding between layers cause the properties of individual crystallites to be highly anisotropic. However, if the crystallites are randomly dispersed then the aggregate becomes isotropic.

The mechanical properties of carbon, especially pyrolytic carbon, are largely dependent on the density. The increased mechanical properties are directly related to the increased density, which indicates that the properties depend mainly on the aggregate structure of the material.

Graphite and the glassy carbons have much lower mechanical strength than pyrolytic carbon, as shown in Table 43-13. However, the average modulus of elasticity is almost the same for all carbons. The strength and toughness of pyrolytic carbon are quite high compared to graphite and the glassy carbons. This is again due to the lesser amount of flaws and unassociated carbons in the aggregate.

As for the ceramics, carbons show excellent compatibility with tissues. The strong compatibility with blood made pyrolytic carbon–deposited heart valve and blood vessel walls widely accepted by surgeons. Because of their high specific strength as fibers and their biocompatibility, they are also being used as a reinforcing component of composite implant materials and tensile loading applications, such as artificial tendon and ligament replacements.

Carbons can be deposited onto finished implants from hydrocarbon gas in a fluidized bed at a controlled temperature. The anisotry, density, crystallite size, and structure of the deposited carbon can be controlled by temperature, composition of the fluidized gas, bed geometry, and residence time of the gas molecules in the bed. The microstructures of deposited carbon should be particularly controlled since the formation of growth features as a

Table 43-13. Properties of Various Types of Carbon

Properties	Types of Carbon		
	Graphite	Glassy	Pyrolytic[a]
Density (g/cm³)	1.5–1.9	1.5	1.5–2.0
Elastic modulus (GPa)	24	24	28
Compressive strength (MPa)	138	172	517 (57[a])
Toughness (m-N/cm³)[b]	6.3	0.6	4.8

[a]1.0 w/o silicone-alloyed pyrolytic carbon, Pyrolite (Carbomedics, Austin, TX).
[b]1 m-N/cm³ = 1.45×10^{-3} in-lb/in³.

result of uneven crystallization can weaken the material. It is also possible to introduce various other elements into the fluidizing gas and codeposit them with carbon. Usually silicon (10 to 20 w/o) is codeposited (or *alloyed*) to increase hardness for applications requiring resistance to abrasion.

Recently pyrolytic carbon was successfully deposited onto the surfaces of blood vessel implants made of polymers. This is called ultra-low-temperature isotropic (ULTI) carbon instead of low-temperature isotropic (LTI) carbon. The deposited carbon is thin enough not to interfere with the flexibility of the grafts yet exhibits excellent blood compatibility.

SELECTED READINGS

Bechtol CO, Ferguson AB, Laing PG: Metals and Engineering in Bone and Joint Surgery. Balliere, Tindall and Cox, London, 1959

Black J: Biological Performance of Materials. Marcel Dekker, New York, 1981

Bloch B, Hastings GW: Plastic Materials in Surgery. 2nd Ed. Charles C Thomas, Springfield, IL, 1972

Bokros JC, Arkins RJ, Shim HS, et al: Carbon in prosthestic devices. In Deviney ML, O'Grady TM (eds): Petroleum Derived Carbons. American Chemical Society Symposium. Series No. 21. American Chemical Society, Washington, DC, 1976

Bruck SD: Blood Compatible Synthetic Polymers: An Introduction. Charles C Thomas, Springfield, IL, 1974

Bruck SD: Properties of Biomaterials in the Physiological Environment. CRC Press, Boca Raton, FL, 1980

Charnley J: Acrylic Cement in Orthopedic Surgery. Churchill Livingstone, Edinburgh, 1970

Dardik H (ed): Graft Materials in Vascular Surgery. Year Book Medical Pub, Chicago, 1978

Ducheyne P, Van der Perre G, Aubert AE (eds): Bioma-

terials and Biomechanics. Elsevier Science Pub, Amsterdam, 1984

Dumbleton JH, Black J: An Introduction to Orthopedic Materials. Charles C Thomas, Springfield, IL, 1975

Edwards WS: Plastic Arterial Grafts. Charles C Thomas, Springfield, IL, 1965

Guidelines for Blood-Material Interactions. Report of the National Heart, Lung, and Blood Institute Working Group, Devices and Technology Branch. NIH Publication No. 80-2185, Revised. US Government Printing Office, Washington, DC, 1985

Guidelines for Physiochemical Characterization of Biomaterials. Report of the National Heart, Lung, and Blood Institute Work Group, Devices and Technology Branch. NIH Publication No. 80-2186. US Government Printing Office, Washington, DC, 1980

Hastings GW, Williams DF (eds): Mechanical Properties of Biomaterials. John Wiley & Sons, New York, 1980

Homsy CA, Armeniades CD (eds): Biomaterials for Skeletal and Cardiovascular Applications. J Biomed Mater Res Symp, No. 3, 1972

Hulbert SF, Young FA, Moyle DD (eds): J Biomed Mater Res Symp, No. 2, 1972

Kronenthal RL, Oser Z (eds): Polymers in Medicine and Surgery. Plenum Press, New York, 1975

Lee H, Neville K: Handbook of Biomedical Plastics. Pasadena Technology Press, Pasadena, CA, 1971

Leinninger RI: Polymers as surgical implants. CRC Crit Rev Bioeng 2:333–360, 1972

Levine SN (ed): Materials in Biomedical Engineering. Ann NY Acad Sci 146(0), 1968

Levine SN (ed): Polymers and Tissue Adhesives. Ann NY Acad Sci 146(4), 1968

Lynch W: Implants: Reconstructing the Human Body. Van Nostrand Reinhold Co, New York, 1982

Mears DC: Materials and Orthopedic Surgery. Williams & Wilkins, Baltimore, 1979

Park JB: Biomaterials: An Introduction. Plenum Pub, New York, 1979

Park JB: Biomaterials Science and Engineering. Plenum Pub, New York, 1984

Rubin LR (ed): Biomaterials in Reconstructive Surgery. CV Mosby, St. Louis, 1983

Schaldach M, Hohmann D (eds): Advances in Artificial Hip and Knee Joint Technology. Springer-Verlag, Berlin, 1976

Schnitman PA, Schulman LB (eds): Dental Implants: Benefits and Risk. A NIH-Harvard Consensus Development Conference. NIH Pub. No. 81–1531. US Department of Health and Human Services, Bethesda, MD, 1980

Syrett BC, Acharya A (eds): Corrosion and Degradation of Implant Materials. ASTM STP 684. American Society for Testing and Materials, Philadelphia, 1979

Szycher M, Robinson WJ (eds): Synthetic Biomedical Polymers, Concepts and Applications. Technomic Pub, Westport CT, 1980

Transactions of the American Society for Artificial Internal Organs. (Published yearly and contains studies related to this chapter.)

Williams DF (ed): Compatibility of Implant Materials. Sector Pub. Ltd, London, 1976

Williams DF (ed): Fundamental Aspects of Biocompatibility. Vol. 1 and 2. CRC Press, Boca Raton, FL, 1981

Williams DF (ed): Systemic Aspects of Blood Compatibility. CRC Press, Boca Raton, FL, 1981

Williams DF (ed): Biocompatibility in Clinical Practice. Vol. I and II. CRC Press, Boca Raton, FL, 1982

Implant Arthroplasty of the First Metatarsophalangeal Joint and Alternatives

44

Vincent J. Hetherington, D.P.M., M.S.
Angel L. Cuesta, D.P.M.

SURGICAL IMPLANTS

The modern types of first metatarsophalangeal joint silicone implants have developed from a long line of design modifications and construction. A brief chronology is presented in Table 44-1. Figure 44-1 shows the appearance of several of these designs in either a photographic or line drawing representation. Of these devices only a few are used clinically. The most commonly used devices are (1) the Swanson design silicone single-stemmed hemi-implant; (2) the Swanson design titanium single-stemmed hemi-implant; (3) the Swanson design double-stemmed total hinged implant; (4) the LaPorta design double-stemmed total hinged implant; and (5) the Lawrence design double-stemmed total hinged implant. The goal, indications, contraindications, and considerations for flexible and titanium implant arthroplasty are outlined in Table 44-2.[13,14]

Swanson Hemi-implant

The first usable silicone elastomeric implant of the great toe specifically described as a joint spacer was introduced by Alfred Swanson along with Dow Corning in 1967.[1] The Swanson design hemi-implant is a silicone intramedullary stemmed implant to replace the base of the proximal phalanx, augmenting the Keller procedure. Although the success with silicone implant arthroplasty is in general favorable, certain problems and complications have developed. Swanson maintained that since the first metatarsal head was not involved in the placing of the hemi-implant, the metatarsal head was still able to transfer flexor power to the great toe and maintain normal propulsion. Force plate analysis has not supported this view. Lack of frontal and transverse plane stability with use of the Swanson hemi-implant has also been described, resulting in hallux varus or valgus in 66 percent of cases in one study.[15] Teich et al. have described the problem of fibrocartilage articulating with the hemi-implant.[15] Reshaping of the head of the first metatarsal may be needed to properly fit a hemi-implant; defects are created that stimulate fibrocartilage proliferation replacing the articular cartilage. Initially the fibrocartilage may be suitable for articulation with the implant, but with time the fibrocartilage deteriorates, and bony irregularities occur in the implant contact area. Recurrence of the deformity has also been observed when the Swanson hemi-implant was used in patients with hallux valgus and rheumatoid arthritis.[7] However, many patients have benefited from its use.

Recently Dow Corning Wright has introduced

Table 44-1. History of Development of Implants for First Metatarsophalangeal Joint Replacement

Author (Ref.)	Year[a]	Material	Design
Swanson[1]	1952	Metallic	Intramedullary stemmed prosthesis for hemispherical cap replacement or metatarsal head
Swanson[1]	1962	Silicone (Dow Corning)	Intramedullary single-stemmed (hemi-) implant (see Fig. 44-1A)
Seeburger[2]	1964	1. Durallium fixated with two vitallium screws 2. Durallium	First metatarsal head replacement Metal cap implant for first metatarsal head (see Fig. 44-1B)
Joplin[3]	1964	Vitallium	1. Single-stemmed prosthesis for base of the proximal phalanx 2. Single-stemmed prosthesis for metatarsal head
Downey[4]	1965	Cobalt chromium alloy	Proposed articulated ball and socket (see Fig. 44-1C)
Kampner[5,6]	1971	Silicone-polyester composite (Cutter Biomedical)	One-piece double-stemmed prosthesis with a hinge design (see Fig. 44-1D)
Swanson et al.[7]	1974	Silicone (Dow Corning)	Double-stemmed flexible hinged toe implant (see Fig. 44-1E)
Weil et al.[8]	1975	Stainless steel metatarsal component, ultra-high molecular weight polyethelene phalangeal component (Richards Medical)	Two-component total design, fixated components using polymethylmethacrylate (see Fig. 44-1F)
Arenson[9]	1977	Silicone, Swanson design—Weil modification (Dow Corning)	Intramedullary single-stemmed (hemi-) implant with 15-degree angulation to accommodate transverse plane alignment of the first metatarsal head (see Fig. 44-1A2)
Johnson and Buck[10]	1981	Stainless steel and polyethelene (DePuy)	Total two-component surface replacement design, fixated with methylmethacrylate
Farnsworth et al.[11]	1983	Silicone LaPorta design (Sutter Biomedical)	Intramedullary double-stemmed hinged total neutral and 15 degree sagittal plane angulation with 10 degree transverse plane angulation (see Fig. 44-1H)
Jarvis et al.[12]	1983	Silicone Lawrence design (Sutter Biomedical)	Intramedullary double-stemmed hinged total; 15 degree sagittal plane angulation. Distal portion of hinge angled (see Fig. 44-1I)
Swanson	1986	Titanium (Dow Corning)	Intramedullary single-stemmed (hemi-) implant (see Fig. 44-1J)

[a]Approximates the year beginning clinical use or is the year of initial publication.

the Swanson design titanium great toe hemi-implant. Because of its combination of strength, light weight, corrosion resistance, and bio-compatibility, titanium is a suitable material for a joint implant.

Dobbs[16] stated that "a diagnosis of active rheumatoid arthritis is a contraindication for any hemi-implant due to the fact that any cartilage that may appear in the joint would act as a nidus for more joint destruction and bony proliferation." It is recommended that the intermetatarsal angle be less than 15 degrees when considering a Swanson hemi-implant. If the intermetatarsal angle is greater than 15 degrees, structural correction by first metatarsal osteotomy may be indicated to reduce this angle. The proximal articular set angle must be within normal limits if considering the

Swanson design hemi-implant but can remain high if the Swanson design/Weil modification hemi-implant is used.

Weil Modification Hemi-implant

Arenson described a "valgus/abductus drift" of the hallux following resectional arthroplasty and use of the Swanson hemi-implant.[9] The tendency of the hallux to drift laterally was seen when the proximal articular set angle was abnormally high. Simply, the implant seeks the least resistant and most congruous position to articulate with the first metatarsal head. This may result in the corrected toe reassuming its preoperative alignment. The collar of this implant is thicker on one side, giving it approximately 15 degrees of angulation. The thicker side of this implant is placed toward the lateral aspect of the first metatarsal, in essence compensating for the proximal articular set angulation. The rest of the Weil design hemi-implant is similar to the standard (Swanson) hemi-implant with two exceptions. A tapered rectangular stem is thought to improve frontal plane rotational stability within the medullary canal, thus preventing hallux varus or valgus. Another modification thought to improve congruency of the implant with the metatarsal head is the smaller radius of curvature of the collar. With a smaller radius of curvature the area the first metatarsal head has to articulate with the implant is less, possibly making the articulation more stable. Whether this is accomplished is speculative.

Swanson Total Hinged Implant

Seven years after the introduction of the hemi-implant a total prosthesis for the first metatarsophalangeal joint was introduced, the Swanson Silastic hinge toe. It is described as a double-stemmed silicone prosthesis with a central U-shaped hinge. Swanson found the best use for his total hinged implant in rheumatoid arthritic feet and in cases of severe arthritic hallux abducto-valgus in elderly patients.[7] In both these conditions maintenance of a normal hallux valgus angle with the Swanson total hinged implant is paramount to predicting its usefulness in these disease states.

Late maintenance of hallux valgus correction was the subject of a study conducted by Swanson in which he compared the ability of the Swanson

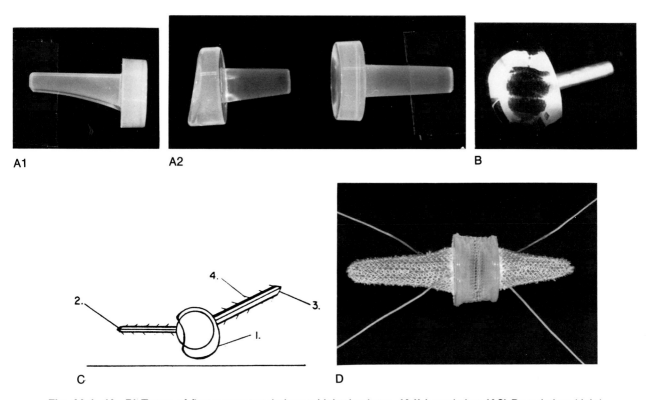

Fig. 44-1. (A–D) Types of first metatarsophalangeal joint implants. **(A1)** lateral view **(A2)** Dorsal view (right) Swanson design silicone single-stemmed hemi-implant and **(A2** left) Weil modification hemi-implant *(right)*. (Dow Corning Wright, Arlington, TN.) **(B)** Durallium first metatarsal head cap. (Austenel Company, New York, NY.) **(C)** Downey articulated ball and socket. *1*, Plantar surface is thicker as a weight-bearing surface; *2*, shaft for proximal phalanx; *3*, shaft for metatarsal; *4*, reverse barbs. (From Downey, with permission.) **(D)** Cutter Biomedical total hinged implant. (Cutter Biomedical, San Diego, CA) *(Figure continues.)*

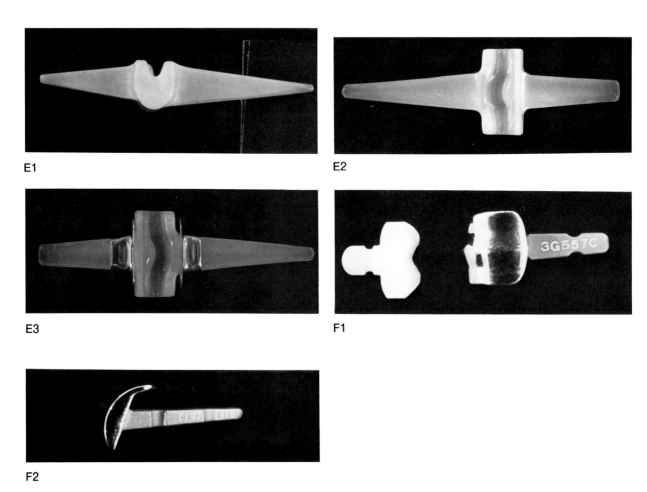

E1

E2

E3

F1

F2

Fig. 44-1. (E–F) *(continued)* Types of first metatarsophalangeal joint implants. **(E)** Swanson design silicone double-stemmed, hinged toe implant. (Dow Corning Wright, Arlington, TN) *Left,* **(E1)** side view; **(E2)** dorsal view; **(E3)** dorsal view with titanium gromets. **(F)** Richards total hinged implant. (Richards Medical Co., Memphis, TN.) **(F1)** Dorsal view; **(F2)** side view of metatarsal component.

hemi-implant and total hinged implant to maintain a normal hallux valgus angle in patients with hallux abductovalgus and rheumatoid arthritis.[7] Swanson's results are shown in Tables 44-3 and 44-4. As Table 44-3 for the standard hemi-implant indicates, in patients with hallux valgus recurrence of the valgus deformity was not a significant problem. However, in the 4- to 30-month follow-up study of 25 rheumatoid arthritic feet the hallux valgus angle showed an average increase of 7 degrees. This, Swanson noted, was evidence of the progressive nature of rheumatoid arthritis, and he believed the total hinged implant was indicated in these cases. Table 44-4 shows postoperative follow-ups, aver-

aging 30 months, of total hinged Silastic implant arthroplasty in 94 rheumatoid and 7 nonrheumatoid feet with severe hallux abductovalgus deformity. There was little or no significant change in the hallux valgus angle postoperatively when using the total hinged implant in either population.

Further results from Swanson's study dealing with postoperative range of motion of single- and double-stemmed implant arthroplasties of the first metatarsophalangeal joint revealed the following information. With the single-stemmed implants, an average 9 degrees of plantar flexion was measured; average dorsiflexion was 50 degrees. Average dorsiflexion with the double-stemmed implant was 42

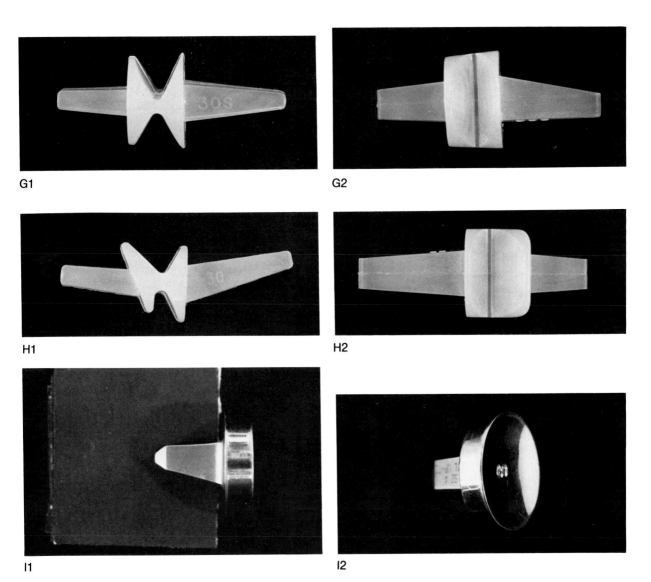

Fig. 44-1. (G–I) *(continued)* Types of first metatarsophalangeal joint implants. **(G)** LaPorta design total hinged implant. (Sutter Biomedical, Inc., San Diego, CA.) *Left,* **(G1)** side view; *right,* **(G2)** top view. **(H)** Lawrence design total hinged implant. (Sutter Biomedical, Inc., San Diego, CA.) *Left,* **(H1)** side view; *right,* **(H2)** dorsal view. **(I)** Swanson design titanium hemi-implant. (Dow Corning Wright, Arlington, TN.) *Left,* **(I1)** side view of mounted implant; *right,* **(I2)** view of articulation surface.

degrees and plantar flexion 10 degrees. Although credited with being able to maintain good correction of the hallux valgus angle, the flexibility and hence range of motion attainable with the Swanson double-stemmed implant came under investigation. This, along with other observations, culminated in Sutter Biomedical introducing two totally new designs in 1982. The first of these was the Lawrence design, followed by the LaPorta design.

Lawrence and LaPorta Design Total Hinged Implants

In both the Lawrence[12] and LaPorta[11] design implants the hinge is H-shaped, designed to allow 85 and 60 degrees of dorsiflexion, respectively (Fig. 44-2). The dorsiflexion permitted by these two implants occurs in the hinge portion alone, without compression of the implant. This is a significant

Table 44-2. Goals, Indications, Contraindications, and Specific Considerations in Implant Arthroplasty of the First Metatarsophalangeal Joint[13,14]

GOALS

Relief of pain
Allow motion
Correct deformity
Provide stability
Cosmesis

INDICATIONS

Degenerative joint disease
    Osteoarthritis
    Hallux limitus
    Post-traumatic arthrosis
Rheumatoid and other forms of inflammatory arthritis
Hallux valgus and deformity
Hallux varus
Salvage procedure with failed primary procedure
Normal neurovascular status
Functional musculotendinous system
Good bone stock
Cooperative patient with realistic postoperative patient goals

CONTRAINDICATIONS

Infection
Open epiphyses
Peripheral neuropathy
Active patients with unrealistic postoperative goals
Prior joint failure

SPECIFIC CONSIDERATIONS

Hemi-joints
    Degenerative changes should be limited to the base of the
        proximal phalanx
    Mild deformity
    Contraindicated in rheumatoid arthritis
    Titanium implant preferred over silicone implant
Total joints
    Joint destruction with deformity of the metatarsal head as
    well as the phalangeal base
    Chronic course of disease
    Marked or severe deformity
    Rheumatoid arthritis

design change from the Swanson double-stemmed implant, which relies heavily on the viscoelastic properties of the silicone rubber for dorsiflexion. The metatarsal stem of both these implants is angulated 15 degrees in the sagittal plane to correspond to the normal metatarsal declination angle. This permits the implant to function without compromising its available range of motion.[12] Other differences in design of the Sutter total hinged implants include broad collars at the hinge portion to allow

good coverage of the cut bone surfaces at the first metatarsal head and proximal phalanx.

With the Lawrence design the distal aspect of the hinge is angled, recognizing the importance of the flexor component and its insertion into the proximal phalangeal base. This allows for angular resection of the proximal phalanx in hopes of maintaining full flexor strength. Finally, the LaPorta implant offers the surgeon three separate designs relative to the 10-degree stem angulation in the transverse plane. Thus there is a right, left, and neutral LaPorta design total hinged implant.

COMPLICATIONS

Some of the complications particular to the most commonly used first metatarsophalangeal joint implants have been described above, and others are illustrated in Figure 44-3. Vanore et al.[17] in 1984 published the results of random retrospective and prospective studies of radiographs, histology, removed implants, clinical photographs, and patient records in which they developed a classification scheme for complications of implant arthroplasty (Table 44-5). Of particular interest is the common complaint of metatarsalgia often reported among patients with implant arthroplasty of the first metatarsophalangeal joint. Because of the decreased weight-bearing function of the hallux and first metatarsal seen in implant arthroplasty, the lateral metatarsals are observed to bear the remaining weight, resulting in metatarsalgia. Mondul et al. noted a difference in the occurrence of metatarsalgia when using hemi- versus total hinged implants, reporting metatarsalgia in 11.3 percent of cases with use of the hemi-implant and in 31.2 percent of cases with use of the total hinged implant.[18]

Biomechanical Complications

In evaluating Silastic arthroplasty of the hallux (total hinged prosthesis), Beverly and co-workers found the increase in peak load under metatarsals two and three to be statistically significant and

Table 44-3. Maintenance of Hallux Valgus Angle Correction by Single-Stemmed (Silicone) Implant

	No. of Patients	Hallux Valgus Angle (Degrees)		
		Preoperative	4 Months Postoperative	30 Months Postoperative
Hallux valgus	10	34	17	18
Rheumatoid arthritis	25	42	18	25

(Data from Swanson et al.[7] with permission.)

quantified it as an increase of 65 percent.[19] Additionally, peak load transmitted by the great toe was reduced by 46 percent. This also resulted in a rise in the peak heel loading, making the foot a less efficient shock absorber. In a similar study on the effects of Silastic arthroplasty on weightbearing using footprints, Arenson and Proner compared weightbearing of the hallux when in quiet stance, active plantar flexion, and ankle equinus.[20] Patients in this study had their first metatarsophalangeal joints replaced with a Swanson total hinged implant. Postoperatively, no weightbearing under the hallux was seen in 100 percent of patients, 62 percent had no weightbearing during active plantar flexion, and 37.5 percent demonstrated no weightbearing with ankle equinus.

Integrity of the first metatarsophalangeal joint may also be crucial during quiet static stance. The term *static stance* refers to a state of bipedal support of body weight during which theoretically all bones of the foot remain motionless.[21] The bipedal support of body weight, also called the base of support, has been defined by Root et al. as that area of ground confined within (1) the lateral margins of both feet, (2) the posterior margins of both feet, and (3) the metatarsophalangeal joints of the feet.[21] It is interesting to note that it is the confines of the ground with the metatarsophalangeal joints and not the metatarsal heads that is a component of the

Table 44-4. Maintenance of Hallux Valgus Angle Correction by Double-Stemmed (Hinged) Implant

	No. of Patients	Hallux Valgus Angle (Degrees)	
		Preoperative	Postoperative[a]
Hallux valgus	7	42	15
Rheumatoid arthritis	94	44	11

(Data from Swanson et al.[7] with permission.)
[a]Average 30 months.

base of support, although it is usually the force under the metatarsal heads that is measured since the force under the joints is difficult to determine. Thus joint stability will become important to having a normal base of support. Furthermore, the first metatarsal head is seen to bear more weight than the lateral metatarsal heads in the normal state,[22] further emphasizing the importance of maintaining a normally functioning first metatarsophalangeal joint.

Studying weight-bearing changes in the rheumatoid foot, Sharma and co-workers determined that in all groups they studied that had rheumatoid arthritis, a reduction in loading under the great toe occurred that was related to the severity of the disease.[23] With increasing metatarsophalangeal joint erosions there was also a significant decrease in loading under the first metatarsal head. It is important to note that this denotes a relative reduction in loading under the hallux and first metatarsal head. Minns and Craxford[22] noted: "The highest pressures under the metatarsal head area in the patient with rheumatoid arthritis are between 2–3 times that of normal subjects." Still, there is a decrease in the loading force under the hallux and metatarsal head because of the much greater increase in loading of the lateral metatarsals. The result of these described changes is the classical type of gait where the foot is used as a platform. Instead of going through the normal heel strike, forefoot loading, and toe-off, the foot is placed on the ground and lifted as a platform without taking the first metatarsophalangeal joint through the range of motion needed for normal toe-off. This antalgic gait pattern is used by the rheumatoid patient to avoid painful pressure points under the metatarsal heads and may become important when considering the use of implants in these patients. Since rheumatoid patients do not take the first metatarsophalangeal joint through the normal range of

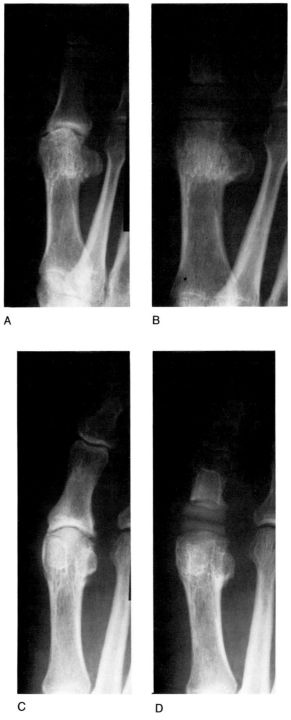

A

B

C

D

Fig. 44-2. Radiographic evaluation of a LaPorta design double-stemmed hinged implant immediately and approximately 18 months postoperatively. **(A)** Obligue view preoperative. **(B)** Obligue view postoperative. **(C)** Dorso-plantarview preoperative. **(D)** Dorsoplantar view postoperative. **(E)** Lateral view preoperative. **(F)** Lateral view postoperative. *(Figure continues.)*

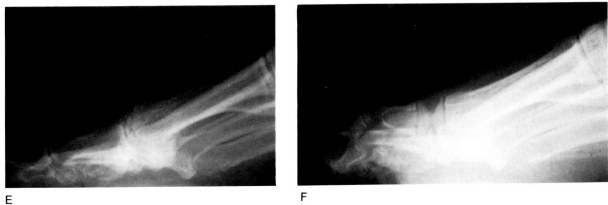

E   F

Fig. 44-2 *(continued).*

motion, Silastic implants placed in these patients experience less cyclic loading with decreased deformation and fatigue, possibly leading to increased success rates in these patients.

The phenomenon of decreased loading of the first metatarsal and hallux in rheumatoid arthritis patients may be particular to that population, and generalizations should not be made. For example,

in reviewing the podiatric and orthopedic literature it is observed the latter tends to stress rheumatoid arthritis whereas the podiatric literature deals more with osteoarthritis. The reason for this is not clear and may be related to the different referral patterns. The difference may become significant when considering first metatarsophalangeal joint Silastic arthroplasty, especially in patients with oc-

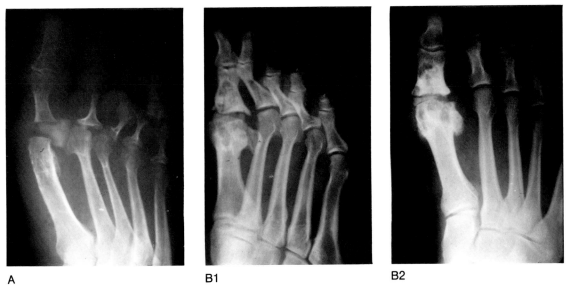

A   B1   B2

Fig. 44-3. Examples of various complications involving implant arthroplasty. **(A)** Displacement of a Swanson design silicone hemi-implant in the immediate postoperative period as a result of insufficient preparation of the implant bed. **(B)** Chondrolysis and bone intolerance secondary to a response to silicone.[77] Note the deformity of the implant. *(Figure continues.)*

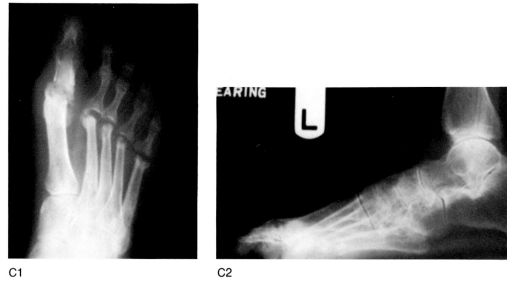

C1   C2

Fig. 44-3 *(continued)*.   **(C)** Dorsal-plantar **(C1)** and lateral **(C2)** views demonstrating several faults: (1) first metatarsal length is excessively long (*left* following pan metatarsal head resection); (2) the implant appears to have been inserted with the metatarsal stem positioned distally **(C1)**; and (3) marked ectopic bone formation (both views). No motion was available at the joint.

cupationally induced osteoarthritis due to excessive loading. In this case, the implant may be required to go through increased loading, possibly increasing the chances of implant failure. Thus when considering implant arthroplasty, it is important to identify the type of patient under consideration. Finally, looking at the foot as a whole, Grundy and co-workers, in studying centers of pressure under the foot while walking, found that the forefoot had what they called a high-force transmitting function when compared to the rearfoot.[24] When quantified, this translated into the fact that the load-bearing function of the forefoot is three times that of the heel. This does not necessarily mean that the forefoot bears more weight, only that it bears it for a longer period of time.

Soft Tissue Complications

Although weightbearing of the first metatarsal is decreased with implant arthroplasty, ground-reactive forces against the implant are enough to cause microfragmentations of the silicone rubber in a number of cases.[25,26] In implant arthroplasty nor-

mal first metatarsal joint motion is altered. With motion in the postoperative condition implant movement, bending, or pistoning occurs. Movement of the implant, the often-referred-to pistoning effect, has recently been described as a necessary action for great toe total joint function in certain implant designs.[27] Abrasive wear of the implant in contact with resected bone surfaces or the endosteal surface contacting the implant results in the formation of particulate silicone. Dow Corning has recently addressed the possible shearing forces that can occur at these bone cut edges by developing thin titanium shields called grommets. Designed for use with the Swanson total hinged implant, they consist of a distal and proximal component to encompass both collars of the implant.

Microfragments or shards of silicone have the ability to initiate certain soft tissue reactions in the host. It seems that the physical form an implanted material takes plays an important role in the type of reaction the host will develop. For example, silicone in particulate form has a greater tendency to trigger an inflammatory response than do pieces in block form.[28]

Table 44-5. Classification of First Metatarsophalangeal Joint Implant Arthroplasty Complications

I. Implant failure
  A. Intrinsic
    1. Deformation
    2. Fatigue fracture
    3. Microfragmentation
  B. Extrinsic
    1. Surgeon modification
    2. Inappropriate usage
II. Alignment abnormalities
  A. Transverse plane instability
    1. Medial subluxation
    2. Lateral subluxation
  B. Sagittal plane instability
    1. Dorsal subluxation
    2. Plantar subluxation
  C. Frontal plane instability — axial malrotation
III. Adjacent bone abnormalities
  A. Aseptic necrosis
    1. Proximal phalanx
    2. First metatarsal head
      a. Cartilage and subchondral bone
      b. Subcortical cancellous bone
  B. Ectopic bone formation
    1. Proximal phalanx
    2. First metatarsal
  C. Bone detritus
  D. Bone cysts
    1. Juxta-articular
    2. Periarticular
  E. Degenerative erosion — bone intolerance to the implant
IV. Soft tissue abnormalities
  A. Reactions to silicone
    1. Reactive synovitis
    2. Foreign body giant cell reaction
    3. Fibrous hyperplasia
  B. Inflammatory reactions extrinsic to silicone
  C. Infection
V. Biomechanical joint failure
  A. Technique error
    1. Excessive metatarsal head resection
    2. Arthrosis of metatarsal-sesamoid complex
    3. Extension and limitation of motion caused by inadequate bone resection
  B. Inherent to joint arthroplasty
    1. Loss of dynamic toe purchase
    2. Metatarsus primus elevatus
    3. Relative decrease of weightbearing function of first metatarsal

(Reprinted with permission of JAPMA)

Local joint reactions to implants have included synovitis and osteitis.[29–33] Lymphadenopathy due to silicone has also been reported.[31] Aptekar et al. believed that, in rheumatoid arthritis patients, inflammation after implantation, or so-called recurrent rheumatoid arthritis, has at least a partial component attributable to silicone.[34] In almost all of the cases reviewed for this chapter an inflammatory reaction was associated with implant failure. Shards or particles of silicone were readily identified in the phagocytic cells, soft tissues, bone, and lymph nodes. Silicone particle size has been demonstrated to be under 1 micron in a patient with a failed great toe prosthesis.[25] Clinical as well as laboratory reports support the role of particulate silicone matter in the development of the inflammatory reaction.[28]

The inflammatory response may be more than just a local foreign body reaction; it may be an immunologically mediated reaction involving both acute and delayed hypersensitivity reactions. Delayed hypersensitivity is a T lymonocyte–mediated immunologic function. Histologic support for this is the marked lymphocytic infiltrate and the demonstration of T cell involvement recognized by electron microscopy in failed implants reported by McCarthy and colleagues.[29]

One of the consequences of prolonged inflammation is calcification. Alterations in local tissue balance may result in dystrophic calcification. One can only speculate at present as to what role this may play in the development of bony overgrowth and ectopic bone formation commonly reported after silicone arthroplasty. Calcification has been reported in soft tissue implants.[35]

It appears that silicone implants may result in the development of immune-mediated complexes and disease in certain patients, and that particulate silicone debris is a consistent associated finding. At present there appears to be no method of identifying the at-risk patients in advance. The practice of reimplantation or exchange of implants should be given careful consideration in patients with implant failure, especially in those with evidence of inflammatory responses of any degree.

Once heralded as the most inert biomaterial implantable, silicone elastomer must be looked at more closely to determine the end result of its interaction with surrounding tissue. Presently, pyrolytic carbon as a biomaterial for first metatarsophalangeal joint implant arthroplasty is under investigation.[36] Pyrolytic carbon's excellent biocompatibility, modulus of elasticity, and ability to withstand cyclical loading show promise, and further studies are being conducted.

Assessment of Complication Incidence

When reviewing the literature on postoperative complications of implant arthroplasty, conclusions must be drawn with caution in light of the publication facts available. With regard to complication rates the literature presents wide variances in patient population, age, volume of procedures, and time of follow-up. Ranges observed are: 10 to 419 for patient population, 15 to 88 years for patient age, 10 to 536 for volume of implant procedures, and 3 months to 12 years for follow-up time. These large variances result in complication rates being reported as unusually high or low depending on the variation in these factors. The discrepancy that exists with complication rates is furthered by the percentage rate of actual types of complications reported. For example, metatarsalgia is reported to occur in as high as 37 percent of cases[8] and as low as 0 percent of cases,[37] and bone encroachment has been reported as occurring as often as 100 percent[38] and as little as 0 percent[39] of the time. This disparity in complication rates makes it difficult for the surgeon to assess the true value of implant arthroplasty on an individual basis. Implant removal and subsequent revision sometimes becomes the only alternative to a failed implant procedure, and removal rates have been reported by Ganley et al. to range from 12 to 36 percent.[40]

ALTERNATIVES TO IMPLANT ARTHROPLASTY

Keller Procedure and Its Modifications

Although originally performed by Davies-Colley in 1887, William L. Keller described a resectional arthroplasty in 1904 commonly known as the Keller procedure.[41] The Keller procedure has been touted as the most universally performed procedure for the correction of hallux abductovalgus deformities.[42] A joint-destructive procedure, the technique involves removal of the base of the prox-

imal phalanx, creating a void between the proximal phalanx and the first metatarsal head. Today the Keller procedure is reserved for patients who show advanced arthritic and degenerative changes of the first metatarsophalangeal joint secondary to hallux abductovalgus deformities, osteoarthritis, and rheumatoid arthritis. The popularity of the Keller procedure is attributed to its technical simplicity, few postoperative complications, and ability to relieve pain. Complications with the Keller procedure are well documented and include metatarsalgia, stress fracture of adjacent metatarsals, loss of toe purchase, recurrence of deformity, and shortening of the hallux. Metatarsalgia and subsequent lesser metatarsal stress fracture are directly related to the inability of the hallux to actively participate in weightbearing postoperatively. In one study, less hallux function was seen when more than one-third of the proximal phalanx had been excised, suggesting decreased weight-bearing function of the hallux.[43]

Designed to prevent the traditional complications of the Keller procedure, the Silastic hemi-implant is now known to have its own set of complications in addition to possessing the typical Keller complications of metatarsalgia, stress fracture, loss of toe purchase, and recurrence of deformity. Stokes, et al. found no statistical difference in the loading of the forefoot in walking when comparing the results of patients with hallux abductovalgus treated with the Keller operation alone and with the Keller operation with Silastic interposition.[44] When used in patients with hallux rigidus, the Swanson design hemi-implant was observed to have more normal foot function and carry near-normal loads.

Attempts to improve the Keller procedure must address the consequences following removal of the base of the proximal phalanx.

Modifications of the Keller procedure dealing with soft tissue interposition usually relate to how the capsule and related structure are handled following resection of the base of the proximal phalanx. Kelikian described a U-shaped flap consisting of the medial joint capsule and the tendon of the abductor hallucis.[45] The flap is split along its length into a dorsal and plantar slip. The plantar slip contains the abductor hallucis tendon and is sutured to the severed end of the flexor hallucis brevis and to the detached common adductor tendon on the lateral side of the joint. This technique covers the head of the first metatarsal, causing a separation between it and the proximal phalanx. For added stability the dorsal slip is sutured to the periosteum in the medial aspect of the remainder of the proximal phalanx. Soren advocated capsular interposition with attachment to the common adductor tendon on the lateral side of the joint.[46] If the medial capsular structure is sufficiently thick it is split lengthwise into a medial and lateral component. The medial component will span the metatarsal head and be attached to the common tendon of the adductor hallucis muscle, while the lateral component will go distally and attach to the remaining portion of the proximal phalanx.

McGlamry et al. have described two modifications to the Keller procedure. The first one deals with the creation of two distal flaps in the joint capsule to be sutured distally around the end of the metatarsal head in hopes of filling the void created by resection of the phalangeal base.[47] In this modification, the distal flaps are created by a T-shaped incision into the joint capsule with the transverse bar of the T usually at the junction of the middle and proximal thirds of the proximal phalanx. The stem of the T-shaped incision begins proximally over the dorsal aspect of the metatarsal neck. Following Z-plasty of the extensor hallucis longus tendon, the tendon must be sutured down to the metatarsal neck to prevent function while fibrous tissue is laid down in the void. According to McGlamry et al., at the time this modification was published it had been found satisfactory in 600 Keller procedures.

An increase in the strength of the hallux was reported by McGlamry et al. in a second modification.[48] Two drill holes placed medially in the remaining proximal phalanx are used to approximate the medial capsular structures with nonabsorbable sutures. A third drill hole is placed plantarly in the proximal phalanx for reattachment of the flexor hallucis brevis tendon.

Hourglassing of the joint capsule has been described by Kaplan and Kaplan and consists of puckering of the joint capsule between the cut end of the proximal phalanx and metatarsal head by nonabsorbable sutures.[42] They reported that fibrous connective tissue reinforced the hourglass configu-

ration, cradling the stump of the proximal phalanx and preventing shortening of the hallux. Simple distraction of the hallux through intramedullary wiring or external stapling has been advocated by Thomas on the grounds that soft tissue healing is hastened by the maintenance of the full length of the hallux, improving end results.[49] In contrast, Sherman et al. noted a marked reduction in passive movement of the interphalangeal joint, with radiographic evidence of degeneration, in those patients treated with a wire.[50] They concluded that there was no advantage in using intramedullary wires following the Keller procedure and identified possible disadvantages.

Fuson believed that proper function is restored if a tenodesis of the flexor hallucis longus tendon with the proximal phalanx is done following the Keller procedure.[51] Two drill holes placed at 5 o'clock and at 7 o'clock in the plantar aspect of the proximal phalanx are used to suture the tendon to the phalanx. Ganley et al. harvested a 3-cm segment of the extensor hallucis brevis tendon and transplanted it to bridge the joint medially, adding stability to the medial repair.[40]

A technique attributed to Le Lievre as reported by Steinbock and Moser includes a capsular revision that attempts to reduce the intermetatarsal angle by repositioning of the sesamoid and the adductor hallucis.[52] The technique is referred to as "circlage fibreux."

Suturing of the intrasesamoidal ligament into the capsular tissue repair and or tenodesis of this ligament to the flexor hallucis longus have also been advocated.[53] The so-called silver dollar Keller, so named because of the thickness of bone resected, has also been described. Poor results were generally encountered as a result of recurrent joint pain.[51] Regnauld described an autogenous graft formed from the resected base of the proximal phalanx and reinserted as a method of improving function postoperatively[54,55] (Fig. 44-4). This procedure is recommended by Regnauld for use in patients with hallux valgus only.

Arthrodesis

Often considered a salvage procedure for degenerative and arthritic joints, arthrodesis of the first metatarsophalangeal joint has consistently yielded

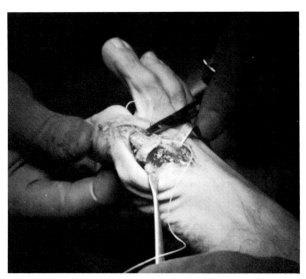

Fig. 44-4. Autogenous bone graft fashioned from the base of the proximal phalanx as described by Regnauld.[54]

good results (Table 44-6). The literature contains numerous reports of surgeons advocating arthrodesis not as a last resort, but as a dependable method of treatment in hallux abductovalgus, hallux rigidus, and rheumatoid arthritis.[56-72] Kelikian cautioned against being too concerned about the motion present in the first metatarsophalangeal joint while forgetting the importance of stability and ability of the joint to bear weight.[45] Henry and Waugh reviewed 170 operations for hallux abductovalgus, consisting of 85 arthrodeses of the first metatarsophalangeal joint and 85 Keller's operations.[43] Footprints were used to assess the pattern of weightbearing of the hallux. After arthrodesis, the hallux bore weight in 80 percent of cases compared with 40 percent after Keller's operation. The researchers concluded that arthrodesis, when correctly performed, is more likely to be followed by weightbearing by the hallux than is Keller's operation.

It is thought by some that the precise operative technique for arthrodesis is not important provided it maintains the position obtained at operation until proper fusion occurs.[56] More important is the angle of fusion between the proximal phalanx and first metatarsal head. McKeever recommended fusion by anticipation of function,[63] but generally the angle of fusion is seen to vary from 15 to 35 degrees in the sagittal plane and 10 to 15 degrees in the transverse plane, depending on how the hallux is positioned with respect to the second toe.

Complications with arthrodesis of the first metatarsophalangeal joint include failure of fusion and malpositioning of the fusion leading to interphalangeal joint arthritis of the hallux. In select patients in whom a Keller-type arthroplasty is indicated, arthrodesis of the first metatarsophalangeal joint may be the superior procedure, providing a strong hallux that will play an active role in weightbearing and ambulation (Fig. 44-5).

Cheilectomy

Cheilectomy in the treatment of hallux rigidus offers the theoretic advantages of preserving the power and motion of the hallux that are lost after resection arthroplasty or arthrodesis while avoiding the potential complications of implant arthroplasty.[73] Originally reported by Nilsonne in 1930,[74] cheilectomy is believed by Hattrap and Johnson to have a definite role in the early management of degenerative joint disease of the first metatarsophalangeal joint. Early on in the pathogenesis of hallux rigidus in the younger patient there is normal joint space, but with a progressive decrease in available dorsiflexion as a result of characteristic chondral and osteochondral lesions observed on the dorsal dome aspect of the first metatarsal head.[75,76] It is important to note that

Table 44-6. Success Rates Reported After First
Metatarsophalangeal Joint Arthrodesis

	Arthrodeses (No. of feet)	Follow-up Time	% Success
Fitzgerald (1969)[56]	100	10 years	91
Riggs and Johnson (1983)[57]	206	15 years	86
Johansson and Barrington (1984)[58]	60	39 months	96
Sussman et al. (1986)[59]	12	17.6 months	92

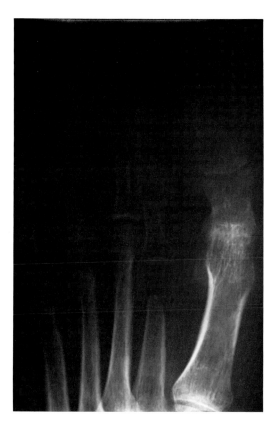

Fig. 44-5. Example of an arthrodesis of the first metatarsophalangeal joint. This patient presented with a painful first metatarsophalangeal joint (MPJ) after a failed primary procedure (chilectomy). The head of the second metatarsal was resected shortly after the primary procedure for a postoperative complication after metatarsal osteotomy performed at the same time as the primary procedure. The patient presented with a painful first MPJ and painful metatarsalgia. Arthrodesis of the first MPJ was performed to retain any weight-bearing function of the hallux. Postoperatively the patient functioned excellently with little foot discomfort.

radiographically these lesions are often missed because they are mainly cartilagenous and later are obscured by secondary degenerative changes. Thus young patients with no radiographic sign of dorsal metatarsal lesions may still derive benefits from a cheilectomy procedure because of the insidiousness of the lesions radiographically (Fig. 44-6).

It is important to create motion in the joint early on through cheilectomy, because with time the limited range of motion results in intra-articular cartilage deterioration with subsequent joint space

Table 44-7. Criteria for Cheilectomy Procedure

1. Young patient
2. Early stage of degenerative joint disease
3. No radiographic sign of significant joint space narrowing
4. Candidate is an active individual (i.e., athlete)
5. Presence of dorsal metatarsal head lesion radiographically

narrowing and subchondral bone eburnation.[75] Unfortunately, however, if allowed to progress to this stage a simple cheilectomy will not alleviate the problem and a joint-destructive procedure may be indicated. To avoid this the authors suggest certain criteria for successful use of cheilectomy in the early management of hallux rigidus (Table 44-7).

Osteotomy in Hallux rigidus

Phalangeal osteotomy for the treatment of hallux rigidus was proposed by Bonney and MacNab[78] in 1952 (Fig. 44-7A). Kessel and Bonney attributed the development of hallux rigidus to metatarsus primus elevatus and demonstrated the usefulness of a dorsiflexory osteotomy of the phalangeal base in those cases in which a plantar-flexory range of motion is preserved.[79] The aim of the operation as described by Citron and Neil is to move the limited arc of movement of the affected joint to a more dorsiflexed position to improve function.[80] They proposed that phalangeal osteotomy was the procedure of choice for hallux rigidus in adolescents with no radiographic evidence of osteoarthritis.

A distal dorsiflexory first metatarsal osteotomy has been attributed to Watermann[81] (Fig. 44-7B). The Watermann osteotomy also relies on a good plantar-flexory range of motion with the presence of viable articular cartilage on the anterior and inferior aspects of the metatarsal head. The Watermann osteotomy is indicated in patients with hallux limitus who are not candidates for joint resection or implant arthroplasty.[82]

The presence of metatarsus primus elevatus can be detected radiographically; however, this may be disputed.[83] Clinically it is evident by an increased dorsiflexory range of motion of the first ray when compared with motion in a plantar-flexory direction. When the first metatarsal head moves a greater distance above than below the plane or

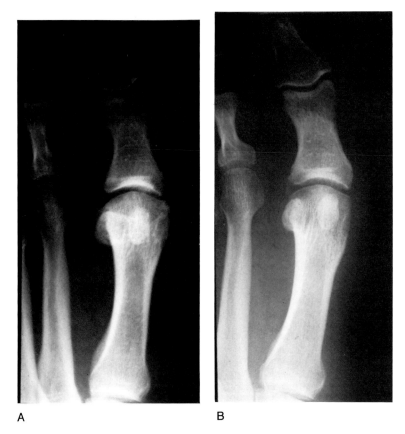

A   B

Fig. 44-6. Pre- **(A and C)** and postoperative **(B and D)** radiographic findings in a patient with degenerative joint disease treated by cheilectomy. *(Figure continues.)*

level of the lesser metatarsals without limitation of motion, the deformity is termed *(congenital) metatarsus primus elevatus.* In acquired deformities limitation of motion occurs with abnormal positioning of the first metatarsal as a result of osseous adaptions or soft tissue restrictions.[84] Metatarsus primus elevatus may also occur after first metatarsal osteotomy for hallux valgus. Treatment of a significant metatarsus primus elevatus is by either distal plantar-flexory osteotomy, such as a modified Austin procedure, or proximal plantar-flexory osteotomy, which may be crestentic, dorsal opening or plantar closing wedge. Drago et al. described a sagittal plane double osteotomy for hallux limitus with a large metatarsus primus elevatus as a primary deforming force[85] (Fig. 44-7C).

CONCLUSION

Implant arthroplasty has its role in the management of disease of the first metatarsophalangeal joint. With proper patient selection this procedure can reduce deformities and relieve pain. However, the implant acts as a joint spacer and should not be expected to provide normal joint function. With this in mind implant arthroplasty becomes a valuable treatment and, with alternative procedures such as the Keller procedure and its modifications, arthrodesis, and cheilectomy, forms an armamentarium for the surgeon to battle painful afflictions of the first metatarsophalangeal joint.

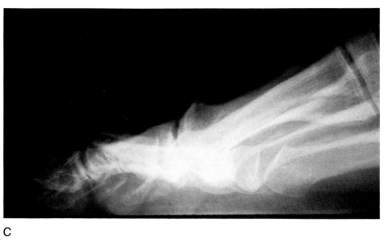

C

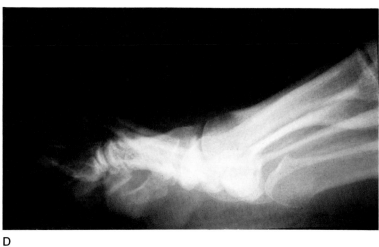

D

Fig. 44-6 *(continued).* **(C, D)**

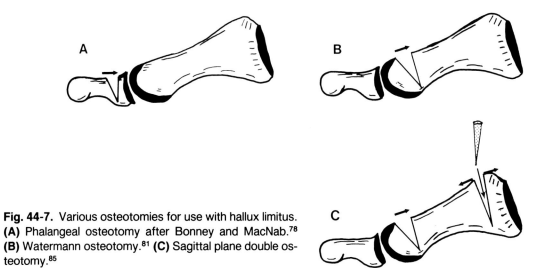

A

B

C

Fig. 44-7. Various osteotomies for use with hallux limitus. **(A)** Phalangeal osteotomy after Bonney and MacNab.[78] **(B)** Watermann osteotomy.[81] **(C)** Sagittal plane double osteotomy.[85]

REFERENCES

1. Swanson AB: Implant arthroplasty for the great toe. Clin Orthop Related Res 85:75, 1972
2. Seeburger RH: Surgical implants of alloyed metal in joints of the feet. J Am Podiatry Assoc 54:391, 1964
3. Joplin RJ: The proper digital nerve, vitallium stem arthroplasty, and some thoughts about foot surgery in general. Clin Orthop Related Res 76:199, 1971
4. Downey MA: A ball and socket metal prosthetic joint replacement as applied to the foot. J Am Podiatry Assoc 55:343, 1965
5. Kampner SL: Total joint replacement in bunion surgery. Orthopedics 1:275, 1978
6. Kampner SL: Total joint prosthetic arthroplasty of the great toe—a 12 year experience. Foot Ankle 4:249, 1984
7. Swanson AB, Lumsden RM, II, Swanson GD: Silicone implant arthroplasty of the great toe. Clin Orthop Related Res 142:30, 1979
8. Weil LS, Pollak RA, Goller WL: Total first joint replacement in hallux valgus and hallux rigidus, long-term results in 484 cases. Clin Podiatry 1:103, 1984
9. Arenson DJ: The angled great toe implant (Swanson design/Weil modification) in the surgical reconstruction of the first metatarsophalangeal joint. Clin Podiatry 1:89, 1984
10. Johnson KA, Buck PG: Total replacement arthroplasty of the first metatarsophalangeal joint. Foot Ankle 1:307, 1981
11. Farnsworth C, Haggard S, Nahmias MC, Dobbs B: The LaPorta great toe implant. J Am Podiatr Med Assoc 76:625, 1986
12. Jarvis BD, Moats DB, Burns A, Gerbert J: Lawrence design first metatarsophalangeal joint prosthesis. J Am Podiatr Med Assoc 76:617, 1986
13. Fenton CF, Gilman RD, Yu GV: Criteria for joint replacement surgery in the foot. J Am Podiatry Assoc 72:535, 1982
14. Swanson AB, Swanson G, deGroot Swanson, and Staff: Treatment Considerations and Resource Materials for Flexible (Silicone) Orthopedic Research Department, Blodgett Memorial Medical Center, Grand Rapids, MI, 1987
15. Teich LJ, Frankel JP, Lipsman S: Silicone hinge replacement arthroplasty. J Am Podiatry Assoc 71:266, 1981
16. Dobbs BM: Hemi-implants in foot surgery. Clin Podiatry 1:79, 1984
17. Vanore J, O'Keefe R, Pikscher I: Silastic implant arthroplasty, complications and their classification. J Am Podiatry Assoc 74:423, 1984
18. Mondul M, Jacobs PM, Caneva RG et al: Implant arthroplasty of the first metatarsophalangeal joint: a 12-year retrospective study. J Foot Surg 24:275, 1985
19. Beverly MC, Horan FT, Hutton WC: Load cell analysis following silastic arthroplasty of the hallux. Int Orthop 9:101, 1985
20. Arenson DJ, Proner SC: A clinical evaluation of the total first metatarsophalangeal joint prosthesis: the use of footprints in assessing foot contact. J Foot Surg 20:117, 1981
21. Root M, Orien W, Weed J: Normal and Abnormal Function of the Foot. p. 56, 357. Clinical Biomechanics Corp, Los Angeles, 1977
22. Minns RJ, Craxford AD: Pressure under the forefoot in rheumatoid arthritis. Clin Orthop Related Res 187:235, 1984
23. Sharma M, Dhanendran M, Corbett M: Changes in load bearing in the rheumatoid foot. Ann Rheum Dis 38:549, 1979
24. Grundy M, Blackburn PA, Tosh RD: An investigation of the centers of pressure under the foot while walking. J Bone Joint Surg [Br] 57:98, 1975
25. Solliton RJ, Shonkweiler W: Silicone shard formation: a product of implant arthroplasty. J Foot Surg 23:363, 1984
26. Lemon RA, Engber WD, McBeath AA: A complication of Silastic hemi arthropathy in bunion surgery. Foot Ankle 4:262, 1984
27. Lauf E, McLaughlin B, McLaughlin E: Swanson great toe flexible hinge endoprosthesis. J Am Podiatr Med Assoc 75:393, 1985
28. Worsing RA, Engber WD, Lange TA: Reactive synovitis from particulate silastic. J Bone Joint Surg [Am] 64:581, 1982
29. McCarthy DJ, Kershisnik W, O'Donnell E: The histopathology of silicone elastomer implant failure in podiatric surgery. J Am Podiatr Med Assoc 76:247, 1986
30. Shiel WC, Jason M: After bilateral metatarsophalangeal joint silicone arthroplasty. Foot Ankle 6:216, 1986
31. Jasim KA, Weerasingne BD: Silicone lymphadenopathy, synovitis and osteitis complicating big toe silastic prostheses. J R Coll Surg Edinburgh 32:29, 1987
32. Bass SJ, Gastwirth CM, Green R et al: Phagocytosis of Silastic material following silastic great toe implant. J Foot Surg 17:70, 1978
33. Weinstock RE, Bass SJ, Wolfson AF, Sorkin BA: Osseous engulfment of a silicone prosthesis with for-

eign body reaction. J Am Podiatry Assoc 72:80, 1984

34. Aptekar RG, Davie JM, Cattell HS: Foreign body reaction to silicone rubber. Clin Orthop Related Res 98:231, 1974

35. Redfern AB, Ryan JJ, Su CT: Calcification of the fibrous capsule about mammary implants. Plast Reconstr Surg 59:249, 1977

36. Hetherington VJ, Kavros SJ, Conway F et al: Pyrolytic carbon as a joint replacement in the foot: a preliminary report. J Foot Surg 21:160, 1982

37. Sethu A, D'Netto DC, Ramakrishna B: Swanson's Silastic implants in great toes. J Bone Joint Surg [Br] 62:83, 1980

38. Gundmundsson G, Robertsson K: Silastic arthroplasty of the first metatarsophalangeal joint. Acta Orthop Scand 51:575, 1980

39. Kravette MA, Baker GI: The Swanson arthroplasty of the great toe: a prospective study. J Foot Surg 17:155, 1978

40. Ganley JV, Lynch FR, Darrigan RD: Keller bunionectomy with fascia and tendon graft. J Am Podiatr Med Assoc 76:602, 1986

41. Keller WJ: Surgical treatment of bunions and hallux valgus. NY Med J 80:741, 1904

42. Kaplan EF, Kaplan GS: The Keller procedure. J Am Podiatry Assoc 64:603, 1974

43. Henry APJ, Waugh W: The use of footprints in assessing the results of operations for hallux valgus. J Bone Joint Surg [Br] 57:478, 1975

44. Stokes IAF, Hutton WC, Stott JRR, Lowe LW: Forces under the hallux valgus foot before and after surgery. Clin Orthop Related Res 142:64, 1979

45. Kelikian H: Hallux Valgus, Allied Deformities of the Forefoot and Metatarsalgia. p. 211, 236. WB Saunders Co, Philadelphia, 1965

46. Soren A: Surgical correction of hallux valgus. Arch Orthop Trauma Surg 96:53, 1980

47. McGlamry ED, Kitting RW, Butlin WE: Keller bunionectomy and hallux valgus correction: an appraisal and current modifications 66 years later. J Am Podiatry Assoc 60:161, 1970

48. McGlamry ED, Kitting RW, Butlin WE: Keller bunionectomy and hallux valgus corrections, further modifications. J Am Podiatry Assoc 63:6, 1973

49. Thomas FB: Keller's arthroplasty modified. J Bone Joint Surg [Br] 44:356, 1962

50. Sherman KP, Douglas DL, Benson MKDA: Keller's arthroplasty: is distraction useful? J Bone Joint Surg [Br] 66:765, 1984

51. Fuson SM: Modification of the Keller operation for increased functional capacity. J Foot Surg 21:292, 1982

52. Steinbock G, Moser M: Die cerclage fibreux als zu-

satzliche mabssnahme dei der operation des hallux valgus. Orthop Praxis 17:840, 1981

53. McCain LR, Nuzzo JJ: The "intersesamoidal ligament" and its employ in the suturing of the Keller bunionectomy procedure. J Am Podiatry Assoc 59:479, 1969

54. Regnauld B: The Foot. Springer-Verlag, Berlin, 1986

55. Kashuk K: Autogenous implant arthroplasty. Podiatry Tracts 1(2):42, 1988

56. Fitzgerald JAW: A review of long-term results of arthrodesis of the first metatarsophalangeal joint. J Bone Joint Surg [Br] 51:488, 1969

57. Riggs SA, Johnson EW: McKeever arthrodesis for the painful hallux. Foot Ankle 3:248, 1983

58. Johansson JE, Barrington TW: Cone arthrodesis of the first metatarsophalangeal joint. Foot Ankle 4:244, 1984

59. Sussman RE, Russo CL, Marquit H, Giorgino R: Arthrodesis of the first metatarsophalangeal joint. J Am Podiatr Med Assoc 76:631, 1986

60. Fitzgerald FAW, Wilkinson JM: Arthrodesis of the metatarsophalangeal joint of the great toe. Clin Orthop Related Res 157:77, 1981

61. Ginsburg AI: Arthrodesis of the first metatarsophalangeal joint. J Am Podiatry Assoc 69:367, 1979

62. Moynihan FJ: Arthrodesis of the metatarsophalangeal joint of the great toe. J Bone Joint Surg [Br] 49:544, 1967

63. McKeever DC: Arthrodesis of the first metatarsophalangeal joint for HV, HR and Metatarsal prima varus. J Bone Joint Surg [Am] 34:129, 1952

64. Lipscomb PR: Arthrodesis of the first MPJ for severe bunions plus HR. Clin Orthop Related Res 142:48, 1979

65. Von Salis-Soglio G, Thomas W: Arthrodesis of the MPJ of the great toe. Arch Orthop Trauma Surg 95:7, 1979

66. Mann RA, Thompson FM: Arthrodesis of the first metatarsophalangeal joint for HV in RA. J Bone Joint Surg [Am] 66:687, 1984

67. Beauchamp CG, Kirby T, Rudge SR et al: Fusion of the first metatarsophalangeal joint in forefoot arthroplasty. Clin Orthop Related Res 190:249, 1984

68. Harrison MHM, Harvey FJ: Arthrodesis of the first metatarsophalangeal joint for hallux valgus and rigidus. J Bone Joint Surg [Am] 45:471, 1963

69. Von Salis-Soglio GF, Gebler-Rothlaenaer B: Die arthrodese des grosszehengrundgelenkes. Arch Orthop 124:288, 1986

70. Marin GA: Arthrodesis of the first MPJ for HV and HR. Guys Hosp Rep 1709:175, 1960

71. Marin GA: Arthrodesis of the MPJ of the big toe for

hallux valgus and hallux rigidus. Int Surg 50:175, 1968

72. Lahz JC: MPJ arthrodesis for HV. J Bone Joint Surg [Br] 55:220, 1973

73. Hattrap SJ, Johnson KA: Subjective results of hallux rigidus following treatment and cheilectomy. Clin Orthop Related Res 228:182, 1988

74. Nilsonne H: Hallux rigidus and its treatment. Acta Orthop Scand 1:295, 1930

75. Gould N: Hallux rigidus: cheilectomy or implant. Foot Ankle 1:315, 1981

76. McMaster MJ: The pathogenesis of hallux rigidus. J Bone Joint Surg [Br] 60:82, 1978

77. Gold RH, Cracchiolo A, Bassett LW: Prosthetic procedures of the joints of the ankle and foot. Semin Roentgenol 21:75, 1986

78. Bonney G, MacNab I: Hallux valgus and hallux rigidus. J Bone Joint Surg [Br] 34:366, 1952

79. Kessel L, Bonney G: Hallux rigidus in the adolescent. J Bone Joint Surg [Br] 40:668, 1958

80. Citron H, Neil M: Dorsal wedge osteotomy of the proximal phalanx for hallux rigidus. J Bone Joint Surg [Br] 69:835, 1987

81. Watermann H: Die arthritis deforman des grosszehengrundege-lenkes als selbstandiges krankheitsbild. Z Chir Orthop Chir 48:346, 1927

82. Cavolo DJ, Cavallaro DC, Arrington LE: The Watermann osteotomy for hallux limitus. J Am Podiatr Assoc 69:52, 1979

83. Meyer JO, Nishon LR, Weiss L, Docs G: Metatarsus primus elevatus and the etiology of hallux rigidus. J Foot Surg 26:237, 1987

84. Root ML, Orien W, Weed JH: Clinical Biomechanics. Vol. II. Normal and Abnormal Function of the Foot. Clinical Biomechanics Corporation, Los Angeles, 1977

85. Drago JJ, Oloff L, Jacobs AM: A comprehensive review of hallux limitus. J Foot Surg 23:213, 1984

Surgical Complications

45

Eric Lauf, D.P.M.

The realm of surgical complications in foot surgery would probably be better suited for a small encyclopedia, cross-referencing all the various interactions and the like, than it is for a chapter in a textbook. Before one can begin to conceptualize the nature of iatrogenic complications, a full understanding of the normal anatomy, structure, biomechanics, and pathomechanics must be understood. Without this knowledge, one cannot hope to understand the mechanisms behind the multitude of problems that can occur during foot surgery, much less conceptualize and implement a plan to correct them. It is the truly wise and talented surgeon who understands the normal structure and interaction of the various body parts, and is best equipped to re-create a properly functioning foot with adequate motion, a smooth and complete weight-bearing surface, and a lever system that is both propulsive and accommodative. The personal rewards of being able to reconstitute a functional foot following iatrogenic complications is almost unparalleled in that it is these patients who require accurate treatment the most, and who most often are, for good reason, least trusting.

The foot and all of its structures are cohesively and completely bound by the skin. The skin encases the foot, and it also provides many functions for the foot, and therefore its interoperative preservation is crucial. While quite important, the skin is very often taken for granted and mishandled intraoperatively. It provides a barrier from desiccation and a protection for the foot against the abnormal stresses of pressure, radiation, trauma, and, of greatest importance to the surgeon, infection. Therefore, proper tissue handling and hydration intraoperatively, as well as skin closure without tension, are essential. Skin closure under tension combined with normal postoperative edema potentiates breakdown, therefore allowing a portal for bacteria to enter the surgically clean area (Fig. 45-1).

Muscles and tendons affect the foot during locomotion and stance as well. They serve three primary functions: stabilization, acceleration, and deceleration. The major muscle function within the foot, however, is to provide joint stability during locomotion. Some of the factors that affect a muscle's ability to contribute to stability and locomotion include its strength, length, phasic activity, mechanical efficiency, and synergistic or antagonistic function. Any surgical procedures that alter a muscle's ability to provide this function will also secondarily affect the function of the foot. These include tendon transfers, transpositioning, and lengthening. Additionally, traumatic episodes such as tendon lacerations that go undetected also affect both propulsion and stability (Fig. 45-2). A thorough knowledge of muscle function is necessary

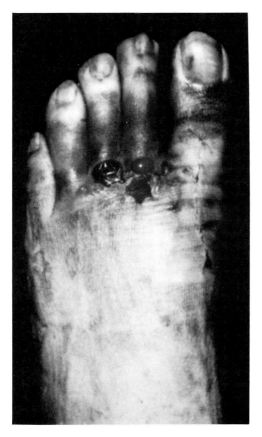

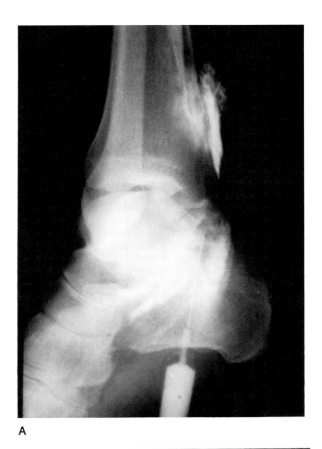

A

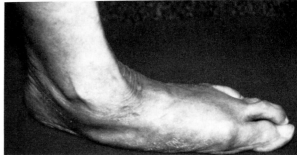

B

Fig. 45-1. Surgical foot 4 days following first metatarso-phalangeal joint implant arthroplasty. Dorsal vesicles and erythema secondary to tight surgical dressings and Beta-dine burn. This increases postoperative pain and likelihood of infection with potentially devastating effects following recent endoprosthesis. The foot was subsequently cleansed thoroughly with saline, the vesicles drained and cultured, prophylactic antibiotics prescribed, and a less constricting dressing applied.

Fig. 45-2. (A) Tenosynoviogram of a 6-month-old posterior tibial tendon laceration. Note the filling defect demonstrated into the posterior tibial tendon sheath. Primary closure of the skin laceration at an emergency room without performing manual muscle testing failed to isolate and repair the injury. **(B)** Instability and weakness with complete collapse of the medial longitudinal arch resulted in additional evaluation and surgery with secondary repair of the tendon laceration, including a free tendon graft from the extensor digitorum longus tendon to the fifth toe, which was restored to function. Primary tendon repair could have been performed had proper examination, which would have elicited the tendon laceration, been done immediately following the initial injury.

when considering surgical alteration of this function, if any hope of achieving a better functional result is to be maintained. Additionally, manual muscle testing should routinely be performed during all physical examinations.

THE VASCULAR TREE

Understanding the vascular tree, including the arterial and venous supply, is paramount to the success of any distal surgical procedure. Failure to evaluate the arterial circulation of the lower extremity, including palpation of the dorsalis pedis, posterior tibial, and popliteal arteries and an assessment of their patency, can doom even a perfectly performed surgical procedure to ischemic changes, which may be irreparable. Patent pedal pulses are a prerequisite to any surgical procedure, and in the moderately obese person, in whom these pulses are not palpable, or the patient with calcified arterial walls, Doppler arterial indexes are mandatory. While a podiatric surgeon cannot be expected to have the expertise of a vascular specialist, a Doppler arterial study may be easily performed and results interpreted. Suffice it to say that a Doppler arterial index of less than 1 should lead to the deferment of an elective procedure with further evaluation by a vascular specialist. Evaluation of the venous system is of equal importance.

Lower extremity surgery, especially that which includes the use of a pneumatic tourniquet in the presence of venous insufficiency, phlebitis, or varicose veins, potentiates thrombophlebitis, pulmonary embolism, and even death. While the mere presence of these systemic conditions does not preclude the performance of surgical procedures, they may necessitate prophylactic antiplatelet therapy or other procedures to minimize the postoperative risk. Unilateral postoperative edema with pain and swelling isolated to the region of the calf is most commonly indicative of phlebitis rather than edema secondary to the surgical procedure. Failure to recognize this may result in thrombophlebitis and/or pulmonary embolism as well, whereas immediate and accurate early detection with follow-up bed rest, warm compresses, and an-

tiplatelet therapy will most often avert a potentially serious surgical complication.

Finally, photoplethysmography, temperature gradients, and the recently developed thermogram may all be utilized to more specifically indicate the variability of the digital circulation following surgical procedures. Most often venous congestion and cyanosis mask normal arterial inflow, simulating ischemia and causing unnecessary great concern. The use of these modalities most often will elicit information that will accurately assess the nature of the digital circulation. Certainly, if any doubt exists, preoperatively or postoperatively, as to the quality of the pedal circulation even after testing, evaluation by a vascular specialist is warranted.

BONE STRUCTURE

The osteology of the foot is very specific, and while the bones and other anatomic structures comprising the foot appear elementary when compared with the surgical procedures themselves, they provide vital surgical references that, when neglected, doom surgical procedures to failure. The foot and its 28 bones are composed of a combination of long bones and flat bones. The tarsus, comprising the majority of flat bones, is biomechanically more stable, therefore helping the body to position itself for either weightbearing or propulsion. The long bones (metatarsals and digits), however, serve as a lever system providing a lattice for forward mobility of the foot. While the diaphysis usually receives the main nutrient artery to the bone, it is the metaphyseal region that contains the vast majority of the vascular supply. Additionally, the diaphysis is principally composed of compact bone, with a smaller surface area, whereas the metaphysis is comprised of a complex trabecular network of cancellous bone. This provides the metaphysis a significantly greater surface area in which an osteotomy may be performed. Additionally, it is this loosely woven nature of cancellous bone, combined with its increased circulation and surface area, that makes it the supreme choice for surgical osteotomies (Fig. 45-3). Deviations from these principles are certain to spell disaster. It is equally important to understand the actual individ-

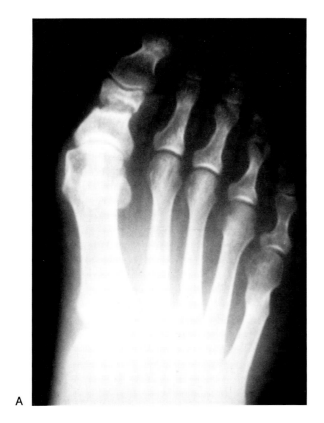

A

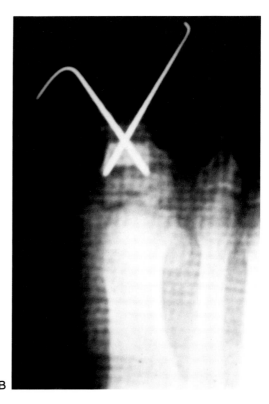

B

Fig. 45-3. The diaphysis of the long bone typically receives the nutrient artery, affording long bones the principal blood supply, yet it is the metaphysis that maintains the more plentiful vascular distribution. This, combined with its more softly woven bone and greater surface area, make it the ideal location for surgical osteotomy placement. **(A)** A midshaft hallux proximal phalangeal osteotomy with inadequate fixation resulted in nonunion. **(B)** Surgical reconstruction involved grafting the base of the proximal phalanx to the distal segment and fixating this graft with obliquely placed Kirschner wires. Additionally, a Dow Corning first metatarsophalangeal joint endoprosthesis was inserted to preserve first metatarsophalangeal joint length, motion, and stability. Initial poor surgical judgment and technique resulted in prolonged disability for this patient.

ual structural characteristics of each bone. The various facets, articular surfaces, and specific anatomic position in which they lie provide significant clues to the surgeon as to the exact structure and, more specifically, the part of the structure that he or she is working on so as to prevent misidentification intraoperatively and the severe consequences that this may potentiate (Fig. 45-4).

The periosteum covers all bones except the areas of hyaline cartilage. It blends with ligaments and tendons at areas of their insertion and consists of two distinct layers, an outer fibrous layer and an inner osteogenic layer. It is this osteogenic layer, the endosteum, that possesses the osteoblasts necessary for bony deposition and growth. It is much more abundant in younger individuals and this is a direct reflection of its increased vascularity and healing potential. It is responsible for fast healing following fractures and surgical osteotomies, and therefore its preservation intraoperatively is paramount. It has been well established that the periosteum receives the majority of its blood supply from the overlying musculature, and therefore surgical dissection should preserve the periosteum in order to promote and expedite postoperative osseous healing.

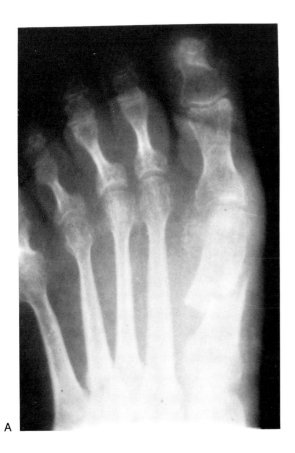

A

Fig. 45-4. An ill-advised midshaft first metatarsal osteotomy resulted in delayed healing, severe shortening of the first metatarsal with its resultant transference of weight to the lesser metatarsals, and severe first metatarsal elevatus with resultant joint jamming. This delayed union increases the likelihood additional surgery with possible grafting, and the metatarsal elevatus certainly dooms this patient to a severe, painful first metatarsophalangeal joint limitation of motion, necessitating additional surgery including repositioning of the first metatarsal shaft and head and possible endoprosthesis.

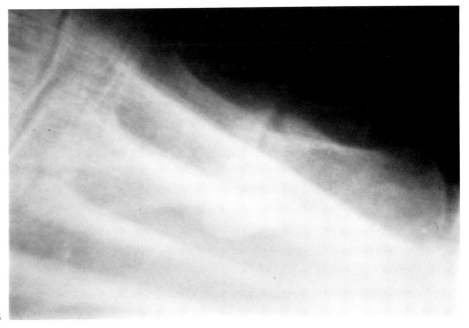

B

BONE PHYSIOLOGY

The homeostasis of the microenvironment maintains the consistency of bone. There are several intrinsic factors that must be equilibrated in order to maintain constancy within bone. These include ion concentration, pH, and a balance between osteocytes, osteoblasts, and osteoclasts. Additionally, the secretion of parathyroid hormone and calcitonin must be balanced. The body maintains several stores within itself and draws upon them as necessary. Bone represents a storage center for calcium, and if serum calcium is depleted the body will draw upon this to fortify itself. The result, however, is a weakening of the bone with other secondary consequences. This translates into delayed osteotomy or fracture healing, bone weakness, pathologic fracture, and the like. Decreased serum calcium results in an increase of parathyroid hormone secretion. This in turn increases osteoclastic activity and increases calcium retention through renal tubular reabsorption.

Increased serum calcium results in secretion of calcitonin. This increases bony deposition of calcium through osteoblasts. Adequate dietary intake and absorption of calcium, phosphorus, and vitamins A, C, and D are also vital for osseous hemostasis. Prolonged dietary deficiency of vitamin D or calcium leads to generalized loss of bone mineral (osteoporosis) with subsequent increased fragility. Vitamin C is essential for the synthesis of collagen and mucopolysaccharides of the bone matrix, and vitamin A is essential for bone growth. A deficiency of these vitamins will result in rickets in children and osteomalacia in the adult.

While these patient factors are seldom explored by the surgeon, except during times of poor bone healing of unknown etiology, an awareness of these factors will certainly help to promote proper healing postoperatively.

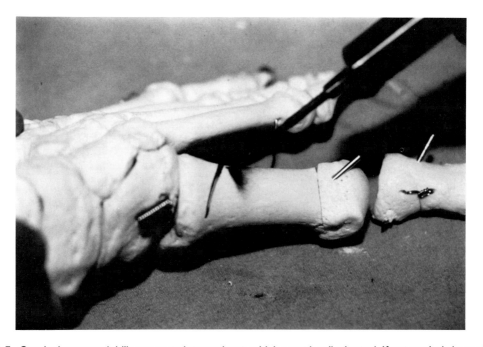

Fig. 45-5. Surgical saws and drills generate intense heat, which must be dissipated. If not cooled via mechanical flushing, this heat is often transferred to the surgical site, resulting in cauterization of bone cells. This increases postoperative inflammation and results in reabsorption of the necrosed bone edges. This in turn potentiates delayed healing of the osteotomy site, pseudoarthrosis, and the like. Mechanical flushing during surgical drilling or osteotomy not only removes bony debris from the surgical site, it cools the site, enhancing the rate of bone healing.

EFFECTS OF POWER INSTRUMENTS ON BONE HEALING

A surgical osteotomy in good alignment and satisfactorily fixated may heal poorly or even demonstrate delayed healing or reabsorption at the osteotomy site with pseudoarthrosis as a result of burning of bone by power instruments. Bone may be cauterized while it is being cut by saws or may be burned by drills and fixation devices such as

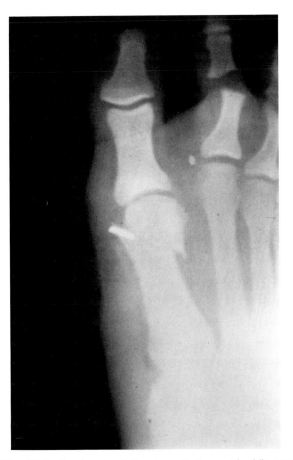

Fig. 45-6. Fractured rotating burr tip incurred while performing metatarsal osteotomy. This occurred as a result of increased metal fatigue secondary to excessive manipulation of the handpiece as well as possible overutilization of the burr without replacement, resulting in metal fatigue. Whatever the cause, the outcome is additional surgery on the patient to retrive the metal fragment.

Kirschner wires. Thermal bone burning results in necrosis, which must be reabsorbed before healing can occur (Fig. 45-5). There are several factors that influence the effect of power instruments on bone healing. These include speed (r.p.m., cycles), temperature, torque, and manipulation. The higher the surgical burr or blade speed the less the inflammatory reaction and the greater the cutting potential or the handpiece. With this increased speed, however, is produced an increase in temperature, which potentiates bone burning. Therefore, continuous mechanical flushing, while serving to remove osseous debris from the surgical field, also cools the bone, thereby decreasing the potential for necrosis.

It is imperative that the temperature of the bone be minimized during osteotomy in order to decrease the potential for thermal necrosis. Osseous cauterization via osteotomy performance may also serve to seal the haversian canals, and with them the microvascularization, thereby delaying bone healing and potentiating delayed union. The increased heat generated in a drill bit at greater speeds also potentiates the fatigue and fracture of the drill bit during usage. Mechanical flushing of the drill bit or saw blade serves to cool the instruments, therefore decreasing the possibility of material failure.

Poor surgical technique, including increased manipulation of the handpiece, enhances the possibility of material failure even more (Fig. 45-6). The slower the speed of a particular handpiece the greater the microfragmentation caused to the bone. This microfragmentation increases debris, thereby enhancing the probability of a foreign body response. Therefore, a surgeon should always employ the maximum speed of a particular handpiece while still maintaining total control of that handpiece in order to increase its cutting potential and minimize microfragmentation of the object being cut. Higher torque, which aids performance of the handpiece, is always preferable. Finally, there is no substitute for good surgical technique, and this axiom is certainly more important than the type of handpiece or fixator used. For example, at higher speeds there is increased bone cutting potential provided to the handpiece. Therefore there is an increased potential for inadvertent wandering and error during osteotomy performance, which

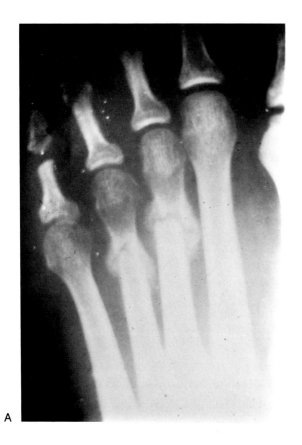

A

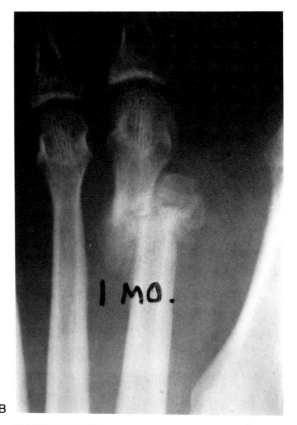

B

Fig. 45-7. (A) Surgical osteotomies to the third and fourth metatarsals placed through the distal metaphysis with no means of fixation, resulting in delayed healing with excessive bone callus and a shortening due to decreased vascularity, excessive movement, and bone necrosis. This translates to increased disability for this patient. Additionally, shortening of the involved metatarsal results in increased weight transferred to the second and fifth metatarsals, potentiating discomfort and deformity to these areas. **(B, C)** Second metatarsal osteotomy without fixation resulting in complete displacement of the surgical site. At 1 month following surgery (B) one can visualize excessive secondary bony formation. Eighteen months following surgery (C) note the lateral shift to the first metatarsal head. Remarkably, however, there is a complete union of the osteotomy site with remodeling of the bone edges, resulting in apparent satisfactory alignment. One should never overlook the body's innate ability to repair itself, although this unique ability should not be counted on as the saviour of surgeons with poor technique.

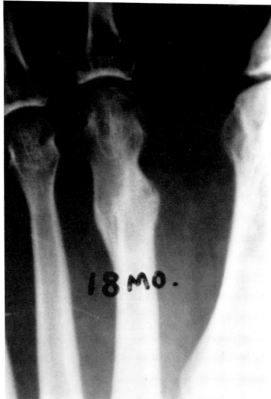

C

should be understood and controlled. Good surgical technique and use of instruments can enhance postoperative results.

BONE FIXATION

Interruption of bone continuity, whether traumatic, intraoperative, or pathologic, is followed by specific reparative processes, all of which delay bone healing and potentiate nonunion or delayed union. Poor fixation or failure to fixate a fracture or osteotomy, can result in subluxation, transfer le-

sion in the case of metatarsal osteotomies, nonunion or delayed union, excessive bone callus, and malalignment (Fig. 45-7), and increases the likelihood of movement at the site. For example, the amount of callus is directly proportional to the relative movement between fracture or osteotomy fragments. Mechanical forces that influence this movement dictate the type of ensuing bone healing. Movement at the bone interface (fracture line) will not occur as long as the static forces (compression) are greater than the dynamic forces (functional load). When the functional load is greater, micromovement will ensue at the contact interface, leading to resorption and loosening. This will convert primary bone healing into secondary healing (Fig. 45-8).

Fracture or osteotomy repair without connective tissue or fibrocartilage formation requires rigid fixation for primary union. The advantages of rigid internal fixation as it concerns bone healing include being able to exactly position an osteotomy or fracture without movement, which provides

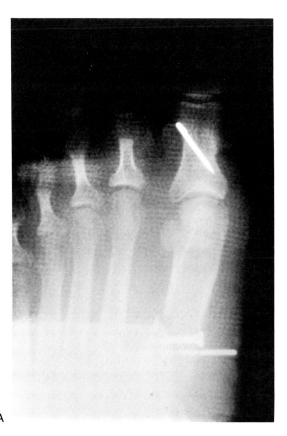

A

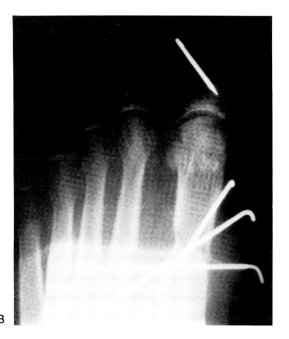

B

Fig. 45-8. (A) First metatarsal base wedge osteotomy, fixated with both cortical bone screw and .062 Kirschner wire, could not withstand the dynamic forces of weightbearing postoperatively, resulting in medial and proximal shifting of the distal segment of the first metatarsal. **(B)** This necessitated additional surgery involving removal of existing hardwear, reconstitution of proper anatomic first metatarsal alignment, and placement of three oblique .062 Kirschner wires.

more accurate anatomic and biomechanical repositioning of the part, thereby yielding more predictable biomechanical results. Additionally, this provides an earlier range of passive motion for physical therapy. Rigid fixation also provides for minimal callus formation, allowing intramedullary callus to bridge bony gaps primarily. External fixators, while providing the same advantages as internal fixators, are more easily removed without additional surgery. They increase the potential for infection, however, via their communication with the outside environment. They also increase the potential for foreign body reactions, and therefore must be completely encased in sterile dressings. Internal fixators require additional surgery for their removal, and the consequences of this must be conceptualized and understood as well. Although the various forms of internal and external fixation potentiate some complications, there is no doubt that the use of these modalities greatly enhances the postoperative benefit and predictability of results.

A surgeon should always physically and intellectually be able to deal with any possible adverse situation before contemplating a surgical procedure. One should be ready to employ an alternative or additional fixator should the first choice not be sufficient or the bone fragment not be capable of supporting it. An inability to adjust for any unforeseen circumstance will in and of itself potentiate iatrogenic complications.

Specific Fixation Modalities and Techniques

Surgical *sutures* are sterile filaments used to approximate and maintain tissues together until healing has endowed the wound with satisfactory strength. In its most basic sense, the mere suturing of a surgical incision provides fixation for the two loose skin edges. This represents perhaps the most age-old and common form of fixation, with the exception of the body's own clotting and splinting mechanisms. A wide and ever-changing variety of suture material exists and a correct selection may make a significant difference in the final result. Absorbable sutures such as silk and cotton elicit the

most tissue reaction because they must be hydrolyzed by the body, thereby potentiating suture rejection and foreign body reaction. Therefore they are seldom used today. Nonabsorbable sutures cause less reactivity. Additionally, synthetic sutures (i.e., polyglycolic acid, dexon, polyglactin, and vicryl) have decreased reactivity as compared to the previously utilized gut-type sutures. Monofilament nylon undergoes significantly minimal hydrolysis and polypropylene is not hydrolyzed at all, thereby making it virtually inert. Stainless steel sutures and fixators are not as inert as some pure synthetic sutures such as Prolene in that they undergo corrosion. Whenever internal metallic sutures are being utilized, this potential must be considered. Finally, characteristics such as tensile strength, elasticity, and knot security must not be overlooked. Stainless steel provides the highest tensile strength and is the strongest of all sutures. Nylon and polypropylene, on the other hand, demonstrate the highest degree of elasticity, making them durable for other reasons. With regard to knots, square knots are strongest and provide the greatest degree of longevity. Knots that are sloppily placed, not tight, or not square potentiate unraveling and thereby enhance the possibility of iatrogenic complications.

While *casts and splints* provide gross immobilization of an extremity, they do not provide complete immobilization of osseous structures. The resulting micromovement of bony fragments potentiates secondary bone healing, thereby delaying the healing process. Additionally, prolonged casting promotes bone demineralization and decreased bone strength (Wolfe's law), thereby supporting the selection of more rigid internal and external fixators to decrease the need for prolonged cast immobilization.

Kirschner wires represent the most widely used type of external fixator in the foot. Although they enhance predictable biomechanical results and are easily removed without additional surgery, they do increase the likelihood of localized infection at the epidermis-pin interface. Antibiotic ointment such as Betadine serves to seal this portal, thereby minimizing inflammation and infection. Kirschner wires may also potentiate necrosis of skin due to the pressure if pins are positioned incorrectly. Finally, if multiple holes are placed within the osseous seg-

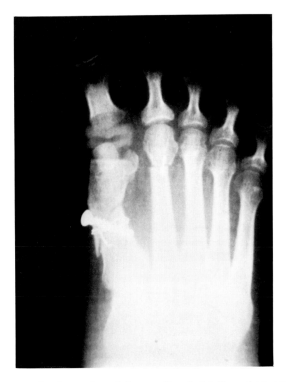

Fig. 45-9. Illustration of the results of violation of several surgical principles. The first metatarsal osteotomy made in the diaphysis potentiated this delayed healing as a result of decreased surface area and vascularity. Additionally, poor judgment in the use of surgical fixators, including the insertion of a cancellous screw and Kirschner wire, resulted in inadequate immobilization that was unable to overcome dynamic forces, resulting in medial and proximal displacement of the first metatarsal osteoeomy. This potentiated first metatarsal elevatus and exuberant bone callus secondary to movement at the osteotomy site, as well as delayed union. Additionally, excessive bone removed from the head of the first metatarsal potentiated transference of weight to lesser metatarsals.

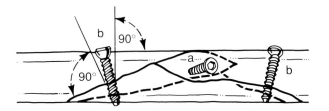

Fig. 45-10. (a) Screw placement 90 degrees to long axis of the bone. (b) Additional screw placement inserted such that they bisect the angles between the perpendicular of the long axis of the bone and the fracture line. This provides rotational stability and increases strength.

ment, the bone may become weakened and unable to support the pin or other method of fixation.

Small fragment fixation, including the use of screws and plates, revolutionized osseous fixation and gave a whole new meaning to the definition of primary bone union. Rigid internal fixation is a prerequisite for specific predictable healing as well as for early postoperative functional rehabilitation. This principle may be applied to fracture care as well as the fixation of surgical osteotomies. However, specific knowledge of AO fixation is essential

for contemplating its usage. The improper use of internal fixators can result in iatrogenic complications far outweighing the failure to fixate a fracture or osteotomy at all (Fig. 45-9). The proper utilization of cortical and cancellous screws where appropriate, as well as the placement of axial or intrafragmentary compression plates, is essential for predictable postoperative results.

When employing bone screws, they must be biomechanically placed in relation to the fracture/osteotomy site in order to provide uniform compression and achieve maximum rigidity. Screws should be inserted in an oblique rather than parallel direction, utilizing at least one screw at right angles to the long axis of the bone. All other screws are inserted so that they bisect the angles between the perpendicular to the long axis of the shaft and the perpendicular to the fracture line (Fig. 45-10). It should also be understood that shear force increases the body weight and with it the stresses placed upon a particular bone. Furthermore, the size of a particular bone or the thickness or site of a particular bone is usually indicative of the stress to that area and is directly proportional. For satisfactory stabilization the number of screw threads in a respective cortex as well as the screw size should increase as the bone size and density increase, with screw threads completely traversing the distal cortex in order to achieve maximal strength. Additionally, although rigid internal fixation enhances earlier passive motion and therapy, it does not necessarily enhance earlier weightbearing, and it is often this principle that, when misunderstood and neglected, potentiates osteotomy subluxation, requiring additional surgery and potentiating delayed healing and increased disability.

STRUCTURAL EQUILIBRIUM OF THE FOOT

The structure and function of the foot is very specific and unforgiving. Deviations from the structural equilibrium and alignment whether congenital or iatrogenically (surgically) induced, are often more deforming and painful than in other areas of the body as a result of the weight-bearing nature of the foot. Combining this with the rigidity of concrete and the confining nature of shoes, it is easy to conceptualize that any structural abnormality would potentially be symptomatic (Fig. 45-11).

The bony architecture of the foot is such that it provides both propulsion and stability. The alignment of the osseous architecture is specific in order to provide the muscles and tendons their maximum advantage. Forces act upon the bones to compress them against each other at the joints. Ligaments

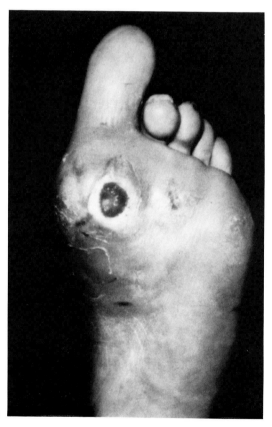
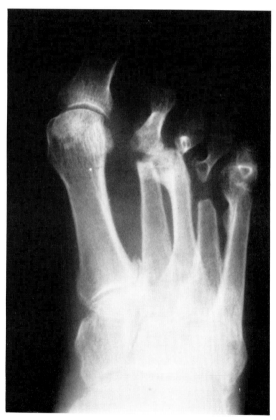

Fig. 45-11. Haphazard and uneven surgical removal of the metatarsal heads in a 51-year-old diabetic patient resulted in excessive weight redistribution to the first metatarsal head. This in turn resulted in a plantar ulceration. Additionally, note the complete lack of understanding and regard for a metatarsal parabola, with complete unevenness in the resection of bone in the lesser metatarsals. Additional surgery was required to remove the first metatarsal head and realign the lesser metatarsal parabola (including the bony bridging between the second digit and third metatarsal), as well as multiple soft tissue lengthenings to create a better functioning foot. The result of such indiscriminate surgery, especially in an insulin-dependent diabetic, could have severe ramifications.

provide tension that resists the tendency for motion to occur at each weight-bearing joint. If the joint does in fact exhibit motion in a direction contrary to its normal plane, hypermobility and instability will occur. If this abnormal hypermobility persists, subluxation with eventual complete dislocation may result.

Weight-bearing stability of the foot bones is particularly dependent upon the osseous restraining mechanism. This mechanism involves the multiarticulated nature of many of the joints, particularly those in the rearfoot. These joints are designed to provide free motion until the end range and then lock, providing stability for the foot during weight-bearing and propulsion. Bones with multiple articular surfaces possessing joints with deeply curved articulations exhibit tendencies toward stronger osseous restraining and a greater tendency for locking in stability than bones with singular, rounder articular surfaces. Therefore the subtalar and midtarsal joints show greater osseous restraining and increased stability, whereas the metatarsophalangeal joints provide more mobility and flexibility.

The metatarsal parabola is smooth and well defined, with the first and fifth metatarsals being the shortest and the second metatarsal achieving the greatest length. Although there is a medial longitudinal arch and a generalized metatarsal declination of approximately 15 to 20 degrees and a slight transverse arch within the metatarsal heads, the general plane of the metatarsal heads from an axial view is smooth and regular, with an even distribution of all the metatarsal heads. The second metatarsal achieves greater length in order to facilitate plantar flexion of the first metatarsal during the propulsive phase of gait. A metatarsus primus adductus angle of between 5 and 8 degrees is normal and expected upon radiographic examination. An increase in this angle does several things. First, it serves to decrease the weight-supporting nature of the first metatarsal head, thereby transferring increased force and pressure to the lesser metatarsals. Additionally, it disturbs the normal stabilizing force of the muscles that attach to the first metatarsal head, thereby leading to hypermobility of the first ray. Hypermobility of the first ray, and in particular first metatarsophalangeal joint elevatus, lends itself to jamming of the first metatarsopha-

langeal joint with secondary first metatarsophalangeal joint stiffness.

Surgical procedures involving the forefoot should be focused on reestablishing the normal metatarsal parabola flexibility, and propulsiveness that ideally should exist. Deviations from this will certainly doom the surgical procedures to failure by adversely increasing stresses to certain parts of the foot while minimizing stresses to others. Surgical extirpation of phalangeal or metatarsal heads without replacement with an endoprosthesis or joint fusion in order to maintain propulsiveness will certainly lead to overpowering of the involved muscle and tendon structures, with secondary contraction and/or dislocation as well as a transference of weight to the additional bones (Fig. 45-12). This transference of weight potentiates fatigue and stress fracture as well as increased stress to the surrounding soft tissues, which can result in hyperkeratosis and pathologic skin lesions.

It has often been said that surgical osteotomy of one metatarsal will lead to a domino effect involving transference of stress to the adjacent metatarsal that necessitates osteotomy of the adjacent metatarsal at some future date. While there is some merit to this opinion, metatarsal osteotomy is often necessary either to relieve pressure from an abnormally declinated or elongated metatarsal, or to compensate for a previous ill-advised surgical procedure. Isolated metatarsal head resections should never be performed with the exception of that of the fifth metatarsal head in a geriatric individual or an individual with poor bone density. Since weight is transferred from the lateral to the medial aspect of the foot during propulsion and weightbearing, often a fifth metatarsal head resection does not result in significantly increased weight to the adjacent fourth metatarsal head. In general, this procedure should be reserved for panmetatarsal head resections in only the most severely arthritic patients who experience extensive metatarsophalangeal joint subluxation, or for cases where no other alternative exists.

Great care must be exercised when performing lesser metatarsal surgery as well. Specific attention to achieving a proper metatarsal parabola should be maintained. Excessive elevation or declination of a metatarsal will certainly lead to abnormally increased stress to adjacent metatarsals, with fur-

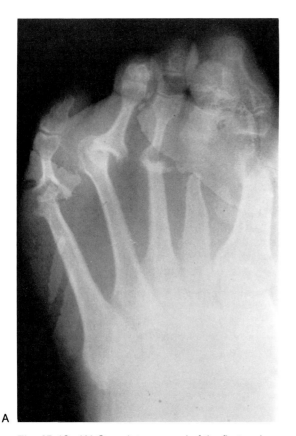 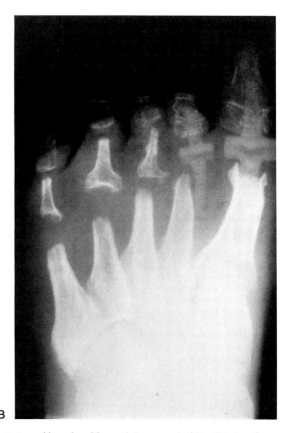

A   B

Fig. 45-12. (A) Complete removal of the first and second metatarsal heads with partial removal of the third and fifth and a completely neglected fourth metatarsal head resulted in excess pressure in the area of the fourth metatarsal with severe pain. Removal of the base of the proximal phalanx of both the first and second toes resulted in additional instability as well. **(B)** Additional surgical revision was necessary to re-create a more normal metatarsal parabola. Insertion of flexible hinge endoprostheses to the first and second metatarsophalangeal joints reconstituted both motion and stability in these areas. Additionally, while the second metatarsal shaft was unable to maintain the proximal stem of the Dow Corning endoprosthesis, the fibrous encapsulation and splinting maintained both length, position, and function, obviating the need for additional surgical replacement.

ther disability being experienced postoperatively. Osteotomies may be placed in the proximal or distal metaphysis but should never be placed within the shaft of the bone. Likewise, rigid internal or external osseous fixation will better ensure more predictive postoperative results.

Lesser digital base resection should almost never be performed regardless of the circumstance. If resected for the correction of a hammertoe deformity, a complete loss of stability is achieved at the metatarsophalangeal joint with an overpowering of the soft tissue structures, thereby actually worsen-

ing the contracture that the base excision was intended to achieve (Fig. 45-13). If excised during the performance of a Hoffman-type procedure, once again stability is compromised. Since the base of the phalange does not possess a weight-bearing component, metatarsal head resection should be the only component necessary besides soft tissue lengthening.

The surgical correction of contracted digits should first involve an accurate assessment of the cause of digital contraction. If the cause of a second digit contraction is severe hallux abductus, then

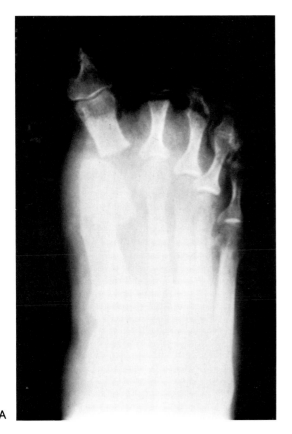 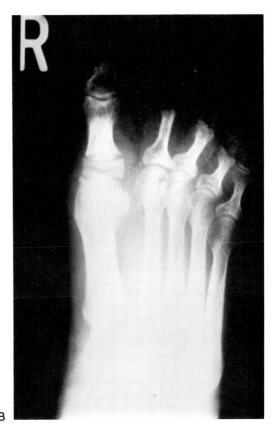

A   B

Fig. 45-13. Surgical removal of the base of the proximal phalanx of the right great toe during the performance of a Keller bunionectomy, without proper closure and postoperative splinting, resulted in instability at the metatarsophalangeal joint and lateral deviation of the phalangeal base into the first metatarsophalangeal joint, with instability and dorsal contracture of the great toe. Additional surgery with insertion of a flexible hinge first metatarsophalangeal joint endoprosthesis created better functional alignment and stability.

the great toe must be realigned before surgically addressing the second toe deformity (Fig. 45-14). If the cause of a fourth toe contracture is an underlying fifth toe, then this deformity must be addressed as well. Once the deformity is addressed, a flexible deformity may be corrected by a variety of tendon-balancing procedures. Rigid deformities that necessitate the removal of a phalangeal head must be followed by either digital fusion or surgical implantation to reconstruct the structural stability of the digit. Failure to achieve this would potentiate continued and possibly worsened digital contraction and/or dislocation with possibilities of deviation extending to the transverse plane as well as the sagittal plane (Fig. 45-15).

Surgical attempts to reduce a bunion deformity must by definition address an increase in the metatarsus primus adductus angle. Failure to reduce this angle will doom the surgical bunion procedure to failure (Fig. 45-16). Reduction of the metatarsus primus adductus angle may be achieved by adductor transfers as well as osseous procedures. The type of osseous procedure selected, if one is indicated, depends on the magnitude of the deformity present, including deviations of the articular surface of the first metatarsal head. Once again, failure to select the appropriate procedures necessary to reduce the metatarsal deviation and redirect the articular cartilage of the head of the first metatarsal will potentiate additional deformity and disability

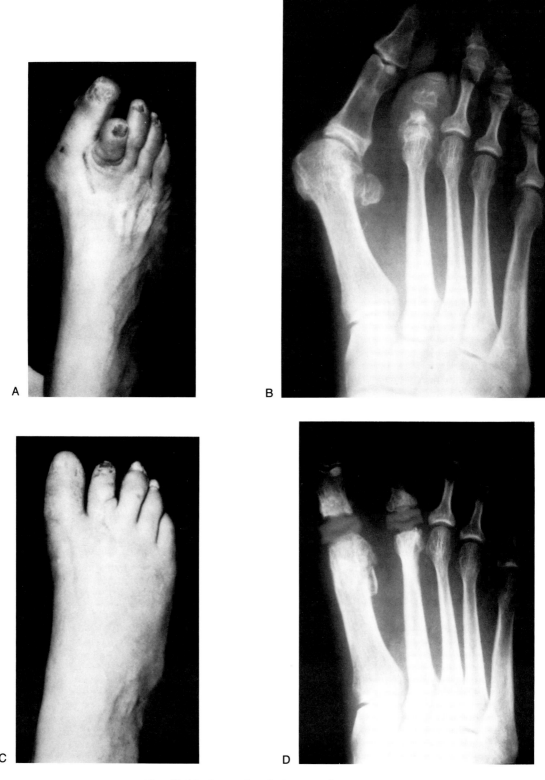

Fig. 45-14. *(Legend on facing page.)*

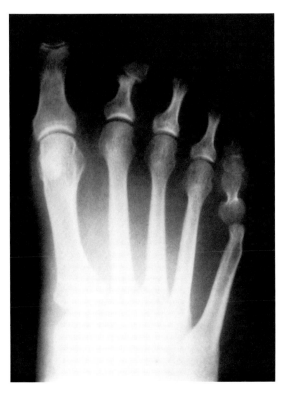

Fig. 45-15. Second toe arthroplasty without fusion or endoprosthesis resulted in abnormal forced, causing malalignment and continued deformity.

gical procedure. Careless resection of excessive bone from the metatarsal head, excision of the fibular sesamoid, and unnecessary adjacent soft tissue lengthenings, including capsule, extensor brevus, and adductor tendon lengthenings, potentiate unwanted deviations of the great toe in adducted, abducted, and hyperextended positions (Fig. 45-17). Only those ancillary procedures necessary to achieve the desired result should be performed intraoperatively. It must be remembered that there is no one procedure that sufficiently addresses all deformities in all circumstances.

Phalangeal osteotomies of the great toe, Akin-type procedures, or interphalangeal joint fusions should be reserved for those instances in which a structural deformity exists to the proximal phalanx. If these procedures are utilized to compensate for deviation in the articular cartilage of the head of the first metatarsal, they will often fail (Fig. 45-18). First metatarsophalangeal joint fusions (McKeever-type procedures) are rarely, if ever, indicated for a first metatarsophalangeal joint reconstruction in the 1980s. While first metatarsophalangeal joint endoprostheses are not without their faults, they provide many advantages, making first metatarsophalangeal joint fusions less desirable (Fig. 45-19).

postoperatively. In addition to addressing the metatarsus primus adductus angle during bunion correction, specific attention should be paid to first metatarsophalangeal joint congruity and motion. Surgical procedures resulting in a rectus and well-aligned first metatarsophalangeal joint must be performed in order to achieve longevity of the sur-

IMPLANTS

Proper functioning of the first ray, including rectus alignment and adequate first metatarsophalangeal joint range of motion, is essential for nor-

Fig. 45-14. (A,B) Surgical correction of a hammered second toe with excessive bone resection in the presence of severe hallux abductus resulted in complete dorsal dislocation of the second toe with severe secondary disability. **(C,D)** Subsequent surgery, including first and second metatarsophalangeal joint endoprosthesis with revisional second toe arthroplasty, reestablished better functional alignment and stability to the first and second metatarsophalangeal joints. Without pressure from the great toe, long-term stability to the second metatarsophalangeal joint is better ensured. Additionally, note the remarkable reduction of the metatarsus primus adductus following insertion of the first metatarsophalangeal joint flexible hinge endoprosthesis without metatarsal osteotomy. Resection of the subluxed first metatarsophalangeal joint with these retrograde forces on the metatarsal oftentimes enables reestablishment of this alignment without the need for metatarsal osteotomy. This becomes most attractive in geriatric patients, in whom metatarsal osteotomy with prolonged immobilization and healing would not be desirable.

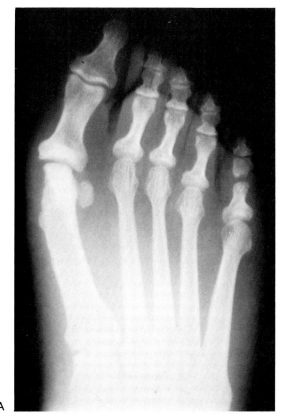 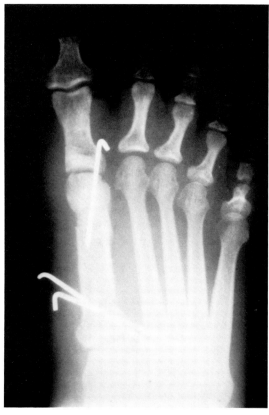

A   B

Fig. 45-16. (A) Attempt to reduce bunion deformity via Silver osteotomy in the presence of metatarsus primus adductus resulted in failure with continued medial protrusion of the metatarsal shaft. **(B)** Surgical revision with double metatarsal osteotomy resulted in a more rectus first metatarsal alignment with better position of the articular cartilage of the first metatarsal as well. Note the reduction of the sesamoid position.

mal gait. Surgeons of the foot have labored throughout the years to modify procedures in an attempt to reapproximate normal anatomic alignment and function of the first ray, because it has become well established that procedures that deviate from this norm are doomed to failure. Before the advent of endoprostheses for the re-creation of the first metatarsophalangeal joint, surgeons were left with only two alternatives when a joint-destructive procedure was necessary: resect the joint without replacement, or fuse the first metatarsophalangeal joint. The former alternative left the patient with a more pain-free yet less propulsive and stable joint. The second alternative often yielded secondary problems that far exceeded the original complaint. Development of a Dow Corn-

ing hemi- and later flexible hinge endoprosthesis afforded surgeons the ability for the first time to replace an arthritic joint and maintain stability and function. While these endoprostheses are no panacea, and occasionally result in secondary problems, they may if utilized properly give very gratifying results. The benefits, if any, of an implant are short lived when failure occurs in any component of the reconstruction essential to success, including the implant material, design, physiologic response from the patient's tissues, or surgical technique. They represent their own "Catch-22": While they are the source of many surgical complications, they often represent the solution to a surgical complication as well.

The Dow Corning flexible hinge first metatarso-

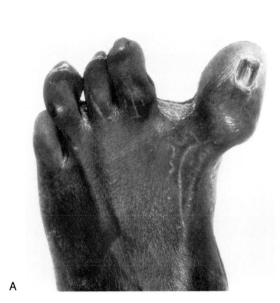

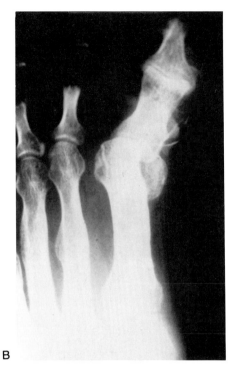

A

B

Fig. 45-17. (A,B) Excessive resection of the medial eminence of the head of the first metatarsal with creation of a negative intermetatarsal angle during first metatarsal osteoeomy, excision of the fibular sesamoid with weakening of the lateral anatomic structures (including the joint capsule), and adductor hallucis tendon resulted in hallux varus complicated with hammering of the hallux-interphalangeal joint.

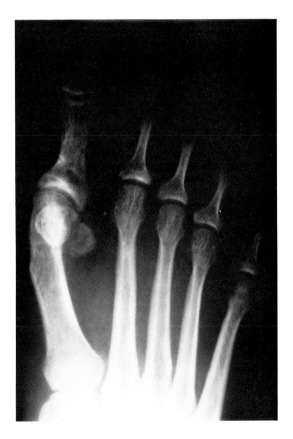

Fig. 45-18. Proximal phalangeal adductory-type osteotomy (Akin) performed to straighten an abducted great toe in the presence of severe malalignment of the articular cartilage of the first metatarsal head. Better surgical technique would involve reduction of the intermetatarsal angle with repositioning of the articular cartilage of the head of the first metatarsal. This would provide both better rectus alignment and improved joint congruity.

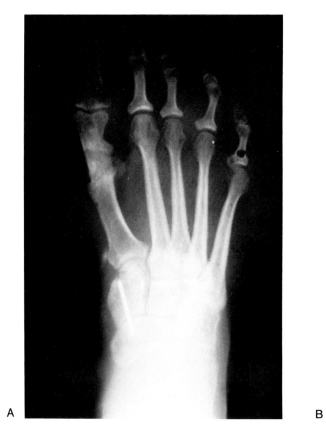
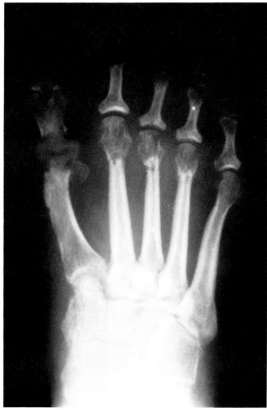

Fig. 45-19. (A) Surgical fusion of the first metatarsophalangeal joint resulted in inability to maintain a normal rectus gait. Transference of weight laterally to the lesser metatarsals resulted in increase of pain and disability. A threaded Stiman pin utilized to accomplish the fusion at the metatarsophalangeal joint was fractured during retrieval and left, bridging the first cuneiform–navicular joint. **(B)** Additional surgery involved the separation of the first metatarsophalangeal joint with the insertion of a first metatarsal joint endoprosthesis, in order to preserve both joint function and stability. Shortening of the lesser metatarsal heads decreased their prominence and created a better metatarsal parabola in view of the shortened first ray. Additionally, removal of the metallic fixator fragment allowed better function at the cuneiform–navicular joint.

phalangeal joint endoprosthesis, Swanson design, is composed of a high-performance silicone elastomer that is relatively nonreactive, nonadherent to tissue, and resistent to degradation by body fluids, thereby demonstrating excellent biocompatibility and biodurability. The silicone elastomer in the implant contains the combined characteristics of elastic memory, structural strength, stability (i.e., hardness), and a long flex life. Each characteristic is necessary in order to obtain a functional implant that will withstand the repeated stress and fatigue factors placed upon the first metatarsophalangeal joint. Elastic memory allows the implant to

return to its original size and shape after repeated flexion and extension. The long flex life provides the ability to withstand repeated loading without the occurrence of fatigue and fracture. A good strength modulus gives the implant lateral stability and prevents distortion in a varus or valgus direction. While the endoprosthesis possesses two intramedullary stems, it is a one-piece implant with the stems connected by a hinge spacer designed to transfer forces across the first metatarsophalangeal joint to the cortical bone. The structure of the hinge was ideally designed to permit dorsiflexion of the toe and stability of the first metatarsophalangeal joint in the lateral direction. The proximal and distal stems are at 90 degrees to the hinge and have a rectangular cross section providing the patient with stability within the medullary canals. The flexible hinge design provides several unique solutions to otherwise clinically frustrating problems in addition to alleviating the discomfort experienced from first metatarsophalangeal joint degenerative joint disease (hallux rigidus and limitus). The double stem design provides transverse plane stability and allows the implant to reduce both hallux valgus and hallux varus. In cases of failed Keller bunionectomies where joint resection has resulted in a flail toe or hallux varus, valgus, or extensus, the flexible hinge endoprosthesis can reconstitute the length of the first ray as well as structural integrity, alignment, and stability (see Figs. 45-12 through 45-14 and 45-19).

While first metatarsophalangeal joint endoprostheses provide numerous beneficial alternatives in forefoot reconstruction, there are several potential negative factors that one must understand before utilization. Approximately 65 degrees of first metatarsophalangeal joint dorsiflexion is necessary for normal ambulation. The Dow Corning first metatarsophalangeal joint endoprosthesis allows for a maximum of 36 degrees of dorsiflexion at its hinge (Fig. 45-20A). Therefore, ideally an addi-

tional 29 degrees of dorsiflexion must be derived when the endoprosthesis has been surgically implanted for normal locomotion to occur. This necessitates bending of the implant stem at the proximal hinge interface if additional motion is to occur. This bending occurs at the proximal stem as a result of the body's attempt to re-create its normal axis of motion within the first metatarsal head (Fig. 45-20B). This increases friction between the implant and the adjoining bone and increases internal stress, thereby decreasing the effectiveness of the hinge and potentiating fatigue and fracture of the implant at the proximal stem-hinge interface (Fig. 45-21). (It should be noted that although this discussion is centered on the Dow Corning endoprosthesis, similar situations exist for the Sutter first metatarsophalangeal joint endoprosthesis.)

Early in the postoperative course essentially all surgically implanted materials undergo a normal physiologic response by the body of encapsulation by fibrous tissue. This fibrous tissue is structurally similar to that found in normal wound healing, and is comprised of collagen, which has a dynamic biology constantly undergoing the process of metabolism and regeneration. However, fibrous tissue is inelastic, possesses a tendency to contract, and can hypertrophy if abnormal stresses are placed upon it. Ideally, implant design should capitalize on the

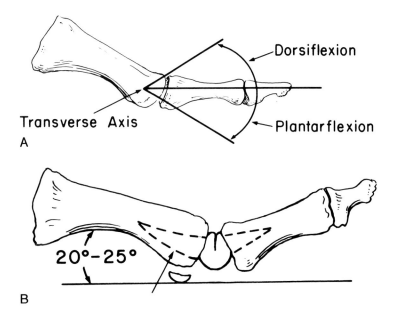

Fig. 45-20. **(A)** First metarsophalangeal and axial motion lies proximal to the joint itself within the metatarsal head. **(B)** The Dow Corning first metatarsophalangeal joint flexible hinge endoprosthesis allows for a maximum of 36 degrees of dorsiflexion at its hinge. The first metatarsophalangeal joint declination averages between 15 and 25 degrees. This allows an additional 11 degrees at the implant hinge before closure. Demands for additional motion at the first metatarsophalangeal joint result in bending of the implant at the proximal stem hinge interface as a result of the body's attempt to attain its normal axis of motion within the first metatarsal head.

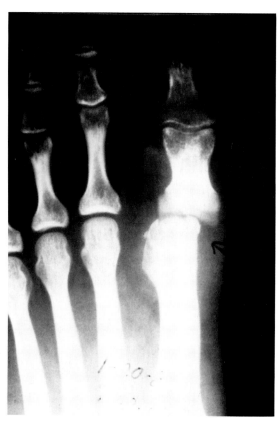

Fig. 45-21. Fracture at the proximal stem-hinge interface of a Dow Corning flexible hinge endoprosthesis secondary to increased stress placed on the implant due to excessive demands for motion and the body's desire to provide this motion within the first metatarsal head. This increases friction at the proximal stem-hinge interface, resulting in fatigue and fracture of the implant at this junction.

fibrous tissue response it elicits postoperatively for its own support, fixation, and longevity. The design of the implant hinge in the Dow Corning and Sutter endoprostheses provides a gap in the joint space that potentiates filling of the space postoperatively with synovium, a fibrous tissue, or the like. This serves to further restrict dorsiflexion of the hinge of the implant postoperatively, possibly resulting in severe limitation of motion at the first metatarsophalangeal joint (Fig. 45-22). Excess fibrous tissue deposition is the reason some individuals experience significantly reduced first meta-

tarsophalangeal joint motion following implant arthroplasty. Gentle range of motion exercises should ensue immediately following implant insertion to minimize this deposition.

The hemi-implant design for first metatarsophalangeal joint replacement was intended to replace only the dystrophic base of the proximal phalanx of the great toe. Additionally, the Weil modification of the Dow Corning hemi-implant provided an angled articular surface designed to compensate for an angled articular surface on the metatarsal head (increased proximal articular set angle). Through its single-stem design, the hemi-implant does not alter the hinge-type motion of the first metatarsophalangeal joint, as is the case with the double-stemmed implant. Additionally, its design provides few gaps for fibrous tissue infiltration, enabling greater joint motion postoperatively. However, its design provides no transverse plane or rotational stability within the first metatarsophalangeal joint. Therefore, it is incapable of reducing hallux varus or valgus. Furthermore since the coefficient of density differs between the silicone elastomer of the hemi-implant and the first metatarsal head, the implant tends to degenerate after varying degrees of time and stress (Fig. 45-23). Conversely, if the implant is utilized with bone of decreased mineralization, the implant might deform the bone, potentially becoming engulfed and incorporated within the medullary canal of the bone itself (Fig. 45-24). Additionally, it is quite rare that the base of the proximal phalanx would be degenerated without significant alteration to the head of the first metatarsal. If the hemi-implant is utilized in the presence of degeneration of the articular surface of the metatarsal head, with its associated irregularities, the longevity and effectiveness of the implant will be greatly reduced. Finally, caution should be exercised when considering these implants in the presence of metatarsus primus varus. A subluxation of the hallux into the interspace and possible dislocation of the implant within the interspace is the most likely result (Fig. 45-25). The angled hemi-implant has displayed an even greater propensity toward lateral displacement. The advent of the flexible hinge implant and publicity regarding the aforementioned complications of the hemi-implant have reduced the utilization of hemi-implants in recent years.

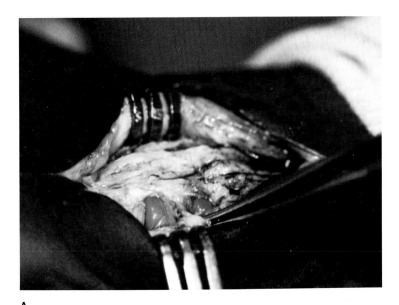

A

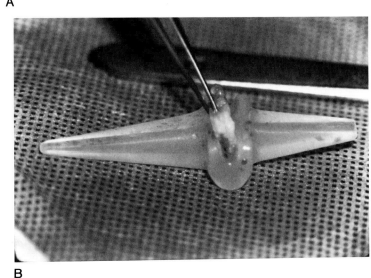

B

Fig. 45-22. (A) Intraoperative inspection of a Dow Corning first metatarsophalangeal joint endoprostheses nine months after insertion. Note the complete fibrous encasement negating all motion for this joint. This translated into stiffness and pain during ambulation by the patient. **(B)** Following implant removal, an elastic plug was removed from the implant hinge.

The Dow Corning and Sutter first metatarsophalangeal joint endoprostheses provide many innate qualities that afford the surgeon many new tools to be utilized during surgical reconstruction when addressing iatrogenic complications. Their design, however, provides many deviations from normal anatomic alignment, thereby raising the potential for complications from the implants. While these complications do not preclude their use, one must be keenly aware of their limitations so as not to create additional complications.

TOURNIQUET USE

Proper understanding of indications and contraindications, application, and usage as well as knowledge of possible complications are essential to tourniquet use for surgical hemostasis. Tourniquets are used in peripheral extremity surgery to render the operative field bloodless so that surgical procedures may be performed with enhanced visi-

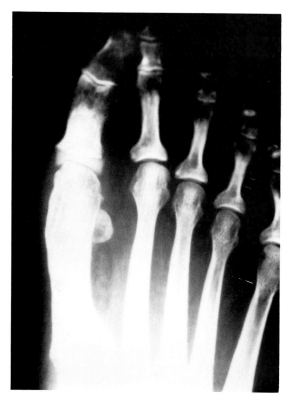

Fig. 45-23. Radiograph demonstrating excessive wear of a hemi-implant secondary to stress from the first metatarsal head, and obliquity at the metatarsal-implant interface.

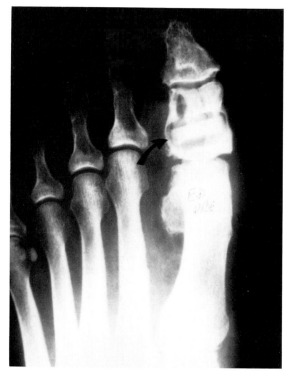

Fig. 45-24. Hemi-implant engulfed within the canal of the proximal phalanx of the great toe secondary to differing coefficients of density between the two substances.

bility, thereby minimizing damage to small vital structures. Sterling Bunnel, the father of modern hand surgery, is reputed to have said that ''Operating on a hand without a tourniquet is like trying to fix a watch in a bottle of ink.'' With a clear bloodless field meticulous anatomic dissection is more easily facilitated and surgical time is reduced tremendously, aiding in reducing surgery fatigue as well as complications of a prolonged open wound such as dessication and infection.

The development of the pneumatic tourniquet with controlled instantaneous hemostasis has made use of pressure elastic band tourniquets such as the Martin's and Esmarch bandages obsolete. These tourniquets do not allow controlled, measurable pressures; therefore, complications of either over-compression or undercompression can occur. Pneumatic tourniquets have not yet been developed for use in digital hemostasis, although a 1/4-

inch Penrose drain applied over a gauze bandage at the base of a digit secured with a hemostat has proven safe and effective.

Preoperative evaluation and examination of a patient before employing a tourniquet should rule out the presence of a peripheral vascular disease, including vasospastic types; past history of or predisposition to thrombophlebitis; and history of and testing for sickle cell disease or trait. The possible complicating factor of vasculitis in arthritic patients should also be considered. Use of tourniquets in patients with arterial compromise can lead to occlusion of existing arteriosclerotic vessels and the possibility of thrombus or embolus formation. The ischemic state created by a tourniquet can result in an irreversible vasospasm in patients with vasospastic disease such as Raynaud's or Berger's disease. Use of a tourniquet in patients with sickle cell disease is contraindicated; use in patients with sickle cell trait is controversial, and it is better to

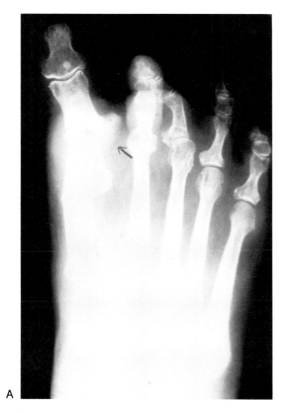

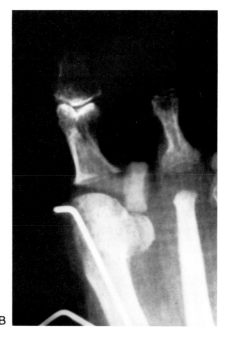

Fig. 45-25. (A) Lateral displacement of a hemi-implant within the intermetatarsal space. **(B)** Displacement of the hemi-implant within the intermetatarsal space following reduction of the intermetatarsal angle. Note the continued obliquity of the articular cartilage at the first metatarsal head potentiating the eventual lateral displacement of the hemi-implant.

not use a tourniquet with this population. Patients with a history of thrombophlebitis or pulmonary embolism or with physical evidence of varicosities are at risk for development of such complications. Preoperative use of heparin with tourniquet use, and avoiding tourniquet use over areas of known varicosities have proven to reduce the incidence of postoperative thrombophlebitis in these patients.

The application of a tourniquet at midthigh level is ideal and is recommended since the circumference of the extremity is greatest at this level, with the greatest amount of soft tissue to protect underlying vital structures from pneumatic pressure. However, a tourniquet at this level is painful and difficult for the patient to tolerate without general or spinal anesthesia. An ankle-level tourniquet placed approximately 5 cm proximal to the distal tip of the medial malleoulus is in primary use today,

aided by local anesthesia and sedation. The tourniquet should never be applied where compression of the underlying superficial nerve tissues can occur; therefore, use of the tourniquet directly at ankle or calf level or directly above or below the knee is contraindicated. Superficial nerve damage from compression may result in paralysis, paresthesia, burning, or exaggerated pain postoperatively. Fortunately, in most cases this is transient and spontaneous recovery occurs within a few days to a few weeks. If not, surgical intervention may be necessary to rule out fibrosis or neuroma formation at the site of compression.

The tourniquet should be applied over a soft, smooth cotton pad with no wrinkles. Wrinkles or folds in the padding may cause pinching of the underlying skin with resultant necrosis and blistering as well as tourniquet discomfort during surgery.

The padding should extend slightly above and below the tourniquet to ensure even distribution of pressure. No operative site preparation liquid should be allowed to remain under the cotton padding, because this may result in a chemical burn or damage to the skin under pressure. A loose tourniquet many times accounts for tourniquet pain, marked hyperemia, postoperative edema, or sensory and motor disturbances. Therefore the surgeon should always examine tourniquet fit, padding, and location before inflation.

Elevation of the limb prior to tourniquet inflation is necessary to exanguinate all venous blood, and has been shown to result in reactive arterial vasospasm, which aids in creating a bloodless field. Elevation at 45 degrees for 3 minutes is recommended to milk the blood from the leg. Along with elevation, use of a Martin's bandage is helpful to exsanguinate the part up to the level of the tourniquet before inflation. Failure to do this may result in increased venous pressure and oozing from the surgical site, with resultant impaired visibility.

The tourniquet should be inflated quickly to allow for rapid occlusion of both arterial and venous vessels. A good arterial tourniquet should put sufficient pressure on tissues surrounding blood vessels to impede blood flow without harm to underlying structures. Recommended pressures are at least 70 to 100 mm Hg above the patient's systolic blood pressure, since it has been shown that the blood pressure may rise during surgery by approximately 70 mm Hg. These values should not exceed 250 mm Hg of pressure in an ankle tourniquet or 500 mm Hg of pressure in a thigh tourniquet.

If sufficient arterial occlusion is not obtained, or if exsanguination of venous blood below the tourniquet level does not occur, venous congestion of the extremity below the tourniquet level may occur. This has been shown to be responsible for microemboli to the vaso nervorum, causing nerve damage, compartment syndrome, and venous clotting with resultant thrombophlebitis. It is also important to remember that some think that development of tourniquet pain is from blood remaining in the venous system because of an inadequate exsanguination before elevation of the tourniquet. This remaining blood builds up lactic acid in the ischemic state, causing discomfort and pain. It should also be realized that under the heat of surgical lights, the ischemic wound should be flushed with frequent irrigations of cool normal saline to maintain viability of the tissues and stable osmolarity.

Ambiguity exists in relation to the maximum length of time for tourniquet application. Bunnel recommended 10 minutes of breathing time (free flow of arterial blood with tourniquet deflated) after 1 to 1.5 hours of tourniquet inflation. Wilgis et al., in a study of venous and arterial blood in human subjects during extremity surgery, found that a profound yet reversible metabolic and respiratory acidosis as well as substantial hypoxia occurs with tourniquet usage. They found that after 1 hour of tourniquet ischemia, it took 5 to 10 minutes of "reactive hyperemia" to reverse the acidosis to normal. After 90 minutes it took greater than 10 minutes, but less than 15 minutes. After 2 hours it took greater than 15 minutes to reverse this acidosis. These guidelines should be used for revascularization during lengthy operative procedures which require multiple tourniquets. Also, Wilgis et al. found that there are no significant myocardial or pulmonary effects from this acid-base shift in normal healthy patients, but there is a possible effect on the myocardium or lungs in patients with preexisting disease of these organs.

Kleneman stated that 3 hours is a safe total tourniquet time based on animal acid-base studies. McGlamry stated that 2 to 3 hours of total tourniquet time is safe, with a breathing time of 5 to 15 minutes after such a period of hemostasis. Most surgeons agree that 1 to 1.5 hours of tourniquet ischemia with 10 to 15 minutes of breathing time is safe for an extremity. No accepted safe duration of tourniquet reinflation after the breathing period exists, although it should not usually exceed three-quarters of an hour for a leg tourniquet. If the proposed procedures necessitate more than 2 hours of tourniquet ischemia, a decision as to whether to continue surgery without the aid of tourniquet, reinflation after a breathing time, or to perform additional procedures at a later date must be made. While there are no absolutes, one thing is certain: tourniquet use in general increases risk of potential complication and prolonged tourniquet use magnifies that risk.

With release of the tourniquet reactive hyperemia and systemic hypotension can occur, especially with the use of bilateral thigh tourniquets. After prolonged occlusion of arterial supply by a tourniquet above systolic blood pressure distal gangrene or postischemic syndrome of edema, coolness of an extremity, and parasthesias consistent with a reflex sympathetic dystrophy can occur. This syndrome is thought to be related primarily to direct damage to the nerve and vascular tissues.

Injury to an artery during an operation with the use of a tourniquet may not be evident until after release of the tourniquet. If suspected, release of the tourniquet before wound and skin closure is necessary. Identification of the involved vessel can then be achieved and the problem accurately addressed. Development of an aneurysm after foot and ankle surgery has been reported with tourniquet use, but is not common.

In summary, the above applications and complications of tourniquet use are an absolute necessity for a surgeon's knowledge. While the tourniquet is a valuable asset during peripheral surgery, it is a potentially dangerous instrument as well, and it is essential to be aware of its adverse potential and to recognize even its delayed complications. Previous planning of the operation as well as proper preoperative evaluation of the patient's medical and physical status will enable the surgeon to use the critical time of tourniquet ischemia maximally. Similarly, frequent postoperative evaluation of the surgical site, the digital circulation, and the tourniquet site may minimize complications related to tourniquet usage.

ANTIBIOTIC PROPHYLAXIS

The need for antibiotic prophylaxis for musculoskeletal surgery arose from the high incidence of postoperative wound infection in otherwise clean orthopedic operations. Numerous studies have shown a pronounced reduction in postoperative infection with the use of perioperative antibiotics, particularly cases involving the implementation of endoprosthetic surgical devices, since risk of prosthetic infection outweighs any risk of the antibiotic.

The choice of antibiotic for prophylaxis should be directed at the most common organisms that occur with the type of surgery being performed. Staphylococci predominate as causative organisms in postoperative wound infections in musculoskeletal surgery. Streptococci, gram-negative organisms, anaerobes, or a mixture have also been known to occur, but at a lower incidence. For this reason a broad-spectrum antibiotic directed at gram-positive organisms is the drug of choice in prophylaxis. The cephalosporin antibiotics have been most frequently prescribed for such use. Cefazolin is recommended because of its spectrum of activity, penetration of soft tissue and bone, and relatively few side effects. Vancomycin or erythromycin are effective as prophylactic agents in patients allergic to penicillins or cephalosporins. Variables such as patient age, surgical procedure, surgeon, hospital, and underlying disease (especially peripheral vascular disease, renal disease, and diabetes mellitus) are also factors to include in the choice of antibiotic for prophylaxis as well as coverage during immediate postoperative period.

It is generally recommended that antimicrobial prophylaxis be administered intravenously within 30 minutes to 1 hour of tourniquet inflation preoperatively. This is done so that peak serum levels may be reached during the surgical period. There is no proven advantage in continuing use of antimicrobial agents after the surgical procedure has been completed. However, it has been this author's experience that administration of one dose of perenteral antibiotic immediately postoperatively has aided in the prevention of postoperative infections. Prophylactic antibiotics may alter the normal flora in any patient, enabling resistant organisms to create infection. Allergic reactions and other adverse effects of many antibiotics used in a prophylactic manner may also occur.

It is important to realize that the use of topical antibiotics in a surgical wound, such as antibiotic flush, is also considered surgical antibiotic prophylaxis. Finally, antibiotic prophylaxis should not result in alteration of precise sterile surgical technique, which in itself is prophylaxis against infection.

CONCLUSION

The subject of surgical complications provides a roller coaster of emotions for a foot surgeon. Every surgeon realizes that even with the greatest attention to detail, circumstances beyond his or her control might arise resulting in iatrogenic morbidity and deformity. This certainly is cause for concern to many lower extremity surgeons. On the other hand, the competent surgeon, often in a strange way, welcomes those patients with obscure surgically induced problems when these problems were caused by another surgeon. By their nature these iatrogenic deformities possess a certain uniqueness, in each case mandating the surgeon to draw from all of his or her experiences and talents to create a more normally functioning and comfortable foot. It is paramount to understand that without a full working knowledge of the normal anatomy, function, and biomechanics of the foot, the surgeon cannot possibly hope to address a surgical complication, or prevent one from occurring.

REFERENCES

1. Lauf E, et al: Swanson great toe flexible hinge endoprosthesis: design, flexibility and function. J Am Podiatr Med Assoc 75:393, 1985
2. Swanson A, Mester W, Swanson G, et al: Durability of silicone implants: an in vivo study. Orthop Clin North Am 4:1097, 1973
3. Frisch E: Functional considerations in implant design. J Med Device Diagn Industries 3:299, 1981
4. Root M, Orien W, Weed J: Normal and Abnormal Function of the Foot. Clinical Biomechanics Corporation, Los Angeles, 1977
5. Gowitzke B: Understanding the Scientific Basis of Human Movement. 2nd Ed. Williams & Wilkins, Baltimore, 1980
6. Teich L, Frankel J, Lipsam S: Silicone hinge replacement arthroplasty. J Am Podiatry Assoc 71:266, 1981
7. Swanson A: Flexible Implant Resection Arthroplasty in the Hands and Extremities: Concepts of Flexible Implant Design. CV Mosby, St. Louis, 1973
8. Thompson HC: The effects of drilling into bone. J Oral Surg 16:22, 1958
9. Griffin KJ: The effect of power instrumentation on bone healing. J Foot Surg 20:301, 1981
10. Whiteside L, Lesker A: The effects of extraperiosteal and subperiosteal dissection. J Bone Joint Surg [Am] 60, 1978
11. Brighton C: The treatment of non unions with electricity. J Bone Surg [Am] 63, 1981
12. McKibbin B: The biology of fracture healing in long bones. J Bone Joint Surg [Br] 60, 1978
13. Connoly J, Hahn H: Fracture healing in weight-bearing and nonweight bearing bones. J Trauma 18, 1978
14. Leighton RL: Complications from mismanagement of fixation devices. Vet Clin North Am 15, 1975
15. Pfeiffer KM: Small Fragment Set Manual. Springer-Verlag, New York, 1974

Surgical Wound Closure in Foot and Ankle Procedures

46

Jose Castillo, M.D.

When form can be translated into terms of function, or states of being into terms of force, we are near the cutting edge of the scimitar of science.

Alan Gregg

A wound is the instantaneous response to injury. Injury involving the cutting or breaking of body tissue, as by violence, accident, or surgery, stimulates repair. Repair as a normal positive reaction to injury is the keystone on which surgery is founded.[1]

CLASSIFICATION OF WOUNDS AND TYPES OF WOUND HEALING

From a clinical point of view surgical wounds have been classified as clean, clean-contaminated, contaminated, and dirty-infected.[2] In approximately 75 percent of cases, the podiatric surgeon is concerned with uninfected operative wounds that are primarily closed and no drainage is necessary; these are clean wounds. When a minimal break in aseptic technique occurs he or she deals with usual flora and therefore there is no unusual contamina-

tion; these wounds are therefore considered clean-contaminated. If a major break in aseptic technique occurs, as may be the case in an operative procedure for excision and/or repair of a fresh traumatic injury or soft tissue laceration, the wound is then classified as contaminated. In the last category, a dirty-infected wound is heavily or clinically infected prior to surgery (such as in abscess, an old traumatic wound with devitalized tissue, osteomyelitis, or the presence of foreign bodies).

From a clinical point of view[3] three basic types of wound healing have been recognized: healing by first, second, and third intention. Healing by first intension, or primary union, is seen in the case of an aseptically incised skin wound that is closed accurately, and takes place with minimal edema; in this wound no discharge or local infection is observed and the end result, in an otherwise healthy individual, will be minimal scar formation with an eventual hairline scar appearance. Healing by second intention is seen when wound healing proceeds from the bottom of the wound toward its outer surface; in this wound scar formation is excessive. Wound contraction rather than primary union is deliberately allowed to take place even in the presence of infection, excessive trauma, and/or tissue loss; approximation of the skin edges is not precise. Healing by third intention has also been referred to as delayed primary closure. The basic rationale for delaying the wound closure is the realignment of the wound surface and lips of a previously contaminated dirty-infected traumatic wound; the optimal time for this type of closure is 4 to 6 days.

Basic Physiologic Knowledge of Wound Healing

Basic physiologic knowledge of wound healing is the central core of surgery.[4] The podiatric surgeon, as in any other surgical subspecialty, has the moral obligation to master this basic knowledge, coupled in turn with a high degree of technical competence, because he or she holds the scalpel in his or her hand. **Local and general factors affect the healing of a wound.**[5] In foot and ankle procedures these factors have response variations that may be grossly depicted in the difference between the healing process of a clean surgical skin incision of a young healthy adult undergoing bunionectomy, and the healing process of a similar procedure in the skin of an elderly diabetic patient with poor circulation and poor nutrition. It is well to remember that in spite of the innumerable studies that have been done at the experimental and clinical levels in an effort to accelerate healing beyond the normal rate, (i.e., the optimal rate observed in a healthy patient), there is not as yet a known method by which this can be accomplished.

Important General Factors

Ascorbic acid is absolutely essential to wound healing. Rare genetic blood coagulation defects such as hemophilia and lack of factor XIII could be deleterious for healing. Severe anemia and severe deficits of serum albumin (below 1.5 g/ml) may repair the healing process considerably. With advanced age the tensile strength of a wound may be slower than in youth; also, on clinical grounds, chronic diseases may interfere with the rate of healing.

Important Local Factors

Adequate local vascularity is critical, because no wound healing takes place in the absence of blood flow. Adequate pressure and tension forces in the wounded area are essential to proper tissue apposition. Abnormal distraction and/or interposition of the lips of a wound may result in unsightly scar appearance and uneven epithelium migration. Avoidance of trauma to the wound edges and judicious use of the appropriate suture materials is always advisable, to negate a predisposition to infection (in the presence of infection no wound heals).

BASIC WOUND HEALING PHASES OF A CLEAN SURGICAL SKIN INCISION[6]

The skin is an organ that heals by scar formation when the papillary dermis is penetrated through its entire thickness. Only the uppermost layer of the skin, that is, the epidermis and/or mucosa, can regenerate. The final appearance of a scar is influenced by a complex series of objective and subjective events that are initiated at the moment that the surgical wound is inflicted and the repair begins. The wound healing process of a surgical skin incision follows the conventional morphologic and histochemical changes, which are initiated with the phase of *hemostasis*. As soon as a clean skin incision is made, the cut vessels are sealed by spasm and by platelet thrombi. There is also a deposition of a fibrin clot that contains trapped erythrocytes and leukocytes.

Within a few hours of wounding, an array of incisional and peri-incisional histochemical reactions occur at the various levels of the wound. The outpouring of tissue fluids, accumulation of cells and fibroblasts, and increase of blood supply to the wound initiate the phase of *traumatic inflammation*, lasting up to 72 hours from the moment of fibrin deposit and capillary engorgement, which is followed by permeability for the exudation of wound edema as ground substance. During this phase vasoactive histamine from mast cells and vasoactive peptides from enzymatic action in plasma proteins build up the wound content with glycoproteins.[7] Meanwhile the leukocytes and macrophages migrating into the wounded tissue engulf and digest debris. In actuality the enzymatic activity for the removal of necrotic tissue is first initiated by polymorphonuclear leukocytes in the first 24 hours of wounding; these are then replaced by macrophages and other monocytes that persist longer in the area as the overlapping *destructive* phase proceeds from inflammation. The physical changes taking place in the ground substance during the phases of inflammation and destruction advance the wound healing process to a phase of *proliferation of capillaries and fibroblasts*. This is coupled with fibrinolysis and a progressive increment in the content of mucopolysaccharides and hydroxyproline for the production of collagen, which results in rapid increase in the tensile strength of the wound lasting ordinarily from 3 to 14 days, to a maximum of 3 weeks.[8] From this point on the phase of *maturation* is initiated, which is basically characterized by a progressive decrease in capillaries and wound cellularity. The increment of collagen slowly increases the tensile strength of the wound as it also undergoes a process of contraction. Maturation in the wound healing process begins during the third week after injury and is not completed for approximately a year or more.

The comprehensive process of the final sealage of a clean surgical wound is initiated within hours of injury. While the inflammatory response goes on, fixed basal cells along the margins of the skin wound produce migrating epithelial cells, which roll down and across fibrin strands and seal off the wound surface.[9]

CLINICAL CORRELATES IN WOUND HEALING[10]

The original interaction of platelets and fibroblasts culminates in a specific control reaction for the biosynthesis of collagen fibers, which are the protein substance that is the chief constituent of connective tissue. The deposition of collagen fibers for scar development reaches its optimal level during the phase of proliferation. The fibers are then loosely arranged and traversed by a rich net of capillaries. Simultaneously there is a progressive subsidence in the inflammatory phase, with changes that give a bulky appearance to the wound margins at the epithelium, stratum papillaris, the denser stratum reticularis, and the subcutaneous level that last until the early onset of the maturation phase. These changes correlate with the clinical appearance of the scar, which is at its worst for approximately 8 to 10 weeks from wounding. As the phase of maturation progresses, 3 to 6 months after injury, there is a decrease in vascularity because the compacted collagen strangles the capillaries. Improvement in the scar appearance is clinically marked as it changes from prominently firm and red to a whitish, discolored, softer consistency after a year or more.[11]

Uncomplicated small wounds seal off by epithelium migration within hours of their being inflicted. Scars may remain metabolically active for years, but in general the progression in the bonding together of newly synthesized scar tissue is one of slow changes in size, shape, color, texture, and strength. Clean surgical skin incisions reapproximated with accuracy and undue tension are bound to result in the type of "hairline" scars nearly unapparent with the passage of time. Contused wound edges result in heavier scars with slow maturing ability. Permanent, unsightly scars usually result from infected wounds. The inflammatory response in these wounds is greatly enhanced, resulting in wider, thicker, and slowly maturing scars. Foreign body reaction may result from excessive unnecessary suture material, as well as excessive devitalized tissue debris, including carbon particles from electrocoagulation. Sanguinous seromata resulting from poorly opposed wound lips may not only be instrumental in enhancing the inflammatory phase of the wound healing process but may stimulate excessive deposition of dermal and subepidermal scar tissue and the eventual formation of pyogenic granulomata if secondary infection takes place.

While objective morphologic and histo-chemical wound healing events[12] are determinative for the color, texture, firmness, and bulk of a scar, there are also subjective events, biochemical in nature, that operate at the scar perimeter as well as in the underlying anatomic structures. Physical changes and alterations in the architecture of the resulting scar were first observed by Dupuytren in 1834 in a patient with three skin puncture wounds inflicted by an owl. Langer in 1861 made a comprehensive study of static biomechanic properties of cadaver skin, and Kocher in 1892 advocated the use of Langer lines for the placement of skin incisions. It was then thought that the healing of clean skin wounds following such lines, would take place with minimal scarring. Experimental and clinical observations in the healing of wounds with various degrees of skin tensions have resulted in the clinical understanding of the so-called relaxed skin tensions lines (RSTLs) of Borges, which are generally at right angles to the underlying tendons and/or muscle pull. The dynamic tensions surrounding surgical skin incisions are related to forces such as gravity and musculoskeletal kinesia (kinetic joint movements and voluntary muscular and tendinous activity). Thus, scars firmly bound to underlying structures may be an unsatisfactory bed for the gliding of tendons. Longitudinal shearing stresses on large thick scars from foot and ankle procedures may influence the dynamics of standing or walking and may even be responsible for remodeling of bone structures. Scar retraction in lax skin areas of the foot may be the direct result of contraction of the wound margins, particularly if associated with inadequate cohesiveness of tissue contact, as is the case in so called "trap door defects."

Correlation of skin tension as a quantitative factor with the integral quality of the cutaneous area bearing the scar surface establishes the need for subtle balance between tension and integrity forces. A combination of words coined in *Architecture Geodesics* by R. Buckminister Fuller in his explorations in the geometry of thinking, "tensegrity structure," seems appropriate. Extrapolating from architecture to the surgical closure of a wound, it may be established that a sound practical objective of a surgeon should be that, in inflicting and primarily closing a clean surgical wound, a subtle balance between skin tension at the suture line and integrity of the overall cutaneous surface should technically prevail, aiming at an eventual satisfactory scar appearance. Finally, it is worth repetitious conventional emphasis to note the need for adequate use of anesthesia, meticulous aseptic techniques, and delicate tissue handling. The efficient cleansing effect of irrigation, coupled with appropriate antimicrobial prophylaxis, is a fundamental tenet. Débridement of devitalized tissue cannot be overemphasized, and avoidance of dead spaces by the natural obliteration, without undue tension, of the subdermally divided tissue is advisable — remembering that excessive surgical sutures impair the wound's ability to resist infection.

TECHNICAL FACTORS IN WOUND MANAGEMENT

Fundamental technical skills are necessary to implement well-devised surgical care.[13] From the moment that a surgeon incises the skin with his or her scalpel, the force, which is shearing in nature, divides the tissue and disrupts the body covering, rendering the once sterile underlying integument exposed to contamination. The cut to the desired depth should be made with a single sweep, so that the resultant wound is uniform and therefore more resistant to infection. Multiple strokes with the knife damage the local defenses and invite infection. The custom of discarding a scalpel following the initial skin incision should not necessarily be a mandatory practice, because experimental studies have demonstrated that the inflammatory response made by a single sweep of the knife is significantly less that in wounds made by multiple strokes.

In traumatic wounds, the injurious forces to the skin are compressive or tensile rather than shearing. The host defenses against these wounds are weaker and suceptible to infection. Use of electrical energy (Bovie use) for either cutting the skin and/or coagulating the dermal and subcutaneous bleeders, also has its place in the technology for skin cutting. Electrosurgical skin incision, however, nearly doubles infection rates and as a result its use has been considerably mitigated. Photonic energy in the form of lasers, particularly carbon dioxide, has also been introduced recently as a tool for skin incision. However, its use is as yet cumbersome because the equipment is difficult and time consuming to maneuver; also it has been experimentally found that photonic skin incisions may have an infection-potentiating effect.

Quantitative bacteriology[14] is the method by which rapid slide technique as well as serial dilution and plating studies may help the surgeon to predict the safety of wound closure, be it primary or delayed, and also predict graft bed receptivity as well as providing information for a possible onset of sepsis, as in burn wounds. Topical antisepsis, sterility, or near-sterility may be achieved in most areas of the body. The surgeon must be familiar with the normal microflora of the skin and mucous membranes. The podiatrist, of course, should be well versed with knowledge about the flora of the interdigital spaces, toenails, and soles of the feet.

BASIC TECHNIQUES FOR WOUND CLOSURE IN FOOT AND ANKLE PROCEDURES[15,16]

The surgical techniques applicable to skin and subcutaneous tissue anywhere in the body are of the utmost specific importance in foot and ankle procedures. Consideration of contour lines and lines of dependency for the placement of skin incisions are helpful to balance, in terms of "tensegrity," between the resultant scar and normal paracicatricial tissue. Elliptical, wedge, "T," or circular excisions of small lesions are best when planned and placed along relaxed skin tension lines. Atraumatic handling of the tissues plus adequate hemostasis by electrocoagulation or ligature of bleeders is of paramount importance. It is worth remembering to avoid excessive deposition of carbon particles or excessive placement of suture material, particularly in the upper dermis. Occasional judicious use of fibrin foam, gelatin foam, or microcrystalline collagen coupled with sustained compression for a few minutes may be beneficial to control capillary oozing.

Sutures

Conventional wound closure requires the use of buried sutures in layers (periostium and/or perichondrium, muscles, fascia, and subcutaneous tissue). Eventually suture material made of collagen or polyglycolic acid is digested by enzymatic action. Suturing remains the preferred method for skin wound closures in foot and ankle procedure (simple interrupted, vertical mattress, horizontal mattress, subcuticular continuous, half-buried horizontal mattress, continuous over-and-over, or continuous interlocking). In foot and ankle sutured skin wounds it is almost imperative to retain stitches for at least 10 to 14 days. However, suturing marks invariably occur when the sutures remain in place for 2 weeks or more. The closure of the skin wound proper may be effected with sutures, steri-strips, skin clips, or wound adhesives, as long as the wound lip apposition is firm and uniform without undue tension or separation. Inversion or overlapping of skin edges is to be avoided, particularly in wounds with edges of unequal thickness. Eversion of the wound edges is occasionally acceptable as long as it is not overdone, because flattening gradually levels the wound surface when sutures are removed. Suturing should be just tight enough to approximate the wound edges, avoiding lateral wound pulling. Keeping the sutures close to the wound edge with the knot placement at the initial point of needle skin entrance is also a sound surgical technique that followed by the progressive removal of the stitches after 7 days, with their replacement by microporous adhesive steri-strips, could be quite helpful in avoiding suture marking in the skin. In this fashion support is provided to the healing wound during the period of tensile strength progression. These methods may also be an aid in the prevention of infection and possible reduction in the tendency, which by idiosyncracy some individuals have, to keloid formation.

Grafts

Following the removal of skin lesions by elliptical, wedge, or circular excision techniques, a soft tissue deficit may result. The most common method to close a defect of this type is with a skin graft. Skin grafts in general serve the overall purpose of coverage of soft tissue defects provided that they have sufficient blood supply from the recipient host site, usually by granulation tissue, which should in turn be healthy. Skin grafts do not take on denuded cortical bone, denuded pericondrium, denuded paratenon, or denuded nerves. Full-thickness grafts, as the name implies, are segments of skin containing the epidermis and entire thickness of dermis, including adnexal structures (sebaceous glands, hair follicles, and sweat glands), as well as capillaries at the level of separation from their blood supply. Partial-thickness grafts contain epidermis and only a portion of dermis. They could be quite thin, intermediate, or relatively thick, varying from 10 to 20 thousands of an inch. The actual thickness of the skin in humans varies with age, sex, and anatomic surfaces of the body. It is a well-known fact that the thickest skin is found on the soles of the feet. The most common sites for obtaining full-thickness skin grafts are the postauricular skin regions, supraclavicular skin, preauricular skin, upper eyelids, antecubital, and inguinal regions. The common surfaces for partial-thickness skin grafts for use on the ankle and foot surfaces are the thighs, where the skin thickness varies, in general, between 20 and 25 thousands of an inch, the calves, and the dorsa of the feet.

A *free graft* is actually a biologic transplant. The classification of free grafts uses the same terminology as proposed and established by Snell in 1964. A skin isograft is a graft between identical twins. A skin autograft is a graft transferred from one place to another in the same individual. An autochthonous graft is a graft replanted on the same site from which it was originally detached in the same individual. A skin allograft is a graft between two individuals of the same species (in this category is cadaver skin). A skin xenograft is a graft between members of different species (in this category is porcine skin).

Skin grafts are totaly detached from the host during transfer. Their vascular and nervous connections are severed. When the transfer of a graft has been technically well accomplished on a host bed with an adequate blood supply, its survival, during the first 24 to 48 hours, is by plasmatic diffusion or imbibition from the host bed nutrients. Revascularization of grafted skin, when it is properly immobilized, is initiated in 12 to 24 hours, becoming progressively strong by 96 hours, at which time "take" is either a success or a failure. The factors operative in the failure of the "take" of a skin graft are collection of fluid and movement between the graft and its bed. The sensory renervation is poorer in split-thickness skin grafts than in full-thickness grafts. The latter in general show fairly good renervation at the periphery but renervation is poor toward the center.

The character and appearance of a skin graft are related to its thickness. Hyperpigmentation of grafted surfaces is a common occurrence that is more prone to happen with split-thickness skin grafting. This problem could be enhanced by exposure to actinic radiation. Full-thickness skin grafts are less prone to hyperpigmentation. Skin anexae (hair follicles, sebaceous glands, and sweat glands) continue to function when included in full-thickness skin grafts as well as thick split-thickness grafts. Full-thickness skin grafts closely resemble normal skin with regard to color, turgor, and hair regrowth and they usually do not contract, as split-thickness grafts do.

A split-thickness skin graft can be obtained by the use of a free knife, humby-knife, and/or dermatomes (the Padget or Brown electrical dermatomes as well as commercial modifications of these). The fixation of a skin graft, depending upon its size and its thickness, can be accomplish by sutures, steri-strips, and/or tie-over dressings. Skin grafting procedures for the lower extremities require a longer time for revascularization and therefore immobilization should be prolonged. It is usually preferred to fix the grafted areas by suturing. In concave surfaces a tie-over or "basket dressing" is the most appropriate modality for graft fixation. The wound sometimes may not be suitable for immediate grafting. In such cases storage of skin grafts can be done "in situ" for up to 10 days. This is a very effective method to store split-thickness grafts. Skin is harvested from the thigh, and immediately replaced on the donor site (autochthonous graft replantation), as an onlay biologic dressing without stitching. Careful immobilizing of the area by a compression circumferential bulky dressing is done. As a rule these grafts can be removed without anesthesia with minimal pain in 2 to 3 days to cover operative soft tissue defects such as may occur on the soles of the feet (i.e., overgrafting procedure following dermabrasion). Storage may also be done by refrigeration of the harvested skin for up to 21 days. Care should be taken in wrapping the skin in moisturized gauze with normal saline solution under sterile conditions.

Following the removal of a skin graft the donor site requires special attention in order to prevent it from becoming infected. The rate and quality of healing is independent of the type of dressing applied next to the wound donor surface. In general nonadherent dressings such as Xerofom gauze are applied, wrapping the area initially with a compression dressing that is removed in approximately 24 hours, leaving the wound covered only with the layer of Xerofom. This wound is then allowed exposure to room air for 2 or 3 days to dry. As epithelization proceeds the Xerofom dressing usually detaches itself spontaneously in about 2 weeks. A heat lamp to increase the temperature of the skin surface of the donor site area usually facilitates smooth reepithelization. Application is done four times a day for 20 minutes at a time.

Flaps

The podiatric surgeon should be encouraged to increase his or her intuitive experiential understanding of the structural skin surface "tensegrity" in order to develop a basic but comprehensive ability to handle soft tissue defects by way of pedicle flaps. If the surgeon is able to rely on flaps it is easier to approach the current gamut of variants in the techniques of soft tissue transfers and microscopic surgery. A flap is an anatomic unit containing skin and subcutaneous tissue, shaped as a tongue, that maintains its blood supply. The vascular supply of a flap may be directionally reversed from one flap side to the opposite, as in simple transplantation maneuvers, or could be connected through segmental vessels to a chosen anatomic area by microvascular techniques. Understanding the anatomy of the blood supply to the skin is basic to planning, development, and transfer of flaps.

Most of the skin is supplied by a pattern in which a large artery from the aorta or a major vessel lies deep to the muscle, from which perforator musculocutaneous branches supply the dermal-subdermal plexus of the skin. A second pattern is provided by direct longitudinal cutaneous arterial vessels located in the subcutaneous tissue. On the basis of this gross anatomical mapping it is possible to visualize segmental, anastomotic, and axial arteries that are in continuity with perfusion pressure gradients from aorta. The podiatric surgeon should be well versed with the axial arteries to the lower extremities, namely, the femoral arteries that come off major branches of the aorta, and lie deep to the muscles proximally and more superficially at the distal segments.

Skin flaps can be classified according to where they are moved and according to their blood supply. Based upon the classification of skin flaps according to their blood supply, there are random pattern skin flaps or simple cutaneous flaps, and axial pattern flaps or arterialized flaps, which in turn can be subdivided into peninsula flaps when they contain a direct cutaneous artery and vein with a bridge of skin and subcutaneous tissue at their base; island flaps, which have a direct cutaneous artery and vein with no skin bridge; and free flaps, also known as free axial pattern skin flaps, for microvascular surgery transfer from a distant site. Free flaps are usually island flaps in which the vessel is divided prior to the transfer and then joined by microvascular techniques to segmental vessels in the recipient site. Classification of flaps according to where they are moved includes local skin flaps and distant skin flaps. *Local skin flaps* can be open or closed. Closure can be accomplished either by skin grafting to the undersurface or by folding the flap over itself as a tube. Local skin flaps can be moved by rotation, transposition, and interpolation, or advanced as a single pedicle by pedicle advancement or by V-Y or Y-V closure. *Distant skin flaps* for lower extremity procedures requiring coverage of soft tissue defects may be subcategorized as direct flaps, often used on the opposite leg to provide coverage of chronic poorly vascularized defects, and indirect flaps which are moved from a distance. This type of flap in podiatric surgery is usually constructed in the thigh as a tubular bipedicle flap.

Z-Plasty

The geometric interchange of two triangular flaps positioned as the letter "Z" permits a gain in length in the direction of the central limb of the Z tracing. The theoretical gain is dependent upon the angles of the Z. In general an angle of 30 degrees provides a gain of 25 percent, a 45 degree angle a gain of 50 percent, and a 75 degree angle a gain of 100 percent. Besides the increase in length of the skin is a desired direction, the use of Z-plasty also permits a change of direction of a given scar because of the rotation of the axis of the "Z" flaps. Multiple Z-plasties are used to attain cosmetically superior scars. Combinations of Y-V closure and advancement with Z-plasty could be quite effective in releasing transverse contractures of interdigital webb spaces. W-plasties are also quite helpful for similar purposes.

REFERENCES

1. Sabiston DC (ed): Textbook of Surgery. p. 300. WB Saunders, Philadelphia, 1986
2. Classifications of operative wounds in relation to contamination and risk of infection. p. 29. In Manual on Control of Infection in Surgical Patients. American College of Surgeons, 1976
3. Hoopps HC: Principles of Pathology, 2nd Ed. p. 305. Meredith Publishing Company, New York 1964
4. Adamson RJ, Musco F, Enquist IF: The chemical dimensions of a healing incision. Surg Gynecol Obstet 135:515, 1966
5. Vander Meulen JC (ed): The management of Infected Wounds. Proceedings of a European Symposium held in The Hague, September 1978. p. 3. Excerpta Medica, Amsterdam, 1978
6. Preston FW, Beal JM: Basic surgical physiology. p. 13. In Donnellan W (ed): Wound Healing. Year Book Medical Publishers, Chicago, 1986
7. Dumphy JE, Udupa KN: Chemical and histochemical sequences in the normal healing of wounds. N Engl J Med 253:841, 1955
8. Howes EL, Sooy JW, Harvey SC: The healing of wounds as determined by their tensile strength. JAMA 92:42, 1929
9. Winter GD: Movement of epidermal cells over the wound surface. In Montagna W, Billingham RE (eds): Wound Healing. Pergamon Press, New York, 1964
10. Ordman LJ, Gillman T: Studies in the healing of cutaneous wounds. Arch Surg 93:857, 1966
11. Weiss P: The biological foundations of wound repair. Harvey Lect 55:13, 1961
12. Chen RW, Postlethwait RW: The biochemistry of wound healing. S Sc 1:215, 1964
13. Dumphy JE: On the nature and care of wounds. Ann R Coll Surg 26:69, 1960
14. Burke JF: Wound infections and early inflammation. S Sc 1:301, 1964
15. Grabb WC, Smith JW (eds): Plastic Surgery, 3rd Ed. p. 1. Little Brown, Boston, 1979
16. Yaremchuk-Burgers, Brumback: Lower extremity salvage and reconstruction. Orthopedic and Plastic Surgery Management. Elsevier Science Publishing Company, New York, 1989

47

Limb Salvage

Edward L. Chairman, D.P.M.

For the past several years life expectancy has increased dramatically. Many reasons account for this phenomenon. With the improvement in communication and education, the public is more aware of the advantages of not smoking, proper diet, and proper exercise. These three components in particular have done more to increase the life expectancy of the average person than almost any other aspect of today's civilization.

Although the quality of life has improved along with the increase in life expectancy, there still comes a time when the quality of life is diminished as a result of various system breakdowns. This chapter pertains to the salvage of the vascular system in the lower extremity.

A significant increase in the number of patients seeking help for complaints of claudication, rest pain, neuropathy, nonhealing ulcers, and gangrene has occurred, necessitating the amalgamation of many different subspecialties of medicine to form a limb salvage team. Limb salvage is an exciting and constantly changing subject. The succession of new advances and techniques is so rapid that newly published articles on the subject seem almost antiquated when released. The practitioner of limb salvage is forced by the very nature of the subject to keep up with the newest literature and also unpublished research. With this in mind, an overview of limb salvage concepts, some of which may be covered more extensively in other chapters of this text, is presented. The reader should keep in mind that concepts and protocols that are acceptable today may in fact be archaic tomorrow. It is incumbent upon the student of this specialty to understand the basic concepts presented in this and other chapters and develop them further in order to continue to improve the various techniques and treatments so far developed. It is our aim to improve the quality of our patients' lives.

In over 80 percent of the cases of lower extremity amputation, the cause is some type of disruption in the circulatory process.[1] Diabetes is involved in 50 to 70 percent of that group.[1] With increased understanding of limb salvage concepts, as much as 50 percent of the amputations done today could be avoided.

Disruption of the circulation to the lower extremity causes devitalization and death of tissue. Revascularization of this limb often requires a vascular surgeon or an invasive radiologist. Removal of devitalized tissue and reconstruction of the foot for maximum function requires a podiatric surgeon, orthopedic surgeon, or vascular surgeon trained in this field.[1]

CLINICAL FINDINGS IN VASCULAR DISEASE

The physician must be able to recognize the signs and symptoms of vascular disease and then properly evaluate them using his or her clinical experience and modern testing techniques to determine the proper treatment for the best results. Intermittent claudication, nocturnal or rest pain, nonhealing ulcers, and gangrene are more obvious signs of problems. However, more insidious signs and symptoms such as cold feet, absent pulses, atrophic skin, hair loss, onychauxic nails, and delayed venous filling time should not be overlooked.

Classification of Ulcers

One of the most common findings in dysvascular limbs is decubitus ulcers. There are two major classifications of ulcers (Table 47-1).

A four-grade classification system was developed by Shea.[2] Grade I presents an intact epidermis. There is sharply defined erythema that is reversible. On occasion, when this is chronic, iron deposits are noted in the intercellular space, causing brown discoloration. Grade II ulcers present as a minor interruption in the dermis that does not affect the subcutaneous tissues. Grade III ulcers penetrate the subcutaneous layers. After debriding the

dry exudate from the ulcer, fatty tissue, muscles, tendons, and even periosteum may be seen. Grade IV decubitus ulcers exhibit deep fistulas. The bone usually has osteomyelitis, which can be diagnosed with routine conventional radiographs or by bone scans when the radiographs are not definitive enough.

A second grading system for ulcers was developed and presented by Wagner.[3] He divided foot lesions into six grades, according to the depth of the ulcer and the presence or absence of infection and gangrene. Grade 0 presents as no open lesion and is most comparable to Shea's grade I classification. Wagner's grade I presents as a very superficial ulcer, possibly over a bony deformity or prominence. Grade I goes deeper through the subcutaneous tissue and exposes tendon, muscle, bone, and possibly joint capsule. Grade III presents as a deep ulcer with a concurrent abscess or osteitis. There are signs of infection, such as erythema, inflammation, and edema. Osteomyelitis and cellulitis may be present. Grade IV ulcers exhibit devitalized tissue in the forefoot or toes. Wet or dry gangrene is present and surgical ablation is needed. Grade V indicates that the foot is beyond functional repair. Gangrene is widespread, and amputation must be done at a higher level.

Using Wagner's system of grading foot lesions, it should be noted that grades I through IV could be reversed back to grade 0 if treatment is successful. Grade V, however, is obviously nonreversible.

Table 47-1. Classification of Ulcers

Shea	Wagner	Description
Grade I	Grade 0	No open lesion; erythema, hemosiderin deposits; bony prominence
Grade II	Grade I	Superficial ulcer not affecting subcutaneous tissue
Grade III	Grade II	Ulcer penetrates subcutaneous tissue; often exposes tendon, muscle, bone, and joint capsule
Grade IV	Grade III	Deeper ulcer with concurrent fistula or abscess; often signs of infection plus osteomyelitis
No grade	Grade IV	Devitalized gangrenous tissue in the forefoot
No grade	Grade V	Widespread gangrene; beyond functional repair

DIAGNOSIS OF VASCULAR PROBLEMS

In attempting to determine the best treatment for a particular vascular problem, nothing surpasses good clinical judgment. One must consider the usual components of a history and physical examination of the patient. Intermittent claudication, nocturnal or rest pain, skin texture, skin color and temperature, hair growth pattern, nail growth pattern, and extent of devitalized tissue are signs and symptoms that must be weighed by the clinician. However, to back up one's clinical judgment, there are many diagnostic tests that can be used.

Radiology

Radiologists are a significant part of the limb salvage team. They are active both in diagnostic testing and in treatment of various etiologies.

Conventional Radiology

Conventional radiographs are used to diagnose osteomyelitis and even malignancies, which must be considered when treating deep ulcerations.

Because much necrotic tissue lies beneath grade III ulcers and is not readily apparent to the naked eye, the use of radiopaque materials in the ulcerated defects to document the extent of the destruction to deeper structures may be considered. However, many other techniques and treatments bypass the need for this technique.

Nuclear Medicine

Although skeletal system imaging with radiopharmaceuticals has been around for more than 20 years, it has only been in the last several years that attention has been given to the foot. Scanning techniques have increased the physician's ability to diagnose underlying osteomyelitis and malignancies long before they show up on a conventional x-ray. The enhanced ability to diagnose osteomyelitis is important because the location of osteomyelitic bone affects the diagnostic and surgical approaches and the treatment of a dysvascular limb.

Technetium-phosphate compounds are commonly used because high doses can be administered without fear of whole body radiation since their half-life is very short (6 hours). Gallium and indium are also used today and are more specific for osteomyelitis than technetium. Technetium-99m phosphate angiogram and blood pool imaging have been used to determine the capability of skin ulcer healing. Lawrence et al., in 1983,[4] and Alazraki et al., in 1985,[5] presented studies that concluded that one could predict whether a skin ulcer would heal by measuring the early blood-pool image of the distribution of technetium-99m phosphate in a radionuclide angiogram. Perfusion of soft tissues (i.e., skin, muscle) and bony structures can be measured quantitatively at 2-second intervals. Osteomyelitis confuses the interpretation because of the hypervascular response of the disease. When osteomyelitis is present the reliability of this technique is diminished.

Angiography

Angiography is most valuable in that by using radiopaque dyes, it allows visualization of the actual stenosis or blockage in various vessels. By being able to create a road map of the vascular anatomy of the lower extremity, the vascular surgeon can plan an aggressive therapeutic approach. New techniques have been developed by the invasive radiologist that can help avoid extensive surgery by using various methods to dilate vascular stenosis in the arterial structures mapped out on the angiogram.

Noninvasive Hemodynamic Techniques

Lassen demonstrated that *induced hypertension* was beneficial in treating ischemic ulcerations, therefore correlating blood pressure and tissue healing.[6] Confusing this evaluation is the fact that patients with calcified, noncompressable arteries give an artificially high pressure. This is common in as many as 50 percent of diabetic patients.[7,8]

Skin perfusion pressure using a radioisotope (^{131}I-labeled antipyrine) method was adapted to the skin by Holstein.[9] Later Lund and Sager found that there is a correlation between skin perfusion pressure and wound healing, but there was no sharp line between perfusion values for amputations that healed or failed.[10] It is therefore a very inexact correlation and not one recommended for widespread usage.

Moore measured *capillary blood flow* using a radioisotope (xenon-133) clearance technique.[11] He injected this isotope intradermally and measured the rate of transport across the membrane. Moore found that he could correlate tissue healing with the capillary blood flow. He was able to determine a value, 2.7 ml/min/100 g tissue, above which 97 percent of the cases healed and below which 100 percent of cases did not heal. Other studies were done with varying results. Kostuik's group determined that a minimum skin blood flow or capillary blood flow of 1.5 ml/min/100 g of tissue was needed.[12] Thus, this particular measurement proved that there was a correlation between the capillary blood flow and healing, but an exact cut-off point could not be determined.

Plethysmography measures changes in limb volume secondary to changes in blood volume. Arterial impedence plethysmography was used by Lee and co-workers to determine whether a below-knee amputation would heal.[13] They also found that photoplethysmography was useful in evaluating the vascular status of the foot but not the leg. A third form of plethysmography is pulse volume recording. This measures the changes in an inflated cuff caused by the pulsation of an artery. Gibbons et al. determined no correlation between the pulse volume recording and healing ability.[8]

Transcutaneous Doppler ultrasound is used to measure the arterial and venous circulation.[1,14] With it systolic pressure at different levels of the foot and leg can be measured and, by dividing this into the brachial artery pressure, an ischemic index can be calculated. The technical components of this test are reviewed in Chapter 17. Healing can be correlated with the ischemic index when it is greater than 0.45 in diabetic patients and 0.35 in other patients. The thickening of the intima of the diabetic's artery is thought to be the cause of this difference in acceptable minimum ischemic index. It should also be noted that one may obtain artificially higher ischemic indices when the artery being measured is calcified and noncompressable.

Comments

It would be very nice if the physician could use a diagnostic test that was consistent in evaluating the healing ability of a limb, thereby giving an absolute direction for treatment. However, no diagnostic studies studied thus far can give an absolute yes or no to a level of viability. Nothing can substitute for experience and clinical evaluation. Diagnostic studies give some objective findings to work with but they do not substitute for experienced clinical evaluation by the physician.

TREATMENT PROTOCOLS

The treatment of the lower extremity for disorders secondary to circulatory problems runs the gamut from very conservative, palliative care to aggressive surgical intervention.

Preventive Measures

The most basic treatment is prevention of problems. Good hygiene, no smoking, lubrication of the skin, padding of bony protuberances, proper shoegear (including Plastazote or Spenco inlays), and appropriate exercise are commonsense preventive measures for all patients with a hint of compromised circulation in the lower extremities.

Not to be overlooked is proper nutrition. Many patients with diabetes mellitus, leg ulcers, and acute infections exhibit decreased zinc blood levels.[15] Lesser quantities of zinc are stored in the diabetic pancreas than in a normal pancreas.[15] Many studies have found that ulcers heal faster in patients with normal zinc levels. A clinically obvious decrease in the time needed for ulcers and other types of skin breaks to heal in the diabetic patient is observed when a dose of 80 mg of zinc is taken three times a day with meals, but this has not yet been documented with controlled studies.

Medication

Symptoms such as claudication and rest pain can be treated in their early states with medication. Diphenhydramine HCl (Benadryl) has been used successfully for rest pain right before the patient goes to bed. The side effect of drowsiness seems to mask the milder discomfort of rest pain and allows the patient a pleasant night's sleep. Quinine sulfate (Quinamm) is used as a skeletal muscle relaxant. By decreasing the excitability of the muscle fiber it decreases the discomfort of the muscle cramping.

In the past, vasodilators were shown to increase circulation in experiments with animals. However, their effectiveness in human patients with peripheral vascular disease is questionable at best.[16] More recently, pentoxifylline (Trental) has come into common use for intermittent claudication. By increasing the flexibility of the red blood cells, it allows them to pass through stenotic vessels. In this author's experience pentoxifylline has proven to be an excellent adjunct to the treatment of intermittment claudication, but it is of little use in resolving rest pain alone. More than 90 percent of all the patients that I started on pentoxifylline have experienced a lessening of their intermittent claudication and were able to walk further without acute pain.

Ideally, it is advantageous to start medication-treated patients on mild to moderate exercise to increase the collateral circulation in their lower extremities. Walking on a daily basis in conjunction with the medication and proper control of all other aspects (e.g., diet, proper shoegear) has proven to be advantageous and sometimes eliminates the ultimate need for definitive surgical intervention.

Invasive Procedures

If the limb salvage team's clinical judgment and results of the diagnostic tests indicate that no amount of local care or medication will prevent the ultimate loss of the limb, an attempt at revascularization by an invasive radiologist or vascular surgeon must be considered.

Invasive Radiology

Balloon angioplasty has become a widely accepted and commonplace procedure. The radiologist attempts to dilate a stenotic vessel by introducing a balloon dilatation catheter. A small increase in the diameter of the lumen will significantly increase the blood flow. If successful, this procedure can eliminate rest pain and intermittent claudication.

It is not uncommon for balloon angioplasty to be successful for a short period of time and then have the vessel lumen close down again. As a result of this phenomenon, there is research going on now into a technique that allows the invasive radiologist to pass a tubelike device into the vessel and lodge it at the site of the angioplasty. When inserted in the proper position, this device opens up and keeps the newly dilated walls in their open position. At the time of this writing, this device is still experimental. In all likelihood it will be a commonplace treatment within a short period of time.

Arterial segments that are occluded by a thrombosis caused by atherosclerotic stenosis, trauma, or a previous angiographic procedure may be cleared by passing a catheter into the thrombus and feeding a thrombolytic agent (e.g., streptokinase) directly into it with the aid of an arterial infusion pump.

At the time of this writing, there is research proceeding rapidly using laser technology and fiber-optics to vaporize atherosclerotic plaque in stenotic vessels. In the hands of a trained practitioner, a 14-cm section of a stenotic femoral artery has been reopened. Laser technology promises to be one of the most important advances in revascularization of stenotic vessels. It could potentially eliminate much of the need for aggressive vascular surgery.

Vascular Bypass Surgery

If it is determined that invasive radiology would not be highly successful for a particular case, more aggressive vascular surgery is necessary.

It is most important that a patient be medically stable prior to surgical intervention. His or her cardiac, renal, and diabetic status should ideally be stable and under control. There are times, however, when this is not possible and the surgeon must proceed without the patient being an ideal candidate.

There are many types of surgical bypasses—for example, femorofemoral, axillo-bifemoral, femoropopliteal, femoro–anterior tibial, and aortico-bifemoral. Success rates of bypass surgery continue to improve,[17] mainly as a result of more experienced surgical judgment and better technique. Our experience and also a review of the literature indicates that bypasses are successfully being done more distally as time goes on. According to Veith et al. the distal aspect of the vessel being bypassed into should not be more than 50 percent stenotic.[17]

Amputation

If a bypass fails as a result of hemorrhage or thrombosis, a reoperation may be indicated. If bypass surgery is not successful, then amputation is the end result. The level of amputation is best determined by a combination of the doctor's clinical evaluation and various testing, including the ischemic index at the different levels of the leg.

Pinzur et al. identified the fact that the success rate of transmetatarsal and partial foot amputations went up dramatically when the surgeon required a minimum lymphocyte count of 1,500 and a 3.0 g/dl serum albumin level along with acceptable (as per Wagner) Doppler ultrasound results.[18] The success rate was substantially higher when taking all three of these factors into consideration over the success rate when considering any one of the factors.

TREATING LOCAL MANIFESTATIONS OF VASCULAR DISEASE

With the successful revascularization of the limb, attention must be directed to the local manifestations of the disease devitalizing the foot. Necrotic tissue cannot be revitalized, and must be removed if healing is to take place.

If there is localized gangrene of the digits and/or forefoot and the limb has been revascularized so that the proximal portion of the foot is viable, then partial amputation is desired. There are many approaches to amputation. One must realize that amputations of the forefoot cannot be standardized, since each case presents its own variations of viability and necrosis.

If the devitalized necrotic tissue is limited in nature and the underlying bone is not affected (e.g., osteomyelitis), then the surgeon should consider surgical débridement of the necrotic tissue followed by an appropriate treatment regimen. This may be conservative and require antisepsis, soaks with an appropriate solution (e.g., acetic acid when *Pseudomonas* is involved), or the application of topical enzymes such as collagenase, fibrinolysin, and proteolytic enzymes. Depending on the results of the culture and sensitivity of the devitalized tissue, the surgeon may combine the use of a systemic antibiotic and possibly even a local antibiotic applied to the area. Another topical treatment uses dextranomer spherical hydrophilic beads (Debrisan), which are able to absorb exudate from secreting lesions. By reducing the exudate in the ulcerated tissue, the tissue is more able to heal.

Determination must be made to differentiate arterial ulcers from venous stasis ulcers. Venous stasis ulcers require treatment that diminishes edema. Therefore, elevation and rest of the affected limb go a long way in decreasing pressure on the venous stasis ulcer but may impair the recovery of an arterial ulcer. Intermittent compression pumps are very successful with venous stasis ulcers and pitting edema in general. In addition, pressure-gradient stockings should be used between treatment with the pump. Other treatments for venous stasis ulcers that have been very successful include a venous heart, a foam-rubber pad applied directly over an ulcer and then incorporated into an Unna boot. The pad creates intermittent compression on the ulcer when the extremity moves, aiding in the return flow of blood in that immediate area.

With the successful revascularization of an extremity followed by the removal of all necrotic tissue one may have a defect in the foot that is too large for normal healing through granulation. At this point the surgeon must consider skin grafts. The most commonly used skin grafts are split-thickness autografts. This is a layer of skin that includes the epidermis and part of the dermis from another site on the patient. There are times when a tissue transfer is necessary. Microvascular surgery can be used to perform a free tissue transfer from one part of the body to the damaged site.[19] This procedure is becoming more commonplace and more successful. It is performed by plastic and reconstructive surgeons who are trained in microvascular surgery. Large defects can also be repaired with peroneal island flaps.[20] There are many pros and cons to this procedure versus the free tissue transfers; however, there are many positive elements to repairing large skin defects that make this procedure attractive.

CONCLUSION

It is obvious from a review of this chapter that a team approach is essential in obtaining the best possible result for the patient. The podiatrist not only provides technical know-how in the form of surgery and various techniques and palliative care, but also serves as the member most likely to identify the problem and alert the other members of the limb salvage team.

Limb salvage protocols and concepts are changing at a rapid pace. New treatments are constantly being developed and improved, but without a basic understanding of the etiology and other aspects of the disease pattern, they cannot be utilized to their maximum potential. Although diagnostic procedures are becoming more definitive, they do not replace good clinical judgment. There is no substitute for experience.

REFERENCES

1. Wagner FW, Jr.: The dysvascular foot: a system for diagnosis and treatment. Foot Ankle 2:66, 1981
2. Shea JD: Pressure sores. Clin Orthop 112:89, 1975
3. Wagner FW, Jr.: The diabetic foot and amputations of the foot. p. 341. In Mann RA (ed): DuVries Surgery of the Foot. 4th Ed. CV Mosby Co, St. Louis, 1978
4. Lawrence P, Syverud J, Disbro M, Alazraki N: Evaluation of technetium 99m phosphate imaging for predicting skin ulcer healing. Am J Surg 146:746, 1983
5. Alazraki N, Dries D, Lawrence P, et al: Assessment of skin ulcer healing capability by technetium-99m phosphate angiogram and blood-pool images. J Nucl Med 26:586, 1985
6. Lassen NA, Larson OA, Sorenson AWS: Conservative treatment of gangrene using mineralocorticoid-induced moderate hypertension. Lancet 1:606, 1968
7. Cheng EY: Lower extremity amputation level: selection using non-invasive hemodynamic methods of evaluation. Arch Phys Med Rehabil 63:475, 1982
8. Gibbons GW, Wheelock FC, Jr., Siembieda C et al: Noninvasive prediction of amputation level in diabetic patients. Arch Surg 114:1253, 1979
9. Holstein P: Distal blood pressure as guidance in choice of amputation level. Scand J Clin Lab Invest 31(Suppl 128):245, 1973
10. Lund P, Sager P: Results of 41 below-knee amputations (sagittal technique) in relation to local skin perfusion pressure (Abstract). Acta Orthop Scand 48:335, 1977
11. Moore WS: Determination of amputation level: measurement of skin blood flow with Xenon (Xe^{133}). Arch Surg 107:798, 1973
12. Kostuik JP, Wood D, Hornby R et al: Measurement of skin blood flow in peripheral vascular disease by epicutaneous application of Xenon^{133}. J Bone Joint Surg [Am] 58:833, 1976
13. Lee BY, Trainor FS, Kavner D et al: Noninvasive hemodynamic evaluation in selection of amputation level. Surg Gynecol Obstet 149:241, 1979
14. Wagner FW, Jr.: Transcutaneous Doppler ultrasound in the prediction of healing and the selection of surgical level for dysvascular lesions of the toes and forefoot. Clin Orthop Related Res 142:110, 1979
15. Engel ED, Erlick NE, Davis RH: Diabetes mellitus impaired wound healing from zinc deficiency. J Am Podiatry Assoc 71:536, 1981
16. Coffman JD: Vasodilator drugs in peripheral vascular disease. N Engl J Med 300:713, 1979
17. Veith FJ, Gupta SK, Samson RH, et al: Progress in limb salvage by reconstructive arterial surgery combined with new or improved adjunctive procedures. Ann Surg 386:386, 1981
18. Pinzur M, Kaminsky M, et al: Amputations at the middle level of the foot. A retrospective and prospective review. J Bone Joint Surg [Am] 68:1061, 1986
19. Allen T, Franklin JD, Withers E, et al: Extremity salvage utilizing microvascular free tissue transfer surgery. Surgery 90:1047, 1981
20. Yoshimura M, Shimada T, Shinichi I, et al: Peroneal island flap for skin defects in the lower extremity. J Bone Joint Surg [Am] 67:935, 1985

Index

Page numbers followed by f denote figures; those followed by t denote tables.